S0-DTC-404

AMERICA'S
TOP DOCTORS

A Castle Connolly Guide

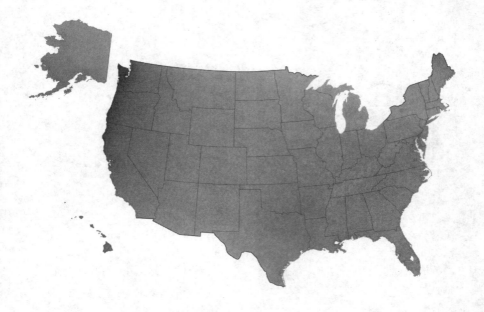

All Rights Reserved   Copyright © 2002, by Castle Connolly Medical Ltd.

Library of Congress Catalog Card Number 2002101282

The selection of medical providers for inclusion in this book was based in part on opinions solicited from physicians, nurs-es, and other health care professionals. The author and publishers cannot assure the accuracy of information provided to them by third parties, since such opinions are necessarily subjective and may be incomplete. The omission from this book of particular health care providers does not mean that such providers are not competent or reputable.

The purpose of this book is educational and informational. It is not intended to replace the advice of your physician or to assist the layman in diagnosing or treating illness, disease, or injury. Following the advice or recommendations set forth in this book is entirely at the reader's own risk. The author and publishers cannot ensure accuracy of, or assume responsibil-ity for, the information in the book as such information is affected by constant change. Liability to any person or organiza-tion for any loss or damage caused by errors or omissions in this book is hereby disclaimed. Whenever possible, readers should consult their own primary care physician when selecting health care providers, including any selection based upon information contained in this book. In order to protect patient privacy the names of patients cited in anecdotes throughout the book have been omitted.

Reproduction in whole or part, or storage in any data retrieval system and reproduction therefrom, is strictly prohibited and violates Federal copyright and trademark laws.

The confidence of our readers in our editorial integrity is crucial to the success of the Castle Connolly Guides. Any use of the Castle Connolly name, or of any list or listing (or portion of either) from any Castle Connolly Guide, for advertising or for any commercial purpose, without prior written consent, is strictly prohibited and may result in legal action.

For more information, please contact Castle Connolly Medical Ltd., 42 West 24th St, New York, New York 10010, 212-367-8400
E-mail: info@castleconnolly.com. Web site: http://www.castleconnolly.com, AOL keyword: Castle Connolly

ISBN 1-883769-26-4 (paperback)
ISBN 1-883769-27-2 (hardcover)

Printed in the United States of America

TABLE OF CONTENTS

HIPPOCRATIC OATH

I swear by Apollo the physician, and Asklepios, and health, and All-Heal and all the gods and goddesses, that, according to my ability and judgement, I will keep this Oath and this stipulation — to reckon him who taught me this Art equally dear to me as my parents, to share my substance with him, and relieve his necessities if required; to look upon his offspring in the same footing as my own brothers, and to teach them this Art, if they should wish to learn it, without fee or stipulation; and that by precept, lecture and every other mode of instruction, I will impart a knowledge of the Art to my own sons, and those of my teachers, and to disciples bound by a stipulation and oath according to the law of medicine, but to none others.

I will follow that system of regimen which, according to my ability and judgement, I consider for the benefit of my patients, and abstain from whatever is deleterious and mischievous. I will give no deadly medicine to anyone if asked nor suggest any such counsel; and in like manner I will not give to a woman a pessary to produce abortion. With purity and wholeness I will pass my life and practice my Art.

I will not cut persons labouring under the stone, but will leave this to be done by men who are practitioners of this work. Into whatever houses I enter, I will go into them for the benefit of the sick, and will abstain from every voluntary act of mischief and corruption; and, further, from the seduction of females or males, of freemen and slaves. Whatever, in connection with my professional practice, or not in connection with it, I see or hear, in the life of men, which ought not to be spoken of abroad, I will not divulge, as reckoning that all such should be kept secret. While I continue to keep this Oath unviolated, may it be granted to me to enjoy life and the practice of the art, respected by all men, in all times! But should I trespass and violate this Oath, may the reverse be my lot!

from Dorland's Illustrated Medical Dictionary. 27th ed. (Philadelphia) W.B. Saunders Co., 1988. Hippocratic Oath. [Hippocrates. Greek physician, 460-377 B.C.]

ABOUT THE PUBLISHERS

John K. Castle, the Chairman of Castle Connolly Medical Ltd., has spent much of the last two decades involved with healthcare institutions and issues. Mr. Castle served as Chairman of the Board of New York Medical College for eleven years, an institution at which he has continued on the Board for more than twenty years.

Mr. Castle has been extensively involved in other healthcare and voluntary activities as well. He served for five years as a public commissioner on the Joint Commission on Accreditation of Healthcare Organizations (JCAHO), the body which accredits most public and private hospitals throughout the United States. Mr. Castle has also served as a trustee of five different hospitals in the metropolitan New York region and is a director emeritus of the United Hospital Fund as well as a trustee of the Whitehead Institute.

In addition to his healthcare activities, Mr. Castle has served on many voluntary boards including the Corporation of the Massachusetts Institute of Technology, as well as numerous corporate boards of directors, including the Equitable Life Assurance Society of the United States. He is chairman of a leading merchant bank and has been chief executive of a major investment bank.

Mr. Castle holds a Bachelor of Science degree from MIT, an MBA with High Distinction from the Harvard Business School, where he was a Baker Scholar, and an honorary doctorate from New York Medical College.

ABOUT THE PUBLISHERS

John J. Connolly, Ed.D., served as President of New York Medical College, the state's largest private medical college, for more than ten years. He is a Fellow of the New York Academy of Medicine, a Fellow of the New York Academy of Sciences, a Director of the New York Business Group on Health, a member of the President's Council of the United Hospital Fund, and a member of the Executive Committee of Funding First. Dr. Connolly has served as a trustee of two hospitals and as Chairman of the Board of one. He is extensively involved in healthcare and community activities, and serves on a number of voluntary and corporate boards. He has served on the Board of the American Lyme Disease Foundation, of which he is a founder and past chairman, and the Board of Advisors of the Whitehead Institute. He holds a Bachelor of Science degree from Worcester State College, a Master's degree from the University of Connecticut, and a Doctor of Education degree in College and University Administration from Teacher's College, Columbia University.

MEDICAL ADVISORY BOARD

We are pleased to have associated with Castle Connolly Medical Ltd. a distinguished group of medical leaders who offer invaluable advice and wisdom in our efforts to assist consumers in making the best healthcare choices. We thank each member of the Medical Advisory Board for their valuable contributions.

Charles Bechert, M.D.
Director
The Sight Foundation
Fort Lauderdale, FL

Roger Bulger, M.D.
President
Association of Academic Health Centers
Washington, DC

Harry J. Buncke, M.D.
Davies Medical Center
San Francisco, CA

Paul T. Calabresi, M.D.
Professor of Medicine and Medical Science
Chairman Emeritus
Department of Medicine
  Brown University
Rhode Island Hospital
Providence, RI

Joseph Cimino, M.D.
Professor and Chairman
Community and Preventive Medicine
  New York Medical College
Valhalla, NY

Jane Clark, M.D.
Ear, Nose, Throat,
  and Hearing Center of Framingham
61 Lincoln St.
Framingham, MA

John C. Duffy, M.D.
Medical Director for Youth Services
Charter Pines Behavioral Health System
Charlotte, NC

J. Richard Gaintner, M.D.
Chief Executive Officer
Shands Health Care
  University of Florida
Gainesville, FL

Menard M. Gertler, M.D., D.Sc.
Clinical Professor of Medicine
Cornell University Medical School
New York, NY

Leo Hennikoff, M.D.
President and CEO
Rush Presbyterian-St.Luke's Medical Center
Chicago, IL

Yutaka Kikkawa, M.D.
Professor and Chairman
Department of Pathology
University of California,
  Irvine College of Medicine
Irvine, CA

Nicholas F. LaRusso, M.D.
Chairman
Division of Gastroenterology
Mayo Medical School Clinic and Foundation
Rochester, MN

MEDICAL ADVISORY BOARD

David Paige, M.D.
Professor
Department of Maternal and Child Health
Johns Hopkins University
Baltimore, MD

Ronald Pion, M.D.
Chairman & CEO
Medical Telecommunications Associates
Los Angeles, CA

Richard L. Reece, M.D.
Editor
Physician Practice Options
Old Saybrook, CT

Leon G. Smith, M.D.
Director of Medicine and Chief of
   Infectious Diseases
St. Michael's Medical Center
Newark, NJ

Helen Smits, M.D.
Visiting Professor
Robert F. Wagner School of Public Service
Former Deputy Director
Centers for Medicare and Medicaid Services
   (CMS)
New York, NY

Ralph Snyderman, M.D.
Chancellor for Health Affairs
Duke University School of Medicine
Durham, NC

FOREWORD

The challenge of finding the best healthcare is a formidable one for most Americans and for others who seek medical care in the United States. While this country offers the best medical care in the world, many people are overwhelmed by its complexity and bureaucracy.

While most of us are fortunate and never need venture beyond our local communities to find medical specialists able to meet our healthcare needs, the needs of many patients cannot be met in their local areas. For them, the search for the top specialists can be as important as life itself!

This great nation is fortunate in possessing some of the world's leading medical centers and specialty hospitals where cutting edge research is conducted and innovative new therapies are practiced daily. These health centers employ and train many of the world's most skilled physicians. My organization, the Association of Academic Health Centers, serves as a forum of exchange for these centers of medical excellence and, therefore, I know them well. However, I also know well the difficulty and challenges that patients and their families face in identifying and locating the tremendous wealth of medical talent and dedication that lies within the walls of these outstanding facilities.

Castle Connolly Medical Ltd. has dedicated extensive time and resources to identifying the best healthcare this nation has to offer. They have done this not to serve physicians or hospitals, but to serve healthcare consumers. Their efforts will be vital and important resources to Americans and others who seek the best medical care available in this country—wherever it is being practiced.

Roger Bulger, M.D.
President, Association of Academic Health Centers
Washington DC

INTRODUCTION

There are times in life when the nature of a disease or medical condition that afflicts you or a loved one warrants identifying the top doctor—the very best specialist anywhere in the nation—to diagnose or treat that particular medical problem. It's at times like these that you need *America's Top Doctors*, the national guide designed to assist you under just these circumstances.

While the overall quality of medical care throughout the United States is generally of very high quality, and in many places is superb, there are still those rare, complex or extremely difficult problems that demand resources beyond the ordinary or that require talents that are exceptional.

This guide identifies those top medical specialists throughout the country who possess the skill and experience to address these problems. Top specialists who provide excellent care tend to be located predominantly, although not exclusively, at major medical centers, specialty hospitals and leading teaching hospitals. These exceptional physicians are acknowledged as such by their peers and are recognized for their expertise by the medical profession.

The top specialists we have identified are not the only excellent physicians who are caring for patients in this nation. Since there are more than 650,000 doctors in the United States, we cannot identify every top specialist. Therefore, we have included narrative to assist those using this guide who may not find the specialist they need within its listings. Clearly, there are many primary care physicians and other well-trained specialists in communities and hospitals throughout the United States.

Most physicians in this guide are board certified not only in a specialty, but also in a subspecialty or in multiple subspecialties. Board or subspecialty certification alone, however, does not distinguish them from excellent specialists at hospitals in your community, many of whom also are board certified in both a specialty and a subspecialty.

INTRODUCTION

However, physicians included in this guide have trained at the top medical centers under medical pioneers who possess state-of-the-art knowledge in a specific disease or problem and have often devised new techniques and therapeutic approaches, many of which are life-saving procedures or cures. These doctors most often practice their science and art at leading hospitals and, more specifically, in programs at hospitals that are recognized for their excellence in a given field. Many others have been trained at leading centers in other nations since the U.S. is not alone in pioneering new medical knowledge, although its position as the leader in "high-tech" medicine is generally acknowledged.

Another major characteristic distinguishing the physicians in this guide from those at local hospitals is their continued focus and training. Rather than practicing at a community hospital (or even at a leading regional hospital) and developing a general, broad-based practice, these physicians continued their training in a particular disease, syndrome or problem to such degree that they developed extensive knowledge and unique skills in treating that particular problem.

Often that focused, advanced training is accompanied by active involvement in clinical research. This is an additional reason why the physicians listed in this guide are located at only a few hundred of the more than six thousand hospitals in the United States. It is difficult, although not impossible, to conduct important clinical research in isolation or without an environment supportive of research. It takes time, money, residents, research associates, technicians, equipment and more to produce significant clinical research. Certainly there have been individuals who have made important and lasting contributions to research with little or none of this support, but those instances are rare. Today, for the most part, major advances in medicine occur in the labs and on the floors of major medical centers and specialty hospitals, in medical schools and in clinical labs created and financed for that purpose by commercial enterprises.

HOW PHYSICIANS WERE SELECTED FOR INCLUSION IN THIS GUIDE

The basis of the Castle Connolly selection process is peer nomination. In some ways, this resembles an enhancement of the process in which a personal physician provides a patient with a referral to another physician for a particular problem. However, if the recommendation of one doctor is good, the recommendation of many doctors is even better. So, we ask many doctors for their recommendations; in fact, over 250,000 doctors!

How do we accomplish this enormous task? Over the years, the Castle Connolly physician-directed research team developed its extensive database of physicians across the nation through periodic mail, telephone and email surveys. This cumulative database is systematically maintained and continuously updated. Surveyed physicians nominate top doctors in both their own and related specialties – especially those to whom they would refer their own patients. Each year this database is supplemented by further mail surveys and telephone interviews with leaders in the various medical specialties and leading physicians at major medical centers. Online surveys also were conducted with members of Physicians' Online (POL), the country's largest community of physicians connected through the Internet.

To augment our large mail, telephone and online samplings, additional surveys are conducted among the following carefully selected groups: directors of graduate medical programs; directors of clinical services at member hospitals of the Council of Teaching Hospitals (COTH); board members of medical specialty academies, associations and societies; and deans and chairs of departments at medical schools.

Building on prior research, thousands of top doctors included in earlier editions of our guides are invited to offer their nominations for *America's Top Doctors*.

INTRODUCTION

Focus then shifted to the 4,254 physicians selected from over 20,112 nominated. Extensive biographical forms were sent to those physicians for completion. After careful review of their professional backgrounds, the Castle Connolly research staff conducted further research to check disciplinary and license histories.

The result is a carefully researched and highly selective list of the top specialists in the nation. This select group of physicians, identified through our extensive research process, constitutes a list of physicians recognized by their peers for their excellence in providing care for specific diseases and problems.

Undoubtedly, there will be comments that we have missed some terrific doctors who should be included. That is inevitable, since this guide is designed to identify only those doctors noted for excellence in diagnosing or treating a specific problem or disease.

What we intentionally have not done is include physicians simply because they have an important title. While a position as a chief of service or a department head at a teaching hospital is an important post, such positions are achieved through a combination of many talents including administrative skills, seniority and factors that are not as important for inclusion in this guide as is skill in clinical care. The same is true of leaders of county medical societies, professional associations or even specialty groups. While these are significant positions and acknowledge leadership among peers, they are not essentially recognition of clinical skills.

The same perspective applies to research expertise. Many physicians listed in the Guide are engaged in clinical research and make significant contributions to their fields, with some devoting a substantial portion of their time to research. However, we avoided including those physicians who solely conduct research and who do not provide patient care.

The result of this extensive research effort is a list of outstanding, highly skilled physicians who are recognized as among the best in their specialties and in the nation; a list which consumers/patients can use to find the very best specialists to meet their particular needs.

Lastly, this book differs from the regional Castle Connolly Guides, *Top Doctors: New York Metro Area, Top Doctors: Chicago Metro Area* and *How to Find the Best Doctors: Florida,* in two important ways. First, **America's Top Doctors** is national, not regional, in scope. Second, the regional Guides are based on the generally accurate premise that healthcare is local and most people find their healthcare where they live and work. However, **America's Top Doctors** is designed to meet the needs of those people who cannot find the right specialists locally but who can and will travel anywhere in the country to be cared for by a top specialist at an outstanding hospital. This guide will assist readers in that important search.

INTRODUCTION

USING THIS GUIDE TO FIND TOP SPECIALISTS

This guide is organized and planned to be as user-friendly as possible. Still, as with anything as complex as medical specialties, subspecialties and the myriad diseases and problems that specialists treat, there needs to be a system to organize the physicians' names, the diseases and problems they manage and their special expertise.

To organize the specialists in this guide, we have followed the American Board of Medical Specialties (ABMS) format. The ABMS is the authoritative body for the recognition of medical specialties. Without the ABMS as the official controlling body there would be hundreds of unregulated medical specialties.

The ABMS recognizes twenty-five specialties and over ninety subspecialties. The listing of ABMS specialties and subspecialties can be found in Appendix A. In addition to ABMS recognized specialties, there are at least one hundred other groups calling themselves "medical specialists" that are not recognized by the ABMS. Some of these groups are working toward recognition and have exams and other standards for membership. Others are organizations of physicians interested in a particular problem or area of medicine that exist to exchange information but have no intention of seeking ABMS recognition. Some groups calling themselves "boards" really have little authority or meaningful standards. Thus, while a physician may state he/she is, for example, a specialist in cosmetic surgery, there is no ABMS recognized specialty by that name. Therefore, you have no idea whether this physician has any special training and expertise or is simply trying to recruit paying patients to a lucrative aspect of surgical practice.

You can get information on a doctor's credentials from the doctor, from the doctor's hospital (Medical Affairs office) or from your health plan if a doctor is in the network. You can also get this information from numerous Web sites, including www.castleconnolly.com. You can check on a physician's board certification by calling the ABMS at (866) 275-2267 or by logging on to its Web site at www.abms.org.

If you seek a particular type of specialist or subspecialist, turn to the section of this guide covering that medical specialty or subspecialty. There you will be able to further restrict your search to a specific geographic region or, if you prefer, to search throughout the nation.

To make your search easier, we have organized the specialties and subspecialties into the following regions: New England, Mid-Atlantic, Midwest, Southeast, Southwest, Great Plains and Mountains, and West Coast and Pacific. To find an outstanding cardiologist in St. Louis, for example, look under cardiology and then under the Midwest region.

A second way to use this guide is to look at the Special Expertise Index, which lists the areas of special expertise of included physicians. This list of special expertises indicates over 2,000 medical topics including diseases, therapeutic approaches and techniques. You can look up the particular disease, problem or technique you are interested in and locate a physician in that manner. We assume that many people using this guide will know what their particular problem is and will begin their exploration with this index. However, we encourage you to read the entire text since it will help you to better understand how to find the right physician for yourself or a family member, especially if one is not found in this guide.

CHOOSING AN APPROPRIATE SPECIALIST

It may seem that choosing the correct specialist to treat a particular medical problem is simply a matter of finding a top doctor in a specific medical specialty. For treatment of a problem with your vision, you would choose an ophthalmologist. A skin or hair problem would require treatment by a dermatologist and a broken bone would need the care of an orthopaedist.

INTRODUCTION

Sometimes, however, the type of specialist needed may not be obvious. For example, back surgery may be performed by either an orthopaedist or a neurosurgeon. Different aspects of sports medicine, as another example, are practiced by orthopaedists who treat sports-related injuries in both adults and children, pediatricians who treat only children or internists and family practitioners whose focus is on prevention of injuries.

In some cases, several specialists with expertise in different areas of medical practice all become involved in treating the same patient's health problem. For example, a person with diabetes might need care from an endocrinologist, a cardiologist and an ophthalmologist. In other situations, doctors trained in different specialties may use varied approaches or differing therapies to manage a disease or condition. Such is the case, for example, with prostate cancer: a patient could be treated by a urologist, a medical oncologist, or a radiotherapist. The urologist might provide the patient with a surgical treatment option, while the medical oncologist would treat the patient with chemotherapy and the radiotherapist would use radiation therapy and/or radioactive seed implantation. All approaches could be successful, or one might be preferable to another, depending on the patient and his condition. Therefore, a wise patient will thoroughly explore all options before making a choice.

Finding the right specialist is also important in terms of the quality of your care. For example, many orthopaedic surgeons will operate on hands, but it is clearly preferable to have someone trained and certified specifically in hand surgery (a subspecialty of both orthopaedics and plastic surgery) to perform that delicate surgery. Similarly, a dermatologist may indicate that his/her practice includes cosmetic surgery, however, there is no approved ABMS dermatology subspecialty or fellowship training in cosmetic surgery. While many dermatologists do pursue additional training in cosmetic surgery, it should be understood that dermatologic practice is limited to cutaneous procedures ranging from the removal of skin tumors to laser resurfacing. On the other hand, some board certified otolaryngologists have additional training that enables them to perform plastic and cosmetic surgery procedures on the head and neck.

Choosing the right type of specialist is as important as selecting the right doctor. For example, the diagnosis of melanoma, a very serious, potentially life threatening form of skin cancer, is missed in many cases. Therefore, if you have a skin lesion that might possibly be melanoma, you should be certain that the pathologist reading your slides is board certified in the subspecialty of dermatopathology.

These examples illustrate this important principle: always seek the best healthcare. Look for the best-trained doctors, not those who simply can do the job. That doesn't mean that you need to consult a doctor listed in this guide every time you have a health problem. It does mean you should be certain that the physicians who care for you, whether in your community or at a world-class medical center, are trained appropriately and are qualified to provide the care you require. Remember, when it comes to healthcare no one wants second best!

Given this complexity, how do you find the right specialist to provide your care? The first and most important person to look to for guidance is your primary care physician. He/she will assess your medical condition, determine the appropriate type of specialist to recommend and perhaps refer you to a specific doctor or doctors. You should always ask your primary care physician why a particular specialist is being recommended, since that specialist may be a colleague in your doctor's medical group or may be the only (or the most conveniently located) specialist of the type in your health plan. Ask how well your primary care physician knows the specialist, whether they have a long-standing professional relationship and if other patients referred to the specialist had successful outcomes. Be sure to ask for several recommendations, if possible, to provide you with some choice among specialists.

INTRODUCTION

If you do not have a primary care doctor, try to learn as much as you can about your medical problem and the type of specialist best suited to treat it. However, keep in mind that many diseases or conditions present with symptoms that often are indistinguishable from those of other diseases or conditions (Lupus and Lyme disease, for example) making them difficult to diagnose precisely even for physicians armed with the results of diagnostic tests.

JUDGING THE QUALIFICATIONS OF A PHYSICIAN

The specialists listed in **America's Top Doctors** are clearly among the best in the nation and have been identified through a rigorous research process and thorough screening by the Castle Connolly research team. Through our extensive surveys and research we have done much of the work in finding a top referral specialist for you. But how do you judge the qualifications of a physician who may not be listed in this Guide? If you are trying to find a specialist on your own, how should you go about it? How can you tell when a physician has the appropriate training in a specialty and how do you distinguish what is meaningful and what is not from among all those plaques and certificates on a doctor's wall?

The following pages will outline that process for you. In fact, what is written here reflects much of the logic that underlies the selection of physicians for this book.

The following material will help you not only in finding a top specialist in this Guide, but it also should be helpful to you in choosing among the many specialists, primary care doctors and other physicians that you will need to consult throughout your life.

The reality is that few of us see only one doctor in our lifetime. Each of us may be cared for by a primary care physician, an ophthalmologist, an orthopaedist, a dermatologist, a surgeon or a number of other specialists. The choices can be many and they can be among the most important choices that we make in our lives.

Education

Your review of your prospective doctor's education and training should begin with medical school. While you may feel that the institution at which someone earned a bachelor's degree could be an indication of the quality of the doctor, most people in the medical field do not believe it plays a major role. A degree from a highly selective undergraduate college or university will help an aspiring doctor gain admission to a medical school, but once there, all students are peers. However, the information on undergraduate colleges, if important to you, is available in the *American Board of Medical Specialties (ABMS) Compendium of Certified Medical Specialists* and other medical directories.

American medical schools are highly standardized, at least in terms of minimal quality. A group known as the Liaison Committee for Medical Education (LCME) accredits all U.S. medical schools that grant medical degrees (MDs) and osteopathic degrees (DOs). Most also are accredited by the appropriate state agency, if one exists, and by regional accrediting agencies that accredit colleges and universities of all kinds.

Furthermore, U.S. medical schools have universally high standards for admission, including success on the undergraduate level and on the Medical College Admissions Tests (MCATs). Although frequently criticized for being slow to change and for training too many specialists, the system of medical education in the United States has insured high quality in medical practice. One recent positive change is a strong effort in most medical schools to diversify the composition of the student body. While these schools have been less successful in enrolling racial minorities, the number of women in U.S. medical schools has increased to the point that women now make up about 40 percent of most classes. In certain specialties preferred by women medical graduates (pediatrics, for example) it is possible that in coming years the majority of specialists will be female.

INTRODUCTION

Most doctors practicing in the United States are graduates of U.S. medical schools, but there are two other groups of doctors who make up a relatively small portion of the total physician population. They are (1) foreign nationals who graduated from foreign schools and (2) U.S. nationals who graduated from foreign schools. (Canadian medical schools are not considered foreign.)

Foreign Medical Graduates

Foreign medical schools vary greatly in quality. Even some of the oldest and finest European schools have become virtually "open door," with huge numbers of unscreened students making teaching and learning difficult. Others are excellent and provided the model for our system of medical education.

The fact that someone graduated from a foreign school does not mean that he/she is a poor doctor. Foreign schools, like U.S. schools, produce good doctors and poor doctors. Foreign medical graduates must pass the same exam taken by U.S. graduates for licensure, but the failure rate for foreign graduates is significantly higher. In the first year of using the new United States Medical Licensing Exam (USMLE), 93 percent of U.S. medical school graduates passed Step II, the clinical exam, as compared with 39 percent of the foreign graduates. It is clear that the quality of foreign schools, if not individual doctors, is not the same as U.S. medical schools, at least as measured by our standards. Nonetheless, many communities and patients have been well served by foreign medical graduates practicing in this country—often in areas where it has been difficult to attract graduates of American schools.

In addition, many foreign medical schools and their teaching hospitals are world renowned for their leadership in medical care, research and teaching and many of the technologies and techniques we utilize in the U.S. today have been developed and perfected in foreign countries.

Residency

Most doctors practicing today have at least three years of postgraduate training (following the MD or DO) in an approved residency program. This not only is an important step in the process of becoming a competent doctor, but it is also a requirement for board (specialty) certification. Most people assume that a prospective doctor needs to complete a three-year residency program to obtain a medical license. That is not an accurate assumption! New York State, for example, requires only one postgraduate year. However, since all approved residencies last at least three years and some, such as those in neurosurgery, general surgery, orthopaedic surgery and urology, may extend for five or more years, it is important to know the details of a doctor's training. Licensure alone is not enough of a basis on which to make a decision.

Without undertaking extensive and detailed research on every residency program, the best assessment you can make of a doctor's residency program is to see if it took place in a large medical center whose name you recognize. The more prestigious institutions tend to attract the best medical students, sometimes regardless of the quality of the individual residency program. If in doubt about a doctor's training, ask the doctor if the residency he/she completed was in the specialty of the practice; if not, ask why not.

It is also important to be certain that a doctor completed a residency that has been approved by the appropriate governing board of the specialty, such as the American Board of Surgery, the American Board of Radiology, or the American Osteopathic Board of Pediatrics. These board groups are listed in Appendices A and B. If you are really concerned about a doctor's training, you should call the hospital that offered the residency and ask if the residency program was approved by the appropriate specialty group. If still in doubt, consult the publication *Directory of Graduate Medical Education Programs*, often called the "green book," found in medical school or hospital libraries, which lists all approved residencies.

Board Certification

With an MD or DO degree and a license, an individual may practice in any medical specialty with or without additional training. For example, doctors with a license but no special training may call themselves cardiologists, pediatricians or gynecologists. This is why board certification is such an important factor. The American Board of Medical Specialties (ABMS) recognizes 25 specialties and over 90 subspecialties. Eighteen boards certify in 106 specialties under the aegis of the American Osteopathic Association (AOA). Doctors who have qualified for such specialization are called board certified; they have completed an approved residency and passed the board's exam. (See Appendix A for an approved ABMS list; see Appendix B for the AOA list. While many doctors who are not board certified do call themselves "specialists," board certification is the best standard by which to measure competence and training. Throughout this Guide a description of each specialty and subspecialty is provided as an introduction to the listing of physicians in that specialty.

You can be confident that doctors who are board certified have, at a minimum, the proper training in their specialty and have demonstrated their proficiency through supervision and testing. While there are many non-board certified doctors who are highly competent, it is more difficult to assess the level of their training. While board certification alone does not guarantee competence, it is a standard that reflects successful completion of an appropriate training program. If it is impossible to find a doctor in your area who is board certified in a particular subspecialty, for example, geriatric medicine or sports medicine, at least be certain the physician is board certified in a related specialty such as internal medicine or orthopaedics.

Board certified doctors are referred to as Diplomates of the Board. Some of the colleges of medical specialties (e.g., the American College of Radiology, the American College of Surgeons) have multiple levels of recognition. The first is basic membership and the second, more prestigious and difficult to obtain, is status as a Fellow. Fellowship status in the colleges is meaningful and is based on experience, professional achievement and recognition by one's peers, including extensive experience in patient care. It should be viewed as a significant professional qualification.

Board Eligibility

Many doctors who have been more recently trained are waiting to take the boards. They are sometimes described as "board eligible," a common term that the ABMS advocates abandoning because of its ambiguity. Board eligible means that the doctor has completed an approved residency and is qualified to sit for the related board's exam.

Each member board of the ABMS has its own policy regarding the use and recognition of the board eligible term. Therefore, the description "board eligible" should not be viewed as a genuine qualification, especially if a doctor has been out of medical school long enough to have taken the certification exam. To the boards, a doctor is either board certified or not. Furthermore, most of the specialty boards permit unlimited attempts to pass the exam and, in some cases, doctors who have failed the exam twice or even ten times continue to call themselves board eligible. In osteopathic medicine, the board eligible status is recognized only for the first six years after completion of a residency.

In addition to the approved lists of specialties and subspecialties of the ABMS and AOA, there are a wide variety of other doctors and groups of doctors who call themselves specialists. At present there are at least 100 such groups called "self-designated medical specialties." They range from doctors who are working to create a recognized body of knowledge and subspecialty training to less formal groups interested in a particular approach to the practice of medicine. These groups may or may not have standards for membership. There is no way to determine the true extent of their members' training and the ABMS or the AOA does not recognize them. While you should be cautious of doctors who claim they are specialists in these areas, many do have advanced training and the groups at least offer a listing of people interested in a particular approach to medical care. Rely on board certification to assure yourself of basic competence, and use membership in one of these groups to indicate strong interest and possible additional training in a particular aspect of medicine. A list of these self-designated medical specialties may be found in Appendix C.

Recertification

A relatively new focus of the specialty boards is the area of recertification. Until recently, board certification lasted for an unlimited time. Now, almost all the boards have put time limits on the certification period. For example, in Internal Medicine and Anesthesiology, the time limit is ten years; in Family Practice, six, and under some circumstances, seven years. These more stringent standards reflect an increasing emphasis on recertification by both the medical boards and state agencies responsible for licensing doctors.

Since the policies of the boards vary widely, it is a good procedure to ask a doctor if certification was awarded and when. If the date was seven to ten years ago, ask if he/she has been recertified. Unfortunately, many boards permit "grandfathering," whereby already certified doctors do not have to be recertified, and recertification requirements apply only to newly certified doctors. Appendix A contains a list of the names and addresses of the boards and the certification period for each board specialty. Even if recertification is not required, it is good professional practice for doctors to undertake the process. It assures you, the patient, that they are attempting to stay current.

Many states have a continuing medical education requirement for doctors. These states typically require a minimum number of continuing medical education (CME) credits for a doctor to maintain a medical license. Twenty-eight states require 150 CME credits over a three-year period. Osteopathic doctors are required to take 150 hours of CME credits within three years to maintain certification.

Fellowships

The purpose of a fellowship is to provide advanced training in the clinical techniques and research of a particular specialty. Fellowships usually, but not always, are designed to lead to board certification in a subspecialty such as cardiology, which is a subspecialty of internal medicine. Many physicians listed in this Guide have had fellowship training. In the U.S. there are a variety of fellowship programs available to doctors, which fall into two broad categories: approved and unapproved. Approved fellowships are those that are approved by the appropriate medical specialty board (e.g., the American Board of Radiology) and lead to subspecialty certificates. Fellowship programs that are unapproved are often in the same areas of training as those that are approved, but they do not lead to subspecialty certificates. Unfortunately, all too often, an unapproved fellowship exists only to provide relatively inexpensive labor for the research and/or patient care activities of a clinical department in a medical school or hospital. In such cases, the learning that takes place is secondary and may be a good deal less than in an approved fellowship. On the other hand, any fellowship is better than none at all and some unapproved fellowships have that status for a valid reason that should not reflect negatively on the program. For example, the fellowship may have been recently created, with approval being sought. To check that a fellowship is an approved one, call the hospital where the training took place or call the medical board for that specialty.

Some physicians may have completed more than one fellowship and may be boarded in two or more subspecialties. Also, some physicians may pursue fellowship training and subspecialty certification, but then choose to practice in their primary field of certification. For example, a doctor who is board certified in internal medicine also may have obtained board certification in cardiology, but may choose to practice primarily internal medicine rather than cardiology. For the most part, the physicians in this Guide practice in their subspecialties.

Professional Reputation

There are doctors who meet every professional standard on paper, but who are simply not good doctors. In all probability the medical community has ascertained that and, while the individual may still practice medicine, his/her reputation will reflect that collective assessment. There are also doctors who are outstanding leaders in their fields because of research or professional activities but who are not particularly strong, or perhaps even active, in patient care. It is important to distinguish that kind of professional reputation from a reputation as a competent, caring doctor in delivering patient care, or in the case of this Guide, as an outstanding practitioner in a given specialty.

Hospital Appointment

Most doctors are on the medical staff of one or more hospitals and are known as "attendings;" some are not. If a doctor does not have admitting privileges or is not on the attending staff of a hospital, you may wish to consider choosing a different doctor. It can be very difficult to ascertain whether or not the lack of hospital appointment is for a good reason. For example, it is understandable that some doctors who are raising families or heading toward retirement choose not to meet the demands (meetings, committees, etc.) of being an attending. However, if you need care in a hospital, the lack of such an appointment means that another doctor will have to oversee that care. In some specialties, such as dermatology and psychiatry, doctors may conduct their entire practice in the office and a hospital appointment is not as essential, or as good a criterion for assessment, as in other specialties.

While mistakes are made, most hospitals are quite careful about admissions to their medical staffs. The best hospitals are highly selective, so a degree of screening (or "credentialing") has been done for you. In other words, the best doctors practice at the best hospitals. Since caring for a patient in a hospital is often a team effort involving a number of specialists, the reputation of the hospital to which the doctor admits patients carries special weight. Hospital medical staffs review their colleagues' credentials and authorize performance of specific procedures. In addition, they typically review and reappoint their medical staff every two or three years. In effect, this is an additional screening to protect patients. It is especially true of hospitals that have what are known as closed staffs, where it is impossible to obtain admitting privileges unless there is a vacancy that the administration and medical staff deem necessary to fill. If you are having a surgical procedure and are concerned about the doctor's skill or experience, it may be worthwhile to call the Medical Affairs office at the doctor's hospital to see if he/she is authorized to perform that procedure in that hospital.

The reasons for a hospital's selectivity are easy to understand: no hospital wishes to expose itself to liability and every hospital wants to have the best reputation possible in order to attract patients. Obviously, the quality of the medical staff is immensely important in creating that reputation. Unfortunately, some hospitals are less diligent when a major group practice of doctors, all of whom have previously been affiliated with the institution, adds new members. In such cases, the hospital may almost automatically grant privileges without conducting the same intensive review given to individual doctors who are not members of a group practice. It is more difficult to obtain admitting privileges when a hospital is operating at full capacity.

A last and very important reason why a hospital appointment is an essential requirement in your choice of doctor is that some states permit doctors to practice without malpractice insurance. If you are injured as a result of a doctor's poor care, you could be without recourse. However, few hospitals permit doctors to practice in them unless they carry malpractice insurance. This not only protects the hospital, but the patient as well.

Medical School Faculty Appointment

Many doctors have appointments on the faculties of medical schools. There is a range of categories from "straight" appointments, meaning full-time appointment as professor, associate professor, assistant professor or instructor, to clinical ranks that may reflect lesser degrees of involvement in teaching or research. If someone carries what is known as a straight academic rank (i.e. "professor of surgery," without clinical in the title), this usually means that the individual is engaged full-time in medical school research, teaching activities and patient care. The title "clinical professor of surgery" usually identifies a part-time or adjunct appointment and less direct involvement in medical school activities such as teaching and research.

Doctors who are full-time academicians may be in the forefront of new techniques and research, but they are not necessarily better doctors. Nonetheless, you would be assured that they have the support of other faculty, residents and medical students.

When you are seeking a subspecialist, a doctor's relationship to a medical school becomes more meaningful since medical school faculties tend to be made up of subspecialists. You are less likely to find large numbers of general or primary care practitioners engaged full-time on a medical school faculty. The newest approaches and techniques in medicine, for the most part, are explored and developed by medical school faculties in their laboratories and clinical practice settings. This is where they practice their subspecialties, as well as teach and perform research. Such leading specialists are not necessarily better doctors than community doctors; rather, they are trained to provide a different kind of medical care. Obviously the type of medical care users of this guide are seeking is that different kind of care available primarily from top subspecialists at leading hospitals and medical centers.

Medical Society Membership

Most medical society memberships sound very prestigious and some are; however, there are many societies that are not selective and which virtually any doctor can join. In addition, membership in many of the more prestigious societies is based on research and publication or on leadership in the field and may have little to do with direct patient care. While it is clearly an honor to be invited to join these groups, membership may be less than helpful in discerning whether a doctor can meet your needs.

Experience

Experience is difficult to assess. Obviously, in most cases, an older doctor has more experience; on the other hand, a younger doctor has been more recently immersed in the challenge of medical school, residency, or even a fellowship, and may be the most up-to-date. If a doctor is board certified, you may assume that assures at least a minimal amount of experience, but since it could be as little as a year, check the date of graduation from medical school or completion of residency to know precisely how long a doctor has been in practice.

There is a good deal of evidence that there is a positive relationship between quantity of experience and quality of care. That is, the more a doctor performs a procedure, the better he/she becomes at it. That is why it is important to ask a doctor about his or her experience with the procedure that you need. Does the doctor see and treat similar cases every day, every week or only rarely? Of course, with some rare diseases, rarely is the only possible answer, but it is relative frequency that is critical. Major metropolitan areas, especially New York and San Francisco, became leaders in the treatment of AIDS because of the number of patients seen in those metropolitan areas. Doctors in the suburbs of New York City (especially in New York's Westchester, Nassau and Suffolk counties) and in Fairfield County, Connecticut became leaders in the research and treatment of Lyme disease because that region is the epicenter of the disease.

In some states, data is available on volume or numbers of certain procedures performed at hospitals. For this information in New York you can call the Center for Medical Consumers, a non-profit advocacy organization, or visit its Web site at www.medicalconsumers.org. For volume and outcome information in other states, visit the Web site of Health Care Choices at www.healthcarechoices.org. There is a good deal of controversy, however, on the validity and usefulness of such data. Opponents cite the fact that some of the data is produced from Medicare patient records only and, thus, is based solely on an elderly population that does not represent the total activity of a hospital or doctor. Proponents of the use of such volume data agree that it is not perfect, but suggest it can be one useful criterion in selecting the best places to receive care for these specific problems. Recognizing the limitations of such data, the healthcare consumer may, nonetheless, find it of interest and use.

The one type of experience you should specifically want to know about is that dealing with any special procedure, particularly a surgical one, that has recently been developed and introduced into practice. For example, in the 1980's many doctors using laparoscopic cholecystectomy, a then new surgical technique for removing gallbladders, experienced a high percentage of problems because they were not properly trained. This prompted the American Board of Surgery to promulgate new standards for the training of surgeons using this technique. Do not hesitate to ask about your doctor's training in a procedure and how frequently and with what degree of success he/she has performed it. Practice may not lead to perfection, but it does improve skills and enhance the probability of success.

In some cases, relatively young doctors have recently completed residency or fellowship training under recognized leaders who have developed new approaches or techniques for dealing with a particular problem. They may have learned the new techniques from their mentors and may be far ahead of the field (and ahead of more senior and distinguished colleagues) in using those approaches. So age and experience must be considered and weighed along with other factors when choosing a physician.

OTHER CONSIDERATIONS

Second Opinions

Second opinions are a valuable medical tool, too infrequently used in many instances and overused in others. Clearly, you do not want to seek another doctor's opinion on every ailment or problem that you face, but a second opinion should be pursued in the following situations:
- before major surgery
- if the diagnosis is serious or life threatening
- if a rare disease is diagnosed

INTRODUCTION

- if a diagnosis is uncertain
- if the number of tests or procedures recommended might be excessive
- if a test result has serious implications (e.g., a positive Pap smear)
- if the treatment suggested is risky or expensive
- if you are uncomfortable with the diagnosis and/or treatment
- if a course of treatment is not successful
- if you question your doctor's competence
- if your insurance company requires it

Most doctors will be supportive if you request a second opinion and many will recommend it. In many cases, insurance companies will pay for second opinions, but check ahead of time to make sure your insurance plan does cover them. In an HMO you may have to be more assertive because one way HMOs control costs is by limiting second opinions. Often, the opinion of a second doctor will confirm the opinion of the first, but the reassurance may be worth the time and extra cost. On the other hand, if the second opinion differs from the first, you have two alternatives: seek the opinion of a third doctor, or educate yourself as much as possible by talking to both doctors, reading up on the problem, and trusting your instincts about which diagnosis is correct.

Office and Practice Arrangements

Although clearly not as important as training or reputation, a specialist's office and practice arrangements often are of significance to patients. Practice arrangements include office hours, office location, billing procedures and accessibility among the many factors that result in how well the office is run.

Some specialists only will see new patients who are referred to them by another doctor. Therefore, you may need to have your treating physician contact the specialist's office to arrange for your initial visit. Your health plan may also require that your primary care doctor provide a referral.

If English is not your first language, it may be advisable to determine whether someone in the specialist's office speaks your primary language or if a translator can be present during appointments. This will ease communication and assure that all questions, responses and instructions are understood.

Accessibility of the specialist's office may be a concern if you are wheelchair-bound, are elderly or cannot climb stairs or negotiate narrow corridors. Convenient parking may also be important to you.

Other arrangements that may need to be made in advance of your first visit or discussed with the specialist's office staff concern payment. You may wish to ask the following:

- Does the specialist accept your health insurance coverage?
- Is the specialist within your plan's network and will you need to pay a co-payment? Or, is the specialist out-of-network and will you have to pay for your care out-of-pocket, meet a deductible or submit a form for reimbursement?
- Are credit cards an acceptable mode of payment?
- Does the specialist accept Medicare, Medicaid or no-fault insurance? Does the specialist treat workers' compensation cases?
- If you are a non-resident of the United States, will you need to arrange for the transfer or exchange of currency to pay the specialist's fee?

When you are choosing a top specialist, these issues may be of lesser or greater importance, depending on the problem and type of care warranted. If you are traveling a great distance to have a specific procedure performed by a top specialist at a major medical center, continuing long-term monitoring or follow-up care by that physician may not be required or may not be feasible and such things as office practice arrangements are of less importance. On the other hand, if you have a chronic problem that needs to be monitored with follow-up care provided by the same top specialist, then such issues as accessibility of the doctor's office, appointment hours, waiting times and courtesy and professionalism of the staff become more significant.

INTRODUCTION

Personal Chemistry

One element of the doctor-patient relationship that we stress in our guides is chemistry between doctor and patient, a part of which is often referred to as a doctor's "bedside manner." While this factor is of major import in a long-term relationship such as one you would have with your primary care physician, it is of less importance when you see a specialist only once or twice. However, since many people using this book may have chronic conditions that require ongoing care, it is important to give the matter some consideration.

It is vital that there is a sense of mutual trust and respect between patient and doctor; a judgment that individuals must make for themselves. Among the many talented doctors listed in this guide, there are very likely some to whom you would relate well and others with whom you may not feel as comfortable.

Patients prefer doctors who listen, demonstrate concern, are responsive to patient needs and spend sufficient time with them. The qualities of physicians in this regard, even the excellent ones in this guide, vary immensely.

You, the patient, are the only one who can assess these qualities because individuals react differently to various personalities. It is important for you to carefully judge your feelings towards a physician, especially if you are embarking on a long-term relationship. You should feel you can be open, trusting and responsive to your physician and that your relationship will be a positive one. Otherwise, find another doctor, since not doing so could adversely affect your care.

Once you have used this guide to identify the top specialist(s) best suited to treat your condition, there is much you can do to maximize the value of your first visit.

MAXIMIZING YOUR FIRST APPOINTMENT WITH A TOP DOCTOR

After your research is done and you've secured an appointment for an initial consultation with a top doctor known for his/her expertise in the diagnosis or treatment of your particular medical condition, what should you do?

Whether your visit to the specialist's office is a car ride or a plane trip away, there undoubtedly will be arrangements to make before your appointment. You may have to take time off from work, arrange for childcare while you are away and make travel plans and hotel reservations, but there are a number of other important steps to take to assure that you and the specialist make the best use of the time you spend together.

Have you done everything you can to prepare yourself and the specialist for the consultation? The following checklist will help you maximize the value of your visit to the specialist and will go a long way toward focusing you on the task at hand—getting the best advice or treatment for your health problem from one of the top doctors in the medical specialty related to your condition.

Gathering the facts
- Does the specialist have all the information needed to make a diagnosis of or treatment plan for your condition?
- Have your medical records, test results and X-rays been sent ahead of time to allow for their review by the specialist in advance of your first appointment?
- Have you written out your medical history emphasizing the particular problem for which you are visiting this specialist?
- Are you prepared with a written list of questions?
- Do you understand the answers?

A specialist becoming newly involved in your care needs to learn as much as possible about the state of your health in a very limited time. Since top doctors are extremely busy people with many demands on their time, you should make certain that all relevant records and case summaries are obtained and sent to the specialist well in advance of your appointment.

Obtaining Your Records

All healthcare providers including hospitals, doctors and their staffs are under legal obligation to maintain the privacy of your medical records. In order to obtain release of those records, you must make a request in writing. If you need to obtain records from a number of providers, you should write one clear and concise letter authorizing release of your records and including your name, address, telephone number, date of birth, social security number and any other identifying information such as a hospital chart number. You then can make photocopies of this letter, but be sure to sign and date each copy as if it were an original. You also may want to specifically name those test results (e.g., pathology slides) or X-ray films (not just written reports or summaries) that must be included in addition to making a general request for your records. It's also a good idea to indicate the date of your appointment so the office staff can respond in a timely manner.

Although state laws require the timely release of medical records, hospital medical records departments and doctors' offices often take several weeks to pull and review patient charts and get them in the mail either to you or to another doctor. In addition to written authorization, you may be asked to pay the costs involved in copying your records, test results and X-ray films because many doctors' offices will not release the originals. Consider placing a call in advance to determine the procedure for releasing your records, how long you can expect it to take and the costs involved so that you can save time by including payment with your release authorization letter. Be sure to allow sufficient time in advance of your consultation appointment for your request to be processed. Since you often must wait several weeks for an appointment with a specialist, allow at least that amount of time to obtain your records.

Even after making your written requests, you should follow up each letter with a telephone call to be sure that your records actually are sent. You should not assume that your request for records will be promptly fulfilled by an often over-burdened, although well-intentioned, office staff.

Remember, the more information the specialist has about your condition, the fewer repeat or additional tests or procedures you will need to undergo, the lower the costs of your consultation and, most important, the more expeditiously the specialist will be able to render an opinion.

THE FACTS AND ONLY THE FACTS

Be thorough and organized in documenting your personal and familial medical histories, the medications you take and in relaying information about your condition. Even seemingly minor bits of information may provide subtle clues to the nature of your medical problem and the optimal way in which to treat it. It's also advisable to bring a list with you of names, addresses and telephone numbers of all physicians who have cared for you, especially those you have seen regarding your current medical problem.

Even though thoroughness is essential to presenting a clear picture of your medical condition, bear in mind that the specialist needs to get to your core health concerns as quickly as possible. Therefore, if you have a complex medical history, you may want to ask your current doctors to provide treatment summaries in addition to copies of your medical records. Hospital records should include your admission history and physical exam, dictated consultation and operation notes and discharge summaries for all hospitalizations. You may also be able to get a cumulative lab and X-ray summary for your hospital stays.

Unlike X-rays, which can be copied at reasonable cost, original pathology slides must be transported by mail or hand-carried. Your specialist may wish to have the pathologist with whom he/she works speak directly with the pathologist who initially interpreted your slides as part of the process of evaluating your case.

BEING PREPARED

You are likely to be a bit nervous when you meet with the specialist you have chosen. Anxiety about your health and concern about your future care may cause you to forget information you should provide or miss hearing or understanding important information that the specialist communicates. Therefore, you may want to write down all relevant information so that you do not leave out anything of importance when you meet with the specialist or complete forms in the office. You also may want to write out your questions in advance so you don't forget anything.

To avoid leaving out important details of your condition or past treatment, prepare a concise, chronological summary before your consultation takes place. You may wish to type it and provide a copy to the specialist for inclusion in your chart. Highlight major medical results or significant events in the course of an illness or treatment if these will enlighten the doctor about your condition. Your personal perspective on the state of your health is vital to a full understanding of your medical problem.

It is possible that the specialist will use language that you do not understand or may speak quickly assuming certain knowledge on your part about your condition or its treatment. Don't hesitate to ask for clarification as often or repeatedly as you may need to in order to fully comprehend what you are being told. If you are concerned that you may forget what the doctor tells you, ask the doctor's permission to take notes or ask if you might bring along a tape recorder so you can later replay what was said, especially any instructions you are given. You may prefer to bring along a relative or close friend to serve as a "second set of ears," but, again, seek the doctor's permission to do so in advance of your appointment.

Following this process will assure that you and the specialist you are consulting get the most from your appointment. After all, you both have the same goal: restoring you to optimal health and well being.

WHAT TO DO IF YOU CAN'T GET AN APPOINTMENT

At times it may be difficult, perhaps even impossible, to secure an appointment with the specific specialist you have identified. There are a number of reasons why this may occur. For example, the specialist may not be taking any new patients or may have such a busy schedule that it takes several weeks or months to get an appointment. He/she may only see patients during very limited hours because of teaching, research or other responsibilities or currently may have other limitations related to the acceptance of new patients.

However, bear in mind that the doctors in this guide are the leaders in their specialties and therefore they work with and train the very best and brightest in their specialties. So, if you are unable to consult with a particular doctor, consider making an appointment with one of his/her outstanding colleagues. You can do this by asking a member of the doctor's office staff to refer you to an associate who is a member of the practice group or to another excellent physician who is specially trained to address your particular medical issue.

You can be comfortable knowing that you will receive high quality care from another specialist who practices in the same top setting.

UTILIZING SPECIAL RESOURCES

The following information on special resources has been included to meet the needs of healthcare consumers who have extraordinarily difficult or unique health problems, and have been unable to identify the resources to address their problems. These patients and their doctors may need to search for very new, cutting-edge, perhaps even experimental and not yet approved therapies. In such cases the search may lead to clinical trials; tests of new drugs and new medical devices or innovative therapeutic approaches. Fortunately, these situations are rare, but when they do occur, they are critical.

In addition to the outstanding private and public hospitals recognized in this guide, the U.S. government maintains its own unique, expert source of patient care and clinical research at the National Institutes of Health (NIH). In fact, the NIH operates its own hospital at which the care provided is usually related to clinical studies its researchers are undertaking.

In addition to those at the NIH, clinical trials also are conducted at leading medical centers and other organizations throughout the country. These facilities may be testing a new drug therapy, a new use for an existing medication or a medical device to deal with a problem that is not being resolved through the use of more traditional approaches.

This section will guide you in utilizing these special resources.

About clinical trials

The Clinical Trial as a Treatment Option

For some patients the best medical treatment may only be available through clinical trials (also called treatment studies), which are designed to develop improved ways to use current medical treatments or to find new medical treatments by studying their effects on humans. Treatments are studied to determine if they are safe, effective and better treatments than conventional or standard therapies. Only if they meet all three of these criteria are they made available to the general public.

Many people are frightened by the term "clinical trial" because it conveys the notion of being a "guinea pig" in an experiment. Contrary to popular belief, however, most new treatments are extensively studied by scientists in the laboratory before they are ever tested by physicians in clinical settings. Among the factors that keep patients from participating in clinical trials are: lack of awareness about clinical trials as a treatment option; fear of side effects or adverse reactions to treatment; refusal of insurance companies to pay for experimental treatments; failure of a physician to inform the patient about clinical trials; difficulty finding suitable clinical trials; unavailability of clinical trials for certain medical problems; distance of the patient from major medical centers conducting clinical trials; disruption of personal and family life; and the decision to stop medical treatment altogether.

Despite these and other obstacles, many people do seek out clinical trials. One of the most pressing reasons to participate is the opportunity to obtain treatment that might not be available otherwise. New medical treatments can offer participants hope for a cure, an extended lifespan, or an improvement in how they feel. Some participants also take comfort in knowing that others may benefit from their contribution to medical knowledge.

Deciding if a clinical trial is the right treatment option for you is no simple matter. Certainly, you will want to talk about it with your doctor(s) and other professionals involved in your care, as well as with family members and friends. But in order to fully benefit from what others have to say — based on either their professional knowledge or personal experience — you need to understand exactly what a clinical trial is and what your role as a volunteer will be.

INTRODUCTION

Understanding Clinical Trials

Clinical trials are conducted for just about every medical condition, including life-threatening diseases such as AIDS or cancer; chronic illnesses such as diabetes and asthma; psychiatric disorders such as depression or anxiety; behavioral problems such as smoking and substance abuse; and even common ailments such as hair loss and acne. Chances are, there is at least one trial (and probably more) that may be appropriate for you.

With more than 100 different types of cancer, it is understandable that a large number of clinical trials are cancer-related. Extensive information about clinical trials for cancer can be found on the Web site of the National Cancer Institute (NCI) which is part of the NIH. CenterWatch, an online clinical trials listing service, identifies 5,200 clinical trials that are actively recruiting patients. Veritas Medicine, another useful online organization, allows individuals to perform personalized searches of its clinical trials database. See "Selected Resources" in Appendix G for more information on clinical trials.

Most clinical trials study new medical treatments, combinations of treatments, or improvements in conventional treatments using drugs, surgery and other medical procedures, medical devices, radiation or other therapies. Newer types of clinical trials, called screening or prevention trials, study how to prevent the incidence or recurrence of disease through the use of medicines, vitamins, minerals or other supplements; and how to screen for disease, especially in its early stages. Another type of trial studies how to improve the quality of life for patients, including both their physical and emotional well-being.

Clinical trials are sponsored both by the federal government (through the National Institutes of Health, the National Cancer Institute and many others) and by private industry through pharmaceutical and biotechnology companies, and through healthcare institutions (hospitals or health maintenance organizations) and community-based physician-investigators. The National Cancer Institute sponsors clinical trials at more than 1000 sites in the United States. Trials are carried out in major medical research centers such as teaching hospitals as well as in community hospitals, specialized medical clinics (for example, those for the treatment of AIDS or Alzheimer's disease) and in doctors' offices.

Though clinical trials often involve hospitalized patients, a fair number of trials are conducted on an outpatient basis. Many trials are part of a cooperative network which may include as few as one or two sites or hundreds of locations, although one center generally assumes responsibility for overall coordination of the research. More than 45 research-oriented institutions, recognized for their scientific excellence, have been designated by the NCI as comprehensive or clinical cancer centers. See "Selected Resources" in Appendix G to find out how to locate these centers.

Clinical research is based on a protocol (established rules or procedures) describing who will be studied, how and when medications, procedures and/or treatments will be administered and how long the study will last. Trials that are conducted simultaneously at different sites use the same protocol to ensure that all patients are treated identically and all data are collected uniformly so that study findings can be compared.

Clinical trials generally are conducted in three phases, as outlined in the study protocol. The first phase begins testing of the treatment on a small group of human subjects after rigorous and successful animal testing has been concluded. The interim phase varies, but usually involves a broader test group and is designed to further evaluate the treatment's safety and more accurately determine appropriate dosage, application methods and side effects. In some trials there may be a fourth phase, conducted after the treatment is in widespread use, to monitor the results of long-term use and the occurrence of any serious side effects.

Some clinical trials test one treatment on one group of subjects, while others compare two or more groups of subjects. In such comparison studies participants are divided into two groups: the control group that receives the standard treatment and the experimental or treatment group which receives the new treatment. For example, the control group may undergo a surgical procedure while the experimental or treatment group undergoes a surgical procedure plus radiation to determine which treatment modality is more effective. To ensure that patient characteristics do not unduly influence the study findings, patients may be randomly assigned to either the control or the experimental group, meaning that each patient's assignment is based purely on chance. In cases in which a standard treatment does not exist for a particular disease, the experimental group of patients receives the new treatment and the control group receives no treatment at all, or receives a placebo, an inactive medicine or procedure that has no treatment value and is sometimes called a "dummy" pill or a "sugar" pill. It is important to keep in mind that patients are never put into a control group without any treatment if there is a known treatment that could help them. Also, whether a patient is receiving an investigational drug or a placebo, he/she receives the same level and quality of medical care as those receiving the investigational treatment.

Questions to ask your doctor and the trial's research team if you are considering participating in a clinical trial:

- Who is sponsoring the trial?
- How many patients will be involved?
- Will the trial be testing a single treatment or a combination of treatments?
- Will there be one treatment group or more than one treatment group?

- If more than one treatment group, how are patients assigned to each group?

- Has this treatment been studied in previous clinical trials? What were the findings?

Protecting the Rights of Participants

The safety of those who participate in clinical trials is a serious matter and is the number one priority of medical investigators. All clinical research, regardless of type of sponsorship, is guided by the same ethical and legal codes that govern the medical profession and the practice of medicine. Most clinical research is federally funded or federally regulated (at least in part) with built-in safeguards for patients. According to federal government regulations (and some state laws), every clinical trial in the United States must be approved and monitored by an Institutional Review Board (IRB), which is an independent committee of physicians, statisticians, community advocates and others (representing at least five distinct disciplines) to ensure that the protocol is being followed.

Government regulations require researchers to fully inform participants about all aspects of a clinical trial before they agree to participate through a process called informed consent. To be sure that you understand your role in a clinical trial, you should jot down any questions beforehand so as not to forget them. You should also consider bringing along a friend or family member for support and additional input, and perhaps even tape recording the conversation (after asking permission to do so) to make sure you do not forget or misunderstand anything. Each participant in a clinical trial must be given a written consent form, which should be available in English and other languages. The consent form explains the following:

- Why the research is being done.

- What the researchers hope to accomplish.

- What types of treatment interventions (and other tests or procedures) will be performed.

37

- How long the study will continue.
- What the expected benefits and the possible risks are.
- What other treatments are available.
- What costs will be covered by the study, by the patient or by third-party payers such as Medicare, Medicaid or private insurance.

Patients also are informed that they may leave the trial, or exclude themselves from any part of it, at any time. Informed consent means exactly what the term implies: you agree to join a clinical trial only after you completely understand exactly what your participation will involve for the duration of the study. By law, each patient must be provided with a copy of the signed consent form, which also must include the name and telephone number of a contact person for questions or additional information. Informed consent is a continuous process, so do not hesitate to ask questions before, during or after the trial.

The investigators must protect the privacy of each participant in a clinical trial by ensuring that all medical records are kept confidential except for inspection by the sponsoring agency, the Food and Drug Administration and other agencies involved in regulating the drug or treatment, and all data are collected anonymously by assigning a numeric code or initials to each individual.

During the course of the trial, participants are regularly seen by members of the research team to monitor their health and well-being. Participants also should be responsible for their own health by following the treatment plan (such as taking the proper dosage of medications on time), keeping all scheduled visits and informing members of the healthcare team about any symptoms that occur. If during the course of the trial, the treatment proves to be ineffective or harmful, the patient is free to leave the study and still obtain conventional care. Conversely, as soon as there is evidence that one treatment modality is better than another, all patients in the trial are given the benefit of the new information.

Questions to ask the sponsors about your rights as a participant in a clinical trial:

- Who is responsible for approving and monitoring this research? Is there an IRB?

- Who informs me about the trial process? Do I sign a consent form? Will I receive a copy?

- May I leave the trial at any time? Have previous patients dropped out? Why?

- Whom do I contact if I am experiencing any difficulty with this trial?

Enrolling in Clinical Trials

Each clinical trial has its own guidelines, called eligibility criteria, for determining who can participate. Treatment studies recruit participants who have a disease or other medical condition, while screening and prevention studies generally recruit healthy volunteers. Inclusion criteria (those that allow you to participate in a study) and exclusion criteria (those that keep you from participating in a study) ensure that the study will answer the research questions posed in the research protocol while maintaining the safety of participants. The disease being studied is a primary factor in selecting suitable patients, but other factors such as the patient's gender, age, treatment history and other diagnosed medical conditions may also be important. Unfortunately, eligibility also may depend upon ability to pay. Many health plans do not cover all of the costs associated with clinical trials because they define these trials as experimental procedures. However, trials sometimes pay volunteers for their time and/or reimburse them for travel, childcare, meals and lodging.

To prevent people who qualify from being excluded from clinical trials for financial reasons, agencies such as the National Cancer Institute are working with health plans to find solutions and a growing number of states require insurance companies to pay for all routine patient care costs in cancer trials. To encourage more senior citizens to participate in cancer trials, Medicare plans to revise its payment policy to cover those trials.

INTRODUCTION

When choosing a clinical trial you should determine the factors that are most important to you. For instance, patients generally prefer to participate in trials near their homes so that they can maintain their usual day-to-day activities, be surrounded by family and friends and avoid travel and lodging costs. If travel or temporary relocation becomes necessary, try to find a trial site that is near to some family member or friend or one that is in a locale similar to your own city or town. Many organizations, such as the National Cancer Institute, will work with patients and their families to identify support networks for them wherever they participate.

Questions to ask the trial's sponsor about eligibility criteria:

- What are the inclusion and exclusion criteria for the clinical trial(s) I am considering?
- How can I improve my chances of being accepted? Can I change my health plan to one that will cover the trial's costs? Can I relocate to another city or state?
- If I am not eligible for one trial, what other trials are being conducted for my condition?
- Will I be paid for my time or reimbursed for my out-of-pocket expenses?

Participating in a Clinical Trial

Clinical trials are conducted by a research team led by a principal investigator (usually a physician) and are comprised of physicians, nurses and other health professionals such as social workers, psychologists and nutritionists. As a participant you may be required to commit a fair amount of time to a clinical trial, often more than with standard treatment. Initially, you will probably be given a physical examination and asked for your medical history. During the trial, you will have regular or periodic visits to the trial site which may include diagnostic and laboratory tests. You also may be asked to follow fixed schedules for medications and other interventions and to keep detailed records of your symptoms and health condition. Generally, clinical trials last from six to twenty-six weeks, though some (called maintenance trials) can last up to a year to determine if a treatment will prevent the relapse of a medical condition.

Participants in clinical trials should remain under the care of their regular physician(s) since clinical trials tend to provide short-term treatment for a specific medical condition and do not generally provide comprehensive primary care. In fact, some trials require that a patient's regular physician sign a consent form before the patient is enrolled. In addition, your regular physician can collaborate with the research team to make sure there are no adverse reactions between your other medications or treatments and the investigational treatment.

Questions to ask the research team or your physician about your role in a clinical trial:

- Who are the members of the health team? Who will be in charge of my care?
- How long will the trial last?
- How does treatment in the trial compare with or differ from the standard treatment?
- Will I be hospitalized? How often? For how long a period of time?
- What will occur during each visit? What treatments or procedures will I be given?
- Will I still be able to see my regular physician(s)? Will my doctor and the research team collaborate?
- Can I be put in touch with other patients who have participated in this trial?

Weighing the Benefits and Risks of a Clinical Trial

If you are considering participation in a clinical trial, you need to consider the medical, emotional and financial ramifications of participation. Of course, the obvious benefit of a clinical trial is the chance that a new treatment may improve your health and prognosis. You will have access to drugs and other medical interventions before they are widely available to the public and you will obtain expert and specialized medical care at leading healthcare facilities. Many patients receive an added psychological benefit by taking an active role in their treatment .

It is important to bear in mind that some medical interventions used in clinical trials may carry potential risks depending upon the type of treatment and the patient's condition. While many side effects or adverse reactions are temporary (such as hair loss and nausea caused by some anticancer drugs), other more serious reactions can be permanent and even life-threatening (for example, heart, liver or kidney damage).

Deciding whether or not to participate in a clinical trial is often a matter of determining if the trial's potential benefits outweigh its possible risks. This is a highly personal decision that may be difficult to make in situations involving experimental treatment in which limited medical information may be available.

Questions to ask the research team about the benefits and risks of a clinical trial:

- What other treatment option(s) do I have at this time? Is there any chance that a more promising treatment may be available soon?

- What are the short and long-term benefits and risks as compared with standard treatment?

- Will I experience any known side effects or adverse reactions? Will these be temporary, long-term or permanent? Relatively minor or perhaps life-threatening?

- If I am harmed in any way by the new treatment, what other treatments will I be entitled to? Who will pay for subsequent treatment?

Getting Information on Clinical Trials

The more information you have about a clinical trial, the easier it will be to make a decision about whether or not it is right for you, and the more confident you will be that you made an appropriate decision. In addition to the "Selected Resources" appendix in this guide, the staff at your local public library, community hospital, or major medical center can assist you in locating the information you need from books, consumer organizations and on the Internet.

LEARNING ABOUT THE NATIONAL INSTITUTES OF HEALTH (NIH)

The National Institutes of Health (NIH) comprise one the world's leading medical research centers and the Federal government's principal agency for biomedical research. An agency of the United States Department of Health, United States Public Health Service, NIH encompasses 25 separate institutions and centers with its main campus located in Bethesda, Maryland. Research is also conducted at several field units across the country and abroad.

PATIENT CARE AT THE NIH

The Warren Grant Magnuson Clinical Center, NIH's principal medical research center and hospital located in Bethesda, Maryland, provides medical care only to patients participating in clinical research programs. Two categories of patients participate in the Clinical Center studies: children and adults who wish to improve their own health, such as those with newly diagnosed medical problems, ongoing medical problems or family history of disease; and healthy volunteers wishing to advance knowledge about the causes, progress and treatment of disease. The patient's case must fit into an ongoing NIH research project for which the patient has the precise kind or stage of illness under investigation. General diagnostic and treatment services common to community hospitals are not available.

The Magnuson Clinical Center is the world's largest biomedical research hospital and ambulatory care facility, housing 1,600 laboratories conducting basic and clinical research. There are 1,200 physicians, dentists and researchers on staff along with 660 nurses and 570 allied healthcare professionals (dieticians, imaging technologists, medical technologists, medical records and clerical staff, pharmacists and therapists).

The Center's hospital is specially designed for medical research and accommodates 540 carefully selected patients who are participating in clinical research programs. Its 350-bed facility has 24 inpatient care units to which 7,000 patients are admitted annually. The Center also has an Ambulatory Care Research Facility (ACRF) that serves 68,000 outpatient visits each year. A new facility, called the Mark O. Hatfield Clinical Research Center, is currently under construction and, when completed in 2002, will include 250 beds for inpatient care and 100 day-hospital stations for outpatient care.

The Clinical Center also maintains a Children's Inn for pediatric outpatients and their families. This family-centered residence operates 24 hours a day, 7 days a week, 365 days a year. Adult outpatients without adequate childcare may make use of a childcare program for their children ages three to seven during the hours of 8:00 AM and 5:00 PM.

In an effort to bring clinical research to the community, NIH supports approximately 77 General Clinical Research Centers (GCRCs) around the country, located within hospitals of major academic medical centers.

It is important to note that, as part of the federal government, the Warren Grant Magnuson Clinical Center provides treatment in clinical trials at no cost to its patients. In some cases, patients receive a stipend to help cover the costs of traveling to Bethesda for treatment and follow-up care. Travel costs for the initial screening visit, however, are not covered.

AREAS OF CLINICAL STUDY AT THE NIH

At the Magnuson Clinical Center alone, NIH physician-scientists conduct about 1,000 studies each year. Among the areas of study are:

- AIDS
- Aging
- Alcohol abuse and alcoholism
- Allergy
- Arthritis, musculoskeletal and- skin diseases
- Cancer
- Child
- Chronic pain
- Deafness and other communic- tion disorders
- Dental and orafacial disorders
- Diabetes
- Digestive and kidney diseases
- Eye disorders
- Heart, lung and blood diseases
- Infectious diseases
- Medical genetics
- Mental health
- Neurological disorders
- Stroke

Not all of these clinical areas are under investigation at any given time, however. The Patient Recruitment and Public Liaison Office (PRPL) at the NIH Clinical Center assists patients, their families and their physicians in obtaining information about participation in NIH clinical trials. Trained nurses are available to answer questions about the research programs and admission procedures.

CANCER CARE AT THE WARREN GRANT MAGNUSON CLINICAL CENTER

The National Cancer Institute (NCI) is the largest of the biomedical research institutes and centers at NIH. There, clinical studies are designed to evaluate new and promising ways to prevent, detect, diagnose and treat cancer. The Warren Grant Magnuson Clinical Center provides a separate outpatient division for cancer patients and also has several designated inpatient units.

INTRODUCTION

If you are interested in entering a cancer study at the Magnuson Clinical Center (or at the General Clinical Research Centers), you should first discuss treatment options with a physician. As a general rule, patients interested in participating in clinical studies must be referred by a physician. However, in some instances, self-referral may be permitted.

If your physician concurs that a clinical study might be appropriate for you, the NIH recommends that the following steps be taken:

- Contact NCI's Clinical Studies Support Center (CSSC), which is staffed by trained oncology (cancer) nurses who can identify appropriate clinical studies for you. Summaries of these trials and other pertinent information about the type of treatment being offered and the type of patients eligible for inclusion can be mailed or faxed to you and/or your physician.

- Review the clinical trials summaries and other information with your physician to decide which study or studies you should consider. Your physician also can contact the CSSC to communicate directly with the investigator in charge of the study.

- In cases in which you meet the initial eligibility requirements, it may be necessary for you to schedule a screening visit at the Clinical Center to learn more about the trial and possibly undergo some medical tests.

- If accepted for a clinical trial, make sure that you understand the details about the treatment and any possible risks and benefits.

Patients with medical problems other than cancer or healthy volunteers who wish to participate in a clinical study should contact the particular NIH institute responsible for the clinical area involved.

Cancer care at the NCI Clinical Centers and Comprehensive Cancer Centers

You may also obtain clinical oncology services (education, screening, diagnosis or treatment) or participate in clinical trials at one of the 11 Clinical Cancer Centers or 41 Comprehensive Cancer Centers designated by the NCI for their scientific excellence and extensive resources devoted to cancer and cancer-related problems. Centers are located in 32 states, with the majority of sites in California, New York and Pennsylvania. You can find out about clinical trials at the NCI-designated centers by contacting NCI's Clinical Studies Support Center (CSSC) or by calling each center directly. Information about other cancer-related services at these centers also may be obtained from the center itself.

GEOGRAPHIC REGIONS AND STATES

To assist you in using *America's Top Doctors* in the most efficient and effective manner, the Guide is divided into seven geographic regions. This will help you to locate a specialist in your local or neighboring region. For example, if you live in Mississippi in the Southeast region and you are willing and able to travel to Louisiana in the Southwest region to consult with a specialist in neurology, you can review just those two regions, under the section headed **"NEUROLOGY."** However, if you prefer to review the information on neurologists *throughout* the country, you can search the entire neurology section. Or, you can consult the **"SPECIAL EXPERTISE INDEX"** in the back of this Guide and choose a neurologist who has specific expertise to meet your particular needs.

The geographic sections are as follows:

> *New England*
> *Mid Atlantic*
> *Southeast*
> *Midwest*
> *Great Plains and Mountains*
> *Southwest*
> *West Coast and Pacific*

The states that are included in each region are listed on the following page and a map of the regions is also provided. Please note that not all regions are represented in all specialties. For example, in **"ADOLESCENT MEDICINE"** there are no listings in the Southwest region.

GEOGRAPHIC REGIONS AND STATES

New England:
Connecticut
Maine
Massachusetts
New Hampshire
Rhode Island
Vermont

Mid Atlantic:
Delaware
Maryland
New Jersey
New York
Pennsylvania
Washington, DC
West Virginia

Southeast:
Alabama
Florida
Georgia
Kentucky
Mississippi
North Carolina
South Carolina
Tennessee
Virginia

Midwest:
Illinois
Indiana
Iowa
Michigan
Minnesota
Missouri
Ohio
Wisconsin

Great Plains and Mountains:
Colorado
Idaho
Kansas
Montana
Nebraska
North Dakota
South Dakota
Utah
Wyoming

Southwest:
Arizona
Arkansas
Louisiana
New Mexico
Oklahoma
Texas

West Coast and Pacific:
Alaska
California
Hawaii
Nevada
Oregon
Washington

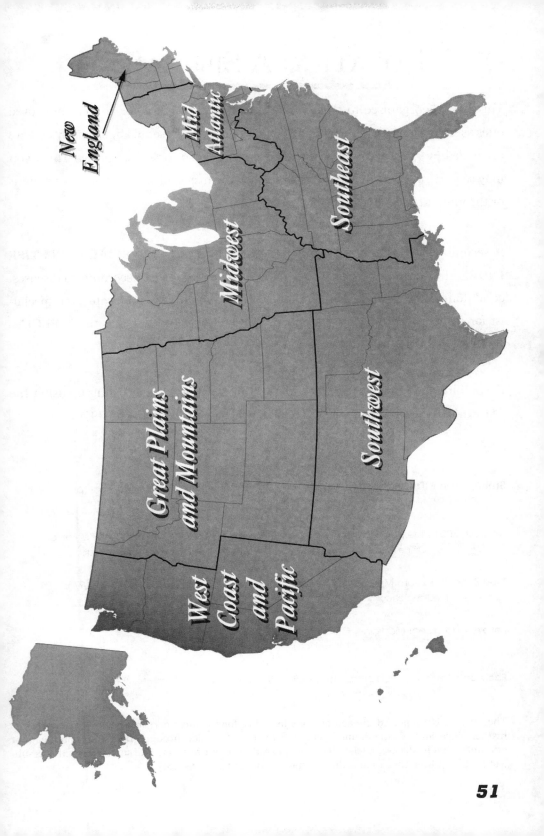

New England

Mid Atlantic

Southeast

Midwest

Great Plains and Mountains

Southwest

West Coast and Pacific

LOCATING A SPECIALIST

This guide is organized to make finding the right specialists for you or your loved ones as simple as possible. Physicians' biographies are presented by specialty and are organized by geographic region within each specialty or subspecialty. Thus, you may search for a particular type of specialist or subspecialist in one or more regions or throughout the nation.

A second way to locate the right specialist is to use the **"SPECIAL EXPERTISE INDEX"** beginning on page 1033. This index is organized according to diseases, conditions and procedures or techniques. For example, you can locate a top specialist for diabetes or for Mohs' surgery by looking for those terms in the **"SPECIAL EXPERTISE INDEX."**

If you already know a specialist's name, you can find his/her listing by using the **"ALPHABETICAL LISTING OF DOCTORS"** beginning on page 1097.

SAMPLE PHYSICIAN LISTING

Smith, John MD (Ped) - *Spec Exp:* Asthma Allergy; **Hospital:** Children's Hospital (page 120);
Name (Specialty)   Special Expertise(s)   Admitting Hospital
                              & Hospital Information Page

Address: 300 Ridge Road Boston, MA 12345; **Phone:** (617) 555-2343; **Board Cert:** Pediatrics 1975;
Office Address   Office Phone   Board Certification(s)

Med School: Harvard Med Sch 1970; **Resid:** Children's Hospital, Boston, MA 1971-1973;
Medical School   Residency(ies)

Fellow: Adolescent Medicine, Children's Hospital, Boston, MA 1973-1974;
Fellowship(s)

Fac Appt: Assoc Prof Pediatrics, The Medical School
Faculty Appointment

The information reported in each doctor's listing is, for the most part, provided by the doctor or his/her office staff. Castle Connolly attempts to verify the data through other sources but cannot guarantee that in all cases all data have been so verified or are accurate. All such information is subject to change from time to time due to changes in physician practices.

HOSPITAL INFORMATION PROGRAM

Among the more than 6,000 acute care and specialty hospitals in the United States, many have extraordinary capabilities for superior patient care. These hospitals, renowned for their use of state-of-the-art equipment and up-to-the-minute technology, also attract outstanding physicians and other healthcare professionals. Many of their physicians are among those in the listings in this Guide.

To further assist you in your search for top specialists and to supplement the information contained in the physician listings that follow, we invited a select group of these fine institutions to profile their services, special programs and centers of excellence in *The Hospital Information Program*. This special section contains pages sponsored by the included hospitals. This paid sponsorship program is totally separate from the physician selection process, which is based upon a completely independent review.

The Hospital Information Program provides an overview of the programs and services offered by the included hospitals with information related to their accreditation and sponsorship. Most also provide their physician referral numbers, should you wish to ask the hospitals for recommendations of doctors not listed in *America's Top Doctors*.

In addition to *The Hospital Information Program*, profiled hospitals were also invited to highlight their special programs or services that focus on a particular disease or medical condition. These can be found in the "Centers of Excellence" sections that are interspersed throughout this book following the medical specialties and/or subspecialties to which they relate. Sponsored pages in the centers of excellence sections reflect the depth of commitment of these hospitals, which provide the staff, resources and financial support necessary to develop these special programs.

We believe you will find this information helpful in your search for the best healthcare—from both physicians and hospitals—throughout the United States!

53

HOSPITAL LISTINGS:

Barnes-Jewish Hospital

BJC HealthCare℠

the primary adult hospital for
Washington University School of Medicine

216 S. Kingshighway
St. Louis, MO 63110
314-TOP-DOCS
(314-867-3627)
or toll free 1-866-867-3627
www.barnesjewish.org

Advancing Medicine. Touching Lives.

A 1,389-bed hospital,
fully accredited by the Joint Commission on Accreditation of Healthcare Organizations.

a leading hospital in the United States

Barnes-Jewish Hospital ranks consistently among the top 10 hospitals nationally in *U.S. News and World Report* ratings. Recognized internationally as a premier teaching and research facility, Barnes-Jewish Hospital:

- is the primary adult teaching hospital of Washington University School of Medicine, one of the top five schools of medicine in the country
- offers more than 10,000 dedicated physicians and staff members who are committed to providing exceptional patient care
- is revered for its hospital-based research programs, which are among the top recipients of funding from the National Institutes of Health.

offering unparalleled clinical excellence

Barnes-Jewish Hospital has a superior reputation for compassionate patient care as well as its exceptional clinical programs including cancer, cardiology, cardiothoracic surgery, dermatology, endocrinology, gastroenterology, general medicine, general surgery, geriatrics, infectious disease, nephrology, neurology, neurosurgery, obstetrics/gynecology, ophthalmology, orthopaedic surgery, otolaryngology, pain management, plastic & reconstructive surgery, psychiatry, pulmonary disease, radiology, rehabilitation, rheumatology, transplantation, trauma, urology and vascular surgery. Today, Barnes-Jewish Hospital:

- is the largest hospital in Missouri with 270,000 inpatient admissions, outpatient visits and emergency department visits from patients around the world
- is home to many clinical firsts, including the world's first successful double lung transplant and the world's first laparoscopic nephrectomy, using a minimally invasive technique developed at the hospital
- is home of the Center for Advanced Medicine, a new, multidisciplinary outpatient center and Siteman Cancer Center, the only NCI-designated cancer center in a 240-mile radius of St. Louis.

"The commitment, compassion and talent of our staff and physicians continue to earn this hospital a world-class reputation."

— Ronald G. Evens, MD, President, Barnes-Jewish Hospital

If you need a physician, go straight to the top.
Call **314-TOP-DOCS** (314-867-3627) or toll free 1-866-867-3627. **www.barnesjewish.org**

CLARIAN HEALTH

Methodist Hospital • Indiana University Hospital • Riley Hospital for Children
Indianapolis, Indiana
317-962-2000

www.clarian.com

Clarian Health and its partners throughout Indiana make up the leading hospital system in the state and one of the busiest and most highly regarded in the nation. There are 8,787 full-time staff at Clarian Health, including 1,269 board-certified specialists and 453 board-certified primary care physicians.

A NEW MODEL FOR CLINICAL CARE

Clarian Health was created in 1997 by bringing together the comprehensive resources of three of the Central Indiana region's strongest medical facilities:
Indiana University Hospital, Methodist Hospital of Indiana, and Riley Hospital for Children. This unique combination offers patients a powerful blending of the highest-quality clinical care, medical education and research, and community health care promotion. Our size and stature—combined, we are one of the busiest hospitals in the nation and the largest in Indiana—enables us to map out new paths in health care.

COMPREHENSIVE PATIENT CARE

We care for the total patient: mind, body and spirit. Our range of services covers virtually every patient need, from complex cardiac procedures and bone marrow transplants to lower-risk outpatient surgeries, primary care visits and patient self-care education.

TURNING RESEARCH INTO TREATMENT

Our superb research capability and our affiliation with Indiana University School of Medicine allow us to move new treatment possibilities from the laboratory bench to the patient's bedside at a remarkable rate. Indiana University School of Medicine educates the second largest medical student body in the country. The School's research efforts—conducted from 18 research centers and institutes—is supported by more than $130 million in grants.

WIDE-RANGING INNOVATION

Clarian stands at the leading edge of innovation in a surprising range of medical specialties. The Indiana University School of Medicine is respected worldwide for its development of innovative approaches to diagnosing and treating the most difficult cardiac conditions. The Indiana University Cancer Center at the School of Medicine received National Cancer Institute designation in 1999 as a Clinical Cancer Center, the first such designated center in the state. Methodist Hospital is one of only two Level I trauma centers in the state.

NATIONAL RECOGNITION, PATIENT SATISFACTION

Clarian Health hospitals have repeatedly been named among the "Best Hospitals in America" by *U.S. News & World Report* magazine, which consistently ranks a number of Clarian's clinical specialties among the top 50 nationwide. Only two other Indiana hospitals were ranked in the report. Also, since 1998, Clarian has set the benchmark standard for exceeding patient expectations among all large hospitals. Ninety-five percent of our patients say that care and treatment is as good or better than expected, and 95% would recommend or use our hospitals again.

THE CLEVELAND CLINIC

9500 Euclid Avenue   Cleveland, OH 44195
Tel. 216/444-CARE (2273) Outside of Cleveland, 800/223-2273
www.clevelandclinic.org

**THE
CLEVELAND
CLINIC**

One of the largest and busiest health centers in America. Number one in heart care. National leaders in Urology and Digestive Diseases. Treating all illnesses and disorders of the body. Second opinions a specialty.

GENERAL OVERVIEW

Founded in 1921, The Cleveland Clinic is a 998-bed hospital that integrates clinical and hospital care with research and education in a private, non-profit group practice. This group practice model provides an environment that allows our physicians to stay at the cutting edge of medical technology. Additionally, there is no financial incentive for any of our physicians to overtreat patients.

VITAL STATISTICS

In 2001, more than 1,100 full-time salaried physicians representing more than 120 medical specialties and subspecialties provided for 2 million outpatient visits, 50,000 hospital admissions and 60,000 surgeries for patients from throughout the United States and more than 80 countries.

ONE OF AMERICA'S BEST

For the past twelve years, The Cleveland Clinic has been named one of the five best hospitals in America in the *U.S.News & World Report* annual "Best Hospitals" survey. In cardiology and cardiac surgery, we lead the nation. Our Heart Center has been ranked number one in America for seven years in a row by *U.S.News & World Report.* The Cleveland Clinic Urological Institute is rated second in the United States, and our Digestive Disease Center is ranked very near the top. Additional specialities rated among America's ten best include Endocrinology, Geriatrics, Nephrology, Neurology and Neurological Surgery, Orthopaedics, Otolaryngology, Pulmonary, and Rheumatology. Other specialties noted for national excellence include Cancer, Gynecology, and Psychiatry.

OUTSTANDING CARE FOR CHILDREN

The Children's Hospital at The Cleveland Clinic offers highly specialized pediatric care in a family-centered atmosphere. It has been ranked the best children's hospital in Ohio by *Child* magazine.

EXPANDING MEDICAL CARE

Over the past several years, The Cleveland Clinic has opened additional state-of-the-art facilities, including the Lerner Research Institute, the Cole Eye Institute, and the Taussig Cancer Center. In Florida, we opened two new campuses combining outpatient clinics with state-of-the-art hospitals in Naples and Weston in 2001.

INTERNATIONAL SERVICES

The Cleveland Clinic's reputation draws patients from all over the world. The International Center is a full-service department dedicated to meeting the needs and requirements of international patients who receive their care at The Cleveland Clinic. The center is staffed by 40 dedicated professionals who offer a variety of services designed to make patients feel welcome and ensure that their visit goes as smoothly as possible.

"The mission of The Cleveland Clinic is threefold: to care for the sick, to educate physicians, and to investigate the causes and treatment of disease."

Sponsored Page

CONTINUUM HEALTH PARTNERS, INC.

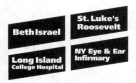

Continuum Health Partners, Inc.

555 West 57th Street
New York, NY 10019
Phone: 800-420-4004
www.WeHealNewYork.org

Sponsorship: Voluntary Not-for-Profit
Beds: 3,048 certified beds
Accreditation: Joint Commission on Accreditation of Healthcare Organizations (JCAHO), Accreditation Council for Graduate Medical Education, Medical Society of New York, in cooperation with the Accreditation Council for Continuing Medical Education

A STRONG PARTNERSHIP WITH A PROUD HERITAGE

Continuum Health Partners, Inc. is a partnership of four venerable health care providers, Beth Israel Medical Center, St. Luke's-Roosevelt Hospital Center, Long Island College Hospital, and the New York Eye and Ear Infirmary. Each of the four partner institutions was established more than a century ago by individuals committed to improving health and health care in their communities. Today, the system represents more than 4,700 physicians and dentists and is superbly equipped to respond to the health care needs of the populations we serve. Continuum providers also see patients in group and private practice settings and in ambulatory centers in New York City and Westchester County.

LOCATIONS

Continuum Health Partners has campuses throughout Manhattan and Brooklyn. Beth Israel Medical Center has three divisions: the Milton and Caroll Petrie Division on the Lower East Side, the Herbert and Nell Singer Division on the Upper East Side, and the Kings Highway Division in Brooklyn. The Phillips Ambulatory Care Center, a state-of-the-art outpatient center, is located at Union Square. St. Luke's-Roosevelt Hospital Center has two campuses on Manhattan's West Side: the St. Luke's Division in Morningside Heights and the Roosevelt Division in Midtown. Long Island College Hospital is located in the Brooklyn Heights/Cobble Hill section of Brooklyn. The New York Eye and Ear Infirmary is located on the Lower East Side.

ACADEMIC AFFILIATIONS

Beth Israel Medical Center is University Hospital and Manhattan Campus for the Albert Einstein College of Medicine. St. Luke's-Roosevelt Hospital Center is University Hospital for Columbia University College of Physicians and Surgeons. Long Island College Hospital is the primary teaching affiliate of the SUNY–Health Science Center at Brooklyn. The New York Eye and Ear Infirmary is the primary teaching center of the New York Medical College and affiliated teaching hospitals in the areas of ophthalmology and otolaryngology.

PHYSICIAN REFERRAL SERVICE: For a referral to a doctor in your neighborhood, call (800) 420-4004. Continuum's Referral Service can help you find a primary care physician or specialist affiliated with Beth Israel, St. Luke's-Roosevelt, Long Island College Hospital, or the New York Eye and Ear Infirmary. Visit our web site at www.WeHealNewYork.org.

DETROIT MEDICAL CENTER

3663 Woodward Ave., Suite 200 • Detroit, Michigan 48201
1-888-DMC-2500
www.dmc.org

Detroit Medical Center
Wayne State University

Southeast Michigan's Largest Health Care Provider.

GENERAL OVERVIEW

The Detroit Medical Center operates seven hospitals and more than 100 outpatient facilities throughout southeast Michigan. The Detroit Medical Center is the region's premier healthcare resource offering the best in research, cutting edge technology, medical education and clinical services.

ACADEMIC & CLINICAL AFFILIATIONS

With over 2,000 licensed beds, the Detroit Medical Center serves as the teaching and clinical research site for Wayne State University School of Medicine and Nursing and Allied Health Services. Wayne State University is the largest single-campus medical school in the country.

BEST AND BRIGHTEST MEDICAL STAFF

The Detroit Medical Center's world-class medical staff consists of 3,000 affiliated physicians, many of whom teach and conduct research at Wayne State University, providing their patients with the most up-to-date and cutting-edge clinical care.

PIONEERING, COMPREHENSIVE MEDICAL CARE

The relationship between the Detroit Medical Center and Wayne State University has already pioneered many treatments for cancer, birth defects, heart disease, and neurological disorders — and innovative diagnostic methods and treatments are being developed every day. The Detroit Medical Center's Children's Hospital of Michigan is the first hospital in the nation to implement computer assisted robot-enhanced surgical system for pediatric patients.

GROWING TO MEET THE COMMUNITY'S NEEDS

Several of the Detroit Medical Center's facilities are growing to meet the community's needs. Sinai-Grace Hospital is undergoing $6.2 million expansion that will house a Comprehensive Heart Center — reviving its open-heart services. Rehabilitation Institute of Michigan has announced a $34.5 million facility project that includes construction of a state-of-the-art, two-story, outpatient therapy and wellness center and a $20 million renovation is underway at Detroit Receiving Hospital's emergency department.

LOCAL AND NATIONAL RECOGNITION

In 2001, the Michigan Minority Business Development Council honored the Detroit Medical Center with its Corporation of the Year — Health Care Sector award in recognition of its excellent minority supplier-purchasing program. Several of the DMC hospitals have garnered national recognition: Children's Hospital of Michigan was named as one of the best children's hospitals in the country by *Child* magazine. Harper University Hospital's stroke program is listed among the Top 100 Stroke Programs in the country. Rehabilitation Institute of Michigan was named as one of "America's Best Hospitals" by *U.S. News and World Report*. Sinai-Grace Hospital's critical care team was recognized as one of the top 100 in the country and the Barbara Ann Karmanos Cancer Institute is Michigan's first National Cancer Institute-designated Comprehensive Cancer Center — one of only two in the state and 40 in the country.

DUKE UNIVERSITY HEALTH SYSTEM

Erwin Road • Durham, NC 27710
1-888-ASK-DUKE • dukehealth.org

Beds: Duke University Hospital: 1,019; Durham Regional Hospital: 391; Raleigh Community Hospital: 205
Accreditation: Accredited by the Joint Commission on Healthcare Accreditation in 2001 for three years

OVERVIEW

Duke University Health System is a world-class health care network dedicated to providing outstanding patient care, educating tomorrow's health care leaders, and discovering better ways to treat disease through biomedical research. Duke offers every level of health service—from wellness and preventive care to the most advanced specialty services—in an atmosphere of caring and compassion.

FACILITIES

The hub of the Health System, Duke University Medical Center is consistently rated among the top medical facilities in the country by *U.S.News & World Report*, and received the 2001 National Research Corporation Consumer Choice Award after local consumers voted it the number-one health care facility in the region. Duke operates one of the country's largest clinical and biomedical research enterprises, and quickly translates advances in technology and medical knowledge into improved patient care. It is the leading medical center in the Southeast, with a medical school ranked among the top three in the nation.

The Health System also provides high-quality clinical services in convenient locations throughout the surrounding region. Included in the Health System are three hospitals, ambulatory surgery centers, primary and specialty care clinics, home care, hospice, skilled nursing care, wellness centers, and community-based clinical partnerships.

CLINICAL PROGRAMS

Duke provides a range of respected clinical programs to meet every patient's needs. Among them are the **Duke Comprehensive Cancer Center**, known for its multidisciplinary approach to treating large tumors and its innovative therapies using bone marrow transplantation and hyperthermia; the **Duke Heart Center**, one of the world's most comprehensive programs, which offers the latest treatments for heart disease; an experienced **organ transplant** team which performs hundreds of transplants each year; **Duke Women's Services**, offering comprehensive care for normal and high-risk pregnancies, reproductive and endocrinology services including the most advanced fertilization techniques, genetic testing, and fetal assessment; a **Children's Hospital & Health Center** offering the full range of primary care and specialty services, including leading programs in bone marrow transplant, pediatric AIDS, and severe combined immunodeficiency syndrome; and an **orthopaedic program** providing expert care in such areas as major joint reconstruction, sports medicine, and reconstructive microsurgery.

In addition, Duke is a leader in the field of **human genetics**. Researchers with Duke's Genomics Institute have helped identify genes associated with obesity and with people's susceptibility to such diseases as breast cancer, colon cancer, Lou Gehrig's disease, and Alzheimer's disease, opening new avenues toward curing and treating these devastating diseases.

To make an appointment with a Duke physician, call 1-888-ASK-DUKE.

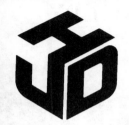

HOSPITAL FOR JOINT DISEASES

301 East 17th Street (at Second Avenue)
New York, NY 10003
212-598-6000
FAX: 212-260-1203
www.jointdiseases.com

Sponsorship:	Mount Sinai NYU Health
Beds:	216
Accreditation:	Joint Commission on Accreditation of Healthcare Organizations (JCAHO), Commission for Accreditation of Rehabilitation Facilities (CARF)

PROFILE
The Hospital for Joint Diseases is one of the nation's leading orthopaedic, rheumatologic, neurologic, and rehabilitation specialty hospitals dedicated to the prevention and treatment of neuromusculoskeletal diseases. HJD is a voluntary, not-for-profit teaching hospital, and part of Mount Sinai NYU Health.

MEDICAL STAFF
The Hospital for Joint Disease has over 500 board certified members of the attending medical staff specializing in orthopaedics, rheumatology, neurology, and rehabilitation medicine.

TEACHING PROGRAMS
The Hospital for Joint Diseases, along with NYU Medical Center, sponsors a fully accredited five-year orthopaedic surgery residency program with twelve residents each year. In addition, seven different fellowships are offered in the subspecialty areas of orthopaedics, hand, foot and ankle, spine, sports medicine, shoulder, and total joint replacement.

SPECIAL PROGRAMS
Orthopaedic Surgery Hip and Knee Replacement Center, Arthroscopic Surgery, Bone Tumor Service, Foot and Ankle Surgery, Hand Surgery, Limb Lengthening and Bone Growth, Occupational and Industrial Orthopaedic Care, Sports Medicine, Pediatric Orthopaedics, Shoulder Institute, Center for Neuromuscular and Developmental Disorders, The Geriatric Hip Fracture Program, Diabetes Foot and Ankle Center, The Scoliosis Program, The Spine Center, The Harkness Center for Dance Injuries, 24-hour Immediate Orthopaedic Care

Center for Arthritis and Autoimmunity Rheumatoid Arthritis, Osteoarthritis, Psoriatic Arthritis, Lupus, Osteoporosis, Fibromyalgia, Scleroderma, Sjogren's Syndrome

Neurology Orthopaedic Neurology, Initiative for Women with Disabilities, Multiple Sclerosis, Neuroimmunology, Neurosurgery, Comprehensive Pain Treatment Center, Clinical Neurophysiology, Movement Disorders, and Neurorehabilitation

Rehabilitation Medicine Comprehensive inpatient (orthopaedic and neurological rehabilitation, pain management) and outpatient rehabilitation services at four locations.

OTHER SERVICES
Managed Care Plans The Hopsital for Joint Diseases participates in over 45 managed care plans covering 72 different products (i.e., HMO, POS, PPO, Medicare, Medicaid, etc.)

Physician Referral The hospital offers a free telephone physician referral service, Monday-Friday, 8:00 am to 4:00 pm. The physician referral service can be reached at 1-888-HJD-DOCS (1-888-453-3627).

HOSPITAL FOR SPECIAL SURGERY

535 East 70th Street, New York, NY 10021
phone: 212-606-1779
web--site: www.hss.edu

Sponsorship:	Private, Non-Profit
Beds:	160
Accreditation:	Awarded Accreditation from the Joint Commission on Accreditation of Healthcare Organizations (JCAHO).

PROFILE

Hospital for Special Surgery is the world's leading orthopedic, rheumatologic and rehabilitation specialty hospital. *US News & World Report* has selected the Hospital as the top ranked hospital in the Northeast for its specialties.

Founded in 1863, the Hospital is dedicated to the prevention and treatment of diseases of the musculoskeletal system. HSS is a voluntary, not for profit teaching hospital, affiliated with the New York Presbyterian Healthcare Network and the Weill Medical College of Cornell University.

MEDICAL STAFF

There are more than 200 board certified attending medical staff at the Hospital. All physicians have appointments at Weill Medical College of Cornell University, and a large number of the staff are actively engaged in groundbreaking research.

TEACHING PROGRAMS

The Hospital for Special Surgery has had a continuous postgraduate training program ("Residency") for more than 100 years. The five -year Orthopedic Surgery Residency has 8 Residents in each class. In addition, HSS postgraduate programs include over 45 fellows from Fellowship programs in Orthopedic Surgery subspecialties, Rheumatic Disease Medicine, Musculoskeletal Radiology and MRI, Neurology, and Anesthesiology. About 100 third year and fourth year medical students rotate through HSS each year, receiving instruction from Residents, Fellows, and Attending Staff.

RESEARCH

The mission of research at Hospital for Special Surgery is to attain the highest level of scientific excellence in orthopedics, rheumatology and related scientific disciplines. Expert scientists and clinicians work in close proximity in three integrated levels of research—basic, applied and clinical—with the goals of discovering the causes of musculoskeletal disease and injury and enhancing the quality of life for those afflicted by them.

SPECIALTIES

The Hospital addresses all problems of the musculoskeletal system. State of the art anesthesia and musculoskeletal radiology are an integral part of patient care. Specialties include: Arthroscopy, Back Pain, Bone Tumors, Carpal Tunnel Syndrome, Cerebral Palsy, Club Foot, Complementary Medicine, Congenital Dislocation of the Hip, Hand Therapy, Joint Replacement Surgery, Juvenile Rheumatoid Arthritis, Ligament Injuries, Limb Lengthening and Deformity, Lyme Disease, Muscular Dystrophy, Orthopedic Trauma, Osteoporosis, Paget's Disease, Pain Management, Pediatric Orthopedics, Pediatric Rheumatology, Physiatry, Podiatry, Rehabilitation (Physical/Occupational Therapy), Rheumatoid Arthritis, Scoliosis, Spina Bifida, Sports Medicine, Systemic Lupus Erythematosus, Women's Sports Medicine.

PHYSICIAN REFERRAL
Call 1.800.854.0071 for a referral to one of our specialists, Monday – Friday 9:00 am – 5:00 pm.

INDIANA UNIVERSITY HOSPITAL

A Part of Clarian Health Partners
550 University Blvd. • Indianapolis, Indiana 46202
317-962-2000

www.clarian.org

As a member of Clarian Health Partners, Indiana University Hospital is part of the leading hospital system in Indiana and one of the busiest and most highly regarded in the nation. It is the home of practice activities for the IU School of Medicine, one of the largest medical schools in the nation.

PUTTING RESEARCH INTO PRACTICE

The physicians at IU Hospital are faculty members of the Indiana University School of Medicine and participate in its extensive teaching and research programs. Their expertise is based on the transfer of research discoveries to clinical trials and into accepted practice. Research is conducted in most basic science and clinical areas, as well as in highly-specialized areas including cancer, arthritis, diabetes, hypertension, medical genetics, alcoholism, Alzheimer's disease, sexually transmitted diseases and general clinical research.

WIDE RANGE OF SPECIALIZED SERVICES

As part of Clarian Health, IU physicians, surgeons, nurses and staff care for more than 57,000 patients a year. The physicians and other health professionals at IU Hospital see patients with complex health problems, including pulmonary diseases, organ failure, all cancers and neurological disorders including Alzheimer's and Parkinson's diseases. Special services and features of IU Hospital include:

- Clinical Trial Site (breast, uterine and testicular cancer treatments).
- Bone Marrow Transplant Program.
- AIDS Research Center.
- Indiana Diabetes Center.
- Coleman Center for Women—research and patient care in treating gynecological cancers and high-risk pregnant women.
- IU Alzheimer's Disease Center, funded by the National Institutes of Health
- Multidisciplinary Prostate Research and Treatment Center.
- Together with IU Department of Radiation Oncology sponsors the Indiana Lions Gamma Knife Center.
- Mark Dyken Neurology Center—one of the country's leading research and patient care centers for epilepsy, stroke and neuromuscular disorders.
- Adult in-patient services and research support for the IU Cancer Center, a National Cancer Institute-designated clinical cancer center.

PIONEERING MEDICAL TREATMENT

IU Hospital has pioneered numerous medical firsts. Significant achievements from IU Hospital include:

- Development of cure for testicular cancer by Lawrence Einhorn, M.D.
- Plays leading role in transplantation research, including first kidney, liver and pancreas transplants in Indiana
- Houses the state's only Positron Emission Tomography (PET) scanner, which is used for patient treatment and research on new applications of PET.

Lenox Hill Hospital

100 East 77th Street, New York, NY 10021
Tel: 212-434-2000   Fax. 212-434-2087
www.lenoxhillhospital.org

Beds: 652
Sponsorship: Voluntary Not-for-Profit
Accreditation: Joint Commission on Accreditation of Healthcare Organizations, College of American Pathologists, American Association of Blood Banks, Accreditation Council for Graduate Medical Education, Accreditation Council for Continuing Medical Education, Commission on Accreditation of Allied Health Education Programs

GENERAL PROFILE

Founded in 1857, Lenox Hill Hospital is an acute care, fully accredited teaching hospital with an excellent reputation for providing the highest quality patient care while pioneering innovative treatments. The hospital offers a wide range of services in medicine, surgery, pediatrics, obstetrics and gynecology and psychiatric services.

Manhattan Eye, Ear & Throat Hospital, a world-renowned specialty hospital serving the community since 1869, is a subsidiary of Lenox Hill Hospital.

MEDICAL STAFF

Lenox Hill Hospital has over 1,300 dedicated physicians on staff, with outstanding national and international reputations in their fields. Over 85% are board certified. Manhattan Eye, Ear & Throat Hospital has 566 physicians on its staff.

TEACHING PROGRAMS

The hospital offers 12 residency programs and 8 fellowship programs and is a major teaching affiliate of New York University School of Medicine.

Lenox Hill Heart & Vascular Insitutue of New York	The Lenox Hill Heart and Vascular Institute is among the leading cardiovascular care programs in the nation. The Institute offers a comprehensive approach to total cardiac and vascular care, providing patients with diagnosis and treatment of simple and complex conditions, as well as rehabilitation and disease prevention. The Institute's internationally renowned team of specialists in cardiology, interventional cardiology, cardiothoracic and vascular surgery, endovascular surgery and radiology treat all types and stages of heart disease.
Orthopedic Surgery	Lenox Hill Hospital is recognized internationally as a leader in orthopedic surgery and sports medicine. The Hospital's Nicholas Institute of Sports Medicine and Athletic Trauma was the first hospital-based center in the U.S. dedicated to the advancement of research in sports medicine. Its expert staff provides treatment and rehabilitation to injured athletes, including players on the NY Jets and Islanders. Lenox Hill Hospital's outstanding orthopedic surgeons are distinguished leaders in total joint replacement surgery, offering the most advanced technology and techniques to increase the durability of hip and knee implants.
Maternal/Child Health	Lenox Hill Hospital is renowned for exceptional obstetrical services, from prenatal care to postpartum care. The hospital's obstetricians/gynecologists manage routine and high-risk obstetrics and gynecological concerns and offer specialized expertise in breast disease, reproductive endocrinology, bladder disorders, infertility and gynecologic oncology.
Otolaryngology - Head & Neck Surgery	Lenox Hill Hospital and Manhattan Eye, Ear & Throat Hospital provide internationally renowned expertise in the diagnosis and treatment of ear, nose, throat and voice disorders in adults and children.
Primary Care & Internal Medicine	A large team of physicians and medical professionals specializing in primary care and internal medicine provides families with comprehensive medical care.

Physician Referral: Need a doctor? Call our 24-hour physician referral service toll free at 1-888-RIGHT MD (1-888-744-4863).

MAIMONIDES MEDICAL CENTER

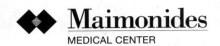

4802 Tenth Avenue
Brooklyn, NY 11219
Phone: (718) 283-6000
Physician Referral: (888) MMC-DOCS
Website: http://www.maimonidesmed.org

Sponsorship: Voluntary Not-for-Profit
Beds: 705 acute, 70 psychiatric
Accreditation: Joint Commission on Accreditation of Healthcare Organizations (JCAHO), American College of Surgeons, American Council of Graduate Medical Education (ACGME)

GENERAL DESCRIPTION

Maimonides Medical Center is the nation's third largest independent teaching hospital. A nonsectarian institution under Jewish auspices, it serves patients from the New York metropolitan area and beyond. Maimonides is a major teaching affiliate of SUNY-Health Science Center at Brooklyn.

MEDICAL STAFF AND TEACHING PROGRAMS

Maimonides Medical Center has nearly 1,200 active physicians, including internationally renowned specialists. The hospital offers 24 residency programs in various areas, including anesthesiology, cardiology, dentistry, emergency medicine, geriatrics, internal medicine, obstetrics and gynecology, orthopaedic surgery, pediatrics, psychiatry, radiology, surgery and urology. The hospital's resident staff is composed of 380 physicians.

CENTERS OF EXCELLENCE

Ambulatory Health Services	25 primary care and specialty sites, including cardiac rehabilitation program and women's healthcare
Genesis Fertility	Comprehensive diagnostic testing and intervention, including hormone replacement therapy, genetic screening, ovulation induction, in-vitro feritilization and other assisted reproductive techniques
The Cardiac Institute	World-renowned excellence in cardiac surgery (1,000+ procedures annually); pioneers many new angiographic techniques (e.g., atherectomy and percutaneous transmyocardial revascularization); leading electrophysiology lab
Infants and Children's Hospital	Pediatric subspecialty services, including adolescent medicine, allergy, behavioral psychology, cardiology, endocrinology, gastroenterology, genetics, hematology/oncology, infectious disease, neonatology, otolaryngology and surgery
Community Mental Health Center	Specialized programs including the Latino Day Program; center for the developmentally disabled; and FACES, an innovative teen theater network
The Orthopaedic Institute	Complex procedures such as limb-lengthening techniques, correction of congenital deformities, endoscopic spinal surgery, repair of traumatic sports injuries. Rehabilitation services include a state-of-the-art center equipped with a full lap pool and advanced exercise equipment
Stella and Joseph Payson Birthing Center	Warm environment with life-saving techniques, 40 physicians and 27 midwives; perinatal testing center with 3-D ultrasound
The Vascular Institute	Comprehensive diagnostic and surgical services for treatment of vascular diseases; largest diagnostic vascular lab in New York State; Wound Treatment Center
Weinberg Emergency Center	More than 80,000 cases annually; heart center; separate pediatric ER

METHODIST HOSPITAL

A Part of Clarian Health Partners
1701 North Senate Blvd.
Indianapolis, Indiana 46202
317-962-2000

www.clarian.org

As a member of Clarian Health Partners, Methodist Hospital is part of the leading hospital system in Indiana and one of the busiest and most highly regarded Level I trauma centers in the nation.

NEARING A CENTURY OF SERVICE

Methodist Hospital opened its doors in 1908 with 65 beds and cared for nearly 900 patients during its first year of operation. Today, Methodist has 775 staffed beds, and Methodist physicians, surgeons, nurses and staff care for more than 57,000 patients a year. It is one of only two regional Level I trauma centers in Indiana and one of the largest teaching hospitals in the area.

WIDE-RANGING EXPERTISE

Methodist specializes in numerous treatment areas, including adult cardiovascular services provided by the Clarian Cardiovascular Center. The hospital is also considered a neurosurgery center of excellence, as well as an expert center for urology, neurology, orthopedics and pediatrics. Methodist also operates two LifeLine helicopter ambulances and houses the Indiana Poison Center. Methodist Hospital also:

- Provides diabetes management educational and support programs at the Methodist Diabetes Center.
- Houses one of the largest neuroscience and neurosurgical programs in the nation.
- Offers comprehensive opthalmological care through the Midwest Eye Institute.
- Provides Indiana's most comprehensive assessment, referrals and inpatient or outpatient treatment options at the Behavioral Health Center.
- Is the campus location for the IU ◆ Methodist Family Practice Center.

A HISTORY OF FIRSTS

Methodist Hospital physicians and staff have contributed to a solid record of medical innovations. Beginning with pioneering work—as one of the primary centers for clinical research—in the use of insulin to treat diabetes mellitus, Methodist has achieved numerous medical "firsts" in a range of areas, including:

- First open-heart surgery and first artificial heart implantation in state.
- First CAT scan system in state, and only the ninth in the nation.
- First heart transplant in a private hospital anywhere in the world.
- First use of an extracorporeal shock wave lithotripter, a device that pulverizes kidney stones using shock waves, in the nation.
- First heart-lung transplant and first double-lung transplant in state.
- First insulin pump implantation for treatment of insulin-dependent diabetes in Midwest.

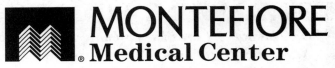

MONTEFIORE
Medical Center

The University Hospital for the Albert Einstein College of Medicine

HENRY AND LUCY MOSES DIVISION	**WEILER/EINSTEIN DIVISION**
111 EAST 210TH STREET	**1825 EASTCHESTER ROAD**
BRONX, NY 10467-2490	**BRONX, NY 10461-2373**
PHONE (718) 920-4321	**PHONE (718) 904-2000**
FAX (718) 920-8543	**FAX (718) 920-2189**

Web Site: www.montefiore.org

Sponsorship	Voluntary Not-for-Profit
Beds	624 acute 20 psych 200 nursing home 106 children's hospital
Accreditation	Joint Commission on Accreditation of Healthcare Organizations (JCAHO), National Committee for Ambulatory Care, American College of Radiology

INNOVATION AND LEADERSHIP IN CLINICAL CARE, TEACHING, RESEARCH AND COMMUNITY OUTREACH

Montefiore Medical Center is internationally recognized as a leader in patient care, education, research and community service. Montefiore serves as a tertiary care referral center offering the most advanced care to patients from the entire New York City metropolitan area and across the nation. The medical center encompasses two acute care hospitals, two new ambulatory specialty care centers, a network of 22 Montefiore Medical Group primary care offices in the Bronx and Westchester County, one of the nation's largest home health agencies, and The Children's Hospital at Montefiore.

Montefiore Medical Center's outstanding, state-of-the-art care includes the following Centers of Excellence: *Montefiore-Einstein Heart Center, Montefiore-Einstein Cancer Center, Neurosciences, The Children's Hospital at Montefiore, Women's Health,* and *Surgery at Montefiore* which includes Montefiore's Institute for Minimally Invasive Surgery.

WESTCHESTER SPECIALTY PROGRAMS

Specialty centers in nearby Westchester County include the Fertility and Hormone Center in Hartsdale, Larchmont Women's Center, Laser & Eye Center in White Plains, and a Multispecialty Center in Eastchester.

INFORMATION

For physician referral or information, call 1-800-MD-MONTE.

THE MOUNT SINAI HOSPITAL

One Gustave L. Levy Place (Fifth Avenue and 98th Street)
New York, NY 10029-6574
Phone: (212) 241-6500

Physician Referral: 1-800-MD-SINAI (637-4624)
www.mountsinai.org

Sponsorship	Voluntary Not-for-Profit
Beds	1,171
Accreditation	Joint Commission on Accreditation of Healthcare Organization (JCAHO)
	Commission for Accreditation of Rehabilitation Facilities (CARF)

Founded in 1852, The Mount Sinai Hospital is one of the country's oldest and largest voluntary teaching hospitals. Mount Sinai is internationally acclaimed for excellence in clinical care, education, and scientific research in nearly every aspect of medicine.

Recognized for excellence in numerous specialties, The Mount Sinai Hospital and its medical staff have been consistently ranked among the best in New York City and the country by such respected magazines as *U.S. News & World Report*, and *New York* magazine. Among the departments and services most frequently singled out for excellence are:

- The **Zena and Michael A. Wiener Cardiovascular Institute**, which provides tertiary and quaternary care for those at risk for heart disease and those who suffer from acute cardiac illnesses. A team of physicians and surgeons works with a full complement of rehabilitation experts and special services designed to help patients live life to the fullest.

- Mount Sinai's new **Cardiothoracic Surgery Center**, brings together one of the nation's most renowned teams of cardiothoracic surgeons, headed by Dr. David Adams. They work in collaboration with their colleagues in cardiovascular care to deliver the best in cardiothoracic surgery, including mitral valve repair, beating heart coronary bypass surgery, minimally invasive valve surgery and pediatric cardiac surgery. Another team member, Dr. Scott Swanson, brings world-class expertise in thoracic surgery to Mount Sinai, including thoracic oncology, swallowing disorders and gastroesophageal reflux disease.

- The **Recanati/Miller Transplantation Institute** is recognized across the country in organ transplantation, and one of the few to successfully provide combined organ transplantation. Renowned for its long-term experience in the field, The Mount Sinai Hospital was the site of the first liver transplant surgery in New York State. The Institute also performs more living-donor liver transplants than any other hospital in the country.

- The **Minimally-Invasive Surgery** program offers an ever-expanding expertise in laparoscopic procedures: aortic valve replacement, mitral valve repair and replacement, abdominal aortic aneurym repair, radical prostatectomy, nephrectomy, cystectomy, gastric bypass, treatments for codometriosis, uterine fibroids, ovarian cysts, as well as for cervical, ovarian, and uterine cancers.

Physician Referral (800) MD-SINAI / (800) 637-4624
The Mount Sinai Hospital provides a free physician referral and health resource service
from 8:30 a.m. to 6 p.m. weekdays, staffed exclusively by registered nurses.
Consumers can also select a Mount Sinai physician by visiting the Find A Doctor section
of our website, www.mountsinai.org.

Sponsored Page

THE NEW YORK EYE & EAR INFIRMARY

310 East Fourteenth St. • New York, New York 10003
Tel.: 212.979.4000 • Fax.: 212.228.0664
Web: www.nyee.edu

NY Eye & Ear Infirmary

Affiliated Teaching
Hospital of New York
Medical College

Continuum Health Partners, Inc.

Sponsorship: Voluntary Not-for-Profit
Beds: 103
Accreditation: Joint Commission on Accreditation of Healthcare Organizations, College of American Pathologists

ABOUT THE NEW YORK EYE AND EAR INFIRMARY

The New York Eye and Ear Infirmary is one of the world's leading facilities for the diagnosis and treatment of diseases of the eyes, ears, nose, throat and related conditions. A voluntary, not-for-profit institution, the Infirmary is an affiliated teaching hospital of New York Medical College and a member of Continuum Health Partners, Inc.

THE MEDICAL STAFF

The Medical Staff includes more than 500 attending physicians and surgeons throughout the metropolitan area. Many are renowned for their breakthrough research introducing widely practiced techniques.

RESEARCH AND EDUCATION

The New York Eye and Ear Infirmary is a national and international leader in research in its specialties, achieving many "firsts" in successful procedures and medical treatments. Laboratories include Cell Culture, Ocular Imaging, and Microsurgical Education.

SPECIALTIES

Ophthalmology: Within this area are subspecialties of cataract, glaucoma, retina, cornea and refractive surgery, ocular plastic surgery, pediatric ophthalmology and strabismus, neuro-ophthalmology and ocular tumor. Laser, photography, fluorescein angiography and electro-physiological testing are among the most advanced services available anywhere.

Otolaryngology: The department is in the forefront of treatment modalities using highly sophisticated endoscopic and laser equipment. Subspecialties include allergy, voice, rhinology, head & neck surgery, otology, neurotology, pediatric otolaryngology, audiology, speech therapy and hearing aid dispensing.

Plastic & Reconstructive Surgery: Microsurgical capabilities and premium patient accommodations provide an optimum environment for facial plasty, liposuction and repair of defects from disease or trauma.

RELATED SERVICES

New York Eye Trauma Center: An advanced program for emergency treatment of eye injuries, it also is the Eye Injury Registry of New York State and leading collector of data which will help develop preventative strategies.

Vision Correction Center: State-of-the-art facility dedicated to all forms of laser refractive surgery performed in an academic medical center in the forefront of teaching and research in vision correction.

Ambulatory Surgery: A comprehensive Ambulatory Surgery Center is designed to expedite admission testing, pre-op preparation and post-op recovery in an efficient and comfortable setting.

Pediatric Specialty Care: The city's only such center coordinating the services of eye and ear, nose and throat specialists with other staff especially sensitive to the youngest patients.

Physician Referral: Call 1-800-449-HOPE (4673)

NewYork-Presbyterian
The University Hospitals of Columbia and Cornell

NewYork Weill Cornell Medical Center
525 East 68th Street
New York, NY 10021

Columbia Presbyterian Medical Center
622 West 168th Street
New York, NY 10032

Sponsorship: Voluntary Not-for-Profit
Beds: 2,369
Accreditation: Joint Commission on Accreditation of Healthcare Organizations (JCAHO), Commission on Accreditation of Rehabilitation Facilities (CARF) and College of American Pathologists (CAP)

The *U.S. News & World Report* has ranked NewYork-Presbyterian Hospital higher in more specialties than any other hospital in the New York area. NewYork-Presbyterian Hospital was named to the *Honor Roll of America's Best Hospitals*.

OVERVIEW:

NewYork-Presbyterian Hospital is the largest hospital in New York and one of the most comprehensive health-care institutions in the world with 5,500 physicians, approximately 96,000 discharges and nearly 1 million out-patient visits annually, and with its affiliated medical schools, more than $330 million in research support.

AMONG ITS RENOWNED CENTERS OF EXCELLENCE ARE:

Children's Hospital of NewYork-Presbyterian – One of the largest, most comprehensive children's hospitals in the world providing highly sophisticated pediatric medical, surgical and intensive care, including a pediatric cardiovascular center, in a compassionate environment.

Columbia Weill Cornell Cancer Centers – Coordinated, multidisciplinary care and the latest therapeutic options and clinical trials available for all types of cancer.

Columbia Weill Cornell Heart Institute – Expert diagnostic capabilities and medical and surgical innovations for simple to complex heart conditions.

Columbia Weill Cornell Neuroscience Centers – Latest research, diagnosis and treatment capabilities in Alzheimer's disease, Multiple Sclerosis, Parkinson's disease, aneurysms, epilepsy, brain tumors, stokes and other neurological disorders.

Columbia Weill Cornell Psychiatry – World-renowned center of excellence in psychiatric treatment, research and education.

Columbia Weill Cornell Transplantation Institute – Adult and pediatric heart, liver, and kidney and adult pancreas and lung transplantation and cutting-edge research.

Columbia Weill Cornell Vascular Care Center – Comprehensive and integrated preventive, diagnostic and treatment program for diverse problems related to arteries and veins throughout the body.

NewYork-Presbyterian Digestive Disease Services – Expert capabilities in the broad range of conditions that affect the organs as well as other components of the digestive system.

Randolph Hearst Burn Center – Largest and busiest burn center in the nation which also conducts research to improve survival and enhance quality of life for burn victims.

In addition, the Hospital offers extraordinary expertise, comprehensive programs and specialized resources in the fields of AIDS, Gene Therapy, Reproductive Medicine and Infertility, Trauma Center and Women's Health Care.

ACADEMIC AFFILIATIONS:

NewYork-Presbyterian is the only hospital in the world affiliated with two Ivy League medical schools; The Joan and Sanford I Weill Medical College of Cornell University and the Columbia University College of Physicians & Surgeons.

Physician Referral: To find a NewYork-Presbyterian Hospital affiliated physician to meet your needs, call toll free 1-877-NYP-WELL (1-877-697-9355) or visit our Web site at www.nyp.org.

NYU MEDICAL CENTER

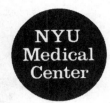

550 First Avenue (at 31st Street)
New York, NY 10016
Physician Referral:
(888) 7–NYU–MED (888–769–8633)
www.nyumedicalcenter.org

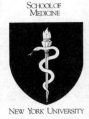

SCHOOL OF MEDICINE

NEW YORK UNIVERSITY

Sponsorship:	**Private, Not-for-Profit**
Beds:	**878 beds**
Accreditation:	**Joint Commission on Accreditation of Healthcare Organizations (JCAHO), Commission for Accreditation of Rehabilitation Facilities (CARF)**

A LEADER IN PATIENT CARE

NYU Medical Center is one of the nation's leading biomedical resources, combining excellence in patient care, research and medical education. A not-for-profit institution, NYU Medical Center includes **Tisch Hospital**, a voluntary 704-bed tertiary care facility serving more than 31,000 inpatients annually, and the **Rusk Institute of Rehabilitation Medicine**, which has 174 beds and serves 2,800 inpatients and more than 53,000 outpatients annually.

The Medical Center maintains close academic and clinical affiliations with the **Hospital for Joint Diseases**, which has 220 beds and is one of the nation's premier hospitals for treating orthopaedic and rheumatological disorders, and **NYU Downtown Hospital**, an excellent 330-bed community hospital.

SPECIAL PROGRAMS AT TISCH HOSPITAL

Cancer One of the country's elite NCI-designated comprehensive cancer centers

Cardiac Surgery A leader in minimally invasive techniques and robotic procedures

Cardiology A full range of diagnostic, prognostic and treatment services for patients of all ages

Epilepsy The largest facility of its kind on the East Coast

Gamma Knife Non-surgical precision treatment for many neurological disorders

Pain Management Specialties: acute cancer and chronic pain management services

Plastic Surgery The largest facility of its kind in the world

Pregnancy (High-Risk) Unparalleled diagnostic techniques and surgical innovations for those with trouble conceiving or with special risks

Skin Diseases Renowned for treating serious and rare skin disorders

Surgery Leading the nation in advancement of minimally invasive procedures and surgical techniques

Transplant Some of the nation's best patient and graft survival techniques

Urology Leaders in treating prostate disorders and other urological problems

THE RUSK INSTITUTE OF REHABILITATION MEDICINE

The world's first and still one of the largest university centers for adult and pediatric rehabilitation, ranked the #1 rehabilitation hospital in New York City by *U.S. News & World Reports* for the last twelve years.

Physician Referral (888) 7-NYU-MED - (888-769-8633)
a free telephone referral service staffed by R.N.s trained to access over 1,500 NYU physicians.

RUSH-PRESBYTERIAN-ST. LUKE'S MEDICAL CENTER

1653 W. CONGRESS PARKWAY   *CHICAGO, IL 60612*
Tel. 312.942.5000   *www.rush.edu*

Beds: 934

Sponsorship/Network Affiliation: Rush-Presbyterian-St. Luke's Medical Center, the heart of the Rush System for Health, is a private, not-for-profit organization.

GENERAL OVERVIEW

For more than 160 years, Rush-Presbyterian-St. Luke's Medical Center has been recognized as a leader in patient care, teaching and research. Located minutes from downtown Chicago on the city's near West Side, Rush is the largest private hospital in Illinois and home of one of the first medical centers in the Midwest. This medical academic center includes the 809-bed Presbyterian-St. Luke's Hospital (including Rush Children's Hospital) and the 154-bed Johnston R. Bowman Health Center for the Elderly as well as Rush University. Its seven Rush institutes draw together patient care and research to address major health problems and offer primary health care services as well as latest treatments for arthritis and orthopedic problems, cancer, heart disease, mental illness, diseases associated with aging and neurological problems.

ACADEMIC & CLINICAL AFFILIATIONS

Integral to the Medical Center is Rush University, which includes Rush Medical College, the College of Nursing, the College of Health Sciences, the Graduate College and a cooperative educational network of 14 liberal arts colleges and universities in six states from Tennessee to Colorado. Rush-Presbyterian-St. Luke's Medical Center is the hub of one of the largest health care networks in the Chicago area, which encompasses five affiliated hospitals in Illinois and a wide range of health services, including alternative health care, hospice services, behavioral health and home health care. These hospitals include, Oak Park Hospital, Riverside HealthCare in Kankakee, Rush-Copley Medical Center in Aurora and Rush North Shore Medical Center in Skokie.

MEDICAL STAFF

Rush-Presbyterian-St. Luke's has 1,241 physicians who represent virtually all medical specialties and sub-specialties. Many of Rush's physicians are also leaders in research, pioneering innovative treatments and improving patient care. The Medical Center's multidisciplinary approach has allowed the development of integrated therapies for patients with diseases such as multiple sclerosis, rheumatoid arthritis and Alzheimer's disease.

COMPREHENSIVE CARE

Rush-Presbyterian-St. Luke's, a major referral center, provides care from the most basic to the most advanced for patients from metropolitan Chicago and across the country. The Medical Center includes six institutes—comprehensive, multidisciplinary centers that offer primary health care services along with leading-edge diagnostic techniques and treatments for a variety of problems, including arthritis and orthopedic problems, heart disease, mental illness, diseases associated with aging and neurological disorders.

PIONEERING RESEARCH

As one of the largest centers for basic and clinical research in the Midwest, Rush is involved in more than 2,000 investigations of promising technologies and therapies aimed at achieving a better understanding of disease, and in fiscal year 2000 Rush researchers received $63.5 million in outside funding. By rapidly transferring knowledge from the laboratory to the bedside, Rush is continually helping patients at Rush and across the country.

ACCREDITATION, COMMENDATIONS & NATIONAL RECOGNITION

Rush-Presbyterian-St. Luke's Medical Center is accredited by the Joint Commission on Accreditation of Healthcare Organizations, the Commission for Accreditation of Rehabilitation Facilities, the Liaison Committee on Medical Education and numerous other organizations. In 2000, *U.S. News & World Report* ranked Rush in the top 50 in 11 medical specialties and tops in heart care in Chicago.

Rush-Presbyterian-St. Luke's Medical Center—Where world-class medicine revolves around you. www.rush.edu

SHANDS AT THE UNIVERSITY OF FLORIDA

1600 SW Archer Road, Gainesville, FL 32610
General information: 352.265.0111
Patient referral: 800.749.7424
Physician-to-physician referral: 800.633.2122
www.shands.org

Sponsorship: Not-for-profit academic medical center affiliated with the University of Florida
Beds: 570
Accreditation: Joint Commission on Accreditation of HealthCare Organizations

A COMPREHENSIVE HEALTHCARE RESOURCE FOR THE SOUTHEAST

Shands at UF is the nationally recognized medical center within the Shands HealthCare system of hospitals and affiliated physician practices located throughout north Florida. The 570-bed private, not-for-profit facility is one of the most comprehensive hospitals in the Southeast, offering highly specialized, complex medical care. The *U.S. News & World Report* "Guide to America's Best Hospitals" ranked Shands at UF in more clinical specialties than any other hospital in Florida.

SPECIALIZED SERVICES

The hospital offers four centers of excellence - in cardiovascular services, neurosurgical/neurological services, cancer care and transplantation - as well as Shands Children's Hospital, nationally recognized for its innovative and family-friendly environmental design.

SPECIALIZED PATIENT CARE

Shands at UF is the flagship academic medical center for the UF Health Science Center, which includes the Colleges of Dentistry, Health Professions, Medicine, Nursing, Pharmacy and Veterinary Medicine. More than 600 UF physicians representing 110 medical specialties work alongside a team of highly skilled nurses and healthcare professionals to provide quality patient care.

Shands at UF is a resource for patients who have complex health problems or are challenged with chronic disease. This high acuity requires advanced technical equipment and state-of-the-art facilities.

PIONEERING RESEARCH

As one of the largest centers for basic and clinical research in the Southeast, Shands at UF is involved in more than 200 investigations of promising technologies and therapies aimed at improving outcomes for disease prevention, diagnosis and treatment. By rapidly transferring knowledge from the "bench to bedside," UF physicians help bring a higher level of care to patients at Shands at UF and medical centers worldwide.

Physician referral
The Shands Consultation Center is your link to more than 600 UF physicians and the numerous programs and services offered by Shands HealthCare. For more information or to schedule an appointment, please call 800.749.7424 or visit our Web site at shands.org.

ST. FRANCIS HOSPITAL
THE HEART CENTER®

100 PORT WASHINGTON BLVD.   ROSLYN, NEW YORK 11576
Tel. 516. 562.6000
www.stfrancisheartcenter.com

Beds: 279
Sponsorship/Network Affiliation: A voluntary not-for-profit organization, St. Francis Hospital is a Member of Catholic Health Services of Long Island.

NEW YORK'S CARDIAC SPECIALTY CENTER

St. Francis Hospital, The Heart Center® is New York State's only specialty designated cardiac center and has the highest cardiac caseload in the Northeast. Founded in 1922 by the Sisters of the Franciscan Missionaries of Mary, St. Francis Hospital is recognized as an innovator in delivering specialized cardiac services in an environment in which excellence and compasssion are emphasized. A range of medical/surgical services are also offered to support cardiac patients. More than 99% of patients would recommend the hospital to a friend.

EXPERIENCED IN CARDIAC CARE AND SURGERY

Open Heart Surgery: Performed 2,476 open heart surgeries in 2001; the only New York hospital with a risk-adjusted mortality rate significantly below the statewide average for coronary bypass surgery, for all three-year periods analyzed by the NY State Department of Health. (1989-1998).

Cardiac Catheterization: Site of 11,646 diagnostic catheterizations and 3,497 coronary angioplasties in 2001 (mortality rate for angioplasty is less than half the statewide average.)

Arrhythmia & Pacemakers: Largest pacemaker and arrhythmia program in the United States; Unparalleled expertise in radiofrequency cardiac ablation. Leading center for off-pump bypass surgery technique and catheter-based treatments for congenital heart defects.

RESEARCH & TECHNOLOGY

Cardiac Research Institute offers leading edge imaging technology and medications, and world renowned researchers in electron beam computed tomography, 3-D echocardiography, MRI and nuclear studies.

INTERNATIONAL PATIENTS

Located 17 miles from JFK International Airport, on Long Island, works with organizations such as the Knights of Malta and Rotary International's Gift of Life program to offer cardiac treatment to individuals from around the world.

ACCREDITATION AND AFFILIATION

Awarded *Accreditation* from the Joint Commission on Accreditation of Healthcare Organizations; Received Consumer Choice Award for Heart Care Service (National Research Corporation, 1999).

St. Francis Hospital, The Heart Center®
The Experience Matters

SAINT VINCENT CATHOLIC MEDICAL CENTERS

Saint Vincent Catholic Medical Centers treats more than 500,000 people each year with services that range from prenatal to hospice care. We are committed to providing exceptional medical care while maintaining a high regard for the dignity of each individual.

Academic Affiliation: We serve as the academic medical center for New York Medical College in New York City.

Sponsorship: The Sisters of Charity and the Diocese of Brooklyn jointly sponsor Saint Vincent Catholic Medical Centers. All our hospitals are accredited by the Joint Commission on Accreditation of Healthcare Organizations.

OUR HOSPITALS

St. Vincent's Hospital Manhattan -- Bayley Seton Hospital – Mary Immaculate Hospital St. John's Queens Hospital – St. Joseph's Hospital – St. Mary's Hospital Brooklyn – St. Vincent's Hospital Staten Island – St. Vincent's Hospital Westchester.

SERVICES OFFERED THROUGHOUT OUR SYSTEM

Behavioral Health Services – Providing a complete array of inpatient and ambulatory treatment choices, we treat people who suffer from mental illness or chemical dependency. We offer one of the few inpatient programs for children in New York City. Our geriatric program offers medical services in addition to treatment for mental illness. We have inpatient and outpatient substance abuse detoxification and rehabilitation programs, and our Latino Treatment Service is both bi-lingual and bi-cultural.

Comprehensive Cancer Centers – Helping patients and their families meet the unique challenges of living with cancer is our focus. We offer the latest technology and the expertise of our world-class cancer specialists – leading physicians who have spearheaded research that has resulted in exciting breakthroughs in the diagnosis and treatment of cancer.

Comprehensive Cardiovascular Center – Offering the most sophisticated diagnostic and treatment methods for every form of heart disease, our cardiologists enjoy international reputations for excellence, and that distinction has been well earned. St. Vincent's Hospital Manhattan, our flagship hospital, maintains one of the oldest and busiest interventional cardiology services in the metropolitan area and has an impressive history of achieving long-term success with these procedures.

Comprehensive HIV Centers – Delivering compassionate care to people with HIV/AIDS since 1981, our team of experienced providers offers medical care and case management services that cover every stage of treatment. Our services cover pediatric to geriatric HIV and include every member of the patient's family.

ADDITIONAL KEY SERVICES

Outstanding emergency care with Level I Trauma Centers at St. Vincent's Hospital Manhattan, St. Vincent's Hospital Staten Island and Mary Immaculate Hospital in Queens – complex and same-day surgery -- advanced diagnostics.

AMBULATORY CARE, SKILLED NURSING FACILITIES AND HOME CARE SERVICES

We also operate ambulatory care sites and skilled nursing facilities and offer traditional and long-term home health services throughout the greater New York metropolitan area.

For more information or to find a physician, call 1-800-CARE-421 or visit us at www.svcmc.org.

THE UNIVERSITY OF CHICAGO HOSPITALS

5841 S. Maryland Avenue • For general information: 1-888-UCH-0200
Chicago, IL 60637-1470 • Web address: www.uchospitals.edu

Beds: 890
Sponsorship: Private. Not-for profit
Accreditation: Joint Commission on Accreditaiton of Healthcare Organizations

AT THE FOREFRONT OF MEDICINE®

We have been at the forefront of medicine for decades -- delivering extraordinary care to patients who come from the Chicago area, as well as from all parts of the world. According to *U.S. News & World Report*'s ranking of America's best hospitals, the University of Chicago Hospitals rank 15th in the nation and first in Illinois. We were named among the best in the country and best in Illinois in eleven specialty areas: cancer, endocrinology, gastroenterology, geriatrics, gynecology, nephrology, orthopaedics, otolaryngology, pulmonary medicine, rheumatology, and urology.

Our mission is to provide superior health care in a compassionate manner, ever mindful of each patient's dignity and individuality. To accomplish our mission, we call upon the skills and expertise of all our medical professionals, who work together to advance biomedical innovation, serve the health needs of the community, and further the knowledge of medical students, physicians, and others dedicated to caring.

WORLD-RENOWNED UNIVERSITY OF CHICAGO PHYSICIANS

All patients are encouraged to establish an ongoing relationship with a personal University of Chicago physician. Should the need arise, this physician will collaborate with or refer to any one of over 400 U of C board-certified specialists, many of whom are world leaders in their areas of expertise. Our faculty physicians see patients at the main Hospitals' campus, as well as at several other locations in the Chicago area. At the main campus, adult inpatient care is provided at Bernard Mitchell Hospital and Chicago Lying-in Hospital.

THE CENTER FOR ADVANCED MEDICINE

The Duchossois Center for Advanced Medicine is home to nearly all specialty clinics of the University of Chicago physicians, along with an unparalleled range of outpatient diagnostic and treatment services. The Center for Advanced Medicine is designed with the patient's best interests in mind. Physician offices are conveniently located next to related diagnostic and treatment suites, enabling patients to receive care for all related medical conditions within the same area of the building.

At the Center, patients have access to significant advances in medical treatment. Our physicians bring to its outpatient setting all of the knowledge and resources of the University of Chicago: virtually every clinical trial available and more research funded by the National Institutes of Health than any other place in the state.

THE UNIVERSITY OF CHICAGO CHILDREN'S HOSPITAL

Staffed by more than 100 faculty physicians, the University of Chicago Children's Hospital is dedicated to helping children with medical problems ranging from the routine to the complex. Our pediatricians provide advanced therapies in virtually all clinical areas. Critically ill or injured children are cared for in the state-of-the-art Frankel Pediatric Intensive Care Unit. In addition, a 53-bassinet neonatal intensive medical care and life support systems. The pediatric liver transplantation program is one of the largest in the country and was the first living-donor program in the world. The University of Chicago Children's Hospital offers every available form of therapy, both conventional and investigational, for a child afflicted with cancer.

WEISS MEMORIAL HOSPITAL AND OTHER OFF-CAMPUS LOCATIONS

Off-campus, care is provided at Louis A. Weiss Memorial Hospital, a 225-bed hospital on Chicago's North Side, and through a network of more than 25 physician offices located throughout Chicago, Chicago's suburbs, and northwest Indiana.

Call 1-888-UCH-0200 for help in choosing a physician suitable to your needs.
Visit our website: www.uchospitals.edu.

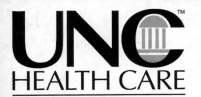

The University of North Carolina Health Care System
101 Manning Drive Chapel Hill, NC 27514
www.unchealthcare.org

Beds: 688
Accreditation: Accredited by JCAHO

GENERAL OVERVIEW

UNC Hospitals – a medical center consisting of four separate hospitals – is the cornerstone of UNC Health Care. People from all 100 North Carolina counties and throughout the Southeast are patients at the 688-bed facility – more than 31,000 each year. More than 2,800 infants are born each year at UNC Hospitals. In 2002, new babies and their families will be welcomed in the new North Carolina Children's Hospital and North Carolina Women's Hospital, which houses an obstetrics and gynecology program ranked as one of the nation's 10 best by *U.S. News & World Report* magazine.

ACADEMIC AND CLINICAL AFFILIATIONS

The University of North Carolina at Chapel Hill School of Medicine relies on UNC Hospitals as its teaching hospital. This partnership has enabled the School of Medicine to become one of only four medical schools in the United States that is ranked in the top 20 percent by the Association of American Medical Colleges both in production of primary care physicians and in receiving research grants from the National Institutes of Health.

MEDICAL STAFF

UNC Hospitals has 966 attending physicians, 53 of whom were listed in the first edition of America's Top Doctors, and 530 residents. Many of the attending physicians also teach and conduct research in the School of Medicine.

UNC Health Care extends beyond Chapel Hill and into the greater Triangle area through its network of primary care and community physician practices located in Orange, Wake, Durham, Chatham Lee, Vance and Alamance counties. These offices, in addition to the UNC Family Practice Center and Ambulatory Care Center, provide the basic health care outpatient services most families need, in convenient neighborhood locations. Nearly a half-million people are cared for at UNC practices and clinics each year.

PIONEERING, COMPREHENSIVE MEDICAL CARE

Specialized patient care services include the Breast Center, Cardiovascular Program, Diabetes Care Center, Lung Center, Rehabilitation Center, Spine Center, Wound Management Program and Comprehensive Transplant Center. The medical center's extensive expertise in arthritis, digestive diseases, endocrinology, ENT, gynecology, hemophilia, infertility, rheumatology, and orthopaedics has achieved both regional and national recognition. And UNC is home to the Lineberger Comprehensive Cancer Center, one of a small number of National Cancer Institute-designated centers in the United States.

ACCREDITATION, COMMENDATIONS AND NATIONAL RECOGNITION

UNC Hospitals is accredited with commendation by the Joint Commission on Accreditation of Healthcare Organizations. Ten of UNC Hospitals' medical specialties were ranked among the top 50 programs of their kind nationwide in *U.S. News & World Report's* annual "America's Best Hospitals" issue.

You can request a physician referral by calling UNC HealthLink at (919) 966-7890, 8:30 a.m. to 5 p.m., Eastern time, Monday through Friday.

UNIVERSITY OF PENNSYLVANIA HEALTH SYSTEM

The Future of Medicine ®

34th and Spruce Streets   *1-800-789-PENN*
Philadelphia, PA 19104   *www.pennhealth.com*

OVERVIEW

For more than two centuries, Penn physicians and scientists have been committed to the highest standards of patient care, education and research. Our commitment has been recognized by our peers and by others throughout the Delaware Valley and across the nation.

U.S. News & World Report has named the Hospital of the University of Pennsylvania to its Honor Roll of the best hospitals in the nation for the fifth straight year. Our hospital is one of just 16 hospitals nationwide – and the only hospital in Pennsylvania, New Jersey and Delaware – named to the list. *U.S. News* also consistently ranks our School of Medicine and School of Nursing among the nation's best.

The University of Pennsylvania Medical Center ranks second nationally in special grant funding from the National Institutes of Health. Four departments – Obstetrics and Gynecology, Physiology, Radiology and Radiation Oncology -- are ranked first nationally.

THE FUTURE OF MEDICINE

Our physicians and scientists are united in the institution's mission to expand the frontiers of medicine through new discoveries in the detection, treatment and prevention of human disease. Because we develop and test new treatments through clinical trials, our patients gain access to the very latest advances, and future generations benefit from the work we do today.

Penn continues to lead the way in discovering new treatment methods for diseases once considered incurable. Groundbreaking research in cancer, neurosciences, genetics and imaging are just a few areas in which Penn has brought the future of medicine closer.

Over the past 30 years, Penn physicians and scientists have participated in many important discoveries, including:

- The first general vaccine against pneumonia
- The introduction of total intravenous feeding
- The development of magnetic resonance imaging and other imaging technologies
- The discovery of the Philadelphia chromosome, which revolutionized cancer research by making the connection between genetic abnormalities and cancer

LOCATIONS

Patients can be seen at University of Pennsylvania Medical Center, Presbyterian Medical Center, Pennsylvania Hospital, Phoenixville Hospital or our outpatient setting at Penn Medicine at Radnor or Penn Medicine at Limerick. Through our primary care physicians and cardiologists, patients can be seen at location close to home either in Bucks, Montgomery and Philadelphia counties in Pennsylvania or in Southern New Jersey. We also provide hospice and homecare services through PennCare at Home and Wissahickon Hospice.

ON THE WEB

Visit **pennhealth.com** for the latest patient education with explanation of surgical procedures and follow-up care, screening tools, drug interactions and descriptions as well as an encyclopedia of information.

For direct connection to one of our Penn physicians, call PennLine **1-800-635-7780**.

UNIVERSITY OF VIRGINIA HEALTH SYSTEM

CHANGING THE FACE OF MEDICINE

University Hospital   1215 Lee Street
Charlottesville, Virginia 22908
www.med.virginia.edu

Beds: 528
Accreditation: Designated Level I Trauma Center, teaching, research and referral center fully accredited by the Joint Commission on Accreditation of Healthcare Organizations (JCAHO)

WHERE INNOVATION AND COMPASSION MERGE

The University of Virginia Health System has earned a reputation as a national healthcare leader through medical research and life-saving discoveries, exceptional patient care, innovative technology and a compassionate environment for patients and their families.

Based in picturesque Central Virginia in the foothills of the Blue Ridge Mountains, UVa was founded by Thomas Jefferson, who inspired a tradition of learning and knowledge that still flourishes today at one of the nation's most renowned academic medical environments.

Patients throughout the mid-Atlantic region and the world come to UVa for a wide array of health care needs, from primary to highly specialized care from our more than 450 specialists and subspecialists.

A COMPREHENSIVE APPROACH

At our state-of the-art Medical Center in Charlottesville, we offer nationally known multidisciplinary specialty centers focused on specific areas and a level I Trauma Center with a Pediatric Emergency Department to give children their own special place. As a pioneer in organ transplant, UVa has given hundreds of patients a new lease on life. Our specialty care centers include the Heart Center, Cancer Center, Women's Place, Children's Medical Center, Neurosciences Center and the Digestive Health Center of Excellence. These centers provide a full range of services, from prevention and wellness to intensive care and rehabilitation. Care is coordinated by teams of physicians, nurses, therapists, nutritionists, pharmacists, chaplains and other professionals. By bringing to the table their own expertise and skill, these professionals give patients the most comprehensive care available.

MAKING MEDICAL BREAKTHROUGHS

UVa physicians are always searching for new and better treatments to enhance care and ultimately cure disease. Some of medicine's major discoveries have taken place at UVa. Whether through pioneering the use of high-tech neurosurgical equipment like the Gamma Knife™ or developing new skin and ovarian cancer treatments by tapping into the body's own immune system, UVa leads the way in the advancement of modern medicine.

In addition to the UVa physicians listed in this year's edition of *America's Top Doctors*, UVa has been featured in *U.S. News & World Report*, *Self*, *Ladies' Home Journal* and *Good Housekeeping* as well as recognized by Solucient as one of the country's Top 100 Hospitals.

To make an appointment with a UVa physician,
call 800 251-3627, locally 434 924-DOCS.

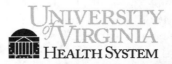

UNIVERSITY *of* VIRGINIA
HEALTH SYSTEM

❖ Vanderbilt Medical Center

1313 21ˢᵗ Avenue South, Suite 405, Nashville, Tennessee 37232-4335
Tel. 615.936.0301 Fax. 615.936.0320 www.mc.vanderbilt.edu

Beds: 661
Vanderbilt University Medical Center (VUMC) is a major not-for-profit academic medical center affiliated with Vanderbilt University located in Nashville, Tennessee. VUMC is a member of the Association of Academic Medical Centers and the University Hospital Consortium.

A History of Excellence

Throughout its history, Vanderbilt University Medical Center (VUMC) has been dedicated to excellence in patient care, medical and nursing education and biomedical research. Since 1875, when the entire newly-founded medical school was housed in a single building, VUMC has grown to become a comprehensive, multi-faceted institution that touches thousands of lives throughout the nation every day.

Comprehensive Medical Care

With a medical staff of 793 physicians, approximately 90% of whom are board certified, and more than 95 specialty services, VUMC offers the most comprehensive range of patient care services of any hospital in the area. VUMC's reputation for excellence has made Vanderbilt a major patient referral center for the Mid-South.

Unique Services

VUMC offers many services that are unique to the region. VUMC has the region's only **Level I trauma center, burn center, voice center, poison control center and liver transplant program**. VUMC's cancer center, the **Vanderbilt-Ingram Cancer Center** is the only National Cancer Institute (NCI)-designated **Comprehensive Cancer Center** in Tennessee and one of only 41 nationwide. Currently located on three floors within Vanderbilt University Hospital, **Vanderbilt Children's Hospital** is the only comprehensive provider of Children's specialty services in Middle Tennessee. The Children's Hospital will be moving to a new freestanding, state-of-the-art facility in the fall of 2003.

Accreditation, Commendations and National Recognition

For the eighth consecutive year, Vanderbilt University Hospital and The Vanderbilt Clinic placed among the nation's *top 50* in **U.S. News & World Report's** annual ranking of American hospitals. Vanderbilt was recognized in 11 of the 17 specialty areas including **Cancer; Digestive Disorders; Ear, Nose and Throat; Gynecology; Heart; Hormonal Disorders; Kidney Disease; Neurology and Neurosurgery; Orthopedics; Respiratory Disorders;** and **Urology**. Vanderbilt is the only Nashville hospital named to the nation's *100 Top Hospitals* list by the **HCIA-Sachs Institute**; and for the third year in a row, VUMC placed in the top tier of the **National Research Corporation's** annual survey and earned the **NRC's Consumer Choice Award**. Vanderbilt is fully accredited by the JCAHO.

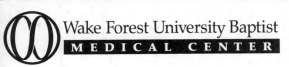

Wake Forest University Baptist
MEDICAL CENTER

Medical Center Boulevard, Winston-Salem, NC 27157-1015
Appointment or Physician Referral: 800-446-2255
Physician-to-physician Consultation: 800-277-7654
www.wfubmc.edu   www.brennerchildrens.org   www.besthealth.com

OVERVIEW

Wake Forest University Baptist Medical Center is composed of N.C. Baptist Hospitals, Inc., an 830-bed tertiary care facility ranked among the nation's top hospitals, and the Wake Forest University School of Medicine, whose reputation for excellence attracts some of the nation's best doctors to its faculty practice. Recognized as a major research center, WFUBMC is renowned for state-of-the-art medical treatment and technology, innovation and teaching excellence.

WORLD-CLASS CARE

U.S.News & World Report ranks N.C. Baptist Hospital of Wake Forest University Baptist Medical Center among the nation's top 50 hospitals in six specialties (July '01). Specialty services include: Brenner Children's Hospital, where young patients receive highly specialized care in a newly built, family-friendly facility; the Heart Center, renowned for the latest diagnostic technologies, innovative treatments and transplant services; the NCI-designated Comprehensive Cancer Center of WFU, where treatment options include gamma knife radiosurgery and gene therapy; the J. Paul Sticht Center on Aging, whose team approach is redefining care for older adults; Neurology and Neurosurgery Services, including Stroke, ALS and Epilepsy Centers and leading edge treatments such as deep brain stimulator implants for Parkinson's disease; and the Women's Health Center, focused on gender-sensitive care and broadening knowledge about diseases affecting women. The Medical Center is home to North Carolina's only Level I Adult and Pediatric Trauma Center accredited by the American College of Surgeons, and handles the most severe trauma cases in the state.

RESEARCH

With outside research funding exceeding $105 million, WFUBMC is expanding the frontiers of medical knowledge. Research centers include: the Comprehensive Cancer Center where over 220 clinical trials are underway, a federally funded, highly active General Clinical Research Center, Human Genomics Center, Centers for Neurobehavioral Study of Alcohol and Neurobiological Investigation of Drug Abuse, Claude D. Pepper Older Americans Center for geriatrics research and the Hypertension and Vascular Disease Center, to name a few.

INNOVATION

Providing patients with the latest technology and treatment – such as North Carolina's only gamma knife -- is a Wake Forest University Baptist Medical Center tradition. WFUBMC experts were first in the U.S. to detect prostate cancer with ultrasound, and first in the world to treat a brain tumor patient with a new GliaSite radiation therapy and to report success with magnetic resonance imaging to diagnose blockages in blood vessels to the heart.

CONSUMER CHOICE

In independent surveys by the National Research Corporation, Greensboro Metropolitan Statistical Area residents name Wake Forest University Baptist Medical Center as their most preferred Triad hospital, citing the best doctors, nurses and overall care (Oct. '01). Outstanding nursing at WFUBMC earned the institution one of the nation's first 15 Magnet Awards for nursing excellence, given in 1999 by the American Nurses Credentialing Center.

WHEN CHOOSING THE BEST MEANS THE MOST

To make an appointment or find a specialist at Wake Forest University Baptist Medical Center, call Health On-Call® at 1-800-446-2255.

WESTCHESTER MEDICAL CENTER

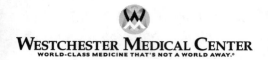

Valhalla Campus
Valhalla, NY 10595
PHONE: (914) 493-7000

www.worldclassmedicine.com

Beds: 1,000
Sponsorship/Network Affiliation: Westchester Medical Center is a public benefit corporation; member of the Pinnacle Healthcare Alliance.

REGIONAL MEDICAL CENTER

As an academic medical center and the region's advanced care and Level 1 Trauma Center, Westchester Medical Center is on the leading edge of medical research and advances in clinical care. Over 3.5 million people in the Hudson Valley region, northern New Jersey and lower Connecticut rely on our services.

FOUR MAJOR FACILITIES

With over 1,000 beds in four facilities—our University Hospital, Behavioral Health Center, Taylor Care Center (for skilled nursing and sub-acute) and Westchester Institute for Human Development (for developmentally disabled)—Westchester Medical Center's renowned specialty services have made us the referral hospital of choice for physicians and patients seeking the highest level and quality of care.

CENTERS OF EXCELLENCE

The academic affiliate of New York Medical College, Westchester Medical Center is home to New York State's largest kidney transplant program, one of only four liver transplant programs and one of only six heart transplant programs in the state. The Children's Hospital at Westchester Medical Center is the only all-specialty children's hospital in the region. Our renowned pediatric specialists treat over 20,000 children each year. The Children's Hospital is also home to the only Level IV regional neonatal intensive care unit and pediatric intensive care unit, as well as a specialized high-risk obstetrics center.

The G.E. Reed Heart Center at Westchester Medical Center boasts one of the most highly regarded cardiology and cardiac surgery programs on the East Coast. With fully equipped medevac helicopters, our STAT Flight team responds in minutes to accidents and other emergencies, and carries critical inter-hospital patient transfers from throughout the region and beyond.

Westchester Medical Center's Trauma and Burn Center features the only burn center between New York City and the Canadian border; our Arlin Cancer Institute offers the latest cancer therapies, including bone marrow and stem cell transplants; and our Neuroscience Center offers neuro-surgical and neurological care, including "knifeless" brain surgery, specialized stroke (brain attack) service and an epilepsy program.

CUTTING-EDGE HEALTHCARE

Westchester Medical Center became the fifth hospital in the U.S. to offer Novalis® Shaped Beam Surgery, the least invasive and most precise treatment option available to patients with cancer, brain tumors, and neurologic and vascular disorders. Other advanced technologies include robotic surgery for minimally invasive surgeries. The DaVinci® Robot allows surgeons more precision, flexibility and visualization similar to traditional surgery, but with better access and faster healing and less scarring for the patient.

Physician Referral: For information on Westchester Medical Center's physicians and surgeons, visit us at www.worldclassmedicine.com or call 914-493-8026 for a copy of our Physician Referral Guide.

THE TRAINING OF A SPECIALIST

Excerpted from "**Which Medical Specialist For You?**"
American Board of Medical Specialties, Evanston, IL, Revised 2000

Everyone knows that a "medical doctor" is a physician who has had years of training to understand the diagnosis, treatment and prevention of disease. The basic training for a physician specialist includes four years of premedical education in a college or university, four years of medical school, and after receiving the M.D. degree, at least three years of specialty training under supervision (called a "residency"). Training in subspecialties can take an additional one to three years.

Some specialists are primary care doctors such as family physicians, general internists and general pediatricians. Other specialists concentrate on certain body systems, specific age groups, or complex scientific techniques developed to diagnose or treat certain types of disorders. Specialties in medicine developed because of the rapidly expanding body of knowledge about health and illness and the constantly evolving new treatment techniques for disease.

A subspecialist is a physician who has completed training in a general medical specialty and then takes additional training in a more specific area of that specialty called a subspecialty. This training increases the depth of knowledge and expertise of the specialist in that particular field. For example, cardiology is a subspecialty of internal medicine and pediatrics, pediatric surgery is a subspecialty of surgery and child and adolescent psychiatry is a subspecialty of psychiatry. The training of a subspecialist within a specialty requires an additional one or more years of full-time education.

The training, or residency, of a specialist begins after the doctor has received the M.D. degree from a medical school. Resident physicians dedicate themselves for three to seven years to full-time experience in hospital and/or ambulatory care settings, caring for patients under the supervision of experienced specialists. Educational conferences and research experience are often part of that training. In years past, the first year of post-medical school training was called an internship, but is now called residency.

Licensure

The legal privilege to practice medicine is governed by state law and is not designed to recognize the knowledge and skills of a trained specialist. A physician is licensed to practice general medicine and surgery by a state board of medical examiners after passing a state or national licensure examination. Each state or territory has its own procedures to license physicians and sets the general standards for all physicians in that state or territory.

Who credentials a specialist and/or subspecialist?

Specialty boards certify physicians as having met certain published standards. There are 24 specialty boards that are recognized by the American Board of Medical Specialties (ABMS) and the American Medical Association (AMA). All of the specialties and subspecialties recognized by the ABMS and the AMA are listed in the brief descriptions that follow. Remember, *a subspecialist first must be trained and certified as a specialist.*

In order to be certified as a medical specialist by one of these recognized boards a physician must complete certain requirements. Generally, these include:
(1) Completion of a course of study leading to the M.D. or D.O. (Doctor of Osteopathy) degree from a recognized school of medicine.

(2) Completion of three to seven years of full-time training in an accredited residency program designed to train specialists in the field.

(3) Many specialty boards require assessments and documentation of individual performance from the residency training director, or from the chief of service in the hospital where the specialist has practiced.

(4) All of the ABMS Member Boards require that a person seeking certification have an unrestricted license to practice medicine in order to take the certification examination.

(5) Finally, each candidate for certification must pass a written examination given by the specialty board. Fifteen of the 24 specialty boards also require an oral examination conducted by senior specialists in that field. Candidates who have passed the exams and other requirements are then given the status of "Diplomate" and are certified as specialists. A similar process is followed for specialists who want to become subspecialists.

All of the ABMS Member Boards now, or will soon, issue only time-limited certificates which are valid for six to ten years. In order to retain certification, diplomates must become "recertified," and must periodically go through an additional process involving continuing education in the specialty, review of credentials and further examination. Boards that may not yet require recertification have provided voluntary recertification with similar requirements.

How to determine if a physician is a certified specialist

Certified specialists are listed in *The Official ABMS Directory of Board Certified Medical Specialists* published by Marquis Who's Who. The *ABMS Directory* can be found in most public libraries, hospital libraries, university libraries and medical libraries, and is also available on CD-ROM. Alternatively, you could ask for that information from your county medical society, the American Board of Medical Specialties, or one of the specialty boards.

The ABMS operates an 800 phone line (1-800-776-2378) to verify the certification status of individual physicians. Additionally, information about the ABMS organization and links to an electronic directory of certified specialists can be accessed through the ABMS Web site at www.abms.org.

Almost all board certified specialists also are members of their medical specialty societies. These societies are dedicated to furthering standards, practice and professional and public education within individual medical specialties. Some, such as the American College of Surgeons and the American College of Obstetricians and Gynecologists, require board certification for full membership. A physician who has attained full membership is called a "Fellow" of the society and is entitled to use this designation in all formal communications such as certificates, publications, business cards, stationery and signage. Thus, "John Doe, M.D., F.A.C.S. (Fellow of the American College of Surgeons) is a board certified surgeon. Similarly, F.A.A.D. (Fellow of the American Academy of Dermatology) following the M.D. or D.O. in a physician's title would likely indicate board certification in that specialty.

PREFACE TO MEDICAL SPECIALTIES

In the pages that follow, each list of doctors in a medical specialty or subspecialty is preceded by a brief description of that specialty (or subspecialty) and the training required for board certification.

A few specialties have not been included since they are specialties for which patients generally do not search beyond their local communities (e.g., Family Practice Medicine) or are specialties for which patients must depend on the expertise of their treating doctors for selection (e.g. Anesthesiology). In addition, Critical Care Medicine (and its subspecialties) has been excluded because in emergency situations there is neither time nor opportunity for choice.

Descriptions of those medical specialties and subspecialties that are not included in the main sections of the Guide may be found in Appendix A.

The following descriptions of medical specialties and subspecialties were provided by the American Board of Medical Specialties (ABMS), an organization comprised of the 24 medical specialty boards that provide certification in 25 medical specialties. A complete listing of all specialists certified by the ABMS can be found in *The Official ABMS Directory of Board Certified Medical Specialists*, published by Marquis Who's Who. It is available (either in a multi-volume directory or on CD-ROM) in most public libraries, hospital libraries, university libraries and medical libraries. The ABMS also operates a toll-free phone line at 1-800-776-2378 to verify the certification status of individual doctors.

The following important policy statement, approved by the ABMS Assembly on March 19, 1987, remains valid.

The Purpose of Certification:
The intent of the certification process, as defined by the member boards of the American Board of Medical Specialties, is to provide assurance to the public that a certified medical specialist has successfully completed an approved educational program and an evaluation, including an examination process designed to assess the knowledge, experience and skills requisite to the provision of high quality patient care in that specialty.

ADOLESCENT MEDICINE

(a subspecialty of either INTERNAL MEDICINE or PEDIATRICS)

An internist or pediatrician who specializes in adolescent medicine is a multi-disciplinary healthcare specialist trained in the unique physical, psychological and social characteristics of adolescents, their healthcare problems and needs.

INTERNAL MEDICINE

A personal physician who provides long-term, comprehensive care in the office and the hospital, managing both common and complex illness of adolescents, adults and the elderly. Internists are trained in the diagnosis and treatment of cancer, infections and diseases affecting the heart, blood, kidneys, joints and digestive, respiratory and vascular systems. They are also trained in the essentials of primary care internal medicine which incorporates an understanding of disease prevention, wellness, substance abuse, mental health and effective treatment of common problems of the eyes, ears, skin, nervous system and reproductive organs.

PEDIATRICS

A physician concerned with the physical, emotional and social health of children from birth to young adulthood. Care encompasses a broad spectrum of health services ranging from preventive healthcare to the diagnosis and treatment of acute and chronic diseases. A pediatrician deals with biological, social and environmental influences on the developing child, and with the impact of disease and dysfunction on development.

Training required: Three years in internal medicine *OR* three years in pediatrics *plus* additional training and examination for certification in adolescent medicine

Physician Listings

Adolescent Medicine

New England

Emans, Sarah Jean Herriot MD (AM) - *Spec Exp:* Pediatric & Adolescent Gynecology; **Hospital:** Children's Hospital - Boston; **Address:** 300 Longwood Avenue, Boston, MA 02115; **Phone:** (617) 355-5482; **Board Cert:** Pediatrics 1975, Adolescent Medicine 1994; **Med School:** Harvard Med Sch 1970; **Resid:** Children's Hospital, Boston, MA 1971-1973; **Fellow:** Adolescent Medicine, Children's Hospital, Boston, MA 1973-1974; **Fac Appt:** Assoc Prof Pediatrics, Harvard Med Sch

Mid Atlantic

Diaz, Angela MD (AM) - *Spec Exp:* Adolescent Medicine - General; **Hospital:** Mount Sinai Hosp (page 68); **Address:** 312 E 94th St, New York, NY 10128-5604; **Phone:** (212) 423-2900; **Board Cert:** Pediatrics 1987, Adolescent Medicine 1994; **Med School:** Columbia P&S 1981; **Resid:** Pediatrics, Mt Sinai Med Ctr, New York, NY 1981-1984; **Fellow:** Adolescent Medicine, Mt Sinai Med Ctr, New York, NY 1984-1985; **Fac Appt:** Assoc Prof Pediatrics, Mount Sinai Sch Med

Schwarz, Donald F. MD (AM) - *Spec Exp:* Adolescent Mothers; Adolescent Chronic Illness; **Hospital:** Chldn's Hosp of Philadelphia; **Address:** 34th St & Civic Center Blvd, 9th Fl, Philadelphia, PA 19104; **Phone:** (215) 590-1462; **Board Cert:** Adolescent Medicine 1994, Pediatrics 1987; **Med School:** Johns Hopkins Univ 1982; **Resid:** Pediatrics, Yale-New Haven Hospital, New Haven, CT 1983-1985; **Fellow:** Adolescent Medicine, Chldn's Hosp, Philadelphia, PA 1985-1987; **Fac Appt:** Prof Pediatrics, Univ Penn

Southeast

Ford, Carol Ann MD (AM) - *Spec Exp:* Adolescent Medicine - General; **Hospital:** Univ of NC Hosp (page 77); **Address:** UNC at Chapel Hill, Dept Ped Adol Med, CB#7225, Wing C, Med School, Chapel Hill, NC 27599-7225; **Phone:** (919) 966-2504; **Board Cert:** Pediatrics 1989, Adolescent Medicine 1994; **Med School:** Univ Fla Coll Med 1983; **Resid:** Internal Medicine, Univ North Carolina Hosp, Chapel Hill, NC 1983-1987; Pediatrics, Univ North Carolina Hosp, Chapel Hill, NC 1983-1987; **Fellow:** Adolescent Medicine, UC San Francisco Med Ctr, San Francisco, CA 1992-1995; **Fac Appt:** Asst Prof Pediatrics, Univ NC Sch Med

Midwest

Blum, Robert W MD/PhD (AM) - *Spec Exp:* Adolescent Medicine - General; **Hospital:** Fairview Southdale Hosp; **Address:** U of Minnesota, Div Ped & Adol Hlth, 216 McNamara Alum Ctr, 200 Oak St SE, Minneapolis, MN 55455; **Phone:** (612) 626-2820; **Board Cert:** Pediatrics 1993, Adolescent Medicine 1994; **Med School:** Howard Univ 1973; **Resid:** Pediatrics, Univ Minn, Minneapolis, MN 1974-1976; **Fellow:** Adolescent Medicine, Univ Minn, Minneapolis, MN 1976-1978; **Fac Appt:** Assoc Prof Pediatrics, Univ Minn

Slap, Gail MD (AM) - *Spec Exp:* Adolescent Medicine; **Hospital:** Cincinnati Chldns Hosp Med Ctr; **Address:** Children's Hosp Med Ctr, Div of Adolescent Med, 3333 Burnet Ave, Bldg PAV, Cincinnati, OH 45229-3039; **Phone:** (513) 636-8602; **Board Cert:** Internal Medicine 1980, Adolescent Medicine 1994; **Med School:** Univ Penn 1977; **Resid:** Internal Medicine, Univ Penn, Philadelphia, PA 1977-1980; **Fellow:** Adolescent Medicine, Children's Hosp, Philadelphia, PA 1980-1982; **Fac Appt:** Prof Pediatrics, Univ Cincinnati

Great Plains and Mountains

Kaplan, David William MD (AM) - *Spec Exp:* Eating Disorders; **Hospital:** Chldn's Hosp - Denver; **Address:** Children's Hospital, 1056 E 19th Ave, Box B025, Denver, CO 80218-1007; **Phone:** (303) 861-6131; **Board Cert:** Pediatrics 1975, Adolescent Medicine 1994; **Med School:** Case West Res Univ 1970; **Resid:** Pediatrics, Univ Colorado Med Ctr, Denver, CO 1970-1972; Pediatrics, Chldns Hosp Med Ctr, Boston, MA 1974-1975; **Fellow:** Public Health & General Preventive Medicine, Harvard Sch Pub Hlth, Boston, MA 1975-1976; **Fac Appt:** Prof Pediatrics, Univ Colo

West Coast and Pacific

Anderson, Martin Mathew MD (AM) - *Spec Exp:* Adolescent Medicine - General; **Hospital:** UCLA Med Ctr; **Address:** UCLA Med Ctr, Dept Pediatrics, 10833 Le Conte Ave, Los Angeles, CA 90095; **Phone:** (310) 825-5803; **Board Cert:** Pediatrics 1986, Adolescent Medicine 1994; **Med School:** UC Davis 1980; **Resid:** Pediatrics, Mott Chldns Hosp, Ann Arbor, MI 1981-1983; **Fellow:** Adolescent Medicine, UCSF, San Francisco, CA 1984-1986; **Fac Appt:** Prof Pediatrics, UCLA

Fuster, Carlos Daniel MD (AM) - *Spec Exp:* Adolescent Medicine - General; **Hospital:** KPH Panorama City Med Ctr; **Address:** Area 108, 13652 Cantara St, Panorama City, CA 91402; **Phone:** (818) 375-2652; **Board Cert:** Adolescent Medicine 1997, Pediatrics 1986; **Med School:** Mount Sinai Sch Med 1980; **Resid:** Pediatrics, Children's Hosp, Los Angeles, CA 1981-1983; **Fellow:** Adolescent Medicine, Children's Hosp, Los Angeles, CA 1983-1985

Irwin Jr, Charles Edwin MD (AM) - *Spec Exp:* Adolescent Medicine - General; **Hospital:** UCSF Med Ctr; **Address:** 3333 California St, Ste 245, San Francisco, CA 94118; **Phone:** (415) 353-2002; **Board Cert:** Pediatrics 1993, Adolescent Medicine 2001; **Med School:** UCSF 1971; **Resid:** Pediatrics, UCSF Med Ctr, San Francisco, CA 1972-1974; **Fellow:** Adolescent Medicine, UCSF Med Ctr, San Francisco, CA 1974-1977; **Fac Appt:** Prof Pediatrics, UCSF

Litt, Iris F MD (AM) - *Spec Exp:* Adolescent Medicine - General; **Hospital:** Stanford Med Ctr; **Address:** Stanford Univ, Div Adolescent Medicine, 750 Welch Rd, Ste 325, Palo Alto, CA 94304; **Phone:** (650) 725-8293; **Board Cert:** Pediatrics 1993, Adolescent Medicine 1994; **Med School:** SUNY Downstate 1965; **Resid:** Pediatrics, NY Hosp, New York, NY 1966-1968; **Fac Appt:** Prof Pediatrics, Stanford Univ

MacKenzie, Richard G MD (AM) - *Spec Exp:* Eating Disorders; Menstrual Disorders; **Hospital:** Chldns Hosp - Los Angeles; **Address:** 5000 Sunset Blvd, Fl 4, Los Angeles, CA 90027-5861; **Phone:** (323) 669-2112; **Med School:** McGill Univ 1966; **Resid:** Internal Medicine, Royal Victoria Hosp, Montreal Canada 1966-1967; **Fellow:** Adolescent Medicine, Childrens Hosp, Los Angeles, CA 1969-1970; **Fac Appt:** Assoc Prof Pediatrics, USC Sch Med

Morris, Robert Edward MD (AM) - *Spec Exp:* Adolescent Medicine - General; **Hospital:** UCLA Med Ctr; **Address:** Pediatric & Adolescent Medicine, 200 UCLA Medical Plaza, Ste 265, Los Angeles, CA 90095; **Phone:** (310) 825-1844; **Board Cert:** Pediatrics 1986, Adolescent Medicine 1997; **Med School:** Temple Univ 1971; **Resid:** Pediatrics, Univ Wash, Seattle, WA 1972-1974; Pediatric Gastroenterology, UCLA, Los Angeles, CA 1981-1982; **Fac Appt:** Prof Pediatrics, UCLA

ALLERGY & IMMUNOLOGY

An allergist-immunologist is trained in evaluation, physical and laboratory diagnosis and management of disorders involving the immune system. Selected examples of such conditions include asthma, anaphylaxis, rhinitis, eczema and adverse reactions to drugs, foods and insect stings as well as immune deficiency diseases (both acquired and congenital), defects in host defense and problems related to autoimmune disease, organ transplantation or malignancies of the immune system. As our understanding of the immune system develops, the scope of this specialty is widening.

Training programs are available at some medical centers to provide individuals with expertise in both allergy/immunology and adult rheumatology, or in both allergy/immunology and pediatric pulmonology. Such individuals are candidates for dual certification.

Training required: Two years in allergy/immunology OR prior certification in internal medicine or pediatrics *plus* additional training and examination.

Physician Listings

Allergy & Immunology

New England

MacLean, James Andrew MD (A&I) - *Spec Exp:* Asthma; Allergy; Urticaria; **Hospital:** MA Genl Hosp; **Address:** Mass Genl Hosp, 55 Fruit St, Bldg Wang - rm 622, Boston, MA 02114; **Phone:** (617) 726-3850; **Board Cert:** Internal Medicine 1988, Allergy & Immunology 1991; **Med School:** McGill Univ 1985; **Resid:** Internal Medicine, Royal Victoria Hosp, Montreal, CN 1986-1989; **Fellow:** Allergy & Immunology, Mass Genl Hosp, Boston, MA 1989-1991; **Fac Appt:** Asst Prof Allergy & Immunology, Harvard Med Sch

Wong, Johnson T MD (A&I) - *Spec Exp:* Asthma; Rhinitis; Sinus Disorders; **Hospital:** MA Genl Hosp; **Address:** 3 Hawthorne Pl, Boston, MA 02114; **Phone:** (617) 726-3850; **Board Cert:** Internal Medicine 1983, Allergy & Immunology 1985; **Med School:** UCSF 1980; **Resid:** Internal Medicine, UCLA-Wadsworth VA Hosp, Los Angeles, CA 1981-1983; **Fellow:** Allergy & Immunology, Mass Genl Hosp, Boston, MA 1983-1986; **Fac Appt:** Asst Prof Medicine, Harvard Med Sch

Mid Atlantic

Adkinson, Franklin MD (A&I) - *Spec Exp:* Drug Sensitivity; Asthma; **Hospital:** Johns Hopkins Hosp - Baltimore; **Address:** 5501 Hopkins Bayview Circle, Baltimore, MD 21224; **Phone:** (410) 550-2051; **Med School:** Johns Hopkins Univ 1969; **Fac Appt:** Prof Medicine, Johns Hopkins Univ

Atkins, Paul C MD (A&I) - *Spec Exp:* Asthma; Sinus Disorders; **Hospital:** Hosp Univ Penn (page 78); **Address:** Hosp Of Univ Penn, Dept A&I, 3400 Spruce St, Fl 3 - Ste G, Philadelphia, PA 19143; **Phone:** (215) 662-2425; **Board Cert:** Internal Medicine 1974, Allergy & Immunology 1975; **Med School:** NY Med Coll 1967; **Resid:** Internal Medicine, NY Med-Metro Hosp Ctr, New York, NY 1968-1970; **Fellow:** Allergy & Immunology, Hosp Univ Penn, Philadelphia, PA 1970-1972; **Fac Appt:** Prof Allergy & Immunology, Univ Penn

Baraniuk, James N MD (A&I) - *Spec Exp:* Asthma and Sinusitis; Immune Deficiency; Neural Regulation of Mucosal Secretion; **Hospital:** Georgetown Univ Hosp; **Address:** GUMC-Lower Level, Gorman Building, 3800 Reservoir Rd NW, Washington, DC 20007; **Phone:** (202) 687-8233; **Board Cert:** Internal Medicine 1984, Allergy & Immunology 1987; **Resid:** Internal Medicine, St Thomas Hosp, Akron, OH 1982-1984; Internal Medicine, Duke Univ, Durham, NC 1984-1985; **Fellow:** Allergy & Immunology, Duke Univ, Durham, NC 1987-1989; Allergy & Immunology, Natnl Heart Lung Instt, London England 1989-1991; **Fac Appt:** Asst Clin Prof Georgetown Univ

Buchbinder, Ellen MD (A&I) - *Spec Exp:* Asthma; Allergy; **Hospital:** Mount Sinai Hosp (page 68); **Address:** 111B E 88th St, New York, NY 10128; **Phone:** (212) 410-3246; **Board Cert:** Internal Medicine 1981, Allergy & Immunology 1983; **Med School:** Tulane Univ 1978; **Resid:** Internal Medicine, New England Deaconess Hosp, Boston, MA 1978-1981; **Fellow:** Allergy & Immunology, Mass Genl Hosp, Boston, MA 1981-1983; **Fac Appt:** Asst Clin Prof Medicine, Mount Sinai Sch Med

Chandler, Michael MD (A&I) - *Spec Exp:* Asthma; Sinus Disorders; **Hospital:** Mount Sinai Hosp (page 68); **Address:** 115 E 61st St, New York, NY 10021-8101; **Phone:** (212) 486-6715; **Board Cert:** Internal Medicine 1984, Allergy & Immunology 1987; **Med School:** Wayne State Univ 1981; **Resid:** Internal Medicine, Northwestern, Chicago, IL 1981-1984; **Fellow:** Allergy & Immunology, Northwestern, Chicago, IL 1984-1986; **Fac Appt:** Clin Inst Medicine, Mount Sinai Sch Med

Cunningham-Rundles, Charlotte MD/PhD (A&I) - *Spec Exp:* Immunotherapy; **Hospital:** Mount Sinai Hosp (page 68); **Address:** 5 E 98th St, New York, NY 10029; **Phone:** (212) 659-9268; **Board Cert:** Internal Medicine 1972; **Med School:** Columbia P&S 1969; **Resid:** Internal Medicine, Bellevue Hosp, New York, NY 1970-1972; **Fellow:** Allergy & Immunology, NYU, New York, NY 1972-1974; **Fac Appt:** Prof Medicine, Mount Sinai Sch Med

Dattwyler, Raymond MD (A&I) - *Spec Exp:* Lyme Disease; **Hospital:** Stony Brook Univ Hosp; **Address:** SUNY Hlth Sci Ctr, Div A & I, Tower 16, , rm 040, Stony Brook, NY 11794-8161; **Phone:** (631) 444-3808; **Board Cert:** Internal Medicine 1977, Allergy & Immunology 1979, Clinical & Laboratory Immunology 1986; **Med School:** SUNY Buffalo 1973; **Resid:** Internal Medicine, Tufts-New England Med Ctr, Boston, MA 1976-1977; **Fellow:** Immunology, Mayo Clinic, Rochester, MN 1974-1976; Clinical Immunology, Mass Genl Hosp-Harvard, Boston, MA 1977-1978; **Fac Appt:** Prof Medicine, SUNY Stony Brook

Levinson, Arnold MD (A&I) - *Spec Exp:* Autoimmune Disease; Immune Deficiency; Allergy; **Hospital:** Hosp Univ Penn (page 78); **Address:** Hosp of Univ Penn, Div A&I, 3400 Spruce St- 3 Ravdin, Ste G, Philadelphia, PA 19104-4219; **Phone:** (215) 662-2425; **Board Cert:** Internal Medicine 1972, Allergy & Immunology 1975; **Med School:** Univ MD Sch Med 1969; **Resid:** Internal Medicine, Baltimore City Hosp, Baltimore, MD 1970-1971; **Fellow:** Clinical Immunology, UCSF, San Francisco, PA 1972-1973; Clinical Immunology, Univ Penn, Philadelphia, PA 1973-1975; **Fac Appt:** Prof Medicine, Univ Penn

Macris, Nicholas T MD (A&I) - *Spec Exp:* Asthma; Autoimmune Disorders; Immune Deficiency; **Hospital:** Lenox Hill Hosp (page 64); **Address:** 1430 2nd Ave, Ste 102, New York, NY 10021-3313; **Phone:** (212) 249-2940; **Board Cert:** Allergy & Immunology 1974; **Med School:** SUNY Hlth Sci Ctr 1958; **Resid:** Internal Medicine, Lenox Hill Hosp, New York, NY 1961-1963; **Fellow:** Allergy & Immunology, Rockefeller Univ, New York, NY 1963-1965; **Fac Appt:** Clin Prof Medicine, Cornell Univ-Weill Med Coll

Mazza, David S MD (A&I) - *Spec Exp:* Asthma-Adult & Pediatric; Sinus Disorders; **Hospital:** St Luke's - Roosevelt Hosp Ctr - Roosevelt Div (page 58); **Address:** 7 Lexington Ave, Ste 3, New York, NY 10010-5517; **Phone:** (212) 677-7170; **Board Cert:** Pediatrics 1983, Allergy & Immunology 1989; **Med School:** Univ VT Coll Med 1977; **Resid:** Pediatrics, New York Univ, New York, NY 1977-1980; **Fellow:** Pediatrics, Bellevue Hosp, New York, NY 1980-1982; Allergy & Immunology, St Luke's-Roosevelt Hosp Ctr, New York, NY 1987-1989; **Fac Appt:** Assoc Prof Columbia P&S

Metcalfe, Dean D MD (A&I) - *Spec Exp:* Mast Cell Diseases; Food Allergy; **Hospital:** Natl Inst of Hlth - Clin Ctr; **Address:** Natl Inst Allergy and Inf Disease, Lab Allergic Dis, 31 Center Drive Bldg 10 - rm 11C205, Bethesda, MD 20892-1881; **Phone:** (301) 496-2165; **Board Cert:** Internal Medicine 1975, Allergy & Immunology 1977; **Med School:** Univ Tenn Coll Med, Memphis 1972; **Resid:** Internal Medicine, Mich Hosp, Ann Arbor, MI 1973-1974; Allergy & Immunology, Natl Inst Allergy & Infectious Dis-NIH, Bethesda, MD 1974-1977; **Fellow:** Rheumatology, Peter Bent Brigham Hosp, Boston, MA 1977-1979

Reisman, Robert E MD (A&I) - *Spec Exp:* Anaphylaxis; Asthma; **Hospital:** Buffalo General Hosp; **Address:** Buffalo Medical Group, 295 Essjay Rd, Williamsville, NY 14221-8216; **Phone:** (716) 630-1130; **Board Cert:** Internal Medicine 1969, Allergy & Immunology 1970; **Med School:** SUNY Buffalo 1956; **Resid:** Internal Medicine, Buffalo Genl Hosp, Buffalo, NY 1957-1959; **Fellow:** Allergy & Immunology, Buffalo Genl Hosp, Buffalo, NY 1959-1961; **Fac Appt:** Clin Prof Medicine, SUNY Buffalo

Shepherd, Gillian M MD (A&I) - *Spec Exp:* Food, Drug & Insect Allergy; Rhinosinusitis & Asthma; Urticaria & Angioedema; **Hospital:** NY Presby Hosp - NY Weill Cornell Med Ctr (page 70); **Address:** 235 E 67th St, Ste 203, New York, NY 10021-6040; **Phone:** (212) 288-9300; **Board Cert:** Internal Medicine 1979, Allergy & Immunology 1981; **Med School:** NY Med Coll 1976; **Resid:** Internal Medicine, Lenox Hill Hosp, New York, NY 1976-1979; **Fellow:** Allergy & Immunology, NY Hosp-Cornell, New York, NY 1979-1981; **Fac Appt:** Assoc Clin Prof Medicine, Cornell Univ-Weill Med Coll

Slankard, Marjorie MD (A&I) - *Spec Exp:* Rhinitis; Asthma; **Hospital:** NY Presby Hosp - Columbia Presby Med Ctr (page 70); **Address:** 16 E 60th St, New York, NY 10022; **Phone:** (212) 326-8410; **Board Cert:** Internal Medicine 1974, Allergy & Immunology 1977; **Med School:** Univ MO-Columbia Sch Med 1971; **Resid:** Internal Medicine, NY Hosp-Cornell Med Ctr, New York, NY 1972-1974; Internal Medicine, Rockefeller Univ Hosp, New York, NY 1973-1974; **Fellow:** Allergy & Immunology, NY Hosp-Cornell Med Ctr, New York, NY 1974-1976; Immunology, Mount Sinai Med Ctr, New York, NY 1976-1980; **Fac Appt:** Assoc Clin Prof Medicine, Columbia P&S

Strober, Warren MD (A&I) - *Spec Exp:* Immune Deficiency; Inflammatory Bowel Disease/Crohn's; **Hospital:** Natl Inst of Hlth - Clin Ctr; **Address:** NIH - Laboratory of Clinical Investigation, Bldg 10 - rm 11-N-238, Bethesda, MD 20892-1890; **Phone:** (301) 496-6810; **Board Cert:** Allergy & Immunology 1977, Internal Medicine 1974; **Med School:** Univ Rochester 1962; **Resid:** Internal Medicine, Strong Meml Hosp, Rochester, NY 1963-1964; Allergy & Immunology, Natl Inst Hlth, Bethesda, MD 1964-1972

Togias, Alkis George MD (A&I) - *Spec Exp:* Asthma; Occupational Asthma; Rhinitis; **Hospital:** Johns Hopkins Bayview Med Ctr; **Address:** Johns Hopkins Asthma & Allergy Ctr, 5501 Hopkins Bayview Circle, rm 3-B-65, Baltimore, MD 21224; **Phone:** (410) 550-2191; **Board Cert:** Allergy & Immunology 1995, Internal Medicine 1990; **Med School:** Greece 1983; **Resid:** Internal Medicine, Johns Hopkins Hosp, Baltimore, MD 1983-1985; Internal Medicine, Johns Hopkins Hosp, Baltimore, MD 1985-1986; **Fellow:** Clinical Immunology, Johns Hopkins Hosp, Baltimore, MD 1986-1988; **Fac Appt:** Assoc Prof Medicine, Johns Hopkins Univ

Southeast

Benenati, Susan MD (A&I) - *Spec Exp:* Asthma; Latex Allergy; Sinus Disorders; **Hospital:** Baptist Hosp - Miami; **Address:** 7000 SW 62nd Ave, Ste 510, South Miami, FL 33143-4721; **Phone:** (305) 665-1623; **Board Cert:** Internal Medicine 1988, Allergy & Immunology 1991; **Med School:** Univ S Fla Coll Med 1984; **Resid:** Internal Medicine, Indiana Univ Med Ctr, Indianapolis, IN 1984-1988; **Fellow:** Allergy & Immunology, Johns Hopkins Hosp, Baltimore, MD 1988-1990; **Fac Appt:** Asst Prof Medicine, Univ Miami Sch Med

Bonner, James Ryan MD (A&I) - *Spec Exp:* Allergy & Immunology - General; **Hospital:** Univ of Ala Hosp at Birmingham; **Address:** Univ of Alabama Hosp, Dept Allergy & Immunology, 2000 Sixth Ave S, Birmingham, AL 35233; **Phone:** (205) 801-8100; **Board Cert:** Internal Medicine 1974, Infectious Disease 1976, Allergy & Immunology 1979; **Med School:** Univ Mich Med Sch 1971; **Resid:** Internal Medicine, Univ Ala Med Ctr, Birmingham, AL 1972-1974; **Fellow:** Allergy & Immunology, Univ Ala Med Ctr, Birmingham, AL 1974-1977; **Fac Appt:** Prof Medicine, Univ Ala

de Shazo, Richard Denson MD (A&I) - *Spec Exp:* Immunodeficiency Disorders; Sinusitis; Rheumatology; **Hospital:** Univ Hosps & Clins - Mississippi; **Address:** Univ Miss Med Ctr, 2500 N State St, Jackson, MS 39216-4505; **Phone:** (601) 984-5600; **Board Cert:** Allergy & Immunology 1977, Geriatric Medicine 1994, Rheumatology 1982, Internal Medicine 1974; **Med School:** Univ Ala 1971; **Resid:** Internal Medicine, Walter Reed Genl Hosp., Washington, DC 1972-1974; Rheumatology, Walter Reed Genl Hosp, Washington, DC 1975-1977; **Fellow:** Clinical Immunology, Walter Reed Genl Hosp., Washington, DC 1974-1975; **Fac Appt:** Prof Medicine, Univ Miss

Fox, Roger W MD (A&I) - *Spec Exp:* Allergy & Immunology - General; **Hospital:** University Comm Hosp; **Address:** U of S FL Asthma, Allergy, Immun Clin Rsch, 13801 Bruce B Downs Blvd, Ste 505, Tampa, FL 33613; **Phone:** (813) 971-9743; **Board Cert:** Internal Medicine 1978, Allergy & Immunology 1981; **Med School:** St Louis Univ 1975; **Resid:** Internal Medicine, Univ S Florida Affil Hosps, Tampa, FL 1976-1978; **Fellow:** Allergy & Immunology, Univ S Florida Affil Hosps, Tampa, FL 1978-1980; **Fac Appt:** Assoc Prof Medicine, Univ S Fla Coll Med

Friedman, Stuart MD (A&I) - *Spec Exp:* Asthma; Sinus Disorders; **Hospital:** Boca Raton Comm Hosp; **Address:** 5162 Linton Blvd #201, Delray Beach, FL 33484-6567; **Phone:** (561) 495-2580; **Board Cert:** Internal Medicine 1980, Allergy & Immunology 1983; **Med School:** Spain 1976; **Resid:** Internal Medicine, Winthrop Univ Hosp, Mineola, NY 1977-1980; **Fellow:** Allergy & Immunology, Univ Cincinnati Med Ctr, Cincinnati, OH 1980-1982

Gluck, Joan MD (A&I) - *Spec Exp:* Asthma in Pregnancy; Asthma/Allergies-Pediatric; Food Allergy; **Hospital:** Baptist Hosp - Miami; **Address:** 8970 SW 87rh Ct, Ste 100, Ste 100, Miami, FL 33176-2207; **Phone:** (305) 279-3366; **Med School:** NYU Sch Med 1972; **Resid:** Pediatrics, Univ Miami-Jackson Meml Hosp, Miami, FL 1972-1974; **Fellow:** Allergy & Immunology, Univ Miami-Jackson Meml Hosp, Miami, FL 1974-1976

Good, Robert MD/PhD (A&I) - *Spec Exp:* Immune Deficiency; Bone Marrow Transplant; Nutrition in Aging-Associated Diseases; **Hospital:** All Children's Hosp; **Address:** 801 Sixth St S, Box 9350, St Petersburg, FL 33701; **Phone:** (727) 892-4470; **Med School:** Univ Minn 1947; **Resid:** Pediatrics, Univ Minn Hosps, Minneapolis, MN 1947-1949; Pediatrics, Univ Minn Hosps, Minneapolis, MN 1950-1951; **Fellow:** Research, Rockefeller Inst, New York, NY 1949-1950; **Fac Appt:** Prof Pediatrics, Univ S Fla Coll Med

Kaplan, Allen MD (A&I) - *Spec Exp:* Urticaria; **Hospital:** Med Univ Hosp Authority; **Address:** Med Univ South Caroline, Div Allergy & Immun, 96 Jonathan Lucas St, Ste 812, CSB, Charleston, SC 29425-2220; **Phone:** (843) 792-3712; **Board Cert:** Internal Medicine 1972, Rheumatology 1972, Allergy & Immunology 1974, Clinical & Laboratory Immunology 1986; **Med School:** SUNY Downstate 1965; **Resid:** Internal Medicine, Strong Meml Hosp, Rochester 1966-1967; **Fac Appt:** Prof Medicine, Univ SC Sch Med

Ledford, Dennis MD (A&I) - *Spec Exp:* Asthma; **Hospital:** University Comm Hosp of Carrollwood; **Address:** U S FL Coll Med, Dept Allergy & Immunology, 13000 Bruce B Downs Blvd, MC 111D, Tampa, FL 33613; **Phone:** (813) 972-7631; **Board Cert:** Rheumatology 1984, Allergy & Immunology 1985; **Med School:** Univ Tenn Coll Med, Memphis 1976; **Resid:** Internal Medicine, City of Memphis Hosp, Memphis, TN 1978-1980; **Fellow:** Rheumatology, NYU Hosp-Bellevue, New York, NY 1980-1982; Allergy & Immunology, Univ South Florida Coll Med, Tampa, FL 1983-1985; **Fac Appt:** Assoc Prof Allergy & Immunology, Univ S Fla Coll Med

Lockey, Richard MD (A&I) - *Spec Exp:* Immune Deficiency; Asthma; Chronic Rhinitis; **Hospital:** University Comm Hosp; **Address:** 13801 Bruce B Downs Blvd, Ste 502, Tampa, FL 33613-3946; **Phone:** (813) 971-9743; **Board Cert:** Internal Medicine 1970, Allergy & Immunology 1974; **Med School:** Temple Univ 1965; **Resid:** Internal Medicine, Univ Mich Hosp, Ann Arbor, MI 1966-1968; **Fellow:** Allergy & Immunology, Univ Mich Hosp, Ann Arbor, MI 1969-1970; **Fac Appt:** Prof Medicine, Univ S Fla Coll Med

Pacin, Michael MD (A&I) - *Spec Exp:* Insect Allergies; **Hospital:** Baptist Hosp - Miami; **Address:** 8970 SW 87th Court, Ste 100, Miami, FL 33176; **Phone:** (305) 279-3366; **Board Cert:** Allergy & Immunology 1979, Internal Medicine 1974; **Med School:** Washington Univ, St Louis 1969; **Resid:** Internal Medicine, Jewish Hosp, St Louis, MO 1970-1971; Internal Medicine, Jackson Meml Hosp, Miami, FL 1971-1972; **Fellow:** Allergy & Immunology, Long Beach VA Hosp 1972-1974

Stein, Mark R MD (A&I) - *Spec Exp:* Asthma; Immune Deficiency; Gastroesopageal Reflux; **Hospital:** Good Samaritan Med Ctr - W Palm Beach; **Address:** 840 US Hwy 1, Ste 235, North Palm Beach, FL 33408-3884; **Phone:** (561) 626-2006; **Board Cert:** Internal Medicine 1975, Allergy & Immunology 1977; **Med School:** Jefferson Med Coll 1968; **Resid:** Internal Medicine, Letterman Army Med Ctr, San Francisco, CA 1972-1975; **Fellow:** Allergy & Immunology, Fitzsimmons Army Med Ctr, Denver, CO 1975-1977

Midwest

Aaronson, Donald W MD (A&I) - *Spec Exp:* Drug Sensitivity; Sinus Disorders; Asthma; **Hospital:** Advocate Lutheran Gen Hosp; **Address:** 3500 Lake Shore Drive, Chicago, IL 60657; **Phone:** (847) 635-7300; **Board Cert:** Allergy & Immunology 1975; **Med School:** Univ IL Coll Med 1961; **Resid:** Internal Medicine, Hines VA Hosp, Chicago, IL 1962-1965; **Fellow:** Allergy & Immunology, Northwestern Univ, Chicago, IL 1965-1966; **Fac Appt:** Clin Prof Medicine, Univ Hlth Sci/Chicago Med Sch

Baker Jr., James Russell MD (A&I) - *Spec Exp:* Immune Deficiency-Thyroid; **Hospital:** Univ of MI Hlth Ctr; **Address:** 1500 E Med Center Drive, Ste 3918, Ann Arbor, MI 48109-0380; **Phone:** (734) 647-2777; **Board Cert:** Internal Medicine 1981, Allergy & Immunology 1983; **Med School:** Loyola Univ-Stritch Sch Med 1978; **Resid:** Internal Medicine, Walter Reed Army Med Ctr, Washington, DC 1979-1981; **Fellow:** Allergy & Immunology, Walter Reed Army Med Ctr/NIAID, Bethesda, MD 1981-1984; **Fac Appt:** Prof Allergy & Immunology, Univ Mich Med Sch

Bush, Robert MD (A&I) - *Spec Exp:* Allergy & Immunology - General; **Hospital:** Univ WI Hosp & Clins; **Address:** 600 Highland Ave, Ste B6-242, Madison, WI 53792; **Phone:** (608) 263-6180; **Board Cert:** Allergy & Immunology 1977, Internal Medicine 1975; **Med School:** W VA Univ 1970; **Resid:** Internal Medicine, Univ Wisc, Madison, WI 1973-1975; Allergy & Immunology, Univ Wisc, Madison, WI 1975-1977; **Fac Appt:** Prof Medicine, Univ Wisc

Busse, William MD (A&I) - *Spec Exp:* Asthma; Autoimmune Disease; **Hospital:** Univ WI Hosp & Clins; **Address:** 600 Highland Ave, rm B6/242, Madison, WI 53792; **Phone:** (608) 263-6180; **Board Cert:** Allergy & Immunology 1974, Internal Medicine 1972; **Med School:** Univ Wisc 1966; **Resid:** Internal Medicine, Cincinnati Genl Hosp, Cincinnati, OH 1967-1968; Internal Medicine, Cincinnati Genl Hosp, Cincinnati, OH 1970-1971; **Fellow:** Allergy & Immunology, Univ Wisc, Madison, WI 1971-1973; **Fac Appt:** Prof Medicine, Univ Wisc

Frigas, Evangelo MD (A&I) - *Spec Exp:* Urticaria; Angioedema; **Hospital:** St Mary's Hosp - Rochester, MN; **Address:** Mayo Clinic, Allergic Diseases Div, 200 First St SW, Rochester, MN 55905; **Phone:** (507) 284-2511; **Board Cert:** Internal Medicine 1978, Allergy & Immunology 1981; **Med School:** Italy 1970; **Resid:** Internal Medicine, Morristown Mem Hosp, Rutger 1976-1978; **Fellow:** Allergy & Immunology, Mayo Clinic, Rochester 1978-1980; **Fac Appt:** Assoc Prof Medicine, Mayo Med Sch

Grammer, Leslie C MD (A&I) - *Spec Exp:* Asthma; Occupational Allergy; **Hospital:** Northwestern Meml Hosp; **Address:** Northwestern Med Faculty Fdn - Ambulatory Care Ctr, 675 N St Clair, Fl 18 - Ste 18-250, Chicago, IL 60611-5975; **Phone:** (312) 695-8624; **Board Cert:** Internal Medicine 1979, Allergy & Immunology 1981, Clinical & Laboratory Immunology 1986, Occupational Medicine 1989; **Med School:** Northwestern Univ 1976; **Resid:** Internal Medicine, Northwestern Univ, Chicago, IL 1977-1979; **Fellow:** Allergy & Immunology, Northwestern Univ, Chicago, IL 1979-1981; **Fac Appt:** Prof Medicine, Northwestern Univ

Greenberger, Paul A MD (A&I) - *Spec Exp:* Asthma; Anaphylaxis; Drug Allergy; **Hospital:** Northwestern Meml Hosp; **Address:** Northwestern Med Faculty Fdn, Ambulatory Care Ctr, 675 N St Clair Fl 18 - Ste 18-250, Chicago, IL 60611; **Phone:** (312) 695-8624; **Board Cert:** Internal Medicine 1976, Allergy & Immunology 1979, Clinical & Laboratory Immunology 1986; **Med School:** Indiana Univ 1973; **Resid:** Internal Medicine, Jewish Hosp, St Louis, MO 1974-1976; **Fellow:** Allergy & Immunology, Northwestern Meml Hosp, Chicago, IL 1976-1978; **Fac Appt:** Prof Medicine, Northwestern Univ

Kaiser, Harold MD (A&I) - *Spec Exp:* Asthma; Rhinitis; Clinical Trials; **Hospital:** Abbott - Northwestern Hosp; **Address:** 825 Nicollett Mall, Ste 1149, Minneapolis, MN 55402-2750; **Phone:** (612) 338-3333; **Board Cert:** Internal Medicine 1963, Allergy & Immunology 1972; **Med School:** Univ Minn 1956; **Resid:** Internal Medicine, Wadsworth VA Hosp, Los Angeles, CA 1957-1958; Allergy & Immunology, VA Hosp-Univ Minn Hosp, Minneapolis, MN 1960-1962; **Fellow:** Allergy & Immunology, UCLA Med Ctr, Los Angeles, CA 1964-1965; **Fac Appt:** Clin Prof Medicine, Univ Minn

Korenblat, Phillip Erwin MD (A&I) - *Spec Exp:* Allergy; Asthma; Anaphylaxis; **Hospital:** Barnes-Jewish Hosp (page 55); **Address:** 1040 N Mason Rd, Ste 115, St. Louis, MO 63141-6361; **Phone:** (314) 542-0606; **Board Cert:** Internal Medicine 1971, Allergy & Immunology 1974; **Med School:** Univ Ark 1960; **Resid:** Internal Medicine, Jewish Hosp, St Louis, MO 1961-1965; **Fellow:** Allergy & Immunology, Scripps Clin Rsch Fdn, La Jolla, CA 1965-1966; **Fac Appt:** Clin Prof Medicine, Washington Univ, St Louis

Sanders, Georgiana MD (A&I) - *Spec Exp:* Asthma; Allergy; Lung Disease-Pediatric; **Hospital:** Univ of MI Hlth Ctr; **Address:** Taubman Ctr, rm 3918, Box 3080, 1500 E Med Ctr Drive, Ann Arbor, MI 48109-0380; **Phone:** (734) 936-5634; **Board Cert:** Pediatrics 1983, Allergy & Immunology 1985; **Med School:** Univ Cincinnati 1975; **Resid:** Pediatrics, Children's Hosp of Mich, Detroit, MI 1975-1978; Pediatrics, Boston City Hospi, Boston, MA 1978-1979; **Fellow:** Allergy & Immunology, Univ of Michigan Hosp, Ann Arbor, MI 1981-1984; **Fac Appt:** Asst Clin Prof Pediatrics, Univ Mich Med Sch

Slavin, Raymond MD (A&I) - *Spec Exp:* Asthma; Sinus Disorders; Immune Deficiency-Lung; **Hospital:** St Louis Univ Hospital; **Address:** St Louis Univ Hlth Scis Ctr, Div Allergy & Immunology, 3635 Vista Ave @Grand Blvd, St.Louis, MO 63110; **Phone:** (314) 577-6070; **Board Cert:** Internal Medicine 1964, Allergy & Immunology 1987; **Med School:** St Louis Univ 1967; **Resid:** Internal Medicine, St Louis Univ Hosp, St Louis, MO 1959-1961; **Fellow:** Allergy & Immunology, Northwestern Univ Med Ctr, Chicago, IL 1961-1964; **Fac Appt:** Prof Medicine, St Louis Univ

Ten, Rosa Maria MD/PhD (A&I) - *Spec Exp:* Immune Deficiency; Asthma; **Hospital:** Mayo Med Ctr & Clin - Rochester, MN; **Address:** Div Allergy & Immunology, 200 1st St SW, Rochester, MN 55905; **Phone:** (507) 284-9077; **Board Cert:** Internal Medicine 1995, Allergy & Immunology 1997; **Med School:** Spain 1982; **Resid:** Internal Medicine, Mayo Clinic, Rochester, MN 1992-1994; **Fellow:** Immunology, Inst Pasteur, Paris France 1989-1991; Allergy & Immunology, Mayo Clinic, Rochester, MN 1995-1996; **Fac Appt:** Assoc Prof Allergy & Immunology, Mayo Med Sch

Wood, John MD (A&I) - *Spec Exp:* Asthma; **Hospital:** Barnes-Jewish Hosp (page 55); **Address:** 22 S Woodsmill Rd, Ste 500S, Chesterfield, MO 63017; **Phone:** (314) 878-6260; **Board Cert:** Pulmonary Disease 1978, Allergy & Immunology 1979; **Med School:** Univ Okla Coll Med 1968; **Resid:** Internal Medicine, Univ Hosp, Oklahoma City, OK 1969-1970; Internal Medicine, Barnes Hosp-Wash Univ Sch Med, St Louis, MO 1970-1971; **Fellow:** Pulmonary Disease, Wash Univ Sch Med, St Louis, MO 1975-1977; Allergy & Immunology, Wash Univ Sch Med, St Louis, MO 1976-1977; **Fac Appt:** Asst Prof Medicine, Washington Univ, St Louis

Great Plains and Mountains

Jones, James F MD (A&I) - *Spec Exp:* Chronic Fatigue Syndrome; **Hospital:** Natl Jewish Med & Rsrch Ctr; **Address:** Nat'l Jewish Med & Rsrch Ctr, 1400 Jackson St, rm K 913, Denver, CO 80206; **Phone:** (303) 398-1195; **Board Cert:** Pediatrics 1974, Allergy & Immunology 1977; **Med School:** Univ Tex Med Br, Galveston 1968; **Resid:** Surgery, Univ Arizona Hosp, Tucson, AZ 1970; Plastic Surgery, Univ Arizona Hosp, Tucson, AZ 1971; **Fellow:** Immunology, Univ Tex Med, TX 1969-1970; Immunology, Univ Arizona Hosp, Tucson, AZ 1971-1975; **Fac Appt:** Assoc Prof Univ Colo

Nelson, Harold MD (A&I) - *Spec Exp:* Asthma; Allergies-Pediatric; **Hospital:** Natl Jewish Med & Rsrch Ctr; **Address:** National Jewish Med & Rsch Ctr, 1400 Jackson St, Denver, CO 80206; **Phone:** (303) 398-1562; **Board Cert:** Internal Medicine 1963, Allergy & Immunology 1983; **Med School:** Emory Univ 1955; **Resid:** Internal Medicine, Letterman Genl Hosp, San Francisco, CA 1959-1962; **Fellow:** Allergy & Immunology, Univ Mich Med Ctr, Ann Arbor, MI 1967-1969; **Fac Appt:** Prof Medicine, Univ Colo

Neustrom, Mark Ray DO (A&I) - *Spec Exp:* Asthma; Rhinitis; **Hospital:** Overland Park Reg Med Ctr; **Address:** 4500 College Blvd, Ste 200, Overland Park, KS 66211; **Phone:** (913) 491-5501; **Board Cert:** Internal Medicine 1991, Allergy & Immunology 1995; **Med School:** Univ Osteo Med & Hlth Sci 1987; **Resid:** Internal Medicine, Univ South Dakota-VA Hosp, Sioux Falls, SD 1987-1990; **Fellow:** Allergy & Immunology, Med Coll Wisc, Milwaukee, WI 1992-1994

Rosenwasser, Lanny J MD (A&I) - *Spec Exp:* Asthma; **Hospital:** Natl Jewish Med & Rsrch Ctr; **Address:** 1400 Jackson St, Ste K 621 B, Denver, CO 80206; **Phone:** (303) 398-1656; **Board Cert:** Internal Medicine 1975, Allergy & Immunology 1977, Clinical & Laboratory Immunology 1990; **Med School:** NYU Sch Med 1972; **Resid:** Univ Calif Affil Hosps, San Francisco, CA 1973-1974; **Fac Appt:** Prof Allergy & Immunology, Univ Colo

Wald, Jeffrey A MD (A&I) - *Spec Exp:* Asthma; Rhinitis; **Hospital:** Overland Park Reg Med Ctr; **Address:** 4500 College Blvd, Ste 200, Overland Park, KS 66211; **Phone:** (913) 491-5501; **Board Cert:** Internal Medicine 1983, Allergy & Immunology 1987; **Med School:** Univ MO-Columbia Sch Med 1980; **Resid:** Internal Medicine, Jewish Hosp, St. Louis, MO 1980-1983; Allergy & Immunology, Natl Jewish Hosp, Denver, CO 1981-1983; **Fellow:** Allergy & Immunology, Natl Jewish Hosp, Denver, CO 1984-1986

Southwest

Freeman, Theodore MD (A&I) - *Spec Exp:* Insect Allergies; **Hospital:** SW Texas Methodist Hosp; **Address:** 8285 Fredericksberg, San Antonio, TX 78229; **Phone:** (210) 614-3923; **Board Cert:** Internal Medicine 1983, Allergy & Immunology 1987; **Med School:** Univ S Fla Coll Med 1980; **Resid:** Internal Medicine, Keesler Med Ctr, Biloxi, MS 1981-1983; Allergy & Immunology, Wilford Hall Med Ctr, San Antonio, TX 1984-1986; **Fellow:** Diagnostic Lab Immunology, Mass Genl Hosp, Boston, MA 1986-1987; **Fac Appt:** Assoc Prof Medicine

West Coast and Pacific

Shapiro, Gail Greenberg MD (A&I) - *Spec Exp:* Asthma & Allergy; **Hospital:** Chldns Hosp and Regl Med Ctr - Seattle; **Address:** NW Asthma & Allergy, 4540 Sand Point Way NE, Ste 200, Seattle, WA 98105-3941; **Phone:** (206) 527-1200; **Board Cert:** Allergy & Immunology 1975, Pediatrics 1975; **Med School:** Johns Hopkins Univ 1970; **Resid:** Pediatrics, Univ Wash, Seattle, WA 1971-1972; **Fellow:** Allergy & Immunology, Univ Wash, Seattle, WA 1972-1974; **Fac Appt:** Clin Prof Pediatrics, Univ Wash

Tamaroff, Marc A MD (A&I) - *Spec Exp:* Sinus Disorders; Asthma; **Hospital:** Long Beach Meml Med Ctr; **Address:** 3816 Woodruff Ave, Ste 209, Long Beach, CA 90808; **Phone:** (562) 496-4749; **Board Cert:** Allergy & Immunology 1983, Internal Medicine 1979; **Med School:** Univ Ariz Coll Med 1974; **Resid:** Internal Medicine, St Mary Med Ctr, Long Beach, CA 1974-1977; **Fellow:** Allergy & Immunology, UCLA Med Ctr, Los Angeles, CA 1977-1979; **Fac Appt:** Assoc Clin Prof Medicine, UCLA

Wasserman, Stephen MD (A&I) - *Spec Exp:* Anaphylaxis; Sinus Disorders; Urticaria; **Hospital:** UCSD Healthcare; **Address:** UCSD Med Ctr, Dept Med, 9500 Gilman Drive, rm 244, Lajolla, CA 92093; **Phone:** (858) 822-4261; **Board Cert:** Internal Medicine 1973, Allergy & Immunology 1975; **Med School:** UCLA 1968; **Resid:** Internal Medicine, Peter Bent Brigham Hosp, Boston, MA 1968-1970; **Fellow:** Allergy & Immunology, R Breck-PB Brigham Hosp, Boston, MA 1972-1974; **Fac Appt:** Prof Medicine, UCSD

CARDIOLOGY

(a subspecialty of INTERNAL MEDICINE)

Cardiology: A cardiologist specializes in diseases of the heart, lungs and blood vessels and manages complex cardiac conditions such as heart attacks and life-threatening, abnormal heartbeat rhythms.

Cardiac Electrophysiology: A field of special interest within the subspecialty of cardiovascular disease which involves intricate technical procedures to evaluate heart rhythms and determine appropriate treatment for them.

Interventional Cardiology: An area of medicine within the subspecialty of cardiology which uses specialized imaging and other diagnostic techniques to evaluate blood flow and pressure in the coronary arteries and chambers of the heart, and uses technical procedures and medications to treat abnormalities that impair the function of the heart.

INTERNAL MEDICINE

A personal physician who provides long-term, comprehensive care in the office and the hospital, managing both common and complex illness of adolescents, adults and the elderly. Internists are trained in the diagnosis and treatment of cancer, infections and diseases affecting the heart, blood, kidneys, joints and digestive, respiratory and vascular systems. They are also trained in the essentials of primary care internal medicine which incorporates an understanding of disease prevention, wellness, substance abuse, mental health and effective treatment of common problems of the eyes, ears, skin, nervous system and reproductive organs.

Training required: Three years in internal medicine *plus* additional training and examination for certification in cardiovascular disease, clinical electrophysiology or interventional cardiology.

Barnes-Jewish Hospital

BJC HealthCare℠

the primary adult hospital for
Washington University School of Medicine

216 S. Kingshighway
St. Louis, MO 63110
314-TOP-DOCS
(314-867-3627)
or toll free 1-866-867-3627
www.barnesjewish.org

HEART SERVICES

advanced technology with compassionate care

As pioneers of many cardiology and cardiothoracic surgery procedures, from ablation therapies to valve repair and replacement, the Washington University heart specialists at Barnes-Jewish Hospital are focused on improving the care of patients with cardiovascular disease. The Heart Services program is noted for:

- maintaining the highest volume heart failure program in the region offering a multidisciplinary approach to patients with advanced heart failure, including transplantation and biventricular pacing
- offering the region's only interventional cardiology program treating patients with the newest angioplasty techniques such as brachytherapy and drug-coated stents
- opening the first Thoracic Aorta Center in the region, offering medical and surgical management of patients with Marfan Syndrome and diseases of the thoracic aorta
- expanding the only regional Center for Adults with Congenital Heart Disease.

latest medical and surgical advancements

Barnes-Jewish Hospital patients have been among the first to benefit from many new procedures as the heart team has helped to pioneer angioplasty techniques, coronary bypass procedures, valvuloplasty, ventricular assist device placement and heart transplantation. Our comprehensive program is recognized for:

- performing more than 1,000 major cardiac surgical cases a year
- continuing the highest volume electrophysiology service in the region offering state-of-the art medical therapy, device therapy and curative, catheter-based ablation procedures for patients with cardiac arrhythmias, including atrial fibrillation
- developing and refining nationally recognized procedures such as off-pump (beating heart) surgery, surgical treatment of atrial fibrillation and endoscopic cardiac surgery
- beginning the first prospective, randomized trial in the world of robotically assisted coronary bypass surgery.

Advancing Medicine. Touching Lives.

"While patients and their families reap the benefits of the clinical and research experience available at Barnes-Jewish Hospital, it is the specialized care that they remember most."

— Michael E. Cain, MD
Director, Cardiovascular Division

— Ralph J. Damiano, Jr., MD
Chief, Cardiac Surgery

If you need a heart specialist, go straight to the top. Call **314-TOP-DOCS** (314-867-3627) or toll free 1-866-867-3627. **www.barnesjewish.org**

THE CLEVELAND CLINIC

9500 Euclid Avenue, Cleveland, OH 44195

Tel. 216/444-6697

www.clevelandclinic.org/heartcenter

AMERICA'S BEST HEART CENTER

The Cleveland Clinic Heart Center, recognized as an international cardiovascular referral center, is one of the largest and busiest heart programs in the United States. Cleveland Clinic Heart Center doctors are leaders in cardiology, cardiac surgery, and research into the heart and its diseases. No heart program has more experience, more knowledge and better access to technology. *U.S.News & World Report* has ranked the Cleveland Clinic Heart Center in the nation's top five since 1990 and best in the nation for heart care since 1995.

Patients come to the Cleveland Clinic Heart Center from across America and from more than 80 countries. In 2000, Heart Center physicians handled more than 58,000 patient visits, completed more than 6,000 cardiac catheterization procedures, and performed nearly 3,700 open heart operations. These numbers, and the outcomes resulting from numerous procedures used to treat each case of heart disease, distinguishes the Cleveland Clinic Heart Center from other institutions.

CLINICAL TRIALS AND RESEARCH

The Cleveland Clinic Heart Center is a recognized leader in multi-center and international trials. An outstanding clinical infrastructure and strong commitment to basic science allow The Cleveland Clinic to remain on the cutting edge of treatment and research in cardiovascular disease. There are nearly 100 trials currently underway at the Cleveland Clinic Heart Center ranging from basic cellular research to the development of a new artificial heart.

HISTORY OF INNOVATIONS

Cleveland Clinic doctors made two major breakthroughs that catapulted the world into the modern era of heart care: coronary angiography and saphenous vein bypass surgery. The development of coronary angiography in 1958 allowed physicians, for the first time, to visualize coronary artery blockages and determine their location and severity. At the time, this innovation represented the single most important advance in modern cardiology, paving the way for the development of saphenous vein bypass surgery, the world's first aortic valve repair and the first minimally invasive surgery for primary repair and replacement of diseased aortic and mitral valves at The Cleveland Clinic.

More recent innovations include circumferential ultrasound vein-ablation to treat atrial fibrillation and bi-ventricular pacing for the treatment of heart failure. Additionally, the Cleveland Clinic Heart Center is the world's most active user of left-ventricular assist devices (LVADs) as a bridge to heart transplant.

LEADING THE BATTLE AGAINST HEART DISEASE

In many cases, Cleveland Clinic Heart Center patients have access to procedures not available elsewhere and many techniques now in use around the world were first performed at the Cleveland Clinic Heart Center. As a result of this leadership, Cleveland Clinic specialists have accumulated the world's largest volume of many highly specialized interventions and an unmatched breadth and depth of experience in treating cardiovascular disease.

Cardiologists and surgeons in the Heart Center treat all conditions affecting the structure or functions of the heart including:

- coronary artery disease (including heart attack)
- valve disease
- abnormal heart rhythms
- heart failure
- congenital heart disease
- hypertrophic cardiomyopathy

CONTINUUM HEALTH PARTNERS, INC.
CONTINUUM HEART INSTITUTE

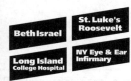

Phone (212) 420-HEART

Continuum Health Partners, Inc.

The Continuum Heart Institute combines the strengths of the cardiac programs at Beth Israel Medical Center, St. Luke's-Roosevelt Hospital Center and Long Island College Hospital for clinical, technological and innovative excellence. The skill and caliber of its cardiologists, cardiovascular surgeons, primary care physicians and other physician specialists is matched only by its state-of-the-art facilities—including the most technologically advanced cardiac care units, catheterization and electrophysiology labs, cardiac surgery suites, open heart recovery units, and cardiopulmonary stepdown telemetry units.

The Continuum Heart Institute offers every heart care service needed to prevent, diagnose, and treat heart disease, including leading-edge cardiac surgery, catheter-based diagnosis and treatment, hypertension diagnosis and treatment, heart failure diagnosis and treatment, and a hypertropic cardiomyopathy program. Strong believers in prevention and early detection, the professionals throughout the Continuum Heart Institute also provide complete medical evaluations, echocardiography, nuclear cardiology services, coronary artery disease prevention, treatment centers for obesity and diabetes, smoking cessation programs, and complementary techniques for relaxation and stress reduction, such as massage therapy and therapeutic touch.

Some of the unique features available at the hospitals of the Continuum Heart Institute include New York City's first robotic surgical suite for closed-chest coronary artery bypass surgery; the Ross procedure—a pulmonary autograft replacement of the aortic valve; and a nationally recognized arrhythmia service.

The program is recognized by the New York State Department of Health as having one of the lowest mortality rates of any New York City hospital, and is consistently ranked among the top five programs in New York State.

CONTINUUM HEART INSTITUTE

In an effort to bridge its many cardiac care programs and provide patients with more streamlined access to its full range of services, the Continuum Heart Institute was established. This interdisciplinary cardiology, cardiac surgery and cardiac rehabilitation team consists of clinicians, surgeons, nurses and nurse practitioners, physician assistants, social workers, complementary care experts and rehabilitation specialists—all working together to give patients a full range of individualized treatment choices and services.

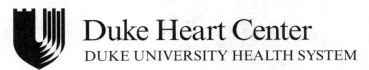

Duke Heart Center

DUKE UNIVERSITY HEALTH SYSTEM

Durham, NC • *1-888-ASK-DUKE* • heartcenter.mc.duke.edu

One of the world's most respected heart programs, Duke Heart Center offers comprehensive cardiac care, from rehabilitation programs to home care to a specialized chest pain unit for 24-hour-a-day diagnosis and emergency treatment.

Highlights include one of the nation's largest and most experienced interventional cardiology programs, with more than 1,700 procedures performed each year; one of the nation's most experienced open heart surgery programs (and one of the few that feature a full team of cardiac anesthesiologists); expertise in minimally invasive surgery; state-of-the-art imaging facilities; and access to the latest medical therapies. Dedicated programs exist for patients with coronary artery disease, valvular heart disease, peripheral vascular disease, arrhythmias, heart failure, and pediatric and adult congenital heart disease.

EXPERIENCE. Studies show that, in heart procedures, greater experience correlates with greater success. Duke far exceeds all nationally recommended volume guidelines for medical facilities and doctors performing angioplasty and open heart surgery. Duke physicians also have access to the Duke Databank for Cardiovascular Disease—the largest and oldest of its kind in the world—enabling them to draw on knowledge of 200,000 cases to determine the best treatment options.

RESULTS. Duke Heart Center's expertise yields better outcomes for our patients. For example, over the past five years Duke bypass surgery patients have had an actual mortality rate of 1.7 percent, less than half of the expected risk-adjusted mortality rate of 3.5 percent (based on risk-adjustment models published in peer-reviewed journals).

RESEARCH. Duke quickly translates new discoveries into treatments that benefit patients. Current studies include hypothermia to protect resuscitated cardiac arrest patients' brains, genetic therapy to reverse cardiac damage, slower normalization of body temperatures after bypass surgery to minimize cognitive declines, radiation to improve angioplasty outcomes, and improved medical management of heart disease.

DUKE HEART CENTER AT A GLANCE

Ranked the #6 heart center in the nation by *U.S.News & World Report*.

Named one of the top 100 cardiovascular hospitals nationwide in *Modern Healthcare*.

More than 80 board-certified cardiologists, cardiac surgeons, and cardiac anesthesiologists care for over 7,000 patients annually.

According to an annual independent survey, 98 percent of Duke heart patients say they would recommend Duke to family and friends.

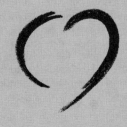

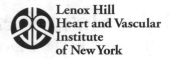

Lenox Hill
Heart and Vascular
Institute
of New York

Lenox Hill Hospital

100 East 77th Street, New York, NY 10021
1-877-HEARTBEAT — www. lenoxhillhospital.org

SETTING THE WORLD STANDARD FOR COMPLEX CARDIOVASCULAR CARE

The Lenox Hill Heart & Vascular Institute is among the leading cardiovascular care programs nationwide. From diagnosis to treatment and recovery, the Institute provides comprehensive care through its distinguished team of cardiologists, interventional cardiologists, cardiothoracic and vascular surgeons, and radiologists.

DEPTH OF EXPERIENCE

The Institute is a major referral center for cardiac care, treating thousands of patients with heart and vascular disease annually. The Institute's physicians perform some 6,000 cardiac catheterizations a year, approximately 3,500 angioplasties, over 1,000 endovascular procedures, and more than 1,000 open heart surgeries. Whether a patient has a simple or complex condition, our physicians have the experience required to provide the best treatment available.

GROUNDBREAKING RESEARCH

Physicians at the Institute constantly seek to broaden the understanding of heart and vascular disease and expand the boundaries of care through research and clinical trials. Our interventional cardiologists are world renowned for clearing blockages in the arteries with balloon angioplasty and stents. Our physicians have been instrumental in obtaining FDA approval of procedures such as applying radiation to stents to interrupt scar tissue growth that can lead to reblockages. The Institute's cardiothoracic surgeons are leaders in the development of minimally invasive surgical techniques, including investigating the role of robotics in cardiac surgery. The Institute is currently leading multiple nationwide studies involving advanced techniques that could change the face of heart and vascular treatment.

STATE-OF-THE-ART FACILITIES

Patients are cared for in modern facilities that are equipped with state-of-the-art technology. There are three operating rooms dedicated to open heart surgery and a new cardiac surgery intensive care unit and step-down unit. The 11th floor of the main hospital building is dedicated to the interventional cardiology and endovascular program, and houses new cardiac catheterization labs with the most technologically advanced equipment available.

LEADERS IN THE FIGHT AGAINST HEART DISEASE

Lenox Hill Heart and Vascular Institute is a pioneer of patient care, research and education. The Institute has set the standard of care nationally and internationally using state-of-the-art technology to treat patients who have simple and complex heart conditions. The Institute's full range of diagnostic and therapeutic services ensures continuity of care from assessment through treatment and rehabilitation. For more information, call the Lenox Hill Heart and Vascular Institute of New York at 1-877-HEARTBEAT.

108   Sponsored Page

THE CARDIAC INSTITUTE
MAIMONIDES MEDICAL CENTER

4802 Tenth Avenue • Brooklyn, NY 11219
Phone (800) 682-5558; (718) 283-8902
Fax (718) 283-8069
www.maimonidesmed.org

CARDIOLOGY

The cardiologists of Maimonides Medical Center are expertly trained to provide cardiac care, from diagnosis to medical treatment. They have at their fingertips the most sophisticated testing and monitoring technology, as well as the most progressive treatments available, including cardiac rehabilitation.

INTERVENTIONAL CARDIOLOGY

When a patient with heart disease needs a more complicated diagnostic workup or therapeutic procedure, they turn to Maimonides Medical Center's interventional cardiology program. New York State statistics and national independent reports have repeatedly confirmed that its catheterization lab yields the best possible outcomes for patients. The Division of Interventional Cardiology's collaboration with the Department of Emergency Medicine ensures that chest pain patients are evaluated immediately—with intervention to stop a heart attack in progress when necessary.

CARDIOTHORACIC SURGERY

With more than 1,000 surgical procedures a year, the Division of Cardiothoracic Surgery has one of the busiest programs in the New York metropolitan area. As a regional training center for cardiac surgeons, it conducts one of the largest residency programs in the country. And as a major research facility, it continually investigates unsolved problems in cardiac surgery. Maimonides' cardiothoracic surgeons not only have the best in mind for their patients—they are guiding the future of cardiac care.

THE CARDIAC INSTITUTE

Heart disease...it can strike suddenly. Its symptoms can be mild or debilitating, intermittent or persistent. It can be diagnosed as a mild, easily treatable condition or it can be found to be life-threatening, requiring major, complex surgery. That is why the best cardiac programs—like the Maimonides Cardiac Institute, directed by Jacob Shani, MD—are those that are prepared for any contingency... from a medical evaluation of chest pain, to intervention to open a blocked artery or surgery to save a life.

MONTEFIORE-EINSTEIN HEART CENTER
Montefiore Medical Center

Address: 111 East 210 Street, Cardiology Department, Bronx NY 10467
Phone: (800) MD-MONTE
www.montefiore.org

NATIONAL LEADER IN CARDIAC CARE

Montefiore enjoys a 60-year tradition in breakthrough research, progressive clinical care and model "quality of life" programs for cardiac patients in the greater New York region and across the nation. This legacy of caring and frontier medical and surgical excellence has evolved into the Montefiore-Einstein Heart Center, which offers patients an approach to cardiac care that is streamlined, state-of-the-art, comprehensive and easily accessible.

Understanding each patient's individual needs is pivotal to the mission of caring at Montefiore, so the Medical Center has carefully developed specific programs for every type of heart disease. The Heart Center has the nation's pre-eminent specialists overseeing programs in: Emergency Chest Pain, Congestive Heart Failure, Non-Invasive Cardiology (Stress Testing, Echocardiography), Interventional Cardiology (Catheterization, Electrophysiology and Arrhythmia), Heart Transplantation, Cardiac and Thoracic Surgery, Pediatric Cardiology and Cardiac Rehabilitation.

Patients have available to them state-of-the-art diagnostic tools, such as PET Scanners and Nuclear Cameras, available in only a few select academic medical centers. This is complemented by an extensive minimally invasive surgery program.

The comfort of easy access to health care is pivotal to consumers today. Montefiore's Heart Center program and experts are available through a vast community network of primary care physicians in the Bronx and Westchester, over 30 primary care centers, and a large staff of full-time and voluntary adult and pediatric cardiologists and cardiothoracic surgeons who have offices at Montefiore's two campuses, the Moses and the Weiler/Einstein Divisions.

Preventive care and early detection are the core of the Heart Center's mission, exemplified in Montefiore's Healthy Heart Program, a community-based screening program to detect and prevent heart disease.

LONG TRADITION OF PIONEERING HEART PROCEDURES

Among many cardiac care milestones, Montefiore cardiologists were the first to develop certain pacing techniques to regulate slow hearts and Montefiore arrhythmia experts pioneered non-surgical procedures to diagnose and cure irregular heart rhythms.

This tradition continues today, with Montefiore Medical Center researchers working to stimulate diseased blood vessels to perform a "natural by-pass," a process called angiogenesis. Other Montefiore researchers are using beta-blockers to defer congestive heart failure, while Montefiore surgeons are developing model programs to improve post-surgical "quality of life."

MONTEFIORE-EINSTEIN HEART CENTER

The Montefiore-Einstein Heart Center is a clinical center of excellence, which offers comprehensive diagnostic and therapeutic cardiac services. It is built on the strengths of two eminent institutions, Montefiore Medical Center and the Albert Einstein College of Medicine, and it is supported by a network of general and specialty cardiologists with practices throughout the region.

The Montefiore-Einstein Heart Center enables physicians to provide patients with access to its full range of adult and pediatric cardiac services for the diagnosis and treatment of acquired and congenital cardiac disease.

Specialty areas include:
* Chest Pain Centers
* Noninvasive and NuclearCardiology Services
* Diagnostic and Interventional Cardiology
* Electrophysiology/ Arrhythmia Services
* Congestive Heart Failure Services
* Cardiothoracic Surgery
* Heart Transplant Center
* Cardiac Rehabilitation

THE MOUNT SINAI HOSPITAL
CARDIOVASCULAR HEALTH

One Gustave L. Levy Place (Fifth Avenue and 98th Street)
New York, NY 10029-6574   Phone: (212) 241-6500
Physician Referral: 1-800-MD-SINAI (637-4624)
www.mountsinai.org

A World Leader in Cardiac Care.

In the 2001 U.S. News & World Report "America's Best Hospitals," cardiac care at The Mount Sinai Hospital was rated as one of the **best in the nation** and **#1 in New York City.**

At Mount Sinai, we take a global view of cardiovascular health. Our system of integrated care produces the best possible results, both for patients and for the future of medicine. Some of the world's most accomplished medical professionals work here, pooling their expertise and building on each other's strengths.

In 2002, Dr. David H. Adams and a team of the nation's most accomplished cardiothoracic and thoracic surgeons. Joined Mount Sinai's world-renowned faculty of physicians and scientists.

From behavioral programs such as smoking cessation and nutritional consulting to the creation of pioneering heart valve repair techniques and less invasive bypass surgical methods, our faculty and staff continually refine what is possible on medicine's most important frontiers.

In addition to **heart and lung transplantation, vascular surgery, noninvasive cardiology, cardiac catheterization,** and an extensive program for **cardiac rhythm disturbances,** we also specialize in the following areas:

Angioplasty: We are ranked as the state's safest center for patients undergoing this procedure.

Valvular heart disease: Integrated assessment includes a full array of diagnostic technologies, opening the door to a wide range of medical and surgical options and long-term follow-up care.

Pediatric cardiology: As children with congenital heart disease successfully reach adulthood, their ongoing cardiac care is seamlessly integrated into Mount Sinai's existing programs.

Minimally invasive cardiac surgery: We perform many procedures using minimally invasive approaches, resulting in less tissue trauma, less scarring, and faster recovery.

Our **Integrative and Behavioral Cardiovascular Health Program** creates a unique synergism, providing unparalleled patient care, while yielding breakthroughs in the prevention and treatment of cardiovascular disease.

THE MOUNT SINAI HOSPITAL

Mount Sinai Medical Center's *Zena and Michael A. Wiener Cardiovascular Institute* is a world leader in mending broken hearts. Under the visionary direction of the internationally renowned cardiologist, Valentin Fuster, MD, PhD, the Institute is recognized worldwide for its expertise in evaluating, managing and preventing cardiovascular disease through the integration of patient care, education and research.

Mount Sinai's Cardiac Catheterization Laboratories offer leading-edge technologies of all kinds, including diagnostic angiography, angioplasty, and biopsy. We can study the heart with the highest degree of precision available anywhere.

We are pioneering new genetic techniques to help hearts with diseased arteries grow new vessels, and to help damaged heart muscle repair itself.

Following are some of the cardiac conditions we treat at Mount Sinai:
- Arrhythmia
- Heart failure
- Coronary Artery Disease
- Heart Attack
- Hypertension
- Mitral Valve Prolapse
- Myocarditis
- Pericarditis
- Pulmonary Hypertension
- Valvula Heart Disease

⅃ NewYork-Presbyterian
┐ The University Hospitals of Columbia and Cornell

Columbia Weill Cornell Heart Institute

Columbia Presbyterian Medical Center
622 West 168th Street
New York, NY 10032

NewYork Weill Cornell Medical Center
525 East 68th Street
New York, NY 10021

OVERVIEW:

The Columbia Weill Cornell Heart Institute has a reputation for treating some of the highest risk cases in the world – healing those patients who cannot be helped anywhere else. We are committed to delivering the finest possible care to adult and pediatric patients by:

- combining the finest minds and cutting-edge technology with the most compassionate care
- helping patients make sense of the complex steps involved in treating their heart condition;
- providing them with a full set of appropriate treatment options for consideration after a complete diagnosis;
- listening, guiding and fully informing patients so that together we can confidently choose the best treatment.

The Columbia Weill Cornell Heart Institute has:

- A well-deserved reputation for clinical excellence – the only heart center in the New York area ranked among the nation's best by *U.S. News & World Report*;
- World-renowned expertise in all areas of cardiac care, including transplantation, open-heart surgery, arrhythmia control, left ventricular assist devices (LVAD) and robotics;
- One of the country's largest and most successful pediatric cardiology, cardiology interventional and cardiac surgery programs.
- The latest heart-imaging technology, including such innovative tools as advanced digital equipment for stress echocardiography SPECT, state-of-the-art MRI, intravascular/intracoronary ultrasound, electrophysiologic studies, nuclear scanning and an outstanding cardiac catheterization laboratory;
- A state-of-the-art Interventional Cardiology Center to diagnose and treat heart disease without surgery, on an inpatient or outpatient basis, including: angioplasty, balloon valvuloplasty, stenting, and intracoronary radiation for restenosis.

Physician Referral: For a physician referral or to learn more about the Columbia Weill Cornell Heart Institute call toll free **1-877-NYP-WELL** (1-877-697-9355) visit our website at **www.nypheart.com**.

HIGHLIGHTS INCLUDE:

- Performed more heart transplants than any other hospital in the world over the last two decades.

- First Robotics-Assisted Coronary Artery Bypass Surgery in the U.S.

- One of the principal investigators (12 institutions throughout the United States) involved in ongoing FDA clinical trials to explore the use and effectiveness of robotics in cardiac surgery.

- Lead medical center in a three-year landmark study of 129 patients – REMATCH (Randomized Evaluation of Mechanical Assistance for the Treatment of Congestive Heart Failure) — which found that implanted heart pumps can extend and improve the quality of life of terminally ill heart failure patients.

- Participating in FDA-approved randomized clinical trial to evaluate use of drug-coated stents versus regular stents on incidence of reoccurrence of renarrowing inside stent.

NYU Medical Center

550 First Avenue (at 31st Street)
New York, NY 10016
Physician Referral: (888) 7-NYU-MED
(888-769-8633) www.nyumedicalcenter.org

SCHOOL OF MEDICINE

NEW YORK UNIVERSITY

ADULT CARDIOVASCULAR SERVICES

MINIMALLY INVASIVE CARDIAC SURGERY

NYU Medical Center's physician-scientists have been at the fore-front of innovation in modern cardiovascular medicine for more than a half-century. In recent years, cardiothoracic surgeons at NYU have pioneered minimally invasive cardiac surgery, dramatically improving treatment of the most common forms of heart disease. More minimally invasive cardiac surgeries have been performed at NYU than at any other hospital in the world.

With the development of minimally invasive technology, surgeons achieve results that are comparable or even superior to those obtained via traditional open-chest surgery. Procedures such as coronary artery bypass grafting (CABG) and mitral valve repair or replacement (MVR) are now performed through a single small incision between the ribs. This approach not only lowers the risk of complications, such as bleeding and infection, but also reduces postoperative pain and scarring, speeds the recovery process, and helps patients resume their normal lives in record time.

THE CARDIAC CATHETERIZATION LABORATORY AND ELECTROPHYSIOLOGY PROGRAM

At the cutting edge of interventional cardiology, the Cardiac Catheterization Laboratory at NYU continues to set the standard of care for catheter-based diagnosis and evaluation of cardiac health. Located at Tisch Hospital, the Cath Lab provides a full range of procedures to evaluate how well the heart muscle and valves are working, whether the heart is beating at regular intervals, detect and measure any narrowing in the coronary arteries, and recommend appropriate treatment if needed.

THE CARDIAC REHABILITATION CENTER

Follow-up care for cardiac patients is all about rehabilitation. What distinguishes cardiac rehab at NYU Medical Center is its quality of organization, rigorousness, and individualized patient care. At the Cardiac Rehab Center, physical rehabilitation takes place in a state-of-the-art gym, replete with spectacular views of the river and the Manhattan skyline. Patients work out to build both aerobic capacity and strength, and are fully supervised to maximize safety. Patient care at the Rehab Center is premised on the powerful idea that it takes a "village" to treat a patient. At NYU, that village is a team of cardiologists, physiatrists, nurses, physical and occupational therapists, psychologists, social workers, exercise physiologists, nutritionists, and other healthcare professionals. The goal is to return patients to their normal lives, rehabilitated and ready to meet the challenges of the world.

NYU MEDICAL CENTER

"The truly remarkable thing about minimally invasive surgery, for me, is that I've had this major heart surgery and I don't even think about it. You can't see my scar. I'm back to my normal life in much better health."
— *Sandy Katz, minimally invasive MVR*

"I'm a millwright welder and use everything from precision instruments to heavy machinery. I don't think I'd be able to do my job now if I had my chest split open. I was able to get home and start moving around right away."
— *Vincent Cirillo, minimally invasive CABG*

Physician Referral
(888) 7-NYU-MED
(888-769-8633)
www.nyumedicalcenter.org

RUSH HEART INSTITUTE
RUSH-PRESBYTERIAN-ST. LUKE'S MEDICAL CENTER

1725 W. Harrison Street, Suite 1159   Chicago, IL 60612
Tel. 312.563.2230   Fax. 312.733.1221

A LEADER IN THE MIDWEST

Staffed by world-renowned physicians, scientists and other health care professionals, the Rush Heart Institute is ranked among the country's top medical centers for the diagnosis and treatment of heart disease.

Serving both adults and children, the Rush Heart Institute provides the most advanced and comprehensive medical and surgical cardiovascular care in the Midwest. The Rush Heart Institute has several programs that are available at only a handful of medical centers in the United States. These include the Rush Heart Failure and Cardiac Transplant Program, which provides innovative medical and surgical treatment for advanced heart failure patients, and the Pulmonary Heart Disease Program, which provides advanced treatment for one of the most deadly and unusual heart diseases. In addition, the Institute has several programs that offer the most innovative, cutting edge therapies available in cardiovascular medicine today; the Rush Interventional Cardiology Program, which provides non-surgical treatments for heart disease; the Rush Preventive Cardiology Program, which offers advanced cholesterol management and risk modification services; and the Rush Electrophysiology Program, which provides advanced treatment for complex cardiac arrhythmias.

COMPREHENSIVE CARDIAC CARE

Cardiovascular surgeons at the Rush Heart Institute are experts in performing all types of heart surgery—from the more routine (bypass surgeries and new minimally invasive procedures) to the more complex (valve repair and replacement procedures and heart transplantation). For patients with chest pain who have not been helped by other treatments, the Rush Heart Institute offers a revolutionary new procedure known as transmyocardial laser revascularization that restores blood flow to damaged areas of the heart. Only a few medical centers in the nation provide this technology.

When time is of the essence, the Rush Emergent Transfer System is available—24 hours a day, 7 days a week—to transport cardiovascular patients in immediate need of advanced therapies and expert care to the Rush Heart Institute by land or air.

RESEARCH & CLINICAL TRIALS

Physicians and scientists at the Institute have received numerous research grants from the National Institutes of Health for pioneering work regarding the causes and treatment of heart disease. More than 60 clinical trials are under way at the Institute to evaluate drugs, devices and technical advances in cardiac care.

CUTTING-EDGE TECHNOLOGY AND TREATMENT

To ensure the accurate diagnosis of cardiac problems, the Rush Heart Institute offers cutting-edge technologies such as the Rush Heart Scan, which uses electron beam computed tomography to detect heart disease long before the onset of problems; three-dimensional and contrast echocardiography, which provides pinpoint accuracy in diagnosing cardiac problems; and positron emission tomography, or PET scanning, which enables physicians to identify damaged, nonfunctioning heart muscle that can be saved with surgical repair.

As a research facility, the Rush Heart Institute has pioneered many innovative treatments. These include procedures performed in the cardiac catheterization laboratory, such as percutaneous (nonsurgical) myocardial channeling for persistent chest pain and low-dose beta radiation to prevent reclosing of coronary vessels after angioplasty. In addition, Rush researchers have investigated the use of DNA to stimulate the growth of healthy new blood vessels in damaged areas of the heart.

To speak to a Rush Heart Institute representative, please call (312) 563-2230.

SHANDS CARDIOVASCULAR CENTER AT THE UNIVERSITY OF FLORIDA

SHANDS AT THE UNIVERSITY OF FLORIDA

1600 SW Archer Road, Gainesville, FL 32610
Patient referral: 800.749.7424
Physician-to-physician referral: 800.633.2122
www.shands.org

SPECIALIZED SERVICES

Shands Cardiovascular Center at UF was among the first in the nation to perform many of the newest medical procedures, some of which were developed by UF physicians. The center offers monitored adult and pediatric care facilities, such as the Cardiac Catheterization Lab, Cardiac Surgical ICU, Medical ICU, Intermediate Care Units, Surgical ICU and Telemetry Care Units.

UF physicians utilize the latest technology for:

- Diagnosing and opening blocked blood vessels in the heart and legs
- Managing heart failure and all phases of heart transplantation, including mechanical support for severe heart failure patients awaiting transplantation, and testing and treating patients with complex arrhythmias
- Using permanent pacemakers and implantable defibrillators
- Correcting complex anomalies with surgical techniques
- Repairing and correcting valve disorders surgically and non-surgically
- Evaluating cardiac function noninvasively

CLINICAL TRIALS AND RESEARCH

The center participates in a variety of clinical trials including National Institutes of Health-sponsored trials in congestive heart failure and ischemic heart disease. Currently Shands Cardiovascular Center at UF is one of 40 centers participating in the Women's Health Initiative, an NIH-sponsored 11-year study evaluating the impact of hormone therapy, dietary change and calcium plus vitamin D supplements on heart disease, cancer and osteoporosis in postmenopausal women.

PHYSICIAN REFERRAL

The Shands Consultation Center is your link to UF physicians at the Shands Cardiovascular Center at UF. For more information or to schedule an appointment, please call 800.749.7424 or visit our Web site at shands.org.

WORLD-CLASS CARDIOVASCULAR CARE

University of Florida physicians at the Shands Cardiovascular Center at UF are leading the fight against heart disease with state-of-the-art diagnosis and advanced surgical and non-surgical techniques. These physicians and surgeons are nationally and internationally recognized leaders in cardiology and thoracic and cardiovascular surgery.

ST. FRANCIS HOSPITAL
THE HEART CENTER®
100 Port Washington Blvd.   Roslyn, New York 11576
516-562-6000   888-HEARTNY
www.stfrancisheartcenter.com

NEW YORK'S SPECIALTY CARDIAC CENTER

New York is home to 33 hospitals that perform open heart surgery, each of which is monitored by the New York State Department of Health for their surgical volume and risk adjusted mortality. Only one, however, reports mortality rates that are consistently below the statewide average and is designated as a cardiac specialty center — St. Francis Hospital, The Heart Center®, located in Roslyn, Long Island, NY.

As a specialty center, approximately three-quarters of St. Francis Hospital's patients are admitted for cardiac-related illess, a contributing factor to The Heart Center's unequalled level of expertise in the diagnosis and treatment of cardiovascular disease.

THE EXPERIENCE MATTERS

- Approximately 2,500 coronary artery bypass surgeries and over 11,000 cardiac catheterizations (to diagnose coronary blockages) are performed each year distinguishing St. Francis Hospital as a national leader

- Experienced in all types of cardiac surgery, including minimally invasive procedures and off-pump coronary artery bypass surgery (OPCAB), designed to minimize trauma and reduce surgical complications.

- Implants more cardiac pacemakers and defibrillators than any center, using the latest pacing devices. Features specialists with over a decade of experience in radiofrequency ablation, a permanent cure for certain types of arrhythmias.

- Fully digital, networked cardiac catheterization and noninvasive cardiac imaging laboratories are among the nation's best equipped and staffed. Services include three-dimensional echocardiography, nuclear SPECT imaging, and ultrafast CT scanning under the leadership of one of the nation's leading cardiac MRI specialists.

- Site of clinical trials designed for detecting early coronary artery disease and evaluating new techniques in clearing coronary blockages and maintaining blood flow, including beta radiaton and new generation stents.

- Largest experience on Long Island with catheter-based techniques designed to treat congenital heart problems, such as repair of atrial septal defects.

"Developments in interventional cardiology have allowed us to treat an increasing percentage of patients who otherwise would require bypass surgery," reports Lawrence A. Reduto, M.D., Executive Vice President, Medical Affairs, St. Francis Hospital.

"St. Francis Hospital performs far more open heart surgical procedures, more than any other hospital in New York City or on Long Island," states Alan D. Guerci, M.D., President and Chief Executive Officer, St. Francis Hospital. "Our large cardiac caseload as a specialty hospital puts us in an excellent position to introduce new surgical techniques that can benefit thousands of people in need of surgery each year."

The University of Chicago Hospitals
Heart Program

5841 S. Maryland Avenue
Chicago, IL 60637-1470
For help finding a physician: 1-888-UCH-0200

AT THE FOREFRONT OF CARDIAC CARE

The University of Chicago Hospitals' cardiac center is among the finest in the nation. Our team of cardiologists and cardiac surgeons at the University of Chicago Hospitals has two goals: to provide state-of-the-art, high quality care to all patients, and to develop new therapies that improve health and prolong lives.

Our team of clinicians, scientists, and medical staff work in the most modern facilities to provide patients with up-to-date treatments often before they are generally available in the community. The new 525,000-square-foot Center for Advanced Medicine houses our outpatient cardiovascular center and offers patients numerous efficiencies, including easier scheduling. And, with all cardiology and related clinics on one floor, multiple tests and procedures can often be performed on the same day.

NEW AND EFFECTIVE TREATMENTS

Our physicians are at the forefront of exciting advances in clinical cardiology:

- New three-dimensional, non-invasive imaging techniques, which enable physicians to better diagnose, evaluate, and treat cardiac conditions.

- Enhanced electrophysiology capabilities for the treatment of abnormal heart rhythms, including the non-surgical implantation of smart defibrillators.

- The use of newly developed interventional techniques to revascularize patients with severe three vessel coronary artery disease without open-heart surgery.

- Innovative medical and surgical therapies for patients with severe ventricular dysfunction and congestive heart failure.

As part of the oldest and most successful National Institutes of Health-funded cardiovascular research program in the country, our physician-scientists benefit from millions of dollars in annual research support to study and cure heart disease. Spanning molecular biology, physiology, pharmacology, and biochemistry of the cardiovascular system, this research helps to develop novel therapies for hyperlipidemias, atherosclerosis, cardiac arrythmias, and heart failure.

**To Find a University of Chicago Heart Specialist,
Call 1-888-UCH-0200
Visit our web site: www.uchospitals.edu**

FINDING NEW THERAPIES FOR HEART DISEASES

University of Chicago experts are unraveling the genetic basis of heart diseases such as hyperlipidemias, atherosclerosis, and congestive heart failure and are devising new genetic and pharmacological therapies for these disorders.

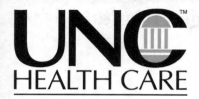
UNC HEART CENTER

The UNC Heart Center is a multidisciplinary team of physicians and nurses with expertise in cardiology, lipid management, lifestyle modification, cardiothoracic surgery and pediatric cardiology. We strive to provide the best possible medical care to the residents of North Carolina and neighboring states, while achieving international recognition for teaching and cardiovascular research.

ADVANCED PATIENT CARE

More than 11,000 patients a year are cared for at the UNC Heart Center. Services available include interventional cardiology, cardiac transplantation, and complex pediatric cardiology and electrophysiology, such as implantable defibrillator and biventricular pacemaker surgeries. The UNC Heart Center has a comprehensive lipids management program and works closely with the UNC Schools of Pharmacy, Public Health and Nursing to define the best therapies for our patients.

CLINICAL LEADERSHIP

Our faculty are leaders in cardiology in the United States. They helped write guidelines for interventional cardiology and chronic heart failure for the American College of Cardiology and American Heart Association. They also participated in writing the definition of myocardial infarction for the European Society of Cardiology and the American College of Cardiology.

RESEARCH

The UNC Heart Center has nationally recognized research programs that focus on understanding the basic mechanisms underlying arteriosclerosis and sudden death. It also has research programs in basic electrophysiology and vascular biology. Clinical trials are focused on heart failure management and all forms of ischemic heart disease.

WOMAN'S HEART PROGRAM

The Woman's Heart Program at UNC provides a full range of educational and clinical services for women who have or are at risk of developing heart disease. Women identified to be at high risk may have a complete cardiovascular evaluation, which includes a consultation with a cardiologist. Participants also receive educational and motivational tools to facilitate health through fitness, nutrition, stress reduction and healthful living habits. The program is designed to help women feel comfortable, confident and informed at every stage of screening and treatment.

PENN CARDIAC CARE
UNIVERSITY OF PENNSYLVANIA
HEALTH SYSTEM

1-800-789-PENN
Philadelphia, PA
www.pennhealth.com

WORLD-CLASS CARDIAC CARE SERVICES

PENN Cardiac Care is the region's most advanced and comprehensive resource for cardiac care, offering referring physicians and patients an array of services throughout the University of Pennsylvania Health System, such as cardiac consultation, arrhythmia management, complex aortic and off-pump bypass surgeries, and heart transplantation. In addition to conducting numerous research studies, we also provide access to state-of-the-art technologies. PENN Cardiac Care physicians and surgeons treat patients experiencing heart problems from the most common to the most complex and work with other specialists in a variety of disciplines to help prolong and enhance the patient's quality of life. Our pursuit of such complicated cases has proven that with experience come better outcomes.

STATE-OF-THE-ART TECHNOLOGY AND RESEARCH

While regionally based, many of our specialists are world-renown, having developed and implemented some of the most progressive cardiac tools and techniques used in cardiology and cardiothoracic surgery, such as minimally invasive robotic surgery, current generation mechanical assist devices, digital echocardiography, and ultrafast CT scanning. PENN Cardiac Care physicians are pioneers of several groundbreaking clinical trials of devices and therapies often not available elsewhere, such as drug-coated stents, new ablative strategies for ventricular tacchycardia and atrial fibrillation, and left ventricular assist devices. The Transplant Center at the University of Pennsylvania Medical Center also has an active team of researchers and participates in many clinical trials, including the investigation of new immunosuppressive drugs and therapies, devices and xenotransplantation.

HEART FAILURE AND CARDIAC TRANSPLANTION PROGRAM

PENN Cardiac Care physicians offer more options than ever before to patients with congestive heart failure and cardiomyopathy. Our multidisciplinary team, available 24 hours a day, includes some of the nation's finest cardiologists, cardiothoracic and transplant surgeons, and specialists in cardiac imaging, electrophysiology, cardiac anesthesia, pulmonary medicine, infectious disease, immunology, and rehabilitation medicine. Our Heart Failure and Cardiac Transplantation team currently provides and continues to investigate the latest intravenous inotropic and surgical therapies for end-stage heart failure. Having performed over 425 cardiac transplants to date, the Transplant Center at the University of Pennsylvania Medical Center is one of the nation's leaders and is the fastest growing center in the Delaware Valley.

NATIONALLY RECOGNIZED FOR EXPERTISE

U.S.News & World Report recently designated the University of Pennsylvania Medical Center as the sixth largest transplant center in the country, as well as one of the nation's top hospitals for excellence in many specialty areas.

For direct connection to one of our Penn physicians, call PennLine **1-800-635-7780** or visit **pennhealth.com**.

PENN CARDIAC CARE LOCATIONS

PENN Cardiac Care has over 100 physicians and surgeons practicing throughout the Delaware Valley, including the 11 following locations in Philadelphia, its suburbs and South Jersey:

- Pennsylvania Hospital
- Phoenixville Hospital
- Presbyterian Medical Center
- University of Pennsylvania Medical Center
- PENN Medicine at Limerick
- PENN Medicine at Radnor
- PENN Cardiac Care at Bucks County
- PENN Cardiac Care at Cherry Hill
- PENN Cardiac Care at Mayfair
- PENN Cardiac Care at Media
- PENN Cardiac Care at Woodbury

THE HEART CENTER
UNIVERSITY OF VIRGINIA HEALTH SYSTEM

(434) 924-DOCS (3627)   (800) 552-3723
Charlottesville, Virginia
www.med.virginia.edu/heart

The University of Virginia Heart Center in Charlottesville, a state-of-the-art treatment and research center, is a widely recognized pioneer in diagnostic and therapeutic cardiology and cardiovascular surgery. Patients are treated with the most innovative options available anywhere. The Heart Center also collaborates with the UVa Children's Medical Center and a network of pediatric cardiologists to offer care to children and young adults with congenital heart disease in a coordinated, statewide program called the Virginia Children's Heart Center.

DIAGNOSTICS, CATHETERIZATION AND ELECTROPHYSIOLOGY

UVa's Heart Center offers a comprehensive array of both non-invasive and invasive diagnostic testing procedures to determine the presence and extent of coronary artery disease. Some of our research includes testing new imaging agents to enhance the sensitivity of nuclear testing and exploring new uses of cardiac magnetic resonance imaging (MRI) to predict recovery of heart muscle function and viability.

The Cardiac Catheterization Laboratory performs more than 4,500 procedures a year, including balloon angioplasty, radial catheterization, stent insertions, atherectomy and rotational atherectomy.

The Electrophysiology Laboratory is renowned for its success in treating a wide range of arrhythmias. The laboratory uses cutting-edge technologies and treatments including catheter ablations, pacemakers, and implantable cardioverter defibrillators, and biventricular pacing for the treatment of severe congestive heart failure.

HEART FAILURE AND TRANSPLANTS

Our Heart Failure and Cardiac Transplant Program is nationally recognized for its comprehensive offerings. Treatments are tailored for each patient and follow a stepwise approach that uses medical and surgical approaches to managing clinical heart failure. We offer drug therapies, intra-aortic balloon pumps and ventricular-assist devices, and surgical alternatives to transplantation.

SURGICAL EXCELLENCE

Our thoracic and cardiovascular surgeons perform more than 1,000 surgeries per year, ranging from traditional coronary bypass surgery to off-pump coronary bypass, complex cardiac reconstruction, laser revascularization, ventricular assist devices and cardiac and lung transplantation. The Heart Center also has expertise in repairing thoracoabdominal aneurysms, which can lead to paralysis if left untreated.

LEADERS IN RESEARCH AND EDUCATION

Because of the numerous clinical trials we conduct, patients often benefit from access to new forms of treatment. We have received more than $37 million in research grant funding over the past three years.

The Heart Center is a partner in a $9.3 million National Institutes of Health grant to explore the connections between diabetes and heart disease. Much of that research will be completed in our Cardiovascular Research Center. More than 80 faculty members with research experience from around the world contribute to UVa's cardiovascular research community.

CardioVillage.com, an award-winning web site created by UVa, provides physicians with comprehensive, clinically relevant and convenient continuing medical education in cardiovascular medicine: www.cardiovillage.com.

The Heart Center at the University of Virginia Health System www.med.virginia.edu/heart

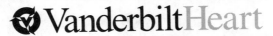

VANDERBILT PAGE-CAMPBELL HEART INSTITUTE

VANDERBILT UNIVERSITY MEDICAL CENTER
2311 PIERCE AVENUE
NASHVILLE, TENNESSEE 37212
PHONE 615.322.2318   FAX 615.323.1786

Comprehensive State-of-the-Art Facility

The Vanderbilt Page-Campbell Heart Institute at Vanderbilt University Medical Center includes inpatient beds and laboratories (invasive and non-invasive) in Vanderbilt Hospital as well as a free-standing, outpatient facility, all dedicated to the delivery of state-of-the-art care for the diagnosis, prevention and treatment of heart disease. The Heart Institute is home to clinical programs that focus on evidence-based, individualized and compassionate patient care, while simultaneously supporting nationally-recognized educational and research programs. Vanderbilt Heart features specialized programs in Cardiac Transplantation, Heart Disease in Women, Atrial Fibrillation, and a comprehensive Vascular Disease Prevention Program. Vanderbilt Heart is consistently ranked in the top 35 in the country according to the national survey recently released in *U.S. News & World Report*, and is the highest ranked program in the state of Tennessee. Vanderbilt supports the largest training and research programs in cardiovascular medicine in the state as well.

Clinical Trials and Research

The Heart Institute supports an innovative and multidisciplinary research program dedicated to discovery in both basic and clinical cardiovascular science. Special areas of strength include a unique program on the mechanisms of coronary development led by Dr. David Bader, and one of 5 national programs on the genetics of coronary and arterial thrombosis led by Dr. Doug Vaughan. There are active clinical research programs in all clinical areas, including congestive heart failure (including left ventricular assist devices), cardiac rhythm disturbances, hyperlipidemia, vascular function, and the genetics of coronary disease. Vanderbilt Heart is currently enrolling patients in more than 30 multi-center clinical trials. Last year, the Vanderbilt Heart research laboratories received more than $7 million in support from the National Institutes of Health.

News from the Heart Institute

The Institute offers the only comprehensive cardiovascular risk assessment program in the region. The program deals with the diverse factors that promote coronary disease, including lipids, inflammation, oxidative stress, thrombosis and genetics and is led by the premiere specialists in the southeast region for management of lipid disorders, MacRae Linton, MD and Sergio Fazio, MD. As part of a multidisciplinary program involving vascular surgery, inter-vention radiology and cardiology faculty members, Vanderbilt Heart has expanded its interventional program to include peripheral vascular disease, led by Dr. Robert Piana, Director of the Cardiac Catheterization laboratories. Vanderbilt Heart just recruited Dr. Mark Lawson as the director of the new program in Cardiac MRI, opening in March 2002.

Our Institute and Leadership

The Program in Adult Cardiovascular Medicine at Vanderbilt celebrated its 30th Anniversary in 2000. The Heart Institute opened its doors in 1999 to offer patients in the region top cardiovascular care services, including nuclear cardiology, echocardiography, exercise testing, and even an outpatient cardiac catheterization laboratory. This 45,000 square-foot facility is located across from the Medical Center and serves over 24,000 outpatient visits annually.

Dr. Douglas E. Vaughan, C. Sidney Burwell Professor of Medicine, Professor of Medicine and Pharmacology, and Chief, Division of Cardiovascular Medicine, directs a multi-disciplinary research program that investigates the role of the plasminogen activator system in cardiovascular disease. His laboratory focuses on the contribution of PAI-1 to arteriosclerosis and thrombosis, and utilizes molecular and cellular models, genetically-modified mice, and human subjects to explore these interactions. He is a member of the American Society of Clinical Investigation, the Association of American Physicians, and is on the Editorial Board of *Circulation*. He serves as the Principal Investigator on research and training grants totaling over $6 million.

WESTCHESTER MEDICAL CENTER
WORLD-CLASS MEDICINE THAT'S NOT A WORLD AWAY.®

Valhalla Campus • Valhalla, NY 10595 • (914) 493-5343

Website: www.worldclassmedicine.com

OVERVIEW

All of Westchester Medical Center's highly regarded heart services are organized within the G. E. Reed Heart Center, which ranks in the top 10 in the state for its cardiac surgery and cardiac catheterization programs. The Heart Center provides advanced cardiac medical diagnosis, treatment and surgery to infants, children and adults from the region and beyond for almost every conceivable heart disorder. Now with its Heart Transplant Program, Westchester Medical Center is home to the only comprehensive heart failure, heart-assist device and heart transplant program between New York City and Albany.

Some of the top cardiologists and cardiac surgeons in the world are at the Medical Center and perform thousands of lifesaving procedures each year, including open-heart surgery and heart transplant, cardiovascular surgery, angioplasty and cardiac catheterizations. The Heart Center is home to a specialized Coronary Care Unit and a dedicated cardiology unit, as well as a state-of-the-art cardiac diagnostic center.

The physicians and surgeons at Westchester Medical Center offer the latest medical and surgical technologies and techniques, from congenital heart defect surgery on babies just hours old to heart transplant and cardiac-assist devices.

Robotics is having an impact on heart surgery at Westchester Medical Center. Considered the next generation of technology in minimally invasive surgery, the robot allows surgeons more precision, better flexibility and 3-D visualization similar to traditional open surgery, and gives patients the benefit of smaller incisions and quicker recovery time. The robot, used at Westchester Medical Center in other surgical specialties, is currently being used during bypass graft surgery and is expected to have wider applications for cardiac surgery in the near future.

As the teaching hospital for New York Medical College, Westchester Medical Center participates in most of the nation's major cardiac studies on new techniques and drug therapies, benefiting cardiac patients at the Medical Center and throughout the world. The Heart Center's catheterization lab is one of the busiest on the East Coast. While treating the most severely ill heart patients, the Heart Center has one of the best records of recovery and one of the shortest average lengths of stay for hospitals in the state.

G.E. REED HEART CENTER

Home to some of the world's top cardiologists and cardiac surgeons, the G.E. Reed Heart Center at Westchester Medical Center offers advanced cardiology services and the latest cardiovascular surgical techniques, including:

- AICD Implants
- Angioplasty
- Atherectomy
- Cardiac Catheterization
- Coronary Artery Bypass Grafting
- Coronary Stents
- Endoscopic Vein Harvesting
- Heart Transplant
- LVAD Implants
- Off-Pump Coronary Artery Bypass
- Minimally Invasive Cardiac Surgery
- Pacemakers
- Radio Frequency Ablation
- Valve Repair

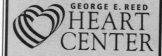

GEORGE E. REED
HEART CENTER

Physician Listings

New England

McGovern, Brian Anthony MD (CE) - *Spec Exp:* Cardiac Electrophysiology - General; **Hospital:** MA Genl Hosp; **Address:** 55 Fruit St Bldg Gray - rm 109, Boston, MA 02114; **Phone:** (617) 726-5557; **Board Cert:** Cardiology (Cardiovascular Disease) 1989, Cardiac Electrophysiology 1992; **Med School:** Ireland 1979; **Resid:** Internal Medicine, Mass Genl Hosp, Boston, MA 1986-1987; **Fellow:** Cardiology (Cardiovascular Disease), Mass Genl Hosp, Boston, MA 1981-1984; **Fac Appt:** Asst Prof Medicine, Harvard Med Sch

Stevenson, William G. MD (CE) - *Spec Exp:* Arrhythmias; **Hospital:** Brigham & Women's Hosp; **Address:** Brigham-Womens Hosp, Cardio Vasc Div, 75 Francis St, Boston, MA 02115; **Phone:** (617) 732-7517; **Board Cert:** Cardiology (Cardiovascular Disease) 1985, Cardiac Electrophysiology 1992; **Med School:** Tulane Univ 1979; **Resid:** Internal Medicine, UCLA Ctr Health Sci, Los Angeles, CA 1980-1982; **Fellow:** Cardiology (Cardiovascular Disease), UCLA Ctr Health Sci, Los Angeles, CA 1982-1984; Cardiac Electrophysiology, UCLA Ctr Health Sci, Los Angeles, CA 1985; **Fac Appt:** Assoc Prof Medicine, Harvard Med Sch

Mid Atlantic

Cohen, Martin MD (CE) - *Spec Exp:* Interventional Cardiology; Pacemakers; Defibrillators; **Hospital:** Westchester Med Ctr (page 82); **Address:** 19 Bradhurst Ave, Ste 700, Hawthorne, NY 10532-2140; **Phone:** (914) 593-7800; **Board Cert:** Cardiac Electrophysiology 1996, Cardiology (Cardiovascular Disease) 1985; **Med School:** SUNY Hlth Sci Ctr 1980; **Resid:** Internal Medicine, Univ Hosp, Brooklyn, NY 1980-1983; **Fellow:** Cardiology (Cardiovascular Disease), Univ Hosp, Brooklyn, NY 1983-1985; Westchester, Valhalla, NY 1985-1986; **Fac Appt:** Assoc Clin Prof Medicine, NY Med Coll

Gomes, J Anthony MD (CE) - *Spec Exp:* Arrhythmias; Heart Attack/Sudden Death; **Hospital:** Mount Sinai Hosp (page 68); **Address:** One Gustave Levy Pl, Box 1054, New York, NY 10029; **Phone:** (212) 241-7272; **Board Cert:** Cardiac Electrophysiology 1994, Cardiology (Cardiovascular Disease) 1975, Internal Medicine 1974; **Med School:** India 1970; **Resid:** Internal Medicine, Mt Sinai Med Ctr, New York, NY 1970-1973; **Fellow:** Cardiology (Cardiovascular Disease), Mt Sinai Med Ctr, New York, NY 1973-1975; **Fac Appt:** Prof Medicine, Mount Sinai Sch Med

Lerman, Bruce MD (CE) - *Spec Exp:* Arrhythmias; **Hospital:** NY Presby Hosp - NY Weill Cornell Med Ctr (page 70); **Address:** 520 E 70th St, New York, NY 10021; **Phone:** (212) 746-2169; **Board Cert:** Cardiology (Cardiovascular Disease) 1985, Cardiac Electrophysiology 1992; **Med School:** Loyola Univ-Stritch Sch Med 1977; **Resid:** Internal Medicine, NorthWestern Univ, Chicago, IL 1977-1980; Internal Medicine, Univ Michigan, Ann Harbor, MI 1980-1981; **Fellow:** Cardiology (Cardiovascular Disease), Univ Penn, Philadelphia, PA 1981-1982; Cardiology (Cardiovascular Disease), Johns Hopkins Hosp, Baltimore, MD 1982-1983; **Fac Appt:** Prof Medicine, Cornell Univ-Weill Med Coll

Levine, Joseph H MD (CE) - *Spec Exp:* Arrhythmias; Pacemakers; **Hospital:** St Francis Hosp - The Heart Ctr (page 74); **Address:** 100 Port Washington Blvd, Roslyn, NY 11576; **Phone:** (516) 562-6672; **Board Cert:** Cardiac Electrophysiology 1992, Cardiology (Cardiovascular Disease) 1987, Internal Medicine 1983; **Med School:** Univ Rochester 1980; **Resid:** Internal Medicine, Yale-New Haven Hosp, New Haven, CT 1980-1983; **Fellow:** Cardiology (Cardiovascular Disease), Johns Hopkins Hosp, Baltimore, MD 1983-1986; Cardiac Electrophysiology, Univ of Pennsylvania Med Ctr, Philadelphia, PA 1984-1986

Marchlinski, Francis Edward MD (CE) - *Spec Exp:* Pacemakers; Arrhythmias; **Hospital:** Hosp Univ Penn (page 78); **Address:** Hosp Univ Penn, Div Cardiology, 3400 Spruce St, Philadelphia, PA 19104; **Phone:** (215) 662-6005; **Board Cert:** Internal Medicine 1979, Cardiology (Cardiovascular Disease) 1981, Cardiac Electrophysiology 1992; **Med School:** Univ Penn 1976; **Resid:** Internal Medicine, Hosp Univ Penn, Philadelphia, PA 1977-1979; **Fellow:** Cardiology (Cardiovascular Disease), Hosp Univ Penn, Philadelphia, PA 1979-1982; **Fac Appt:** Prof Medicine, Univ Penn

Rothman, Steven Alan MD (CE) - *Spec Exp:* Arrhythmias; **Hospital:** Temple Univ Hosp; **Address:** Temple Univ Hosp, 3401 N Broad St, Bldg Parkinson - Ste 9, Philadelphia, PA 19140; **Phone:** (215) 707-4724; **Board Cert:** Cardiology (Cardiovascular Disease) 1995, Cardiac Electrophysiology 1996; **Med School:** Temple Univ 1988; **Resid:** Internal Medicine, Univ Maryland Med System, Baltimore, MD 1988-1991; Cardiology (Cardiovascular Disease), Temple Univ Hosp, Philadelphia, PA 1991-1995

Southeast

Anderson, Mark MD (CE) - *Spec Exp:* Arrhythmias; **Hospital:** Vanderbilt Univ Med Ctr (page 80); **Address:** Vanderbilt Univ Med Ctr, 315 Med Rsch Bldg II, Nashville, TN 37232-6300; **Phone:** (615) 322-2318; **Board Cert:** Internal Medicine 1992, Cardiology (Cardiovascular Disease) 1995, Cardiac Electrophysiology 1996; **Med School:** Univ Minn 1989; **Resid:** Internal Medicine, Stanford Univ Sch Med, Stanford, CA 1990-1991; **Fellow:** Cardiology (Cardiovascular Disease), Stanford Univ Sch Med, Stanford, CA 1991-1994; Cardiac Electrophysiology, Stanford Univ Sch Med, Stanford, CA 1994-1996; **Fac Appt:** Assoc Prof Medicine, Vanderbilt Univ

Curtis, Anne B MD (CE) - *Spec Exp:* Pacemakers; Arrhythmias; Ablation; **Hospital:** Shands Hlthcre at Univ of FL (page 73); **Address:** Shands Healthcare, Univ FL, Dept Med, PO Box 100277, Gainesville, FL 32610-0277; **Phone:** (352) 392-2469; **Board Cert:** Cardiology (Cardiovascular Disease) 1985, Cardiac Electrophysiology 1992; **Med School:** Columbia P&S 1979; **Resid:** Internal Medicine, NY Presby Hosp, New York, NY 1979-1982; **Fellow:** Cardiology (Cardiovascular Disease), Duke Univ Med Ctr, Durham, NC 1982-1986; **Fac Appt:** Prof Medicine, Univ Fla Coll Med

DiMarco, John Philip MD/PhD (CE) - *Spec Exp:* Arrhythmias; Pacemakers; Defibrillators; **Hospital:** Univ of VA Hlth Sys (page 79); **Address:** Univ Virginia Hlth Scis Ctr, PO Box 800158, Charlottesville, VA 22908-0158; **Phone:** (434) 924-2031; **Board Cert:** Cardiology (Cardiovascular Disease) 1981, Cardiac Electrophysiology 1998; **Med School:** Case West Res Univ 1975; **Resid:** Internal Medicine, Mass Genl Hosp, Boston, MA 1975-1977; Critical Care Medicine, Case West Res Univ, Cleveland, OH 1977-1978; **Fellow:** Cardiology (Cardiovascular Disease), Mass Genl Hosp, Boston, MA 1978-1981; **Fac Appt:** Prof Medicine, Univ VA Sch Med

Ellenbogen, Kenneth A. MD (CE) - *Spec Exp:* Arrhythmias; Pacemakers; Defibrillators; **Hospital:** Med Coll of VA Hosp; **Address:** Med College of Virginia/ Electrophysiology, P.O.Box 980053, Box 980053, Richmond, VA 23219; **Phone:** (804) 828-7565; **Board Cert:** Cardiology (Cardiovascular Disease) 1985, Cardiac Electrophysiology 1992; **Med School:** Johns Hopkins Univ 1980; **Resid:** Internal Medicine, Johns Hopkins Hosp, Baltimore, MD 1981-1983; **Fellow:** Cardiology (Cardiovascular Disease), Duke Univ Med Ctr, Durham, NC 1983-1986; **Fac Appt:** Assoc Prof Cardiology (Cardiovascular Disease), Med Coll VA

Epstein, Andrew Ernest MD (CE) - *Spec Exp:* *Arrhythmias; Defibrillators; Ablation;* **Hospital:** Univ of Ala Hosp at Birmingham; **Address:** Univ of Alabama @ Birmingham, 1530 3rd Ave S Bldg THT 321, Birmingham, AL 35294-0006; **Phone:** (205) 934-7114; **Board Cert:** Cardiac Electrophysiology 1996, Cardiology (Cardiovascular Disease) 1983, Internal Medicine 1980; **Med School:** Univ Rochester 1977; **Resid:** Internal Medicine, Barnes Hosp, St Louis, MO 1977-1980; **Fellow:** Cardiology (Cardiovascular Disease), Univ Ala Hosp, Birmingham, AL 1980-1982; **Fac Appt:** Prof Medicine, Univ Ala

Interian Jr, Alberto MD (CE) - *Spec Exp:* *Cardiac Electrophysiology - General;* **Hospital:** Univ of Miami - Jackson Meml Hosp; **Address:** Bldg Central - rm 401, 1611 NW 12th Ave, Miami, FL 33136; **Phone:** (305) 585-5532; **Board Cert:** Cardiology (Cardiovascular Disease) 1987, Internal Medicine 1985; **Med School:** Univ Miami Sch Med 1982; **Resid:** Internal Medicine, Univ Miami Project to Cure Paralysis, Miami, FL; **Fellow:** Cardiology (Cardiovascular Disease), Univ Miami Project to Cure Paralysis, Miami, FL 1986-1988; **Fac Appt:** Prof Medicine, Univ Miami Sch Med

Sorrentino, Robert A. MD (CE) - *Spec Exp:* *Pacemakers;* **Hospital:** Duke Univ Med Ctr (page 60); **Address:** 7623 Erwing Rd, Box 3330, Durham, NC 27710; **Phone:** (919) 681-4358; **Board Cert:** Cardiology (Cardiovascular Disease) 1991, Cardiac Electrophysiology 1996; **Med School:** Albany Med Coll 1985; **Resid:** Internal Medicine, Duke Univ Med Ctr, Durham, NC 1985-1988; **Fellow:** Cardiology (Cardiovascular Disease), Duke Univ Med Ctr, Durham, NC 1988-1991; Cardiac Electrophysiology, Duke Univ Med Ctr, Durham, NC 1988-1991; **Fac Appt:** Asst Prof Medicine, Duke Univ

Midwest

Cain, Michael Edwin MD (CE) - *Spec Exp:* *Arrhythmias;* **Hospital:** Barnes-Jewish Hosp (page 55); **Address:** Washington Univ, 660 S Euclid Ave, Box 8086, St Louis, MO 63110-1010; **Phone:** (314) 747-3032; **Board Cert:** Cardiology (Cardiovascular Disease) 1983, Cardiac Electrophysiology 1992; **Med School:** Geo Wash Univ 1975; **Resid:** Internal Medicine, Barnes Hosp, St Louis, MO 1976-1977; **Fellow:** Cardiology (Cardiovascular Disease), Barnes Hosp, St Louis, MO 1977-1979; Cardiac Electrophysiology, U Penn, Philadelphia, PA 1979-1981; **Fac Appt:** Prof Medicine, Washington Univ, St Louis

Hammill, Stephen Charles MD (CE) - *Spec Exp:* *Pacemakers;* **Hospital:** Mayo Med Ctr & Clin - Rochester, MN; **Address:** Div Cardiovascular Diseases, 200 1st St SW, Rochester, MN 55905; **Phone:** (507) 284-4888; **Board Cert:** Cardiology (Cardiovascular Disease) 1981, Cardiac Electrophysiology 1992; **Med School:** Univ Colo **Resid:** Internal Medicine, Univ Colorado Hlth Sci Ctr, Denver, CO 1974-1977; **Fellow:** Cardiology (Cardiovascular Disease), Duke Univ Med Ctr, Durham, NC 1978-1981; **Fac Appt:** Prof Medicine, Mayo Med Sch

Morady, Fred MD (CE) - *Spec Exp:* *Arrhythmias-Atrial; WPW Syndrome; Arrhythmias;* **Hospital:** Univ of MI Hlth Ctr; **Address:** 1500 E Med Ctr Drive, rm B1-F245, Box 0022, Ann Arbor, MI 48109-0022; **Phone:** (734) 647-7321; **Board Cert:** Cardiology (Cardiovascular Disease) 1981, Cardiac Electrophysiology 1994; **Med School:** UCSF 1975; **Resid:** Internal Medicine, UC-San Francisco, San Francisco, CA 1976-1978; **Fellow:** Cardiology (Cardiovascular Disease), UC-San Francisco, San Francisco, CA 1978-1980; **Fac Appt:** Prof Cardiology (Cardiovascular Disease), Univ Mich Med Sch

Prystowsky, Eric Neal MD (CE) - *Spec Exp:* *Arrhythmias;* **Hospital:** St Vincent's Hosp and Hlth Ctr - Indianapolis; **Address:** 8333 Naab Rd, Ste 200, Indianapolis, IN 46260; **Phone:** (317) 338-6024; **Board Cert:** Cardiology (Cardiovascular Disease) 1979, Cardiac Electrophysiology 1992; **Med School:** Mount Sinai Sch Med 1973; **Resid:** Internal Medicine, Mt. Sinai Hosp., New York, NY 1974-1976; **Fellow:** Cardiology (Cardiovascular Disease), Duke U. Med Ctr., Durham, NC 1976-1979; **Fac Appt:** Prof Medicine, Duke Univ

CARDIAC ELECTROPHYSIOLOGY *Midwest*

Schuger, Claudio David MD (CE) - *Spec Exp:* Cardiac Electrophysiology - General; **Hospital:** Henry Ford Hosp; **Address:** 2799 W Grand Blvd, rm B1451, Detroit, MI 48202-2608; **Phone:** (313) 916-2417; **Board Cert:** Cardiology (Cardiovascular Disease) 1997, Cardiac Electrophysiology 1998; **Med School:** Argentina 1977; **Resid:** Internal Medicine, Hacarmel Hosp, Haifa, Israel 1980-1982; **Fellow:** Cardiology (Cardiovascular Disease), Bikur Cholim Hosp, Jerusalem, Israel 1983-1985; Cardiac Electrophysiology, Harper Hosp-Wayne State Univ, Detroit, MI 1987-1990; **Fac Appt:** Asst Prof Medicine, Wayne State Univ

Waldo, Albert MD (CE) - *Spec Exp:* Arrhythmias-Atrial; Arrhythmias-Ventricular; Syncope; **Hospital:** Univ Hosp of Cleveland; **Address:** Univ Hosp Cleveland- Dept Cardiology, 11100 Euclid Ave, Cleveland, OH 44106-1736; **Phone:** (216) 844-7690; **Board Cert:** Internal Medicine 1971, Cardiology (Cardiovascular Disease) 1975, Cardiac Electrophysiology 1992; **Med School:** SUNY Downstate 1962; **Resid:** Internal Medicine, Baltimore City Hosp, Baltimore, MD 1963-1965; Internal Medicine, Kings Co Hosp, Brooklyn, MD 1965-1966; **Fellow:** Cardiac Electrophysiology, Columbia Presby Med Ctr, New York, NY 1966-1968; Cardiology (Cardiovascular Disease), Columbia Presby Med Ctr, New York, NY 1968-1969; **Fac Appt:** Prof Medicine, Case West Res Univ

Wilber, David James MD (CE) - *Spec Exp:* Arrhythmias; Defibrillators; **Hospital:** Loyola Univ Med Ctr; **Address:** 2160 S First Ave Bldg 107 - rm 1861, Maywood, IL 60153; **Phone:** (708) 216-9449; **Board Cert:** Internal Medicine 1980, Cardiology (Cardiovascular Disease) 1985, Cardiac Electrophysiology 1992; **Med School:** Northwestern Univ 1977; **Resid:** Internal Medicine, Northwestern Meml Hosp, Chicago, IL 1978-1980; **Fellow:** Cardiology (Cardiovascular Disease), Univ Mich Med Sch, Ann Arbor, MI 1982-1984; Cardiac Electrophysiology, Mass Genl Hosp, Boston, MA 1984-1986; **Fac Appt:** Prof Medicine, Univ Chicago-Pritzker Sch Med

Southwest

Jackman, Warren MD (CE) - *Spec Exp:* Cardiac Electrophysiology - General; **Hospital:** Univ OK Hlth Sci Ctr; **Address:** 1200 Everett Drive, MC UH6E103, Oklahoma City, OK 73104; **Phone:** (405) 271-8764; **Board Cert:** Internal Medicine 1979, Cardiology (Cardiovascular Disease) 1981, Cardiac Electrophysiology 1992; **Med School:** Univ Fla Coll Med 1976; **Resid:** Internal Medicine, Wake Fores Univ Hosp, Winston-Salem, NC 1977-1979; **Fellow:** Cardiology (Cardiovascular Disease), Indiana Univ Hosp, Indianapolis, IN 1979-1981; **Fac Appt:** Prof Medicine, Univ Okla Coll Med

West Coast and Pacific

Cannom, David S MD (CE) - *Spec Exp:* Cardiac Electrophysiology - General; **Hospital:** Good Samaritan Hosp - Los Angeles; **Address:** 1245 Wilshire Blvd, Ste 703, Los Angeles, CA 90017-4806; **Phone:** (213) 977-0419; **Board Cert:** Cardiology (Cardiovascular Disease) 1975, Internal Medicine 1980; **Med School:** Univ Minn 1967; **Resid:** Internal Medicine, Yale- New Haven Hosp, New Haven, CT 1968-1969; **Fellow:** Cardiology (Cardiovascular Disease), Stanford Unv, Palo Alto, CA 1971-1973; **Fac Appt:** Clin Prof Medicine, UCLA

Gang, Eli Shimshon MD (CE) - *Spec Exp:* Cardiac Electrophysiology - General; **Hospital:** Cedars-Sinai Med Ctr; **Address:** 414 N Camden Drive, Ste 1100, Beverly Hills, CA 90210; **Phone:** (310) 278-3400; **Board Cert:** Cardiac Electrophysiology 1996, Cardiology (Cardiovascular Disease) 1981; **Med School:** Columbia P&S 1975; **Resid:** Internal Medicine, Roosevelt Hosp, New York, NY 1976-1978; **Fellow:** Cardiology (Cardiovascular Disease), Columbia Presby Hosp, New York, NY 1978; **Fac Appt:** Clin Prof Medicine, UCLA

Swerdlow, Charles Dennis MD (CE) - *Spec Exp:* Defibrillators; Arrhythmias; **Hospital:** Cedars-Sinai Med Ctr; **Address:** 8635 W 3rd St, Ste 1190W, Los Angeles, CA 90048-6101; **Phone:** (310) 652-4600; **Board Cert:** Cardiac Electrophysiology 1994, Cardiology (Cardiovascular Disease) 1981; **Med School:** Harvard Med Sch 1976; **Resid:** Internal Medicine, LA Co- Harbor Genl Hosp, Los Angeles, CA 1977-1979; **Fellow:** Cardiac Electrophysiology, Stanford Med Ctr, Stanford, CA 1979-1981; **Fac Appt:** Clin Prof Medicine, UCLA

CARDIOLOGY (CARDIOVASCULAR DISEASE)

New England

Balady, Gary MD (Cv) - *Spec Exp: Preventive Cardiology;* **Hospital:** Boston Med Ctr; **Address:** Dept Cardiology, 88 East Newton St, Bldg C8, Boston, MA 02118; **Phone:** (617) 638-7490; **Board Cert:** Cardiology (Cardiovascular Disease) 1985, Internal Medicine 1982; **Med School:** Rutgers Univ 1979; **Resid:** Internal Medicine, Univ Hosp-Boston Univ, Boston, MA 1980-1982; **Fellow:** Cardiology (Cardiovascular Disease), Boston Univ Med Ctr, Boston, MA 1982-1985; **Fac Appt:** Prof Medicine, Boston Univ

Batsford, William P MD (Cv) - *Spec Exp: Cardiac Electrophysiology;* **Hospital:** Yale - New Haven Hosp; **Address:** Yale Univ Sch Med, Dept Cardio Vascular Med, 333 Cedar St, 3 FMP, Box 208017, New Haven, CT 06520-8017; **Phone:** (203) 785-4126; **Board Cert:** Cardiology (Cardiovascular Disease) 1977, Internal Medicine 1972; **Med School:** Albany Med Coll 1969; **Resid:** Internal Medicine, Hosp Univ Penn, Pennsylvalnia, PA 1969-1972; **Fac Appt:** Prof Medicine, Yale Univ

Braunwald, Eugene MD (Cv) - *Spec Exp: Cardiology Research;* **Hospital:** Brigham & Women's Hosp; **Address:** Dept Medicine, 75 Francis St, Boston, MA 02115; **Phone:** (617) 278-1086; **Board Cert:** Cardiology (Cardiovascular Disease) 1965, Internal Medicine 1960; **Med School:** NYU Sch Med 1952; **Resid:** Internal Medicine, Johns Hopkins Hosp, Baltimore, MD 1957-1958; **Fellow:** Cardiology (Cardiovascular Disease), Bellvue Hosp, New York, NY 1954-1955; Cardiology (Cardiovascular Disease), Natl Inst Health, Bethesda, MD 1957; **Fac Appt:** Prof Medicine, Harvard Med Sch

Cohen, Lawrence Sorel MD (Cv) - *Spec Exp: Cardiology (Cardiovascular Disease) - General;* **Hospital:** Yale - New Haven Hosp; **Address:** Yale Univ Sch Med, Dept Med, 333 Cedar St, Ste FMP 313, New Haven, CT 06520-8017; **Phone:** (203) 785-4128; **Board Cert:** Internal Medicine 1966, Cardiology (Cardiovascular Disease) 1967; **Med School:** NYU Sch Med 1958; **Resid:** Internal Medicine, Yale-New Haven Hosp, New Haven, CT 1958-1960; Internal Medicine, Yale-New Haven Hosp, New Haven, CT 1964-1965; **Fellow:** Research, Peter Bent Brigham Hosp, Boston, MA 1962-1964; **Fac Appt:** Prof Medicine, Yale Univ

De Sanctis, Roman MD (Cv) - *Spec Exp: Cardiology (Cardiovascular Disease) - General;* **Hospital:** MA Genl Hosp; **Address:** 15 Parkman St, Bldg WACC - Ste 467, Boston, MA 02114; **Phone:** (617) 726-2889; **Board Cert:** Internal Medicine 1962, Cardiology (Cardiovascular Disease) 1971; **Med School:** Harvard Med Sch 1955; **Resid:** Internal Medicine, Mass Genl Hosp, Boston, MA 1958-1960; **Fellow:** Cardiology (Cardiovascular Disease), Mass Genl Hosp, Boston, MA 1960-1962; **Fac Appt:** Prof Medicine, Harvard Med Sch

Dzau, Victor J MD (Cv) - *Spec Exp: Vascular Medicine;* **Hospital:** Brigham & Women's Hosp; **Address:** 75 Francis St, Boston, MA 02115-6195; **Phone:** (617) 732-6340; **Board Cert:** Internal Medicine 1976, Cardiology (Cardiovascular Disease) 1981; **Med School:** McGill Univ 1972; **Resid:** Internal Medicine, PB Brigham Hosp, Boston, MA 1974-1976; PB Brigham Hospital, Boston, MA 1978-1979; **Fellow:** Research, Mass Genl Hosp, Boston, MA 1976-1978; Cardiology (Cardiovascular Disease), Mass Genl Hosp, Boston, MA 1979-1980; **Fac Appt:** Prof Medicine, Harvard Med Sch

Hutter Jr, Adolph M MD (Cv) - *Spec Exp:* Cardiology (Cardiovascular Disease) - General; **Hospital:** MA Genl Hosp; **Address:** 55 Fruit St, Bldg ACC - Ste 467, Boston, MA 02114-3139; **Phone:** (617) 726-2884; **Board Cert:** Internal Medicine 1969, Cardiology (Cardiovascular Disease) 1971; **Med School:** Univ Wisc 1963; **Resid:** Internal Medicine, Strong Meml Hosp, Rochester, MN 1966-1968; **Fellow:** Cardiology (Cardiovascular Disease), Mass Genl Hosp, Boston, MA 1968-1970; **Fac Appt:** Assoc Prof Medicine, Harvard Med Sch

Josephson, Mark Eric MD (Cv) - *Spec Exp:* Cardiac Electrophysiology; Arrhythmias; **Hospital:** Beth Israel Deaconess Med Ctr - Boston; **Address:** 185 Pilgrim Rd, Ste Baker 4, Boston, MA 02215; **Phone:** (617) 632-7393; **Board Cert:** Cardiology (Cardiovascular Disease) 1975, Cardiac Electrophysiology 1992; **Med School:** Columbia P&S 1969; **Resid:** Internal Medicine, Mt Sinai Med Ctr, New York, NY 1970-1971; **Fellow:** Cardiology (Cardiovascular Disease), Hosp Univ Penn, Philadelphia, PA 1973-1975; **Fac Appt:** Prof Medicine, Harvard Med Sch

Kirshenbaum, James M MD (Cv) - *Spec Exp:* Cardiac Catheterization/Angioplasty; Coronary Artery Disease; Congestaive Heart Failure; **Hospital:** Brigham & Women's Hosp; **Address:** Brigham & Womens Hosp, Div Cardiology, 75 Francis St, Boston, MA 02115-6106; **Phone:** (617) 732-7173; **Board Cert:** Internal Medicine 1982, Cardiology (Cardiovascular Disease) 1985; **Med School:** Harvard Med Sch 1979; **Resid:** Internal Medicine, Peter Bent Brigham Hosp, Boston, MA 1980-1982; **Fellow:** Cardiology (Cardiovascular Disease), Brigham & Womens Hosp, Boston, MA 1982-1985; **Fac Appt:** Assoc Prof Medicine, Harvard Med Sch

Konstam, Marvin Amnon MD (Cv) - *Spec Exp:* Transplant Medicine-Heart; Congestive Heart Failure; Coronary Angioplasty; **Hospital:** New England Med Ctr - Boston; **Address:** New England Med Ctr, Div Card, 750 Washington St, Boston, MA 02111; **Phone:** (617) 636-6293; **Board Cert:** Internal Medicine 1979, Cardiology (Cardiovascular Disease) 1981; **Med School:** Columbia P&S 1975; **Resid:** Diagnostic Radiology, Mass Genl Hosp, Boston, MA 1976-1978; Internal Medicine, Mass Genl Hosp, Boston, MA 1978-1979; **Fellow:** Cardiology (Cardiovascular Disease), Brigham & Women's Hosp, Boston, MA 1979-1981; **Fac Appt:** Prof Medicine, Tufts Univ

Libby, Peter MD (Cv) - *Spec Exp:* Atherosclerosis; **Hospital:** Brigham & Women's Hosp; **Address:** Brigham & Women's Hosp, Cardiovascular Div, 75 Francis St, Boston, MA 02115-5822; **Phone:** (617) 732-8086; **Board Cert:** Internal Medicine 1976, Cardiology (Cardiovascular Disease) 1981; **Med School:** UCSD 1973; **Resid:** Internal Medicine, Peter Bent Brigham Hosp, Boston, MA 1974-1976; **Fellow:** Physiology, Harvard Med Sch, Boston, MA 1976-1979; Cardiology (Cardiovascular Disease), Brigham & Woman's Hosp, Boston, MA 1979-1980; **Fac Appt:** Prof Medicine, Harvard Med Sch

Loscalzo, Joseph MD (Cv) - *Spec Exp:* Cardiology (Cardiovascular Disease) - General; **Hospital:** Boston Med Ctr; **Address:** 88 E Newton St, Boston, MA 02118-2394; **Phone:** (617) 638-7254; **Board Cert:** Cardiology (Cardiovascular Disease) 1983, Internal Medicine 1981; **Med School:** Univ Penn 1978; **Resid:** Internal Medicine, Peter Bent Brigham Hosp., Boston, MA 1979-1981; **Fellow:** Cardiology (Cardiovascular Disease), Brigham & Women's Hosp, Boston, MA 1981-1983; **Fac Appt:** Prof Medicine, Boston Univ

Manning, Warren MD (Cv) - *Spec Exp:* Arrhythmias-Atrial; Echocardiography; **Hospital:** Beth Israel Deaconess Med Ctr - Boston; **Address:** Beth Israel Deaconess Med Ctr, Dept Cardiology, 330 Brookline Ave, Boston, MA 02215-5400; **Phone:** (617) 667-2192; **Board Cert:** Cardiology (Cardiovascular Disease) 1989, Internal Medicine 1986; **Med School:** Harvard Med Sch 1983; **Resid:** Internal Medicine, Beth Israel Hosp., Boston, MA 1984-1986; **Fellow:** Cardiology (Cardiovascular Disease), Beth Israel Hosp., Boston, MA 1986-1989; **Fac Appt:** Assoc Prof Medicine, Harvard Med Sch

O'Gara, Patrick Thomas MD (Cv) - *Spec Exp:* Heart Valve Disease; Coronary Artery Disease; **Hospital:** Brigham & Women's Hosp; **Address:** Brigham & Womens Hosp, Cardiovascular Div, 75 Francis St, Boston, MA 02115; **Phone:** (617) 732-8380; **Board Cert:** Internal Medicine 1981, Cardiology (Cardiovascular Disease) 1983; **Med School:** Northwestern Univ 1978; **Resid:** Internal Medicine, Mass Genl Hosp, Boston, MA 1978-1981; **Fellow:** Cardiology (Cardiovascular Disease), Mass Genl Hosp, Boston, MA 1981-1983; **Fac Appt:** Assoc Prof Medicine, Harvard Med Sch

Palacios, Igor F MD (Cv) - *Spec Exp:* Interventional Cardiology; **Hospital:** MA Genl Hosp; **Address:** Mass Gen Hosp, 55 Fruit St Bldg Bulfinch - rm 105, Boston, MA 02114; **Phone:** (617) 726-8424; **Board Cert:** Internal Medicine 1979, Cardiology (Cardiovascular Disease) 1981; **Med School:** Venezuela 1969; **Resid:** Cardiology (Cardiovascular Disease), Hosp. U de Caracas, Venezuela 1972-1973; **Fac Appt:** Assoc Prof Medicine, Harvard Med Sch

Ridker, Paul M. MD (Cv) - *Spec Exp:* Coronary Artery Disease; Preventive Medicine; **Hospital:** Brigham & Women's Hosp; **Address:** Div Preventive Medicine, 900 Commonwealth Ave E, 3rd Fl, Boston, MA 02115-6110; **Phone:** (617) 278-0869; **Board Cert:** Internal Medicine 1989, Cardiology (Cardiovascular Disease) 1991; **Med School:** Harvard Med Sch 1986; **Resid:** Internal Medicine, Brigham-Womens Harvard, Boston, MA 1987-1989; **Fellow:** Cardiology (Cardiovascular Disease), Brigham-Womens Harvard, Boston, MA 1989-1991; **Fac Appt:** Assoc Prof Medicine, Harvard Med Sch

Stevenson, Lynne W MD (Cv) - *Spec Exp:* Congestive Heart Failure; **Hospital:** Brigham & Women's Hosp; **Address:** Brigham & Women's Hosp, Tower 3, 75 Francis St, Boston, MA 02115; **Phone:** (617) 732-7406; **Board Cert:** Internal Medicine 1982, Cardiology (Cardiovascular Disease) 1985; **Med School:** Stanford Univ 1979; **Resid:** Internal Medicine, UCLA Med Ctr, Los Angeles, CA 1980-1982; **Fellow:** Cardiology (Cardiovascular Disease), UCLA Med Ctr, Los Angeles, CA 1982-1984; **Fac Appt:** Assoc Prof Medicine, Harvard Med Sch

Weyman, Arthur Edward MD (Cv) - *Spec Exp:* Echocardiography; **Hospital:** MA Genl Hosp; **Address:** Mass Genl Hosp, Cardiac Ultrasound Lab, 55 Fruit St, Boston, MA 02114; **Phone:** (617) 724-7738; **Board Cert:** Internal Medicine 1973, Cardiology (Cardiovascular Disease) 1975; **Med School:** UMDNJ-NJ Med Sch, Newark 1966; **Resid:** Internal Medicine, St Vincent's Hosp, New York, NY 1971-1973; **Fellow:** Cardiology (Cardiovascular Disease), Indiana Univ Med Ctr, Bloomington, IN 1973-1974; Cardiology (Cardiovascular Disease), Indiana Univ Med Ctr, Bloomington, IN 1974-1975; **Fac Appt:** Prof Medicine, Harvard Med Sch

Williams, David MD (Cv) - *Spec Exp:* Interventional Cardiology; **Hospital:** Rhode Island Hosp; **Address:** Rhode Island Hosp, Div Cardiology, 593 Eddy St, Providence, RI 02903; **Phone:** (401) 444-4581; **Board Cert:** Internal Medicine 1972, Cardiology (Cardiovascular Disease) 1975; **Med School:** Hahnemann Univ 1969; **Resid:** Internal Medicine, Hahnemann Univ Hosp, Philadelphia, PA 1970-1972; **Fellow:** Cardiology (Cardiovascular Disease), UC Davis Med Ctr, Sacramento, CA 1972-1974; **Fac Appt:** Prof Medicine, Brown Univ

Zaret, Barry L. MD (Cv) - *Spec Exp:* Nuclear Cardiology; Heart Failure; Coronary Artery Disease; **Hospital:** Yale - New Haven Hosp; **Address:** 333 Cedar St, 3-FMP, New Haven, CT 06520-8017; **Phone:** (203) 785-4127; **Board Cert:** Internal Medicine 1973, Cardiology (Cardiovascular Disease) 1973; **Med School:** NYU Sch Med 1966; **Resid:** Internal Medicine, Bellevue Hosp Ctr, New York, NY 1967-1969; **Fellow:** Cardiology (Cardiovascular Disease), Johns Hopkins Hosp, Baltimore, MD 1969-1971; **Fac Appt:** Prof Medicine, Yale Univ

Mid Atlantic

Abittan, Meyer H MD (Cv) - *Spec Exp:* Angiography-Coronary; **Hospital:** St Francis Hosp - The Heart Ctr (page 74); **Address:** 100 Port Washington Blvd, Ste G-03, Roslyn, NY 11576; **Phone:** (516) 365-6444; **Board Cert:** Interventional Cardiology 1999, Cardiology (Cardiovascular Disease) 1991, Internal Medicine 1989; **Med School:** Mount Sinai Sch Med 1986; **Resid:** Internal Medicine, Brookdale Univ Hosp Med Ctr, Brooklyn, NY 1986-1989; Cardiology (Cardiovascular Disease), Mt Sinai Med Ctr, New York, NY 1989-1990; **Fellow:** Cardiology (Cardiovascular Disease), Mt Sinai Med Ctr, New York, NY 1989-1990

Achuff, Stephen Charles MD (Cv) - *Spec Exp:* Angina; Heart Valve Disease; **Hospital:** Johns Hopkins Hosp - Baltimore; **Address:** 600 N Wolfe St, Carnegie Bldg, rm 568, Baltimore, MD 21287-0005; **Phone:** (410) 955-7670; **Board Cert:** Internal Medicine 1974, Cardiology (Cardiovascular Disease) 1977; **Med School:** Univ MO-Columbia Sch Med 1969; **Resid:** Internal Medicine, Johns Hopkins Hosp, Baltimore, MD 1969-1971; Internal Medicine, Johns Hopkins Hosp, Baltimore, MD 1973-1974; **Fellow:** Cardiology (Cardiovascular Disease), Johns Hopkins Hosp, Baltimore, MD 1971-1973; Cardiology (Cardiovascular Disease), Royal Infirmary, Scotland 1974-1975; **Fac Appt:** Prof Medicine, Johns Hopkins Univ

Ambrose, John MD (Cv) - *Spec Exp:* Cardiac Catheterization; Coronary Artery Disease; **Hospital:** St Vincent Cath Med Ctr - Staten Island (page 75); **Address:** 170 W 12th St, New York, NY 10011; **Phone:** (212) 604-2818; **Board Cert:** Internal Medicine 1975, Cardiology (Cardiovascular Disease) 1977; **Med School:** NY Med Coll 1972; **Resid:** Internal Medicine, Mount Sinai, New York, NY 1972-1975; **Fellow:** Cardiology (Cardiovascular Disease), Mount Sinai, New York, NY 1975-1977; **Fac Appt:** Prof Medicine, NY Med Coll

Baughman, Kenneth MD (Cv) - *Spec Exp:* Congestive Heart Failure; Cardiomyopathy; **Hospital:** Johns Hopkins Hosp - Baltimore; **Address:** Johns Hopkins Hosp, Dept Cardiology, 600 N Wolfe St, Baltimore, MD 21287; **Phone:** (410) 955-3097; **Board Cert:** Internal Medicine 1975, Cardiology (Cardiovascular Disease) 1979; **Med School:** Univ MO-Columbia Sch Med 1972; **Resid:** Internal Medicine, Johns Hopkins Hosp, Baltimore, MD 1973-1975; Internal Medicine, Johns Hopkins Hosp, Baltimore, MD 1975-1977; **Fellow:** Cardiology (Cardiovascular Disease), Mass Genl Hosp, Boston, MA 1977-1979; **Fac Appt:** Prof Medicine, Johns Hopkins Univ

Blumenthal, David S MD (Cv) - *Spec Exp:* Heart Valve Disease; Stress Test; Preventive Cardiology; **Hospital:** NY Presby Hosp - NY Weill Cornell Med Ctr (page 70); **Address:** 407 E 70th St, Fl 1, New York, NY 10021-5302; **Phone:** (212) 861-3222; **Board Cert:** Internal Medicine 1978, Cardiology (Cardiovascular Disease) 1981; **Med School:** Cornell Univ-Weill Med Coll 1975; **Resid:** Internal Medicine, NY Hosp-Cornell Univ, New York, NY 1975-1978; Internal Medicine, NY Hosp-Cornell Univ, New York, NY 1980-1981; **Fellow:** Cardiology (Cardiovascular Disease), Johns Hopkins Hosp, Baltimore, MD 1978-1980; **Fac Appt:** Clin Prof Medicine, Cornell Univ-Weill Med Coll

Borer, Jeffrey MD (Cv) - *Spec Exp:* Heart Valve Disease; Heart Failure; **Hospital:** NY Presby Hosp - NY Weill Cornell Med Ctr (page 70); **Address:** 525 E 68th St, New York, NY 10021; **Phone:** (212) 746-4646; **Board Cert:** Internal Medicine 1973, Cardiology (Cardiovascular Disease) 1975; **Med School:** Cornell Univ-Weill Med Coll 1969; **Resid:** Internal Medicine, Mass Genl Hosp, Boston, MA 1969-1970; Internal Medicine, Mass Genl Hosp, Boston, MA 1970-1971; **Fellow:** Cardiology (Cardiovascular Disease), Nat Heart, Lung & Blood Inst, Bethesda, MD 1971-1974; Cardiology (Cardiovascular Disease), Guy's Hosp Univ of London, London, England 1974-1975; **Fac Appt:** Prof Cardiology (Cardiovascular Disease), Cornell Univ-Weill Med Coll

Brozena, Susan Celia MD (Cv) - *Spec Exp:* Transplant Medicine-Heart; Congestive Heart Failure; **Hospital:** Hosp Univ Penn (page 78); **Address:** Univ Penn Med Ctr, Div Cardiovascular Med, 3400 Spruce St, 6 Penn Tower, Philadelphia, PA 19104; **Phone:** (800) 789-7366; **Board Cert:** Internal Medicine 1984, Cardiology (Cardiovascular Disease) 1987; **Med School:** Temple Univ 1981; **Resid:** Internal Medicine, Temple Univ Hosp, Philadelphia, PA 1981-1984; **Fellow:** Cardiology (Cardiovascular Disease), Temple Univ Hosp, Philadelphia, PA 1984-1986; **Fac Appt:** Assoc Prof Medicine, Univ Penn

Cerqueira, Manuel MD (Cv) - *Spec Exp:* Cardiac Imaging; **Hospital:** Georgetown Univ Hosp; **Address:** Georgetown Univ Hosp, Dept Cardiology, 3800 Reservoir Rd NW, Fl 5-PHC, Washington, DC 20007-2197; **Phone:** (202) 687-7190; **Board Cert:** Nuclear Medicine 1984, Cardiology (Cardiovascular Disease) 1989; **Med School:** NYU Sch Med 1976; **Resid:** Cardiology (Cardiovascular Disease), Yale-New Haven Hosp, CT 1980-1982; Internal Medicine, Bellvue Hosp Ctr, New York, NY 1979-1980; **Fellow:** Nuclear Medicine, Yale-New Haven Hosp, CT 1982-1983; **Fac Appt:** Prof Medicine, Georgetown Univ

Cohen, Howard A MD (Cv) - *Spec Exp:* Interventional Cardiology; **Hospital:** UPMC - Presbyterian Univ Hosp; **Address:** UPP-Cardiovascular Institute, 200 Lothrop St, Bldg S566 - Scaife Hall, Pittsburgh, PA 15213; **Phone:** (412) 647-6000; **Board Cert:** Internal Medicine 1974, Cardiology (Cardiovascular Disease) 1977; **Med School:** NYU Sch Med 1970; **Resid:** Internal Medicine, Bellevue Hosp Ctr, New York, NY 1971-1974; **Fellow:** Cardiology (Cardiovascular Disease), Johns Hopkins Hosp, Baltimore, MD 1974-1976

Coppola, John MD (Cv) - *Spec Exp:* Cardiac Catheterization; **Hospital:** St Vincent Cath Med Ctrs - Manhattan (page 75); **Address:** 32 W 18th St, FL 4, New York, NY 10011; **Phone:** (212) 647-6420; **Board Cert:** Cardiology (Cardiovascular Disease) 1983, Interventional Cardiology 1999; **Med School:** NY Med Coll 1978; **Resid:** Internal Medicine, St Vincent's Hosp, New York, NY 1979-1981; **Fellow:** Cardiology (Cardiovascular Disease), St Vincent's Hosp, New York, NY 1982-1983

Eisen, Howard J MD (Cv) - *Spec Exp:* Transplant Medicine-Heart; Congestive Heart Failure; **Hospital:** Temple Univ Hosp; **Address:** Temple Univ Cardi Transpl Prgm, 3401 N Broad St, Ste 320, Philadelphia, PA 19140; **Phone:** (215) 707-5900; **Board Cert:** Internal Medicine 1984, Cardiology (Cardiovascular Disease) 1987; **Med School:** Univ Penn 1981; **Resid:** Internal Medicine, Hosp Univ Penn, Philadelphia, PA 1982-1984; **Fellow:** Cardiology (Cardiovascular Disease), Barnes Hosp-Wash Univ, St Louis, MO 1984-1987; **Fac Appt:** Prof Medicine, Temple Univ

Follansbee, William MD (Cv) - *Spec Exp:* Cardiology (Cardiovascular Disease) - General; **Hospital:** UPMC - Presbyterian Univ Hosp; **Address:** 200 Lothrop St, Scaife Hall, Ste A382, Pittsburgh, PA 15213; **Phone:** (412) 647-3437; **Board Cert:** Internal Medicine 1977, Cardiology (Cardiovascular Disease) 1981; **Med School:** Univ Penn 1974; **Resid:** Internal Medicine, Hosp Univ Penn, Philadelphia, PA 1975-1979; **Fellow:** Cardiology (Cardiovascular Disease), Hosp Univ Penn, Philadelphia, PA 1977-1978

Fuster, Valentin MD (Cv) - *Spec Exp:* Heart Disease-Congenital; Atherosclerosis; Coronary Artery Disease; **Hospital:** Mount Sinai Hosp (page 68); **Address:** One Gustave Levy Pl, Box 1030, New York, NY 10029; **Phone:** (212) 241-7911; **Board Cert:** Cardiology (Cardiovascular Disease) 1977, Internal Medicine 1976; **Med School:** Spain 1967; **Resid:** Internal Medicine, Mayo Clinic, Rochester, MN 1971-1972; Cardiology (Cardiovascular Disease), Mayo Clinic, Rochester, MN 1972-1974; **Fellow:** Cardiology (Cardiovascular Disease), Univ Edinburgh, Scotland, UK 1968-1971; **Fac Appt:** Prof Medicine, Mount Sinai Sch Med

Gliklich, Jerry MD (Cv) - *Spec Exp:* *Heart Valve Disease;* **Hospital:** NY Presby Hosp - Columbia Presby Med Ctr (page 70); **Address:** 161 Fort Washington Ave, Ste 645, New York, NY 10032-3713; **Phone:** (212) 305-5588; **Board Cert:** Internal Medicine 1978, Cardiology (Cardiovascular Disease) 1981; **Med School:** Columbia P&S 1975; **Resid:** Internal Medicine, New York Hosp-Cornell, New York, NY 1975-1978; **Fellow:** Cardiology (Cardiovascular Disease), Columbia-Presby Hosp, New York, NY 1978-1981; **Fac Appt:** Clin Prof Medicine, Columbia P&S

Gottdiener, John MD (Cv) - *Spec Exp:* *Invasive Cardiology;* **Hospital:** St Francis Hosp - The Heart Ctr (page 74); **Address:** St Francis Hosp, Dematteis Ctr for Research, 100 Port Washington Blvd, Roslyn, NY 11576; **Phone:** (516) 622-4555; **Board Cert:** Internal Medicine 1975, Cardiology (Cardiovascular Disease) 1979; **Med School:** Georgetown Univ 1970; **Resid:** Internal Medicine, UNC Hosp, Chapel Hill, NC 1971-1972; **Fellow:** Cardiology (Cardiovascular Disease), Georgetown Univ Hosp, Washington, DC 1974-1976

Gulotta, Stephen J MD (Cv) - *Spec Exp:* *Cardiac Catheterization;* **Hospital:** St Francis Hosp - The Heart Ctr (page 74); **Address:** 100 Port Washington Blvd, Roslyn, NY 11576; **Phone:** (516) 365-5599; **Board Cert:** Internal Medicine 1965, Cardiology (Cardiovascular Disease) 1968; **Med School:** SUNY Hlth Sci Ctr 1958; **Resid:** Internal Medicine, Montefiore Hosp, Bronx, NY 1959-1961; **Fellow:** Cardiology (Cardiovascular Disease), New York Hosp/Cornell, New York, NY 1961-1962

Halperin, Jonathan MD (Cv) - *Spec Exp:* *Peripheral Vascular Disease;* **Hospital:** Mount Sinai Hosp (page 68); **Address:** 5 E 98th St, Fl 3, New York, NY 10029; **Phone:** (212) 427-1540; **Board Cert:** Internal Medicine 1980, Cardiology (Cardiovascular Disease) 1981; **Med School:** Boston Univ 1975; **Resid:** Internal Medicine, Mass Genl Hosp, Boston, MA 1975-1977; **Fellow:** Peripheral Vascular Disease, Boston Univ, Boston, MA 1977-1978; Cardiology (Cardiovascular Disease), Boston Univ, Boston, MA 1978-1980; **Fac Appt:** Prof Medicine, Mount Sinai Sch Med

Herling, Irving M MD (Cv) - *Spec Exp:* *Cholesterol/Lipid Disorders; Heart Valve Disease; Aortic Diseases;* **Hospital:** Hosp Univ Penn (page 78); **Address:** Hosp Univ Penn, Dept Card Med, 3400 Spruce St, Penn Tower, Ste 800, Philadelphia, PA 19104-4219; **Phone:** (215) 662-6020; **Board Cert:** Internal Medicine 1977, Cardiology (Cardiovascular Disease) 1979; **Med School:** Univ Penn 1974; **Resid:** Internal Medicine, Hosp Univ Penn, Philadelphia, PA 1975-1977; **Fellow:** Cardiology (Cardiovascular Disease), Hosp Univ Penn, Philadelphia, PA 1977; **Fac Appt:** Assoc Prof Medicine, Univ Penn

Killip, Thomas MD (Cv) - *Spec Exp:* *Coronary Artery Disease; Heart Valve Disease;* **Hospital:** Beth Israel Med Ctr - Petrie Division (page 58); **Address:** Heart Institute, 1st Ave and 16th St, New York, NY 10003; **Phone:** (212) 420-4010; **Board Cert:** Internal Medicine 1977, Cardiology (Cardiovascular Disease) 1968; **Med School:** Cornell Univ-Weill Med Coll 1952; **Resid:** Internal Medicine, NY Hospital, New York, NY 1957-1958; Cardiology (Cardiovascular Disease), NY Hospital, New York, NY 1954-1955; **Fellow:** Cardiac Respiratory Physiology, NY Hospital, New York, NY 1955-1957; **Fac Appt:** Prof Medicine, Albert Einstein Coll Med

Klapholz, Marc MD (Cv) - *Spec Exp:* *Congestive Heart Failure; Angioplasty;* **Hospital:** St Vincent Cath Med Ctrs - Manhattan (page 75); **Address:** 153 W 11th St Fl 790, Spellman Bldg, New York, NY 10011-8305; **Phone:** (212) 604-7380; **Board Cert:** Internal Medicine 1989, Cardiology (Cardiovascular Disease) 1991, Interventional Cardiology 1999; **Med School:** Albert Einstein Coll Med 1986; **Resid:** Internal Medicine, Bronx Municipal Hosp, Bronx, NY 1986-1989; **Fellow:** Cardiology (Cardiovascular Disease), Bronx Municipal Hosp, Bronx, NY 1989-1992

Kostis, John B MD (Cv) - *Spec Exp: Hypertension;* **Hospital:** Robert Wood Johnson Univ Hosp @ New Brunswick; **Address:** 125 Paterson St, Ste 5100, New Brunswick, NJ 08903-0019; **Phone:** (732) 235-7208; **Board Cert:** Internal Medicine 1973, Cardiology (Cardiovascular Disease) 1973; **Med School:** Greece 1960; **Resid:** Internal Medicine, Evanglismos Hosp, Athens, Greece 1963-1964; Internal Medicine, Cumberland Med Ctr, Brooklyn, NY 1965-1967; **Fellow:** Cardiology (Cardiovascular Disease), Philadelphia Genl Hosp, Philadelphia, PA 1967-1969; **Fac Appt:** Prof Medicine, UMDNJ-RW Johnson Med Sch

Liang, Bruce T MD (Cv) - *Spec Exp: Ischemic Heart Disease;* **Hospital:** Hosp Univ Penn (page 78); **Address:** Univ Penn Med Ctr, Dept Cardiology, 3400 Spruce St, Philadelphia, PA 19104; **Phone:** (215) 662-7355; **Board Cert:** Infectious Disease 1985, Cardiac Electrophysiology 1987; **Med School:** Harvard Med Sch 1982; **Resid:** Internal Medicine, Univ Penn Med Ctr, Philadelphia, PA 1983-1985; **Fellow:** Cardiology (Cardiovascular Disease), Brigham & Womens Hosp, Boston, MA 1985-1987; **Fac Appt:** Assoc Prof Medicine, Univ Penn

Lindsay Jr, Joseph MD (Cv) - *Spec Exp: Cardiology (Cardiovascular Disease) - General;* **Hospital:** Washington Hosp Ctr; **Address:** 110 Irving St NW, Washington, DC 20010; **Phone:** (202) 877-7597; **Board Cert:** Internal Medicine 1966, Cardiology (Cardiovascular Disease) 1968; **Med School:** Emory Univ 1958; **Resid:** Internal Medicine, Grady Meml Hosp, Atlanta, GA 1959-1960; Cardiology (Cardiovascular Disease), Grady Meml Hosp, Atlanta, GA 1963-1966; **Fac Appt:** Prof Medicine, Geo Wash Univ

Moses, Jeffrey W MD (Cv) - *Spec Exp: Angiography-Coronary; Angioplasty; Vascular Medicine;* **Hospital:** Lenox Hill Hosp (page 64); **Address:** 130 E 77th St, New York, NY 10021-1851; **Phone:** (212) 434-2606; **Board Cert:** Internal Medicine 1977, Cardiology (Cardiovascular Disease) 1981, Interventional Cardiology 1999; **Med School:** Univ Penn 1974; **Resid:** Internal Medicine, Presby Univ Med Ctr, Philadelphia, PA 1975-1977; **Fellow:** Cardiology (Cardiovascular Disease), Presby Univ Penn Med Ctr, Philadelphia, PA 1978-1980; **Fac Appt:** Clin Prof Medicine, NYU Sch Med

Naccarelli, Gerald V MD (Cv) - *Spec Exp: Cardiac Electrophysiology; Pacemakers; Arrhythmias;* **Hospital:** Penn State Univ Hosp - Milton S Hershey Med Ctr; **Address:** Penn State Univ Coll Med, 500 University Drive, Box 850, Hershey, PA 17033; **Phone:** (717) 531-3907; **Board Cert:** Internal Medicine 1979, Cardiology (Cardiovascular Disease) 1981, Cardiac Electrophysiology 1992; **Med School:** Penn State Univ-Hershey Med Ctr 1976; **Resid:** Internal Medicine, NC Bapt Hosp, Winston-Salem, NC 1977-1978; **Fellow:** Cardiology (Cardiovascular Disease), Penn State Univ-Hershey Med Ctr, Hershey, PA 1978-1979; Cardiac Electrophysiology, Indiana Univ Med Ctr, Indianapolis, IN 1980-1981; **Fac Appt:** Prof Cardiology (Cardiovascular Disease), Penn State Univ-Hershey Med Ctr

Packer, Milton MD (Cv) - *Spec Exp: Congestive Heart Failure;* **Hospital:** NY Presby Hosp - Columbia Presby Med Ctr (page 70); **Address:** 177 Fort Washington Ave Bldg Milstein Fl 5, New York, NY 10032-3713; **Phone:** (212) 305-9260; **Board Cert:** Internal Medicine 1976, Cardiology (Cardiovascular Disease) 1979; **Med School:** Jefferson Med Coll 1973; **Resid:** Internal Medicine, Bronx Muni Hosp Ctr, Bronx, NY 1973-1976; **Fellow:** Cardiology (Cardiovascular Disease), Mount Sinai Hosp, New York, NY 1976-1978

Parrillo, Joseph E MD (Cv) - *Spec Exp: Septic Shock;* **Hospital:** Cooper Med Ctr; **Address:** 1 Cooper Plaza Fl 4, Camden, NJ 08103; **Phone:** (856) 342-2604; **Board Cert:** Cardiology (Cardiovascular Disease) 1981, Critical Care Medicine 1995; **Med School:** Cornell Univ-Weill Med Coll 1972; **Resid:** Allergy & Immunology, Natl Inst Hlth, Bethesda, MD 1974-1977; Internal Medicine, NY Hosp-Cornell Med Ctr, New York, NY 1977-1978; **Fellow:** Cardiology (Cardiovascular Disease), Mass Genl Hosp, Boston, MA 1978-1980; **Fac Appt:** Prof Cardiology (Cardiovascular Disease), Rush Med Coll

Plehn, Jonathan MD (Cv) - *Spec Exp:* Echocardiography; Congestive Heart Failure; **Hospital:** St Francis Hosp - The Heart Ctr (page 74); **Address:** St Francis Hosp, Div Research and Education, 100 Port Washington Blvd, Roslyn, NY 11576; **Phone:** (516) 622-4550; **Board Cert:** Internal Medicine 1981, Cardiology (Cardiovascular Disease) 1983; **Med School:** NYU Sch Med 1977; **Resid:** Internal Medicine, Montefiore Hosp, Pittsburgh, PA 1978-1980; Cardiology (Cardiovascular Disease), Montefiore Hosp, Pittsburgh, PA 1980-1981; **Fellow:** Cardiology (Cardiovascular Disease), St Lukes Hosp, Chicago, IL 1981-1983; **Fac Appt:** Assoc Prof Medicine, SUNY Stony Brook

Sacchi, Terrence J MD (Cv) - *Spec Exp:* Arrhythmias; Cardiac Catheterization; Coronary Angioplasty/Stents; **Hospital:** Long Island Coll Hosp (page 58); **Address:** 339 Hicks St, Brooklyn, NY 11201-5509; **Phone:** (718) 780-4626; **Board Cert:** Internal Medicine 1979, Cardiology (Cardiovascular Disease) 1981; **Med School:** Albany Med Coll 1976; **Resid:** Internal Medicine, St Vincent's Hosp & Med Ctr, New York, NY 1976-1979; **Fellow:** Cardiology (Cardiovascular Disease), Georgetown Univ Hosp, Washington, DC 1979-1981; Interventional Cardiology, Mercy Hospital, Des Moines, IA 1986; **Fac Appt:** Assoc Prof Medicine, SUNY Downstate

Schulman, Steven Paul MD (Cv) - *Spec Exp:* Cardiology (Cardiovascular Disease) - General; **Hospital:** Johns Hopkins Hosp - Baltimore; **Address:** 600 N Wolfe St Bldg Carnegie - rm 568, Baltimore, MD 21287; **Phone:** (410) 955-7378; **Board Cert:** Cardiology (Cardiovascular Disease) 1989, Internal Medicine 1986; **Med School:** Johns Hopkins Univ 1981; **Resid:** Internal Medicine, Johns Hopkins Hosp, Baltimore, MD 1982-1984; **Fellow:** Cardiology (Cardiovascular Disease), Johns Hopkins Hosp, Baltimore, MD 1984-1985; Cardiology (Cardiovascular Disease), Johns Hopkins Hops, Baltimore, MD 1986-1988; **Fac Appt:** Assoc Prof Medicine, Johns Hopkins Univ

Schwartz, Allan MD (Cv) - *Spec Exp:* Interventional Cardiology; Cardiac Catheterization; **Hospital:** NY Presby Hosp - Columbia Presby Med Ctr (page 70); **Address:** 161 Ft Washington Ave, Ste 551, New York, NY 10032-3713; **Phone:** (212) 305-5367; **Board Cert:** Internal Medicine 1977, Cardiology (Cardiovascular Disease) 1979; **Med School:** Columbia P&S 1974; **Resid:** Internal Medicine, Columbia-Presby Med Ctr, New York, NY 1975-1976; **Fellow:** Cardiology (Cardiovascular Disease), Mass Genl Hosp, Boston, MA 1976-1978

Segal, Bernard L MD (Cv) - *Spec Exp:* Stroke; Heart Disease; Non-Invasive Cardiology; **Hospital:** Thomas Jefferson Univ Hosp; **Address:** 111 S 11th St, rm 6215, Philadelphia, PA 19107; **Phone:** (215) 955-5050; **Board Cert:** Cardiology (Cardiovascular Disease) 1964, Internal Medicine 1962; **Med School:** McGill Univ 1955; **Resid:** Internal Medicine, Johns Hopkins Hosp, Baltimore, MD 1956-1957; Internal Medicine, Beth Israel Hosp, Boston, MA 1957-1958; **Fellow:** Cardiology (Cardiovascular Disease), Georgetown Univ Hosp, Washington, DC 1958-1959; Cardiology (Cardiovascular Disease), St George's Hosp, London, England 1959-1960; **Fac Appt:** Prof Medicine, Jefferson Med Coll

Shani, Jacob MD (Cv) - *Spec Exp:* Cardiac Catheterization; Angioplasty; Interventional Cardiology; **Hospital:** Maimonides Med Ctr (page 65); **Address:** Maimonides Med Ctr, Cardiac Cath Lab, 4802 10th Ave, Brooklyn, NY 11219-2844; **Phone:** (718) 283-7480; **Board Cert:** Internal Medicine 1981, Cardiology (Cardiovascular Disease) 1983, Interventional Cardiology 1999; **Med School:** Israel 1977; **Resid:** Internal Medicine, Maimonides Med Ctr, Brooklyn, NY 1977-1981; **Fellow:** Cardiology (Cardiovascular Disease), Beth Israel Hosp-Harvard, Boston, MA 1981-1983; **Fac Appt:** Clin Prof Medicine, SUNY Downstate

Shlofmitz, Richard A MD (Cv) - *Spec Exp:* Heart Disease; Hypertension; **Hospital:** St Francis Hosp - The Heart Ctr (page 74); **Address:** 100 Port Washington Blvd, Ste 105, Roslyn, NY 11576-1353; **Phone:** (516) 390-9640; **Board Cert:** Internal Medicine 1984, Cardiology (Cardiovascular Disease) 1987; **Med School:** NYU Sch Med 1980; **Resid:** Internal Medicine, North Shore Univ Hosp, Manhasset, NY 1980-1984; Cardiology (Cardiovascular Disease), Columbia Presby Med Ctr, New York, NY 1984-1987

Sonnenblick, Edmund MD (Cv) - *Spec Exp:* Hypertension; Congestive Heart Failure; **Hospital:** Montefiore Med Ctr - Weiler-Einstein Div (page 67); **Address:** 1825 Eastchester Rd, Bronx, NY 10461-2301; **Phone:** (718) 904-2932; **Board Cert:** Internal Medicine 1968; **Med School:** Harvard Med Sch 1958; **Resid:** Internal Medicine, Columbia-Presby Med Ctr, New York, NY 1959-1963; **Fellow:** Cardiology (Cardiovascular Disease), Natl Heart Inst, Bethesda, MD 1963-1967; **Fac Appt:** Prof Medicine, Albert Einstein Coll Med

Sutton, Martin G St John MD (Cv) - *Spec Exp:* Congental Heart Disease-Adult; Cardiovascular Imaging; **Hospital:** Hosp Univ Penn (page 78); **Address:** Hosp Univ Penn, Div Cardiovascular Med, 3400 Spruce St, Philadelphia, PA 19104; **Phone:** (215) 662-7355; **Med School:** England 1970; **Resid:** Internal Medicine, Cambridge Univ Hosp, Cambridge, England; **Fellow:** Cardiology (Cardiovascular Disease), Royal Brompton Hosp, London, England; **Fac Appt:** Prof Medicine, Univ Penn

Tenenbaum, Joseph MD (Cv) - *Spec Exp:* Heart Valve Disease; Coronary Artery Disease; **Hospital:** NY Presby Hosp - Columbia Presby Med Ctr (page 70); **Address:** 161 Ft Washington Ave, New York, NY 10032; **Phone:** (212) 305-5288; **Board Cert:** Internal Medicine 1977, Cardiology (Cardiovascular Disease) 1979; **Med School:** Harvard Med Sch 1974; **Resid:** Internal Medicine, Columbia-Presby Med Ctr, New York, NY 1974-1977; **Fellow:** Cardiology (Cardiovascular Disease), Mt Sinai Hosp, New York, NY 1977-1979; **Fac Appt:** Prof Medicine, Columbia P&S

Thames, Marc MD (Cv) - *Spec Exp:* Coronary Artery Disease; Congestive Heart Failure; **Hospital:** Temple Univ Hosp; **Address:** Dept Cardiology, 3401 N Broad St, Fl 9, Philadelphia, PA 19140; **Phone:** (215) 707-3346; **Board Cert:** Cardiology (Cardiovascular Disease) 1979, Internal Medicine 1974; **Med School:** Med Coll VA 1970; **Resid:** Internal Medicine, Peter Bent Brigham Hosp, Boston, MA 1971-1974; **Fellow:** Cardiology Research, Peter Bent Brigham Hosp, Boston, MA 1974-1975; Cardiology (Cardiovascular Disease), Mayo Clinic, Rochester, MN 1975-1977; **Fac Appt:** Prof Medicine, Temple Univ

Southeast

Bashore, Thomas MD (Cv) - *Spec Exp:* Heart Valve Disease; Pulmonary Hypertension; Congenital Heart Disease-Adult; **Hospital:** Duke Univ Med Ctr (page 60); **Address:** Duke Univ Med Ctr, PO Box 3012, Durham, NC 27710; **Phone:** (919) 681-2407; **Board Cert:** Internal Medicine 1975, Cardiology (Cardiovascular Disease) 1977; **Med School:** Ohio State Univ 1972; **Resid:** NC Meml Hosp, Chapel Hill, NC 1973-1975; **Fellow:** Cardiology (Cardiovascular Disease), Duke Univ Med Ctr, Durham, NC 1975-1977; **Fac Appt:** Prof Medicine, Duke Univ

Bass, Theodore Adam MD (Cv) - *Spec Exp:* Cardiology (Cardiovascular Disease) - General; **Hospital:** Shands Jacksonville; **Address:** 655 W 8th St, Bldg ACC - Fl 5, Jacksonville, FL 32209; **Phone:** (904) 244-2655; **Board Cert:** Cardiology (Cardiovascular Disease) 1981, Internal Medicine 1979; **Med School:** Brown Univ 1976; **Resid:** Internal Medicine, Mayo Clinic, Rochester, NY 1977-1979; **Fellow:** Cardiology (Cardiovascular Disease), Univ Hosp, Boston, MA 1979-1981; **Fac Appt:** Prof Medicine, Univ Fla Coll Med

Behar, Victor Samuel MD (Cv) - *Spec Exp:* Cardiac Catheterization; Angioplasty; **Hospital:** Duke Univ Med Ctr (page 60); **Address:** Duke Univ Med Center, Box 3126, Durham, NC 27710-3126; **Phone:** (919) 684-4295; **Board Cert:** Internal Medicine 1968, Cardiology (Cardiovascular Disease) 1973; **Med School:** Duke Univ 1961; **Resid:** Internal Medicine, Duke Univ Med Ctr, Durham, NC 1962-1963; Internal Medicine, Duke Univ Med Ctr, Durham, NC 1967-1968; **Fellow:** Cardiology (Cardiovascular Disease), Duke Univ Med Ctr, Durham, NC 1965-1967; **Fac Appt:** Prof Medicine, Duke Univ

Beller, George Allan MD (Cv) - *Spec Exp:* Coronary Artery Disease; Nuclear Cardiology; **Hospital:** Univ of VA Hlth Sys (page 79); **Address:** UVA Health Systems, Cardiology Dept, Box 800158, Charlottesville, VA 22908-0158; **Phone:** (804) 924-2134; **Board Cert:** Cardiology (Cardiovascular Disease) 1977, Internal Medicine 1971; **Med School:** Univ VA Sch Med 1966; **Resid:** Internal Medicine, Wisc Hosps, Madison, WI 1967-1968; Cardiology (Cardiovascular Disease), Boston City Hosp, Boston, MA 1968-1970; **Fellow:** Cardiology (Cardiovascular Disease), Mass Genl Hosp, Boston, MA 1973-1974

Borzak, Steven MD (Cv) - *Spec Exp:* Myocardial Infarction; Angina-Unstable; **Hospital:** JFK Med Ctr - Atlantis; **Address:** 110 JFK Drive, Ste 110, Atlantis, FL 33462; **Phone:** (561) 641-9541; **Board Cert:** Internal Medicine 1987, Cardiology (Cardiovascular Disease) 1991; **Med School:** Univ IL Coll Med 1984; **Resid:** Internal Medicine, Michael Reese Hosp, Chicago, IL 1985-1988; **Fellow:** Cardiology (Cardiovascular Disease), Brigham & Women's Hosp, Boston, MA 1988-1991

Bourge, Robert Charles MD (Cv) - *Spec Exp:* Transplant Medicine-Heart; Heart Failure; **Hospital:** Univ of Ala Hosp at Birmingham; **Address:** 1900 University Blvd, Bldg 311, Birmingham, AL 35294-0006; **Phone:** (205) 934-4011; **Board Cert:** Internal Medicine 1982, Cardiology (Cardiovascular Disease) 1985; **Med School:** Louisiana State Univ 1979; **Resid:** Internal Medicine, Univ Alabama Hosp, Birmingham, AL 1979-1982; **Fellow:** Cardiology (Cardiovascular Disease), Univ Alabama Hosp, Birmingham, AL 1982-1984; **Fac Appt:** Prof Medicine, Univ Ala

Byrd III, Benjamin F MD (Cv) - *Spec Exp:* Heart Disease-Congenital; Echocardiography; **Hospital:** Vanderbilt Univ Med Ctr (page 80); **Address:** 2311 Pierce Ave, Div Cardiology, Nashville, TN 37232-8802; **Phone:** (615) 322-2318; **Board Cert:** Internal Medicine 1981, Cardiology (Cardiovascular Disease) 1983; **Med School:** Vanderbilt Univ 1977; **Resid:** Psychiatry, Harvard Univ, Boston, MA 1978-1979; Internal Medicine, Vanderbilt Univ Hosp, Nashville, TN 1979-1981; **Fellow:** Cardiology (Cardiovascular Disease), Vanderbilt Univ Hosp, Nashville, TN 1981-1983; Cardiology (Cardiovascular Disease), UCSF, San Francisco, CA 1983-1984; **Fac Appt:** Assoc Prof Cardiology (Cardiovascular Disease), Vanderbilt Univ

Califf, Robert M MD (Cv) - *Spec Exp:* Interventional Cardiology; Heart Failure; **Hospital:** Duke Univ Med Ctr (page 60); **Address:** 2400 Pratt St, Ste 0311, Durham, NC 27705; **Phone:** (919) 681-5816; **Board Cert:** Internal Medicine 1984, Cardiology (Cardiovascular Disease) 1985; **Med School:** Duke Univ 1978; **Resid:** Internal Medicine, UCSF, San Francisco, CA 1979-1980; **Fellow:** Cardiology (Cardiovascular Disease), Duke Univ Med Ctr, Durham, NC 1978; Cardiology (Cardiovascular Disease), Duke Univ Med Ctr, Durham, NC 1980-1983; **Fac Appt:** Prof Medicine, Duke Univ

Clements Jr, Stephen MD (Cv) - *Spec Exp:* Cardiac Catheterization; Echocardiography; **Hospital:** Emory Univ Hosp; **Address:** Emory Clinic, 1365 Clifton Rd NE Bldg A, Atlanta, GA 30322; **Phone:** (404) 778-3468; **Board Cert:** Internal Medicine 1971, Cardiology (Cardiovascular Disease) 1975; **Med School:** Med Coll GA 1966; **Resid:** Internal Medicine, Grady Meml Hosp, Atlanta, GA 1967-1970; **Fellow:** Cardiology (Cardiovascular Disease), Emory Univ Sch Med, Atlanta, GA 1969-1971; **Fac Appt:** Prof Cardiology (Cardiovascular Disease)

139

Conti, Charles Richard MD (Cv) - *Spec Exp:* Angioplasty; Myocardial Infarction; **Hospital:** Shands Hlthcre at Univ of FL (page 73); **Address:** Shands Healthcare Univ FL, Dept Cardio, 1600 SW Archer Rd, rm M438, Gainesville, FL 32610; **Phone:** (352) 392-4383; **Board Cert:** Internal Medicine 1967, Cardiology (Cardiovascular Disease) 1971; **Med School:** Johns Hopkins Univ 1960; **Resid:** Internal Medicine, Johns Hopkins, Baltimore, MD 1961-1965; Internal Medicine, Johns Hopkins, Baltimore, MD 1967-1968; **Fellow:** Cardiology (Cardiovascular Disease), Johns Hopkins, Baltimore, MD 1965-1967

Del Negro, Albert Anthony MD (Cv) - *Spec Exp:* Irregular Heartbeat; **Hospital:** Inova Fairfax Hosp; **Address:** 3020 Hamaker Ct, Ste 401, Fairfax, VA 22031; **Phone:** (703) 849-0770; **Board Cert:** Cardiac Electrophysiology 1994, Cardiology (Cardiovascular Disease) 1981; **Med School:** Georgetown Univ 1969; **Resid:** Internal Medicine, DC Genl Hosp, Washington, DC 1970-1972; **Fellow:** Cardiology (Cardiovascular Disease), Georgetown Univ Med Ctr, Washington, DC 1972-1973; Cardiology (Cardiovascular Disease), VA Med Ctr, Washington, DC 1973-1974; **Fac Appt:** Asst Clin Prof Medicine, Georgetown Univ

Douglas Jr, John Simonton MD (Cv) - *Spec Exp:* Interventional Cardiology; Cardiac Catheterization; Coronary Artery Disease; **Hospital:** Emory Univ Hosp; **Address:** Emory University Hospital, 1364 Clifton Rd, rm F606, Atlanta, GA 30322; **Phone:** (404) 727-7040; **Board Cert:** Cardiology (Cardiovascular Disease) 1975, Interventional Cardiology 1999; **Med School:** Washington Univ, St Louis 1967; **Resid:** Internal Medicine, Grady Mem Hosp, Atlanta, GA 1971-1972; Internal Medicine, NC Mem Hosp, Chapel Hill, NC 1968-1969; **Fellow:** Cardiology (Cardiovascular Disease), Emory Affil Hosps, Atlanta, GA 1972-1974; **Fac Appt:** Prof Medicine, Emory Univ

Harrison, John Kevin MD (Cv) - *Spec Exp:* Interventional Cardiology; Heart Valve Disease; **Hospital:** Duke Univ Med Ctr (page 60); **Address:** Duke Univ Med Ctr, PO Box 3331, Durham, NC 27710; **Phone:** (919) 681-3763; **Board Cert:** Internal Medicine 1988, Cardiology (Cardiovascular Disease) 1991; **Med School:** NYU Sch Med 1984; **Resid:** Internal Medicine, Johns Hopkins Hosp, Baltimore, MD 1984-1987; **Fellow:** Cardiology (Cardiovascular Disease), Duke Univ Med Ctr, Durham, NC 1988-1990; **Fac Appt:** Assoc Prof Cardiology (Cardiovascular Disease), Duke Univ

Margolis, James MD (Cv) - *Spec Exp:* Cardiac Catheterization; Invasive Cardiology; **Hospital:** Miami Heart Inst - North Campus; **Address:** Miami Intl Cardiac Consultants, 4701 N Meridian Ave, Bldg Adams - Ste 440, Miami Beach, FL 33140-2910; **Phone:** (305) 674-3117; **Board Cert:** Cardiology (Cardiovascular Disease) 1975, Interventional Cardiology 1999; **Med School:** Univ IL Coll Med 1968; **Resid:** Internal Medicine, Barnes Hosp, St Louis, MO 1971-1972; **Fellow:** Cardiology (Cardiovascular Disease), Duke Med Ctr, Durham, NC 1972-1974; **Fac Appt:** Clin Prof Medicine, Univ Miami Sch Med

Myerburg, Robert MD (Cv) - *Spec Exp:* Cardiac Electrophysiology; Arrhythmias-Defibrillators/Pacemakers; Sudden Cardiac Death; **Hospital:** Univ of Miami - Jackson Meml Hosp; **Address:** Univ Miami Sch Med Div Cardio Fl D-39, Box 016960, Miami, FL 33101-6960; **Phone:** (305) 585-5523; **Board Cert:** Cardiology (Cardiovascular Disease) 1970, Cardiac Electrophysiology 1998; **Med School:** Univ MD Sch Med 1961; **Resid:** Internal Medicine, Charity Hosp, New Orleans, LA 1964-1966; **Fellow:** Cardiology (Cardiovascular Disease), Grady Meml Hosp, Atlanta, GA 1966-1968; Cardiac Electrophysiology, Columbia Univ Coll P & S, New York, NY 1968-1970; **Fac Appt:** Prof Medicine, Univ Miami Sch Med

Nocero, Michael MD (Cv) - *Spec Exp:* Nuclear Cardiology; **Hospital:** Florida Hosp; **Address:** Central Fla Cardi Group, 500 E Colonial Drive, Orlando, FL 32803-4504; **Phone:** (407) 841-7151; **Board Cert:** Internal Medicine 1972, Cardiology (Cardiovascular Disease) 1976; **Med School:** NYU Sch Med 1966; **Resid:** Internal Medicine, Bellevue Hosp Ctr NYU, New York, NY 1967-1968; Internal Medicine, Bellevue Hosp Ctr NYU, New York, NY 1970-1971; **Fellow:** Cardiology (Cardiovascular Disease), Bellevue Hosp Ctr NYU, New York, NY 1971-1973

Pepine, Carl J MD (Cv) - *Spec Exp:* Heart Disease-Ischemic; **Hospital:** Shands Hlthcre at Univ of FL (page 73); **Address:** Div Cardiovascular Medicine, 1600 Archer Rd, Box 100277, Gainesville, FL 32610-0277; **Phone:** (352) 846-0620; **Board Cert:** Cardiology (Cardiovascular Disease) 1973, Internal Medicine 1971; **Med School:** UMDNJ-NJ Med Sch, Newark 1966; **Resid:** Internal Medicine, Jefferson Univ Hosp, Philadelphia, PA 1967-1968; Internal Medicine, Naval Hosp-Thomas Jefferson Univ, Philadelphia, PA 1968-1969; **Fellow:** Cardiology (Cardiovascular Disease), Naval Hosp-Thomas Jeff Univ, Philadelphia, PA 1969-1971; **Fac Appt:** Prof Medicine, Univ Fla Coll Med

Phillips III, Harry Rissler MD (Cv) - *Spec Exp:* Angioplasty; Cardiac Catheterization; **Hospital:** Duke Univ Med Ctr (page 60); **Address:** 7412 Hospital N, Box 3126, Durham, NC 27710; **Phone:** (919) 681-4804; **Board Cert:** Internal Medicine 1978, Cardiology (Cardiovascular Disease) 1979; **Med School:** Duke Univ 1975; **Resid:** Internal Medicine, Mass Genl Hosp, Boston, MA 1976-1977; **Fellow:** Cardiology (Cardiovascular Disease), Mass Genl Hosp, Boston, MA 1977-1979

Powers, Eric Randall MD (Cv) - *Spec Exp:* Heart Valve Disease; Interventional Cardiology; **Hospital:** Univ of VA Hlth Sys (page 79); **Address:** UVA Health System, Cardiology Div, PO Box 800662, Charlottesville, VA 22908; **Phone:** (804) 924-5204; **Board Cert:** Cardiology (Cardiovascular Disease) 1979, Internal Medicine 1977; **Med School:** Harvard Med Sch 1974; **Resid:** Internal Medicine, Mass Genl Hosp, Boston, MA 1974-1976; **Fellow:** Cardiology (Cardiovascular Disease), Mass Genl Hosp, Boston, MA 1976-1979; **Fac Appt:** Prof Medicine, Univ VA Sch Med

Robertson, Rose Marie MD (Cv) - *Spec Exp:* Autonomic Disorders; Syncope; **Hospital:** Vanderbilt Univ Med Ctr (page 80); **Address:** Vanderbilt Univ Med Ctr, Div Cardiology, 2311 Pierce Ave, Nashville, TN 37232-6300; **Phone:** (615) 322-2318; **Board Cert:** Internal Medicine 1974, Cardiology (Cardiovascular Disease) 1975; **Med School:** Harvard Med Sch 1970; **Resid:** Internal Medicine, Mass Genl Hosp, Boston, MA 1971-1972; **Fellow:** Cardiology (Cardiovascular Disease), Johns Hopkins Hosp, Baltimore, MD 1973-1975; **Fac Appt:** Prof Medicine, Vanderbilt Univ

Russell Jr, Richard O MD (Cv) - *Spec Exp:* Mitral Valve Disease; Coronary Artery Disease; Congestive Heart Failure; **Hospital:** Montclair - Baptist Med Ctr; **Address:** 880 Monclair Rd Fl 1, Birmingham, AL 35213-1971; **Phone:** (205) 599-3500; **Board Cert:** Internal Medicine 1965, Cardiology (Cardiovascular Disease) 1967; **Med School:** Vanderbilt Univ 1956; **Resid:** Internal Medicine, Peter Bent Brigham Hosp, Boston, MA 1959-1960; Internal Medicine, Peter Bent Brigham Hosp, Boston, MA 1963-1964; **Fellow:** Cardiology (Cardiovascular Disease), Med Coll Alabama Hosp, Birmingham, AL 1960-1962; **Fac Appt:** Clin Prof Medicine, Univ Ala

Smith Jr, Sidney C MD (Cv) - *Spec Exp:* Cardiology (Cardiovascular Disease) - General; **Hospital:** Univ of NC Hosp (page 77); **Address:** Univ NC-Div Cardiology, 324 Barnett-Womack Bldg, Box CB7075, Chapel Hill, NC 27599-7075; **Phone:** (919) 966-0732; **Board Cert:** Internal Medicine 1972, Cardiology (Cardiovascular Disease) 1973; **Med School:** Yale Univ 1967; **Resid:** Internal Medicine, Peter Bent Brigham Hosp, Boston, MA 1968-1969; **Fellow:** Cardiology (Cardiovascular Disease), Peter Bent Brigham Hosp, Boston, MA 1969-1971; Research, Harvard Med Sch, Boston, MA 1969-1971; **Fac Appt:** Prof Medicine, Univ NC Sch Med

CARDIOLOGY

Vetrovec, George MD (Cv) - *Spec Exp:* Interventional Cardiology; **Hospital:** Med Coll of VA Hosp; **Address:** 1200 E Broad St, Fl 6th, Box 980036, Richmond, VA 23298; **Phone:** (804) 828-8885; **Board Cert:** Internal Medicine 1974, Cardiology (Cardiovascular Disease) 1977, Interventional Cardiology 1999; **Med School:** Univ VA Sch Med 1970; **Resid:** Internal Medicine, Med Coll Virginia Hosp, Richmond, VA 1971-1974; **Fellow:** Cardiology (Cardiovascular Disease), Med Coll Virginia Hosp, Richmond, VA 1974-1976; **Fac Appt:** Prof Medicine, Med Coll VA

Vignola, Paul MD (Cv) - *Spec Exp:* Interventional Cardiology; **Hospital:** Mount Sinai Med Ctr; **Address:** 4300 Alton Rd, Miami Beach, FL 33140-2800; **Phone:** (305) 674-2533; **Board Cert:** Cardiology (Cardiovascular Disease) 1977, Interventional Cardiology 1999; **Med School:** Yale Univ 1971; **Resid:** Internal Medicine, Yale-New Haven Hosp, New Haven, CT 1972-1974; **Fellow:** Cardiology (Cardiovascular Disease), Mass Genl Hospital-Harvard, Boston, MA 1974-1976

Wenger, Nanette Kass MD (Cv) - *Spec Exp:* Heart Disease in Women; Heart Disease in the Elderly; Cardiac Rehabilitation; **Hospital:** Grady Hlth Sys; **Address:** Emory Univ Sch of Med, 69 Butler St SE, Atlanta, GA 30303; **Phone:** (404) 616-4420; **Med School:** Harvard Med Sch 1954; **Resid:** Internal Medicine, Mount Sinai Med Ctr, New York, NY 1954-1957; Cardiology (Cardiovascular Disease), Mount Sinai Med Ctr, New York, NY 1957-1958; **Fellow:** Cardiology (Cardiovascular Disease), Emory Univ Sch Med, Atlanta, GA 1958-1959; **Fac Appt:** Prof Medicine, Emory Univ

Midwest

Armstrong, William F MD (Cv) - *Spec Exp:* Non-Invasive Cardiology; **Hospital:** Univ of MI Hlth Ctr; **Address:** 1500 E Med Center Drive, Ste L3119, Ann Arbor, MI 48108-0273; **Phone:** (734) 936-9678; **Board Cert:** Internal Medicine 1979, Cardiology (Cardiovascular Disease) 1981; **Med School:** Va Commonwealth Univ 1976; **Resid:** Internal Medicine, Med Coll of Virginia Hosp, VA 1977-1979; **Fellow:** Cardiology (Cardiovascular Disease), Indiana University Hosp 1979-1982; **Fac Appt:** Prof Medicine, Univ Mich Med Sch

Bonow, Robert O MD (Cv) - *Spec Exp:* Nuclear Cardiology; Heart Valve Disease; Coronary Artery Disease; **Hospital:** Northwestern Meml Hosp; **Address:** 201 E Huron Bldg Galter Fl 10 - Ste 240, Chicago, IL 60611; **Phone:** (312) 695-1052; **Board Cert:** Internal Medicine 1976, Cardiology (Cardiovascular Disease) 1981; **Med School:** Univ Penn 1973; **Resid:** Internal Medicine, Hosp Univ Penn, Philadelphia, PA 1974-1976; **Fellow:** Cardiology (Cardiovascular Disease), Nat Heart Inst, Bethesda, MD 1976-1979; **Fac Appt:** Prof Medicine, Northwestern Univ

Braverman, Alan Charles MD (Cv) - *Spec Exp:* Marfan's Syndrome; Aortic Diseases & Dissection; **Hospital:** Barnes-Jewish Hosp (page 55); **Address:** Barnes-Jewish Hosp, 1 Barnes Hospital Plaza, Ste 16419, St Louis, MO 63110; **Phone:** (314) 362-1291; **Board Cert:** Internal Medicine 1988, Cardiology (Cardiovascular Disease) 1991; **Med School:** Univ MO-Kansas City 1985; **Resid:** Internal Medicine, Brigham-Women's Hosp, Boston, MA 1985-1988; Internal Medicine, Brigham-Women's Hosp, Boston, MA 1990-1991; **Fellow:** Cardiology (Cardiovascular Disease), Brigham-Women's Hosp/Harvard, Boston, MA 1988-1990; **Fac Appt:** Assoc Prof Medicine, Washington Univ, St Louis

Burket, Mark W. MD (Cv) - *Spec Exp:* Peripheral Vascular Intervention; **Hospital:** Med Coll of Ohio Hosps; **Address:** 3000 Arlington Ave, Ste 1192, Toledo, OH 43614-5809; **Phone:** (419) 383-3697; **Board Cert:** Internal Medicine 1982, Cardiology (Cardiovascular Disease) 1985; **Med School:** Ohio State Univ 1979; **Resid:** Internal Medicine, Ohio State Univ, Columbus, OH 1980-1982; **Fellow:** Cardiology (Cardiovascular Disease), Med Coll Ohio, Toledo, OH 1982-1985

Chaitman, Bernard R. MD (Cv) - *Spec Exp:* Nuclear Cardiology; Echocardiography; **Hospital:** St Louis Univ Hospital; **Address:** University Club Tower, 1034 S Brentwood Blvd, Ste 1120, St.Louis, MO 63117; **Phone:** (314) 726-1612; **Board Cert:** Internal Medicine 1973, Cardiology (Cardiovascular Disease) 1975; **Med School:** McGill Univ 1969; **Resid:** Internal Medicine, Royal Victoria Hosp, Montreal Canada 1970-1972; **Fellow:** Cardiology (Cardiovascular Disease), Univ Oregon Hosp, Portland, OR 1972-1974; **Fac Appt:** Prof Medicine, St Louis Univ

Cody Jr., Robert James MD (Cv) - *Spec Exp:* Congestive Heart Failure; Transplant Medicine-Heart; **Hospital:** Univ of MI Hlth Ctr; **Address:** 1500 E Med Ctr Dr, Bldg Women's - Ste L3622, Ann Arbor, MI 48109-0271; **Phone:** (734) 936-5255; **Board Cert:** Internal Medicine 1977, Cardiology (Cardiovascular Disease) 1981; **Med School:** Penn State Univ-Hershey Med Ctr 1974; **Resid:** Internal Medicine, Cleveland Clinic Hospital, Cleveland, OH 1974-1978; **Fellow:** Cardiology (Cardiovascular Disease), Mass Genl Hosp, Boston, MA 1978-1980; **Fac Appt:** Prof Cardiology (Cardiovascular Disease), Univ Mich Med Sch

Cooper, Christopher MD (Cv) - *Spec Exp:* Radial Artery Catherization; **Hospital:** Med Coll of Ohio Hosps; **Address:** 3000 Arlington Ave, Toledo, OH 43614; **Phone:** (419) 383-3925; **Board Cert:** Internal Medicine 1991, Cardiology (Cardiovascular Disease) 1995; **Med School:** Univ Cincinnati 1988; **Resid:** Internal Medicine, Brigham & Womens Hosp, Boston, MA 1989-1991; **Fellow:** Cardiology (Cardiovascular Disease), Brigham & Women's Hosp-Harvard Med Sch, Boston, MA 1991-1994

De Franco, Anthony MD (Cv) - *Spec Exp:* Interventional Cardiology; Preventive Cardiology; **Hospital:** McLaren Reg Med Ctr; **Address:** McLaren Regional Med Ctr, 401 S Ballenger Hwy, Flint, MI 48532-3685; **Phone:** (810) 342-3029; **Board Cert:** Internal Medicine 1989, Cardiology (Cardiovascular Disease) 1993, Interventional Cardiology 2000; **Med School:** Tufts Univ 1985; **Resid:** Internal Medicine, Univ Chicago Med Ctr, Chicago, IL 1986-1988; **Fellow:** Cardiology (Cardiovascular Disease), Cleveland Clinic, Cleveland, OH 1990-1993; Interventional Cardiology, Cleveland Clinic, Cleveland, OH 1993-1994; **Fac Appt:** Assoc Prof Medicine, Mich State Univ

Douglas, Pamela S MD (Cv) - *Spec Exp:* Non-Invasive Cardiology; **Hospital:** Univ WI Hosp & Clins; **Address:** Univ Wisconsin Hosp, 600 Highland Ave Bldg CSC 3248 - Ste H6-352, Madison, WI 53792; **Phone:** (608) 263-1527; **Board Cert:** Internal Medicine 1981, Cardiology (Cardiovascular Disease) 1983; **Med School:** Med Coll VA 1978; **Resid:** Internal Medicine, Univ Penn Hosp, Philadelphia, PA 1978-1981; **Fellow:** Cardiology (Cardiovascular Disease), Univ Penn Hosp, Philadelphia, PA 1981-1984; **Fac Appt:** Prof Medicine, Univ Wisc

Eagle, Kim A MD (Cv) - *Spec Exp:* Aortic Dissection; **Hospital:** Univ of MI Hlth Ctr; **Address:** 1500 E Med Center Drive, Ste 3910, Ann Arbor, MI 48109-0366; **Phone:** (734) 936-5275; **Board Cert:** Internal Medicine 1982, Cardiology (Cardiovascular Disease) 1987; **Med School:** Tufts Univ 1979; **Resid:** Internal Medicine, Yale New Haven Hosp-Yale Univ, New Haven, CT 1980-1983; **Fellow:** Cardiology (Cardiovascular Disease), Mass Genl Hosp-Harvard, Boston, MA 1983-1986; **Fac Appt:** Asst Prof Medicine, Univ Mich Med Sch

Faxon, David P MD (Cv) - *Spec Exp:* Interventional Cardiology; **Hospital:** Univ of Chicago Hosps (page 76); **Address:** 5841 S Maryland Ave, MC 6080, Chicago, IL 60637; **Phone:** (773) 702-1919; **Board Cert:** Internal Medicine 1974, Cardiology (Cardiovascular Disease) 1977; **Med School:** Boston Univ 1971; **Resid:** Internal Medicine, Mary Hitchcock Meml Hosp 1972-1974; **Fellow:** Cardiology (Cardiovascular Disease), Mary Hitchcock Meml Hosp 1974-1976; **Fac Appt:** Assoc Prof Medicine

Feinstein, Steven B MD (Cv) - *Spec Exp:* Echocardiography; **Hospital:** Rush-Presby - St Luke's Med Ctr (page 72); **Address:** 1725 W Harrison St, Ste 1159, Chicago, IL 60612; **Phone:** (312) 563-2230; **Board Cert:** Internal Medicine 1980; **Med School:** Univ Minn 1977; **Resid:** Internal Medicine, Michael Reese Hosp, Chicago, IL 1978-1980; **Fellow:** Cardiology (Cardiovascular Disease), Wadsworth VA Hosp-UCLA, Los Angeles, LA 1981-1983; **Fac Appt:** Prof Medicine, Rush Med Coll

Gardin, Julius Markus MD (Cv) - *Spec Exp:* Echocardiography; Geriatric Cardiology; **Hospital:** St John Hosp and Med Ctr; **Address:** St John Hosp & Med Ctr, 22201 Moross Rd, PB II, Ste 470, Detroit, MI 48236; **Phone:** (313) 343-6390; **Board Cert:** Internal Medicine 1975, Cardiology (Cardiovascular Disease) 1977; **Med School:** Univ Mich Med Sch 1972; **Resid:** Internal Medicine, Univ Mich Hosp, Ann Arbor, MI 1972-1975; **Fellow:** Cardiology (Cardiovascular Disease), Georgetown Univ Hosp, Washington, DC 1975-1977; **Fac Appt:** Prof Medicine, Wayne State Univ

Gibbons, Raymond John MD (Cv) - *Spec Exp:* Nuclear Cardiology; Myocardial Infarction; **Hospital:** Mayo Med Ctr & Clin - Rochester, MN; **Address:** Div Cardio Diseases, 200 1st St SW, Rochester, MN 55905; **Phone:** (507) 284-2541; **Board Cert:** Internal Medicine 1979, Cardiology (Cardiovascular Disease) 1981; **Med School:** Harvard Med Sch 1976; **Resid:** Internal Medicine, Mass Genl Hosp, Boston, MA 1977-1978; **Fellow:** Cardiology (Cardiovascular Disease), Duke Univ Med Ctr, Durham, NC 1978-1981; **Fac Appt:** Prof Medicine, Mayo Med Sch

Grubb, Blair Paul MD (Cv) - *Spec Exp:* Autonomic Disorders; Cardiac Electrophysiology; **Hospital:** Med Coll of Ohio Hosps; **Address:** Medical College of Ohio - Cardiac Clinic, 3000 Arlington Ave, rm 1192, Toledo, OH 43614-2598; **Phone:** (419) 383-3697; **Board Cert:** Internal Medicine 1985, Cardiology (Cardiovascular Disease) 1987, Cardiac Electrophysiology 1994; **Med School:** Dominican Republic 1980; **Resid:** Internal Medicine, Grtr Baltimore Med Ctr, Baltimore, MD 1982-1985; **Fellow:** Cardiology (Cardiovascular Disease), MS Hershey Med Ctr/Penn State, PA 1985-1988; Cardiac Electrophysiology; **Fac Appt:** Prof Medicine, Univ SD Sch Med

Heroux, Alain MD (Cv) - *Spec Exp:* Transplant Medicine-Heart; Heart Failure; **Hospital:** Rush-Presby - St Luke's Med Ctr (page 72); **Address:** Rush Presby-St Lukes Med Ctr, Cardiac Transplant Unit, 1725 W Harrison St, rm 439, Chicago, IL 60612; **Phone:** (312) 563-2121; **Med School:** Canada 1981; **Resid:** Internal Medicine, Laval Univ Med Ctr, Quebec, Canada 1982-1985; Cardiology (Cardiovascular Disease), Royal Victory Hosp, Quebec, Canada 1986-1987; **Fellow:** Heart Transplant Medicine, Univ Virginia Med Coll, Charlottesville, VA 1988-1989; **Fac Appt:** Asst Prof Medicine, Rush Med Coll

Jaffe, Allan S. MD (Cv) - *Spec Exp:* Cardiology (Cardiovascular Disease) - General; **Hospital:** Mayo Med Ctr & Clin - Rochester, MN; **Address:** Div Cardiovascular Disease, 200 First St SW, Rochester, MN 55905; **Phone:** (507) 284-9325; **Board Cert:** Internal Medicine 1976, Cardiology (Cardiovascular Disease) 1979; **Med School:** Univ MD Sch Med 1973; **Resid:** Internal Medicine, Barnes Hosp, St Louis, MO 1974-1975; Internal Medicine, Washington Univ, St Louis, MO 1976; **Fellow:** Cardiology (Cardiovascular Disease), Barnes Hosp, St Louis, MO 1976-1978

Johnson, Maryl R MD (Cv) - *Spec Exp:* Congestive Heart Failure; Transplant Medicine-Heart; **Hospital:** Northwestern Meml Hosp; **Address:** 201 E Huron, Ste 11-240, Chicago, IL 60611; **Phone:** (312) 695-0008; **Board Cert:** Internal Medicine 1981, Cardiology (Cardiovascular Disease) 1983; **Med School:** Univ Iowa Coll Med 1977; **Resid:** Internal Medicine, Univ Iowa Hosp, Iowa City, IA 1978-1981; **Fellow:** Cardiology (Cardiovascular Disease), Univ Iowa Hosp, Iowa City, IA 1979-1982; **Fac Appt:** Assoc Prof Medicine, Northwestern Univ

Kereiakes, Dean J MD (Cv) - *Spec Exp:* Interventional Cardiology; **Hospital:** Christ Hospital; **Address:** 2123 Auburn Ave, Ste 136, Cincinnati, OH 45219-2966; **Phone:** (513) 721-8881; **Board Cert:** Cardiology (Cardiovascular Disease) 1985, Internal Medicine 1981; **Med School:** Univ Cincinnati 1978; **Resid:** Internal Medicine, Mass Genl Hospital, Boston, MA 1980-1981; Internal Medicine, UC San Francisco, San Francisco, CA 1981-1982; **Fellow:** Cardiology (Cardiovascular Disease), UC San Francisco, San Francisco, CA 1982-1984; **Fac Appt:** Clin Prof Medicine, Univ Cincinnati

Mehlman, David J MD (Cv) - *Spec Exp:* Echocardiography; Prosthetic Valves; Congestive Heart Failure; **Hospital:** Northwestern Meml Hosp; **Address:** Northwestern Univ Med Ctr, 675 N St Clair Galter 19-100, Chicago, IL 60611; **Phone:** (312) 695-4965; **Board Cert:** Internal Medicine 1976, Cardiology (Cardiovascular Disease) 1979; **Med School:** Johns Hopkins Univ 1973; **Resid:** Internal Medicine, Johns Hopkins Hosp, Baltimore, MD 1974-1976; **Fellow:** Cardiology (Cardiovascular Disease), Univ Chicago Hosps, Chicago, IL 1976-1978; **Fac Appt:** Assoc Prof Medicine, Northwestern Univ

Messer, Joseph V MD (Cv) - *Spec Exp:* Coronary Artery Disease; Congestive Heart Failure; Preventive Cardiology; **Hospital:** Rush-Presby - St Luke's Med Ctr (page 72); **Address:** 1725 W Harrison St, Ste 1138, Chicago, IL 60612; **Phone:** (312) 243-6800; **Board Cert:** Internal Medicine 1972; **Med School:** Harvard Med Sch 1956; **Resid:** Internal Medicine, Peter Bent Brigham Hosp, Boston, MA 1957-1958; Internal Medicine, Peter Bent Brigham Hosp, Boston, MA 1960-1961; **Fellow:** Cardiology (Cardiovascular Disease), Peter Bent Brigham Hosp/Harvard Univ, Boston, MA 1958-1960; Biochemistry, Brandeis U, Boston, MA 1963-1964; **Fac Appt:** Prof Medicine, Rush Med Coll

Moran, John MD (Cv) - *Spec Exp:* Coronary Artery Disease; **Hospital:** Loyola Univ Med Ctr; **Address:** 2160 S 1st Ave, Bldg 110 - Ste 6210, Maywood, IL 60153; **Phone:** (708) 327-3600; **Board Cert:** Internal Medicine 1971, Cardiology (Cardiovascular Disease) 1973; **Med School:** Loyola Univ-Stritch Sch Med 1964; **Resid:** Internal Medicine, Univ Ill Rsch Ed Hosp, Chicago, IL 1965-1967; **Fellow:** Cardiology (Cardiovascular Disease), Univ Ill Rsch Ed Hosp, Chicago, IL 1967-1969; **Fac Appt:** Prof Medicine, Loyola Univ-Stritch Sch Med

Nemickas, Rimgaudas MD (Cv) - *Spec Exp:* Valvular Heart Disease; Cholesterol/Lipid Disorder; **Hospital:** Advocate IL Masonic Med Ctr; **Address:** 6417 W 87th St, Oaklawn, IL 60653; **Phone:** (708) 233-5630; **Board Cert:** Internal Medicine 1969, Cardiology (Cardiovascular Disease) 1973; **Med School:** Loyola Univ-Stritch Sch Med 1961; **Resid:** Internal Medicine, Univ Illinois Med Clinic, Chicago, IL 1966-1967; **Fellow:** Cardiology (Cardiovascular Disease), Cook County Hosp, Chicago, IL 1962-1963; Cardiology (Cardiovascular Disease), Univ Chicago Hosp, Chicago, IL 1967-1969; **Fac Appt:** Clin Prof Medicine, Loyola Univ-Stritch Sch Med

O'Neill, William MD (Cv) - *Spec Exp:* Interventional Cardiology; **Hospital:** William Beaumont Hosp; **Address:** 3601 W 13 Mile Rd, Fl 3, Royal Oak, MI 48073; **Phone:** (248) 551-4163; **Board Cert:** Internal Medicine 1980, Cardiology (Cardiovascular Disease) 1983; **Med School:** Wayne State Univ 1977; **Resid:** Internal Medicine, Wayne State U Affil Hosps, Detroit, MI 1978-1980

Rahko, Peter MD (Cv) - *Spec Exp:* Congestive Heart Failure; Heart Valve Disease; Echocardiography; **Hospital:** Univ WI Hosp & Clins; **Address:** Univ Wisc Hosp & Clin, 600 Highland Ave, Ste 86, Madison, WI 53792-0001; **Phone:** (608) 263-1530; **Board Cert:** Internal Medicine 1982, Cardiology (Cardiovascular Disease) 1985; **Med School:** Univ Minn 1979; **Resid:** Internal Medicine, Indiana Univ Med Ctr, Indianapolis, IN 1979-1982; **Fellow:** Cardiology (Cardiovascular Disease), Univ Pittsburgh, Pittsburgh, PA 1982-1985; **Fac Appt:** Assoc Prof Medicine, Univ Wisc

Reiss, Craig MD (Cv) - *Spec Exp:* *Heart Disease-Ischemic; Coronary Artery Disease;* **Hospital:** Barnes-Jewish Hosp (page 55); **Address:** 1020 N Mason Rd, St Louis, MO 63141; **Phone:** (314) 362-1291; **Board Cert:** Internal Medicine 1986, Cardiology (Cardiovascular Disease) 1989; **Med School:** Univ MO-Kansas City 1983; **Resid:** Internal Medicine, Brigham & Women's Hosp, Boston, MA 1984-1986; Internal Medicine, Brigham & Women's Hosp, Boston, MA 1988-1989; **Fellow:** Cardiology (Cardiovascular Disease), Brigham& Women's Hosp, Boston, MA 1986-1988; **Fac Appt:** Assoc Prof Medicine, Washington Univ, St Louis

Rich, Stuart MD (Cv) - *Spec Exp:* *Pulmonary Hypertension; Heart Failure;* **Hospital:** Rush-Presby - St Luke's Med Ctr (page 72); **Address:** Center for Pulmonary & Heart Disease, 1725 W Harrison St, Ste 020, Chicago, IL 60612; **Phone:** (312) 563-2169; **Board Cert:** Cardiology (Cardiovascular Disease) 1981, Internal Medicine 1978; **Med School:** Loyola Univ-Stritch Sch Med 1974; **Resid:** Internal Medicine, Jewish Hosp, St Louis, MO 1975-1978; **Fellow:** Cardiology (Cardiovascular Disease), Univ Chicago, Chicago, IL 1978-1980; **Fac Appt:** Prof Medicine, Rush Med Coll

Rogers, Joseph MD (Cv) - *Spec Exp:* *Congestive Heart Failure; Transplant Medicine-Heart;* **Hospital:** Barnes-Jewish Hosp (page 55); **Address:** 660 S Euclid Ave, Box 8086, St Louis, MO 63110; **Phone:** (314) 454-7687; **Board Cert:** Internal Medicine 1991, Cardiology (Cardiovascular Disease) 1995; **Med School:** Univ Nebr Coll Med 1988; **Resid:** Internal Medicine, Univ Nebraska Med Ctr, Omaha, NE 1988-1991; **Fellow:** Cardiology (Cardiovascular Disease), Wash Univ Med Ctr, St Louis, MO 1991-1995; **Fac Appt:** Assoc Prof Medicine, Washington Univ, St Louis

Rosenbush, Stuart MD (Cv) - *Spec Exp:* *Coronary artery disease; Angioplasty & stents;* **Hospital:** Rush-Presby - St Luke's Med Ctr (page 72); **Address:** Associates In Cardiology Ltd, 1725 W Harrison St, Ste 1138, Chicago, IL 60612-3835; **Phone:** (312) 243-6800; **Board Cert:** Cardiology (Cardiovascular Disease) 1981, Internal Medicine 1979; **Med School:** Univ IL Coll Med 1976; **Resid:** Internal Medicine, Michael Reese Hosp, Chicago, IL 1976-1979; **Fellow:** Cardiology (Cardiovascular Disease), Rush Presby, Chicago, IL 1979-1981; **Fac Appt:** Asst Prof Cardiology (Cardiovascular Disease), Rush Med Coll

Ruggie, Neal MD (Cv) - *Spec Exp:* *Mitral Valve Prolapse; Congenital Heart Disease-Adult;* **Hospital:** Rush-Presby - St Luke's Med Ctr (page 72); **Address:** 1725 W Harrison St, Ste 1138, Associates In Cardiology Ltd, Chicago, IL 60612-3835; **Phone:** (312) 243-6800; **Board Cert:** Internal Medicine 1976, Cardiology (Cardiovascular Disease) 1979; **Med School:** Johns Hopkins Univ 1973; **Resid:** Internal Medicine, Rush Presby St Lukes, Chicago, IL 1974-1976; **Fellow:** Cardiology (Cardiovascular Disease), Rush Presby St Lukes, Chicago, IL 1976-1978; **Fac Appt:** Assoc Prof Cardiology (Cardiovascular Disease), Rush Med Coll

Safian, Robert D MD (Cv) - *Spec Exp:* *Interventional Cardiology;* **Hospital:** William Beaumont Hosp; **Address:** 3601 W 13 Mile Rd Bldg Heart Ctr Fl 3, Royal Oak, MI 48073; **Phone:** (248) 551-5482; **Board Cert:** Internal Medicine 1983, Cardiology (Cardiovascular Disease) 1987; **Med School:** Univ Fla Coll Med 1979; **Resid:** Pathology, Univ Miami Med Ctr, Miami, FL 1980-1981; Internal Medicine, UC San Diego Med Ctr, San Diego, CA 1981-1983; **Fellow:** Cardiology (Cardiovascular Disease), Beth Israel Hosp-Harvard, Boston, MA 1984-1987

Seward, James Bernard MD (Cv) - *Spec Exp:* *Cardiology-Pediatric; Echocardiography;* **Hospital:** Mayo Med Ctr & Clin - Rochester, MN; **Address:** Div Cardiovascular Diseases, 200 First St SW, Rochester, MN 55905; **Phone:** (507) 284-3581; **Board Cert:** Internal Medicine 1974, Cardiology (Cardiovascular Disease) 1975; **Med School:** Univ Mich Med Sch 1968; **Resid:** Internal Medicine, Boston City Hosp, Boston, MA 1968-1971; Internal Medicine, Mayo Clinic, Rochester, MN 1972; **Fellow:** Cardiology (Cardiovascular Disease), Mayo Clinic, Rochester, MN 1973-1975; **Fac Appt:** Prof Pediatrics, Mayo Med Sch

Stewart, William MD (Cv) - *Spec Exp:* Heart Valve Disease; Heart Valve Surgery-Aortic & Mitral; **Hospital:** Cleveland Clin Fdn (page 57); **Address:** 9500 Euclid Ave, Ste F15, Dept Cardiovascular Disease, Cleveland, OH 44195; **Phone:** (216) 444-5923; **Board Cert:** Internal Medicine 1980, Cardiology (Cardiovascular Disease) 1983; **Med School:** Univ Cincinnati 1977; **Resid:** Internal Medicine, Univ Mich Hosp, Ann Arbor, MI 1977-1980; **Fellow:** Cardiology (Cardiovascular Disease), Boston Med Ctr, Boston, MA 1980-1982; Cardiology (Cardiovascular Disease), Mass Genl Hosp, Boston, MA 1982-1984; **Fac Appt:** Assoc Prof Medicine, Ohio State Univ

Topol, Eric Jeffrey MD (Cv) - *Spec Exp:* Coronary Artery Disease; Interventional Cardiology; **Hospital:** Cleveland Clin Fdn (page 57); **Address:** Cleveland Clinic Heart Ctr, 9500 Euclid Ave, Cleveland, OH 44195; **Phone:** (216) 445-9490; **Board Cert:** Internal Medicine 1982, Cardiology (Cardiovascular Disease) 1985; **Med School:** Univ Rochester 1979; **Resid:** Internal Medicine, Univ California Sch Med, San Francisco, CA 1979-1982; **Fellow:** Cardiology (Cardiovascular Disease), Johns Hopkins Hospital, Baltimore, MD 1982-1985; **Fac Appt:** Prof Cardiology (Cardiovascular Disease), Ohio State Univ

Vander Ark, Condon R MD (Cv) - *Spec Exp:* Congestive Heart Failure; **Hospital:** Univ WI Hosp & Clins; **Address:** 600 Highland Ave Bldg CSC - rm H6/356, Madison, WI 53792; **Phone:** (608) 263-1530; **Board Cert:** Internal Medicine 1971; **Med School:** Univ Mich Med Sch 1961; **Resid:** Internal Medicine, Butterworth Hosp, Grand Rapids, MI 1962-1963; Internal Medicine, Mich Med Ctr, Ann Arbor, MI 1965-1966; **Fellow:** Cardiology (Cardiovascular Disease), Mich Med Ctr, Ann Arbor, MI 1966-1968; **Fac Appt:** Assoc Prof Medicine, Univ Wisc

Vander Laan, Ronald Lee MD (Cv) - *Spec Exp:* Cardiac Rehabilitation; **Hospital:** Spectrum Health East; **Address:** 1900 Wealthy St SE, Ste 200, Grand Rapids, MI 49506; **Phone:** (616) 454-5551; **Board Cert:** Internal Medicine 1985, Cardiology (Cardiovascular Disease) 1987; **Med School:** Univ Mich Med Sch 1982; **Resid:** Internal Medicine, Blodgett Meml Hosp, Grand Rapids, MI 1982-1985; **Fellow:** Cardiology (Cardiovascular Disease), Cleveland Clinic Fdn, Cleveland, OH 1985-1987

Whitlow, Patrick Lee MD (Cv) - *Spec Exp:* Cardiology (Cardiovascular Disease) - General; **Hospital:** Cleveland Clin Fdn (page 57); **Address:** Dept Cardiology and Vascular Med, 9500 Euclid Ave, Cleveland, OH 44195; **Phone:** (216) 444-1746; **Board Cert:** Internal Medicine 1979, Cardiology (Cardiovascular Disease) 1981, Interventional Cardiology 1999; **Med School:** Duke Univ 1976; **Resid:** Internal Medicine, Parkland Meml Hosp, Dallas, TX 1977-1979; **Fellow:** Cardiology (Cardiovascular Disease), Univ Alabama Hosp, Birmingham, AL 1979

Williams, Kim A MD (Cv) - *Spec Exp:* Nuclear Cardiology; Heart Disease-Ischemic; **Hospital:** Univ of Chicago Hosps (page 76); **Address:** 5758 S Maryland Ave, Ste 5C, MC-9025, Chicago, IL 60637; **Phone:** (773) 702-9461; **Board Cert:** Cardiology (Cardiovascular Disease) 1985, Internal Medicine 1982; **Med School:** Univ Chicago-Pritzker Sch Med 1975; **Resid:** Internal Medicine, Emory Univ, Atlanta, GA 1980-1982; **Fellow:** Cardiology (Cardiovascular Disease), Univ Chicago, Chicago, IL 1982-1984; Nuclear Medicine, Univ Chicago, Chicago, IL 1984-1986; **Fac Appt:** Assoc Prof Cardiology (Cardiovascular Disease), Univ Chicago-Pritzker Sch Med

Young, James B MD (Cv) - *Spec Exp:* Transplant Medicine-Heart; Heart Failure; **Hospital:** Cleveland Clin Fdn (page 57); **Address:** 9500 Euclid Ave, Ste F25, Cleveland, OH 44195; **Phone:** (216) 444-2270; **Board Cert:** Internal Medicine 1977, Cardiology (Cardiovascular Disease) 1979; **Med School:** Baylor Coll Med 1974; **Resid:** Internal Medicine, Baylor Affl Hosp, Houston, TX 1975-1977; Internal Medicine, Methodist Hosp, Houston, TX 1980; **Fellow:** Cardiology (Cardiovascular Disease), Baylor Affl Hosp, Houston, TX 1977-1979

Zipes, Douglas P MD (Cv) - *Spec Exp:* Arrhythmias; **Hospital:** Methodist Hosp - Indianapolis (page 66); **Address:** 1800 N Capitol, Ste E475, Indianapolis, IN 46202; **Phone:** (317) 962-0555; **Board Cert:** Cardiac Electrophysiology 1998, Cardiology (Cardiovascular Disease) 1972, Internal Medicine 1970; **Med School:** Harvard Med Sch 1964; **Resid:** Internal Medicine, Duke Univ Hosp, Durham, NC 1965-1966; **Fellow:** Cardiology (Cardiovascular Disease), Duke Univ Hosp, Durham, NC 1966-1968; **Fac Appt:** Prof Medicine, Indiana Univ

Great Plains and Mountains

Anderson, Jeffrey L MD (Cv) - *Spec Exp:* Arrhythmias; **Hospital:** Univ Utah Hosp and Clin; **Address:** Univ Utah Div Cardiology, 50 N Medical Drive, Salt Lake City, UT 84132; **Phone:** (801) 581-7715; **Board Cert:** Internal Medicine 1975, Cardiology (Cardiovascular Disease) 1979, Cardiac Electrophysiology 1992; **Med School:** Harvard Med Sch 1972; **Resid:** Internal Medicine, Mass Genl Hosp, Boston, MA 1973-1974; **Fellow:** Research, Natl Inst Hlth, Bethesda, MD 1974-1976; Cardiology (Cardiovascular Disease), Stanford Univ Med Ctr, Stanford, CA 1976-1978; **Fac Appt:** Prof Medicine, Univ Utah

Lindenfeld, JoAnn MD (Cv) - *Spec Exp:* Congestive Heart Failure; Transplant Medicine-Heart; **Hospital:** Univ Colo HSC - Denver; **Address:** 4200 E 9th Ave, Box B 130, Denver, CO 80262; **Phone:** (303) 315-4410; **Board Cert:** Cardiology (Cardiovascular Disease) 1979, Internal Medicine 1976; **Med School:** Univ Mich Med Sch 1973; **Resid:** Internal Medicine, University California, San Diego, CA 1973-1977; Cardiology (Cardiovascular Disease), University Texas, San Antonio, TX 1977-1979; **Fac Appt:** Prof Medicine, Univ Colo

Southwest

Freeman, Gregory Lane MD (Cv) - *Spec Exp:* Interventional Cardiology; **Hospital:** Univ of Texas Hlth & Sci Ctr; **Address:** Univ Texas Hlth Sci Ctr, Dept Cardiology, 7703 Floyd Curl, MC 7872, San Antonio, TX 78229; **Phone:** (210) 567-4600; **Board Cert:** Internal Medicine 1979, Cardiology (Cardiovascular Disease) 1983; **Med School:** Loyola Univ-Stritch Sch Med 1976; **Resid:** Internal Medicine, Cook County Hosp, Chicago, IL 1977-1979; **Fellow:** Cardiology (Cardiovascular Disease), Loyola Univ Med Ctr, Maywood, IL 1979-1981; Research, UCSD Sch Med, San Diego, CA 1981-1983; **Fac Appt:** Prof Medicine, Univ Tex, San Antonio

Garcia-Gonzalez, Efrain MD (Cv) - *Spec Exp:* Cardiac Catheterization; **Hospital:** St Luke's Episcopal Hosp - Houston; **Address:** 6624 Fannin St, Ste 2480, Houston, TX 77030-2309; **Phone:** (713) 529-5530; **Board Cert:** Internal Medicine 1963, Cardiology (Cardiovascular Disease) 1964; **Med School:** Univ Puerto Rico 1955; **Resid:** Internal Medicine, Brooke Army Genl Hosp, Ft Sam Houston, TX 1957-1959; **Fellow:** Cardiology (Cardiovascular Disease), Brooke Army Genl Hosp, Ft. Sam Houston, TX 1960-1961; **Fac Appt:** Clin Prof Medicine, Baylor Coll Med

Gould, K Lance MD (Cv) - *Spec Exp:* Preventive Cardiology; PET Imaging; **Hospital:** Meml Hermann Hosp; **Address:** Univ Texas Med Sch - PET Imaging Ctr, 6431 Fannin, Rm 4256 MSB, Houston, TX 77030; **Phone:** (713) 500-6611; **Board Cert:** Cardiology (Cardiovascular Disease), Internal Medicine; **Med School:** Case West Res Univ 1964; **Resid:** Internal Medicine, U Washington Med Ctr, Seattle, WA 1965-1967; Cardiology (Cardiovascular Disease), U Washington Med Ctr, Seattle, WA 1964-1964; **Fellow:** Cardiology (Cardiovascular Disease), U Washington Med Ctr, Seattle, WA 1969-1971; **Fac Appt:** Prof Medicine, Univ Tex, Houston

Massin, Edward Krauss MD (Cv) - *Spec Exp:* *Congestive Heart Failure; Transplant Medicine-Heart; Coronary Artery Disease;* **Hospital:** St Luke's Episcopal Hosp - Houston; **Address:** Cardiology Consultants of Houston, 6624 Fannin St, Fl 2310, Houston, TX 77030-2335; **Phone:** (713) 796-2668; **Board Cert:** Internal Medicine 1973, Cardiology (Cardiovascular Disease) 1973; **Med School:** Washington Univ, St Louis 1965; **Resid:** Internal Medicine, Barnes Hosp, St Louis, MO 1966-1967; **Fellow:** Cardiology (Cardiovascular Disease), Univ Colo Med Ctr, Denver, CO 1969-1971; **Fac Appt:** Clin Prof Medicine, Baylor Coll Med

Ramee, Stephen Robert MD (Cv) - *Spec Exp:* *Angiography-Coronary;* **Hospital:** Ochsner Found Hosp; **Address:** Ochsner Clinic, Cath Lab, 1514 Jefferson Hwy, New Orleans, LA 70121; **Phone:** (504) 842-4135; **Board Cert:** Internal Medicine 1983, Cardiac Electrophysiology 1985, Interventional Cardiology 1999; **Med School:** Geo Wash Univ 1980; **Resid:** Internal Medicine, Letterman Army Med Ctr, San Francisco, CA 1981-1983; **Fellow:** Cardiology (Cardiovascular Disease), Letterman Army Med Ctr, San Francisco, CA 1983-1985

Willerson, James Thorton MD (Cv) - *Spec Exp:* *Cardiology (Cardiovascular Disease) - General;* **Hospital:** St Luke's Episcopal Hosp - Houston; **Address:** 7000 Fannin St, rm UCT 1707, Houston, TX 77030; **Phone:** (713) 500-6500; **Board Cert:** Internal Medicine 1972, Cardiology (Cardiovascular Disease) 1974; **Med School:** Baylor Coll Med 1965; **Resid:** Internal Medicine, Mass Genl Hosp, Boston, MA 1966-1967; **Fellow:** Cardiology (Cardiovascular Disease), Mass Genl Hosp, Boston, MA 1966-1967; **Fac Appt:** Prof Medicine, Univ Tex, Houston

West Coast and Pacific

Barr, Mark Lee MD (Cv) - *Spec Exp:* *Transplant-Lung; Transplant-Heart; Transplant-Heart & Lung;* **Hospital:** USC Univ Hosp - R K Eamer Med Plz; **Address:** 1510 San Pablo St, Ste #415, Los Angeles, CA 90033-4612; **Phone:** (323) 442-5849; **Board Cert:** Infectious Disease 1984, Anesthesiology 1987, Critical Care Medicine 1987, Cardiology (Cardiovascular Disease) 1989; **Med School:** Mount Sinai Sch Med 1981; **Resid:** Surgery, Bellevue Hosp Ctr, New York, NY 1983-1984; Surgical Critical Care, Columbia Presby Med Ctr, New York, NY 1984-1985; **Fellow:** Cardiothoracic Transplantation, Colum-Presby Med, New York, NY 1985-1987; Cardiology (Cardiovascular Disease), Colum-Presby Med, New York, NY 1987-1990; **Fac Appt:** Assoc Prof Thoracic Surgery, USC Sch Med

Bleifer, Selvyn Burton MD (Cv) - *Spec Exp:* *Non-Invasive Cardiology;* **Hospital:** Cedars-Sinai Med Ctr; **Address:** 414 N Camden Drive, Ste 1100, Beverly Hills, CA 90210-4532; **Phone:** (310) 278-3400; **Board Cert:** Internal Medicine 1962, Cardiology (Cardiovascular Disease) 1975; **Med School:** UCSF 1955; **Resid:** Internal Medicine, VA Hosp, Boston, MA 1956-1958; Cardiology (Cardiovascular Disease), Mt Sinai Hosp, New York, NY 1958; **Fac Appt:** Assoc Clin Prof Medicine, UCLA

Brindis, Ralph Gerard MD (Cv) - *Spec Exp:* *Cardiology (Cardiovascular Disease) - General;* **Hospital:** Kaiser Permanente Med Ctr - SF; **Address:** 2350 Geary Blvd, rm 218, San Francisco, CA 94115; **Phone:** (415) 202-2616; **Board Cert:** Internal Medicine 1980, Cardiology (Cardiovascular Disease) 1999; **Med School:** Emory Univ 1977; **Resid:** Internal Medicine, Fort Miley VA Hosp, San Francisco, CA 1980-1981; Internal Medicine, Herbert C Moffitt Hosp, San Francisco, CA 1978-1980; **Fellow:** Cardiology (Cardiovascular Disease), Herbert C Moffitt Hosp, San Francisco, CA 1981-1983; **Fac Appt:** Prof Medicine, UCSF

Chatterjee, Kanu MD (Cv) - *Spec Exp:* Coronary Artery Disease; Congestive Heart Failure; **Hospital:** UCSF Med Ctr; **Address:** 1182 Moffitt Hospital, 505 Parnassus Ave, Box 0124, San Francisco, CA 94143-0327; **Phone:** (415) 476-1326; **Board Cert:** Internal Medicine 1973, Cardiology (Cardiovascular Disease) 1975; **Med School:** India 1956; **Fellow:** Cardiology (Cardiovascular Disease), Brompton Hosp, London, England 1969-1971; **Fac Appt:** Prof Cardiology (Cardiovascular Disease), UCSF

Choe, Soo-Sang MD (Cv) - *Spec Exp:* Cardiology (Cardiovascular Disease) - General; **Hospital:** Loma Linda Univ Med Ctr; **Address:** 903 E Devovshire Ave, Ste A, Hemet, CA 92543; **Phone:** (909) 925-0571; **Board Cert:** Internal Medicine 1984, Cardiology (Cardiovascular Disease) 1995; **Med School:** South Korea 1967; **Resid:** Internal Medicine, Hahnemann Med Coll Hosp Hosp, Philadelphia, PA 1972-1974; Cardiology (Cardiovascular Disease), Sloan-Kettering Meml Hosp, New YorK, NY 1974-1975; **Fellow:** Cardiology (Cardiovascular Disease), Bronx VA Hosp, New York, NY 1975-1977

Criley, John Michael MD (Cv) - *Spec Exp:* Cardiac Catheterization; **Hospital:** LAC - Harbor - UCLA Med Ctr; **Address:** 21840 S Normandy Ave, Ste 70, Torrance, CA 90502; **Phone:** (310) 222-5101; **Med School:** Stanford Univ 1956; **Resid:** Internal Medicine, Johns Hospkins Hosp, Baltimore, MD 1956-1960; **Fac Appt:** Prof Medicine, UCLA

Elkayam, Uri MD (Cv) - *Spec Exp:* Congestive Heart Failure; **Hospital:** LAC & USC Med Ctr; **Address:** 1200 N State St, rm 7621, Los Angeles, CA 90033; **Phone:** (323) 226-7541; **Board Cert:** Cardiology (Cardiovascular Disease) 1991, Internal Medicine 1989; **Med School:** Israel 1973; **Resid:** Internal Medicine, Ichilov Hosp, Tel-Aviv, Israel 1976; **Fellow:** Cardiology (Cardiovascular Disease), Albert Einstein Hosp, New York, NY 1978; Cardiology (Cardiovascular Disease), Cedars Sinai Med Ctr, Los Angeles, CA 1978-1979; **Fac Appt:** Prof Medicine, Univ SC Sch Med

Fishbein, Daniel P MD (Cv) - *Spec Exp:* Congestive Heart Failure; Transplant Medicine-Heart; **Hospital:** Univ WA Med Ctr; **Address:** Div Cardiology, 1959 NE Pacific St, Box 356422, Seattle, WA 98195; **Phone:** (206) 598-4300; **Board Cert:** Cardiology (Cardiovascular Disease) 1987, Internal Medicine 1983; **Med School:** Albert Einstein Coll Med 1980; **Resid:** Internal Medicine, Lankenau Hosp, Wynnewood, PA 1980-1981; Internal Medicine, Univ Wash Med Ctr, Seattle, WA 1981-1983; **Fellow:** Cardiology (Cardiovascular Disease), Univ Wash Med Ctr, Seattle, WA 1984-1987

Gershengorn, Kent N MD (Cv) - *Spec Exp:* Cardiology (Cardiovascular Disease) - General; **Hospital:** UCSF Med Ctr; **Address:** 350 Parnassus Ave, Ste 701, San Francisco, CA 94117; **Phone:** (415) 476-6388; **Board Cert:** Internal Medicine 1973, Cardiology (Cardiovascular Disease) 1973; **Med School:** SUNY Buffalo 1965; **Resid:** Internal Medicine, Mt Sinai Hosp, New York, NY 1968-1970; Cardiology (Cardiovascular Disease), Mt Sinai Hosp, New York, NY 1970-1971; **Fellow:** Cardiology (Cardiovascular Disease), Herbert C Moffitt Hosp-UCSF, San Francisco, CA 1971-1972; **Fac Appt:** Clin Prof Medicine, UCSF

Goldschlager, Nora F MD (Cv) - *Spec Exp:* Cardiology (Cardiovascular Disease) - General; **Hospital:** San Francisco Gen Hosp; **Address:** San Francisco Genl Hosp, Dept Cardiology, 1001 Potrero Ave, rm 5G1, San Franciscxo, CA 94110-2897; **Phone:** (415) 206-3503; **Board Cert:** Internal Medicine 1973, Cardiac Electrophysiology 1973; **Med School:** NYU Sch Med 1965; **Resid:** Infectious Disease, Montefiore Med Ctr, Bronx, NY 1966-1967; Internal Medicine, Henry Ford Hosp, Detroit MI, 67 1968; **Fellow:** Cardiology (Cardiovascular Disease), Wayne State Univ Med Ctr, Detroit MI, 68 1969; Cardiology (Cardiovascular Disease), Pacific Med Ctr, San Francisco, CA 1969-1970; **Fac Appt:** Clin Prof Medicine, UCSF

Heger, Joel William MD (Cv) - *Spec Exp:* Cardiology (Cardiovascular Disease) - General; **Hospital:** LAC & USC Med Ctr; **Address:** 10 Congress St, Ste 507, Passadena, CA 91105-3023; **Phone:** (626) 792-5300; **Board Cert:** Cardiology (Cardiovascular Disease) 1979, Interventional Cardiology 1999; **Med School:** USC Sch Med 1972; **Resid:** Internal Medicine, USC Med Ctr, Los Angeles, CA 1973-1975; **Fellow:** Cardiology (Cardiovascular Disease), USC Med Ctr, Los Angeles, CA 1975-1976; Cardiology (Cardiovascular Disease), UCLA Med Ctr, Torrance, CA 1976-1978; **Fac Appt:** Clin Prof Medicine, USC Sch Med

Hunt, Sharon Ann MD (Cv) - *Spec Exp:* Transplant Medicine-Heart; **Hospital:** Stanford Med Ctr; **Address:** 300 Pasteur Dr, Falk Bldg, Ste CVRC213, Stanford, CA 94305-5406; **Phone:** (650) 498-6605; **Board Cert:** Internal Medicine 1977, Cardiology (Cardiovascular Disease) 1979; **Med School:** Stanford Univ 1972; **Resid:** Internal Medicine, Stanford Univ Hosp, Stanford, CA 1972-1974; **Fellow:** Cardiology (Cardiovascular Disease), Stanford Univ Hosp, Stanford, CA 1974-1976; **Fac Appt:** Prof Medicine, Stanford Univ

Kobashigawa, Jon Akira MD (Cv) - *Spec Exp:* Transplant Medicine-Heart; **Hospital:** UCLA Med Ctr; **Address:** 100 UCLA Med Plaza, Ste 630, Los Angeles, CA 90095; **Phone:** (310) 794-1200; **Board Cert:** Internal Medicine 1983, Cardiology (Cardiovascular Disease) 1987; **Med School:** Mount Sinai Sch Med 1980; **Resid:** Internal Medicine, UCLA Med Ctr, Los Angeles, CA 1981-1983; **Fellow:** Cardiology (Cardiovascular Disease), UCLA Med Ctr, Los Angeles, CA 1984-1986; **Fac Appt:** Assoc Clin Prof Cardiology (Cardiovascular Disease), UCLA

Parmley, William Watts MD (Cv) - *Spec Exp:* Coronary Artery Disease; Heart Failure; **Hospital:** UCSF Med Ctr; **Address:** UCSF-Moffit Long Hosp, 505 Parnassus Ave, rm 1180, San Francisco, CA 94143-0124; **Phone:** (415) 476-1326; **Board Cert:** Internal Medicine 1970, Cardiology (Cardiovascular Disease) 1972; **Med School:** Johns Hopkins Univ 1963; **Resid:** Internal Medicine, Johns Hopkins Hosp, Baltimore, MD 1963-1965; **Fellow:** Cardiology (Cardiovascular Disease), Natl Heart Institute, Bethesda, MD 1965-1967; Cardiology (Cardiovascular Disease), Peter Bent Brigham, Boston, MA 1967-1969; **Fac Appt:** Prof Medicine, UCSF

Perloff, Joseph Kayle MD (Cv) - *Spec Exp:* Heart Disease-Congenital; **Hospital:** UCLA Med Ctr; **Address:** UCLA Med Ctr, 650 Charles E. Young Drive S, rm 47-123 CHS, Box 951679, Los Angeles, CA 90095-1679; **Phone:** (310) 825-2019; **Board Cert:** Internal Medicine 1960, Cardiology (Cardiovascular Disease) 1967; **Med School:** Louisiana State Univ 1951; **Resid:** Internal Medicine, Mt Sinai Hosp, New York, NY 1951-1954; Internal Medicine, Georgetown Univ Hosp, Washington, DC 1955-1956; **Fellow:** Cardiology (Cardiovascular Disease), Natl Heart Hosp, London, England 1954-1955; **Fac Appt:** Prof Pediatric Cardiology, UCLA

Scheinman, Melvin M MD (Cv) - *Spec Exp:* Cardiac Electrophysiology; Heart Rhythm Abnormalities; **Hospital:** UCSF Med Ctr; **Address:** 500 Parnassus Ave, Ste MU436 East Tower, San Francisco, CA 94143-1354; **Phone:** (415) 476-5706; **Board Cert:** Cardiology (Cardiovascular Disease) 1971, Cardiac Electrophysiology 1992; **Med School:** Albert Einstein Coll Med 1960; **Resid:** Internal Medicine, NC Meml Hosp, Chapel Hill, NC 1963-1965; **Fellow:** Cardiology (Cardiovascular Disease), UCSF, San Francisco, CA 1965-1967; **Fac Appt:** Prof Medicine, UCSF

Schnittger, Ingela MD (Cv) - *Spec Exp:* Cardiovascular Imaging-Non-Invasive; **Hospital:** Stanford Med Ctr; **Address:** 300 Pasteur Drive, Ste H2157, Stanford, CA 94305-5233; **Phone:** (650) 723-5196; **Board Cert:** Internal Medicine 1980, Cardiology (Cardiovascular Disease) 1983; **Med School:** Sweden 1975; **Resid:** Internal Medicine, Stanford Univ Hosp, Stanford, CA 1979-1980; **Fellow:** Cardiology (Cardiovascular Disease), Stanford Univ Hosp, Stanford, CA 1980-1983; **Fac Appt:** Assoc Prof Medicine, Stanford Univ

Schroeder, John S MD (Cv) - *Spec Exp:* Congestive Heart Failure; Coronary Artery Disease; **Hospital:** Stanford Med Ctr; **Address:** 300 Pasteur Dr, Bldg CVRC 293, Stanford, CA 94305-5406; **Phone:** (650) 723-5561; **Board Cert:** Internal Medicine 1969, Cardiology (Cardiovascular Disease) 1973; **Med School:** Univ Mich Med Sch 1962; **Resid:** Internal Medicine, Stanford Univ Med Ctr, Stanford, CA 1965-1967; **Fellow:** Cardiology (Cardiovascular Disease), Stanford Univ Med Ctr, Stanford, CA 1967-1969; **Fac Appt:** Prof Cardiology (Cardiovascular Disease), Stanford Univ

Shah, Prediman K MD (Cv) - *Spec Exp:* Coronary Artery Disease; Cardiomy Oparthy; **Hospital:** Cedars-Sinai Med Ctr; **Address:** Cedars-Sinai Med Ctr, 8700 Beverly Blvd, rm 5347, Los Angeles, CA 90048-1865; **Phone:** (310) 423-3884; **Board Cert:** Internal Medicine 1975, Cardiology (Cardiovascular Disease) 1977; **Med School:** India 1969; **Resid:** All India Inst Med Scis, New Delhi, India 1970-1971; Internal Medicine, Montefiore Hosp, New York, NY 1973-1974; **Fellow:** Cardiology (Cardiovascular Disease), Montefiore Hosp, New York, NY 1974-1976; **Fac Appt:** Prof Medicine, UCLA

Wilansky, Susan MD (Cv) - *Spec Exp:* Heart Disease in Women; Heart Disease in Pregnancy; **Hospital:** Kaiser Foundation Hosp - Anaheim; **Address:** Southern California Permanente Med Grp, 411 N Lakeview Ave, Anaheim, CA 92807; **Phone:** (888) 988-2800; **Board Cert:** Cardiology (Cardiovascular Disease) 1989; **Med School:** McMaster Univ 1979; **Resid:** Internal Medicine, Toronto Hosp-Univ Toronto, Toronto Canada 1980-1983; Cardiology (Cardiovascular Disease), Toronto Hosp-Univ Toronto, Toronto Canada 1983-1985; **Fellow:** Electrocardiograph, Toronto Hosp-Univ Toronto, Toronto Canada 1985-1986

INTERVENTIONAL CARDIOLOGY

New England

Diver, Daniel Joseph MD (IC) - *Spec Exp:* Angioplasty; Coronary Artery Disease; **Hospital:** St Francis Hosp & Med Ctr; **Address:** 114 Woodland St, Hartford, CT 06105; **Phone:** (860) 714-5900; **Board Cert:** Interventional Cardiology 1999, Cardiology (Cardiovascular Disease) 1989; **Med School:** Johns Hopkins Univ 1981; **Resid:** Internal Medicine, Johns Hopkins Hosp, Baltimore, MD 1982-1984; **Fellow:** Cardiology (Cardiovascular Disease), Beth Israel Hosp/Harvard, Boston, MA 1984-1987; **Fac Appt:** Prof Medicine, Univ Conn

Jacobs, Alice K MD (IC) - *Spec Exp:* Cardiac Catheterization; **Hospital:** Boston Med Ctr; **Address:** Boston Univ Med Ctr, Dept Cardiology, 88 E Newton St, Boston, MA 02118; **Phone:** (617) 638-7490; **Board Cert:** Internal Medicine 1978, Cardiology (Cardiovascular Disease) 1985; **Med School:** St Louis Univ 1975; **Resid:** Internal Medicine, St Louis Univ Hosp, St Louis, MO 1976-1978; **Fellow:** Endocrinology, UCSD Med Ctr, San Diego, Ca 1978-1980; Cardiology (Cardiovascular Disease), Boston Univ Med Ctr, Boston, MA 1980-1982; **Fac Appt:** Prof Medicine, Boston Univ

Weiner, Bonnie H MD (IC) - *Spec Exp:* Interventional Cardiology - General; **Hospital:** U Mass Meml Hlth Care - Worcester; **Address:** 55 Lake Ave N, Worcester, MA 01655-0002; **Phone:** (508) 856-3691; **Board Cert:** Internal Medicine 1977, Cardiology (Cardiovascular Disease) 1979, Interventional Cardiology 1999; **Med School:** Oregon Hlth Scis Univ 1974; **Resid:** Internal Medicine, Norwalk Hosp, Norwalk, CT 1975-1977; **Fellow:** Cardiology (Cardiovascular Disease), Univ Mass, Worcester, MA

Mid Atlantic

Leon, Martin MD (IC) - *Spec Exp:* Interventional Cardiology - General; **Hospital:** Lenox Hill Hosp (page 64); **Address:** 130 E 77th St Fl 9, New York, NY 10021; **Phone:** (212) 434-6300; **Board Cert:** Internal Medicine 1979, Cardiology (Cardiovascular Disease) 1983; **Med School:** Yale Univ 1975; **Resid:** Internal Medicine, Yale-New Haven Hosp, New Haven, CT 1976-1978; **Fellow:** Cardiology (Cardiovascular Disease), Yale-New Haven Hosp, New Haven, CT 1980

Pichard, Augusto MD (IC) - *Spec Exp:* Angioplasty; **Hospital:** Washington Hosp Ctr; **Address:** 110 Irving St NW, Ste 4B1, Washington, DC 20010; **Phone:** (202) 877-5975; **Board Cert:** Internal Medicine 1975, Cardiology (Cardiovascular Disease) 1977, Interventional Cardiology 1999; **Med School:** Chile 1969; **Resid:** Internal Medicine, Catholic U, Washington, DC 1970-1971; Internal Medicine, U Chile 1969-1970; **Fellow:** Cardiology (Cardiovascular Disease), Cleveland Clin, Cleveland, OH 1971-1973

Reiner, Jonathan S MD (IC) - *Spec Exp:* Interventional Cardiology - General; **Hospital:** G Washington Univ Hosp; **Address:** 2150 Penn Ave NW, Washington, DC 20037; **Phone:** (202) 994-5400; **Board Cert:** Interventional Cardiology 1999, Cardiology (Cardiovascular Disease) 1993; **Med School:** Georgetown Univ 1986; **Resid:** Internal Medicine, North Shore Univ Hosp, Manhasset, NY 1987-1989; **Fellow:** Cardiology (Cardiovascular Disease), George Wash Sch Med, Washington, DC 1990-1993; **Fac Appt:** Asst Prof Medicine, Geo Wash Univ

Roubin, Gary MD/PhD (IC) - *Spec Exp:* Endovascular Surgery; Stroke-Carotid Artery Stent; **Hospital:** Lenox Hill Hosp (page 64); **Address:** Lenox Hill Hosp, Black Hall 9FL, 130 E 77th St, New York, NY 10021; **Phone:** (212) 434-2606; **Med School:** Australia 1975; **Resid:** Internal Medicine, Royal Prince Albert Hosp, Sidney, Australia 1976-1989; Cardiology (Cardiovascular Disease), Hallstrom Inst of Cardiology, Sidney, Australia 1979-1981; **Fellow:** Cardiology Research, Natl Heart Fdn, Sidney, Australia 1981-1983; Interventional Cardiology, Emory Univ, Atlanta, GA 1984-1985; **Fac Appt:** Clin Prof Medicine, NYU Sch Med

Southeast

Applegate, Robert Joseph MD (IC) - *Spec Exp:* Cardiac Catheterization; Angioplasty; **Hospital:** Wake Forest Univ Baptist Med Ctr (page 81); **Address:** Wake Forest Univ Baptist Med Ctr, Cardiology Sect, Medical Center Blvd, Winston-Salem, NC 27157; **Phone:** (336) 716-6674; **Board Cert:** Interventional Cardiology 1999, Cardiology (Cardiovascular Disease) 1987; **Med School:** Univ VA Sch Med 1980; **Resid:** Internal Medicine, Oregon Hlth Sci Univ Hosp, Portland, OR 1981-1983; **Fellow:** Pharmacology, Univ Texas Hlth Sci Ctr, San Antonio, TX 1983-1984; Cardiology (Cardiovascular Disease), Univ Texas Hlth Sci Ctr, San Antonio, TX 1984-1986; **Fac Appt:** Prof Medicine, Wake Forest Univ Sch Med

Braden, Gregory Alan MD (IC) - *Spec Exp:* Cardiac Catheterization; **Hospital:** Forsyth Med Ctr; **Address:** 1381 Westgate Center Drive, Winston Salem, NC 27103; **Phone:** (336) 718-0113; **Board Cert:** Cardiology (Cardiovascular Disease) 1989, Interventional Cardiology 1999; **Med School:** Wake Forest Univ Sch Med 1982; **Resid:** Internal Medicine, Univ Texas Med Br Hosp, Galveston, TX 1982-1985; **Fellow:** Cardiology (Cardiovascular Disease), Vanderbilt Univ Med, Nashville, TN 1986-1989

King III, Spencer MD (IC) - *Spec Exp:* Interventional Cardiology - General; **Hospital:** Promina Piedmont Hosp; **Address:** 95 Collier Rd NW, Ste 2075, Atlanta, GA 30309; **Phone:** (404) 351-4353; **Board Cert:** Interventional Cardiology 1999, Cardiology (Cardiovascular Disease) 1971; **Med School:** Med Coll GA 1963; **Resid:** Internal Medicine, Emory Univ Hosp, Atlanta, GA 1966-1968; **Fellow:** Cardiology (Cardiovascular Disease), Emory U Sch Med, Atlanta, GA 1968-1970

Matar, Fadi MD (IC) - *Spec Exp:* Angioplasty; **Hospital:** Tampa Genl Hosp; **Address:** 508 South Habana, Ste 340, Tampa, FL 33609-3568; **Phone:** (813) 353-1515; **Board Cert:** Cardiology (Cardiovascular Disease) 1993, Interventional Cardiology 1999; **Med School:** Lebanon 1987; **Resid:** Internal Medicine, Maryland Genl Hosp, Baltimore, MD 1987-1990; **Fellow:** Cardiology (Cardiovascular Disease), Wash Hosp Ctr, Washington DC, WA 1990-1994; **Fac Appt:** Asst Prof Medicine, Univ S Fla Coll Med

Morris, Douglas MD (IC) - *Spec Exp:* Interventional Cardiology; **Hospital:** Emory Univ Hosp; **Address:** Heart Center, 1365 Clifton Rd NE, Bldg A, Atlanta, GA 30322; **Phone:** (404) 778-5310; **Board Cert:** Interventional Cardiology 1999, Cardiology (Cardiovascular Disease) 1975; **Med School:** Baylor Coll Med 1968; **Resid:** Internal Medicine, Vanderbilt Univ, Nashville, TN 1969-1970; Internal Medicine, Vanderbilt Univ, Nashville, TN 1972-1973; **Fellow:** Cardiology (Cardiovascular Disease), Emory University, Atlanta, GA 1973-1975; **Fac Appt:** Prof Cardiology (Cardiovascular Disease), Emory Univ

Midwest

Clark, Vivian MD (IC) - *Spec Exp:* Coronary Angioplasty; Cardiac Catheterization; **Hospital:** Henry Ford Hosp; **Address:** 2799 W Grand Blvd, Ste K14, Detroit, MI 48202; **Phone:** (313) 876-2737; **Board Cert:** Internal Medicine 1982, Cardiology (Cardiovascular Disease) 1985, Interventional Cardiology 1999; **Med School:** Ohio State Univ 1979; **Resid:** Internal Medicine, Akron City Hospital, Akron, OH 1980-1982; **Fellow:** Cardiology (Cardiovascular Disease), Henry Ford Hospital, Detroit, MI 1982-1984

Ellis, Stephen Geoffrey MD (IC) - *Spec Exp:* Angioplasty; Angiogenesis; **Hospital:** Cleveland Clin Fdn (page 57); **Address:** Cleveland Clinic, 9500 Euclid Ave, Ste F25, Cleveland, OH 44195-0002; **Phone:** (216) 445-6712; **Board Cert:** Internal Medicine 1981, Cardiology (Cardiovascular Disease) 1985; **Med School:** UCLA 1978; **Resid:** Internal Medicine, Cedars-Sinai Med Ctr, Los Angeles, CA 1978-1981; **Fellow:** Cardiology (Cardiovascular Disease), Stanford University, Stanford, CA 1982-1985; Interventional Cardiology, Emory University, Atlanta, GA 1985-1986; **Fac Appt:** Prof Medicine, Ohio State Univ

Feldman, Ted MD (IC) - *Spec Exp:* Interventional Cardiology - General; **Hospital:** Evanston Hosp; **Address:** 9977 Woods Drive, Skokie, IL 60077-1057; **Phone:** (847) 663-8410; **Board Cert:** Cardiology (Cardiovascular Disease) 1985, Interventional Cardiology 1999; **Med School:** Indiana Univ 1978; **Resid:** Internal Medicine, Rush-Presby-St Lukes, Chicago, IL 1978-1982; **Fellow:** Cardiology (Cardiovascular Disease), Univ Chicago, Chicago, IL 1982-1985; **Fac Appt:** Prof Medicine, Univ Chicago-Pritzker Sch Med

Holmes Jr., David Richard MD (IC) - *Spec Exp:* Interventional Cardiology; Myocardial Infarction; **Hospital:** Mayo Med Ctr & Clin - Rochester, MN; **Address:** Div Cardiovascular Diseases, 200 1st St SW, Rochester, MN 55905; **Phone:** (507) 255-2504; **Board Cert:** Internal Medicine 1974, Cardiology (Cardiovascular Disease) 1977, Interventional Cardiology 1999; **Med School:** Med Coll Wisc 1971; **Resid:** Cardiology (Cardiovascular Disease), Mayo Clinic, Rochester, MN 1972; **Fac Appt:** Prof Medicine, Mayo Med Sch

Klein, Lloyd MD (IC) - *Spec Exp:* Coronary Disease-Complex; Coronary Angiography & Interventions; **Hospital:** Rush-Presby - St Luke's Med Ctr (page 72); **Address:** Rush Presby-St Luke's Med Ctr, 1653 W Congress Pkwy, Ste 1035, Chicago, IL 60612-3835; **Phone:** (312) 942-2985; **Board Cert:** Cardiology (Cardiovascular Disease) 1983, Interventional Cardiology 1999; **Med School:** Univ Cincinnati 1977; **Resid:** Internal Medicine, Albert Einstein-Bronx Muni Hosp, Bronx, NY 1977-1980; **Fellow:** Cardiology (Cardiovascular Disease), Mt Sinai Med Ctr, New York, NY 1980-1982; **Fac Appt:** Prof Medicine, Rush Med Coll

Pitt, Bertram MD (IC) - *Spec Exp:* Interventional Cardiology - General; **Hospital:** Univ of MI Hlth Ctr; **Address:** Univ Mich Med Ctr, Div Cardiology, 1500 E Med Ctr Dr, Ann Arbor, MI 48109-0366; **Phone:** (734) 936-5260; **Board Cert:** Internal Medicine 1973, Cardiology (Cardiovascular Disease) 1975; **Med School:** Switzerland 1959; **Resid:** Internal Medicine, Beth Israel Hosp, Boston, MA 1960-1963; **Fellow:** Cardiology (Cardiovascular Disease), Johns Hopkins Hosp, Baltimore, MD 1966-1968; **Fac Appt:** Prof Medicine, Univ Mich Med Sch

Weaver, Wayne Douglas MD (IC) - *Spec Exp:* Myocardial Infarction; Angioplasty; Cholesterol/Lipid Disorders; **Hospital:** Henry Ford Hosp; **Address:** Henry Ford Hosp, K-14, 2799 W Grand Blvd, Detriot, MI 48202-2689; **Phone:** (313) 916-2737; **Board Cert:** Internal Medicine 1974, Cardiology (Cardiovascular Disease) 1977; **Med School:** Tufts Univ 1971; **Resid:** Internal Medicine, Univ Wash Hosp, Seattle, WA 1972-1974; **Fellow:** Cardiology (Cardiovascular Disease), Univ Wash Hosp, Seattle, WA 1974-1976

INTERVENTIONAL CARDIOLOGY

White, Carl W MD (IC) - *Spec Exp:* Interventional Cardiology - General; **Hospital:** Fairview-Univ Med Ctr - Univ Campus; **Address:** Cardiovascular Div, Dept Med, Univ of MN, 420 Delaware St, Minneapolis, MN 55455; **Phone:** (612) 625-9100; **Board Cert:** Cardiology (Cardiovascular Disease) 1973, Interventional Cardiology 1999; **Med School:** Univ Nebr Coll Med 1964; **Resid:** Internal Medicine, Univ Iowa Hosp, Des Moines, IA 1967-1970; **Fellow:** Cardiology (Cardiovascular Disease), Univ Iowa Hosp, Des Moines, IA 1970-1972; **Fac Appt:** Prof Medicine, Univ Minn

Southwest

Bailey, Steven Roderick MD (IC) - *Spec Exp:* Interventional Cardiology - General; **Hospital:** Univ of Texas Hlth & Sci Ctr; **Address:** 7703 Floyd Curl Drive, MC 7872, San Antonio, TX 78229-3900; **Phone:** (210) 567-4601; **Board Cert:** Internal Medicine 1981, Cardiology (Cardiovascular Disease) 1983, Interventional Cardiology 1999; **Med School:** Oregon Hlth Scis Univ 1978; **Resid:** Internal Medicine, Fitzsimmons AMC, Denver, CO 1979-1981; **Fellow:** Cardiology (Cardiovascular Disease), Fitzsimmons AMC, Denver, CO 1981-1983; **Fac Appt:** Prof Medicine, Univ Tex, San Antonio

Kleiman, Neal Stephen MD (IC) - *Spec Exp:* Angioplasty; **Hospital:** Methodist Hosp - Houston; **Address:** 6565 Fannin St Bldg F - Ste 1090, Houston, TX 77030; **Phone:** (713) 790-4952; **Board Cert:** Interventional Cardiology 1999, Cardiology (Cardiovascular Disease) 1987; **Med School:** Columbia P&S 1981; **Resid:** Internal Medicine, Baylor Coll Med, Houston, TX 1981-1984; **Fellow:** Interventional Cardiology, Baylor Coll Med, Houston, TX 1984-1987; **Fac Appt:** Assoc Prof Medicine, Baylor Coll Med

Smalling, Richard Warren MD/PhD (IC) - *Spec Exp:* Stroke; **Hospital:** Meml Hermann Hosp; **Address:** 6431 Fannin St, MS 1246, Houston, TX 77030-1501; **Phone:** (713) 500-6559; **Board Cert:** Internal Medicine 1978, Cardiology (Cardiovascular Disease) 1981, Interventional Cardiology 1999; **Med School:** Univ Tex, Houston 1975; **Resid:** Internal Medicine, UCSD Med Ctr, San Diego, CA 1975-1978; **Fellow:** Cardiology (Cardiovascular Disease), UCSD Med Ctr, San Diego, CA 1978-1980; **Fac Appt:** Prof Medicine, Univ Tex, Houston

West Coast and Pacific

Buchbinder, Maurice MD (IC) - *Spec Exp:* Cardiac Catheterization; **Hospital:** Sharp Mem Hosp; **Address:** 9834 Genesee Ave, Ste 312, La Jolla, CA 92037; **Phone:** (858) 625-4488; **Board Cert:** Internal Medicine 1981, Cardiology (Cardiovascular Disease) 1983; **Med School:** Canada 1978; **Resid:** Internal Medicine, Jewish Genl Hosp, Montreal, Canada 1979-1980; Internal Medicine, Stanford Univ Hosp, Stanford, CA 1980-1982; **Fellow:** Cardiology (Cardiovascular Disease), Stanford Univ Hosp, Stanford, CA 1982-1983

Teirstein, Paul Shepherd MD (IC) - *Spec Exp:* Coronary Angioplasty; Stent Placement; Coronary Radiation Therapy; **Hospital:** Green Hosp - Scripps Clinic; **Address:** Scripps Clinic - Torrey Pines, 10666 N Torrey Pines Rd, La Jolla, CA 92037; **Phone:** (858) 554-9905; **Board Cert:** Cardiology (Cardiovascular Disease) 1987, Interventional Cardiology 1999; **Med School:** Mount Sinai Sch Med 1980; **Resid:** Internal Medicine, Brigham & Women's Hosp, Boston, MA 1981-1983; **Fellow:** Cardiology (Cardiovascular Disease), Stanford Univ, Stanford, CA 1983-1986; Cardiology (Cardiovascular Disease), Mid-Amer Heart Inst, Kansas City, MO 1986-1987

CHILD NEUROLOGY

(a subspecialty of NEUROLOGY)

A neurologist specializes in the diagnosis and treatment of all types of disease or impaired function of the brain, spinal cord, peripheral nerves, muscles and autonomic nervous system, as well as the blood vessels that relate to these structures. A child neurologist has special skills in the diagnosis and management of neurologic disorders of the neonatal period, infancy, early childhood and adolescence.

Training required: Four years

Physician Listings

New England

Darras, Basil Theodore MD (ChiN) - *Spec Exp:* Neuromuscular Disorders; **Hospital:** Children's Hospital - Boston; **Address:** 300 Longwood Ave, Boston, MA 02115; **Phone:** (617) 355-8235; **Board Cert:** Pediatrics 1988, Neurology 1992; **Med School:** Greece 1977; **Resid:** Pediatrics, Nassau County Med Ctr, East Meadow, NY 1980-1982; Child Neurology, Tufts-New England Med Ctr, Boston, MA 1982-1985; **Fellow:** Clinical Genetics, Yale Univ Sch Med, New Haven, CT 1985-1988; **Fac Appt:** Assoc Prof Neurology, Harvard Med Sch

Holmes, Gregory Lawrence MD (ChiN) - *Spec Exp:* Epilepsy/Seizure Disorders; Neurologic Disorders; **Hospital:** Children's Hospital - Boston; **Address:** 300 Longwood Ave, Boston, MA 02115-5724; **Phone:** (617) 355-8461; **Board Cert:** Pediatrics 1979, Neurology 1980; **Med School:** Univ VA Sch Med 1974; **Resid:** Pediatrics, Yale-New Haven Hosp, New Haven, CT 1975-1976; **Fellow:** Pediatric Neurology, Univ Va, Charlottesville, VA 1976-1979; **Fac Appt:** Prof Harvard Med Sch

Shaywitz, Bennett MD (ChiN) - *Spec Exp:* Learning Disorders; Dyslexia; **Hospital:** Yale - New Haven Hosp; **Address:** Dept Pediatrics, 333 Cedar St, rm LMP-3089, New Haven, CT 06520; **Phone:** (203) 785-4641; **Board Cert:** Child Neurology 1973, Pediatrics 1968; **Med School:** Washington Univ, St Louis 1963; **Resid:** Pediatrics, Bronx Muni Hosp Ctr, Bronx, NY 1964-1967; **Fellow:** Child Neurology, Albert Einstein Coll Med, Bronx, NY 1967-1970; **Fac Appt:** Prof Child Neurology, Yale Univ

Volpe, Joseph J. MD (ChiN) - *Spec Exp:* Neonatal Neurology; Cerebral Palsy; **Hospital:** Children's Hospital - Boston; **Address:** 300 Longwood Ave, Bldg Segan Fl 11, Boston, MA 02115-5724; **Phone:** (617) 355-6386; **Board Cert:** Pediatrics 1970, Neurology 1974; **Med School:** Harvard Med Sch 1964; **Resid:** Pediatrics, Mass Genl Hosp, Boston, MA 1965-1966; Neurology, Mass Genl Hosp, Boston, MA 1968-1971; **Fellow:** Natl Inst Child Hlth Human Dev, Bethesda, MD 1966-1968; **Fac Appt:** Prof Neurology, Harvard Med Sch

Mid Atlantic

Aron, Alan MD (ChiN) - *Spec Exp:* Neurofibromatosis; Seizure Disorders; **Hospital:** Mount Sinai Hosp (page 68); **Address:** 5 E 98th St, New York, NY 10029; **Phone:** (212) 831-4393; **Board Cert:** Pediatrics 1963, Neurology 1967; **Med School:** Columbia P&S 1958; **Resid:** Pediatrics, Babies Hosp-Columbia Presby, New York, NY 1959-1961; **Fellow:** Child Neurology, Babies Hosp-Columbia Presby, New York, NY 1961-1964; **Fac Appt:** Prof Pediatric Endocrinology, Mount Sinai Sch Med

Chutorian, Abraham MD (ChiN) - *Spec Exp:* Autoimmune Disease-Nervous System; Movement Disorders; **Hospital:** NY Presby Hosp - NY Weill Cornell Med Ctr (page 70); **Address:** 525 E 68th St, Box 91, New York, NY 10021-4870; **Phone:** (212) 746-3278; **Board Cert:** Pediatrics 1962, Neurology 1965; **Med School:** Univ Manitoba 1957; **Resid:** Pediatrics, Children's Hosp, Los Angeles, CA 1958-1960; **Fellow:** Neurology, Columbia-Presby Med Ctr, New York, NY 1960-1963; **Fac Appt:** Prof Neurology, Cornell Univ-Weill Med Coll

Crawford, Thomas Owen MD (ChiN) - *Spec Exp:* Neuromuscular Disorders; Muscular Dystrophy; **Hospital:** Johns Hopkins Hosp - Baltimore; **Address:** 600 N Wolfe St Bldg Jefferson - rm 123, Baltimore, MD 21287-8811; **Phone:** (410) 955-4259; **Board Cert:** Pediatrics 1986, Neurology 1990; **Med School:** USC Sch Med 1980; **Resid:** Neurology, Children's Hosp, Los Angeles, CA 1984-1987; Pediatrics, LAC-USC Med Ctr, Los Angeles, CA 1981-1984; **Fellow:** Neurology, Johns Hopkins Hosp, Baltimore, MD 1987-1988; **Fac Appt:** Asst Prof Neurology, Johns Hopkins Univ

De Vivo, Darryl C MD (ChiN) - *Spec Exp:* Child Neurology - General; **Hospital:** NY Presby Hosp - Columbia Presby Med Ctr (page 70); **Address:** 710 W 168th St, rm 201, New York, NY 10032; **Phone:** (212) 305-5244; **Board Cert:** Child Neurology 1972; **Med School:** Univ VA Sch Med 1964; **Resid:** Pediatrics, Mass Genl Hosp, Boston, MA 1965-1966; Neurology, Mass Genl Hosp, Boston, MA 1966-1967; **Fellow:** Neurology, Natl Inst Hlth, Bethesda, MD 1967-1969; Child Neurology, Children's Hosp-Wash Univ, St Louis, MO 1969-1970; **Fac Appt:** Prof Neurology, Columbia P&S

Eviatar, Lydia MD (ChiN) - *Spec Exp:* Balance Disorders; Tourette's Syndrome; Seizure Disorders; **Hospital:** Long Island Jewish Med Ctr; **Address:** 269-01 76th Ave, rm 267, New Hyde Park, NY 11040-1433; **Phone:** (718) 470-3450; **Board Cert:** Pediatrics 1968, Child Neurology 1977; **Med School:** Israel 1961; **Resid:** Pediatrics, Israel 1961-1966; **Fellow:** Child Neurology, UCLA Med Ctr, Los Angeles, CA 1966-1967; Neurology, UCLA Med Ctr, Los Angeles, CA 1967-1969; **Fac Appt:** Prof Neurology, Albert Einstein Coll Med

Freeman, John M MD (ChiN) - *Spec Exp:* Epilepsy/Seizure Disorders; Ketogenic Diet; **Hospital:** Johns Hopkins Hosp - Baltimore; **Address:** Johns Hopkins Hospital, 600 N Wolfe St, Meyer Bldg 2-130, Baltimore, MD 21287; **Phone:** (410) 955-9100; **Board Cert:** Pediatrics 1963, Child Neurology 1969; **Med School:** Johns Hopkins Univ 1958; **Resid:** Pediatrics, Johns Hopkins Hosp, Baltimore, MD 1959-1961; **Fellow:** Child Neurology, Columbia-Presby Med Ctr, New York, NY 1961-1964; **Fac Appt:** Prof Pediatrics, Johns Hopkins Univ

Lell, Mary-Elizabeth MD (ChiN) - *Spec Exp:* Neonatal Neurology; Learning Disorders; **Hospital:** St Vincent Cath Med Ctrs - Manhattan (page 75); **Address:** 153 W 11th St, Ste 457, New York, NY 10011; **Phone:** (212) 604-7494; **Board Cert:** Child Neurology 1976, Pediatrics 1980; **Med School:** Univ Penn 1968; **Resid:** Neurology, Univ Vermont, Burlington, VT 1969-1971; Pediatrics, St Louis Univ-Chldns Hosp, St Louis, MO 1971-1972; **Fellow:** Child Neurology, Columbia Presby Hosp, New York, NY 1972-1974; **Fac Appt:** Assoc Clin Prof Neurology, NY Med Coll

Maytal, Joseph MD (ChiN) - *Spec Exp:* Epilepsy/Seizure Disorders; Migraine; **Hospital:** Schneider's Chldns Hosp; **Address:** 269-01 76th Ave Fl 2nd - rm 267, New Hyde Park, NY 11040-1434; **Phone:** (718) 470-3450; **Board Cert:** Pediatrics 1986, Child Neurology 1988; **Med School:** Israel 1978; **Resid:** Pediatrics, Brookdale Hosp, Brooklyn, NY 1982-1983; Child Neurology, Albert Einstein Coll Med, Bronx, NY 1983-1986; **Fellow:** Neurological Physiology, Albert Einstein Med Coll, Bronx, NY 1986-1987; **Fac Appt:** Clin Prof Neurology, Albert Einstein Coll Med

Packer, Roger MD (ChiN) - *Spec Exp:* Brain Tumors; Neurofibromatosis-Type 1; **Hospital:** Chldns Natl Med Ctr - DC; **Address:** Division of Neurology, 111 Michigan Ave NW, Washington, DC 20010-2978; **Phone:** (202) 884-2120; **Board Cert:** Child Neurology 1982, Pediatrics 1982; **Med School:** Northwestern Univ 1976; **Resid:** Pediatrics, Chldns Med Ctr, Cincinnati, OH 1976-1978; Neurology, Univ Pennsylvania Chldns Hosp, Philadelphia, PA 1978-1981; **Fac Appt:** Prof Neurology, Geo Wash Univ

Patterson, Marc MD (ChiN) - *Spec Exp:* Neurogenetics; Developmental Delay; Metabolic Disease-Neurologic; **Hospital:** NY Presby Hosp; **Address:** Division of Pediatric Neurology, 180 Fort Washington Ave, Ste 542, New York, NY 10032-3710; **Phone:** (212) 305-6038; **Board Cert:** Child Neurology 1994; **Med School:** Australia 1981; **Resid:** Neurology, Univ Queenland, Brisbane, Australia 1986-1988; Child Neurology, Mayo Clinic, Rochester, MN 1988-1990; **Fellow:** Metabolic Neurology, Natl Inst Health, Bethesda, MD 1990-1992; Pediatrics, Mayo Clinic, Rochester, MN 1992-1993; **Fac Appt:** Prof Child Neurology, Columbia P&S

Southeast

Fenichel, Gerald M MD (ChiN) - *Spec Exp:* Amyotrophic Lateral Sclerosis(ALS); Neuromuscular Disorders; **Hospital:** Vanderbilt Univ Med Ctr (page 80); **Address:** Vanderbuilt Univ Sch Med, Dept Neurology, 2100 Pierce Ave, rm 351, Nashville, TN 37212; **Phone:** (615) 936-2024; **Board Cert:** Neurology 1966, Child Neurology 1968; **Med School:** Yale Univ 1959; **Resid:** Neurology, Natnl Inst Neuro Disorders-NIH, Bethesda, MD 1961-1963; Neurology, Yale-New Haven Hosp, New Haven, CT 1963-1964; **Fac Appt:** Prof Neurology, Vanderbilt Univ

Greenwood, Robert Samuel MD (ChiN) - *Spec Exp:* Child Neurology; Neurofibromatosis; Epilepsy; **Hospital:** Univ of NC Hosp (page 77); **Address:** U NC Sch Med Dept. Neurology, 751 Burnett Womack, MC-CB 7025, Chapel Hill, NC 27599; **Phone:** (919) 966-2528; **Board Cert:** Neurology 1979, Pediatrics 1974; **Med School:** Univ Tex Med Br, Galveston 1968; **Resid:** Child Neurology, Chldns Hosp., St. Louis, MO 1973-1975; Pediatrics, Chldns Hosp, St. Louis, MO 1970-1971; **Fellow:** Child Neurology, Childrens Hosp, St Louis, MO 1976-1977; **Fac Appt:** Prof Neurology, Univ NC Sch Med

Turk, William MD (ChiN) - *Spec Exp:* Epilepsy/Seizure Disorders; Headache; **Hospital:** Wolfson Children's Hosp @ Baptist Med Cen; **Address:** 807 Children's Way, Jacksonville, FL 32207; **Phone:** (904) 390-3780; **Board Cert:** Pediatrics 1981, Child Neurology 1984; **Med School:** Case West Res Univ 1976; **Resid:** Pediatrics, NC Meml Hosp, Chapel Hill, NC 1977-1979; Neurology, Barnes Hospital, St Louis, MO 1979-1980; **Fellow:** Child Neurology, St Louis Chldns Hosp, St Louis, MO 1980-1983; **Fac Appt:** Asst Prof Neurology, Univ Fla Coll Med

Midwest

Epstein, Leon G MD (ChiN) - *Spec Exp:* AIDS/HIV; **Hospital:** Children's Mem Hosp; **Address:** 2300 Childrens Plaza, Box 51, Div Neurology, Chicago, IL 60614; **Phone:** (773) 880-4352; **Board Cert:** Child Neurology 1979; **Med School:** Wayne State Univ 1973; **Resid:** Neurology, St Joseph's Mercy-Univ Michigan, Ann Arbor, MI 1973-1974; Neurology, Univ Arizona, Tucson, AZ 1974-1976; **Fellow:** Neurology, Columbia Presby Med Ctr, New York, NY 1976-1978; **Fac Appt:** Prof Pediatrics, Northwestern Univ

Nigro, Michael A DO (ChiN) - *Spec Exp:* Neurologic Disorders; Neuromuscular Disorders; **Hospital:** Chldns Hosp of Michigan (page 59); **Address:** Michigan Inst for Neur Disorders, 28595 Orchard Lake Rd, Ste 200, Farmington Hill, MI 48334; **Phone:** (248) 553-0010; **Board Cert:** Neurology 1975, Clinical Neurophysiology 1996; **Med School:** Philadelphia Coll Osteo Med 1966; **Resid:** Neurology, Detroit Osteo Hosp, Highland Park, MI 1967-1970; Child Neurology, Childrens Hosp/Univ Penn, Philadelphia, PA 1970-1972; **Fac Appt:** Prof Child Neurology, Wayne State Univ

Noetzel, Michael MD (ChiN) - *Spec Exp:* Cerebral Palsy; Epilepsy/Seizure Disorders; Movement Disorders; **Hospital:** St Louis Children's Hospital; **Address:** 1 Children's Pl, Ste 12E25, St Louis, MO 63110; **Phone:** (314) 454-6120; **Board Cert:** Child Neurology 1984, Pediatrics 1984; **Med School:** Univ VA Sch Med 1977; **Resid:** Pediatrics, St Louis Chldns Hosp, St Louis, MO 1978-1979; Neurology, Barnes Hosp, St Louis, MO 1979-1980; **Fellow:** Child Neurology, St Louis Chldns Hosp, St Louis, MO 1980-1982; **Fac Appt:** Assoc Prof Child Neurology, Washington Univ, St Louis

Prensky, Arthur MD (ChiN) - *Spec Exp:* Headache; **Hospital:** St Louis Children's Hospital; **Address:** 1 Children's Pl, Ste 12E25, St Louis, MO 63110; **Phone:** (314) 454-6120; **Board Cert:** Neurology 1966, Child Neurology 1969; **Med School:** NYU Sch Med 1955; **Resid:** Neurology, Mass Genl Hosp, Boston, Ma 1960-1963; **Fellow:** Neurology, Mass Genl Hosp, Boston, Ma 1963-1966; **Fac Appt:** Prof Neurology, Washington Univ, St Louis

CHILD NEUROLOGY

Stumpf, David A MD (ChiN) - *Spec Exp:* Ataxia; Epilepsy/Seizure Disorders; **Hospital:** Northwestern Meml Hosp; **Address:** 675 N St Clair St Fl 20 - Ste 100, Chicago, IL 60611; **Phone:** (312) 695-7950; **Board Cert:** Child Neurology 1979, Pediatrics 1978; **Med School:** Univ Colo 1972; **Resid:** Pediatrics, Strong Meml Hosp, Rochester, NY 1973-1974; Neurology, Childrens Hosp, Boston, MA 1974-1977; **Fac Appt:** Prof Neurology, Northwestern Univ

Wyllie, Elaine MD (ChiN) - *Spec Exp:* Epilepsy/Seizure Disorders; **Hospital:** Cleveland Clin Fdn (page 57); **Address:** 9500 Euclid Ave, Desk S51, Cleveland, OH 44195; **Phone:** (216) 444-2095; **Board Cert:** Pediatrics 1982, Child Neurology 1986; **Med School:** Indiana Univ 1978; **Resid:** Pediatrics, Indiana Univ Sch Med, Indianapolis, IN 1978-1980; Pediatrics, Case West Res Med Sch, Cleveland, OH 1980-1981; **Fellow:** Child Neurology, Cleveland Clinic Fdn, Cleveland, OH 1981-1984; Clinical Neurophysiology, Cleveland Clinic Fdn, Cleveland, OH 1984-1985

Great Plains and Mountains

Bale Jr, James MD (ChiN) - *Spec Exp:* Epilepsy/Seizure Disorders; **Hospital:** Primary Children's Med Ctr; **Address:** Primary Chldns Med Ctr, 100 N Medical , Ste 2700, Salt Lake City, UT 84113; **Phone:** (801) 588-3385; **Board Cert:** Child Neurology 1982, Pediatrics 1993; **Med School:** Univ Mich Med Sch 1975; **Resid:** Pediatrics, Univ Utah, Salt Lake City, UT 1975-1977; Neurology, Univ Utah, Salt Lake City, UT 1977-1980; **Fellow:** Infectious Disease, Univ Utah, Salt Lake City, UT 1980-1981; Neurological Virus, UC San Fran-VAMC, San Francisco, CA 1981-1982; **Fac Appt:** Prof Neurology, Univ Utah

Southwest

Edgar, Terence MD (ChiN) - *Spec Exp:* Neuromuscular Disorders; Cerebral Palsy; **Hospital:** Arkansas Chldns Hosp; **Address:** Dept Neurology, 800 Marshall St, Box 512, Little Rock, AR 72202; **Phone:** (501) 320-1850; **Board Cert:** Child Neurology 1997, Pediatrics 1995; **Med School:** South Africa 1984; **Resid:** Pediatrics, Univ of Pretoria, Pretoria, South Africa 1989-1992; Pediatrics, Univ Wisconsin Hosp & Clin, Madison, WI 1992-1993; **Fellow:** Child Neurology, Univ Wisconsin Hosp & Clin, Madison, WI 1993-1996; **Fac Appt:** Asst Prof Pediatrics, Univ Ark

Fishman, Marvin Allen MD (ChiN) - *Spec Exp:* Child Neurology - General; **Hospital:** TX Chldns Hosp - Houston; **Address:** 6621 Fannin St, CC1710, Houston, TX 77030; **Phone:** (832) 822-1750; **Board Cert:** Pediatrics 1966, Child Neurology 1972; **Med School:** Univ IL Coll Med 1961; **Resid:** Pediatrics, Michael Reese Hosp, Chicago, IL 1962-1964; Child Neurology, Mass Genl Hosp, Boston, MA 1966-1967; **Fellow:** Child Neurology, Chldns Hosp, St Louis, MO 1967-1969; **Fac Appt:** Prof Child Neurology, Baylor Coll Med

Iannaccone, Susan MD (ChiN) - *Spec Exp:* Neuromuscular Disorders; **Hospital:** Texas Scottish Rite Hosp for Children - Dallas; **Address:** 2222 Welborn St, Dallas, TX 75219-3924; **Phone:** (214) 559-7830; **Board Cert:** Pediatrics 1975, Child Neurology 1976; **Med School:** SUNY Hlth Sci Ctr 1969; **Resid:** Pediatrics, St Louis Childrens Hosp-Washington 1971-1972; Neurology, Strong Meml Hosp, Rochester, NY 1972-1975; **Fellow:** Neurology, Strong Meml Hosp, Rochester, NY 1972-1975; **Fac Appt:** Assoc Prof Neurology, Univ Cincinnati

West Coast and Pacific

Ashwal, Stephen MD (ChiN) - *Spec Exp:* Child Neurology - General; **Hospital:** Loma Linda Univ Med Ctr; **Address:** 11370 Anderson St, Ste B100, Loma Linda, CA 92354; **Phone:** (909) 558-2848; **Board Cert:** Pediatrics 1975, Child Neurology 1978; **Med School:** NYU Sch Med 1970; **Resid:** Pediatrics, Bellevue Hosp, New York, NY 1971-1973; **Fellow:** Child Neurology, Univ Minn, Minneapolis, MN 1973-1976; **Fac Appt:** Prof Pediatrics, Loma Linda Univ

Ferriero, Donna Marie MD (ChiN) - *Spec Exp:* *Neuro-Endocrinology;* **Hospital:** UCSF Med Ctr; **Address:** Box 0136, 500 Parnassus Ave, San Francisco, CA 94143; **Phone:** (415) 353-2605; **Board Cert:** Child Neurology 1987, Pediatrics 1986; **Med School:** UCSF 1979; **Resid:** Pediatrics, Mass Genl Hosp, Boston, MA 1981-1982; Child Neurology, UCSF, San Francisco, CA 1982-1985; **Fellow:** Neurological Endocrinology, UCSF, San Francisco, CA 1985-1987

Haas, Richard H MD (ChiN) - *Spec Exp:* *Mitochondrial Disorders;* **Hospital:** UCSD Healthcare; **Address:** 9500 Gilman Drive, La Jolla, CA 92093-0935; **Phone:** (858) 587-4004; **Board Cert:** Child Neurology 1983, Pediatrics 1985; **Med School:** England 1972; **Resid:** Pediatrics, Univ London, London, UK 1976-1979; Child Neurology, Univ Colorado, Denver, CO 1979-1981; **Fellow:** Biochemical Mental Retardation, Univ Colorado, Denver, CO 1979-1981; **Fac Appt:** Assoc Prof Child Neurology, UCSD

Lott, Ira T MD (ChiN) - *Spec Exp:* *Down Syndrome;* **Hospital:** UCI Med Ctr; **Address:** UC Irvine Med Ctr, Pavilion 1, Dept Ped/Neurology, 101 City Dr S, Orange, CA 92868-3201; **Phone:** (714) 456-7002; **Board Cert:** Pediatrics 1975, Child Neurology 1977; **Med School:** Ohio State Univ 1967; **Resid:** Pediatrics, Mass Genl Hosp, Boston, MA 1967-1969; **Fellow:** Research, Natl Inst Hlth, Bethesda, MD 1969-1971; Neurology, Harvard-Mass Genl Hosp, Boston, MA 1971-1974; **Fac Appt:** Prof Child Neurology, UC Irvine

Menkes, John H MD (ChiN) - *Spec Exp:* *Genetic Disorders; Movement Disorders;* **Hospital:** Cedars-Sinai Med Ctr; **Address:** 9320 Wilshire Blvd, Ste 202, Beverly Hills, CA 90212-3216; **Phone:** (310) 246-6582; **Board Cert:** Pediatrics 1958, Neurology 1962; **Med School:** Johns Hopkins Univ 1952; **Resid:** Pediatrics, Boston Children's Hosp, Boston, MA 1952-1954; Pediatrics, Bellevue Hosp Ctr, New York, NY 1956-1957; **Fellow:** Child Neurology, Neurological Inst, New York, NY 1957-1960; **Fac Appt:** Prof Emeritus Child Neurology, UCLA

Mitchell, Wendy Gayle MD (ChiN) - *Spec Exp:* *Epilepsy/Seizure Disorders; Developmental Disorders, Autism; Cysticercosis;* **Hospital:** Chldns Hosp - Los Angeles; **Address:** Children's Hosp Los Angeles, Dept Neuro, 4650 Sunset Blvd, Box 82, Los Angeles, CA 90027; **Phone:** (323) 669-2471; **Board Cert:** Pediatrics 1978, Child Neurology 1983; **Med School:** UCSF 1973; **Resid:** Pediatrics, Moffit Hosp-UCSF, San Francisco, CA 1973-1975; Child Neurology, Univ NC, Chapel Hill, NC 1978-1981; **Fellow:** Child Psychiatry, Mt Zion Hosp, San Francisco, CA 1975-1976; **Fac Appt:** Prof Neurology, USC Sch Med

Mobley, William Charles MD (ChiN) - *Spec Exp:* *Child Neurology - General;* **Hospital:** Stanford Med Ctr; **Address:** 1201 Welch Rd, MSLS Bldg, rm P205, Palo Alto, CA 94305; **Phone:** (650) 723-6424; **Board Cert:** Pediatrics 1983, Child Neurology 1987; **Med School:** Stanford Univ 1976; **Resid:** Pediatrics, Stanford Univ Schl Med, Stanford, CA 1977-1979; Neurology, Johns Hopkins Hosp, Baltimore, MD 1979-1982; **Fac Appt:** Prof Neurology, UCSF

Shields, William Donald MD (ChiN) - *Spec Exp:* *Epilepsy/Seizure Disorders;* **Hospital:** UCLA Med Ctr; **Address:** UCLA Med Ctr, Dept Ped/Neurology, 10833 Le Conte Ave, Los Angeles, CA 90095; **Phone:** (310) 825-6196; **Board Cert:** Child Neurology 1977, Pediatrics 1978; **Med School:** Univ Utah 1971; **Resid:** Pediatrics, USC Med Ctr, Los Angeles, CA 1971-1973; Neurology, Univ Utah Med Ctr, Salt Lake City, UT 1973-1976; **Fac Appt:** Prof Pediatrics, UCLA

Trauner, Doris Ann MD (ChiN) - *Spec Exp:* *Autism; Speech Disorders;* **Hospital:** UCSD Healthcare; **Address:** UCSD Med Ctr, Div Ped Neuro, 9500 Gilman Dr, MC-0935, La Jolla, CA 92093-0935; **Phone:** (858) 587-4004; **Board Cert:** Pediatrics 1978, Child Neurology 1979; **Med School:** Med Coll VA 1972; **Resid:** Neurology, UCSD Med Ctr, San Diego, CA 1974-1975; Pediatrics, UCSD Med Ctr, San Diego, CA 1973-1974; **Fellow:** Child Neurology, Univ Chicago, Chicago, IL 1975-1977; **Fac Appt:** Prof Pediatrics, UCSD

163

CLINICAL GENETICS

A specialist trained in diagnostic and therapeutic procedures for patients with genetically-linked diseases. This specialist uses modern cytogenetic, radiologic and biochemical testing to assist in specialized genetic counseling, implements needed therapeutic interventions and provides prevention through prenatal diagnosis.

A clinical geneticist demonstrates competence in providing comprehensive diagnostic, management and counseling services for genetic disorders.

A medical geneticist plans and coordinates large scale screening programs for inborn errors of metabolism, hemoglobinopathies, chromosome abnormalities and neural tube defects.

Training required: Two or four years

THE MOUNT SINAI HOSPITAL

Human Genetics

One Gustave L. Levy Place (Fifth Avenue and 98th Street)
New York, NY 10029-6574   Phone: (212) 241-6500
Physician Referral: 1-800-MD-SINAI (637-4624)
www.mountsinai.org

The Department of Human Genetics at the Mount Sinai Hospital is one of the largest medical genetics units in the country, providing expert diagnostic, therapeutic, and counseling services for patients and families with genetic disorders, birth defects, and pregnancy loss. The Department performs sophisticated diagnostic tests in its state-of-the-art DNA, biochemical, and cytogenetics laboratories.

The Department has over 30 internationally recognized physician and scientist faculty, ten experienced genetic counselors, and a full support and research staff of over 150 people who provide expert clinical services.

Programs offered by the Department include:

- Comprehensive Genetic Diagnostic and Counseling Services:

    Genetic Screening Program

    Prenatal Diagnostic Services

    Cancer Genetic Counseling Program

- The Center for Jewish Genetic Disease- the first such center in the world.
- Program for Inherited Metabolic Diseases
- The Comprehensive Gaucher Disease Treatment Program
- The International Center for Fabry Disease
- The International Center for Types A and B Niemann-Pick Disease

Groundbreaking Research and New Forms of Treatment
Almost everyone has a disease or condition that runs in the family, in fact, there are over 10,000 known genetic disorders, and current research is identifying the genetic susceptibilities or predispositions for many common diseases and cancers. Towards this goal, the Department Of Human Genetics is performing research to develop new or improved methods for the diagnosis, prevention, and treatment of these diseases and disorders. The Human Genome Project and the advances in gene therapy have accelerated this research.

THE MOUNT SINAI HOSPITAL

Advances in Diagnosis and Disease Treatment
In the past two years alone, Mount Sinai researchers have had remarkable success identifying the genes responsible for seven genetic diseases and in developing new treatments for two inherited disorders.

Following are some examples:

Research pioneered by Mount Sinai's Department of Human Genetics has developed a safe and effective treatment for **Fabry Disease,** an inherited metabolic disorder that results in kidney failure, heart disease, strokes, and premature death.

In addition, our department has made remarkable progress toward the development of treatment for **Niemann-Pick Type B Disease,** a hereditary disorder that results in death in childhood or early adulthood.

We have recently identified the genes responsible for a several diseases, including a debilitating juvenile arthritis syndrome. The identification of this gene may lead to greater understanding and new treatments for arthritis.

Because our researchers have identified the gene causing **Noonan Syndrome,** a common genetic disorder that causes congenital heart defects, affected families can now receive early diagnosis and prevention.

PHYSICIAN LISTINGS

Clinical Genetics

New England

Holmes, Lewis B MD (CG) - *Spec Exp:* Birth Defects; Inherited Diseases; **Hospital:** MA Genl Hosp; **Address:** 55 Fruit St, Bldg Warren 801, Boston, MA 02114-2696; **Phone:** (617) 726-1742; **Board Cert:** Pediatrics 1968, Clinical Genetics 1982; **Med School:** Duke Univ 1963; **Resid:** Pediatrics, Mass Genl Hosp, Boston, MA; **Fac Appt:** Prof Pediatrics, Harvard Med Sch

Korf, Bruce MD/PhD (CG) - *Spec Exp:* Inherited Diseases; Neuro-Genetics; **Hospital:** Brigham & Women's Hosp; **Address:** Partners Center for Human Genetics, 77 Avenue Louis Pasteur, Bldg HIM - Fl 6 - Ste 642, Boston, MA 02115; **Phone:** (617) 525-5750; **Board Cert:** Clinical Genetics 1984, Child Neurology 1986; **Med School:** Cornell Univ-Weill Med Coll 1980; **Resid:** Pediatrics, Chldns Hosp, Boston, MA 1981-1982; Neurology, Chldns Hosp, Boston, MA 1982-1985; **Fellow:** Clinical Genetics, Chldns Hosp, Boston, MA 1982-1985; **Fac Appt:** Assoc Prof Neurology, Harvard Med Sch

Mahoney, Maurice J MD (CG) - *Spec Exp:* Clinical Genetics - General; **Hospital:** Yale - New Haven Hosp; **Address:** Yale Genetics Consultation Serv, 333 Cedar St, rm WWW330, New Haven, CT 06520-3206; **Phone:** (203) 785-2661; **Board Cert:** Pediatrics 1967, Clinical Genetics 1982, Clinical Biochemical Genetics 1982; **Med School:** Univ Pittsburgh 1962; **Resid:** Pediatrics, Johns Hopkins Hosp, Baltimore, MD 1963-1965; Pediatrics, Childrens Hosp, Pittsburgh, PA 1965-1966; **Fellow:** Clinical Genetics, Yale Univ Sch Med, New Haven, CT 1968-1970; **Fac Appt:** Prof Clinical Genetics, Yale Univ

Seashore, Margretta MD (CG) - *Spec Exp:* Inherited Metabolic Disorders; **Hospital:** Yale - New Haven Hosp; **Address:** Yale Univ Sch Med, Dept Genetics, 333 Cedar St, rm 305, New Haven, CT 06520; **Phone:** (203) 785-2660; **Board Cert:** Clinical Genetics 1982, Pediatrics 1970; **Med School:** Yale Univ 1965; **Resid:** Pediatrics, Yale-New Haven Hosp, New Haven, CT 1966-1968; **Fellow:** Clinical Genetics, Yale-New Haven Hosp, New Haven, CT 1968-1970; **Fac Appt:** Prof Clinical Genetics, Yale Univ

Mid Atlantic

Anyane-Yeboa, Kwame MD (CG) - *Spec Exp:* Syndromology; Prenatal Genetic Diagnosis; **Hospital:** NY Presby Hosp - Columbia Presby Med Ctr (page 70); **Address:** Babies and Childrens Hosp, 3959 Broadway Fl 6 - Ste 601A, New York, NY 10032; **Phone:** (212) 305-6731; **Board Cert:** Clinical Genetics 1982, Pediatrics 1979; **Med School:** Ghana 1972; **Resid:** Pediatrics, Harlem Hosp, New York, NY 1974-1977; **Fellow:** Clinical Genetics, Babies Hosp-Columbia, New York, NY 1977-1980; **Fac Appt:** Assoc Prof Pediatrics, Columbia P&S

Biesecker, Leslie Glenn MD (CG) - *Spec Exp:* Clinical Genetics - General; **Hospital:** Natl Inst of Hlth - Clin Ctr; **Address:** 9000 Rockville Pike, Bldg 49, Ste 4A80, Bethesda, MD 20892; **Phone:** (301) 402-2041; **Board Cert:** Pediatrics 1987, Clinical Genetics 1990; **Med School:** Univ IL Coll Med 1983; **Resid:** Pediatrics, Univ Wisc Hosp, Madison, WI 1984-1986; **Fellow:** Clinical Genetics, Univ Mich Med Ctr, Ann Arbor, MI 1988-1990

Davis, Jessica S MD (CG) - *Spec Exp:* Marfan's Syndrome; Mental Retardation; Neurofibromatosis; **Hospital:** NY Presby Hosp - NY Weill Cornell Med Ctr (page 70); **Address:** 525 E 68th St Bldg HT150, Box 28, New York, NY 10021; **Phone:** (212) 746-1496; **Board Cert:** Clinical Genetics 1984; **Med School:** Columbia P&S 1959; **Resid:** Pediatrics, St Luke's Hosp, New York, NY 1961-1962; **Fellow:** Clinical Genetics, Albert Einstein Coll Med, Bronx, NY 1961-1965; Cytogenetics, Albert Einstein Col Med, Bronx, NY 1965-1966; **Fac Appt:** Assoc Clin Prof Pediatrics, Cornell Univ-Weill Med Coll

Desnick, Robert J MD/PhD (CG) - *Spec Exp:* Porphyria; Fabry's Disease, Gaucher Disease; Inherited Metabolic Disorders; **Hospital:** Mount Sinai Hosp (page 68); **Address:** Mt Sinai Sch Med, Box 1498, Fifth Ave @ 100th Street, New York, NY 10029; **Phone:** (212) 659-6700; **Board Cert:** Clinical Genetics 1982, Clinical Molecular Genetics 1999, Clinical Biochemical Genetics 1982; **Med School:** Univ Minn 1971; **Resid:** Pediatrics, Univ Minn Hosps, Minneapolis, MN 1972-1973; **Fac Appt:** Prof Clinical Genetics, Mount Sinai Sch Med

Desposito, Franklin MD (CG) - *Spec Exp:* Birth Defects; Genetic Disorders; **Hospital:** UMDNJ-Univ Hosp-Newark; **Address:** MSB-F540, 185 S Orange Ave, Newark, NJ 07103; **Phone:** (973) 972-3300; **Board Cert:** Pediatrics 1986, Clinical Genetics 1982; **Med School:** Univ Hlth Sci/Chicago Med Sch 1957; **Resid:** Pediatrics, Long Island Jewish Hosp, New Hyde Park, NY 1958-1961; **Fellow:** Hematology, Univ Wisc Sch Med, Milwaukee, WI 1961-1963; **Fac Appt:** Prof Pediatrics, UMDNJ-NJ Med Sch, Newark

Marion, Robert MD (CG) - *Spec Exp:* Genetic Disorders; **Hospital:** Montefiore Med Ctr (page 67); **Address:** 111 E 210th St, Bronx, NY 10467; **Phone:** (718) 920-4300; **Board Cert:** Pediatrics 1985, Clinical Genetics 1987; **Med School:** Albert Einstein Coll Med 1979; **Resid:** Pediatrics, Montefiore Med Ctr, Bronx, NY 1980-1982; **Fellow:** Clinical Genetics, Montefiore Med Ctr, Bronx, NY 1982-1984; **Fac Appt:** Prof Pediatrics, Albert Einstein Coll Med

Nussbaum, Robert MD (CG) - *Spec Exp:* Genetic Disorders; **Hospital:** Natl Inst of Hlth - Clin Ctr; **Address:** Natl Human Gen Res Inst, 49 Convent Dr MSC 4472, Bethesda, MD 20892; **Phone:** (301) 402-2039; **Board Cert:** Internal Medicine 1978, Clinical Genetics 1982; **Med School:** Harvard Med Sch 1975; **Resid:** Internal Medicine, Barnes Hospital, St Louis, MO 1976-1978; **Fellow:** Clinical Genetics, Baylor, Houston, TX 1978-1983; **Fac Appt:** Prof Clinical Genetics, Univ Penn

Rosenbaum, Kenneth MD (CG) - *Spec Exp:* Clinical Genetics - General; **Hospital:** Chldns Natl Med Ctr - DC; **Address:** 111 Michigan Ave NW, Washington, DC 20010; **Phone:** (202) 884-2187; **Board Cert:** Pediatrics 1976, Clinical Genetics 1982; **Med School:** Univ Louisville Sch Med 1971

Shapiro, Lawrence R MD (CG) - *Spec Exp:* Clinical Genetics - General; **Hospital:** Westchester Med Ctr (page 82); **Address:** Regional Med Genetics Ctr, 19 Bradhurst Ave, Ste 1600, Hawthorne, NY 10532; **Phone:** (914) 347-3010; **Board Cert:** Pediatrics 1967, Clinical Genetics 1982; **Med School:** NYU Sch Med 1962; **Resid:** Pediatrics, Los Angeles Chldns Hosp, Los Angeles, CA 1962-1964; Pediatrics, Bellevue Hosp, New York, NY 1964-1965; **Fellow:** Clinical Genetics, NYU, New York, NY 1965; Clinical Genetics, Mount Sinai Med Ctr, New York, NY 1967-1968; **Fac Appt:** Prof Pediatrics, NY Med Coll

Willner, Judith P MD (CG) - *Spec Exp:* Dysmorphology; Birth Defects; Metabolic Genetic Disorders; **Hospital:** Mount Sinai Hosp (page 68); **Address:** 1 Gustave Levy Pl, Box 1497, New York, NY 10029; **Phone:** (212) 241-6947; **Board Cert:** Pediatrics 1977, Clinical Genetics 1982; **Med School:** NYU Sch Med 1971; **Resid:** Pediatrics, Children's Hosp Natl Med Ctr, Washington, DC 1972-1973; **Fellow:** Clinical Genetics, Mount Sinai Hosp, New York, NY 1974-1977; **Fac Appt:** Prof Clinical Genetics, Mount Sinai Sch Med

Zackai, Elaine MD (CG) - *Spec Exp:* Craniosynostosis; Cytogenetic Disorders; **Hospital:** Chldn's Hosp of Philadelphia; **Address:** Dept Clinical Genetics, 34th & Civic Center Blvd, Rm 2150, Philadelphia, PA 19104; **Phone:** (215) 590-2920; **Board Cert:** Clinical Genetics 1982, Pediatrics 1977; **Med School:** NYU Sch Med 1968; **Resid:** Pediatrics, Albert Einstein Med Sch, Bronx, NY 1968-1969; Pediatrics, Chldns Hosp, St Louis, MO 1969-1970; **Fellow:** Clinical Genetics, Chldns Hosp, St Louis, MO 1970-1971; Clinical Genetics, Yale Univ Med Sch, New Haven, CT 1971-1972; **Fac Appt:** Prof Pediatrics, Univ Penn

Southeast

Driscoll, Daniel J MD (CG) - *Spec Exp:* Angelman Syndrome; Prader-Willi Syndrome; Obesity; **Hospital:** Shands Hlthcre at Univ of FL (page 73); **Address:** Univ Florida-Pediatric Genetics, 1600 SW Archer Rd, Box 100296, Gainesville, FL 32610-0296; **Phone:** (352) 392-4104; **Board Cert:** Pediatrics 1987, Clinical Genetics 1990; **Med School:** Albany Med Coll 1983; **Resid:** Pediatrics, Johns Hopkins Hosp, Baltimore, MD 1983-1986; **Fellow:** Clinical Genetics, Johns Hopkins Hosp, Baltimore, MD 1986-1989; **Fac Appt:** Assoc Prof Pediatrics, Univ Fla Coll Med

Elsas II, Louis Jacob MD (CG) - *Spec Exp:* Urine Maple Syrup Disease; **Hospital:** Chldn's Hlthcre of Atlanta - Scottish Rite; **Address:** Div Med Genetics, 2040 Ridgewood Drive, Atlanta, GA 30322; **Phone:** (404) 727-5863; **Board Cert:** Clinical Molecular Genetics 1996, Clinical Genetics 1982, Clinical Biochemical Genetics 1982, Internal Medicine 1972; **Med School:** Univ VA Sch Med 1962; **Resid:** Internal Medicine, Yale-New Haven Hosp, New Haven, CT 1963-1965; **Fellow:** Clinical Genetics, New HAven Hosp-Yale, New Haven, CT 1965-1968; **Fac Appt:** Prof Pediatrics, Emory Univ

Saul, Robert MD (CG) - *Spec Exp:* Birth Defects; **Hospital:** Self Regional Healthcare; **Address:** Greenwood Genetic Ctr, One Gregor Mendel Cir, Greenwood, SC 29646-2307; **Phone:** (864) 941-8100; **Board Cert:** Pediatrics 1981, Clinical Genetics 1982; **Med School:** Univ Colo 1976; **Resid:** Pediatrics, Duke Med Ctr, Durham, NC 1976-1979; **Fellow:** Clinical Genetics, Greenwood Genetics Ctr, Greenwood, SC 1979-1981

Seaver, Laurie Heron MD (CG) - *Spec Exp:* Fetal Pathology; Fetal Alcohol Syndrome; **Hospital:** Self Regional Healthcare; **Address:** Greenwood Genetic Ctr, One Gregor Mendel Cir, Greenwood, SC 29646; **Phone:** (864) 941-8100; **Board Cert:** Pediatrics 1998, Clinical Genetics 1993; **Med School:** Univ Ariz Coll Med 1987; **Resid:** Pediatrics, Univ Ariz, Tucson, AZ 1988-1990; **Fellow:** Clinical Genetics, Univ Ariz Coll Med, Tucson, AZ 1990-1993

Stevenson, Roger E MD (CG) - *Spec Exp:* Birth Defects; Mental Retardation; **Hospital:** Self Regional Healthcare; **Address:** Greenwood Genetic Ctr, One Gregor Mendel Cir, Greenwood, SC 29646-2307; **Phone:** (864) 941-8100; **Board Cert:** Pediatrics 1971, Clinical Genetics 1982, Clinical Cytogenetics 1984; **Med School:** Wake Forest Univ Sch Med 1966; **Resid:** Pediatrics, Johns Hopkins Hosp, Baltimore, MD 1967-1969; **Fellow:** Clinical Genetics, Johns Hopkins Hosp, Baltimore, MD 1971-1972

Midwest

Charrow, Joel MD (CG) - *Spec Exp:* Biochemical Genetics; Lysosomal Diseases; Neurofibromatosis; **Hospital:** Children's Mem Hosp; **Address:** Chldns Meml. Hosp. - Div. Genetics, 2300 Chldn Plaza, MS 59, Chicago, IL 60614-3318; **Phone:** (773) 880-4462; **Board Cert:** Clinical Biochemical Genetics 1987, Clinical Genetics 1982, Pediatrics 1980; **Med School:** Mount Sinai Sch Med 1976; **Resid:** Pediatrics, Chldns Meml Hosp-Northwestern U., Chicago, IL 1977-1979; **Fellow:** Clinical Genetics, Chldns Meml Hosp-Northwestern U., Chicago, IL 1979-1981; **Fac Appt:** Assoc Prof Pediatrics, Northwestern Univ

Gray, Diana Lee MD (CG) - *Spec Exp:* Prenatal Diagnosis; **Hospital:** Barnes-Jewish Hosp (page 55); **Address:** Barnes-Jewish Hosp, Dept ObGyn, 216 S Kingshighway Blvd, Ste 5300, MS 90-31-644, St Louis, MO 63110; **Phone:** (314) 454-8135; **Board Cert:** Obstetrics & Gynecology 1996, Clinical Genetics 1993; **Med School:** Univ IL Coll Med 1981; **Resid:** Obstetrics & Gynecology, Wash Univ, St Louis, MO 1982-1985; Obstetrics & Gynecology, Wash Univ, St Louis, MO 1985-1987; **Fellow:** Obstetrics & Gynecology, Wash Univ, St Louis, MO 1985-1987; Clinical Genetics, Wash Univ, St Louis, MO 1988-1990; **Fac Appt:** Assoc Prof Clinical Genetics, Washington Univ, St Louis

Martin, Rick A MD (CG) - *Spec Exp:* Dysmorphology; **Hospital:** St Louis Children's Hospital; **Address:** 1 Children's Pl, Ste 4S30, St Louis, MO 63110; **Phone:** (314) 454-6093; **Board Cert:** Pediatrics 1998, Clinical Genetics 1993; **Med School:** Univ Utah 1987; **Resid:** Pediatrics, UCSD, San Diego, CA 1988-1990; **Fellow:** Clinical Genetics, UCSD, San Diego, CA 1990-1992; **Fac Appt:** Assoc Prof Clinical Genetics, Washington Univ, St Louis

Saal, Howard MD (CG) - *Spec Exp:* Craniofacial Disorders; Cleft Palate/Lip; Neurofibromatosis; **Hospital:** Cincinnati Chldns Hosp Med Ctr; **Address:** 3333 Burnett Ave, Box MLC 4006, Cinncinnati, OH 45219; **Phone:** (513) 636-4760; **Board Cert:** Clinical Genetics 1984, Pediatrics 1985; **Med School:** Wayne State Univ 1979; **Resid:** Pediatrics, Univ Conn Hlth Ctr, Farmington, CT 1979-1982; **Fellow:** Clinical Genetics, Univ Wash, Seattle, WA 1982-1984; **Fac Appt:** Prof Pediatrics, Univ Cincinnati

Weaver, David Dawson MD (CG) - *Spec Exp:* Inherited Bone Disorders; Genetic Disorders; Prenatal Diagnosis; **Hospital:** IN Univ Hosp (page 63); **Address:** 975 W Walnut St, Bldg IB - Ste 130, Indianapolis, IN 46202-5251; **Phone:** (317) 274-2241; **Board Cert:** Pediatrics 1978, Clinical Genetics 1982; **Med School:** Oregon Hlth Scis Univ 1966; **Resid:** Pediatrics, Oregon Hlth Scis Univ Sch Med, Portland, OR 1970-1972; **Fellow:** Metabolic Diseases, Oregon Hlth Scis Univ Sch Med, Portland, OR 1974-1976; Clinical Genetics, Univ WA Sch Med, Seattle, WA; **Fac Appt:** Prof Clinical Genetics, Indiana Univ

Whelan, Alison MD (CG) - *Spec Exp:* Clinical Genetics - General; **Hospital:** Barnes-Jewish Hosp (page 55); **Address:** 660 S Euclid Ave, Box 8073, St Louis, MO 63110; **Phone:** (314) 454-6093; **Board Cert:** Clinical Genetics 1996; **Med School:** Washington Univ, St Louis 1986; **Resid:** Internal Medicine, Barnes Hosp, St Louis, MO 1987-1989; Pediatrics, Wash U Sch Med, St Louis, MO 1992-1994; **Fellow:** Research, Wash U Sch Med, St Louis, MO 1989-1991; Clinical Genetics, Wash U Sch Med, St Louis, MO 1993-1994; **Fac Appt:** Asst Prof Medicine, Washington Univ, St Louis

Great Plains and Mountains

Carey, John MD (CG) - *Spec Exp:* Neurofibromatosis; Birth Defects; **Hospital:** Univ Utah Hosp and Clin; **Address:** Univ Utah Med Ctr-Div of Med Gen, 50 N Med Dr, 2C412SOM, Salt Lake City, UT 84132-0001; **Phone:** (801) 581-8943; **Board Cert:** Pediatrics 1979, Clinical Genetics 1982; **Med School:** Georgetown Univ 1972; **Resid:** Pediatrics, UCSF Med Ctr, San Francisco, CA 1973-1975; **Fellow:** Clinical Genetics, UCSF Med Ctr, San Francisco, CA 1976-1979; **Fac Appt:** Prof Medicine, Univ Utah

Southwest

Craigen, William MD (CG) - *Spec Exp:* Biochemical Genetics; Mitochondrial Diseases; **Hospital:** TX Chldns Hosp - Houston; **Address:** Dept Molecular & Human Genetics, 1 Baylor Plaza, S-821, Houston, TX 77030; **Phone:** (713) 798-8305; **Board Cert:** Pediatrics 1992, Clinical Genetics 1993, Clinical Biochemical Genetics 1993; **Med School:** Baylor Coll Med 1988; **Resid:** Pediatrics, Baylor Coll Med, Houston, TX 1988-1990; Pediatrics, Baylor Coll Med, Houston, TX 1990-1992; **Fellow:** Clinical Genetics, Baylor Coll Med, Houston, TX 1988-1990; **Fac Appt:** Assoc Prof Clinical Genetics, Baylor Coll Med

Cunniff, Christopher MD (CG) - *Spec Exp:* Birth Defects; **Hospital:** Univ Med Ctr; **Address:** U Ariz Coll Med-Dept Ped, Sect Med Genetics, 1501 N Campbell Ave, Box 24-5073, Tucson, AZ 85724; **Phone:** (520) 626-5175; **Board Cert:** Pediatrics 1996, Clinical Genetics 1990; **Med School:** Univ Ala 1984; **Resid:** Pediatrics, MC Hosp Vermont, Burlington, VT 1985-1987; **Fellow:** Clinical Genetics, UCSD Med Ctr, San Diego, CA 1987-1989; **Fac Appt:** Assoc Prof Pediatrics, Univ Ariz Coll Med

Huff, Robert Whitley MD (CG) - *Spec Exp:* Genetic Disorders; Obstetrics & Gynecology; **Hospital:** Univ of Texas Hlth & Sci Ctr; **Address:** UT Hlth Scis, Dept OB/GYN, 7703 Floyd Curl Drive, San Antonio, TX 78229-3901; **Phone:** (210) 567-4999; **Board Cert:** Obstetrics & Gynecology 1974, Maternal & Fetal Medicine 1979, Clinical Genetics 1990; **Med School:** Baylor Coll Med 1966; **Resid:** Obstetrics & Gynecology, Bexar Co Hosp, San Antonio, TX 1969-1972; **Fac Appt:** Prof Obstetrics & Gynecology, Univ Tex, San Antonio

Northrup, Hope MD (CG) - *Spec Exp:* Biochemical Genetics; Neuro-Genetics; Dysmorphology; **Hospital:** Meml Hermann Hosp; **Address:** Univ TX Med Sch-Houston-Dept Peds-Div Med Genetics, 6431 Fannin St, Houston, TX 77030-1501; **Phone:** (713) 500-5760; **Board Cert:** Pediatrics 1988, Clinical Genetics 1990, Clinical Biochemical Genetics 1990; **Med School:** Med Univ SC 1983; **Resid:** Pediatrics, Children's MC-Southwestern Med Sch, Dallas, TX 1983-1986; **Fellow:** Clinical Genetics, Baylor Coll Med, Houston, TX 1986-1989; **Fac Appt:** Prof Pediatrics, Univ Tex, Houston

West Coast and Pacific

Boles, Richard Gregory MD (CG) - *Spec Exp:* Mitochondrial Disorders; Mitochondrial Dis/Maternal Inheritance; **Hospital:** Chldns Hosp - Los Angeles; **Address:** 4650 Sunset Blvd, MS 90, Los Angeles, CA 90027; **Phone:** (323) 669-2178; **Board Cert:** Pediatrics 1994, Clinical Genetics 1993; **Med School:** UCLA 1987; **Resid:** Pediatrics, Harbor-UCLA Med Ctr, Torrance, CA 1988-1990; **Fellow:** Genetics and Metabolism, Yale Univ Sch Med, New Haven, CT 1991-1993; **Fac Appt:** Asst Prof Pediatrics, USC Sch Med

Cassidy, Suzanne MD (CG) - *Spec Exp:* Prader-Willi Syndrome; Connective Tissue Disorders; Neurocutaneous Disorders; **Hospital:** UCI Med Ctr; **Address:** 101 The City Drive, Bldg2- Fl 3, Orange, CA 92868-3298; **Phone:** (714) 456-5791; **Board Cert:** Pediatrics 1983, Clinical Genetics 1982; **Med School:** Vanderbilt Univ 1976; **Resid:** Pediatrics, Univ Wash Affil Prgms, Seattle, WA 1978-1979; **Fellow:** Clinical Genetics, Univ Wash, Seattle, WA 1979-1981; **Fac Appt:** Prof Pediatrics, UC Irvine

Cederbaum, Stephen D MD (CG) - *Spec Exp:* Inborn Errors of Metabolism; **Hospital:** UCLA Med Ctr; **Address:** 760 Westwood Ave Bldg NPI - rm 68230, Los Angeles, CA 90095; **Phone:** (310) 825-0402; **Board Cert:** Clinical Genetics 1982, Clinical Biochemical Genetics 1982; **Med School:** NYU Sch Med 1964; **Resid:** Internal Medicine, Barnes Hosp, St. Louis, MO 1965-1966; **Fellow:** Clinical Genetics, Univ Wash, Seattle, WA 1968-1970; **Fac Appt:** Prof Pediatrics, UCLA

Curry, Cynthia J MD (CG) - *Spec Exp:* Clinical Genetics - General; **Hospital:** Valley Chldns Hosp; **Address:** 9300 Valley Childrens Pl, MS FC 21, Madera, CA 93638; **Phone:** (559) 353-6626; **Board Cert:** Clinical Genetics 1982, Pediatrics 1973; **Med School:** Yale Univ 1967; **Resid:** Pediatrics, Univ Minn Hosp, Seattle, WA 1968-1969; Pediatrics, Univ Wash Orth Chldns Hosp, Minneapolis, MN 1969-1970; **Fellow:** Clinical Genetics, UCSF Med Ctr, San Francisco, CA 1975-1976; **Fac Appt:** Prof Clinical Genetics, UCSF

Falk, Rena Ellen MD (CG) - *Spec Exp:* Prenatal Diagnosis; Mental Retardation; Prenatal Genetic Diagnosis; **Hospital:** Cedars-Sinai Med Ctr; **Address:** 444 S San Vicente Blvd, Ste 1001, Los Angeles, CA 90048; **Phone:** (310) 423-9942; **Board Cert:** Clinical Genetics 1982, Pediatrics 1976; **Med School:** UCLA 1971; **Resid:** Pediatrics, Cedars-Sinai Med Ctr, Los Angeles, CA 1971-1973; **Fellow:** Clinical Genetics, UCLA Med School, Los Angeles, CA 1973-1975; UCLA, Los Angeles, CA 1975-1977; **Fac Appt:** Prof Pediatrics, UCLA

Graham Jr, John M MD (CG) - *Spec Exp: Dysmorphology; Craniofacial Disorders; Mental Retardation;* **Hospital:** Cedars-Sinai Med Ctr; **Address:** 444 S San Vicente Blvd, Ste 1001, Los Angeles, CA 90048-4175; **Phone:** (310) 423-9914; **Board Cert:** Pediatrics 1982, Clinical Genetics 1982; **Med School:** Med Univ SC 1975; **Resid:** Pediatrics, Boston Chldns Hosp-Harvard Med Sch, Boston, MA 1976-1977; **Fellow:** Developmental Pediatrics, Boston Chldns Hosp, Boston, MA 1977-1978; Dysmorphology, Univ Wash, Seattle, WA 1978-1980; **Fac Appt:** Prof Pediatrics, UCLA

Grody, Wayne W MD/PhD (CG) - *Spec Exp: Genetic Disorders; Familial Cancer;* **Hospital:** UCLA Med Ctr; **Address:** 10833 Le Conte Ave, Los Angeles, CA 90095-1732; **Phone:** (310) 825-5648; **Board Cert:** Clinical Genetics 1990, Anatomic Pathology 1987, Clinical Biochemical Genetics 1990; **Med School:** Baylor Coll Med 1977; **Resid:** Pathology, UCLA Med Ctr, Los Angeles, CA 1982-1986; **Fellow:** Clinical Genetics, UCLA Med Ctr, Los Angeles, CA 1985-1987; **Fac Appt:** Prof Clinical Genetics, UCLA

Hoyme, Harold Eugene MD (CG) - *Spec Exp: Fetal Alcohol Syndrome; Cytogenetic Disorders; Dysmorphology;* **Hospital:** Stanford Med Ctr; **Address:** 300 Pasteur Drive, rm H315, Stanford, CA 94305-5208; **Phone:** (650) 723-6858; **Board Cert:** Pediatrics 1980, Clinical Genetics 1984; **Med School:** Univ Chicago-Pritzker Sch Med 1976; **Resid:** Pediatrics, UCSD Med Ctr, San Diego, CA 1977-1979; **Fac Appt:** Prof Clinical Genetics, Stanford Univ

Hudgins, Louanne MD (CG) - *Spec Exp: Congenital Abnormalities-Limb;* **Hospital:** Stanford Med Ctr; **Address:** 300 Pasteur Drive, Ste H315, Stanford, CA 94305-5208; **Phone:** (650) 723-6858; **Board Cert:** Pediatrics 1997, Clinical Genetics 1993; **Med School:** Univ Kans 1984; **Resid:** Pediatrics, Univ Conn Hlth Ctr, Farmington, CT 1984-1987; **Fellow:** Clinical Genetics, Univ Conn Hlth Ctr, Farmington, CT 1987-1990; **Fac Appt:** Assoc Prof Pediatrics, Stanford Univ

Jonas, Adam Jonathan MD (CG) - *Spec Exp: Biochemical Genetics; Inherited Diseases;* **Hospital:** LAC - Harbor - UCLA Med Ctr; **Address:** 1000 W Carson St, Box 17, Torrance, CA 90509-2910; **Phone:** (310) 222-2301; **Board Cert:** Pediatrics 1982, Clinical Genetics 1990; **Med School:** UCSD 1976; **Resid:** Pediatrics, Chldns Ortho Hosp, Seattle, WA 1976-1978; Pediatrics, Univ Hosp, San Diego, CA 1978-1979; **Fellow:** Genetics and Metabolism, UCSD Sch Med, San Diego, CA 1979-1982; **Fac Appt:** Prof Pediatrics, UCLA

Jones, Marilyn MD (CG) - *Spec Exp: Dysmorphology; Craniofacial Disorders;* **Hospital:** Children's Hosp and Hlth Ctr - San Diego; **Address:** 3020 Children's Way, MC 5031, San Diego, CA 92123-2746; **Phone:** (858) 576-5840; **Board Cert:** Pediatrics 1979, Clinical Genetics 1982; **Med School:** Columbia P&S 1974; **Resid:** Internal Medicine, UCSD Med Ctr, San Diego, CA 1975-1977; Pediatrics, UCSD Med Ctr, San Diego, CA 1977; **Fellow:** Dysmorphology, UCSD Med Ctr, San Diego, CA 1977-1979; **Fac Appt:** Adjct Prof Pediatrics, UCSD

Morris, Colleen A. MD (CG) - *Spec Exp: Williams Syndrome; Inherited Diseases; Fetal Alcohol Syndrome;* **Hospital:** Univ Med Ctr-Las Vegas; **Address:** Univ of Nevada Sch of Medicine, Dept Pediatrics, 2040 W Charleston, Ste 401, Las Vegas, NV 89102; **Phone:** (702) 671-2200; **Board Cert:** Clinical Genetics 1987, Pediatrics 1986; **Med School:** Loyola Univ-Stritch Sch Med 1981; **Resid:** Pediatrics, Phoenix Hosp Affil Ped Prgm, Phoenix, AZ 1981-1984; **Fellow:** Clinical Genetics, Univ Utah Sch Med, Salt Lake City, UT 1984-1986; **Fac Appt:** Prof Pediatrics, Univ Nevada

Pagon, Roberta Anderson MD (CG) - *Spec Exp: Eye Diseases-Hereditary; Sexual Differentiation Disorders;* **Hospital:** Chldns Hosp and Regl Med Ctr - Seattle; **Address:** Chldns Hosp Med Ctr.-Div Med Genetics CH-25, 4800 Sand Point Way NE, Seattle, WA 98105-0371; **Phone:** (206) 526-2056; **Board Cert:** Pediatrics 1978, Clinical Genetics 1982; **Med School:** Harvard Med Sch 1972; **Resid:** Pediatrics, Univ Wash Affil Hosp, Seattle, WA 1973-1975; **Fellow:** Clinical Genetics, Univ Wash, Seattle, WA 1976-1979; **Fac Appt:** Prof Pediatrics, Univ Wash

Rimoin, David L MD/PhD (CG) - *Spec Exp:* Skeletal Dysplasias; Marfan's Syndrome; Birth Defects; **Hospital:** Cedars-Sinai Med Ctr; **Address:** Cedars-Sinai Med Ctr, 444 S San Vicente, Ste 1001, Los Angeles, CA 90048-4174; **Phone:** (310) 423-4461; **Board Cert:** Internal Medicine 1968, Clinical Genetics 1984; **Med School:** McGill Univ 1961; **Resid:** Internal Medicine, Royal Victoria Hosp, Montreal, Canada 1962-1963; Internal Medicine, Johns Hopkins Hosp, Baltimore, MD 1963-1964; **Fellow:** Clinical Genetics, Johns Hopkins Hosp, Baltimore, MD 1964-1967; **Fac Appt:** Prof Pediatrics, UCLA

Weitzel, Jeffrey Nelson MD (CG) - *Spec Exp:* Breast Cancer; Ovarian Cancer; Familial Cancer; **Hospital:** City of Hope Natl Med Ctr & Beckman Rsch; **Address:** City of Hope Cancer Ctr, 1500 E Duarte Rd, Duarte, CA 91010; **Phone:** (626) 359-8111; **Board Cert:** Internal Medicine 1986, Medical Oncology 1989, Hematology 1990, Clinical Genetics 1996; **Med School:** Univ Minn 1983; **Resid:** Internal Medicine, Univ Minn Hosps, Minneapolis, IN 1984-1986; Hematology, Hammersmith Hosp, London, England 1986-1987; **Fellow:** Hematology, Tufts U-New England Hosps, Boston, MA 1987-1992; Clinical Genetics, Tufts U-New England Hosps, Boston, MA 1994-1994; **Fac Appt:** Assoc Clin Prof Preventive Medicine, USC Sch Med

Wilcox, William MD (CG) - *Spec Exp:* Inborn Errors of Metabolism; Skeletal Dysplasias; **Hospital:** Cedars-Sinai Med Ctr; **Address:** Cedars Sinai Med Ctr, Dept Med Genetics, 444 S San Vincente Blvd, Ste 1001, Los Angeles, CA 90048; **Phone:** (310) 423-9914; **Board Cert:** Pediatrics 1999, Clinical Genetics 1993; **Med School:** UCLA 1988; **Resid:** Pediatrics, UCLA Med Ctr, Los Angeles, CA 1989-1991; **Fellow:** Clinical Genetics, Cedars-Sinai Med Ctr, Los Angeles, CA 1991; **Fac Appt:** Asst Prof Pediatrics, UCLA

Colon & Rectal Surgery

A colon and rectal surgeon is trained to diagnose and treat various diseases of the intestinal tract, colon, rectum, anal canal and perianal area by medical and surgical means. This specialist also deals with other organs and tissues (such as the liver, urinary and female reproductive system) involved with primary intestinal disease.

Colon and rectal surgeons have the expertise to diagnose and often manage anorectal conditions such as hemorrhoids, fissures (painful tears in the anal lining), abscesses and fistulae (infections located around the anus and rectum) in the office setting. They also treat problems of the intestine and colon and perform endoscopic procedures to evaluate and treat problems such as cancer, polyps (precancerous growths) and inflammatory conditions.

Training required: Six years (including general surgery)

NYU Medical Center

SCHOOL OF MEDICINE

550 First Avenue (at 31st Street)
New York, NY 10016
Physician Referral: (888) 7-NYU-MED
(888-769-8633)
www.mininvasive.med.nyu.edu

NEW YORK UNIVERSITY

COLON AND RECTAL SURGERY

Removal of a segment of the colon is a major operation. When performed by conventional surgery, a large incision and 5-8 days hospitalization is necessary. At NYU Medical Center, surgeons use laparoscopic techniques to perform the same operation through a number of tiny incisions.

The advantages of laparoscopic surgery come from minimizing the trauma of access to internal organs. By avoiding a long incision through the muscles, many post-operative problems are eliminated and pain is markedly reduced. Patients can breathe and cough better after surgery. The need for strong pain medications is drastically reduced so the drowsiness, fatigue, and unsteadiness they cause are virtually eliminated. It is possible to return to normal activities in a fraction of the time necessary after regular surgery.

Minimally invasive techniques are used to treat:

• Diverticulitis of the colon

• Inflammatory stricture of the small intestine near the colon

• Large polyps that cannot be removed during a colonoscopy

• Tumors

Most patients will need a colonoscopy before they can be seen by a surgeon. NYU Medical Center is one of the few centers in New York City to offer the virtual colonscopy, a minimally invasive alternative to traditional colonoscopy. With significantly less discomfort than the traditional colonscopy, many patients choose our less invasive test year after year.

NYU MEDICAL CENTER

Colon cancer is one of the most prevalent, yet easily detectable cancers in existence today. In addition to conducting clinical trials on the best treatments for colon cancer, NYU Medical Center offers patients the virtual colonoscopy, a new piece of technology designed to eliminate the old, invasive procedure. Patients report a significant difference in comfort. Call today to schedule your virtual colonoscopy. Anyone over 50 should have one each year.

Physician Referral
(888) 7-NYU-MED
(888-769-8633)
www.mininvasive.med.nyu.edu

PHYSICIAN LISTINGS

Colon & Rectal Surgery

New England

Bleday, Ronald MD (CRS) - *Spec Exp:* Colon Cancer; **Hospital:** Brigham & Women's Hosp; **Address:** Brigham & Women's Hosp, 45 Francis St, Bldg ASB2, Boston, MA 02115; **Phone:** (617) 732-8460; **Board Cert:** Surgery 1999, Colon & Rectal Surgery 1992; **Med School:** McGill Univ 1982; **Resid:** Surgery, Brown Univ-RI Hosp, Providence, RI 1982-1989; Surgical Oncology, Brigham & Women's Hosp, Boston, MA 1984-1986; **Fellow:** Endoscopy, Mass Genl Hosp, Boston, MA 1990; Colon & Rectal Surgery, Univ Minn, Minneapolis, MN 1990-1991; **Fac Appt:** Asst Prof Surgery, Harvard Med Sch

Coller, John MD (CRS) - *Spec Exp:* Colon Cancer; **Hospital:** Lahey Cli.; **Address:** 41 Mall Rd, Burlington, MA 01805; **Phone:** (781) 744-8581; **Board Cert:** Surgery 1973, Colon & Rectal Surgery 1973; **Med School:** Univ Penn 1965; **Resid:** Surgery, Hosp Univ Penn, Philadelphia, PA 1966-1972; **Fellow:** Colon & Rectal Surgery, Lahey Clinic Fdtn, Boston, MA 1972-1973

Littlejohn, Charles MD (CRS) - *Spec Exp:* Colon & Rectal Cancer; **Hospital:** Stamford Hosp; **Address:** 70 Mill River St, Stamford, CT 06902-3725; **Phone:** (203) 323-8989; **Board Cert:** Surgery 1994, Colon & Rectal Surgery 1985; **Med School:** Dartmouth Med Sch 1978; **Resid:** Surgery, Univ Rochester Affil Hosps, Rochester, NY 1979-1980; Surgery, UMDNJ-Rutgers Affil Hosp, Newark, NJ 1980-1983; **Fellow:** Colon & Rectal Surgery, UMDNJ-Rutgers Affil Hosp, Newark, NJ 1983-1984; **Fac Appt:** Asst Clin Prof Surgery, NY Med Coll

Roberts, Patricia L MD (CRS) - *Spec Exp:* Diverticulitis; Colon Cancer; **Hospital:** Lahey Cli.; **Address:** 41 Mall Rd, Burlington, MA 01805; **Phone:** (781) 744-8243; **Board Cert:** Colon & Rectal Surgery 1988, Surgery 1996; **Med School:** Boston Univ 1981; **Resid:** Surgery, Boston Univ-Boston City Hosp, Boston, MA 1981-1986; **Fellow:** Colon & Rectal Surgery, Lahey Clinic, Burlington, MA 1986-1988; **Fac Appt:** Asst Clin Prof Colon & Rectal Surgery, Tufts Univ

Schoetz, David MD (CRS) - *Spec Exp:* Inflammatory Bowel Disease/Crohn's; Colon & Rectal Cancer; Incontinence-Fecal; **Hospital:** Lahey Cli.; **Address:** Lahey Clinic Medical Center, Dept of Colon Rectal Surgery, 41 Mall Rd, Burlington, MA 01805; **Phone:** (781) 744-8889; **Board Cert:** Colon & Rectal Surgery 1983, Surgery 1991; **Med School:** Med Coll Wisc 1974; **Resid:** Surgery, Boston Univ Med Ctr., Boston, MA 1975-1981; **Fellow:** Colon & Rectal Surgery, Lahey Clin Med Ctr., Burlington, MA 1981-1982; **Fac Appt:** Prof Surgery, Tufts Univ

Shellito, Paul C MD (CRS) - *Spec Exp:* Colon & Rectal Cancer; Ulcerative Colitis; Anorectal Disorders; **Hospital:** MA Genl Hosp; **Address:** 15 Parkman St, Ste 336, Boston, MA 02114; **Phone:** (617) 724-0365; **Board Cert:** Colon & Rectal Surgery 1994, Surgery 1992; **Med School:** Harvard Med Sch 1977; **Resid:** Surgery, Mass Genl Hosp., Boston, MA 1982-1983; Surgery, Auckland U Med Sch. 1981; **Fellow:** Colon & Rectal Surgery, U Minn., Minneapolis, MN 1984-1985; **Fac Appt:** Asst Prof Surgery, Harvard Med Sch

Mid Atlantic

Forde, Kenneth MD (CRS) - *Spec Exp:* Colon & Rectal Cancer; **Hospital:** NY Presby Hosp - Columbia Presby Med Ctr (page 70); **Address:** Columbia Presbyterian Med Ctr, Atchley Pavilion, 161 Fort Washington Ave, rm 812, New York, NY 10032-3713; **Phone:** (212) 305-5394; **Board Cert:** Surgery 1967; **Med School:** Columbia P&S 1959; **Resid:** Surgery, Bellevue Hosp Ctr, New York, NY 1960-1964; Surgery, Columbia Presby Hosp, New York, NY 1961-1963; **Fac Appt:** Clin Prof Surgery, Columbia P&S

Fry, Robert Dean MD (CRS) - *Spec Exp:* Rectal Cancer; Inflammatory Bowel Disease/Crohn's; **Hospital:** Thomas Jefferson Univ Hosp; **Address:** Thomas Jefferson Univ Hosp, 1100 Walnut St, Ste 702, Philadelphia, PA 19107; **Phone:** (215) 955-5869; **Board Cert:** Surgery 1996, Colon & Rectal Surgery 1998; **Med School:** Washington Univ, St Louis 1972; **Resid:** Surgery, Jewish Hosp, St Louis, MO 1973-1977; **Fellow:** Colon & Rectal Surgery, Cleveland Clin Fdn, Cleveland, OH 1977-1978; **Fac Appt:** Prof Surgery

Gingold, Bruce MD (CRS) - *Spec Exp:* Colostomy Avoidance; Inflammatory Bowel Disease/Crohn's; Colonoscopy; **Hospital:** St Vincent Cath Med Ctrs - Manhattan (page 75); **Address:** 36 7th Ave, Ste 507, New York, NY 10011-6600; **Phone:** (212) 675-2997; **Board Cert:** Colon & Rectal Surgery 1976, Surgery 1977; **Med School:** Jefferson Med Coll 1970; **Resid:** Surgery, St Vincent's Hosp & Med Ctr, New York, NY 1970-1975; **Fellow:** Colon & Rectal Surgery, Cleveland Clinic, Cleveland, OH 1975-1976; **Fac Appt:** Assoc Clin Prof Surgery, NY Med Coll

Golub, Richard MD (CRS) - *Spec Exp:* Colon & Rectal Cancer; Laparoscopic Surgery; Hemorrhoid Surgery; **Hospital:** Univ Hosp - Brklyn; **Address:** 450 Clarkson Ave, Box 40, Brooklyn, NY 11203-2012; **Phone:** (718) 270-3349; **Board Cert:** Surgery 2000, Colon & Rectal Surgery 2000; **Med School:** Albert Einstein Coll Med 1984; **Resid:** Surgery, Univ Hosp Stony Brook, Stony Brook, NY 1984-1990; **Fellow:** Colon & Rectal Surgery, Grant Medical Center, Columbus, OH 1990-1991; **Fac Appt:** Assoc Prof Surgery, SUNY Downstate

Gorfine, Stephen MD (CRS) - *Spec Exp:* Anal Fissure; Hemorrhoids; Rectal Cancer; **Hospital:** Mount Sinai Hosp (page 68); **Address:** 25 E 69th St, New York, NY 10021-4925; **Phone:** (212) 517-8600; **Board Cert:** Surgery 1987, Colon & Rectal Surgery 1988; **Med School:** Univ Mass Sch Med 1978; **Resid:** Internal Medicine, Mount Sinai Hosp, New York, NY 1978-1981; Surgery, Mount Sinai Hosp, New York, NY 1981-1985; **Fellow:** Colon & Rectal Surgery, Ferguson Hosp, Grand Rapids, MI 1986-1987; **Fac Appt:** Assoc Clin Prof Surgery, Mount Sinai Sch Med

Medich, David MD (CRS) - *Spec Exp:* Rectal Cancer; Ulcerative Colitis; Inflammatory Bowel Disease/Crohn's; **Hospital:** Allegheny General Hosp; **Address:** 320 E North Ave, Ste 312, Pittsburgh, PA 15212; **Phone:** (412) 359-3901; **Board Cert:** Surgery 1994, Colon & Rectal Surgery 1995; **Med School:** Ohio State Univ 1987; **Resid:** Surgery, Univ of Pittsburgh, Pittsburgh, PA 1987-1990; **Fellow:** Research, Univ of Pittsburgh, Pittsburgh, PA 1990-1993; Colon & Rectal Surgery, Cleveland Clin Fdn, Cleveland, OH 1993-1994; **Fac Appt:** Assoc Prof Surgery

Milsom, Jeffrey W MD (CRS) - *Spec Exp:* Laparoscopic Gastrointestinal Surgery; Colon & Rectal Cancer; **Hospital:** NY Presby Hosp; **Address:** Weill Medical College, Div Colon & Rectal Surgery, 525 E 68th St, Payson 717A, Box 172, New York, NY 10021; **Phone:** (212) 746-6030; **Board Cert:** Colon & Rectal Surgery 1986, Surgery 1992; **Med School:** Univ Pittsburgh 1979; **Resid:** Surgery, Roosevelt Hosp, New York, NY 1980-1981; Surgery, Univ Virginia Med Ctr, Charlottesville, VA 1981-1984; **Fellow:** Colon & Rectal Surgery, Ferguson Hosp, Grand Rapids, MI 1984-1985; **Fac Appt:** Prof Surgery, Mount Sinai Sch Med

Salvati, Eugene MD (CRS) - *Spec Exp:* Colon & Rectal Surgery - General; **Hospital:** Muhlenberg Regional Med Ctr; **Address:** 3900 Park Ave, Ste 101, Edison, NJ 08820-3032; **Phone:** (732) 494-6640; **Board Cert:** Colon & Rectal Surgery 1956, Surgery 1962; **Med School:** Univ MD Sch Med 1947; **Resid:** Surgery, St Vincent Hosp, Indianapolis, IN 1950-1951; Surgery, Veterans Hosp, Indianapolis, IN 1951-1952; **Fellow:** Colon & Rectal Surgery, Allentown Genl Hosp, Allentown, PA 1954-1956; **Fac Appt:** Clin Prof Surgery, UMDNJ-RW Johnson Med Sch

Smith, Lee MD (CRS) - *Spec Exp:* Colon & Rectal Cancer; Inflammatory Bowel Disease/Crohn's; **Hospital:** Washington Hosp Ctr; **Address:** 110 Irving St NW, Ste 3B-31, Washington, DC 20010-2975; **Phone:** (202) 877-8484; **Board Cert:** Surgery 1971, Colon & Rectal Surgery 1973; **Med School:** UCSF 1962; **Resid:** Surgery, Naval Hosp, San Diego, CA 1966-1970; Colon & Rectal Surgery, Univ Minn, Minneapolis, MN 1972-1973; **Fac Appt:** Prof Surgery, Geo Wash Univ

Steinhagen, Randolph MD (CRS) - *Spec Exp:* Diverticulitis; Colon & Rectal Cancer; Inflammatory Bowel Disease/Crohn's; **Hospital:** Mount Sinai Hosp (page 68); **Address:** 5 E 98th St Fl 11, Box 1263, New York, NY 10029-6501; **Phone:** (212) 241-3336; **Board Cert:** Colon & Rectal Surgery 1985, Surgery 1992; **Med School:** Wayne State Univ 1977; **Resid:** Surgery, Mount Sinai Hosp, New York, NY 1977-1982; **Fellow:** Colon & Rectal Surgery, Cleveland Clinic, Cleveland, OH 1982-1983; **Fac Appt:** Assoc Prof Surgery, Mount Sinai Sch Med

Whelan, Richard MD (CRS) - *Spec Exp:* Laparoscopic Surgery; Colon Cancer; **Hospital:** NY Presby Hosp - Columbia Presby Med Ctr (page 70); **Address:** 161 Ft Washington Ave, Rm 817, New York, NY 10032; **Phone:** (212) 305-6136; **Board Cert:** Surgery 1988, Colon & Rectal Surgery 1990; **Med School:** Columbia P&S 1982; **Resid:** Surgery, Columbia Presby, New York, NY 1982-1987; **Fellow:** Colon & Rectal Surgery, Univ Minn Med Ctr, Minneapolis, MN 1987-1988; **Fac Appt:** Assoc Clin Prof Surgery, Columbia P&S

Wong, Westley Douglas MD (CRS) - *Spec Exp:* Endorectal Ultrasonography; Artificial Anal Sphincter; Rectal Cancer-Sphincter Saving Surgery; **Hospital:** Mem Sloan Kettering Cancer Ctr; **Address:** Meml Sloan Kettering Cancer Ctr, 1275 York Ave, rm C991, New York, NY 10021-6094; **Phone:** (212) 639-5117; **Board Cert:** Surgery 1997, Colon & Rectal Surgery 1985; **Med School:** Canada 1972; **Resid:** Surgery, Univ Manitoba Hosp, Canada 1973-1977; **Fellow:** Colon & Rectal Surgery, Univ Minn Med Ctr, Minneapolis, MN 1983-1984; **Fac Appt:** Assoc Clin Prof Surgery, Cornell Univ-Weill Med Coll

Southeast

Carbonell, Manuel MD (CRS) - *Spec Exp:* Colon & Rectal Surgery - General; **Hospital:** Mercy Hosp - Miami, FL; **Address:** 3661 S Miami Ave, Ste 1006, Miami, FL 33133-4214; **Phone:** (305) 854-2432; **Board Cert:** Colon & Rectal Surgery 1971; **Med School:** Med Coll Wisc 1958; **Resid:** Surgery, Jackson Meml Hosp, Miami, FL 1959-1963; **Fellow:** Colon & Rectal Surgery, Mercy Hosp, Miami, FL 1963-1965

Christie, John MD (CRS) - *Spec Exp:* Endoscopy; **Hospital:** Baptist Hosp - Miami; **Address:** Gastroenterology Care Center, 7500 SE 87th Ave, Ste 200, Miami, FL 33173-2131; **Phone:** (305) 913-0666; **Board Cert:** Surgery 1971; **Med School:** Univ Cincinnati 1965; **Resid:** Surgery, Wadsworth VA Hosp-UCLA, Los Angeles, CA 1966-1970; **Fellow:** Endoscopy, Beth Israel Med Ctr, New York, NY 1972; **Fac Appt:** Assoc Clin Prof Colon & Rectal Surgery, Univ Miami Sch Med

Cohen, Alfred M MD (CRS) - *Spec Exp:* Colorectal Cancer-Liver Metastasis; **Hospital:** Univ Kentucky Med Ctr; **Address:** Markey Cancer Center, 800 Rose St, Ste 140, Lexington, KY 40536; **Phone:** (859) 323-6556; **Board Cert:** Surgery 1976; **Med School:** Johns Hopkins Univ 1967; **Resid:** Surgical Oncology, Surg Branch Natl Cancer Inst, Bethesda, MD 1969-1971; Surgery, Mass Genl Hosp, Boston, MA 1972-1975; **Fac Appt:** Prof Surgery, Univ KY Coll Med

Foley, Eugene F MD (CRS) - *Spec Exp:* Colon & Rectal Surgery; Ulcerative Colitis; **Hospital:** Univ of VA Hlth Sys (page 79); **Address:** PO Box 800709, Charlottesville, VA 22908; **Phone:** (804) 924-9304; **Board Cert:** Surgery 1994, Colon & Rectal Surgery 1993; **Med School:** Harvard Med Sch 1985; **Resid:** Surgery, New England Deaconess Hosp, Boston, MA; **Fellow:** Colon & Rectal Surgery, Lahey Clinic, Burlington, MA; **Fac Appt:** Assoc Prof Surgery, Univ VA Sch Med

Galandiuk, Susan MD (CRS) - *Spec Exp:* Colon & Rectal Cancer; Inflammatory Bowel Disease/Crohn's; **Hospital:** Univ Louisville Hosp; **Address:** Dept Surgery, 550 S Jackson, Ambulatory Care Bldg, Louisville, KY 40292; **Phone:** (502) 852-4568; **Board Cert:** Surgery 1998, Colon & Rectal Surgery 1991; **Med School:** Germany 1982; **Resid:** Surgery, Cleveland Clinic Fdtn, Cleveland, OH 1984-1988; **Fellow:** Surgery, Univ Louisville Hosp, Louisville, KY 1988-1989; Colon & Rectal Surgery, Mayo Clinic, Rochester, MN 1989-1990; **Fac Appt:** Assoc Prof Surgery, Univ Louisville Sch Med

Hartmann, Rene MD (CRS) - *Spec Exp:* Colon & Rectal Surgery - General; **Hospital:** Baptist Hosp - Miami; **Address:** 9195 Sunset Drive, Ste 230, Miami, FL 33173-3488; **Phone:** (305) 271-0300; **Board Cert:** Surgery 1978, Colon & Rectal Surgery 1994; **Med School:** Venezuela 1971; **Resid:** Surgery, Jackson Meml Hoso, Miami, FL 1973-1976; Surgery, Orange Meml Hosp, Orlando, FL 1976-1977; **Fellow:** Colon & Rectal Surgery, Grant Hosp, Columbus, OH 1977-1978; **Fac Appt:** Assoc Clin Prof Surgery, Univ Miami Sch Med

Larach, Sergio MD (CRS) - *Spec Exp:* Colon Cancer; Inflammatory Bowel Disease/Crohn's; **Hospital:** Orlando Reg Med Ctr; **Address:** Colon & Rectal Clin of Orlando, 110 W Underwood St, Ste A, Orlando, FL 32806; **Phone:** (407) 422-3790; **Board Cert:** Colon & Rectal Surgery 1979; **Med School:** Chile 1968; **Resid:** Surgery, Hosp de Salvador, Santiago, Chile 1968-1973; Surgery, Orlando Reg Med Ctr, Orlando, FL 1973-1976; **Fellow:** Colon & Rectal Surgery, Univ Texas Med Sch, Houston, TX 1976-1977; **Fac Appt:** Assoc Prof Surgery, Univ Fla Coll Med

Nogueras, Juan Jose MD (CRS) - *Spec Exp:* Colorectal Cancer; Inflammatory Bowel Disease/Crohn's; Incontinence; **Hospital:** Cleveland Clin FL; **Address:** 2950 Clevland Clinic Blvd, Weston, FL 33331; **Phone:** (954) 659-5251; **Board Cert:** Surgery 1997, Colon & Rectal Surgery 1993; **Med School:** Jefferson Med Coll 1982; **Resid:** Surgery, Columbia Presby Med Ctr, New York, NY 1983-1987; **Fellow:** Colon & Rectal Surgery, Univ Minn, Minneapolis, MN 1990-1991

Wexner, Steven MD (CRS) - *Spec Exp:* Rectal Cancer; Inflammatory Bowel Disease/Crohn's; Laparoscopic Surgery; **Hospital:** Cleveland Clin FL; **Address:** 2950 Cleveland Clinic Blvd, Weston, FL 33331; **Phone:** (954) 659-6020; **Board Cert:** Surgery 1996, Colon & Rectal Surgery 1989; **Med School:** Cornell Univ-Weill Med Coll 1982; **Resid:** Surgery, Roosevelt Hosp, New York, NY 1982-1987; **Fellow:** Colon & Rectal Surgery, Univ Minn, Minneapolis, MN 1987-1988; **Fac Appt:** Prof Surgery, Univ S Fla Coll Med

Midwest

Abcarian, Herand MD (CRS) - *Spec Exp:* Rectal Cancer/Sphincter Preservation; Laparoscopic Surgery; Anorectal Disorders; **Hospital:** Univ of IL at Chicago Med Ctr; **Address:** 30 N Michigan Ave, Ste 1118, Chicago, IL 60602; **Phone:** (312) 782-4828; **Board Cert:** Colon & Rectal Surgery 1972, Surgery 1972; **Med School:** Iran 1965; **Resid:** Surgery, Cook County Hosp, Chicago, IL 1967-1971; Colon & Rectal Surgery, Cook County Hosp, Chicago, IL 1971-1972; **Fac Appt:** Prof Surgery, Univ IL Coll Med

Dozois, Roger R MD (CRS) - *Spec Exp:* Inflammatory Bowel Disease/Crohn's; Polyposis Syndromes; **Hospital:** Mayo Med Ctr & Clin - Rochester, MN; **Address:** Div Colon & Rectal Surg, 200 1st St SW, Rochester, MN 55905; **Phone:** (507) 284-2622; **Board Cert:** Surgery 1974, Colon & Rectal Surgery 1984; **Med School:** Laval Univ, Quebec 1965; **Resid:** Surgery, Mayo Clinic, Rochester, MN 1966-1971

Fazio, Victor MD (CRS) - *Spec Exp:* Inflammatory Bowel Disease/Crohn's; Colon & Rectal Cancer; **Hospital:** Cleveland Clin Fdn (page 57); **Address:** Cleveland Clinic, Dept Colorectal Surg, 9500 Euclid Ave, Box A111, Cleveland, OH 44195; **Phone:** (216) 444-6672; **Board Cert:** Colon & Rectal Surgery 1976; **Med School:** Australia 1964; **Resid:** Surgery, St Vincents Hosp, Sidney, Australia 1967-1971; Surgery, Lahey Clinic, Boston, MA 1972; **Fellow:** Colon & Rectal Surgery, Cleveland Clinic, Cleveland, OH 1973

Fleshman, James MD (CRS) - *Spec Exp:* Colon & Rectal Cancer; Laparoscopic Surgery; **Hospital:** Barnes-Jewish Hosp (page 55); **Address:** Washington Univ Sch Med, 660 S Euclid Ave, Box 8109, St Louis, MO 63110; **Phone:** (314) 454-7177; **Board Cert:** Colon & Rectal Surgery 1988, Surgery 1996; **Med School:** Washington Univ, St Louis 1980; **Resid:** Surgery, Jewish Hospital, St. Louis, MO 1980-1986; **Fellow:** Colon & Rectal Surgery, Univ Toronto, Toronto, CN 1986-1987; **Fac Appt:** Prof Surgery, Washington Univ, St Louis

Goldberg, Stanley MD (CRS) - *Spec Exp:* Diverticulitis; **Hospital:** Abbott - Northwestern Hosp; **Address:** 1731 Medical Arts Bldg-Div Colorectal Surgery, 825 Nicollet Mall, Minneapolis, MN 55402-2606; **Phone:** (612) 339-4534; **Board Cert:** Colon & Rectal Surgery 1963, Surgery 1964; **Med School:** Univ Minn 1956; **Resid:** Surgery, Minneapolis VA Hosp, Minneapolis, MN 1957-1960; Colon & Rectal Surgery, Univ Minnesota Hosps, Minneapolis, MN 1960-1963; **Fac Appt:** Clin Prof Surgery, Univ Minn

Kodner, Ira Joe MD (CRS) - *Spec Exp:* Colon & Rectal Cancer; Inflammatory Bowel Disease/Crohn's; Laparoscopic Surgery; **Hospital:** Barnes-Jewish Hosp (page 55); **Address:** 660 S Euclid Ave, Ste 14102, Box 8109, St. Louis, MO 63110; **Phone:** (314) 454-7177; **Board Cert:** Colon & Rectal Surgery 1975, Surgery 1975; **Med School:** Washington Univ, St Louis 1967; **Resid:** Surgery, Barnes-Jewish Hosp, St. Louis, MO 1971-1974; **Fellow:** Colon & Rectal Surgery, Cleveland Clinic, Cleveland, OH 1974-1975; **Fac Appt:** Prof Surgery, Washington Univ, St Louis

Lowry, Ann C MD (CRS) - *Spec Exp:* Anal Sphincter Repair; Rectovaginal Fistula; **Hospital:** Abbott - Northwestern Hosp; **Address:** 6545 France Avenue S, Ste 474, Edina, MN 55435; **Phone:** (651) 312-1700; **Board Cert:** Colon & Rectal Surgery 1988, Surgery 1993; **Med School:** Tufts Univ 1977; **Resid:** Surgery, New England Med Ctr Hosps, Boston, MA 1978-1982; **Fellow:** Colon & Rectal Surgery, Univ Minn Affil Hosps, Minneapolis, MN 1986-1987; **Fac Appt:** Clin Prof Surgery, Univ Minn

MacKeigan, John MD (CRS) - *Spec Exp:* Rectal Cancer; Anal Surgery; Ulcerative Colitis; **Hospital:** Spectrum Health East; **Address:** The Ferguson Clinic, 4100 Lake Dr SE, Ste 205, Grand Rapids, MI 49546; **Phone:** (616) 356-4100; **Board Cert:** Colon & Rectal Surgery 1974; **Med School:** Dalhousie Univ 1969; **Resid:** Surgery, Dalhousie Univ, Halifax, Nova Scotia 1969-1973; Colon & Rectal Surgery, Ferguson Hosp, Grand Rapids, MI 1973-1974; **Fac Appt:** Assoc Prof Surgery, Mich State Univ

Nelson, Heidi MD (CRS) - *Spec Exp:* Colon & Rectal Cancer; **Hospital:** Mayo Med Ctr & Clin - Rochester, MN; **Address:** Div Colon & Rectal Surg, 200 First St SW, Fl E6A, Rochester, MN 55905; **Phone:** (507) 284-3329; **Board Cert:** Colon & Rectal Surgery 1989, Surgery 1995; **Med School:** Univ Wash 1981; **Resid:** Surgery, Oregan Hlth Sci Univ Hosp, Portland, OR 1981-1987; Colon & Rectal Surgery, Oregan Hlth Sci Univ Hosp, Portland, OR 1984-1985; **Fellow:** Colon & Rectal Surgery, Mayo Clinic, Rochester, MN 1987-1988; **Fac Appt:** Prof Surgery, Mayo Med Sch

Nivatvongs, Santhat MD (CRS) - *Spec Exp:* Colon & Rectal Cancer; Anorectal Disorders; Inflammatory Bowel Disease; **Hospital:** Mayo Med Ctr & Clin - Rochester, MN; **Address:** Mayo Clinic, CRS Sect, 200 First St SW, Rochester, MN 55905-0002; **Phone:** (507) 284-4985; **Board Cert:** Colon & Rectal Surgery 1971, Surgery 1971; **Med School:** Thailand 1964; **Resid:** Surgery, Harper Hosp, Detroit, MI 1966-1967; Surgery, United Hosp, St Paul, MN 1967-1970; **Fellow:** Colon & Rectal Surgery, Univ Minn, Minneapolis, MN 1970-1971; **Fac Appt:** Prof Surgery, Mayo Med Sch

Pemberton, John MD (CRS) - *Spec Exp:* Rectal Surgery; Inflammatory Bowel Disease/Crohn's; **Hospital:** Mayo Med Ctr & Clin - Rochester, MN; **Address:** Div Colon & Rectal Surgery, 200 First St SW, Rochester, MN 55905; **Phone:** (507) 284-2359; **Board Cert:** Surgery 1984, Colon & Rectal Surgery 1985; **Med School:** Tulane Univ 1976; **Resid:** Surgery, Mayo Clinic, Rochester, MN 1977-1983; **Fellow:** Colon & Rectal Surgery, Mayo Clinic, Rochester, MN 1983-1984; **Fac Appt:** Prof Surgery, Mayo Med Sch

Rothenberger, David MD (CRS) - *Spec Exp:* Colon & Rectal Cancer; **Hospital:** Fairview-Univ Med Ctr - Univ Campus; **Address:** 420 Delaware St SE, MC-450, Minneapolis, MN 55455; **Phone:** (612) 625-3288; **Board Cert:** Surgery 1979, Colon & Rectal Surgery 1979; **Med School:** Tufts Univ 1973; **Resid:** Surgery, St Paul-Ramsey Med Ctr, St Paul, MN 1974-1978; **Fellow:** Colon & Rectal Surgery, Univ Minnesota Hosps, Minneapolis, MN 1978-1979; **Fac Appt:** Clin Prof Surgery, Univ Minn

Saclarides, Theodore John MD (CRS) - *Spec Exp:* Rectal Cancer-Sphincter Preservation; Incontinence-Fecal; Inflammatory Bowel Disease; **Hospital:** Rush-Presby - St Luke's Med Ctr (page 72); **Address:** University Surgeons, 1725 W Harrison St, Ste 810, Chicago, IL 60612-3832; **Phone:** (312) 942-6543; **Board Cert:** Colon & Rectal Surgery 1989, Surgery 1996; **Med School:** Univ Miami Sch Med 1982; **Resid:** Surgery, Rush Presby-St Luke's Hosp, Chicago, IL 1982-1987; **Fellow:** Colon & Rectal Surgery, Mayo Clinic, Rochester, MN 1987-1988; **Fac Appt:** Prof Surgery, Rush Med Coll

Senagore, Anthony MD (CRS) - *Spec Exp:* Laparoscopic Surgery; Colon & Rectal Cancer; **Hospital:** Cleveland Clin Fdn (page 57); **Address:** Cleveland Clinic, 9500 Euclid Ave, rm A111, Cleveland, OH 44195-0002; **Phone:** (216) 445-7882; **Board Cert:** Surgery 1995, Colon & Rectal Surgery 2001; **Med School:** Mich State Univ 1981; **Resid:** Surgery, Butterworth Hospital-Michigan State Univ, Grand Rapids, MI 1982-1987; Colon & Rectal Surgery, Ferguson Hospital, Grand Rapids, MI 1987-1989

Stryker, Steven J MD (CRS) - *Spec Exp:* Colon & Rectal Cancer; Inflammatory Bowel Disease/Crohn's; Laparoscopic Colectomy; **Hospital:** Northwestern Meml Hosp; **Address:** Northwestern Meml Hosp, 676 N Saint Clair St, Ste 1525, Chicago, IL 60611; **Phone:** (312) 943-5427; **Board Cert:** Surgery 1992, Colon & Rectal Surgery 1986; **Med School:** Northwestern Univ 1978; **Resid:** Surgery, Northwestern Meml Hosp, Chicago, IL 1978-1983; **Fellow:** Colon & Rectal Surgery, Mayo Clinic, Rochester, MN 1983-1985; **Fac Appt:** Assoc Clin Prof Surgery, Northwestern Univ

Wolff, Bruce MD (CRS) - *Spec Exp:* Inflammatory Bowel Disease; Crohn's Disease; Colon & Rectal Cancer; **Hospital:** Mayo Med Ctr & Clin - Rochester, MN; **Address:** Mayo Clinic, Div Colon & Rectal Surgery, 200 First St SW, Rochester, MN 55905; **Phone:** (507) 284-2472; **Board Cert:** Colon & Rectal Surgery 1983, Surgery 1990; **Med School:** Duke Univ 1973; **Resid:** Surgery, Cornell Med Ctr, New York, NY 1977-1981; **Fellow:** Colon & Rectal Surgery, Mayo Med Sch, Rochester, NY 1981-1982; **Fac Appt:** Prof Surgery, Mayo Med Sch

Great Plains and Mountains

Thorson, Alan MD (CRS) - *Spec Exp:* Colorectal Cancer; Crohn's Disease and Ulcerative Colitis; Incontinence-Fecal; **Hospital:** Clarkson Bishop Mem Hosp; **Address:** 8712 W Dodge Rd, Ste 240, Omaha, NE 68114-3419; **Phone:** (402) 343-1122; **Board Cert:** Surgery 1994, Colon & Rectal Surgery 1999; **Med School:** Univ Nebr Coll Med 1979; **Resid:** Surgery, Univ of Nebraska, Omaha, NE 1979-1984; Colon & Rectal Surgery, University of Minnesota, Minneaplis, MN 1984-1985; **Fac Appt:** Assoc Prof Surgery, Creighton Univ

Southwest

Bailey, Harold Randolph MD (CRS) - *Spec Exp:* Endometriosis-Intestine; Rectal Cancer-Sphincter Preservation; Inflammatory Bowel Disease; **Hospital:** Methodist Hosp - Houston; **Address:** Colon & Rectal Clinic, Smith Tower, 6550 Fannin St, Ste 2307, Houston, TX 77030-2717; **Phone:** (713) 790-9250; **Board Cert:** Surgery 1974, Colon & Rectal Surgery 1994; **Med School:** Univ Tex SW, Dallas 1968; **Resid:** Surgery, Hermann Hosp-Univ Tex Med Sch, Houston, TX 1969-1973; **Fellow:** Colon & Rectal Surgery, Ferguson-Droste Hosp, Grand Rapids, MI 1973-1974; **Fac Appt:** Clin Prof Surgery, Univ Tex, Houston

Beck, David MD (CRS) - *Spec Exp:* Colon & Rectal Cancer; Minimally Invasive Surgery; **Hospital:** Ochsner Found Hosp; **Address:** Ochsner Cancer Institute, 1514 Jefferson Hwy, 4th Fl, New Orleans, LA 70121; **Phone:** (504) 842-4060; **Board Cert:** Colon & Rectal Surgery 1987; **Med School:** Univ Miami Sch Med 1979; **Resid:** Surgery, Wilford Hall USAF Med Ctr, Lackland AFB, TX 1980-1984; **Fellow:** Colon & Rectal Surgery, Cleveland Clinic Fdn, Cleveland, OH 1985-1986; **Fac Appt:** Assoc Prof Surgery, F Edward Herbert Sch Med

Huber, Philip MD (CRS) - *Spec Exp:* Colon & Rectal Cancer; Inflammatory Bowel Disease; Obesity/Bariatric Surgery; **Hospital:** St Paul Univ Hosp; **Address:** St Paul Hosp, Dept Surg Ste 530, 5939 Harry Hines Blvd, Dallas, TX 75235-6246; **Phone:** (214) 879-3787; **Board Cert:** Colon & Rectal Surgery 1993, Surgery 1997; **Med School:** Columbia P&S 1972; **Resid:** Surgery, Parkland Hosp, Dallas, TX 1973-1977; Colon & Rectal Surgery, Presby Hosp, Dallas, TX 1978; **Fac Appt:** Prof Surgery, Univ Tex SW, Dallas

Opelka, Frank MD (CRS) (relocated to Boston, MA) - *Spec Exp:* Colon Cancer; **Hospital:** Beth Israel Deaconess Med Ctr; **Address:** Beth Israel Deaconess Med Ctr, Colon & Rectal Surgery, 330 Brookline Ave, Bldg Stoneman 932, Boston, MA 02215; **Phone:** (617) 667-4159; **Board Cert:** Colon & Rectal Surgery 2002; **Med School:** Univ Hlth Sci/Chicago Med Sch 1981; **Resid:** Surgery, Eisenhower AMC, Augusta, GA 1982-1986; Colon & Rectal Surgery, Ochsner Clinic, New Orleans, LA 1989-1990

West Coast and Pacific

Beart Jr, Robert W MD (CRS) - *Spec Exp:* Colon & Rectal Cancer; Inflammatory Bowel Disease/Crohn's; **Hospital:** USC Norris Cancer Comp Ctr; **Address:** 1450 San Pablo St, Ste 5400, Los Angeles, CA 90033-4612; **Phone:** (323) 442-5751; **Board Cert:** Surgery 1993, Colon & Rectal Surgery 1995; **Med School:** Harvard Med Sch 1971; **Resid:** Surgery, Univ Colorado Medical Center, Denver, CO 1972-1976; Colon & Rectal Surgery, Mayo Clinic, Rochester, MN 1977-1978; **Fellow:** Transplant Surgery, Univ Colorado Medical Center, Denver, CO 1974-1975; **Fac Appt:** Prof Surgery, USC Sch Med

Coutsoftides, Theodore MD (CRS) - *Spec Exp:* Colon & Rectal Surgery - General; **Hospital:** St Joseph's Hosp - Orange; **Address:** 1310 W Stewart, Ste 605, Orange, CA 92868-3857; **Phone:** (714) 532-2544; **Board Cert:** Colon & Rectal Surgery 1977, Surgery 1987; **Med School:** Israel 1970; **Resid:** Surgery, Cleveland Clinic, Cleveland, OH 1971-1973; Surgery, Royal Victoria Hosp, Montreal, Canada 1973-1976; **Fellow:** Colon & Rectal Surgery, Cleveland Clinic, Cleveland, OH 1976-1977; **Fac Appt:** Assoc Prof Surgery, UC Irvine

Schrock, Theodore R MD (CRS) - *Spec Exp:* Colon & Rectal Surgery - General; **Hospital:** UCSF Med Ctr; **Address:** 500 Parnassus Ave, MUE 505, San Francisco, CA 94143-0296; **Phone:** (415) 353-2760; **Board Cert:** Surgery 1972; **Med School:** UCSF 1964; **Resid:** Surgery, UCSF-Moffit Hosp, San Francisco, CA 1965-1967; Surgery, UCSF-Moffit Hosp, San Francisco, CA 1969-1971; **Fellow:** Surgery, Mass Genl Hosp, Boston, MA 1967-1969

Stamos, Michael J MD (CRS) - *Spec Exp:* Colon & Rectal Cancer; Laparoscopic Surgery; Colonic Volvulus; **Hospital:** LAC - Harbor - UCLA Med Ctr; **Address:** 3400 Lomita Blvd, Ste 500, Torrance, CA 90505; **Phone:** (310) 539-2630; **Board Cert:** Surgery 1991, Colon & Rectal Surgery 1992; **Med School:** Case West Res Univ 1985; **Resid:** Surgery, Jackson Meml Hosp, Miami, Fl 1985-1990; Colon & Rectal Surgery, Ochsner Clinic, New Orleans, LA 1990-1991; **Fac Appt:** Assoc Prof Surgery, UCLA

Volpe, Peter Anthony MD (CRS) - *Spec Exp:* Colon Cancer; **Hospital:** CA Pacific Med Ctr - Pacific Campus; **Address:** 3838 California St, Ste 616, San Francisco, CA 94118; **Phone:** (415) 668-0411; **Board Cert:** Surgery 1970, Colon & Rectal Surgery 1971; **Med School:** Ohio State Univ 1961; **Resid:** Surgery, UCSF Hosp, San Francisco, CA 1964-1969; **Fac Appt:** Clin Prof Surgery, UCSF

DERMATOLOGY

A dermatologist is trained to diagnose and treat pediatric and adult patients with benign and malignant disorders of the skin, mouth, external genitalia, hair and nails, as well as a number of sexually transmitted diseases. The dermatologist has had additional training and experience in the diagnosis and treatment of skin cancers, melanomas, moles and other tumors of the skin, the management of contact dermatitis and other allergic and nonallergic skin disorders, and in the recognition of the skin manifestations of systemic (including internal malignancy) and infectious diseases. Dermatologists have special training in dermatopathology and in the surgical techniques used in dermatology. They also have expertise in the management of cosmetic disorders of the skin such as hair loss and scars, and the skin changes associated with aging.

Training required: Four years

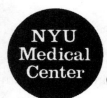

550 First Avenue (at 31st Street)
New York, NY 10016
Physician Referral: (888) 7-NYU-MED
(888-769-8633) www.nyumedicalcenter.org

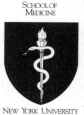

SCHOOL OF MEDICINE

NEW YORK UNIVERSITY

DERMATOLOGY:
TAKING CARE OF SKIN PROBLEMS

The Ronald O. Perelman Department of Dermatology at NYU Medical Center is recognized nationally and internationally as a leader in dermatology. Through the **Charles C. Harris Skin and Cancer Pavilion**, the Medical Center's general and specialty clinics and affiliated hospital facilities, the staff members of the Department provide primary and consultative dermatologic care for over 100,000 ambulatory and hospitalized patients yearly. In addition, faculty members of the Department train many students, residents and fellows each year, and conduct major research projects aimed at the most significant dermatologic problems of our day.

The expertise of NYU Medical Center's dermatologists encompasses all facets of medical, surgical, pediatric and cosmetic dermatology, including diseases of the hair, nails, and mucuous membranes. Laser surgery is performed for a wide variety of pigmented and nonpigmented skin lesions, and Mohs micrographic surgery is available for cutaneous tumors. Dermatologists at NYU Medical Center work closely with researchers trying to better understand and help alleviate dermatologic conditions, so their care of even the most common dermatological problems such as acne, eczema, psoriasis, and warts takes advantage of the most up-to-date breakthroughs in medicine and science.

Research for the purpose of discovering the causes of and developing new treatments for dermatologic diseases goes hand in hand with patient care and teaching. The Department conducts a strong and diversified research program in the basic and applied sciences, studying fundamental processes that have a bearing on clinical practice, as well as new and different methods of therapy. Over 30 members of the full-time faculty are engaged in laboratory and clinical research and active participation in their research projects forms an integral part of the residency program.

AREAS OF BASIC AND CLINICAL RESEARCH

AIDS: Kaposi's sarcoma and skin infections

Allergic Diseases: Hives and vasculitis

Bullous Diseases: Epidermolysis bullosa and pemphigus

Dermatopharmacology

Dermatopathology

Dermatologic Manifestations of Systemic Diseases

Epithelial Biology: Psoriasis, eczema and ichthyosis

Hair: Alopecia and hirsutism

Immunodermatology: Contact dermatitis

Laser: Birthmarks, skin tumors, pigmentary disorders

Mycology: Superficial and deep fungal infections

Oncology: Melanoma, basal cell carcinoma, squamous cell carcinoma, cutaneous lymphoma

Pediatric Dermatology: Inherited pigmentary disorders and birthmarks

Photomedicine: Psoriasis, vitiligo, eczema and lymphoma of the skin

Surgery: Cosmetic and cancer surgery

Viral Diseases: AIDS and herpes

PHYSICIAN LISTINGS

Dermatology

New England

Anderson, Richard Rox MD (D) - *Spec Exp:* *Skin Laser Surgery; Skin Cancer;* **Hospital:** MA Genl Hosp; **Address:** 275 Cambridge St, Ste 501, Boston, MA 02114; **Phone:** (617) 724-6960; **Board Cert:** Dermatology 1991; **Med School:** Harvard Med Sch 1984; **Resid:** Dermatology, Mass Genl Hosp, Boston, MA 1988-1991; **Fellow:** Dermatologic Research, Mass Genl Hosp, Boston, MA 1986-1988; **Fac Appt:** Assoc Prof Dermatology, Harvard Med Sch

Arndt, Kenneth MD (D) - *Spec Exp:* *Skin Laser Surgery; Cosmetic Dermatology; Dermatologic Therapeutics;* **Hospital:** Beth Israel Deaconess Med Ctr - Boston; **Address:** Skincare Phys of Chestnut Hill, 1244 Boylston St, Route 9, Ste 302, Chestnut Hill, MA 02467; **Phone:** (617) 731-1600; **Board Cert:** Dermatology 1966; **Med School:** Yale Univ 1961; **Resid:** Dermatology, Mass Genl Hosp-Harvard Med Sch, Boston, MA 1962-1965; **Fellow:** Dermatology, Harvard Med Sch, Boston, MA 1964-1965; **Fac Appt:** Prof Dermatology, Harvard Med Sch

Braverman, Irwin MD (D) - *Spec Exp:* *Psoriasis/Lupus; Skin Diseases; Cutaneous T-Cell Lymphoma;* **Hospital:** Yale - New Haven Hosp; **Address:** Yale Faculty Practice - Yale Phys Bldg, 800 Ave, Fl 4th, New Haven, CT 06520-8059; **Phone:** (203) 785-4092; **Board Cert:** Dermatology 1963, Dermatopathology 1982; **Med School:** Yale Univ 1955; **Resid:** Internal Medicine, Yale-New Haven Hosp, New Haven, CT 1955-1956; Internal Medicine, Yale-New Haven Hosp, New Haven, CT 1958-1959; **Fellow:** Dermatology, Yale-New Haven Hosp, New Haven, CT 1959-1962; **Fac Appt:** Prof Dermatology, Yale Univ

Dover, Jeffrey MD (D) - *Spec Exp:* *Skin Laser Surgery-Resurfacing; Photomedicine;* **Hospital:** Beth Israel Deaconess Med Ctr - Boston; **Address:** Skin Care Physicians of Chestnut Hill, 1244 Boylston St, Ste 302, Chestnut Hill, MA 02467; **Phone:** (617) 731-1600; **Board Cert:** Dermatology 1985; **Med School:** Univ Ottawa 1981; **Resid:** Dermatology, Univ Toronto, Toronto, Canada 1982-1984; Dermatology, St Johns Hosp, London 1984-1985; **Fellow:** Dermatology, Mass Genl Hosp-Harvard, Boston, MA 1985-1987; **Fac Appt:** Assoc Prof Dermatology, Dartmouth Med Sch

Edelson, Richard MD (D) - *Spec Exp:* *Skin Cancer; Skin Diseases-Immunologic;* **Hospital:** Yale - New Haven Hosp; **Address:** 800 Howard Ave, 800 Howard Ave, New Haven, CT 06519; **Phone:** (203) 785-4632; **Board Cert:** Dermatology 1977; **Med School:** Yale Univ 1970; **Resid:** Dermatology, Mass Genl Hosp, Boston, MA 1971-1972; Dermatology, Natl Inst Hlth, Bethesda, MD 1972-1975; **Fac Appt:** Prof Dermatology, Yale Univ

Gilchrest, Barbara MD (D) - *Spec Exp:* *Photoaging; Melanoma;* **Hospital:** Boston Med Ctr; **Address:** 609 Albany St, Ste 507, Boston, MA 02118-2394; **Phone:** (617) 638-5538; **Board Cert:** Internal Medicine 1975, Dermatology 1978; **Med School:** Harvard Med Sch 1971; **Resid:** Internal Medicine, Boston City Hosp, Boston, MA 1972-1973; Dermatology, Harvard Med Sch, Boston, MA 1973-1976; **Fellow:** Photo Biology, Harvard Med Sch, Boston, MA 1974-1975; **Fac Appt:** Prof Dermatology, Boston Univ

Leffell, David MD (D) - *Spec Exp:* *Mohs' Surgery; Melanoma & Skin Cancer; Laser Skin Surgery;* **Hospital:** Yale - New Haven Hosp; **Address:** 800 Howard Ave Fl 4 - rm 483, Dept of Dermatology, New Haven, CT 06519-1369; **Phone:** (203) 785-3466; **Board Cert:** Internal Medicine 1984, Dermatology 1987; **Med School:** McGill Univ 1981; **Resid:** Internal Medicine, New York Hosp, New York, NY 1981-1984; Dermatology, Yale-New Haven Hosp, New Haven, CT 1984-1986; **Fellow:** Dermatologic Surgery, Univ Michigan Med Ctr, Ann Arbor, MI 1987-1988; Dermatology, Yale-New Haven Hosp, New Haven, CT 1986-1987; **Fac Appt:** Prof Dermatology, Yale Univ

Maloney, Mary MD (D) - *Spec Exp:* Mohs' Surgery; Skin Laser Surgery; **Hospital:** U Mass Meml Hlth Care - Worcester; **Address:** Univ Mass Med Ctr, 281 Lincoln St, Ste 4, Worcester, MA 01605; **Phone:** (508) 334-5962; **Board Cert:** Dermatology 1982; **Med School:** Univ VT Coll Med 1977; **Resid:** Internal Medicine, Hartford Hospital, Hartford, CT 1978-1979; Dermatology, Dartmouth Med Ctr, Lebanon, NH 1979-1982; **Fellow:** Dermatologic Surgery, UCSF, San Francisco, CA 1983; **Fac Appt:** Prof Medicine, Univ Mass Sch Med

McDonald, Charles J MD (D) - *Spec Exp:* Lymphoma; Autoimmune Disease-Treatment; Psoriasis; **Hospital:** Rhode Island Hosp; **Address:** RI Hosp Dept Derm, 593 Eddy St APC 10, Providence, RI 02903; **Phone:** (401) 444-7816; **Board Cert:** Dermatology 1966; **Med School:** Howard Univ 1960; **Resid:** Internal Medicine, Hosp St Raphael, New Haven, CT 1961-1963; Dermatology, Yale New Haven Hosp, New Haven, CT 1963-1965; **Fellow:** Clinical Oncology, Yale New Haven Hosp, New Haven, CT 1965-1966; **Fac Appt:** Prof Dermatology, Brown Univ

Mihm Jr., Martin C. MD (D) - *Spec Exp:* Melanoma; Vascular Birthmarks; Dermatopathology; **Hospital:** MA Genl Hosp; **Address:** Mass General Hospital, 55 Fruit St Bldg Warren 827, Boston, MA 02114; **Phone:** (617) 724-1350; **Board Cert:** Dermatology 1969, Dermatopathology 1974, Anatomic Pathology 1974; **Med School:** Univ Pittsburgh 1961; **Resid:** Internal Medicine, Mt Sinai Hosp, New York, NY 1962-1964; Dermatology, Mass General Hosp, Boston, MA 1964-1967; **Fellow:** Anatomic Pathology, Mass General Hosp, Boston, MA 1969-1972; **Fac Appt:** Clin Prof Pathology, Harvard Med Sch

Mid Atlantic

Ackerman, A Bernard MD (D) - *Spec Exp:* Dermatopathology; Melanoma; Inflammatory Diseases of Skin; **Hospital:** St Luke's - Roosevelt Hosp Ctr - Roosevelt Div (page 58); **Address:** 145 E 32nd St Fl 10, New York, NY 10016; **Phone:** (212) 889-6225; **Board Cert:** Dermatology 1970, Dermatopathology 1974; **Med School:** Coll Physicians & Surgeons 1962; **Resid:** Dermatology, Univ Penn, Philadelphia, PA 1966-1967; Dermatology, Mass Genl Hosp, Boston, MA 1967-1968; **Fellow:** Dermatopathology, Mass Genl Hosp, Boston, MA 1968-1969

Alster, Tina MD (D) - *Spec Exp:* Skin Laser Surgery-Resurfacing; Scar Revision; Birthmark Elimination; **Hospital:** Georgetown Univ Hosp; **Address:** Washington Inst. Derm Laser Surg., 2311 M St NW, Ste 200, Washington, DC 20037-1445; **Phone:** (202) 785-8855; **Board Cert:** Dermatology 1990; **Med School:** Duke Univ 1986; **Resid:** Dermatology, Yale Univ, New Haven, CT 1987-1989; **Fellow:** Dermatologic Laser Surgery, Boston Univ Hosp, Boston, MA 1989-1990; **Fac Appt:** Asst Clin Prof Dermatology, Georgetown Univ

Anhalt, Grant James MD (D) - *Spec Exp:* Blistering Diseases; Pemphigus; **Hospital:** Johns Hopkins Hosp - Baltimore; **Address:** 720 Rutlend Ave, Ste 771, Baltimore, MD 21205-2196; **Phone:** (410) 955-2992; **Board Cert:** Dermatology 1980; **Med School:** Canada 1975; **Resid:** Internal Medicine, Hlth Scis Ctr, Winnipeg, Canada 1976-1977; Dermatology, Univ Mich Med Ctr, Ann Arbor, MI 1977-1980; **Fellow:** Allergy & Immunology, Univ Mich Med Ctr, Ann Arbor, MI 1980-1981; **Fac Appt:** Prof Dermatology, Johns Hopkins Univ

Bernstein, Robert M MD (D) - *Spec Exp:* Hair Restoration/Transplant; **Hospital:** NY Presby Hosp - Columbia Presby Med Ctr (page 70); **Address:** 2159 Center Ave, Fort Lee, NJ 07024; **Phone:** (212) 826-2400; **Board Cert:** Dermatology 1982; **Med School:** UMDNJ-NJ Med Sch, Newark 1978; **Resid:** Dermatology, Albert Einstein Med Ctr, Bronx, NY 1979-1982; **Fac Appt:** Assoc Clin Prof Dermatology, Columbia P&S

Bystryn, Jean-Claude MD (D) - *Spec Exp:* Skin Cancer-Melanoma; Blistering Diseases; Pemphigus; **Hospital:** NYU Med Ctr (page 71); **Address:** 530 1st Ave, Ste 7F, New York, NY 10016-6402; **Phone:** (212) 889-3846; **Board Cert:** Dermatology 1970, Clinical & Laboratory Dermatologic Immunology 1984; **Med School:** NYU Sch Med 1962; **Resid:** Internal Medicine, Montefiore Hosp, Bronx, NY 1963-1964; Dermatology, New York Univ, New York, NY 1966-1969; **Fellow:** Immunology, New York Univ, New York, NY 1969-1972; **Fac Appt:** Prof Dermatology, NYU Sch Med

DeLeo, Vincent A. MD (D) - *Spec Exp:* Photosensitivity; Contact Dermatitis; Eczema; **Hospital:** St Luke's - Roosevelt Hosp Ctr - Roosevelt Div (page 58); **Address:** 425 W 59th St, Ste 5C, New York, NY 10019-1104; **Phone:** (212) 523-6003; **Board Cert:** Dermatology 1976; **Med School:** Louisiana State Univ 1969; **Resid:** Dermatology, Columbia U-USPHS, New York, NY 1972-1976; **Fac Appt:** Assoc Prof Dermatology, Columbia P&S

Dzubow, Leonard MD (D) - *Spec Exp:* Mohs' Surgery; Skin Laser Surgery; **Hospital:** Hosp Univ Penn (page 78); **Address:** 3400 Spruce St, Bldg Rhodes Pavillion Fl 2, Philadelphia, PA 19104-4211; **Phone:** (215) 662-6534; **Board Cert:** Internal Medicine 1978, Dermatology 1980; **Med School:** Univ Penn 1975; **Resid:** Internal Medicine, Upstate Med Ctr, Syracuse, NY 1976-1977; Internal Medicine, Hosp Penn, Philadelphia, PA 1977-1978; **Fellow:** Dermatology, NYU-Skin Cancer Unit, New York, NY 1978-1980; **Fac Appt:** Prof Dermatology, Univ Penn

Fisher, Michael MD (D) - *Spec Exp:* Dermatology - General; **Hospital:** Montefiore Med Ctr - Weiler-Einstein Div (page 67); **Address:** 1575 Blondell Ave, Ste 200, Bronx, NY 10461; **Phone:** (718) 405-8300; **Board Cert:** Dermatology 1970; **Med School:** SUNY Hlth Sci Ctr 1963; **Resid:** Dermatology, Mass Genl Hosp-Harvard, Boston, MA 1966-1969; **Fac Appt:** Prof Dermatology, Albert Einstein Coll Med

Freedberg, Irwin M MD (D) - *Spec Exp:* Psoriasis; **Hospital:** NYU Med Ctr (page 71); **Address:** 530 1st Ave, Ste 7R, New York, NY 10016; **Phone:** (212) 263-5889; **Board Cert:** Dermatology 1963; **Med School:** Harvard Med Sch 1956; **Resid:** Internal Medicine, Beth Israel Hosp, Boston, MA 1957-1958; Dermatology, Mass Genl Hosp., Boston, MA 1959-1961; **Fellow:** Internal Medicine, Beth Israel Hosp, Boston, MA 1958-1959; **Fac Appt:** Prof Dermatology, NYU Sch Med

Geronemus, Roy MD (D) - *Spec Exp:* Skin Laser Surgery; Mohs' Surgery; Cosmetic Dermatology; **Hospital:** NYU Med Ctr (page 71); **Address:** 317 E 34 St, Ste 11N, New York, NY 10016-4974; **Phone:** (212) 686-7306; **Board Cert:** Dermatology 1983; **Med School:** Univ Miami Sch Med 1979; **Resid:** Dermatology, NYU-Skin Cancer Unit, New York, NY 1980-1983; **Fellow:** Mohs Surgery, NYU-Skin Cancer Unit, New York, NY 1983-1984; **Fac Appt:** Clin Prof Dermatology, NYU Sch Med

Gordon, Marsha MD (D) - *Spec Exp:* Cosmetic Dermatology; Acne; Skin Cancer; **Hospital:** Mount Sinai Hosp (page 68); **Address:** 5 E 98th St, Fl 12, Box 1048, New York, NY 10029-6501; **Phone:** (212) 831-4119; **Board Cert:** Dermatology 1988; **Med School:** Univ Penn 1984; **Resid:** Dermatology, Mount Sinai Hosp, New York, NY 1985-1988; **Fac Appt:** Assoc Clin Prof Dermatology, Mount Sinai Sch Med

Granstein, Richard MD (D) - *Spec Exp:* Acne; Immune Deficiency-Skin; Skin Cancer; **Hospital:** NY Presby Hosp - NY Weill Cornell Med Ctr (page 70); **Address:** 520 E 70th St Fl 3 - Ste 326, New York, NY 10021; **Phone:** (212) 746-2007; **Board Cert:** Clinical & Laboratory Dermatologic Immunology 1985, Dermatology 1983; **Med School:** UCLA 1978; **Resid:** Dermatology, Mass Genl Hosp, Boston, MA 1979-1981; **Fellow:** Research, Natnl Cancer Inst-Frederick Cancer Resch Facilitys, Frederick, MD 1981-1982; Dermatology, Mass Genl Hosp, Boston, MA 1982-1983; **Fac Appt:** Prof Dermatology, Cornell Univ-Weill Med Coll

Grossman, Melanie MD (D) - *Spec Exp:* Skin Laser Surgery; Photoaging; **Hospital:** NY Presby Hosp - Columbia Presby Med Ctr (page 70); **Address:** 161 Madison Ave, Ste 4NW, New York, NY 10016-5405; **Phone:** (212) 725-8600; **Board Cert:** Dermatology 1999; **Med School:** NYU Sch Med 1988; **Resid:** Internal Medicine, Yale-New Haven Hosp, New Haven, CT 1988-1989; Dermatology, Columbia/Presby Hosp, New York, NY 1989-1992; **Fellow:** Laser Surgery, Mass Genl Hosp/Harvard, Boston, MA 1992-1994; **Fac Appt:** Dermatology, Columbia P&S

Katz, Stephen MD (D) - *Spec Exp:* Immune Deficiency-Skin; **Hospital:** Natl Inst of Hlth - Clin Ctr; **Address:** NIH- Dermatology Branch, Bldg 10 - rm 12N238, Bethesda, MD 20892; **Phone:** (301) 496-2481; **Board Cert:** Dermatology 1971, Clinical & Laboratory Dermatologic Immunology 1985; **Med School:** Tulane Univ 1966; **Resid:** Dermatology, Univ Miami Project to Cure Paralysis, Miami, FL 1967-1970; **Fellow:** Research, London, England 1972-1974

Kopf, Alfred MD (D) - *Spec Exp:* Skin Cancer-Melanoma; Dysplastic Moles; **Hospital:** NYU Med Ctr (page 71); **Address:** 350 5th Ave, Ste 7805, New York, NY 10118; **Phone:** (212) 689-5050; **Board Cert:** Dermatology 1957; **Med School:** Cornell Univ-Weill Med Coll 1951; **Resid:** Dermatology, NYU Sch Med, New York, NY 1952-1955; **Fac Appt:** Clin Prof Dermatology, NYU Sch Med

Lebwohl, Mark MD (D) - *Spec Exp:* Psoriasis; Skin Cancer; **Hospital:** Mount Sinai Hosp (page 68); **Address:** 5 E 98th St, Fl 12, New York, NY 10029-6501; **Phone:** (212) 876-7199; **Board Cert:** Internal Medicine 1981, Dermatology 1983; **Med School:** Harvard Med Sch 1978; **Resid:** Internal Medicine, Mount Sinai Hosp, New York, NY 1979-1981; **Fellow:** Dermatology, Mount Sinai Hosp, New York, NY 1981-1983; **Fac Appt:** Prof Dermatology, Mount Sinai Sch Med

Leyden, James MD (D) - *Spec Exp:* Infectious Disease; Acne; **Hospital:** Hosp Univ Penn (page 78); **Address:** University of Pennsylvania Hospital, 3600 Spruce St, Bldg Rhoads - Fl 2nd, Philadelphia, PA 19104; **Phone:** (215) 662-6151; **Board Cert:** Dermatology 1973; **Med School:** Univ Penn 1966; **Resid:** Dermatology, Univ Penn, Philadelphia, PA 1967-1968; Dermatology, Univ Penn, Philadelphia, PA 1970-1971; **Fac Appt:** Prof Dermatology, Univ Penn

Miller, Stanley MD (D) - *Spec Exp:* Dermatologic Surgery; Skin Cancer; **Hospital:** Johns Hopkins Hosp - Baltimore; **Address:** John Hopkins Outpat Ctr, 601 N Caroline St Fl 6, Baltimore, MD 21287-0900; **Phone:** (410) 955-3345; **Board Cert:** Dermatology 1989; **Med School:** Univ VT Coll Med 1984; **Resid:** Dermatology, UC San Diego, San Diego, CA 1986-1989; **Fellow:** Surgery, U Penn, Philadelphia, PA 1989-1991; **Fac Appt:** Prof Dermatology, Johns Hopkins Univ

Nigra, Thomas P MD (D) - *Spec Exp:* Hair Problems; Vitiligo; Melanoma; **Hospital:** Washington Hosp Ctr; **Address:** Washington Hosp Ctr, 110 Irving St NW, Fl 2B-44, Washington, DC 20010-2976; **Phone:** (202) 877-6227; **Board Cert:** Dermatology 1973; **Med School:** Univ Penn 1967; **Resid:** Dermatology, Mass Genl Hosp, Boston, MA 1968-1969; Dermatology, Mass Genl Hosp, Boston, MA 1972-1973; **Fac Appt:** Clin Prof Dermatology, Geo Wash Univ

Orlow, Seth MD (D) - *Spec Exp:* Dermatology-Pediatric; Hemangiomas/Birthmarks; Psoriasis/Eczema; **Hospital:** NYU Med Ctr (page 71); **Address:** 530 1st Ave, Ste 7R, New York, NY 10016; **Phone:** (212) 263-5889; **Board Cert:** Dermatology 1990; **Med School:** Albert Einstein Coll Med 1986; **Resid:** Pediatrics, Mt Sinai Hosp, New York, NY 1986-1987; Dermatology, Yale Med Sch, New Haven, CT 1987-1989; **Fellow:** Dermatology, Yale Med Sch, New Haven, CT 1989-1990; **Fac Appt:** Prof Dermatology, NYU Sch Med

Rigel, Darrell MD (D) - *Spec Exp:* Melanoma; Skin Cancer; Cosmetic Dermatology; **Hospital:** NYU Med Ctr (page 71); **Address:** 35 E 35th Street, Ste 208, New York, NY 10016-3823; **Phone:** (212) 684-5964; **Board Cert:** Dermatology 1983; **Med School:** Geo Wash Univ 1978; **Resid:** Dermatology, New York Univ, New york, NY 1979-1982; **Fellow:** Dermatology, New York Univ, New York, NY 1982-1983; **Fac Appt:** Clin Prof Dermatology, NYU Sch Med

Robins, Perry MD (D) - *Spec Exp:* *Mohs' Surgery; Skin Cancer-Melanoma;* **Hospital:** NYU Med Ctr (page 71); **Address:** 530 First Ave, Ste 7H, New York, NY 10016; **Phone:** (212) 263-7222; **Board Cert:** Dermatology 1991; **Med School:** Germany 1960; **Resid:** Dermatology, VA Med Ctr, Bronx, NY 1961-1962; Dermatology, NYU Med Ctr, New York, NY 1963; **Fac Appt:** Prof Dermatology, NYU Sch Med

Safai, Bijan MD (D) - *Spec Exp:* *Dermatologic Surgery; Cosmetic Dematology; Skin Cancer;* **Hospital:** Westchester Med Ctr (page 82); **Address:** NY Med Coll, rm 217, Vosburgh Pavillion, Valhalla, NY 10595; **Phone:** (914) 594-4566; **Board Cert:** Dermatology 1974; **Med School:** Iran 1965; **Resid:** Internal Medicine, VA Med Ctr, New York, NY 1969-1970; Dermatology, NYU Med Ctr, New York, NY 1970-1973; **Fellow:** Immunology, Mem Sloan-Kettering Cancer Ctr, New York, NY 1973-1974; **Fac Appt:** Prof Dermatology, NY Med Coll

Scher, Richard K MD (D) - *Spec Exp:* *Nail Surgery; Nail Diseases; Acne;* **Hospital:** NY Presby Hosp - Columbia Presby Med Ctr (page 70); **Address:** 16 E 60th St, New York, NY 10022; **Phone:** (212) 326-8465; **Board Cert:** Dermatology 1960; **Med School:** Howard Univ 1955; **Resid:** Dermatology, NYU Med Ctr, New York, NY 1956-1959; **Fac Appt:** Prof Dermatology, Columbia P&S

Shalita, Alan MD (D) - *Spec Exp:* *Acne; Rosacea;* **Hospital:** Univ Hosp - Brklyn; **Address:** Downstate Derm Assoc, 450 Clarkson Ave, Box 46, Brooklyn, NY 11203-2012; **Phone:** (718) 270-1230; **Board Cert:** Dermatology 1971; **Med School:** Wake Forest Univ Sch Med 1964; **Resid:** Dermatology, NYU Med Ctr, New York, NY 1967-1970; **Fellow:** Dermatologic Research, NYU Med Ctr, New York, NY 1970-1973; **Fac Appt:** Prof Dermatology, SUNY Hlth Sci Ctr

Shupack, Jerome L MD (D) - *Spec Exp:* *Rare Skin Disorders; Psoriasis; Dermatologic Pharmacology;* **Hospital:** NYU Med Ctr (page 71); **Address:** 530 1st Ave, New York, NY 10016-6497; **Phone:** (212) 263-7344; **Board Cert:** Dermatology 1970; **Med School:** Columbia P&S 1963; **Resid:** Internal Medicine, Mt Sinai Hosp, New York, NY 1964-1965; Dermatology, NYU Hosp, New York, NY 1967-1970; **Fac Appt:** Prof Dermatology, NYU Sch Med

Stanley, John R MD (D) - *Spec Exp:* *Blistering Diseases; Pemphigus;* **Hospital:** Hosp Univ Penn (page 78); **Address:** Dept Dermatology, 3600 Spruce St, 2 Rhoads Pavilion, Philadelphia, PA 19104; **Phone:** (215) 662-3626; **Board Cert:** Clinical & Laboratory Dermatologic Immunology 1985, Dermatology 1978; **Med School:** Harvard Med Sch 1974; **Resid:** Dermatology, NYU Med Ctr, New York, NY 1975-1978; **Fac Appt:** Prof Dermatology, Univ Penn

Zitelli, John MD (D) - *Spec Exp:* *Mohs' Surgery; Skin Cancer;* **Hospital:** UPMC - Presbyterian Univ Hosp; **Address:** Shadyside Med Ctr, 5200 Centre Ave, Ste 303, Pittsburgh, PA 15232; **Phone:** (412) 681-9400; **Board Cert:** Dermatology 1980; **Med School:** Univ Pittsburgh 1976; **Resid:** Dermatology, Univ Hlth Ctr Hosp, Pittsburgh, PA 1977-1979; **Fellow:** Mohs Surgery, Univ Wisconsin, Madison, WI 1980

Southeast

Amonette, Rex A MD (D) - *Spec Exp:* *Skin Cancer; Mohs' Surgery;* **Hospital:** Univ of Tenn Bowld Hosp; **Address:** Memphis Derm Clinic, 1455 Union Ave, Memphis, TN 38104-6727; **Phone:** (901) 726-6655; **Board Cert:** Dermatology 1974; **Med School:** Univ Ark 1966; **Resid:** Dermatology, Univ Tenn, Memphis, TN 1969-1971; **Fellow:** Mohs Surgery, NYU Med Ctr, New York, NY 1971-1972; **Fac Appt:** Clin Prof Dermatology, Univ Tenn Coll Med, Memphis

DERMATOLOGY

Burton III, Claude Shreve MD (D) - *Spec Exp:* Leg Ulcers; Wound Healing/Care; Hemangioma; **Hospital:** Duke Univ Med Ctr (page 60); **Address:** Duke Univ Med Ctr, Box 3511, Durham, NC 27702-3511; **Phone:** (919) 681-5421; **Board Cert:** Internal Medicine 1982, Dermatology 1984; **Med School:** Duke Univ 1979; **Resid:** Internal Medicine, Duke Univ, Durham, NC 1980-1982; Dermatology, Duke Univ, Durham, NC 1982-1984; **Fac Appt:** Assoc Prof Medicine, Duke Univ

Callen, Jeffrey P MD (D) - *Spec Exp:* Lupus Dermatomysitis Vasculitis; **Hospital:** Jewish Hosp HlthCre Svcs Inc; **Address:** 310 E Broadway, Ste 200, Louisville, KY 40202; **Phone:** (502) 583-1749; **Board Cert:** Dermatology 1977, Internal Medicine 1975; **Med School:** Univ Mich Med Sch 1972; **Resid:** Internal Medicine, Univ Michigan Med Ctr, Ann Arbor 1972-1975; Dermatology, Univ Michigan Med Ctr, Ann Arbor 1975-1977; **Fac Appt:** Prof Medicine, Univ Louisville Sch Med

Camisa, Charles MD (D) - *Spec Exp:* Dermatology - General; **Hospital:** Cleveland Clin FL; **Address:** 6101 Pine Ridge Rd, Naples, FL 34119; **Phone:** (941) 348-4335; **Board Cert:** Dermatology 1981, Clinical & Laboratory Dermatologic Immunology 1987; **Med School:** Mount Sinai Sch Med 1981; **Resid:** Dermatology, NYU Hospital, New York, NY 1978-1981; **Fac Appt:** Assoc Prof Medicine, Ohio State Univ

Cohen, Bernard H MD (D) - *Spec Exp:* Hair Loss & Restoration Surgery; Cosmetic Dermatology; Skin Surgery; **Hospital:** Baptist Hosp - Miami; **Address:** 2800 Ponce de Leon Blvd, Ste 140, Coral Gables, FL 33134; **Phone:** (305) 444-0120; **Board Cert:** Dermatology 1972; **Med School:** Columbia P&S 1967; **Resid:** Dermatology, NYU Med Ctr, New York, NY 1968-1971; **Fac Appt:** Clin Prof Dermatology, Univ Miami Sch Med

Eaglstein, William MD (D) - *Spec Exp:* Wound Healing/Care; **Hospital:** Univ of Miami - Jackson Meml Hosp; **Address:** 1444 NW Ninth Ave, Miami, FL 33136; **Phone:** (305) 243-6704; **Board Cert:** Dermatology 1971; **Med School:** Univ MO-Kansas City 1965; **Resid:** Dermatology, Univ Miami/Jackson Meml, Miami, FL 1966-1969; **Fac Appt:** Prof Dermatology, Univ Miami Sch Med

Eichler, Craig MD (D) - *Spec Exp:* Skin Cancer; Dermatologic Surgery; Dermatologic Infectious Disease; **Hospital:** Cleveland Clin FL; **Address:** 6101 Pine Ridge Rd, Naples, FL 34119; **Phone:** (877) 675-7223; **Board Cert:** Dermatology 1993; **Med School:** Univ Fla Coll Med 1989; **Resid:** Dermatology, Univ Texas, Galveston, TX 1989-1993

Fenske, Neil MD (D) - *Spec Exp:* Skin Cancer; Aging Skin; Psoriasis; **Hospital:** Tampa Genl Hosp; **Address:** 12901 Bruce B Downs Blvd MDC-33, Tampa, FL 33612-4742; **Phone:** (813) 974-2920; **Board Cert:** Dermatology 1977, Dermatopathology 1984; **Med School:** St Louis Univ 1973; **Resid:** Dermatology, Wisc Hlth Sci Ctr, Madison, WI 1974-1977; **Fac Appt:** Prof Medicine, Univ S Fla Coll Med

Flowers, Franklin P MD (D) - *Spec Exp:* Mohs' Surgery; Dermatopathology; **Hospital:** Shands Hlthcre at Univ of FL (page 73); **Address:** 2000 SW Archer Rd, Ste 3151, Gainesville, FL 32610; **Phone:** (352) 265-8001; **Board Cert:** Dermatology 1976, Dermatopathology 1981; **Med School:** Univ Fla Coll Med 1971; **Resid:** Dermatology, Ohio State Univ, Columbus, OH 1972-1975; **Fellow:** Mohs Surgery, Univ Alabama, Birmingham, AL 1992-1993; **Fac Appt:** Prof Medicine, Univ Fla Coll Med

Green, Howard MD (D) - *Spec Exp:* Mohs' Surgery; **Hospital:** St Mary's Med Ctr - W Palm Bch; **Address:** 120 Butler St, West Palm Beach, FL 33401; **Phone:** (561) 659-1510; **Board Cert:** Dermatology 1992; **Med School:** Boston Univ 1985; **Resid:** Internal Medicine, Jefferson Univ Hosp, Philadelphia, PA 1986-1988; Dermatology, Harvard Med Sch, Boston, MA 1988-1992; **Fellow:** Mohs Surgery, Boston Univ Med Ctr, Boston, MA 1992-1993

198

Johr, Robert MD (D) - *Spec Exp:* *Skin Cancer;* **Hospital:** Boca Raton Comm Hosp; **Address:** 1050 NW 15th St, Ste 201A, Boca Raton, FL 33486-1341; **Phone:** (561) 368-4545; **Board Cert:** Dermatology 1981; **Med School:** Mexico 1975; **Resid:** Dermatology, Roswell Pk Cancer, Cleveland, NY 1976-1977; Dermatology, Metro Med Ctr, Buffalo, NY 1977-1979; **Fac Appt:** Assoc Clin Prof Dermatology, Univ Miami Sch Med

Jorizzo, Joseph L. MD (D) - *Spec Exp:* *Dermatology; Rheumatologic Dermatology; Dermatologic Immunology;* **Hospital:** Wake Forest Univ Baptist Med Ctr (page 81); **Address:** Wake Forest Univ Sch Med, Dept Derm, Med Ctr Blvd, Winston-Salem, NC 27157; **Phone:** (336) 716-3926; **Board Cert:** Dermatology 1979; **Med School:** Boston Univ 1975; **Resid:** Dermatology, Univ NC, Chapel Hill, NC 1976-1979; **Fellow:** Dermatology, Derm Inst, London, England 1979-1980; **Fac Appt:** Prof Dermatology, Wake Forest Univ Sch Med

Leshin, Barry MD (D) - *Spec Exp:* *Dermatologic Surgery; Mohs' Surgery;* **Hospital:** Forsyth Med Ctr; **Address:** 125 Sunnynoll, Ste 100, Winston-Salem, NC 27106; **Phone:** (336) 724-2434; **Board Cert:** Dermatology 1985; **Med School:** Univ Tex, Houston 1981; **Resid:** Dermatology, Univ IA Hosp, Iowa City, IA 1982-1985; **Fellow:** Dermatologic Surgery, Univ IA Hosp, Iowa City, IA 1985-1986

Pinnell, Sheldon MD (D) - *Spec Exp:* *Skin & Collagen Disorders; Melanoma/Skin Cancer;* **Hospital:** Duke Univ Med Ctr (page 60); **Address:** Trent Drive S, Box 3135, Durham, NC 27710; **Phone:** (919) 684-5337; **Board Cert:** Dermatology 1971; **Med School:** Yale Univ 1963; **Resid:** Internal Medicine, Minn Hosp, Minneapolis, MN 1964-1965; **Fellow:** Dermatology, Mass Genl Hosp, Boston, MA 1968-1971; **Fac Appt:** Prof Dermatology, Duke Univ

Sherertz, Elizabeth F MD (D) - *Spec Exp:* *Dermatitis;* **Hospital:** Wake Forest Univ Baptist Med Ctr (page 81); **Address:** Wake Forest Baptist Med Center, Med Center Blvd, Winston Salem, NC 27157-1071; **Phone:** (336) 716-3203; **Board Cert:** Dermatology 1982; **Med School:** Univ VA Sch Med 1978; **Resid:** Internal Medicine, Univ VA Hosp, Charlottesville, VA 1978-1979; Dermatology, Duke Univ, Durham, NC 1979-1982; **Fac Appt:** Prof Dermatology, Wake Forest Univ Sch Med

Sobel, Stuart MD (D) - *Spec Exp:* *Skin Cancer; Blistering Diseases;* **Hospital:** Mem Reg Hosp - Hollywood; **Address:** 4340 Sheridan St, Ste 101, Hollywood, FL 33021-3511; **Phone:** (954) 983-5533; **Board Cert:** Dermatology 1977; **Med School:** Tufts Univ 1972; **Resid:** Dermatology, Mt Sinai Hosp, New York, NY 1973-1976

Sokoloff, Daniel MD (D) - *Spec Exp:* *Dermatology - General;* **Hospital:** St Mary's Med Ctr - W Palm Bch; **Address:** 1000 45th St, Ste 1, West Palm Beach, FL 33407-2416; **Phone:** (561) 863-1000; **Board Cert:** Dermatology 1982; **Med School:** Geo Wash Univ 1977; **Resid:** Dermatology, Baylor Coll Med, Houston, TX 1979

Midwest

Bailin, Philip Lawrence MD (D) - *Spec Exp:* *Mohs' Surgery; Skin Laser Surgery;* **Hospital:** Cleveland Clin Fdn (page 57); **Address:** 9500 Euclid Ave, MC A61, Cleveland, OH 44195; **Phone:** (216) 444-2115; **Board Cert:** Dermatology 1975; **Med School:** Northwestern Univ 1968; **Resid:** Dermatology, Cleveland Clinic Fdn, Cleveland, OH 1971-1974; **Fellow:** Dermatopathology, AFIP, Washignton, DC 1974-1975

Cornelius, Lynne A MD (D) - *Spec Exp:* *Melanoma;* **Hospital:** Barnes-Jewish Hosp (page 55); **Address:** 969 N Mason St, Ste 220, St Louis, MO 63141; **Phone:** (314) 362-8187; **Board Cert:** Dermatology 1989; **Med School:** Univ MO-Columbia Sch Med 1984; **Resid:** Dermatology, Wash Univ, St Louis, MO 1986-1989; **Fellow:** Dermatology, Emory, Atlanta, GA 1989-1992; **Fac Appt:** Asst Prof Dermatology, Washington Univ, St Louis

DERMATOLOGY

Fivenson, David MD (D) - *Spec Exp:* Blistering Diseases; Wound Healing/Care; Lupus/SLE; **Hospital:** Henry Ford Hosp; **Address:** Dept of Dermatology, 2799 W Grand Blvd, Detroit, MI 48202-2689; **Phone:** (313) 876-2972; **Board Cert:** Dermatology 1989, Clinical & Laboratory Dermatologic Immunology 1991; **Med School:** Univ Mich Med Sch 1984; **Resid:** Dermatology, Univ Cincinnati Med Ctr, Cincinnati, OH 1986-1989; **Fellow:** Immunological Dermatology, Univ California San Diego Med Ctr, San Diego, CA 1985-1986

Garden, Jerome MD (D) - *Spec Exp:* Skin Laser Surgery; **Hospital:** Northwestern Meml Hosp; **Address:** 150 E Huron St, Ste 910, Chicago, IL 60611-2946; **Phone:** (312) 280-0890; **Board Cert:** Dermatology 1984; **Med School:** Northwestern Univ 1980; **Resid:** Internal Medicine, Northwestern Univ, Chicago, IL 1980-1981; Dermatology, Northwestern Univ, Chicago, IL 1981-1984; **Fac Appt:** Assoc Clin Prof Dermatology, Northwestern Univ

Hanke, C William MD (D) - *Spec Exp:* MOHS Surgery; Laser Surgery; Cosmetic Surgery; **Hospital:** St Vincent's Hosp - Carmel; **Address:** Laser & Skin Surgery Center of Indiana, 13450 N Meridian St, Ste 355, Carmel, IN 46032-1486; **Phone:** (317) 582-8484; **Board Cert:** Dermatology 1978, Dermatopathology 1982; **Med School:** Univ Iowa Coll Med 1971; **Resid:** Dermatology, Cleveland Clinic, Cleveland, OH 1975-1978; Dermatopathology, Indiana Univ, Indianapolis, IN 1981-1982; **Fellow:** Cutaneous Oncology, Cleveland Clinic, Cleveland, OH 1978-1979

Hruza, George J MD (D) - *Spec Exp:* Skin Laser Surgery; Mohs' Surgery; Cosmetic Surgery; **Hospital:** St Lukes Hosp; **Address:** Laser & Derm Surg Ctr, 14377 Woodlake Dr., Ste 111, St. Louis, MO 63017; **Phone:** (314) 878-3839; **Board Cert:** Dermatology 1986; **Med School:** NYU Sch Med 1982; **Resid:** Internal Medicine, New York Hosp-Cornell Univ, New York City, NY 1982-1983; Dermatology, NYU Med Ctr-Skin Cancer Unit, New York City, NY 1983-1986; **Fellow:** Surgery, Mass Genl Hosp-Harvard, Boston, MA 1986-1987; Surgery, Univ Wisc Med Sch, Madison, WI 1987-1988; **Fac Appt:** Assoc Clin Prof Dermatology, St Louis Univ

Johnson, Timothy M MD (D) - *Spec Exp:* Melanoma; Cosmetic Surgery-Face; **Hospital:** Univ of MI Hlth Ctr; **Address:** 1147 Cancer Ctr, Univ Hosp, 1500 E Medical Center Drive, Ann Arbor, MI 48109-0314; **Phone:** (734) 936-4068; **Board Cert:** Dermatology 1988; **Med School:** Univ Tex, Houston 1984; **Resid:** Surgery, Univ Mich, Ann Arbor, MI 1988-1989; Dermatology, Univ Texas, Houston, TX 1985-1988; **Fellow:** Surgery, Univ Oregon, Portland, OR 1989-1990; **Fac Appt:** Assoc Prof Dermatology, Univ Mich Med Sch

Neuberg, Marcy MD (D) - *Spec Exp:* Mohs' Surgery; Skin Cancer; Pigmented Lesions; **Hospital:** Froedtert Meml Lutheran Hosp; **Address:** Dept Dermatology, 9200 West Wisconsin Avenue, Milwaukee, WI 53226; **Phone:** (414) 805-3666; **Med School:** Oregon Hlth Scis Univ 1982; **Resid:** Internal Medicine, Georgetown Univ, Washington, DC 1982-1985; Dermatology, Boston Univ Sch of Med Ctr, Boston, MA 1985-1988; **Fellow:** Mohs Surgery, Tufts New England Med Ctr, Boston, MA 1988-1990; **Fac Appt:** Assoc Prof Dermatology, Med Coll Wisc

Paller, Amy Susan MD (D) - *Spec Exp:* Genetic Skin Disorders; Immune Disorders of Skin; Atopic Dermatitis; **Hospital:** Children's Mem Hosp; **Address:** Children's Meml Hosp, 2300 Chldns Plaza #107, Chicago, IL 60614-3394; **Phone:** (773) 880-4698; **Board Cert:** Pediatrics 1982, Dermatology 1983; **Med School:** Stanford Univ 1978; **Resid:** Pediatrics, Chldns Meml Hosp, Chicago, IL 1979-1981; Dermatology, Northwestern Meml Hosp, Chicago, IL 1981-1983; **Fellow:** Research, Univ NC Hosp, Chapel Hill, NC 1983-1984; **Fac Appt:** Prof Dermatology, Northwestern Univ

Shwayder, Tor A MD (D) - *Spec Exp:* Dermatology-Pediatric; Skin Laser Surgery-Birthmarks; **Hospital:** Henry Ford Hosp; **Address:** Henry Ford Hosp, Dept Derm, 2799 W Grand Blvd, Detroit, MI 48202-2689; **Phone:** (313) 916-2161; **Board Cert:** Pediatrics 1986, Dermatology 1987; **Med School:** Univ Mich Med Sch 1980; **Resid:** Pediatrics, Univ of Michigan Hlth Sys, Ann Arbor, MI 1980-1983; Dermatology, Strong Meml Hosp-Univ of Rochester, Rochester, MI 1984-1987; **Fac Appt:** Asst Prof Dermatology, Wayne State Univ

Sontheimer, Richard MD (D) - *Spec Exp:* Dermatologic Immunology; Lupus/SLE; **Hospital:** Univ of IA Hosp and Clinics; **Address:** Dept Dermatology, 200 Hawkins, rm 2045-BT, Iowa City, IA 52242-1090; **Phone:** (319) 356-7500; **Board Cert:** Clinical & Laboratory Dermatologic Immunology 1985, Dermatology 1979; **Med School:** Univ Tex SW, Dallas 1972; **Resid:** Internal Medicine, Univ Utah Affil Hosps, Salt Lake City, UT 1974-1976; Dermatology, Parkland Meml Hosp, Dallas, TX 1978-1979; **Fellow:** Research, Southwestern Med Sch, Dallas, TX 1976-1978; **Fac Appt:** Prof Dermatology, Univ Iowa Coll Med

Treadwell, Patricia MD (D) - *Spec Exp:* Dermatology-Pediatric; Birthmarks; **Hospital:** Riley Chldrn's Hosp (page 588); **Address:** 550 N University Blvd, Ste UH3240, Indianapolis, IN 46202; **Phone:** (317) 274-7744; **Board Cert:** Pediatrics 1982, Dermatology 1983; **Med School:** Cornell Univ-Weill Med Coll 1977; **Resid:** Pediatrics, James Whitcomb Riley Hosp, Indianapolis, IN 1978-1980; Dermatology, Indiana Univ Med Ctr, Indianapolis, IN 1980-1983

Voorhees, John MD (D) - *Spec Exp:* Aging Skin; Psoriasis; Photoaging; **Hospital:** Univ of MI Hlth Ctr; **Address:** Taubman Hlth Care Ctr, 1500 E Med Ctr Dr, rm 1910, Box 0314, Ann Arbor, MI 48109-0314; **Phone:** (734) 936-4054; **Board Cert:** Dermatology 1970; **Med School:** Univ Mich Med Sch 1963; **Resid:** Dermatology, Univ Mich Hosp, Ann Arbor, MI 1966-1969; **Fac Appt:** Prof Dermatology, Univ Mich Med Sch

Zelickson, Brian D MD (D) - *Spec Exp:* Skin Laser Surgery; **Hospital:** Abbott - Northwestern Hosp; **Address:** 825 Nicollet Ave, Med Arts Bldg, Ste 1002, Minneapolis, MN 55402; **Phone:** (612) 338-0711; **Board Cert:** Dermatology 1999; **Med School:** Mayo Med Sch 1986; **Resid:** Dermatology, Mayo Clinic, Rochester, MN 1988-1990; **Fac Appt:** Asst Prof Dermatology, Univ Minn

Great Plains and Mountains

Krueger, Gerald MD (D) - *Spec Exp:* Psoriasis; **Hospital:** Univ Utah Hosp and Clin; **Address:** Univ Utah Hlth Sci Ctr, Dept Derm, 50 N Medical Dr, Ste 4B454, Salt Lake City, UT 84132; **Phone:** (801) 581-6465; **Board Cert:** Dermatology 1973; **Med School:** Loma Linda Univ 1966; **Resid:** Dermatology, Univ Colorado Med Ctr, Denver, Co 1969-1972; **Fac Appt:** Prof Dermatology, Univ Utah

Weston, William L MD (D) - *Spec Exp:* Lupus/SLE-Neonatal; **Hospital:** Univ Colo HSC - Denver; **Address:** 1665 N Ursula St, Aurora, CO 80010; **Phone:** (720) 848-0500; **Board Cert:** Dermatology 1973, Pediatrics 1970; **Med School:** Univ Colo 1965; **Resid:** Dermatology, Colo Med Ctr, Denver, CO 1970-1972; Pediatrics, UCSF, San Francisco, CA 1967-1968; **Fac Appt:** Prof Dermatology, Univ Colo

Southwest

Butler, David F MD (D) - *Spec Exp:* Skin Cancer; **Hospital:** Univ Med Ctr - Lubbock; **Address:** UMC-Dept Dermatology, 3601 4th St, rm 48-100, Lubbock, TX 79430; **Phone:** (806) 743-1842; **Board Cert:** Dermatology 1985; **Med School:** Univ Tex Med Br, Galveston 1980; **Resid:** Dermatology, Walter Reed Army Med Ctr, Washington, DC 1982-1985; **Fac Appt:** Assoc Prof Medicine, Texas Tech Univ

DERMATOLOGY

Cockerell, Clay J MD (D) - *Spec Exp:* Dermatopathology; **Hospital:** Zale Lipshy Univ Hosp; **Address:** Dermatopath Labs, 2330 Butler St, Ste 115, Dallas, TX 75235; **Phone:** (214) 638-2222; **Board Cert:** Dermatology 1999, Dermatopathology 1986; **Med School:** Baylor Coll Med 1981; **Resid:** Dermatology, NYU Med Ctr, New York, NY 1982-1985; **Fellow:** Dermatopathology, NYU Med Ctr, New York, NY 1985-1986; **Fac Appt:** Prof Dermatopathology, Univ Tex SW, Dallas

Duvic, Madeleine MD (D) - *Spec Exp:* Cutaneous T-Cell Lymphoma; Skin Cancer; **Hospital:** Univ of TX MD Anderson Cancer Ctr, The; **Address:** MD Anderson Cancer Ctr, Dept Derm, 1515 Holcombe Blvd, Box 434, Houston, TX 77030; **Phone:** (713) 745-1113; **Board Cert:** Dermatology 1981, Internal Medicine 1982; **Med School:** Duke Univ 1977; **Resid:** Dermatology, Duke Univ, Durham, NC 1978-1980; Internal Medicine, Duke Univ, Durham, NC 1980-1982; **Fellow:** Geriatric Medicine, Duke Univ, Durham, NC 1982-1984; **Fac Appt:** Prof Dermatology, Univ Tex, Houston

Hansen, Ronald MD (D) - *Spec Exp:* Dermatology-Pediatric; **Hospital:** Univ Med Ctr; **Address:** Univ Arizona Hlth Sci Ctr, Dept Dermatology, 1501 N Campbell St, Box 245038, Tucson, AZ 85724; **Phone:** (520) 626-7783; **Board Cert:** Pediatrics 1974, Dermatology 1980; **Med School:** Univ Iowa Coll Med 1968; **Resid:** Pediatrics, Childrens Hosp, Los Angeles, CA 1969-1970; Pediatrics, Stanford Univ Med Ctr, Stanford, CA 1970-1972; **Fellow:** Dermatology, U of Arizona, Tuscon, AZ 1978-1980; **Fac Appt:** Prof Dermatology, Univ Hlth Sci/Chicago Med Sch

Horn, Thomas MD (D) - *Spec Exp:* Graft vs. Host Disease; Skin Cancer; **Hospital:** UAMS; **Address:** Univ Arkansas Med Scis, 4301 W Markham Dr, MS 576, Little Rock, AR 72205; **Phone:** (501) 686-5110; **Board Cert:** Dermatology 1987, Dermatopathology 1988; **Med School:** Univ VA Sch Med 1982; **Resid:** Dermatology, Univ Maryland, Baltimore, MD 1984-1987; **Fellow:** Dermatopathology, Johns Hopkins Hosp, Baltimore, MD 1987-1989

Levy, Moise MD (D) - *Spec Exp:* Dermatology-Pediatric; Vascular Malformations; **Hospital:** TX Chldns Hosp - Houston; **Address:** 6621 Fannin St, CC 620.16, Houston, TX 77030; **Phone:** (832) 822-3720; **Board Cert:** Pediatrics 1985, Dermatology 1986; **Med School:** Univ Tex, Houston 1979; **Resid:** Pediatrics, Univ Texas Affil Hosp, Houston, TX 1980-1983; Dermatology, Baylor Coll Med, Houston, TX 1983-1986; **Fac Appt:** Prof Dermatology, Baylor Coll Med

Menter, M Alan MD (D) - *Spec Exp:* Psoriasis; **Hospital:** Baylor Univ Medical Ctr; **Address:** 5310 Harvest Hill Rd, Ste 260, Dallas, TX 75230-5891; **Phone:** (972) 386-7546; **Board Cert:** Dermatology 1978; **Med School:** Africa 1978; **Resid:** Dermatology, Pretoria General Hospital 1968-1971; Dermatology, Guys Hospital, London, England 1972; **Fellow:** Dermatology, St Johns Hospital, London, England 1973; Dermatology, Univ Texas-Southwestern, Dallas, TX 1977; **Fac Appt:** Clin Prof Dermatology, Univ Tex SW, Dallas

Taylor, R Stan MD (D) - *Spec Exp:* Mohs' Surgery; Melanoma; Skin Cancer; **Hospital:** Zale Lipshy Univ Hosp; **Address:** Univ Tex SW Med Sch, 5323 Harry Hines Blvd, DF3 608, Dallas, TX 75390-9192; **Phone:** (214) 648-0628; **Board Cert:** Dermatology 1989; **Med School:** Univ Tex Med Br, Galveston 1985; **Resid:** Dermatology, Univ Mich, Ann Arbor, MI 1986-1989; **Fellow:** Immunological Dermatology, Univ Mich, Ann Arbor, MI 1989-1990; Mohs Surgery, Oreg Hlth Sci Univ, Portland, OR 1990-1991; **Fac Appt:** Assoc Prof Dermatology, Univ Tex SW, Dallas

Wheeland, Ronald MD (D) - *Spec Exp:* Skin Laser Surgery; Mohs' Surgery; Cosmetic Dematology; **Hospital:** Univ NM Hosp; **Address:** 1651 Galisteo St, Ste 8, Santa Fe, NM 87505-4752; **Phone:** (505) 992-3400; **Board Cert:** Dermatology 1977, Dermatopathology 1978; **Med School:** Univ Ariz Coll Med 1973; **Resid:** Dermatology, Univ Oklahoma Hlth Sci Ctr, Oklahoma City, OK 1974-1977; **Fellow:** Dermatopathology, Univ Oklahoma Hlth Sci Ctr, Oklahoma City, OK 1977-1978; Dermatologic Surgery, Cleveland Clin Fnd, Cleveland, OH 1983-1984; **Fac Appt:** Prof Dermatology, Univ New Mexico

West Coast and Pacific

Berg, Daniel MD (D) - *Spec Exp:* Skin Laser Surgery; Skin Cancer; **Hospital:** Univ WA Med Ctr; **Address:** Univ Washington Med Ctr, Box 356166, Seattle, WA 98195; **Phone:** (206) 598-2112; **Board Cert:** Dermatology 1991; **Med School:** Univ Toronto 1985; **Resid:** Internal Medicine, Sunnybrook Med Ctr, Toronto, CN 1987-1988; Dermatology, Duke Univ Med Ctr, Durham, NC 1988-1991; **Fellow:** Dermatologic Surgery, Univ Toronto, Toronto, CN 1992-1993; **Fac Appt:** Prof Dermatology, Univ Wash

Conant, Marcus A MD (D) - *Spec Exp:* AIDS/HIV-Kaposi's Sarcoma; **Hospital:** UCSF Med Ctr; **Address:** 350 Parnassus Ave, Ste 808, San Francisco, CA 94117; **Phone:** (415) 661-2613; **Board Cert:** Dermatology 1969; **Med School:** Duke Univ 1961; **Resid:** Dermatology, UCSF Med Ctr, San Francisco, CA 1964-1967; **Fac Appt:** Clin Prof Dermatology, UCSF

Fitzpatrick, Richard MD (D) - *Spec Exp:* Hair Transplantation & Laser Surgery; Photoaging; **Hospital:** Scripps Meml Hosp - La Jolla; **Address:** 477 N El Camino Real, Ste B303, Encinitas, CA 92024; **Phone:** (760) 753-1027; **Board Cert:** Dermatology 1978; **Med School:** Emory Univ 1970; **Resid:** Dermatology, UCLA, Los Angeles, CA 1975-1978

Frieden, Ilona J MD (D) - *Spec Exp:* Dermatology-Pediatric; Vascular Birthmarks; Hemangioma; **Hospital:** UCSF - Mount Zion Med Ctr; **Address:** 1701 Divisadero St, Box 0316, Department of Dermatology, San Francisco, CA 94143-0316; **Phone:** (415) 353-7800; **Board Cert:** Dermatology 1983, Pediatrics 1983; **Med School:** UCSF 1977; **Resid:** Pediatrics, UCSF Med Ctr, San Francisco, CA 1978-1980; Dermatology, UCSF Med Ctr, San Fransisco, CA 1980-1983; **Fac Appt:** Clin Prof Dermatology

Glogau, Richard Gordon MD (D) - *Spec Exp:* Mohs' Surgery; Cosmetic Dermatology; **Hospital:** UCSF Med Ctr; **Address:** 350 Parnassus Ave, Ste 400, San Francisco, CA 94117; **Phone:** (415) 564-1261; **Board Cert:** Dermatopathology 1982, Dermatology 1978; **Med School:** Harvard Med Sch 1973; **Resid:** Dermatology, UCSF Med Ctr, San Francisco, CA 1974-1977; **Fellow:** Chemosurgery, UCSF Med Ctr, San Francisco, CA 1977-1978; **Fac Appt:** Clin Prof Dermatology, UCSF

Grimes, Pearl E MD (D) - *Spec Exp:* Pigment Disorders; **Hospital:** UCLA Med Ctr; **Address:** 321 N Larchment Blvd, Ste 609, Los Angeles, CA 90004-6405; **Phone:** (323) 467-4389; **Board Cert:** Dermatology 1979; **Med School:** Washington Univ, St Louis 1974; **Resid:** Dermatology, Howard Univ, Washington, DC 1976-1979; **Fac Appt:** Assoc Prof Dermatology, UCLA

Gurevitch, Arnold William MD (D) - *Spec Exp:* Blistering Diseases; Atopic Dermatitis; Pediatric Dermatology; **Hospital:** USC Univ Hosp - R K Eamer Med Plz; **Address:** USC Ambulatory Health Center, 1355 San Pablo St, Los Angeles, CA 90033-1026; **Phone:** (323) 442-5100; **Board Cert:** Dermatology 1967; **Med School:** UCLA 1962; **Resid:** Dermatology, Harbor-UCLA Med Ctr, Torrance, CA 1963-1966; **Fac Appt:** Prof Dermatology, Univ SC Sch Med

Kane, Bryna MD (D) - *Spec Exp:* Cosmetic Dematology; Dermatology-Pediatric; **Hospital:** Long Beach Meml Med Ctr; **Address:** 701 E 28th St, Ste 418, Long Beach, CA 90806; **Phone:** (562) 989-5512; **Board Cert:** Dermatology; **Med School:** UC Davis 1980; **Resid:** Pediatrics, UCLA, Los Angeles, CA 1981-1983; **Fellow:** Dermatology, LAC-Harbor UCLA, Los Angeles, CA 1983-1986

Kilmer, Suzanne L MD (D) - *Spec Exp:* Skin Laser Surgery; **Hospital:** Univ CA - Davis Med Ctr; **Address:** 3835 J St, Sacramento, CA 95816; **Phone:** (916) 456-0400; **Board Cert:** Dermatology 1999; **Med School:** UC Davis 1987; **Resid:** Dermatology, UC Davis Med Ctr, Sacramento, CA 1988-1991; **Fellow:** Laser Surgery, Mass Genl Hosp, Boston, MA 1991-1992; **Fac Appt:** Asst Clin Prof Dermatology, UC Davis

DERMATOLOGY

West Coast and Pacific

Lask, Gary P MD (D) - *Spec Exp:* Skin Laser Surgery-Resurfacing; Cosmetic Dermatology; **Hospital:** UCLA Med Ctr; **Address:** 16260 Ventura Blvd, Ste 530, Encino, CA 91436-4603; **Phone:** (818) 788-4022; **Board Cert:** Dermatology 1983; **Med School:** Mexico 1977; **Resid:** Dermatology, Martin Luther King Jr Hosp, Los Angeles, CA 1980-1983; **Fac Appt:** Clin Prof Dermatology, UCLA

Lowe, Nicholas J MD (D) - *Spec Exp:* Psoriasis; **Hospital:** UCLA Med Ctr; **Address:** S Calif Derm/Psoriasis Ctr Inc, 2001 Santa Monica Blvd, Ste 490w, Santa Monica, CA 90404-2104; **Phone:** (310) 264-2434; **Board Cert:** Dermatology 1978; **Med School:** England 1968; **Resid:** Dermatology, Univ Southhampton, England, UK 1972-1974; Dermatology, Liverpool Univ, England, UK 1974-1977; **Fellow:** Dermatology, Scripps Clin, La Jolla, CA 1975-1976; **Fac Appt:** Clin Prof Dermatology, UCLA

Tabak, Brian MD (D) - *Spec Exp:* Skin Cancer; **Hospital:** Long Beach Meml Med Ctr; **Address:** 2865 Atlantic Ave, Ste 152, Long Beach, CA 90806; **Phone:** (562) 595-7581; **Board Cert:** Dermatology 1981; **Med School:** McGill Univ 1977; **Resid:** Dermatology, USC Med Ctr, Los Angeles, CA 1978-1981; **Fac Appt:** Asst Clin Prof Medicine, USC Sch Med

ENDOCRINOLOGY, DIABETES & METABOLISM

(a subspecialty of INTERNAL MEDICINE)

An internist who concentrates on disorders of the internal (endocrine) glands such as the thyroid and adrenal glands. This specialist also deals with disorders such as diabetes, metabolic and nutritional disorders, pituitary diseases, menstrual and sexual problems.

INTERNAL MEDICINE

An internist is a personal physician who provides long-term, comprehensive care in the office and the hospital, managing both common and complex illness of adolescents, adults and the elderly. Internists are trained in the diagnosis and treatment of cancer, infections and diseases affecting the heart, blood, kidneys, joints and digestive, respiratory and vascular systems. They are also trained in the essentials of primary care internal medicine which incorporates an understanding of disease prevention, wellness, substance abuse, mental health and effective treatment of common problems of the eyes, ears, skin, nervous system and reproductive organs.

Training required: Three years in internal medicine *plus* additional training and examination for certification in endocrinology, diabetes and metabolism

Physician Listings

Endocrinology, Diabetes & Metabolism

New England

Axelrod, Lloyd MD (EDM) - *Spec Exp:* Diabetes; Geriatric Endocrinology; **Hospital:** MA Genl Hosp; **Address:** 50 Staniford St Fl 3 - Ste 340, Boston, MA 02114; **Phone:** (617) 726-8722; **Board Cert:** Internal Medicine 1973, Endocrinology, Diabetes & Metabolism 1973; **Med School:** Harvard Med Sch 1967; **Resid:** Internal Medicine, Peter Bent Brigham Hosp, Boston, MA 1968-1969; Internal Medicine, Mass Genl Hosp, Boston, MA 1970-1971; **Fellow:** Endocrinology, Diabetes & Metabolism, Peter Bent Brigham Hosp, Boston, MA 1969-1970; Endocrinology, Diabetes & Metabolism, Mass Genl Hosp, Boston, MA 1971-1972; **Fac Appt:** Assoc Prof Medicine, Harvard Med Sch

Biller, Beverly M K MD (EDM) - *Spec Exp:* Pituitary Disorders; Cushing's Syndrome; Acromegaly; **Hospital:** MA Genl Hosp; **Address:** 15 Parkman St Bldg WAC - Ste 730-S, Boston, MA 02114; **Phone:** (617) 726-3870; **Board Cert:** Endocrinology, Diabetes & Metabolism 1989, Internal Medicine 1986; **Med School:** Univ Okla Coll Med 1983; **Resid:** Internal Medicine, Beth Israel Deaconness Hosp, Boston, MA 1983-1986; **Fellow:** Endocrinology, Diabetes & Metabolism, Mass Genl Hosp, Boston, MA 1989

Cushing, Gary W MD (EDM) - *Spec Exp:* Thyroid Disorders; **Hospital:** Lahey Cli.; **Address:** Lahey Clinic, 4 East Endocrinology, 41 Mall Rd, Burlington, MA 01805; **Phone:** (781) 273-8492; **Board Cert:** Internal Medicine 1983, Endocrinology 1985; **Med School:** Univ Mass Sch Med 1980; **Resid:** Internal Medicine, St Vincent Hosp, Worcester, MA 1981-1983; **Fellow:** Endocrinology, Beth Israel Hosp, Boston, MA 1983-1985; **Fac Appt:** Assoc Clin Prof Medicine, Tufts Univ

Daniels, Gilbert MD (EDM) - *Spec Exp:* Thyroid Disorders; Parathyroid Disease; Pituitary Disorders; **Hospital:** MA Genl Hosp; **Address:** 15 Parkman St, Bldg WACC - Ste 730, Boston, MA 02114; **Phone:** (617) 726-8430; **Board Cert:** Internal Medicine 1972, Endocrinology, Diabetes & Metabolism 1975; **Med School:** Harvard Med Sch 1966; **Resid:** Internal Medicine, Mass Genl Hosp, Boston, MA 1972; **Fellow:** Biochemistry, Natl Inst Hlth, Bethesda, MD 1970; Endocrinology, Diabetes & Metabolism, UCSF Med Ctr, San Francisco, CA 1971; **Fac Appt:** Assoc Prof Medicine, Harvard Med Sch

Godine, John Elliott MD/PhD (EDM) - *Spec Exp:* Diabetes; **Hospital:** MA Genl Hosp; **Address:** 50 Staniford St, Ste 340, Boston, MA 02114; **Phone:** (617) 726-8722; **Board Cert:** Internal Medicine 1979, Endocrinology, Diabetes & Metabolism 1981; **Med School:** Harvard Med Sch 1976; **Resid:** Internal Medicine, Mass Genl Hosp, Boston, MA 1977-1978; **Fellow:** Endocrinology, Diabetes & Metabolism, Mass Genl Hosp, Boston, MA 1978-1981; **Fac Appt:** Asst Prof Medicine, Harvard Med Sch

Hare, John W MD (EDM) - *Spec Exp:* Diabetes; **Hospital:** Beth Israel Deaconess Med Ctr - Boston; **Address:** One Joslin Pl, Boston, MA 02215; **Phone:** (617) 732-2645; **Board Cert:** Internal Medicine 1972, Endocrinology, Diabetes & Metabolism 1975; **Med School:** Indiana Univ 1965; **Resid:** Internal Medicine, VA Rsch Hosp, Chicago, IL 1969-1970; Internal Medicine, New England Deaconess Hosp, Boston, MA 1966-1967; **Fellow:** Endocrinology, Diabetes & Metabolism, Northwestern Univ, Chicago, IL 1970-1973; **Fac Appt:** Assoc Clin Prof Medicine, Harvard Med Sch

Klibanski, Anne MD (EDM) - *Spec Exp:* Pituitary Disorders; Prolactin Disorders; **Hospital:** MA Genl Hosp; **Address:** Mass Genl Hosp, Neuro-endocrine Ctr, 55 Fruit St Bldg BUL - Ste 457B, Boston, MA 02114; **Phone:** (617) 726-3870; **Board Cert:** Internal Medicine 1978, Endocrinology, Diabetes & Metabolism 1981; **Med School:** NYU Sch Med 1975; **Resid:** Internal Medicine, Bellevue Hosp Ctr, New York, NY 1976-1978; **Fellow:** Endocrinology, Mass Genl Hosp-Harvard, Boston, MA 1978-1981; **Fac Appt:** Assoc Prof Endocrinology, Diabetes & Metabolism, Harvard Med Sch

Lechan, Ronald MD/PhD (EDM) - *Spec Exp:* Pituitary Disorders; Hypothalamic Dysfunction; **Hospital:** New England Med Ctr - Boston; **Address:** 750 Washington St, Box 268, Boston, MA 02111-1854; **Phone:** (617) 636-5689; **Board Cert:** Internal Medicine 1979, Endocrinology, Diabetes & Metabolism 1981; **Med School:** Univ VA Sch Med 1976; **Resid:** Internal Medicine, Beth Israel Hosp, Boston, MA 1977-1978; **Fellow:** Endocrinology, Diabetes & Metabolism, Tufts-New England Med Ctr., Boston, MA 1978-1981; **Fac Appt:** Prof Medicine, Tufts Univ

Moses, Alan Charles MD (EDM) - *Spec Exp:* Diabetes; Metabolic Disorders; **Hospital:** Beth Israel Deaconess Med Ctr - Boston; **Address:** Joslin Diabetes Center, One Joslin Pl, Boston, MA 02215; **Phone:** (617) 732-2501; **Board Cert:** Internal Medicine 1976, Endocrinology, Diabetes & Metabolism 1981; **Med School:** Washington Univ, St Louis 1973; **Resid:** Internal Medicine, Barnes Hosp, St Louis, MO 1974-1975; **Fellow:** Endocrinology, Diabetes & Metabolism, National Cancer Inst 1975-1978; Endocrinology, Diabetes & Metabolism, Tufts-NEMC, Boston, MA 1978-1979; **Fac Appt:** Assoc Prof Medicine, Harvard Med Sch

Seely, Ellen Wells MD (EDM) - *Spec Exp:* Endocrinology, Diabetes & Metabolism - General; **Hospital:** Brigham & Women's Hosp; **Address:** Brigham and Womens Hosp, Endocrine Div - rm 277, 221 Longwood Ave, Boston, MA 02115-5804; **Phone:** (617) 732-5661; **Board Cert:** Internal Medicine 1984, Endocrinology, Diabetes & Metabolism 1987; **Med School:** Columbia P&S 1981; **Resid:** Internal Medicine, Brigham & Womens Hosp, Boston, MA 1982-1984; **Fellow:** Endocrinology, Diabetes & Metabolism, Brigham & Womens Hosp, Boston, MA 1984-1987; **Fac Appt:** Assoc Prof Medicine, Harvard Med Sch

Sherwin, Robert MD (EDM) - *Spec Exp:* Diabetes; **Hospital:** Yale - New Haven Hosp; **Address:** Sect Endocrinology, 333 Cedar St Bldg Fitkin - rm 101, Box 208020, New Haven, CT 06520-8020; **Phone:** (203) 785-4183; **Board Cert:** Internal Medicine 1972; **Med School:** Albert Einstein Coll Med 1967; **Resid:** Internal Medicine, Mt Sinai Hosp, New York, NY 1968-1969; Internal Medicine, Mt Sinai Hosp, New York, NY 1971-1972; **Fellow:** Metabolism, Yale-New Haven Hosp, New Haven, CT 1972-1973; **Fac Appt:** Prof Medicine, Yale Univ

Williams, Gordon H MD (EDM) - *Spec Exp:* Hypertension; Pituitary Disorders; **Hospital:** Brigham & Women's Hosp; **Address:** 221 Longwood Ave, Boston, MA 02115-5817; **Phone:** (617) 732-5666; **Board Cert:** Internal Medicine 1970, Endocrinology, Diabetes & Metabolism 1975; **Med School:** Harvard Med Sch 1963; **Resid:** Internal Medicine, Peter Bent Brigham Hosp, Boston, MA 1966-1967; **Fellow:** Endocrinology, Diabetes & Metabolism, Peter Bent Brigham Hosp, Boston, MA 1967-1970; **Fac Appt:** Prof Medicine, Harvard Med Sch

Mid Atlantic

Bilezikian, John P MD (EDM) - *Spec Exp:* Osteoporosis; Bone Disorders-Metabolic; Parathyroid Disease; **Hospital:** NY Presby Hosp - Columbia Presby Med Ctr (page 70); **Address:** 630 W 168th St, New York, NY 10032-3702; **Phone:** (212) 305-6238; **Board Cert:** Internal Medicine 1975, Endocrinology, Diabetes & Metabolism 1977; **Med School:** Columbia P&S 1969; **Resid:** Internal Medicine, Columbia-Presby Hosp, New York, NY 1973-1975; **Fellow:** Endocrinology, Diabetes & Metabolism, Natl Inst Health, Bethesda, MD; **Fac Appt:** Prof Medicine, Columbia P&S

Blum, Manfred MD (EDM) - *Spec Exp:* Thyroid Disorders; Parathyroid Disease; **Hospital:** NYU Med Ctr (page 71); **Address:** 530 1st Ave, Ste 4E, New York, NY 10016; **Phone:** (212) 263-7444; **Board Cert:** Internal Medicine 1974, Endocrinology 1975; **Med School:** NYU Sch Med 1957; **Resid:** Internal Medicine, Montefiore Hosp, New York, NY 1958-1959; Internal Medicine, Bellevue Hosp, New York, NY 1959-1960; **Fellow:** Endocrinology, Harvard-Beth Israel Hosp, Boston, MA 1960-1961; **Fac Appt:** Clin Prof Medicine, NYU Sch Med

Bockman, Richard MD/PhD (EDM) - *Spec Exp:* Bone Disorders-Metabolic; Osteoporosis; **Hospital:** Hosp For Special Surgery (page 62); **Address:** 519 E 72nd St, New York, NY 10021; **Phone:** (212) 606-1458; **Board Cert:** Internal Medicine 1975; **Med School:** Yale Univ 1968; **Resid:** Internal Medicine, NYU, New York, NY 1973-1975; **Fellow:** Internal Medicine, Weill Med Coll-Cornell, New York, NY 1971-1973; **Fac Appt:** Prof Medicine, Cornell Univ-Weill Med Coll

Cooper, David Stephen MD (EDM) - *Spec Exp:* Thyroid Disorders; **Hospital:** Sinai Hosp - Baltimore; **Address:** Sinai Hospital, Div Endo, 2401 W Belvedere Ave, Baltimore, MD 21215-5270; **Phone:** (410) 601-5961; **Board Cert:** Internal Medicine 1987, Endocrinology, Diabetes & Metabolism 1979; **Med School:** Tufts Univ 1973; **Resid:** Internal Medicine, Barnes Hosp, St Louis, MO 1974-1976; **Fellow:** Endocrinology, Diabetes & Metabolism, Mass Genl Hosp, Boston, MA 1976-1979; **Fac Appt:** Prof Medicine, Johns Hopkins Univ

Davies, Terry MD (EDM) - *Spec Exp:* Thyroid Disorders; Graves' Disease; Hashimoto's Disease; **Hospital:** Mount Sinai Hosp (page 68); **Address:** 1 Gustave Levy Pl, Box 1055, New York, NY 10029-6500; **Phone:** (212) 241-7975; **Med School:** England 1971; **Resid:** Internal Medicine, Univ of Newcastle, England, UK 1971-1975; **Fellow:** Endocrinology, Diabetes & Metabolism, Univ of Newcastle, England, UK 1975-1977; Endocrinology, Diabetes & Metabolism, Natl Inst Hlth, Bethesda, MD 1977-1979; **Fac Appt:** Prof Medicine, Mount Sinai Sch Med

Dobs, Adrian Sandra MD (EDM) - *Spec Exp:* Hormonal Disorders; **Hospital:** Johns Hopkins Hosp - Baltimore; **Address:** Johns Hopkins Hosp, 1830 E Monument St, Fl 3 - Ste 328, Baltimore, MD 21287-4904; **Phone:** (410) 955-2130; **Board Cert:** Internal Medicine 1981, Endocrinology, Diabetes & Metabolism 1987; **Med School:** Albany Med Coll 1978; **Resid:** Internal Medicine, Montefiore Hosp, Bronx, NY 1979-1982; **Fellow:** Endocrinology, Diabetes & Metabolism, Johns Hopkins Hosp, Baltimore, MD 1982-1984; **Fac Appt:** Assoc Prof Medicine, Johns Hopkins Univ

Drexler, Andrew Jay MD (EDM) - *Spec Exp:* Diabetes; Diabetes in Pregnancy; **Hospital:** Mount Sinai Hosp (page 68); **Address:** 1200 5th Ave, New York, NY 10029-6574; **Phone:** (212) 241-2000; **Board Cert:** Internal Medicine 1977, Endocrinology, Diabetes & Metabolism 1981; **Med School:** NYU Sch Med 1972; **Resid:** Internal Medicine, Barnes Hosp, St Louis, MO 1975-1976; **Fellow:** Endocrinology, Diabetes & Metabolism, Wash Univ Med Ctr, St Louis, MO 1976-1978; **Fac Appt:** Assoc Clin Prof Medicine, Mount Sinai Sch Med

Felig, Philip MD (EDM) - *Spec Exp:* Diabetes; Thyroid Disease; **Hospital:** Lenox Hill Hosp (page 64); **Address:** 1056 5th Ave, New York, NY 10028-0112; **Phone:** (212) 534-5900; **Board Cert:** Internal Medicine 1968; **Med School:** Yale Univ 1961; **Resid:** Internal Medicine, Yale-New Haven Hosp, New Haven, CT 1961-1967; **Fellow:** Endocrinology, Diabetes & Metabolism, Peter Bent Brigham Hosp-Harvard, Boston, MA 1967-1969

Fleischer, Norman MD (EDM) - *Spec Exp:* Thyroid Disorders; Adrenal Disorders; **Hospital:** Montefiore Med Ctr - Weiler-Einstein Div (page 67); **Address:** 1575 Blondell Ave, Ste 200, Bronx, NY 10461-2601; **Phone:** (718) 405-8260; **Board Cert:** Internal Medicine 1968, Endocrinology, Diabetes & Metabolism 1973; **Med School:** Vanderbilt Univ 1961; **Resid:** Internal Medicine, Bronx Muni Hosp Ctr, Bronx, NY 1961-1964; **Fellow:** Endocrinology, Diabetes & Metabolism, Vanderbilt Univ, Nashville, TN 1964-1966; **Fac Appt:** Prof Medicine, Albert Einstein Coll Med

Greene, Loren Wissner MD (EDM) - *Spec Exp:* Diabetes; Thyroid Disorders; Osteoporosis; **Hospital:** NYU Med Ctr (page 71); **Address:** 530 1st Ave, Ste 4B, New York, NY 10016-6402; **Phone:** (212) 263-7449; **Board Cert:** Internal Medicine 1978, Endocrinology, Diabetes & Metabolism 1981; **Med School:** NYU Sch Med 1975; **Resid:** Internal Medicine, Bellevue Hosp Ctr-NYU, New York, NY 1976-1978; **Fellow:** Endocrinology, Diabetes & Metabolism, Bellevue Hosp Ctr-NYU, New York, NY 1978-1980; **Fac Appt:** Assoc Clin Prof Medicine, NYU Sch Med

Hurley, James R MD (EDM) - *Spec Exp:* Thyroid Disorders; Graves' Disease; Thyroid Cancer; **Hospital:** NY Presby Hosp - NY Weill Cornell Med Ctr (page 70); **Address:** 525 E 68th St, Box 136, New York, NY 10021-4870; **Phone:** (212) 746-6290; **Board Cert:** Internal Medicine 1968, Nuclear Medicine 1972; **Med School:** Cornell Univ-Weill Med Coll 1961; **Resid:** Internal Medicine, New York Hosp, New York, NY 1962-1964; **Fellow:** Endocrinology, Diabetes & Metabolism, New York Hosp, New York, NY 1964-1965; **Fac Appt:** Assoc Prof Medicine, Cornell Univ-Weill Med Coll

Jacobs, Thomas MD (EDM) - *Spec Exp:* Adrenal Disorders; Pituitary Disorders; Bone-Calcium Problems; **Hospital:** NY Presby Hosp - Columbia Presby Med Ctr (page 70); **Address:** 161 Fort Washington Ave, rm 210, New York, NY 10032-3713; **Phone:** (212) 305-5578; **Board Cert:** Internal Medicine 1973, Endocrinology, Diabetes & Metabolism 1975; **Med School:** Johns Hopkins Univ 1968; **Resid:** Internal Medicine, Columbia Presby Hosp, New York, NY 1968-1973; **Fellow:** Endocrinology, Diabetes & Metabolism, Univ Wash Med Ctr, Seattle, WA 1973-1975; **Fac Appt:** Clin Prof Medicine, Columbia P&S

Korytkowski, Mary T MD (EDM) - *Spec Exp:* Diabetes; Polycystic Ovary Disease; Thyroid Disorders; **Hospital:** UPMC - Presbyterian Univ Hosp; **Address:** Univ of Pittsburgh Physicians - Div Endocrinology, 3601 Fifth Ave, Falk Bldg, Ste 2B, Pittsburgh, PA 15213; **Phone:** (412) 383-8700; **Board Cert:** Endocrinology, Diabetes & Metabolism 1989, Internal Medicine 1985; **Med School:** Univ NC Sch Med 1982; **Resid:** Internal Medicine, Francis Scott Key Med Ctr, Baltimore, MD 1982-1985; **Fellow:** Endocrinology, Diabetes & Metabolism, Sinai Hosp, Baltimore, MD 1986-1988; Endocrinology, Johns Hopkins Hosp, Baltimore, MD 1986-1988; **Fac Appt:** Assoc Prof Medicine, Univ Pittsburgh

Ladenson, Paul William MD (EDM) - *Spec Exp:* Thyroid Disorders; **Hospital:** Johns Hopkins Hosp - Baltimore; **Address:** Johns Hopkins, Dept Endocrin & Metab, 1830 E Monument St, rm 333, Baltimore, MD 21287-0003; **Phone:** (410) 955-3663; **Board Cert:** Internal Medicine 1978, Endocrinology, Diabetes & Metabolism 1981; **Med School:** Harvard Med Sch 1975; **Resid:** Internal Medicine, Mass Genl Hosp, Boston, MA 1975-1978; **Fellow:** Endocrinology, Diabetes & Metabolism, Mass Genl Hosp, Boston, MA 1978-1980; **Fac Appt:** Prof Medicine, Johns Hopkins Univ

Mahler, Richard J MD (EDM) - *Spec Exp:* Thyroid Disorders; **Hospital:** NY Presby Hosp - NY Weill Cornell Med Ctr (page 70); **Address:** 220 E 69th St, New York, NY 10021; **Phone:** (212) 879-4073; **Board Cert:** Internal Medicine 1987; **Med School:** NY Med Coll 1959; **Resid:** Internal Medicine, NY Med-Metro Med, New York, NY 1960-1962; Endocrinology, Diabetes & Metabolism, NY Med Coll, New York, NY 1962-1963; **Fellow:** Endocrinology, Diabetes & Metabolism, Univ Durham, Durham, NC 1963-1964; **Fac Appt:** Assoc Clin Prof Medicine, Cornell Univ-Weill Med Coll

Mandel, Susan MD (EDM) - *Spec Exp:* Thyroid Disorders; Calcium Disorders; **Hospital:** Hosp Univ Penn (page 78); **Address:** Hospital of Univ of Pa-Dept Endocrinology, 3400 Spruce St, Philadelphia, PA 19104; **Phone:** (215) 662-2300; **Board Cert:** Internal Medicine 1989, Endocrinology 1991; **Med School:** Columbia P&S 1986; **Resid:** Internal Medicine, Columbia Presby Hosp, New York, NY 1987-1989; **Fellow:** Endocrinology, Barigham & Womens Hosp, Boston, MA 1989-1992; **Fac Appt:** Asst Prof Medicine, Univ Penn

McConnell, Robert John MD (EDM) - *Spec Exp:* Thyroid Disorders; **Hospital:** NY Presby Hosp - Columbia Presby Med Ctr (page 70); **Address:** 161 Fort Washington Ave, New York, NY 10032-3713; **Phone:** (212) 305-5579; **Board Cert:** Endocrinology, Diabetes & Metabolism 1981, Internal Medicine 1978; **Med School:** Columbia P&S 1973; **Resid:** Wash-Barnes Hosp., St. Louis, MO 1974-1975; **Fellow:** Endocrinology, Diabetes & Metabolism, Colum-Presby Hosp., New York, NY 1975-1978; **Fac Appt:** Assoc Prof Medicine, Columbia P&S

Mersey, James Harris MD (EDM) - *Spec Exp:* Diabetes; **Hospital:** Greater Baltimore Med Ctr; **Address:** 6565 N Charles St, Ste 411, Baltimore, MD 21204-5803; **Phone:** (410) 828-7417; **Board Cert:** Internal Medicine 1975, Endocrinology, Diabetes & Metabolism 1977; **Med School:** Johns Hopkins Univ 1972; **Resid:** Internal Medicine, Johns Hopkins Hosp, Baltimore, MD 1973-1974; Internal Medicine, Johns Hopkins Hosp, Baltimore, MD 1976-1977; **Fellow:** Endocrinology, Diabetes & Metabolism, Peter Bent Brigham Hosp., Boston, MA 1974-1976; **Fac Appt:** Asst Prof Medicine, Johns Hopkins Univ

Ratner, Robert MD (EDM) - *Spec Exp:* Diabetes in Pregnancy; Thyroid/Lipid Disorders; *Diabetes;* **Hospital:** Washington Hosp Ctr; **Address:** 650 Pennsylvania Ave SE, Ste 50, Washington, DC 20003; **Phone:** (202) 675-1042; **Board Cert:** Internal Medicine 1980, Endocrinology, Diabetes & Metabolism 1983; **Med School:** Baylor Coll Med 1977; **Resid:** Internal Medicine, Baylor Affil Hosps, Houston, TX 1978-1980; **Fellow:** Endocrinology, Diabetes & Metabolism, Lahey Clin/Joslin Clin, Boston, MA 1980-1982; **Fac Appt:** Assoc Prof Endocrinology, Diabetes & Metabolism, Geo Wash Univ

Resnick, Lawrence MD (EDM) - *Spec Exp:* Hypertension; **Hospital:** NY Presby Hosp - NY Weill Cornell Med Ctr (page 70); **Address:** 520 E 70th St Fl 4, New York, NY 10021; **Phone:** (212) 746-2210; **Board Cert:** Internal Medicine 1973, Endocrinology, Diabetes & Metabolism 1975; **Med School:** Northwestern Univ 1970; **Resid:** Internal Medicine, Univ Chicago Hosps, Chicago, IL 1971-1973; **Fellow:** Endocrinology, Diabetes & Metabolism, Columbia-Presby Hosp, New York, NY 1973-1974; Cardiology (Cardiovascular Disease), Peter Bent Brigham Hosp, Boston, MA 1979-1980; **Fac Appt:** Prof Medicine, Cornell Univ-Weill Med Coll

Saudek, Christopher D MD (EDM) - *Spec Exp:* Diabetes; **Hospital:** Johns Hopkins Hosp - Baltimore; **Address:** 600 N Wolfe Bldg Osler - Ste 576, Baltimore, MD 21287; **Phone:** (410) 955-2132; **Board Cert:** Internal Medicine 1972; **Med School:** Cornell Univ-Weill Med Coll 1967; **Resid:** Internal Medicine, Rush-Presby-St Lukes Hosp, Chicago, IL 1968-1969; Internal Medicine, Boston City Hosp-Harvard, Boston, MA 1969-1970; **Fellow:** Endocrinology, Diabetes & Metabolism, Thorndale Lab-Harvard Med Sch, Boston, MA 1970-1972; **Fac Appt:** Prof Medicine

Schwartz, Stanley MD (EDM) - *Spec Exp:* Diabetes; **Hospital:** Hosp Univ Penn (page 78); **Address:** Univ Penn Med Ctr, EDM Division, 3400 Spruce St, Ravdin Bldg, 3rd Fl, Philadelphia, PA 19104; **Phone:** (215) 662-2517; **Board Cert:** Internal Medicine 1976, Endocrinology, Diabetes & Metabolism 1979; **Med School:** Univ Chicago-Pritzker Sch Med 1973; **Resid:** Internal Medicine, Hosp Univ Penn, Philadelphia, PA 1974-1976; **Fellow:** Endocrinology, Diabetes & Metabolism, Univ Chicago, Chicago, IL 1976-1978; **Fac Appt:** Assoc Prof Medicine, Univ Penn

Shuldiner, Alan Rodney MD (EDM) - *Spec Exp:* Diabetes; Eating Disorders-Obesity; **Hospital:** University of MD Med Sys; **Address:** Div Endocrinology, Diabetes & Metabolism, 660 W Redwood St, rm HH-494, Baltimore, MD 21201; **Phone:** (410) 706-1623; **Board Cert:** Endocrinology, Diabetes & Metabolism 1989, Internal Medicine 1988; **Med School:** Harvard Med Sch 1984; **Resid:** Internal Medicine, Columbia-Presbyterian Hosp, New York, NY 1984-1986; **Fellow:** Endocrinology, Diabetes & Metabolism, Natl Inst Hlth, Bethesda, MD 1986-1990; **Fac Appt:** Prof Medicine, Univ MD Sch Med

Snyder, Peter Joseph MD (EDM) - *Spec Exp:* Pituitary Tumors; Reproductive Endocrinology-Male; **Hospital:** Hosp Univ Penn (page 78); **Address:** Univ Penn Med Grp, 3400 Spruce St, Philadelphia, PA 19104; **Phone:** (215) 898-0208; **Board Cert:** Internal Medicine 1972, Endocrinology, Diabetes & Metabolism 1972; **Med School:** Harvard Med Sch 1965; **Resid:** Internal Medicine, Beth Israel Hosp, Boston, MA 1966-1967; Internal Medicine, Beth Israel Hosp, Boston, MA 1969-1970; **Fellow:** Endocrinology, Diabetes & Metabolism, Penn Hosp, Philadelphia, PA 1970-1971; **Fac Appt:** Prof Medicine, Univ Penn

Surks, Martin MD (EDM) - *Spec Exp:* Thyroid Disorders; **Hospital:** Montefiore Med Ctr (page 67); **Address:** 111 E 210th St, Bronx, NY 10467-2401; **Phone:** (718) 920-4331; **Board Cert:** Internal Medicine 1967, Endocrinology, Diabetes & Metabolism 1977; **Med School:** NYU Sch Med 1960; **Resid:** Internal Medicine, Montefiore Hosp Med Ctr, Bronx, NY 1961-1962; Internal Medicine, VA Hosp, Bronx, NY 1963-1964; **Fellow:** Research, NIMAS, Bethesda, MD 1963-1964; **Fac Appt:** Prof Pathology, Albert Einstein Coll Med

Wartofsky, Leonard MD (EDM) - *Spec Exp:* Thyroid Cancer; **Hospital:** Washington Hosp Ctr; **Address:** 110 Irving St NW, Washington, DC 20010-2975; **Phone:** (202) 877-3109; **Board Cert:** Internal Medicine 1971, Endocrinology, Diabetes & Metabolism 1972; **Med School:** Geo Wash Univ 1964; **Resid:** Internal Medicine, Barnes Hosp, New York, NY 1965-1966; Internal Medicine, Bronx Muni Hosp Ctr, New York, NY 1966-1967; **Fellow:** Endocrinology, Diabetes & Metabolism, Boston City Hosp, Boston, MA 1967-1969; **Fac Appt:** Prof Medicine, Uniformed Srvs Univ, Bethesda

Young, Iven MD (EDM) - *Spec Exp:* Thyroid Disorders; Osteoporosis; Pituitary Disorders; **Hospital:** St Vincent Cath Med Ctrs - Manhattan (page 75); **Address:** 130 W 12th St, Ste 7D, New York, NY 10011-8270; **Phone:** (212) 675-9332; **Board Cert:** Internal Medicine 1966, Endocrinology, Diabetes & Metabolism 1973; **Med School:** NYU Sch Med 1959; **Resid:** Internal Medicine, VA Med Ctr, New York, NY 1960-1963; **Fellow:** Endocrinology, Diabetes & Metabolism, NYU Med Ctr, New York, NY 1963-1966; **Fac Appt:** Assoc Clin Prof Medicine, NY Med Coll

Southeast

Barrett, Eugene Joseph MD (EDM) - *Spec Exp:* Diabetes; Cholesterol/Lipid Disorders; **Hospital:** Univ of VA Hlth Sys (page 79); **Address:** UVA Hosp, Endocrinology, PO Box 801390, Charlottesville, VA 22908; **Phone:** (804) 924-1175; **Board Cert:** Endocrinology, Diabetes & Metabolism 1995, Internal Medicine 1978; **Med School:** Univ Rochester 1975; **Resid:** Internal Medicine, Strong Meml Hosp, Rochester, NY 1975-1977; **Fellow:** Endocrinology, Diabetes & Metabolism, Yale Univ Hosp, New Haven, CT 1977; **Fac Appt:** Prof Medicine, Univ VA Sch Med

Bell, David S H MD (EDM) - *Spec Exp:* Diabetes-Insulin-dependent; Diabetes-Insulin Pump Therapy; **Hospital:** Univ of Ala Hosp at Birmingham; **Address:** Univ Alabama-Boshell Diabetes Rsch Bldg, 1808 7th Avenue South, Birmingham, AL 35294-0001; **Phone:** (205) 975-2404; **Board Cert:** Internal Medicine 1987, Endocrinology, Diabetes & Metabolism 1981; **Med School:** Ireland 1970; **Resid:** Internal Medicine, Royal Victoria Hosp, Belfast, Northern Ireland 1972-1973; Endocrinology, Diabetes & Metabolism, Univ Saskatchewan Hosp, Saskatchewan, Canada 1973-1975; **Fellow:** Endocrinology, Diabetes & Metabolism, Greater Baltimore Med Ctr, Baltimore, MD 1975-1976; **Fac Appt:** Prof Medicine, Univ Ala

Dalkin, Alan Craig MD (EDM) - *Spec Exp:* Bone Disorders-Metabolic; Osteoporosis; **Hospital:** Univ of VA Hlth Sys (page 79); **Address:** PO Box 801387, Charlottesville, VA 22908; **Phone:** (804) 924-5629; **Board Cert:** Endocrinology, Diabetes & Metabolism 1989, Internal Medicine 1987; **Med School:** Univ Mich Med Sch 1984; **Resid:** Internal Medicine, Univ Chicago, Chicago, IL 1985-1987; **Fellow:** Endocrinology, Diabetes & Metabolism, Univ Michigan Med Ctr, Ann Harbor, MI 1987-1990; **Fac Appt:** Assoc Prof Endocrinology, Diabetes & Metabolism, Univ VA Sch Med

Earp III, Henry Shelton MD (EDM) - *Spec Exp:* Cancer-Hormonal Influences; **Hospital:** Univ of NC Hosp (page 77); **Address:** 5316 Highgate Drive, Ste 125, Durham, NC 27713; **Phone:** (919) 484-1015; **Board Cert:** Internal Medicine 1976, Endocrinology, Diabetes & Metabolism 1977; **Med School:** Univ NC Sch Med 1970; **Resid:** Internal Medicine, NC Meml Hosp, Chapel Hill, NC 1974-1975; **Fellow:** Endocrinology, Diabetes & Metabolism, Univ North Carolina, Chapel Hill, NC 1975-1977; **Fac Appt:** Prof Medicine, Univ NC Sch Med

Ellis III, George John MD (EDM) - *Spec Exp:* *Endocrinology, Diabetes & Metabolism - General;* **Hospital:** Duke Univ Med Ctr (page 60); **Address:** Duke Univ Med Ctr, Box 2924, Durham, NC 27710; **Phone:** (919) 684-5568; **Board Cert:** Internal Medicine 1969; **Med School:** Harvard Med Sch 1963; **Resid:** Internal Medicine, Duke Med Ctr, Durham, NC 1965-1968; **Fellow:** Endocrinology, Diabetes & Metabolism, Duke Med Ctr, Durham, NC 1964-1967; **Fac Appt:** Assoc Prof Medicine, Duke Univ

Feinglos, Mark MD (EDM) - *Spec Exp:* *Diabetes;* **Hospital:** Duke Univ Med Ctr (page 60); **Address:** Duke Univ Med Ctr, Box 3921, Durham, NC 27710; **Phone:** (919) 684-3208; **Board Cert:** Internal Medicine 1976, Endocrinology, Diabetes & Metabolism 1977; **Med School:** McGill Univ 1973; **Resid:** Internal Medicine, Duke Univ, Durham, NC 1973-1975; **Fellow:** Endocrinology, Diabetes & Metabolism, Duke Univ, Durham, NC 1975-1978; **Fac Appt:** Prof Medicine, Duke Univ

Graber, Alan MD (EDM) - *Spec Exp:* *Diabetes; Thyroid Disorders;* **Hospital:** Vanderbilt Univ Med Ctr (page 80); **Address:** Vanderbilt Univ Med Ctr, Div Endocrinology, 2220 Pierce Ave, rm 715 PRB, Nashville, TN 37232; **Phone:** (615) 322-4752; **Board Cert:** Internal Medicine 1968, Endocrinology, Diabetes & Metabolism 1972; **Med School:** Washington Univ, St Louis 1961; **Resid:** Internal Medicine, Vanderbilt Univ Hosp, Nashville, TN 1962-1963; Internal Medicine, Univ Washington Hosp, Seattle, WA 1965-1966; **Fellow:** Endocrinology, Diabetes & Metabolism, Vanderbilt Univ Hosp, Nashville, TN 1963-1964; Endocrinology, Diabetes & Metabolism, Univ Washington Hosp, Seattle, WA 1964-1965; **Fac Appt:** Prof Medicine, Vanderbilt Univ

Kreisberg, Robert Alan MD (EDM) - *Spec Exp:* *Diabetes; Cholesterol/Lipid Disorders; Osteoporosis;* **Hospital:** Univ of S Ala Med Ctr; **Address:** Univ Southern Alabama, 307 University Blvd, Bldg CSAB 170, Mobile, AL 36688-3053; **Phone:** (334) 460-7189; **Board Cert:** Internal Medicine 1987, Endocrinology 1972; **Med School:** Northwestern Univ 1958; **Resid:** Internal Medicine, Northwestern Univ, Chicago, IL 1959-1962; **Fellow:** Endocrinology, Diabetes & Metabolism, Peter Bent Brigham Hosp, Boston, MA 1962-1964; **Fac Appt:** Prof Medicine, Univ S Ala Coll Med

Marshall, John Crook MD/PhD (EDM) - *Spec Exp:* *Neuroendocrinology; Hypothalamic Dysfunction; Reproductive Endocrinology;* **Hospital:** Univ of VA Hlth Sys (page 79); **Address:** Univ VA Hlth System, Hospital Dr, Box 800612, Charlottesville, VA 22908-0612; **Phone:** (434) 924-2431; **Board Cert:** Internal Medicine 1978, Endocrinology, Diabetes & Metabolism 1981; **Med School:** England 1973; **Resid:** Neurology, Natl Hosp Queen Square, London, England 1967-1968; Cardiology (Cardiovascular Disease), Natl Heart Hosp, London, England 1968-1969; **Fellow:** Endocrinology, Diabetes & Metabolism, Hammersmith Hospital, London, England; Endocrinology, Diabetes & Metabolism, Harbor Genl Hosp-UCLA, Los Angeles, CA 1973-1974; **Fac Appt:** Prof Medicine, Univ VA Sch Med

Ontjes, David A MD (EDM) - *Spec Exp:* *Osteoporosis; Thyroid & Pituitary Disorders; Adrenal Disorders;* **Hospital:** Univ of NC Hosp (page 77); **Address:** Univ of NC Chapel Hill, Dept of Medicine - CB 7527, Chapell Hill, NC 27599-7527; **Phone:** (919) 966-3336; **Board Cert:** Internal Medicine 1972, Endocrinology, Diabetes & Metabolism 1972; **Med School:** Harvard Med Sch 1964; **Resid:** Internal Medicine, Boston City Hosp, Boston, MA 1964-1966; **Fac Appt:** Prof Medicine, Univ NC Sch Med

Ovalle, Fernando MD (EDM) - *Spec Exp:* *Diabetes;* **Hospital:** Univ of Ala Hosp at Birmingham; **Address:** UAB Sch Med, 1808 Seventh Ave S, Bldg BDB - rm 813, Birmingham, AL 35294; **Phone:** (205) 975-2422; **Board Cert:** Internal Medicine 1995, Endocrinology, Diabetes & Metabolism 1997; **Med School:** Mexico 1989; **Resid:** Internal Medicine, Henry Ford Hosp, Detroit, MI 1991-1995; **Fellow:** Endocrinology, Diabetes & Metabolism, Barnes Hosp-Wash U Sch Med, St Louis, MO 1995-1997; **Fac Appt:** Asst Prof Medicine, Univ Ala

Powers, Alvin C MD (EDM) - *Spec Exp: Diabetes;* **Hospital:** Vanderbilt Univ Med Ctr (page 80); **Address:** Vanderbilt Univ Med Ctr, Div Endocrinology, 2220 Pierce Ave, rm 715 PRB, Nashville, TN 37232; **Phone:** (615) 936-1653; **Board Cert:** Internal Medicine 1982, Endocrinology, Diabetes & Metabolism 1985; **Med School:** Univ Tenn Coll Med, Memphis 1979; **Resid:** Internal Medicine, Duke Univ Med Ctr, Durham, NC 1980-1982; **Fellow:** Endocrinology, Diabetes & Metabolism, Mass Genl Hosp, Boston, MA 1983-1985; **Fac Appt:** Assoc Prof Medicine, Vanderbilt Univ

Quinn, Suzanne Lorraine MD (EDM) - *Spec Exp: Endocrinology, Diabetes & Metabolism - General;* **Hospital:** Shands Hlthcre at Univ of FL (page 73); **Address:** Shands at Univ Florida, Dept Endocrinology, 1600 SW Archer Rd, Gainesville, FL 32610; **Phone:** (352) 392-2612; **Board Cert:** Internal Medicine 1988, Endocrinology, Diabetes & Metabolism 1993; **Med School:** Univ Fla Coll Med 1985; **Resid:** Internal Medicine, Univ Fla Coll Med, Gainesville, FL 1985-1988; **Fellow:** Endocrinology, Diabetes & Metabolism, Univ Fla Coll Med, Gainesville, FL 1989-1992; **Fac Appt:** Assoc Prof Medicine, Univ Fla Coll Med

Skyler, Jay S MD (EDM) - *Spec Exp: Diabetes;* **Hospital:** Univ of Miami - Jackson Meml Hosp; **Address:** Univ Miami, PO Box 16960 D-110, Miami, FL 33101-6960; **Phone:** (305) 243-6146; **Board Cert:** Internal Medicine 1972, Endocrinology, Diabetes & Metabolism 1973; **Med School:** Jefferson Med Coll 1969; **Resid:** Internal Medicine, Duke Med Ctr, Durham, NC 1969-1971; **Fellow:** Endocrinology, Diabetes & Metabolism, Duke Med Ctr, Durham, NC 1971-1973; **Fac Appt:** Prof Medicine, Univ Miami Sch Med

Veldhuis, Johannes D MD (EDM) - *Spec Exp: Reproductive Endocrinology; Pituitary Disorders; Adrenal & Gonadal Disorders;* **Hospital:** Univ of VA Hlth Sys (page 79); **Address:** Jordan Hall, Dept Internal Med, PO Box 800202, Charlottesville, VA 22908; **Phone:** (434) 924-1825; **Board Cert:** Endocrinology, Diabetes & Metabolism 1979, Internal Medicine 1977; **Med School:** Penn State Univ-Hershey Med Ctr 1974; **Resid:** Internal Medicine, Mayo Grad Sch Med, Rochester, MN 1975-1977; **Fellow:** Endocrinology, Diabetes & Metabolism, Penn State Univ Hosp, Hershey, PA 1977-1978; **Fac Appt:** Prof Medicine, Univ VA Sch Med

Weissman, Peter MD (EDM) - *Spec Exp: Diabetes;* **Hospital:** Baptist Hosp - Miami; **Address:** 8940 SW 88th St, Ste 804E, Miami, FL 33176-2148; **Phone:** (305) 595-0777; **Board Cert:** Internal Medicine 1972, Endocrinology, Diabetes & Metabolism 1972; **Med School:** NYU Sch Med 1966; **Resid:** Internal Medicine, Barnes Hosp/Wash Univ, St Louis, MO 1966-1968; **Fellow:** Geriatric Medicine, Gerontology Rsch Ctr, Baltimore, MD 1968-1970; Endocrinology, Diabetes & Metabolism, Univ Mich Hosp, Ann Arbor, MI 1970-1972; **Fac Appt:** Assoc Clin Prof Endocrinology, Diabetes & Metabolism, Univ Miami Sch Med

Midwest

Bahn, Rebecca Sue MD (EDM) - *Spec Exp: Thyroid Disorders; Graves' Disease;* **Hospital:** Mayo Med Ctr & Clin - Rochester, MN; **Address:** Division of Endocrinology, 200 1st St SW, Rochester, MN 55905; **Phone:** (507) 284-1600; **Board Cert:** Internal Medicine 1985, Endocrinology, Diabetes & Metabolism 1987; **Med School:** Mayo Med Sch 1981; **Resid:** Internal Medicine, Mayo Clinic, Rochester, MN 1982-1984; **Fellow:** Endocrinology, Diabetes & Metabolism, Mayo Clinic, Rochester, MN 1984-1986; **Fac Appt:** Prof Medicine, Mayo Med Sch

Brennan, Michael Desmond MD (EDM) - *Spec Exp: Thyroid Disorders; Diabetes;* **Hospital:** Mayo Med Ctr & Clin - Rochester, MN; **Address:** Mayo Clinic - Div Endo, 200 1st St SW, Rochester, MN 55905; **Phone:** (507) 284-1600; **Board Cert:** Internal Medicine 1975, Endocrinology, Diabetes & Metabolism 1977; **Med School:** Ireland 1969; **Resid:** Internal Medicine, Mayo Clinic, Rochester, MN 1972-1975; Internal Medicine, Henry Ford Hosp, Detroit, MI 1971-1972; **Fellow:** Endocrinology, Diabetes & Metabolism, Mayo Clinic, Rochester, MN 1975-1977; **Fac Appt:** Assoc Prof Medicine, Mayo Med Sch

Burke, Susan F MD (EDM) - *Spec Exp:* Diabetes; Thyroid Disorders; Osteoporosis; **Hospital:** Northwestern Meml Hosp; **Address:** 676 N Saint Clair St, Ste 2020, Chicago, IL 60611-2941; **Phone:** (312) 280-4700; **Board Cert:** Internal Medicine 1981, Endocrinology, Diabetes & Metabolism 1983; **Med School:** Northwestern Univ 1978; **Resid:** Internal Medicine, Northwestern Meml Hosp, Chicago, IL 1979-1981; **Fellow:** Endocrinology, Diabetes & Metabolism, Northwestern Univ Med Sch, Chicago, IL 1981-1984; **Fac Appt:** Clin Inst Medicine, Northwestern Univ

Collins, Francis M MD (EDM) - *Spec Exp:* Hormonal Disorders; Diabetes; Thyroid; **Hospital:** Good Samaritan Hosp - Cincinnati; **Address:** 463 Ohio Pike, Ste 300, Cincinnati, OH 45255; **Phone:** (513) 528-5600; **Board Cert:** Internal Medicine 1978, Endocrinology, Diabetes & Metabolism 1981; **Med School:** Univ Chicago-Pritzker Sch Med 1975; **Resid:** Internal Medicine, Univ Pittsburgh, Pittsburgh, PA 1978-1978; **Fellow:** Endocrinology, Diabetes & Metabolism, Ohio State Univ, Columbus, OH 1978-1980; **Fac Appt:** Asst Clin Prof Endocrinology, Diabetes & Metabolism, Univ Cincinnati

Cryer, Philip E MD (EDM) - *Spec Exp:* Diabetes; **Hospital:** Barnes-Jewish Hosp (page 55); **Address:** Washington Univ Med School, Div Endocrinology, Diabetis, Metabolism, 660 S Euclid, Box 8127, St Louis, MO 63110; **Phone:** (314) 362-7617; **Board Cert:** Internal Medicine 1972, Endocrinology, Diabetes & Metabolism 1972; **Med School:** Northwestern Univ 1962; **Resid:** Internal Medicine, Barnes Jewish Hosp, St Louis, MO 1966-1972; **Fellow:** Endocrinology, Diabetes & Metabolism, Wash Univ Sch Med, St Louis, MO 1967-1968; **Fac Appt:** Prof Medicine, Washington Univ, St Louis

De Groot, Leslie MD (EDM) - *Spec Exp:* Thyroid Cancer; Graves' Disease; **Hospital:** Univ of Chicago Hosps (page 76); **Address:** 5841 S Maryland Ave, MC 9015, Div Endocrinology, Chicago, IL 60637; **Phone:** (773) 702-6138; **Board Cert:** Internal Medicine 1960; **Med School:** Columbia P&S 1952; **Resid:** Internal Medicine, Columbia-Presby, New York, NY 1952-1954; Internal Medicine, Mass Genl Hosp, Boston, MA 1957; **Fellow:** Endocrinology, Diabetes & Metabolism, Mass Genl Hosp, Boston, MA 1957-1959; **Fac Appt:** Prof Medicine, Univ Chicago-Pritzker Sch Med

Ehrmann, David Alan MD (EDM) - *Spec Exp:* Polycystic Ovary Disease; Diabetes; **Hospital:** Univ of Chicago Hosps (page 76); **Address:** 8541 S Maryland Ave, MC 1027, Chicago, IL 60637; **Phone:** (773) 702-9653; **Board Cert:** Internal Medicine 1985, Endocrinology, Diabetes & Metabolism 1987; **Med School:** Univ Mich Med Sch 1985; **Resid:** Internal Medicine, Univ Mich Med Ctr, Ann Arbor, MI 1983-1985; **Fellow:** Endocrinology, Diabetes & Metabolism, Univ Chicago Hosps, Chicago, IL 1985-1988; **Fac Appt:** Assoc Prof Endocrinology, Diabetes & Metabolism, Univ Chicago-Pritzker Sch Med

Emanuele, Mary Ann MD (EDM) - *Spec Exp:* Diabetes; **Hospital:** Loyola Univ Med Ctr; **Address:** Loyola Univ Hlth Sys, 2160 S 1st Ave Bldg 117 - rm 11, Maywood, IL 60153-3304; **Phone:** (708) 216-6200; **Board Cert:** Internal Medicine 1978, Endocrinology, Diabetes & Metabolism 1983; **Med School:** Loyola Univ-Stritch Sch Med 1975; **Resid:** Internal Medicine, Northwestern Univ, Chicago, IL 1975-1976; Internal Medicine, Univ Hawaii, Honolulu, HI 1976-1978; **Fellow:** Endocrinology, Edward Hines Jr VA Hosp, Hines, IL 1978-1980; **Fac Appt:** Prof Medicine, Loyola Univ-Stritch Sch Med

Emanuele, Nicholas Victor MD (EDM) - *Spec Exp:* Endocrinology, Diabetes & Metabolism - General; **Hospital:** Loyola Univ Med Ctr; **Address:** Loyola Univ Med Ctr, Dept Endocrinology, 2160 S First Ave Bldg 117 - rm 11, Maywood, IL 60153; **Phone:** (708) 216-6200; **Board Cert:** Internal Medicine 1975, Endocrinology 1979; **Med School:** Northwestern Univ 1967; **Resid:** Internal Medicine, Hines VA Hosp, Chicago, IL 1972-1974; **Fellow:** Endocrinology, Northwestern Univ, Chicago, IL 1974-1976

Heinecke, Jay W MD (EDM) - *Spec Exp:* Atherosclerosis; Cholesterol/Lipid Disorders; **Hospital:** Barnes-Jewish Hosp (page 55); **Address:** Wash Univ Sch Med, Div Atherosclerosis, Nutr & Lipid Rsch, 660 S Euclid Ave, Box 8046, St Louis, MO 63110; **Phone:** (314) 362-3500; **Board Cert:** Internal Medicine 1986, Endocrinology 1987; **Med School:** Washington Univ, St Louis 1981; **Resid:** Internal Medicine, Univ Washington, Seattle, WA 1982-1983; **Fellow:** Endocrinology, Univ Washington, Seattle, WA 1984-1987; **Fac Appt:** Prof Medicine, Washington Univ, St Louis

Herman, William H MD (EDM) - *Spec Exp:* Diabetes; **Hospital:** Univ of MI Hlth Ctr; **Address:** 1500 E Medical Center Drive, 3920 Taubman Center, Box 0354, Ann Arbor, MI 48109; **Phone:** (734) 647-5922; **Board Cert:** Internal Medicine 1982, Endocrinology, Diabetes & Metabolism 1989; **Med School:** Boston Univ 1979; **Resid:** Internal Medicine, Univ Michigan, Ann Arbor, MI 1980-1982; Preventive Medicine, Ctrs Dis Control, Atlanta, GA 1984-1985; **Fellow:** Endocrinology, Diabetes & Metabolism, Univ Michigan, Ann Arbor, MI 1985-1988; **Fac Appt:** Assoc Prof Medicine, Univ Mich Med Sch

Jensen, Michael D. MD (EDM) - *Spec Exp:* Eating Disorders-Obesity; Eating Disorders; Diabetes; **Hospital:** Mayo Med Ctr & Clin - Rochester, MN; **Address:** Div Endocrinology, 200 W 1st St, Fl 18, Rochester, MN 55905; **Phone:** (507) 284-1600; **Board Cert:** Internal Medicine 1982, Endocrinology, Diabetes & Metabolism 1985; **Med School:** Univ MO-Kansas City 1979; **Resid:** Internal Medicine, Mayo Clinic, Rochester, MN 1980-1982; **Fellow:** Endocrinology, Diabetes & Metabolism, Mayo Clinic, Rochester, MN 1982-1985; **Fac Appt:** Prof Medicine, Mayo Med Sch

Khosla, Sundeep MD (EDM) - *Spec Exp:* Osteoporosis; Bone Disorders-Metabolic; **Hospital:** Mayo Med Ctr & Clin - Rochester, MN; **Address:** Mayo Clinic - Div Endo, 200 1st St SW, Rochester, MN 55905; **Phone:** (507) 284-3707; **Board Cert:** Internal Medicine 1985, Endocrinology 1987; **Med School:** Harvard Med Sch 1982; **Resid:** Internal Medicine, Mass Genl Hosp, Boston, MA 1983-1985; **Fellow:** Endocrinology, Diabetes & Metabolism, Mass Genl Hosp, Boston, MA 1985-1988; **Fac Appt:** Asst Prof Medicine, Mayo Med Sch

Licata, Angelo A MD (EDM) - *Spec Exp:* Bone Disorders-Metabolic; **Hospital:** Cleveland Clin Fdn (page 57); **Address:** 9500 Euclid Ave, Ste A53, Cleveland, OH 44195; **Phone:** (216) 444-6248; **Board Cert:** Internal Medicine 1983; **Med School:** Univ Rochester 1973; **Resid:** Internal Medicine, Georgetown Univ Hosps, Washigton, DC 1976; **Fellow:** Endocrinology, Diabetes & Metabolism, Natl Inst Hlth, Washington, DC 1974; **Fac Appt:** Asst Clin Prof Medicine, Case West Res Univ

Mazzone, Theodore MD (EDM) - *Spec Exp:* Cholesterol/Lipid Disorders; Type 2 Diabetes; **Hospital:** Rush-Presby - St Luke's Med Ctr (page 72); **Address:** 1725 W Harrison St, Ste 250, Chicago, IL 60612; **Phone:** (312) 942-6163; **Board Cert:** Internal Medicine 1980, Endocrinology, Diabetes & Metabolism 1983; **Med School:** Northwestern Univ 1977; **Resid:** Internal Medicine, UCLA Med Ctr, Los Angeles, CA 1977-1980; **Fellow:** Endocrinology, Diabetes & Metabolism, Univ Wash Med Ctr, Seattle, WA 1980-1983; **Fac Appt:** Prof Medicine, Rush Med Coll

McMahon, Marion MD (EDM) - *Spec Exp:* Nutrition; Diabetes; **Hospital:** Mayo Med Ctr & Clin - Rochester, MN; **Address:** Div Endocrinology, 200 1st St SW, Rochester, MN 55902; **Phone:** (507) 284-1600; **Board Cert:** Internal Medicine 1985, Endocrinology, Diabetes & Metabolism 1987; **Med School:** Univ Wisc 1981; **Resid:** Internal Medicine, Med Coll Wisconsin, Milwaukee, WI 1981-1984; **Fellow:** Endocrinology, Diabetes & Metabolism, Mayo Clinic, Rochester, MN 1984-1987; Nutrition, New England Deaconess Hosp, Boston, MA 1987-1988

Polonsky, Kenneth S MD (EDM) - *Spec Exp:* Diabetes; **Hospital:** Barnes-Jewish Hosp (page 55); **Address:** CB8066 660 S Euclid Ave, St Louis, MO 63110; **Phone:** (314) 362-8061; **Board Cert:** Internal Medicine 1978; **Med School:** South Africa 1973; **Resid:** Internal Medicine, Michael Reese Hosp & Med Ctr, Chicago, IL 1976; Internal Medicine, VA Hosp, Hines, IL 1976; **Fellow:** Internal Medicine, Univ Chicago, Chicago, IL 1978; **Fac Appt:** Prof Med, Washington Univ, St Louis, MO

Rizza, Robert Alan MD (EDM) - *Spec Exp:* Diabetes-Lipid Disorders; Hypoglycemia; **Hospital:** St Mary's Hosp - Rochester, MN; **Address:** Mayo Clinic - Div Endo, 200 First St SW, Fl W18B, Rochester, MN 55905; **Phone:** (507) 284-1600; **Board Cert:** Internal Medicine 1976, Endocrinology, Diabetes & Metabolism 1979; **Med School:** Univ Fla Coll Med 1971; **Resid:** Internal Medicine, Johns Hopkins Hosp, Baltimore, MD 1971-1973; **Fellow:** Endocrinology, Diabetes & Metabolism, Mayo Clinic, Rochester, MN 1976-1979; **Fac Appt:** Prof Medicine, Mayo Med Sch

Robertson, Gary Lee MD (EDM) - *Spec Exp:* Diabetes Insipidus; Pituitary/Hypothalamic Disease; **Hospital:** Northwestern Meml Hosp; **Address:** 675 N St Claire, Ste 250, Chicago, IL 60611; **Phone:** (312) 695-7970; **Med School:** Harvard Med Sch 1961; **Resid:** Internal Medicine, Univ Louisville Hosp, Louisville, KY 1961-1964; **Fellow:** Internal Medicine, Brigham & Women's Hosp, Boston, MA 1964-1967

Semenkovich, Clay F MD (EDM) - *Spec Exp:* Cholesterol/Lipid Disorders; Diabetes; **Hospital:** Barnes-Jewish Hosp (page 55); **Address:** 4570 Children's Pl, St Louis, MO 63110; **Phone:** (314) 362-3500; **Board Cert:** Internal Medicine 1984, Endocrinology, Diabetes & Metabolism 1987; **Med School:** Washington Univ, St Louis 1981; **Resid:** Internal Medicine, Barnes Hosp, St Louis, MO 1981-1984; **Fellow:** Endocrinology, Diabetes & Metabolism, Wash Univ, St Louis, MO 1984-1986; **Fac Appt:** Assoc Prof Medicine, Washington Univ, St Louis

Werner, Phillip Ladd MD (EDM) - *Spec Exp:* Diabetes; **Hospital:** Advocate Lutheran Gen Hosp; **Address:** Nesset Pavilion, 1775 Ballard Rd, Park Ridge, IL 60068; **Phone:** (847) 318-2400; **Board Cert:** Endocrinology, Diabetes & Metabolism 1977, Internal Medicine 1975; **Med School:** Univ IL Coll Med 1972; **Resid:** Internal Medicine, Univ IL Affl Hosp, Chicago, IL 1973-1974; **Fellow:** Endocrinology, Diabetes & Metabolism, Univ Washington, Seattle, WA 1975-1977; **Fac Appt:** Prof Medicine, Univ Hlth Sci/Chicago Med Sch

Great Plains and Mountains

Eckel, Robert MD (EDM) - *Spec Exp:* Diabetes; Eating Disorders-Obesity; **Hospital:** Univ Colo HSC - Denver; **Address:** Univ Colorado Hlth Scis Ctr, 4200 E 9th Ave, MS B141, Denver, CO 80262; **Phone:** (303) 315-8443; **Board Cert:** Internal Medicine 1976, Endocrinology, Diabetes & Metabolism 1979; **Med School:** Univ Cincinnati 1973; **Resid:** Internal Medicine, University Wisc Hosp, Madison, WI 1974-1976; **Fellow:** Endocrinology, Diabetes & Metabolism, Univ Washington, Seattle, WA 1976-1979; **Fac Appt:** Prof Medicine, Univ Colo

Ridgway, E Chester MD (EDM) - *Spec Exp:* Thyroid Cancer; Thyroid Disorders; Pituitary Disorders; **Hospital:** Univ Colo HSC - Denver; **Address:** 1635 N Ursula St, PO, Box 6510, Aurora, CO 80015; **Phone:** (720) 848-2650; **Board Cert:** Internal Medicine 1972, Endocrinology 1973; **Med School:** Univ Colo 1968; **Resid:** Internal Medicine, Mass Genl Hosp, Boston, MA 1969-1970; **Fellow:** Endocrinology, Mass Genl Hosp, Boston, MA 1970-1972; **Fac Appt:** Prof Medicine, Univ Colo

Southwest

Gagel, Robert F MD (EDM) - *Spec Exp:* Thyroid Cancer; **Hospital:** Univ of TX MD Anderson Cancer Ctr, The; **Address:** MD Anderson Cancer Ctr, 1515 Holcombe Blvd, Box 433, Houston, TX 77030; **Phone:** (713) 792-2351; **Board Cert:** Internal Medicine 1975, Endocrinology 1977; **Med School:** Ohio State Univ 1971; **Resid:** Internal Medicine, New England Med Ctr, Boston, MA 1971-1973; **Fellow:** Endocrinology, New England Med Ctr, Boston, MA 1973-1975; Endocrinology Research, Harvard Med Sch, Boston, MA 1977-1981; **Fac Appt:** Prof Medicine, Univ Tex, Houston

Griffin, James Emmet MD (EDM) - *Spec Exp:* Hypogonadism-Male; Thyroid Disorders; **Hospital:** Parkland Mem Hosp; **Address:** Univ Texas SW Med Ctr, Dept Med, 5323 Harry Hines Blvd, Dallas, TX 75390-8857; **Phone:** (214) 648-3494; **Board Cert:** Endocrinology, Diabetes & Metabolism 1977, Internal Medicine 1975; **Med School:** Univ Kans 1970; **Resid:** Internal Medicine, Univ Kansas Med Ctr, Kansas City, KS 1971-1972; **Fellow:** Endocrinology, Diabetes & Metabolism, Univ Texas Hlth Sci Ctr, Dallas, TX 1974-1976; **Fac Appt:** Prof Medicine, Univ Tex SW, Dallas

Lavis, Victor Ralph MD (EDM) - *Spec Exp:* Diabetes; **Hospital:** Meml Hermann Hosp; **Address:** Adult Diabetes and Endo Ctr, 6410 Fannin, Bldg Hermann Prof - Fl 6, Houston, TX 77030; **Phone:** (713) 704-6661; **Board Cert:** Endocrinology, Diabetes & Metabolism 1998, Internal Medicine 1969; **Med School:** Stanford Univ 1962; **Resid:** Internal Medicine, Boston Cty Hosp Harvard, Boston, MA 1962-1964; Internal Medicine, UCLA, Los Angeles, CA 1966-1967; **Fellow:** Endocrinology, Diabetes & Metabolism, Univ Washington, Washington, DC 1967-1970; **Fac Appt:** Prof Endocrinology, Diabetes & Metabolism, Univ Tex, Houston

Levy, Philip MD (EDM) - *Spec Exp:* Diabetes; Thyroid Disorders; **Hospital:** Good Samaritan Regl Med Ctr - Phoenix; **Address:** Phoenix Endocrinology Clin, 1300 N 12th St, Ste 600, Phoenix, AZ 85006-2850; **Phone:** (602) 252-3699; **Board Cert:** Internal Medicine 1963, Endocrinology 1972, Neuroradiology 1976; **Med School:** Univ Pittsburgh 1956; **Resid:** Internal Medicine, Michael Reese Hosp, Chicago, IL 1957-1960; Endocrinology, Diabetes & Metabolism, Guys Hosp Med Sch, London, England 1961-1962; **Fellow:** Endocrinology, Diabetes & Metabolism, Michael Reese Hosp, Chicago, IL 1960-1961; **Fac Appt:** Clin Prof Medicine, Univ Ariz Coll Med

Mundy, Gregory Robert MD (EDM) - *Spec Exp:* Osteoporosis; Bone Disorders-Metabolic; **Hospital:** Univ of Texas Hlth & Sci Ctr; **Address:** 14960 Omicron Drive, San Antonio, TX 78229-3217; **Phone:** (210) 567-4900; **Board Cert:** Endocrinology, Diabetes & Metabolism 1977, Internal Medicine 1975; **Med School:** Australia 1973; **Resid:** Internal Medicine, Royal Hobart Hosp, Tasmania, Australia 1968-1970; **Fac Appt:** Prof Medicine, Univ Tex, San Antonio

Raskin, Philip MD (EDM) - *Spec Exp:* Diabetes; **Hospital:** Zale Lipshy Univ Hosp; **Address:** Univ Tex SW Med Ctr, 5323 Harry Hines Blvd, Ste G5.238, Dallas, TX 75390-8858; **Phone:** (214) 648-2017; **Board Cert:** Internal Medicine 1972, Endocrinology 1973; **Med School:** Univ Pittsburgh 1966; **Resid:** Internal Medicine, Hlth Ctr Hosps-Univ Pittsburgh, Pittsburgh, PA 1967-1968; **Fellow:** Endocrinology, Diabetes & Metabolism, Southwestern Med Sch, Dallas, TX 1970-1972; **Fac Appt:** Prof Medicine, Univ Tex SW, Dallas

Reasner, Charles A MD (EDM) - *Spec Exp:* Thyroid Disorders; **Hospital:** Univ of Texas Hlth & Sci Ctr; **Address:** Texas Diabetes Inst, 701 S Zarzamora St, San Antonio, TX 78207; **Phone:** (210) 358-7402; **Board Cert:** Internal Medicine 1983, Endocrinology 1985; **Med School:** Loma Linda Univ 1979; **Resid:** Internal Medicine, USAF Med Ctr, Keesler AFB, MS 1981-1983; **Fellow:** Endocrinology, Diabetes & Metabolism, Wilford Hall Med Ctr, Lackland AFB, TX 1983-1985; **Fac Appt:** Assoc Prof Medicine, Univ Tex, San Antonio

West Coast and Pacific

Berkson, Richard Alan MD (EDM) - *Spec Exp:* *Diabetes; Thyroid Disorders;* **Hospital:** St Mary's Med Ctr; **Address:** 1868 Pacific Ave, Long Beach, CA 90806-6113; **Phone:** (562) 595-4718; **Board Cert:** Internal Medicine 1975, Endocrinology, Diabetes & Metabolism 1977; **Med School:** SUNY Buffalo 1972; **Resid:** Internal Medicine, Univ Program, Buffalo, NY 1972-1975; **Fellow:** Endocrinology, Diabetes & Metabolism, Joslin Clinic, Boston, MA 1975-1976; Endocrinology, Diabetes & Metabolism, UCLA Ctr Hlth Scis, Los Angeles, CA 1976-1977; **Fac Appt:** Assoc Clin Prof Medicine, UCLA

Chait, Alan MD (EDM) - *Spec Exp:* *Cholesterol/Lipid Disorders; Diabetes; Nutrition;* **Hospital:** Univ WA Med Ctr; **Address:** Univ Washington Med Ctr, 1959 NE Pacific St, Box 356426, Seattle, WA 98195; **Phone:** (206) 598-5068; **Med School:** South Africa 1967; **Resid:** Internal Medicine, Hammersmith Hosp, London, England 1969-1971; **Fellow:** Endocrinology, Diabetes & Metabolism, Hammersmith Hosp, London, England 1971-1973; Endocrinology, Diabetes & Metabolism, Univ Washington, Seattle, WA 1975-1977; **Fac Appt:** Prof Medicine, Univ Wash

Chopra, Inder Jit MD (EDM) - *Spec Exp:* *Endocrinology, Diabetes & Metabolism - General;* **Hospital:** UCLA Med Ctr; **Address:** 900 Veteran Ave Bldg Warren Hall - rm 24-130, Los Angeles, CA 90095-7073; **Phone:** (310) 825-2346; **Board Cert:** Internal Medicine 1972, Endocrinology, Diabetes & Metabolism 1973; **Med School:** India 1961; **Resid:** Internal Medicine, Queens Medical Center, Honolulu, HI 1962; Internal Medicine, Inst Med Sci, New Delhi India 1967; **Fellow:** Endocrinology, Diabetes & Metabolism, Harbor-UCLA, Torrance, CA 1968-1971; **Fac Appt:** Prof Medicine, UCLA

Fitzgerald, Paul Anthony MD (EDM) - *Spec Exp:* *Diabetes; Thyroid Disorders; Pituitary Disorders;* **Hospital:** UCSF Med Ctr; **Address:** 350 Parnassus Ave, Ste 710, San Francisco, CA 94117; **Phone:** (415) 665-1136; **Board Cert:** Endocrinology, Diabetes & Metabolism 1981, Internal Medicine 1975; **Med School:** Jefferson Med Coll 1972; **Resid:** Internal Medicine, Presby Med Ctr-Univ Colo, Denver, CO 1973-1975; **Fellow:** Endocrinology, Diabetes & Metabolism, UC San Francisco Med Ctr, San Francisco, CA 1976-1978; **Fac Appt:** Clin Prof Medicine, UCSF

Gonzalez, Martha MD (EDM) - *Spec Exp:* *Osteoporosis/ Menopause; Thyroid Disorders; Diabetes;* **Hospital:** Comm Mem Hosp - San Buena Ventura; **Address:** 116 N Brent St, Ventura, CA 93003; **Phone:** (805) 656-4311; **Board Cert:** Internal Medicine 1995, Endocrinology, Diabetes & Metabolism 1997; **Med School:** UCLA 1986; **Resid:** Internal Medicine, UCLA-Wadsworth VA Med Ctr, West Los Angeles, CA 1988-1990; **Fellow:** Endocrinology, Diabetes & Metabolism, LA Co-USC Med Ctr, Los Angeles, CA 1990-1992

Greenspan, Francis S MD (EDM) - *Spec Exp:* *Endocrinology, Diabetes & Metabolism - General;* **Hospital:** UCSF Med Ctr; **Address:** 350 Parnassus Ave, Ste 609, San Francisco, CA 94117; **Phone:** (415) 476-1121; **Board Cert:** Internal Medicine 1977, Endocrinology, Diabetes & Metabolism 1972; **Med School:** Cornell Univ-Weill Med Coll 1943; **Resid:** Internal Medicine, New York Hosp, New York, NY 1944-1947; Internal Medicine, Stanford Univ Hosp, Stanford, CA 1947-1948; **Fellow:** Endocrinology, Diabetes & Metabolism, Univ Calif, Berkeley, CA 1947-1948; **Fac Appt:** Clin Prof Medicine, UCSF

Hoffman, Andrew R MD (EDM) - *Spec Exp:* *Pituitary Disorders; Pituitary Tumors; Neuroendocrinology;* **Hospital:** Stanford Med Ctr; **Address:** 3801 Miranda Ave, Palo Alto, CA 94304; **Phone:** (650) 858-3930; **Board Cert:** Internal Medicine 1979, Endocrinology, Diabetes & Metabolism 1981; **Med School:** Stanford Univ 1976; **Resid:** Internal Medicine, Mass Genl Hosp, Boston, MA 1977-1978; **Fellow:** Pharmacology, Mass Genl Hosp, Boston, MA 1978-1980; Endocrinology, Diabetes & Metabolism, Mass Genl Hosp, Boston, MA 1980-1982; **Fac Appt:** Prof Medicine, Stanford Univ

Hsueh, Willa Ann MD (EDM) - *Spec Exp:* Diabetes; Hypertension; **Hospital:** UCLA Med Ctr; **Address:** 900 Veteran Ave, Ste 24-130, Los Angeles, CA 90095-7073; **Phone:** (310) 794-7555; **Board Cert:** Internal Medicine 1976, Endocrinology, Diabetes & Metabolism 1977; **Med School:** Ohio State Univ 1973; **Resid:** Internal Medicine, Johns Hopkins Hosp, Baltimore, MD 1974-1975; **Fellow:** Endocrinology, Diabetes & Metabolism, Johns Hopkins Hosp, Baltimore, MD 1975-1976; **Fac Appt:** Prof Medicine, UCLA

Ipp, Eli MD (EDM) - *Spec Exp:* Diabetes; **Hospital:** LAC - Harbor - UCLA Med Ctr; **Address:** 21840 S Normandy Ave, Ste 700, Torrance, CA 90502; **Phone:** (310) 222-5101; **Board Cert:** Internal Medicine 1979, Endocrinology, Diabetes & Metabolism 1981; **Med School:** South Africa 1968; **Resid:** Internal Medicine, Tel Hashomer Hosp, Tel Aviv, Israel 1970-1974; **Fellow:** Endocrinology, Diabetes & Metabolism, Univ Tex SW, Dallas, TX 1976-1978; **Fac Appt:** Prof Medicine, UCLA

Kamdar, Vikram V MD (EDM) - *Spec Exp:* Diabetes; Diabetic Leg/Foot Problems; **Hospital:** Rancho Los Amigos Natl Rehab Ctr; **Address:** 7601 E Imperial Hwy, Ste 145HB, Downey, CA 90242; **Phone:** (562) 401-7225; **Board Cert:** Internal Medicine 1978, Endocrinology, Diabetes & Metabolism 1979; **Med School:** India 1971; **Resid:** Internal Medicine, Lemuel Shattuck Hosp, Boston, MA 1972; Endocrinology, Diabetes & Metabolism, Cedars-Sinai Med Ctr, Los Angeles, CA 1975-1977; **Fellow:** Endocrinology, Diabetes & Metabolism, LA Co-USC Med Ctr, Los Angeles, CA 1973-1975; **Fac Appt:** Assoc Clin Prof Medicine, USC Sch Med

Melmed, Shlomo MD (EDM) - *Spec Exp:* Pituitary Tumors; Acromegaly; **Hospital:** Cedars-Sinai Med Ctr; **Address:** Cedars Sinai Med Ctr, Pituitary Ctr, 8700 Beverly Blvd, Los Angeles, CA 90048; **Phone:** (310) 423-4691; **Board Cert:** Internal Medicine 1979, Endocrinology, Diabetes & Metabolism 1983; **Med School:** South Africa 1970; **Resid:** Internal Medicine, Sheba Med Ctr, Tel Hashomer 1972-1976; **Fellow:** Endocrinology, Diabetes & Metabolism, Wadsworth VA Hosp, Los Angeles, CA 1978-1980; **Fac Appt:** Prof Medicine, UCLA

Rudnick, Paul Arthur MD (EDM) - *Spec Exp:* Diabetes; **Hospital:** Cedars-Sinai Med Ctr; **Address:** 8920 Wilshire Blvd, Ste 635, Beverly Hills, CA 90211-2007; **Phone:** (310) 652-3870; **Board Cert:** Endocrinology, Diabetes & Metabolism 1973, Internal Medicine 1977; **Med School:** Yale Univ 1958; **Resid:** Internal Medicine, Peter Bent Brigham Hosp, Boston, MA 1961-1962; **Fellow:** Endocrinology, Diabetes & Metabolism, Mass Genl Hosp, Boston, MA 1962-1963

Singer, Peter Albert MD (EDM) - *Spec Exp:* Thyroid Disorders; **Hospital:** LAC & USC Med Ctr; **Address:** 1355 San Pablo St, rm 120, Los Angeles, CA 90033; **Phone:** (323) 442-5575; **Board Cert:** Internal Medicine 1972, Endocrinology, Diabetes & Metabolism 1973; **Med School:** UCSF 1965; **Resid:** Internal Medicine, LA Co-USC Med Ctr, Los Angeles, CA 1968-1971; **Fellow:** Endocrinology, Diabetes & Metabolism, LA Co-USC Med Ctr, Los Angeles, CA 1971-1973; **Fac Appt:** Clin Prof Medicine, USC Sch Med

Swerdloff, Ronald Sherwin MD (EDM) - *Spec Exp:* Andrology; Pituitary Tumors; **Hospital:** LAC - Harbor - UCLA Med Ctr; **Address:** 1000 W Carson St, Box 446, Torrance, CA 90502-2059; **Phone:** (310) 222-1867; **Board Cert:** Internal Medicine 1968, Endocrinology, Diabetes & Metabolism 1972; **Med School:** UCSF 1962; **Resid:** Internal Medicine, Univ Washington, Seattle, WA 1963-1964; Endocrinology, Diabetes & Metabolism, NIH Geron Branch, Baltimore, MD 1964-1966; **Fellow:** Endocrinology, Diabetes & Metabolism, Harbor-UCLA Med Ctr, Torrance, CA 1967-1969; **Fac Appt:** Prof Medicine, UCLA

Woeber, Kenneth Alois MD (EDM) - *Spec Exp:* Thyroid Disorders; **Hospital:** UCSF Med Ctr; **Address:** 1600 Divisadero St Fl 4 - rm C-432, San Francisco, CA 94115; **Phone:** (415) 885-7574; **Board Cert:** Internal Medicine 1980, Endocrinology, Diabetes & Metabolism 1973; **Med School:** South Africa 1957; **Resid:** Internal Medicine, Jackson Miami Hosp, Miami, FL 1959-1962; **Fellow:** Endocrinology, Diabetes & Metabolism, Harvard Med Unit-Boston City Hosp, Boston, MA 1962-1964; **Fac Appt:** Prof Medicine, UCSF

GASTROENTEROLOGY

(a subspecialty of INTERNAL MEDICINE)

An internist who specializes in diagnosis and treatment of diseases of the digestive organs including the stomach, bowels, liver and gallbladder. This specialist treats conditions such as abdominal pain, ulcers, diarrhea, cancer and jaundice and performs complex diagnostic and therapeutic procedures using endoscopes to see internal organs.

INTERNAL MEDICINE

An internist is a personal physician who provides long-term, comprehensive care in the office and the hospital, managing both common and complex illness of adolescents, adults and the elderly. Internists are trained in the diagnosis and treatment of cancer, infections and diseases affecting the heart, blood, kidneys, joints and digestive, respiratory and vascular systems. They are also trained in the essentials of primary care internal medicine which incorporates an understanding of disease prevention, wellness, substance abuse, mental health and effective treatment of common problems of the eyes, ears, skin, nervous system and reproductive organs.

Training required: Three years in internal medicine *plus* additional training and examination for certification in gastroenterology

THE MOUNT SINAI HOSPITAL
GASTROINTESTINAL AND SURGICAL SPECIALTIES

One Gustave L. Levy Place (Fifth Avenue and 98th Street)
New York, NY 10029-6574   Phone: (212) 241-6500
Physician Referral: 1-800-MD-SINAI (637-4624)
www.mountsinai.org

Mount Sinai's Division of Gastroenterology is renowned for its delivery of patient care, research, and education in diseases of the gastrointestinal tract.

In 1958, the National Institute of Health recognized the importance of Mount Sinai as a research center, with a grant for gastroenterology fellowship training. This prestigious grant was re-awarded in 2000 as a combined GI/Liver training grant, making Mount Sinai currently the only medical school in the New York metropolitan area with this award.

Eminent physicians, surgeons, radiologists, hepatologists, and pathologists have provided a rich body of knowledge in the diagnosis and management of inflammatory bowel disease, peptic ulcer disease, esophageal disorders, gastrointestinal cancer, and liver, biliary, and pancreatic diseases.

One of our more publicized successes was a breakthrough for people suffering from ulcerative colitis, a disease of the large intestine. Mount Sinai physicians perfected the Kock pouch, an internal reservoir for collecting waste created form the patient's own healthy small intestine.

Mount Sinai's Gastrointestinal and Surgical Specialties Care Center is a comprehensive center that unites the medical disciplines of gastroenterology, urology, and their related surgical specialties, as well as an array of minimally-invasive surgical programs.

The Care Center houses renowned programs for the treatment of inflammatory bowel diseases, colorectal, head, and neck cancers, and sinus diseases as well as for reconstructive surgery, bariatric surgery for obesity, and end-stage renal disease.

The Division of Pediatric Gastroenterology, Nutrition, and Liver Diseases provides consultative services and treatment for the full range of children's digestive and nutritional diseases.

THE MOUNT SINAI HOSPITAL

Some of the many medical conditions treated at Mount Sinai's Gastroenterology Care Center:

- Colon and Rectal Disorders

- Inflammatory Bowel Diseases (Crohn's Disease, Ulcerative Colitis)

- Irritable Bowel

- Syndrome

- Gastrointestinal, liver, and pancreatic cancers

- Male Infertility and Erectile Dysfunction

- Obesity

- Urologic Disorders

NewYork-Presbyterian
The University Hospitals of Columbia and Cornell
NewYork-Presbyterian Digestive Disease Services

NewYork Weill Cornell Medical Center
525 East 68th Street
New York, NY 10021

Columbia Presbyterian Medical Center
622 West 168th Street
New York, NY 10032

OVERVIEW:

The Digestive Disease Services of NewYork-Presbyterian Hospital provide expert capabilities in research, education and clinical care of patients with gastrointestinal, liver and bile duct, pancreatic and nutritional disorders.

The Hospital offers a wide range of diagnostic tests including,
- Routine procedures, such as endoscopy, capsule endoscopy, colonoscopy and flexible sigmoidoscopy.
- Endoscopic retrograde cholangiopancreatography (ERCP) to evaluate the ducts of the gallbladder, pancreas and liver
- Endoscopic ultrasonography (EUS)to provide detailed images of the upper and lower gastrointestinal tract and for the staging of patients with esophageal, gastric and rectal cancers. The Hospital is one of the few centers using EUS for needle aspiration of pancreatic cysts and tumors.
- Laparoscopy for direct examination of the liver, gallbladder and spleen and in the diagnosis, staging and treatment of pancreatic, gastric, esophageal and colorectal cancer.

The Hospital is a leader in treating gastrointestinal (GI) conditions. For example,
- The Minimal Access Surgery Center (MASC) is at the forefront of developing and applying new technologies, such as robotics, computerized image processing and enhanced optics. It is improving the outcomes of GI surgical patients and speeding their recovery from conditions such as GERD, gallbladder disease, and benign and malignant colon and rectal disease.
- Our surgeons also perform endoscopic sewing (endocinch) and radiofrequency treatment (Stretta procedure) for GERD.
- Our surgeons are internationally renowned in the use of laparoscopic methods for cancer and other colorectal conditions. They are highly experienced with the Whipple procedure to remove a pancreas tumor, which improves the survival rates and life expectancies of patients with pancreatic cancer and other less common pancreas problems.

Additionally, our physicians are involved in numerous clinical trials, including studies on Cox-2 inhibitors for preventing colorectal cancer and familial polyposis (a precursor to colorectal cancer), and antiviral therapy for chronic hepatitis C.

Physician Referral: For a physician referral or to learn more about the NewYork-Presbyterian Digestive Disease Services call toll free **1-877-NYP-WELL** (1-877-697-9355) or visit our Web Site at **www.nyp.org**.

COMPREHENSIVE CARE

Patients benefit from the collaboration of gastroenterologists, hepatologists, surgeons and diagnostic and pathology experts who develop optimal treatment plans. Areas of expertise include:

- GI Cancer, including esophageal, colorectal, liver, pancreatic and gastric tumors
- Inflammatory Bowel Diseases (Ulcerative Colitis and Crohn's Disease)
- Liver Diseases. The Hospital has a comprehensive Hepatitis C Center and the Center for Liver Disease and Transplantation
- Esophageal Disorders, including gastroesophageal reflux disease (GERD) and Barrett's esophagus
- Pancreatic and Biliary Disorders
- Celiac Disease
- Polyps of the Colon
- Peptic Ulcer Disease/Helicobacter Pylori Infections
- Gallbladder and Bile Duct Disorders
- Restorative surgery to avoid colostomies in diseases like rectal cancer, Crohn's disease, ulcerative colitis, and incontinence
- Anal diseases, such as hemorrhoids, fistulas, vascular tumors, abscesses and others

NYU Medical Center

SCHOOL OF MEDICINE

550 First Avenue (at 31st Street)
New York, NY 10016
Physician Referral: (888) 7-NYU-MED
(888-769-8633) www.nyumedicalcenter.org

NEW YORK UNIVERSITY

GASTROENTEROLOGY

The mission of the Division of Gastroenterology at NYU Medical Center is excellence in the delivery of patient care, research, and education in diseases of the gastrointestinal tract. Its physicians bring with them a rich body of knowledge in the diagnosis and management of inflammatory bowel disease, peptic ulcer disease, esophageal disorders, gastrointestinal cancer, and liver, biliary, and pancreatic diseases. Their multidisciplinary approach insures the greatest possible patient care at NYU's three acclaimed, academically-integrated teaching hospitals: Tisch Hospital (New York University Hospital), Bellevue Hospitals Center, and the New York Harbor Health Care System (Manhattan Veterans Hospital).

Members of the Division of Gastroenterology are nationally recognized leaders who are involved in numerous studies in the field of gastroenterology and hepatology, including clinical research in liver diseases (especially hepatitis C), endoscopy, colon cancer screening, acute and chronic GI bleeding, and Helicobacter pylori.

Always at the forefront of new technologies, NYU's gastroenterologists work side-by-side with radiologists to perform virtual colonoscopies, a new minimally invasive technique for finding early-stage cancers in the colon.

Virtual colonoscopy is a new screening test in which a radiologist uses a CAT (Computer Assisted Tomography) scanner and sophisticated image processing computers to actually recreate and evaluate the inner surface of the colon. The CAT scanner provides the x-ray images; the image-processing computers create the 3-D display for the final interpretation by the referring gastroenterologist. The study gives a complete evaluation of the entire surface of the colon and can be performed quickly, with little discomfort and extremely accurate readings.

NYU MEDICAL CENTER

The colon and the rectum are the final sections of the large intestine. In the United States, approximately 150,000 people are diagnosed with colorectal cancer every year and of these, approximately 55,000 will die of the disease. Cancer of the colon is the second leading cause of cancer death in the United States. Most experts agree that it is preventable, and NYU is on the cutting edge of 21st century research into quicker, safer, and more accurate diagnosis and treatment, with its fiberoptic colonoscopy that examines the entire colon with the use of fiber optics.

Physician Listings

Gastroenterology

New England

Banks, Peter Alan MD (Ge) - *Spec Exp:* Inflammatory Bowel Disease/Crohn's; Pancreatic Disease; **Hospital:** Brigham & Women's Hosp; **Address:** Brigham & Women's Hosp, Div Gastro, 45 Francis St, Bldg ASBII - Fl 2, Boston, MA 02115; **Phone:** (617) 732-6389; **Board Cert:** Internal Medicine 1968, Gastroenterology 1970; **Med School:** Columbia P&S 1961; **Resid:** Internal Medicine, Beth Israel Hosp, Boston, MA 1962-1963; **Fellow:** Gastroenterology, Mt Sinai Hosp, New York, NY 1965-1967; **Fac Appt:** Assoc Prof Medicine, Harvard Med Sch

Bonkovsky, Herbert MD (Ge) - *Spec Exp:* Porphyria; Liver Disease; Nutrition; **Hospital:** U Mass Meml Hlth Care - Worcester; **Address:** 55 Lake Ave N, Worcester, MA 01655; **Phone:** (508) 856-2846; **Board Cert:** Gastroenterology 1977, Internal Medicine 1973; **Med School:** Case West Res Univ 1967; **Resid:** Internal Medicine, MetroHealth Med Ctr, Cleveland, OH 1968-1969; Internal Medicine, Dartmouth-Hitchcock Med Ctr, Lebanon, NH 1971-1973; **Fellow:** Gastroenterology, Dartmouth Med Sch, Lebanon, NH 1971-1973; Hepatology, Yale Univ Sch Med, New Haven, CT 1973-1974; **Fac Appt:** Prof Medicine, Emory Univ

Carr-Locke, David L MD (Ge) - *Spec Exp:* Pancreatic/Biliary Endoscopy(ERCP); Pancreatic & Biliary Disease; Therapeutic Endoscopy; **Hospital:** Brigham & Women's Hosp; **Address:** Endoscopy Center, 75 Francis St, Boston, MA 02115-6106; **Phone:** (617) 732-7414; **Board Cert:** Internal Medicine 1974; **Med School:** England 1972; **Resid:** Obstetrics & Gynecology, Orsett Hosp, Essex, England 1974; Internal Medicine, Leicester Hosp, Leicester, England 1976-1978; **Fellow:** Gastroenterology, New England Baptist Hosp, Boston, MA 1978-1982; Gastroenterology, New England Baptist Hosp, Boston, MA 1979; **Fac Appt:** Assoc Prof Medicine, Harvard Med Sch

Chuttani, Ram MD (Ge) - *Spec Exp:* Pancreatic/Biliary Endoscopy(ERCP); Gastrointestinal Cancer; **Hospital:** Brigham & Women's Hosp; **Address:** 330 Brookline Ave, Ste 116, Boston, MA 02215; **Phone:** (617) 667-0162; **Board Cert:** Gastroenterology 1991, Internal Medicine 1990; **Med School:** India 1983; **Resid:** Internal Medicine, Norwalk Hosp-Yale Univ, New Haven, CT 1984-1987; **Fellow:** Gastroenterology, Brigham & Women's Hosp, W Roxbury, VA 1987-1990; **Fac Appt:** Asst Prof Medicine, Boston Univ

Dienstag, Jules Leonard MD (Ge) - *Spec Exp:* Liver Disease; Hepatitis; Transplant Medicine-Liver; **Hospital:** MA Genl Hosp; **Address:** Gastroenterology Unit, 55 Fruit St - GRJ 825, Boston, MA 02114-2696; **Phone:** (617) 726-7450; **Board Cert:** Internal Medicine 1975; **Med School:** Columbia P&S 1972; **Resid:** Internal Medicine, University of Chicago Hospitals/Clinics, Chicago, IL 1972-1974; **Fellow:** Infectious Disease, Natl Inst Hlth, Bethesda, MD 1974-1976; Gastroenterology, Mass Genl Hosp, Boston, MA 1976-1978; **Fac Appt:** Assoc Prof Medicine, Harvard Med Sch

Friedman, Lawrence S. MD (Ge) - *Spec Exp:* Liver Disease; **Hospital:** MA Genl Hosp; **Address:** Mass Genl Hosp, Gastro Unit, 55 Fruit St Blake 456D, Boston, MA 02114; **Phone:** (617) 724-6005; **Board Cert:** Internal Medicine 1981, Gastroenterology 1983; **Med School:** Johns Hopkins Univ 1978; **Resid:** Internal Medicine, Johns Hopkins Hosp, Baltimore, MD 1979-1981; **Fellow:** Gastroenterology, Mass Genl Hosp, Boston, MA 1981-1984; **Fac Appt:** Prof Medicine, Harvard Med Sch

Peppercorn, Mark MD (Ge) - *Spec Exp:* Inflammatory Bowel Disease/Crohn's; **Hospital:** Beth Israel Deaconess Med Ctr - Boston; **Address:** Beth Israel Deconess Med Ctr, 330 Brookline Ave, Boston, MA 02215; **Phone:** (617) 667-2153; **Board Cert:** Internal Medicine 1974, Gastroenterology 1977; **Med School:** Harvard Med Sch 1968; **Resid:** Internal Medicine, Beth Israel Hosp, Boston, MA 1969-1974; Metabolic Diseases, Natl Inst Hlth, Bethesda, MD 1970-1972; **Fellow:** Gastroenterology, Beth Israe Hospl, Boston, MA 1972-1973; **Fac Appt:** Prof Medicine, Harvard Med Sch

Mid Atlantic

Aronchick, Craig A MD (Ge) - *Spec Exp:* Barrett's Esophagus; Pancreatic/Biliary Endoscopy(ERCP); **Hospital:** Pennsylvania Hosp (page 78); **Address:** 800 Spruce St, Philadelphia, PA 19107; **Phone:** (215) 829-3561; **Board Cert:** Internal Medicine 1981, Gastroenterology 1983; **Med School:** Temple Univ 1978; **Resid:** Internal Medicine, Temple Univ Hosp, Philadelphia, PA 1978-1981

Bayless, Theodore MD (Ge) - *Spec Exp:* Inflammatory Bowel Disease/Crohn's; Ulcerative Colitis; **Hospital:** Johns Hopkins Hosp - Baltimore; **Address:** 600 N Wolfe St, Blalock Bldg, Ste 461, Baltimore, MD 21287; **Phone:** (410) 955-4166; **Board Cert:** Internal Medicine 1966; **Med School:** Univ Hlth Sci/Chicago Med Sch 1957; **Resid:** Internal Medicine, Memorial Sloan Kettering Hosp, New York, NY 1958-1960; **Fellow:** Gastroenterology, Johns Hopkins Hospl, Baltimore, MD 1960-1962; **Fac Appt:** Prof Medicine, Johns Hopkins Univ

Bodenheimer Jr, Henry MD (Ge) - *Spec Exp:* Hepatitis; Transplant Medicine-Liver; Cirrhosis; **Hospital:** Mount Sinai Hosp (page 68); **Address:** 5 E 98th St, New York, NY 10029-6501; **Phone:** (212) 241-0034; **Board Cert:** Internal Medicine 1978, Gastroenterology 1981; **Med School:** Tufts Univ 1975; **Resid:** Internal Medicine, Mount Sinai Hosp, New York, NY 1975-1978; **Fellow:** Gastroenterology, Mount Sinai Hosp, New York, NY 1978-1979; Gastroenterology, Rhode Island Hosp, Providence, RI 1979-1981; **Fac Appt:** Prof Medicine, Mount Sinai Sch Med

Brandt, Lawrence MD (Ge) - *Spec Exp:* AIDS/HIV; Ischemic Bowel Disease; **Hospital:** Montefiore Med Ctr (page 67); **Address:** 111 E 210th St, Bronx, NY 10467-2401; **Phone:** (718) 920-4476; **Board Cert:** Internal Medicine 1972, Gastroenterology 1975; **Med School:** SUNY Downstate 1968; **Resid:** Internal Medicine, Mount Sinai Hosp, New York, NY 1968-1972; **Fellow:** Gastroenterology, Mount Sinai Hosp, New York, NY 1971-1972; **Fac Appt:** Prof Medicine, Albert Einstein Coll Med

Cohen, Jonathan MD (Ge) - *Spec Exp:* ERCP; Pancreatic & Liver Disease; Colonoscopy; **Hospital:** NYU Med Ctr (page 71); **Address:** 232 E 30th St, New York, NY 10016-8202; **Phone:** (212) 889-5544; **Board Cert:** Internal Medicine 1993, Gastroenterology 1995; **Med School:** Harvard Med Sch 1990; **Resid:** Internal Medicine, Beth Israel Hosp, Boston, MA 1991-1993; **Fellow:** Gastroenterology, UCLA, Los Angeles, CA 1993-1995; Gastroenterology, Wellesley Hosp Univ Toronto, Toronto, Canada; **Fac Appt:** Asst Clin Prof Medicine, NYU Sch Med

Deren, Julius J MD (Ge) - *Spec Exp:* Inflammatory Bowel Disease/Crohn's; **Hospital:** Univ Penn - Presby Med Ctr; **Address:** Bldg Wright Saunders - Ste 218, 39th & Market St, Philadelphia, PA 19104; **Phone:** (215) 662-8900; **Board Cert:** Internal Medicine 1968, Gastroenterology 1970; **Med School:** SUNY Downstate 1958; **Resid:** Gastroenterology, Boston City Hosp/Harvard, Boston, MA 1961-1962; Internal Medicine, Maimonides Hosp, Brooklyn, NY 1959-1961; **Fellow:** Physiology, Harvard, Boston, MA 1962-1964; **Fac Appt:** Prof Medicine, Univ Penn

Dieterich, Douglas MD (Ge) - *Spec Exp:* Hepatitis; AIDS/HIV; Liver Disease; **Hospital:** Cabrini Med Ctr; **Address:** 232 E 20th St, Fl 2, New York, NY 10003-1802; **Phone:** (212) 995-6904; **Board Cert:** Internal Medicine 1981, Gastroenterology 1987; **Med School:** NYU Sch Med 1978; **Resid:** Internal Medicine, Bellevue Hosp Ctr-NYU, New York, NY 1978-1981; **Fellow:** Gastroenterology, Bellevue Hosp Ctr-NYU, New York, NY 1981-1983; **Fac Appt:** Assoc Prof Medicine, NYU Sch Med

Farmer, Richard G MD (Ge) - *Spec Exp:* Inflammatory Bowel Disease/Crohn's; **Hospital:** Georgetown Univ Hosp; **Address:** GUMC - Second Floor, Main Hospital, 3800 Reservoir Rd NW, Ste 2207, Washington, DC 20007; **Phone:** (202) 687-8035; **Board Cert:** Gastroenterology 1968, Internal Medicine 1963; **Med School:** Univ Minn 1960; **Resid:** Internal Medicine, Mayo Clinic, Rochester, MN 1957-1960; **Fellow:** Gastroenterology, Mayo Clinic, Rochester, MN 1960; **Fac Appt:** Clin Prof Medicine, Georgetown Univ

Fleischer, David MD (Ge) - *Spec Exp:* Barrett's Esophagus; Esophageal Cancer; **Hospital:** Georgetown Univ Hosp; **Address:** GUMC-Main Hospital, 3800 Reservoir Rd NW, Fl 2nd - Ste 2122, Washington, DC 20007-2197; **Phone:** (202) 687-8741; **Board Cert:** Internal Medicine 1975, Gastroenterology 1977; **Med School:** Vanderbilt Univ 1970; **Resid:** Internal Medicine, Wellington Hosp 1973-1974; Internal Medicine, Metro General Hosp CWRU, Cleveland, OH 1974-1975; **Fellow:** Gastroenterology, LA Co Harbor-UCLA Medical Center, Torrance, CA 1975-1977; **Fac Appt:** Prof Medicine, Georgetown Univ

Holt, Peter R MD (Ge) - *Spec Exp:* Diarrhea; Ulcerative Colitis/Crohn's; Celiac Disease; **Hospital:** St Luke's - Roosevelt Hosp Ctr - Roosevelt Div (page 58); **Address:** 1111 Amsterdam Ave, Ste 1216, New York, NY 10025-1716; **Phone:** (212) 523-3680; **Board Cert:** Internal Medicine 1966; **Med School:** England 1954; **Resid:** Internal Medicine, London Hosp, London, England 1954-1955; Internal Medicine, St Luke's Hosp, New York, NY 1957-1959; **Fellow:** Gastroenterology, Mass Genl Hosp, Boston, MA 1959-1961; **Fac Appt:** Prof Emeritus Medicine, Columbia P&S

Jacobson, Ira MD (Ge) - *Spec Exp:* Pancreatic Disease; Hepatitis; Endoscopy; **Hospital:** NY Presby Hosp - NY Weill Cornell Med Ctr (page 70); **Address:** 50 E 69th St, New York, NY 10021-5016; **Phone:** (212) 746-2115; **Board Cert:** Internal Medicine 1982, Gastroenterology 1985; **Med School:** Columbia P&S 1979; **Resid:** Internal Medicine, Univ Cal San Francisco, San Francisco, CA 1979-1982; **Fellow:** Gastroenterology, Mass Genl Hosp, Boston, MA 1982-1984; **Fac Appt:** Prof Medicine, Cornell Univ-Weill Med Coll

Kalloo, Anthony Nicholas MD (Ge) - *Spec Exp:* Endoscopy; **Hospital:** Johns Hopkins Hosp - Baltimore; **Address:** 1830 E Monument St, rm 419, Baltimore, MD 21205; **Phone:** (410) 955-9697; **Board Cert:** Internal Medicine 1985, Gastroenterology 1987; **Med School:** Jamaica 1979; **Resid:** Internal Medicine, Howard Univ Hosp, Washington, DC 1983-1985; **Fellow:** Gastroenterology, VA Med Ctr/Georgetown Univ Hosp, Washington, DC 1985; **Fac Appt:** Assoc Prof Gastroenterology, Johns Hopkins Univ

Kodsi, Baroukh MD (Ge) - *Spec Exp:* Endoscopy; Gastroesophageal Reflux; **Hospital:** Maimonides Med Ctr (page 65); **Address:** 925 48th St, Brooklyn, NY 11219; **Phone:** (718) 851-6767; **Med School:** Egypt 1945; **Resid:** Internal Medicine, Boston Med Ctr, Boston, MA 1959-1961; **Fellow:** Gastroenterology, Boston Med Ctr, Boston, MA 1961-1963; **Fac Appt:** Assoc Clin Prof Medicine, SUNY Downstate

Korelitz, Burton I MD (Ge) - *Spec Exp:* Inflammatory Bowel Disease/Crohn's; **Hospital:** Lenox Hill Hosp (page 64); **Address:** 45 E 85th St, Ste 1E, New York, NY 10028-0957; **Phone:** (212) 988-3800; **Board Cert:** Internal Medicine 1958, Gastroenterology 1961; **Med School:** Boston Univ 1951; **Resid:** Internal Medicine, VA Hosp, Boston, MA 1952-1953; Gastroenterology, Beth Israel Hosp, Boston, MA 1953-1954; **Fellow:** Gastroenterology, Mt Sinai Hosp, New York, NY 1956; **Fac Appt:** Clin Prof Medicine, NYU Sch Med

Kotler, Donald P MD (Ge) - *Spec Exp:* Esophageal Disorders; AIDS/HIV-Nutrition; Malnutrition; **Hospital:** St Luke's - Roosevelt Hosp Ctr - Roosevelt Div (page 58); **Address:** 421 W 113th St, Ste 1301, New York, NY 10025; **Phone:** (212) 523-3670; **Board Cert:** Internal Medicine 1976, Gastroenterology 1979; **Med School:** Albert Einstein Coll Med 1973; **Resid:** Internal Medicine, Jacobi Med Ctr, Bronx, NY 1973-1976; **Fellow:** Gastroenterology, Hosp of Univ of Penn, Philadelphia, PA 1976-1978; **Fac Appt:** Assoc Prof Medicine, Columbia P&S

Lichtenstein, Gary R MD (Ge) - *Spec Exp:* Inflammatory Bowel Disease; **Hospital:** Hosp Univ Penn (page 78); **Address:** Hosp of Univ Penn, Div Gastroenterology, 3400 Spruce St, Philadelphia, PA 19104-4283; **Phone:** (215) 349-8222; **Board Cert:** Internal Medicine 1987, Gastroenterology 1989; **Med School:** Mount Sinai Sch Med 1984; **Resid:** Internal Medicine, Duke Univ Med Ctr, Durham, NC 1984-1987; **Fellow:** Gastroenterology, Univ Penn Hosp, Philadelphie, PA 1987-1990; **Fac Appt:** Assoc Prof Medicine, Univ Penn

Lightdale, Charles MD (Ge) - *Spec Exp:* Barrett's Esophagus; Photodynamic Therapy; Endoscopic Ultrasonography; **Hospital:** NY Presby Hosp - Columbia Presby Med Ctr (page 70); **Address:** Columbia-Presbyterian Medical Center, 161 Fort Washington Ave Bldg Irving Pavilion - rm 812, New York, NY 10032; **Phone:** (212) 305-3423; **Board Cert:** Internal Medicine 1972, Gastroenterology 1973; **Med School:** Columbia P&S 1966; **Resid:** Internal Medicine, Yale-New Haven Hosp, New Haven, CT 1966-1968; Internal Medicine, NY Hosp-Cornell Med Ctr, New York, NY 1968-1969; **Fellow:** Gastroenterology, NY Hosp-Cornell Med Ctr, New York, NY 1971-1973; **Fac Appt:** Prof Medicine, Columbia P&S

Lipshutz, William H. MD (Ge) - *Spec Exp:* Inflammatory Bowel Disease/Crohn's; Colon Cancer; Esophageal Disorders; **Hospital:** Pennsylvania Hosp (page 78); **Address:** 800 Spruce St, Philadelphia, PA 19107; **Phone:** (215) 829-3561; **Board Cert:** Gastroenterology 1973, Internal Medicine 1972; **Med School:** Univ Penn 1967; **Resid:** Internal Medicine, Pennsylvania Hospital, Philadelphia, PA 1971-1972; Internal Medicine, Penn Hospital, Philadelphia, PA 1968-1969; **Fellow:** Gastroenterology, Univ Pennsylvania Med Ctr, Philadelphia, PA 1969-1971; **Fac Appt:** Clin Prof Medicine, Univ Penn

Markowitz, David MD (Ge) - *Spec Exp:* Gastroesophageal Reflux (GERD); Esophageal Disorders; **Hospital:** NY Presby Hosp - Columbia Presby Med Ctr (page 70); **Address:** 161 Ft Washington Ave, New York, NY 10032; **Phone:** (212) 305-1024; **Board Cert:** Internal Medicine 1988, Gastroenterology 1991; **Med School:** Columbia P&S 1985; **Resid:** Internal Medicine, Columbia-Presby, New York, NY 1985-1988; **Fellow:** Gastroenterology, Columbia-Presby, New York, NY 1988-1991

Mayer, Lloyd MD (Ge) - *Spec Exp:* Inflammatory Bowel Disease/Crohn's; Ulcerative Colitis; **Hospital:** Mount Sinai Hosp (page 68); **Address:** 1425 Madison Ave, Box 1089, New York, NY 10029; **Phone:** (212) 659-9266; **Board Cert:** Internal Medicine 1979, Gastroenterology 1981; **Med School:** Mount Sinai Sch Med 1976; **Resid:** Internal Medicine, Bellevue Hosp, New York, NY 1976-1979; **Fellow:** Gastroenterology, Mount Sinai Med Ctr, New York, NY 1979-1981; **Fac Appt:** Prof Medicine, Mount Sinai Sch Med

Metz, David C. MD (Ge) - *Spec Exp:* Peptic Acid Disorders; Neuroendocrine Tumors; Gastroesophageal Reflux; **Hospital:** Hosp Univ Penn (page 78); **Address:** Univ of Penn MC, Gastro Div, 3400 Spruce St, 3 Dulles, Philadelphia, PA 19104; **Phone:** (215) 662-3541; **Board Cert:** Internal Medicine 1989, Gastroenterology 1991; **Med School:** South Africa 1982; **Resid:** Internal Medicine, Albert Einstein Med Center, Philadelphia, PA 1986-1988; **Fellow:** Gastroenterology, Natl Naval Med Ctr, Bethesda, MD 1989-1991; **Fac Appt:** Assoc Prof Medicine, Univ Penn

Miskovitz, Paul MD (Ge) - *Spec Exp:* Endoscopy; Irritable Bowel Syndrome; **Hospital:** NY Presby Hosp - NY Weill Cornell Med Ctr (page 70); **Address:** 50 E 70th St, New York, NY 10021-4928; **Phone:** (212) 717-4966; **Board Cert:** Internal Medicine 1978, Gastroenterology 1981; **Med School:** Cornell Univ-Weill Med Coll 1975; **Resid:** Internal Medicine, NY Hosp, New York, NY 1975-1978; **Fellow:** Gastroenterology, NY Hosp, New York, NY 1978-1980; **Fac Appt:** Clin Prof Medicine, Cornell Univ-Weill Med Coll

Present, Daniel MD (Ge) - *Spec Exp:* Inflammatory Bowel Disease/Crohn's; Ulcerative Colitis; **Hospital:** Mount Sinai Hosp (page 68); **Address:** 12 E 86th St, New York, NY 10028-0506; **Phone:** (212) 861-2000; **Board Cert:** Internal Medicine 1966, Gastroenterology 1970; **Med School:** SUNY Downstate 1959; **Resid:** Internal Medicine, Mount Sinai Med Ctr, New York, NY 1962-1964; **Fellow:** Gastroenterology, Mount Sinai Med Ctr, New York, NY 1964-1966; **Fac Appt:** Clin Prof Medicine, Mount Sinai Sch Med

Ravich, William Jay MD (Ge) - *Spec Exp:* Dysphagia; Achalasia; **Hospital:** Johns Hopkins Hosp - Baltimore; **Address:** Johns Hopkins Hospital, Div Gastroenterology, 600 N Wolfe St Bldg Blalock - rm 465, Baltimore, MD 21287; **Phone:** (410) 955-4910; **Board Cert:** Gastroenterology 1981, Internal Medicine 1978; **Med School:** Univ Hlth Sci/Chicago Med Sch 1975; **Resid:** Gastroenterology, Montefiore Hosp., Bronx, NY 1977-1978; Internal Medicine, Montefiore Hosp., Bronx, NY 1976-1978; **Fellow:** Gastroenterology, Johns Hopkins Hosp., Baltimore, MD 1978-1981; **Fac Appt:** Assoc Prof Gastroenterology, Johns Hopkins Univ

Sachar, David MD (Ge) - *Spec Exp:* Inflammatory Bowel Disease/Crohn's; Ulcerative Colitis; **Hospital:** Mount Sinai Hosp (page 68); **Address:** 5 E 98th St, Ste 11, New York, NY 10029-6501; **Phone:** (212) 241-4299; **Board Cert:** Gastroenterology 1972, Internal Medicine 1969; **Med School:** Harvard Med Sch 1963; **Resid:** Internal Medicine, Beth Israel Hosp, Boston, MA 1964-1965; Internal Medicine, Beth Israel Hosp, Boston, MA 1967-1968; **Fellow:** Gastroenterology, Mount Sinai Hosp, New York, NY 1968-1970; **Fac Appt:** Clin Prof Medicine, Mount Sinai Sch Med

Shike, Moshe MD (Ge) - *Spec Exp:* Gastrointestinal Cancer; Nutrition; **Hospital:** Mem Sloan Kettering Cancer Ctr; **Address:** 1275 York Ave, rm S-536, New York, NY 10021; **Phone:** (212) 639-7230; **Board Cert:** Internal Medicine 1977, Gastroenterology 1981; **Med School:** Israel 1975; **Resid:** Internal Medicine, Mt Auburn, Boston, MA 1975-1976; **Fellow:** Gastroenterology, Univ of Toronto, Toronto, Canada 1978-1981; **Fac Appt:** Prof Medicine, Cornell Univ-Weill Med Coll

Siegel, Jerome MD (Ge) - *Spec Exp:* Pancreatic/Biliary Endoscopy (ERCP); **Hospital:** Beth Israel Med Ctr - Petrie Division (page 58); **Address:** 60 E End Ave, New York, NY 10028-7907; **Phone:** (212) 734-8874; **Board Cert:** Internal Medicine 1978, Gastroenterology 1979; **Med School:** Med Coll GA 1960; **Resid:** Internal Medicine, NY VA Med Ctr, New York, NY 1963-1965; Gastroenterology, NY VA Med Ctr, New York, NY 1965-1966; **Fellow:** Gastroenterology, Royal Free Hosp, London, England 1973-1975; **Fac Appt:** Assoc Clin Prof Medicine, Albert Einstein Coll Med

Wald, Arnold MD (Ge) - *Spec Exp:* Constipation; Gastrointestinal Motility Disorders; Irritable Bowel Syndrome; **Hospital:** UPMC - Presbyterian Univ Hosp; **Address:** Univ Pitt Med Ctr, Dept Gastro, 200 Lothrop St, Pittsburgh, PA 15213; **Phone:** (412) 648-9241; **Board Cert:** Internal Medicine 1972, Gastroenterology 1975; **Med School:** SUNY Downstate 1968; **Resid:** Internal Medicine, SUNY - Downstate Med Ctr, Brooklyn, NY 1968-1971; **Fellow:** Gastroenterology, Johns Hopkins Hosp, Baltimore, MD 1973-1975; **Fac Appt:** Prof Medicine, Univ Pittsburgh

Waye, Jerome MD (Ge) - *Spec Exp:* Endoscopy; Colon Cancer; Colonoscopy; **Hospital:** Mount Sinai Hosp (page 68); **Address:** 650 Park Ave, New York, NY 10021-6115; **Phone:** (212) 439-7779; **Board Cert:** Internal Medicine 1965, Gastroenterology 1970; **Med School:** Boston Univ 1958; **Resid:** Internal Medicine, Mount Sinai Hosp, New York, NY 1959-1961; **Fellow:** Gastroenterology, Mount Sinai Hosp, New York, NY 1961-1962; **Fac Appt:** Clin Prof Medicine, Mount Sinai Sch Med

Winawer, Sidney J MD (Ge) - *Spec Exp:* Endoscopy; Colon Cancer; **Hospital:** Mem Sloan Kettering Cancer Ctr; **Address:** 1275 York Ave, Box 90, New York, NY 10021-6094; **Phone:** (212) 639-7678; **Board Cert:** Internal Medicine 1965, Gastroenterology 1973; **Med School:** SUNY Hlth Sci Ctr 1956; **Resid:** Internal Medicine, VA Med Ctr, New York, NY 1959-1961; Internal Medicine, Maimonides Hosp, Brooklyn, NY 1961-1962; **Fellow:** Gastroenterology, Boston City Hosp, Boston, MA 1962-1964; **Fac Appt:** Prof Medicine, Cornell Univ-Weill Med Coll

Southeast

Barkin, Jamie MD (Ge) - *Spec Exp:* Pancreatic & Biliary Disease; Gastrointestinal Cancer; **Hospital:** Mount Sinai Med Ctr; **Address:** Mount Sinai Medical Center, 4300 Alton Rd, Ste G22, Miami Beach, FL 33140-2800; **Phone:** (305) 674-2240; **Board Cert:** Internal Medicine 1973, Gastroenterology 1975; **Med School:** Univ Miami Sch Med 1970; **Resid:** Internal Medicine, Univ Miami Hosp, Miami, FL 1971-1973; **Fellow:** Gastroenterology, Univ Miami Hosp, Miami, FL 1973-1975; **Fac Appt:** Prof Medicine, Univ Miami Sch Med

Bloomer, Joseph MD (Ge) - *Spec Exp:* Porphyria; Liver Disease; **Hospital:** Univ of Ala Hosp at Birmingham; **Address:** Univ of Ala at Birmingham, 284 MCLM, 1918 University Blvd, Birmingham, AL 35294; **Phone:** (205) 975-9699; **Board Cert:** Internal Medicine 1972, Gastroenterology 1985; **Med School:** Case West Res Univ 1966; **Resid:** Internal Medicine, UC/San Francisco Med Ctr, San Francisco, CA 1966-1968; **Fac Appt:** Prof Medicine, Univ Ala

Boyce Jr, H Worth MD (Ge) - *Spec Exp:* Swallowing Disorders; Barrett's Esophagus; **Hospital:** H Lee Moffitt Cancer Ctr & Research Inst; **Address:** Ctr for Swallowing Disorders, 12901 Bruce B Downs Blvd, MC-72, Tampa, FL 33612; **Phone:** (813) 974-3374; **Board Cert:** Internal Medicine 1977, Gastroenterology 1965; **Med School:** Wake Forest Univ Sch Med 1955; **Resid:** Internal Medicine, Brooke Army Hosp, Fort Sam Houston, TX 1956-1959; Gastroenterology, Brooke Army Hosp, Fort Sam Houston, TX 1959-1960; **Fac Appt:** Prof Medicine, Univ S Fla Coll Med

Brazer, Scott Robert MD (Ge) - *Spec Exp:* Gastroesophageal Reflux; Colorectal Cancer; Chest Pain; **Hospital:** Duke Univ Med Ctr (page 60); **Address:** Duke Univ Med Center, Box 3662, Durham, NC 27710; **Phone:** (919) 684-1817; **Board Cert:** Internal Medicine 1984, Gastroenterology 1987; **Med School:** Case West Res Univ 1981; **Resid:** Internal Medicine, Duke Univ, Durham, NC 1982-1984; Internal Medicine, Duke Univ, Durham, NC 1987-1988; **Fellow:** Gastroenterology, Duke Unic, Durham, NC 1985-1987; **Fac Appt:** Assoc Prof Medicine, Duke Univ

Brenner, David Allen MD (Ge) - *Spec Exp:* Porphyria; **Hospital:** Univ of NC Hosp (page 77); **Address:** 156 Glaxo Bldg, CB#7038, Chapel Hill, NC 27599-7038; **Phone:** (919) 966-0650; **Board Cert:** Internal Medicine 1982, Gastroenterology 1986; **Med School:** Yale Univ 1979; **Resid:** Internal Medicine, Yale, New Haven, CT 1979-1982; **Fellow:** Research, Natl Inst Hlth, Bethesda, MD 1982-1985; Gastroenterology, Univ California, San Diego, CA 1985-1986; **Fac Appt:** Prof Emeritus Medicine, Univ NC Sch Med

Castell, Donald O MD (Ge) - *Spec Exp: Esophageal Disorders; Gastroesophageal Reflux; Motility Disorders;* **Hospital:** Med Univ Hosp Authority; **Address:** 96 Jonathan Lucas St, Ste 210, Box 250327, Charleston, SC 29425; **Phone:** (843) 792-7522; **Board Cert:** Internal Medicine 1977, Gastroenterology 1970; **Med School:** Geo Wash Univ 1960; **Resid:** Internal Medicine, US Naval Hosp, Bethesda, MA 1962-1965; **Fellow:** Gastroenterology, Tufts Univ, Boston, MA 1967-1969; **Fac Appt:** Prof Medicine, Univ SC Sch Med

Cominelli, Fabio MD/PhD (Ge) - *Spec Exp: Inflammatory Bowel Disease/Crohn's; Ulcerative Colitis;* **Hospital:** Univ of VA Hlth Sys (page 79); **Address:** PO Box 800708, Charlottesville, VA 22908; **Phone:** (804) 243-6400; **Board Cert:** Gastroenterology 1986; **Med School:** Italy 1983; **Resid:** Gastroenterology, Careggi Hosp-Univ of Italy, Florence, Italy 1983-1986; **Fellow:** Gastroenterology, Harbor-UCLA Med Ctr, Torrance, CA 1987-1989; **Fac Appt:** Prof Medicine, Univ VA Sch Med

Cotton, Peter MD (Ge) - *Spec Exp: Pancreatc Disease; Biliary Disease;* **Hospital:** Med Univ Hosp Authority; **Address:** MUSC - Digestive Disease Center - 210 CSB, 96 Jonathan Lucas St, Box 250327, Charleston, SC 29425; **Phone:** (843) 792-6865; **Med School:** England 1963; **Resid:** Internal Medicine, St Thomas' Hosp, London, UK 1966-1970; Gastroenterology, St Thomas' Hosp, London, UK 1970-1973; **Fac Appt:** Prof Medicine, Med Univ SC

Davis, Gary L MD (Ge) - *Spec Exp: Liver Disease; Hepatitis; Transplant Medicine-Liver;* **Hospital:** Shands Hlthcre at Univ of FL (page 73); **Address:** University of Florida, 1600` SW Archer Rd, Ste MSB 440, Gainesville, FL 32610-0214; **Phone:** (352) 392-7353; **Board Cert:** Internal Medicine 1979, Gastroenterology 1983; **Med School:** Univ Minn 1976; **Resid:** Internal Medicine, Mayo Grad Sch Med, Minneapolis, MN 1977-1979; **Fellow:** Gastroenterology, Mayo Grad Sch Med, Minneapolis, MN 1979-1981; Natl Inst of Hlth, Bethesda, MD 1982-1984; **Fac Appt:** Prof Medicine, Univ Fla Coll Med

Diamond, Jeffrey MD (Ge) - *Spec Exp: Inflammatory Bowel Disease/Crohn's; Ulcerative Colitis; Gastroesophageal Reflux;* **Hospital:** Mem Reg Hosp - Hollywood; **Address:** 4700 Sheridan St, Ste M, Hollywood, FL 33021; **Phone:** (954) 961-8400; **Board Cert:** Internal Medicine 1972, Gastroenterology 1993; **Med School:** NYU Sch Med 1965; **Resid:** Internal Medicine, Kings County Hosp, Brooklyn, NY 1966-1968; Gastroenterology, Univ of Miami Jackson Mem Hosp, Miami, FL 1968-1969; **Fellow:** Gastroenterology, Jackson Mem Hosp, Miami, FL 1968-1969; **Fac Appt:** Clin Prof Medicine, Univ Miami Sch Med

Drossman, Douglas Arnold MD (Ge) - *Spec Exp: Gastrointestinal Motility Disorders; Psychiatric Aspects of GI Disorders;* **Hospital:** Univ of NC Hosp (page 77); **Address:** 726 Burnett Womack , Box CB 7080, Chapel Hill, NC 27599-7080; **Phone:** (919) 966-0141; **Board Cert:** Internal Medicine 1973, Gastroenterology 1979; **Med School:** Albert Einstein Coll Med 1970; **Resid:** Internal Medicine, NC Meml Hosp-UNC, Chapel Hill, NC 1971-1972; Internal Medicine, Bellevue Hosp Ctr-NYU, New York, NY 1972-1973; **Fellow:** Psychiatry, Univ Rochester, Rochester, NY 1975-1976; Gastroenterology, NC Meml Hosp-UNC, Chapel, NY 1976-1978; **Fac Appt:** Prof Medicine, Univ NC Sch Med

Forsmark, Christopher MD (Ge) - *Spec Exp: AIDS/HIV-Gastrointestinal Complications; Gastrointestinal Cancer; Pancreatitis;* **Hospital:** Shands Hlthcre at Univ of FL (page 73); **Address:** University of Florida, 1600 SW Archer Rd, Box 100214, Gainesville, FL 32610-0214; **Phone:** (352) 392-2877; **Board Cert:** Internal Medicine 1986, Gastroenterology 1989; **Med School:** Johns Hopkins Univ 1983; **Resid:** Internal Medicine, Univ Calif-San Fran, San Francisco, CA 1984-1987; **Fellow:** Gastroenterology, Univ Calif-San Fran, San Francisco, CA 1987-1990; **Fac Appt:** Assoc Prof Gastroenterology, Univ Fla Coll Med

Hawes, Robert H MD (Ge) - *Spec Exp:* Endoscopic Ultrasound; Pancreatic/Biliary Endoscopy (ERCP); **Hospital:** Med Univ Hosp Authority; **Address:** 96 Jonathan Lucas St, Ste 210, Box 250327, Charleston, SC 29425; **Phone:** (843) 792-7896; **Board Cert:** Internal Medicine 1985, Gastroenterology 1987; **Med School:** Indiana Univ 1980; **Fac Appt:** Prof Medicine, Med Univ SC

Hoffman, Brenda MD (Ge) - *Spec Exp:* Liver & Biliary Disease; Endoscopic Ultrasound; **Hospital:** Med Univ Hosp Authority; **Address:** Digestive Disease Center, 210 CSB, 96 Jonathan Lucas St, Box 250327, Charleston, SC 29425; **Phone:** (843) 792-6865; **Board Cert:** Internal Medicine 1986, Gastroenterology 1989; **Med School:** Univ KY Coll Med 1993; **Resid:** Internal Medicine, MUSC Med Ctr, Charleston, SC 1984-1987; **Fellow:** Gastroenterology, MUSC Med Ctr, Charleston, SC 1987-1989; **Fac Appt:** Asst Prof Medicine, Univ SC Sch Med

Lambiase, Louis MD (Ge) - *Spec Exp:* Pancreatitis; **Hospital:** Shands Jacksonville; **Address:** GI Div, 3rd FL, 653 W 8th St, Jacksonville, FL 32209; **Phone:** (904) 244-3273; **Board Cert:** Gastroenterology 1993, Internal Medicine 1990; **Med School:** Univ Miami Sch Med 1987; **Resid:** Internal Medicine, Univ Pittsburgh-Presby VA, Pittsburgh, PA 1987-1990; **Fellow:** Gastroenterology, Univ Fla Coll Med, Gainsville, Fl 1990; **Fac Appt:** Assoc Prof Medicine, Univ Fla Coll Med

Liddle, Rodger Alan MD (Ge) - *Spec Exp:* Gastrointestinal Cancer; **Hospital:** Duke Univ Med Ctr (page 60); **Address:** Duke Univ Med Ctr, Dept Gastroenterology, Box 3913, Durham, NC 27710; **Phone:** (919) 684-5066; **Board Cert:** Internal Medicine 1981, Gastroenterology 1983; **Med School:** Vanderbilt Univ 1978; **Resid:** Internal Medicine, UCSF Med Ctr, San Francisco, CA 1979-1981; **Fellow:** Gastroenterology, UCSF Med Ctr, San Francisco, CA 1981-1984; **Fac Appt:** Prof Medicine, Duke Univ

Raiford, David S MD (Ge) - *Spec Exp:* Liver Disease; Drug Hepatotoxicity; Liver Tumors; **Hospital:** Vanderbilt Univ Med Ctr (page 80); **Address:** The Vanderbilt Clinic, Div Gastroenterology, Box 1501, Nashville, TN 37232; **Phone:** (615) 322-0128; **Board Cert:** Internal Medicine 1989, Gastroenterology 1991; **Med School:** Johns Hopkins Univ 1985; **Resid:** Internal Medicine, Johns Hopkins Hosp, Baltimore, MD 1985-1988; **Fac Appt:** Prof Medicine, Vanderbilt Univ

Roche, James Kenneth MD/PhD (Ge) - *Spec Exp:* Inflammatory Bowel Disease/Crohn's; Diarrhea; **Hospital:** Univ of VA Hlth Sys (page 79); **Address:** UVA Health Systems, Div Gastroenterology, PO Box 801317, Charlottesville, VA 22908; **Phone:** (804) 243-2655; **Board Cert:** Internal Medicine 1975; **Med School:** Univ Penn 1969; **Resid:** Internal Medicine, Univ Hlth Ctr Penn, Pittsburgh, PA 1970-1971; Internal Medicine, Duke Univ Med Ctr, Durham, NC 1973-1974; **Fellow:** Gastroenterology, Duke Univ Med Ctr, Durham, NC 1974-1977; **Fac Appt:** Assoc Prof Gastroenterology, Univ VA Sch Med

Rogers, Arvey MD (Ge) - *Spec Exp:* Endoscopy; Inflammatory Bowel Disease/Crohn's; **Hospital:** Univ of Miami - Jackson Meml Hosp; **Address:** Univ Miami Hosp and Clinics, 1425 NW 12th Ave, Ste D1007, Miami, FL 33136-1002; **Phone:** (305) 585-5120; **Board Cert:** Internal Medicine 1965, Gastroenterology 1968; **Med School:** Univ Tex Med Br, Galveston 1958; **Resid:** Internal Medicine, Jackson Meml Hosp, Miami, FL 1959-1961; Infectious Disease, Jackson Meml Hosp, Miami, FL 1961-1962; **Fellow:** Gastroenterology, Coral Gables VA Med Ctr, Miami, FL 1962-1964; **Fac Appt:** Prof Medicine, Univ Miami Sch Med

Schiff, Eugene MD (Ge) - *Spec Exp:* Hepatitis C; Liver Disease; **Hospital:** Cedars Med Ctr - Miami; **Address:** Univ Miami Ctr for Liver Disease, 1500 NW 12th Ave, Ste 1101, Miami, FL 33136-3877; **Phone:** (305) 243-5787; **Board Cert:** Internal Medicine 1980, Gastroenterology 1972; **Med School:** Columbia P&S 1962; **Resid:** Internal Medicine, Cincinnati Genl Hosp, Cincinati, OH 1963-1964; Internal Medicine, Parkland Meml Hosp, Dallas, TX 1966-1967; **Fellow:** Gastroenterology, Univ Tex Med Ctr, Dallas, TX 1967-1969; **Fac Appt:** Prof Medicine, Univ Miami Sch Med

Scudera, Peter MD (Ge) - *Spec Exp:* Transplant Medicine-Liver; **Hospital:** Inova Fair Oaks Hosp; **Address:** 3700 Joseph Siewick Dr, Ste 308, Fairfax, VA 22033; **Phone:** (703) 716-8700; **Board Cert:** Gastroenterology 1989, Internal Medicine 1987; **Med School:** Cornell Univ-Weill Med Coll 1984; **Resid:** Internal Medicine, New York Hosp-Cornell, New York, NY 1985-1987; **Fellow:** Gastroenterology, NewYork Hosp-Cornell, New York, NY 1987-1989

Shenk, Ian MD (Ge) - *Spec Exp:* Irritable Bowel Syndrome; **Hospital:** Inova Fairfax Hosp; **Address:** 3027 Javier Rd, Fairfax, VA 22031; **Phone:** (703) 435-8535; **Board Cert:** Gastroenterology 1973, Internal Medicine 1970; **Med School:** Johns Hopkins Univ 1965; **Resid:** Internal Medicine, Johns Hopkins Hosp, Baltimore, MD 1965-1967; Surgery, Yale-New Haven Hosp, New Haven, CT 1967-1968

Shiffman, Mitchell MD (Ge) - *Spec Exp:* Transplant Medicine-Liver; Hepatitis C; **Hospital:** Univ of VA Hlth Sys (page 79); **Address:** VCU Health Systems, Div Hepatology, Box 980341, Richmond, VA 23298-0711; **Phone:** (804) 828-4060; **Board Cert:** Internal Medicine 1986, Gastroenterology 1989; **Med School:** SUNY Syracuse 1983; **Resid:** Internal Medicine, Med Coll Va, Richmond, VA 1984-1986; **Fellow:** Gastroenterology, Med Coll Va, Richmond, VA 1986-1988; **Fac Appt:** Assoc Prof Medicine, Univ VA Sch Med

Toskes, Phillip MD (Ge) - *Spec Exp:* Nutrition; Malabsorption; Pancreatitis; **Hospital:** Shands Hlthcre at Univ of FL (page 73); **Address:** Univ of FLA, 1600 SW Archer Rd, Box 100277, Gainesville, FL 32610-0214; **Phone:** (352) 392-2877; **Board Cert:** Internal Medicine 1970, Gastroenterology 1973; **Med School:** Univ MD Sch Med 1965; **Resid:** Internal Medicine, Univ of Maryland Hosp, Baltimore, MD 1966-1968; **Fellow:** Gastroenterology, Hosp Univ Penn, Philadelphia, PA 1968-1970; **Fac Appt:** Prof Medicine, Univ Fla Coll Med

Midwest

Achkar, Edgar MD (Ge) - *Spec Exp:* Esophageal Disorders; Motility Disorders; **Hospital:** Cleveland Clin Fdn (page 57); **Address:** 9500 Euclid Ave, Ste S40, Cleveland, OH 44195; **Phone:** (216) 444-6523; **Board Cert:** Internal Medicine 1978, Gastroenterology 1979; **Med School:** France 1964; **Resid:** Internal Medicine, Lahey Clin, Boston, MA 1965-1967; **Fellow:** Gastroenterology, Lahey Clin, Boston, MA 1967-1968; Gastroenterology, Clevland Clin, Cleveland, OH 1968-1969; **Fac Appt:** Asst Prof Medicine, Ohio State Univ

Bacon, Bruce MD (Ge) - *Spec Exp:* Hepatitis C; Hepatic Iron Metabolism; Liver Disease; **Hospital:** St Louis Univ Hospital; **Address:** 3660 Vista Ave, St Louis, MO 63110; **Phone:** (314) 577-6150; **Board Cert:** Internal Medicine 1978, Gastroenterology 1983; **Med School:** Case West Res Univ 1975; **Resid:** Internal Medicine, Metro Genl Hosp, Cleveland, OH 1976-1979; **Fellow:** Gastroenterology, Metro Genl Hosp, Cleveland, OH 1979-1982; **Fac Appt:** Prof Medicine, St Louis Univ

Blei, Andres T MD (Ge) - *Spec Exp:* Hepatitis C; Liver Disease; **Hospital:** Northwestern Meml Hosp; **Address:** 675 N Sinclair, Ste 17-250, Chicago, IL 60611; **Phone:** (312) 695-5620; **Board Cert:** Internal Medicine 1981, Gastroenterology 1985; **Med School:** Argentina 1973; **Resid:** Internal Medicine, Police Posadas, Buenos Aires, Argentina 1974-1976; Hepatology, Yale Univ Sch Med, New Haven, CT 1976-1978; **Fellow:** Gastroenterology, Univ Chicago Hosp, Chicago, IL 1978-1980; **Fac Appt:** Prof Medicine, Northwestern Univ

Bresalier, Robert MD (Ge) - *Spec Exp:* Gastrointestinal Cancer; Peptic Acid Disorders; **Hospital:** Henry Ford Hosp; **Address:** Dept of Gastroenterology, 2799 W Grand Blvd, Detroit, MI 48202-2689; **Phone:** (313) 916-9452; **Board Cert:** Internal Medicine 1981, Gastroenterology 1983; **Med School:** Univ Chicago-Pritzker Sch Med 1978; **Resid:** Internal Medicine, Barnes Hosp-Washington Univ, Saint Louis, MO 1978-1981; **Fellow:** Gastroenterology, Univ California San Francisco Med Ctr, San Francisco, CA 1981-1983; **Fac Appt:** Assoc Prof Medicine, Univ Mich Med Sch

Brown, Kimberly A MD (Ge) - *Spec Exp:* Liver Disease; Transplant-Liver; **Hospital:** Henry Ford Hosp; **Address:** 2799 W Grand Blvd, Gastro K-7, Detroit, MI 48202; **Phone:** (313) 916-2393; **Board Cert:** Internal Medicine 1988, Gastroenterology 1991; **Med School:** Wayne State Univ 1985; **Resid:** Internal Medicine, Univ Michigan, Ann Arbor, MI 1985-1988; Internal Medicine, Univ Michigan, Ann Arbor, MI 1988-1989; **Fellow:** Gastroenterology, Univ Michigan, Ann Arbor, MI 1989-1992

Clouse, Ray Eugene MD (Ge) - *Spec Exp:* Gastroesophageal Reflux; Esophageal Disorders; **Hospital:** Barnes-Jewish Hosp (page 55); **Address:** 4921 Park View Pl 8, St Louis, MO 63110; **Phone:** (314) 747-2066; **Board Cert:** Internal Medicine 1979; **Med School:** Indiana Univ 1976; **Resid:** Internal Medicine, Barnes Hosp/Washington Univ Sch Med, Saint Louis, MO 1976-1978; **Fellow:** Gastroenterology, Barnes Hosp/Washington Univ Sch Med, Saint Louis, MO 1978-1979; **Fac Appt:** Prof Medicine, Washington Univ, St Louis

Craig, Robert M MD (Ge) - *Spec Exp:* Inflammatory Bowel Disease/Crohn's; Gallbladder Disorders; Swallowing Disorders; **Hospital:** Northwestern Meml Hosp; **Address:** 233 E Erie St Ste 206, Chicago, IL 60611; **Phone:** (312) 908-9644; **Board Cert:** Internal Medicine 1972, Gastroenterology 1975; **Med School:** Northwestern Univ 1967; **Resid:** Internal Medicine, VA Rsch Hosp, Chicago, IL 1968-1969; Internal Medicine, VA Rsch Hosp, Chicago, IL 1971-1972; **Fellow:** Gastroenterology, Northwestern Univ Med Ctr, Chicago, IL 1972-1974; **Fac Appt:** Prof Medicine, Northwestern Univ

Di Magno, Eugene MD (Ge) - *Spec Exp:* Pancreatic Disease; **Hospital:** Mayo Med Ctr & Clin - Rochester, MN; **Address:** Div of Gastroenterology, 200 1st St SW, Rochester, MN 55905; **Phone:** (507) 284-2407; **Board Cert:** Gastroenterology 1972, Internal Medicine 1969; **Med School:** Univ Penn 1962; **Resid:** Internal Medicine, Mayo Clinic, Rochester, MN 1966-1968; **Fellow:** Gastroenterology, Mayo Clinic, Rochester, MN 1968-1970; **Fac Appt:** Prof Medicine, Mayo Med Sch

Edmundowicz, Steven MD (Ge) - *Spec Exp:* Endoscopy; Biliary Disease; **Hospital:** Barnes-Jewish Hosp (page 55); **Address:** Washington Univ Sch Medicine, Div Gastroenterology, 4921 Parkview Pl Fl 8, St. Louis, MO 63110; **Phone:** (314) 747-2066; **Board Cert:** Internal Medicine 1986, Gastroenterology 1989; **Med School:** Jefferson Med Coll 1983; **Resid:** Internal Medicine, Barnes Hosp/Wash Univ, St Louis, MO 1984-1986; **Fellow:** Gastroenterology, Barnes Hosp/Wash Univ, St Louis, MO 1986; **Fac Appt:** Asst Clin Prof Medicine, Jefferson Med Coll

Elliott, David MD (Ge) - *Spec Exp:* Celiac Disease; Inflammatory Bowel Disease/Crohn's; Intestinal Parasites; **Hospital:** Univ of IA Hosp and Clinics; **Address:** Dept Digestive Diseases, 200 Hawkins Drive, rm 4611-JCP, Iowa City, IA 52242; **Phone:** (319) 356-4901; **Board Cert:** Gastroenterology 1993, Internal Medicine 1991; **Med School:** Wayne State Univ 1988; **Resid:** Internal Medicine, Johns Hopkins Hosp, Baltimore, MD 1989-1991; **Fellow:** Gastroenterology, Univ Iowa Hosps, Iowa City, IA 1991; **Fac Appt:** Asst Prof Medicine, Univ Iowa Coll Med

Gostout, Christopher John MD (Ge) - *Spec Exp:* Gastroscopy; Endoscopy; **Hospital:** Mayo Med Ctr & Clin - Rochester, MN; **Address:** Div of Gastroenterology, 200 First St SW, Rochester, MN 55905; **Phone:** (507) 266-6932; **Board Cert:** Internal Medicine 1979, Gastroenterology 1981; **Med School:** SUNY Downstate 1976; **Resid:** Internal Medicine, Mayo Clinic, Rochester, MN 1977-1979; **Fellow:** Gastroenterology, Mayo Clinic, Rochester, MN 1979-1981

Hanauer, Stephen MD (Ge) - *Spec Exp:* Inflammatory Bowel Disease/Crohn's; Crohn's Disease; Ulcerative Colitis; **Hospital:** Univ of Chicago Hosps (page 76); **Address:** Univ Chicago Hosps, 5758 S Maryland Ave, MC-9028, Chicago, IL 60637; **Phone:** (773) 702-1466; **Board Cert:** Internal Medicine 1980, Gastroenterology 1983; **Med School:** Univ IL Coll Med 1977; **Resid:** Internal Medicine, Univ Chicago Hosps, Chicago, IL 1978-1980; **Fellow:** Gastroenterology, Univ Chicago Hosps, Chicago, IL 1980-1982; **Fac Appt:** Prof Gastroenterology, Univ Chicago-Pritzker Sch Med

Jensen, Donald MD (Ge) - *Spec Exp:* Transplant Medicine-Liver; Hepatitis C; Cirrhosis; **Hospital:** Rush-Presby - St Luke's Med Ctr (page 72); **Address:** 1725 W Harrison St, Ste 306, University Hepatologists, Chicago, IL 60612-3828; **Phone:** (312) 942-8910; **Board Cert:** Internal Medicine 1975, Gastroenterology 1981; **Med School:** Univ IL Coll Med 1972; **Resid:** Internal Medicine, Rush Presby, Chicago, IL 1972-1975; Gastroenterology, Rush Presby, Chicago, IL 1975-1976; **Fellow:** Gastroenterology, King's Coll, London, England 1976-1978; **Fac Appt:** Prof Medicine, Rush Med Coll

Kahrilas, Peter MD (Ge) - *Spec Exp:* Esophageal Disorders; Swallowing Disorders; **Hospital:** Northwestern Meml Hosp; **Address:** 675 N St Clair, Fl 17 - Ste 250, Chicago, IL 60611; **Phone:** (312) 695-0606; **Board Cert:** Internal Medicine 1982, Gastroenterology 1987; **Med School:** Univ Rochester 1979; **Resid:** Internal Medicine, Univ Hosp, Cleveland, OH 1979-1982; **Fellow:** Gastroenterology, Northwestern Univ, Chicago, IL 1982-1984; Research, Med Coll Wisc, Milwaukee, WI 1984-1986; **Fac Appt:** Prof Medicine, Northwestern Univ

Klamut, Michael MD (Ge) - *Spec Exp:* Gastroenterology - General; **Hospital:** Loyola Univ Med Ctr; **Address:** 2160 S 1st Ave Bldg 117 - Ste 20A, Maywood, IL 60153-5500; **Phone:** (708) 216-8563; **Board Cert:** Internal Medicine 1976; **Med School:** Loyola Univ-Stritch Sch Med 1973; **Resid:** Internal Medicine, Loyola Univ Med, Maywood, IL 1974-1976; **Fellow:** Gastroenterology, Loyola Univ Med, Maywood, IL 1976-1978; **Fac Appt:** Assoc Prof Medicine, Loyola Univ-Stritch Sch Med

Konicek, Frank MD (Ge) - *Spec Exp:* Gastroenterology - General; **Hospital:** Advocate IL Masonic Med Ctr; **Address:** 3004 N Ashland Ave, Chicago, IL 60657; **Phone:** (773) 871-4600; **Board Cert:** Internal Medicine 1977, Gastroenterology 1975; **Med School:** Loyola Univ-Stritch Sch Med 1963; **Resid:** Internal Medicine, St Francis Hosp, Evanston, IL 1964-1965; Internal Medicine, Hines VA Hosp, Hines, IL 1967-1969; **Fellow:** Gastroenterology, Hines VA Hosp, Hines, IL 1969-1971; **Fac Appt:** Clin Prof Medicine, Loyola Univ-Stritch Sch Med

Kwo, Paul Y MD (Ge) - *Spec Exp:* Hepatitis C; **Hospital:** IN Univ Hosp (page 63); **Address:** 975 W Walnut St Bldg 1B - Ste 327, Indianapolis, IN 46202-5121; **Phone:** (317) 274-3090; **Board Cert:** Internal Medicine 1991, Gastroenterology 1995; **Med School:** Wayne State Univ 1988; **Resid:** Internal Medicine, Univ Maryland, Baltimore, MD 1989-1991; **Fellow:** Gastroenterology, Mayo Clinic, Rochester, MN; **Fac Appt:** Assoc Clin Prof Medicine, Indiana Univ

La Russo, Nicholas Francis MD (Ge) - *Spec Exp:* Transplant Medicine-Liver; Liver & Biliary Disease; **Hospital:** Mayo Med Ctr & Clin - Rochester, MN; **Address:** Mayo Medical Center, 200 1st St SW, Rochester, MN 55905-0001; **Phone:** (507) 284-8700; **Board Cert:** Gastroenterology 1979, Internal Medicine 1972; **Med School:** NY Med Coll 1969; **Resid:** Internal Medicine, Mayo Clinic, Rochester, MN 1970-1972; **Fellow:** Gastroenterology, Mayo Clinic, Rochester, MN 1972-1975; **Fac Appt:** Prof Medicine, Mayo Med Sch

Levitan, Ruven MD (Ge) - *Spec Exp:* Malabsorption; Inflammatory Bowel Disease; Esophageal Disorders; **Hospital:** Advocate Lutheran Gen Hosp; **Address:** 4709 Golf Rd, Ste 1000, Skokie, IL 60076-1260; **Phone:** (847) 677-1170; **Board Cert:** Internal Medicine 1980, Gastroenterology 1968; **Med School:** Israel 1953; **Resid:** Internal Medicine, Mount Sinai Med Ctr, New York, NY 1956-1957; Gastroenterology, Beth Israel Med Ctr, Boston, MA 1958-1959; **Fellow:** Internal Medicine, Mem Sloan Kettering Cancer Ctr, New York, NY 1957-1958; **Fac Appt:** Clin Prof Medicine, Univ IL Coll Med

Lindor, Keith Douglas MD (Ge) - *Spec Exp:* Liver Disease/Biliary Cirrhosis; Sclerosing Cholangitis; **Hospital:** Mayo Med Ctr & Clin - Rochester, MN; **Address:** Div of Gastroenterology, 200 1st St SW, Rochester, MN 55905; **Phone:** (507) 284-2511; **Board Cert:** Gastroenterology 1987, Internal Medicine 1983; **Med School:** Mayo Med Sch 1979; **Resid:** Internal Medicine, North Carolina Baptist Hosp, Winston-Salem, NC 1979-1982; **Fellow:** Gastroenterology, Mayo Clinic, Rochester, MN 1983-1986; **Fac Appt:** Prof Medicine, Mayo Med Sch

Luxon, Bruce MD (Ge) - *Spec Exp:* Liver Disease; Hepatitis C; **Hospital:** St Louis Univ Hospital; **Address:** St Louis Univ Hosp, 3635 Vista Ave, St Louis, MO 63110-0250; **Phone:** (314) 577-8764; **Board Cert:** Internal Medicine 1989, Gastroenterology 1991; **Med School:** Univ MO-Columbia Sch Med 1985; **Fac Appt:** Assoc Prof Medicine, St Louis Univ

Meiselman, Mick Scott MD (Ge) - *Spec Exp:* Gastroenterology - General; **Hospital:** Evanston Hosp; **Address:** 506 Green Bay Rd, Kenilworth, IL 60043-1002; **Phone:** (847) 256-3495; **Board Cert:** Internal Medicine 1982, Gastroenterology 1985; **Med School:** Northwestern Univ 1979; **Resid:** Internal Medicine, Cedars-Sinai/UCLA, Los Angeles, CA 1979-1982; **Fellow:** Gastroenterology, UCSF Med Ctr, San Francisco, CA 1982-1984; **Fac Appt:** Asst Clin Prof Medicine, Northwestern Univ

Owyang, Chung MD (Ge) - *Spec Exp:* Motility Disorders; Digestion; **Hospital:** Univ of MI Hlth Ctr; **Address:** 1500 E Med Ctr, rm 3912, Box 0362, Taubman Health Care Center, Ann Arbor, MI 48109-0362; **Phone:** (888) 229-7408; **Board Cert:** Internal Medicine 1976, Gastroenterology 1981; **Med School:** McGill Univ 1972; **Resid:** Internal Medicine, Montreal Genl-Hosp, Montreal, CN 1973-1975; **Fellow:** Gastroenterology, Mayo Grad Sch., Rochester, MN 1975-1978; **Fac Appt:** Prof Medicine, Univ Mich Med Sch

Rao, Satish S C MD (Ge) - *Spec Exp:* Constipation; Incontinence-Fecal; Non-Cardiac Chest Pain; **Hospital:** Univ of IA Hosp and Clinics; **Address:** Univ Iowa Coll Med, Div Gastroenterology, 4612 JCP, 200 Hawkins Drive, Iowa City, IA 52242; **Phone:** (319) 353-6602; **Board Cert:** Internal Medicine 1996, Gastroenterology 1998; **Med School:** India 1978; **Resid:** Internal Medicine, Sunderland Hosps, Sunderland, England 1980-1982; Internal Medicine, York Dist Hosp, York, England 1982-1984; **Fellow:** Royal Hallamshire Hosp, Sheffield, England 1984-1986; Gastroenterology, Royal Liverpool Hosp, Liverpool, England 1987-1988; **Fac Appt:** Assoc Prof Medicine, Univ Iowa Coll Med

Reichelderfer, Mark MD (Ge) - *Spec Exp:* Endoscopy; **Hospital:** Univ WI Hosp & Clins; **Address:** 600 Highland Ave, rm H6/516, Madison, WI 53792; **Phone:** (608) 263-8094; **Board Cert:** Gastroenterology 1979, Internal Medicine 1977; **Med School:** Coll Physicians & Surgeons 1974; **Resid:** Internal Medicine, Mary Imogene Bassett Hosp, Cooperstown, NY 1975-1977; **Fellow:** Gastroenterology, Univ Wisc Hosps & Clin, Madison, WI 1977-1979; **Fac Appt:** Prof Medicine, Univ Wisc

Rex, Douglas Kevin MD (Ge) - *Spec Exp:* Endoscopy; **Hospital:** IN Univ Hosp (page 63); **Address:** 550 N University Blvd, Ste 2300, Indianapolis, IN 46202-5203; **Phone:** (317) 274-0912; **Board Cert:** Internal Medicine 1985, Gastroenterology 1987; **Med School:** Indiana Univ 1980; **Resid:** Internal Medicine, Indiana Univ Med Ctr, Indianapolis, IN 1981-1982; Internal Medicine, Indiana Univ Hosp, Indianapolis, IN 1984-1985; **Fellow:** Gastroenterology, Indiana Univ Med Ctr, Indianapolis, IN 1982-1984; **Fac Appt:** Assoc Prof Medicine, Indiana Univ

Richter, Joel MD (Ge) - *Spec Exp:* Gastroesophageal Reflux; Esophageal Disorders; **Hospital:** Cleveland Clin Fdn (page 57); **Address:** 9500 Euclid Ave, Ste A30, Cleveland, OH 44195; **Phone:** (216) 445-9102; **Board Cert:** Internal Medicine 1978, Gastroenterology 1981; **Med School:** Univ Tex SW, Dallas 1975; **Resid:** Internal Medicine, Natl Naval Med Ctr, Bethesda, MD 1976-1978; **Fellow:** Gastroenterology, Natl Naval Med Ctr, Bethesda, MD 1978-1980; **Fac Appt:** Prof Medicine, Ohio State Univ

Sandborn, William Jeffery MD (Ge) - *Spec Exp:* Inflammatory Bowel Disease/Crohn's; Ulcerative Colitis; Crohn's Disease; **Hospital:** Mayo Med Ctr & Clin - Rochester, MN; **Address:** Mayo Clinic, 200 First St SW, Rochester, MN 55905; **Phone:** (507) 284-0959; **Board Cert:** Infectious Disease 1990, Gastroenterology 1993; **Med School:** Loma Linda Univ 1987; **Resid:** Internal Medicine, Loma Linda U., Loma Linda, CA 1987-1990; **Fellow:** Gastroenterology, Mayo Clinic, Rochester, MN 1990-1993; **Fac Appt:** Assoc Prof Medicine, Mayo Med Sch

Schmidt, Warren Norman MD (Ge) - *Spec Exp:* Liver Disease; **Hospital:** Univ of IA Hosp and Clinics; **Address:** Dept Gastroenterology, 200 Hawkins Drive, 4544 JCP, Iowa City, IA 52242; **Phone:** (319) 356-4060; **Board Cert:** Gastroenterology 1997, Internal Medicine 1993; **Med School:** Univ Tenn Coll Med, Memphis 1989; **Resid:** Internal Medicine, U Tenn Ctr Hlth Sci, Memphis, TN 1990-1992; **Fellow:** Gastroenterology, U Iowa Hosp & Clin, Iowa City, IA 1992

Schulze, Konrad S MD (Ge) - *Spec Exp:* Gastroesophageal Reflux; Gastric Diseases; Gastroparesis; **Hospital:** Univ of IA Hosp and Clinics; **Address:** Digestive Disease Clinic, 200 Hawkins Drive Bldg Colloton - rm 4-JC, Iowa City, IA 52242; **Phone:** (319) 356-4060; **Board Cert:** Internal Medicine 1987, Gastroenterology 1975; **Med School:** Germany 1968; **Resid:** Psychiatry, Boston City Hosp, Boston, MA 1970-1971; Internal Medicine, Montreal General Hosp, Montreal, Canada 1971-1974; **Fellow:** Gastroenterology, Univ IA, Iowa City, IA 1975-1977

Silverman, William Bruce MD (Ge) - *Spec Exp:* Liver Disease; Pancreatic/Biliary Endoscopy(ERCP); **Hospital:** Univ of IA Hosp and Clinics; **Address:** Div GI/Hepatology, 200 Hawkins Drive Bldg JCP - rm 4553, Iowa City, IA 52242; **Phone:** (319) 384-9995; **Board Cert:** Gastroenterology 1997, Internal Medicine 1988; **Med School:** Belgium 1984; **Resid:** Internal Medicine, Lutheran Hosp-Univ Ill, Chicago, IL 1985-1987; **Fellow:** Gastroenterology, Univ Hosp-Case West Res, Cleveland, OH 1988-1989; Gastroenterology, Univ Brussels, Brussels, Belgium 1989-1990; **Fac Appt:** Assoc Prof Medicine, Univ Iowa Coll Med

Sivak, Michael MD (Ge) - *Spec Exp:* Endoscopy; Endoscopic Ultrasound; **Hospital:** Univ Hosp of Cleveland; **Address:** 11100 Euclid Ave, Cleveland, OH 44106-5066; **Phone:** (216) 844-7344; **Board Cert:** Internal Medicine 1977; **Med School:** Hahnemann Univ 1969; **Resid:** Internal Medicine, Cleveland Clinic, Cleveland, OH 1970-1972; **Fellow:** Gastroenterology, Cleveland Clinic, Cleveland, OH 1972-1974; **Fac Appt:** Prof Medicine, Case West Res Univ

Tremaine, William John MD (Ge) - *Spec Exp:* Inflammatory Bowel Disease/Crohn's; Ulcerative Colitis; **Hospital:** St Mary's Hosp - Rochester, MN; **Address:** Mayo Clinic, 200 1st St SW, Rochester, MN 55905-0002; **Phone:** (507) 284-2469; **Board Cert:** Internal Medicine 1979, Gastroenterology 1981; **Med School:** Univ Miss 1976; **Resid:** Internal Medicine, Mayo Clinic, Rochester, MN 1978-1980; **Fellow:** Gastroenterology, Mayo Clinic, Rochester, MN 1980-1981; **Fac Appt:** Prof Medicine, Mayo Med Sch

Van Thiel, David MD (Ge) - *Spec Exp:* Transplant Medicine-Liver; Hepatitis; **Hospital:** Loyola Univ Med Ctr; **Address:** 2160 S First Ave Bldg 114 - rm 54, Maywood, IL 60153; **Phone:** (708) 216-0364; **Board Cert:** Gastroenterology 1975, Internal Medicine 1972; **Med School:** UCLA 1967; **Resid:** Internal Medicine, NY Cornell Med Ctr, New York, NY 1968-1969; Gastroenterology, Univ Hosp, Boston, MA 1971-1972; **Fellow:** Gastroenterology, Univ Hosp, Boston, MA 1972-1974; **Fac Appt:** Prof Medicine, Loyola Univ-Stritch Sch Med

Wiesner, Russell MD (Ge) - *Spec Exp:* Transplant Medicine-Liver; **Hospital:** Mayo Med Ctr & Clin - Rochester, MN; , Rochester, MN 55905; **Board Cert:** Infectious Disease 1978, Gastroenterology 1981; **Med School:** Med Coll Wisc 1975

Winans, Charles MD (Ge) - *Spec Exp:* Esophageal & Swallowing Disorders; Gastroesophageal Reflux; Swallowing Disorders; **Hospital:** Univ of Chicago Hosps (page 76); **Address:** Univ Chicago Hosps, 5758 S Maryland Ave, MC-9028, Chicago, IL 60637; **Phone:** (773) 702-6137; **Board Cert:** Internal Medicine 1968, Gastroenterology 1970; **Med School:** Case West Res Univ 1961; **Resid:** Internal Medicine, Univ Hosp, Cleveland, OH 1962-1964; **Fellow:** Gastroenterology, Boston Univ Med Ctr, Boston, MA 1964-1966; **Fac Appt:** Prof Medicine, Univ Chicago-Pritzker Sch Med

Great Plains and Mountains

Fitz, J Gregory MD (Ge) - *Spec Exp:* Gastroenterology - General; **Hospital:** Univ Colo HSC - Denver; **Address:** 4200 E 9th Ave, MS RW 6412, Gastroenterology and Hepatology, Denver, CO 80262; **Phone:** (303) 315-2536; **Board Cert:** Internal Medicine 1982, Gastroenterology 1985; **Med School:** Duke Univ 1979; **Resid:** Internal Medicine, Univ Calif Med Ctr, San Francisco, CA 1979-1982; **Fellow:** Gastroenterology, Univ Calif Med Ctr, San Francisco, CA 1982-1985; **Fac Appt:** Prof Gastroenterology, Univ Colo

Hunter, Ellen B MD (Ge) - *Spec Exp:* Hepatitis; **Hospital:** St. Luke's Reg Med Ctr - Boise; **Address:** 425 W Vannock, Boise, ID 83702; **Phone:** (208) 343-6458; **Board Cert:** Internal Medicine 1986, Gastroenterology 1989; **Med School:** Georgetown Univ 1983; **Resid:** Internal Medicine, Vanderbilt Univ Med Ctr, Nashville, TN 1984-1986; **Fellow:** Gastroenterology, Mayo Clinic, Rochester, MN 1986-1989

Sorrell, Michael MD (Ge) - *Spec Exp:* Transplant Medicine-Liver; Hepatitis; **Hospital:** Nebraska Hlth Sys; **Address:** 983285 Nebraska Medical Center, Omaha, NE 68198-3285; **Phone:** (402) 559-7912; **Board Cert:** Internal Medicine 1972; **Med School:** Univ Nebr Coll Med 1959; **Resid:** Internal Medicine, Univ Nebr Hosp, Omaha, NE 1966-1968; Gastroenterology, Univ Nebr Hosp, Omaha, NE 1968-1969; **Fac Appt:** Prof Medicine, Univ Nebr Coll Med

Southwest

Anderson, Karl MD (Ge) - *Spec Exp:* Porphyria; **Hospital:** Univ of TX Med Brch Hosps at Galveston; **Address:** Univ Tex Med Br-Ewing Hall, 700 Harborside Dr, Galveston, TX 77555-1109; **Phone:** (409) 772-4661; **Board Cert:** Internal Medicine 1972, Gastroenterology 1972; **Med School:** Johns Hopkins Univ 1965; **Resid:** Internal Medicine, Vanderbilt Univ Hosp, Nashville, TN 1966-1967; Internal Medicine, NY Hosp-Cornell Med Ctr, New York, NY 1967-1968; **Fellow:** Gastroenterology, NY Hosp-Cornell Med Ctr, New York, NY 1968-1970; **Fac Appt:** Prof Medicine, Univ Tex Med Br, Galveston

Balart, Luis A MD (Ge) - *Spec Exp:* Hepatitis C; **Hospital:** Louisiana State Univ Hosp; **Address:** 2820 Napoleon Ave, Ste 700, New Orleans, LA 70115; **Phone:** (504) 899-8401; **Board Cert:** Internal Medicine 1976, Gastroenterology 1981; **Med School:** Cuba 1972

Brady III, Charles Elmer MD (Ge) - *Spec Exp:* *Esophageal Disorders;* **Hospital:** Univ of Texas Hlth & Sci Ctr; **Address:** Univ Texas Hlth Sci Ctr, Div Gastroenterology, 7703 Floyd Curl Drive, MC 7878, San Antonio, TX 78229-3900; **Phone:** (210) 567-4876; **Board Cert:** Internal Medicine 1974, Gastroenterology 1977; **Med School:** Med Coll VA 1971; **Resid:** Internal Medicine, Wilford Hall Med Ctr, Lackland AFB, TX 1972-1974; **Fellow:** Gastroenterology, Univ Tex, Dallas, TX 1974-1976; **Fac Appt:** Assoc Prof Medicine, Univ Tex, San Antonio

Cunningham, John MD (Ge) - *Spec Exp:* *Sphincter of Oddi Dysfunction; Pancreatitis; Bleeding-Gastrointestinal;* **Hospital:** Univ Med Ctr; **Address:** Univ Arizona, Div Gastroenterology, 1501 N Campbell Ave, Tuscon, AZ 85724-5028; **Phone:** (520) 626-6119; **Board Cert:** Internal Medicine 1975, Gastroenterology 1977; **Med School:** Med Coll VA 1970; **Resid:** Internal Medicine, Med Univ SC, Charleston, SC 1973-1975; **Fellow:** Gastroenterology, Med Univ SC, Charleston, SC 1975-1977; **Fac Appt:** Prof Medicine, Univ SC Sch Med

Feldman, Mark MD (Ge) - *Spec Exp:* *Peptic Acid Disorders;* **Hospital:** Presby Hosp - Dallas; **Address:** 8200 Walnut Hill Ln, Dept Internal Med, Dallas, TX 75231; **Phone:** (214) 345-7883; **Board Cert:** Internal Medicine 1976, Gastroenterology 1989; **Med School:** Temple Univ 1972; **Resid:** Internal Medicine, Temple Univ, Philadelphia, PA 1972-1977; **Fellow:** Gastroenterology, Univ SW Texas, Dallas, TX 1975-1976; **Fac Appt:** Prof Medicine, Univ Tex SW, Dallas

Fordtran, John MD (Ge) - *Spec Exp:* *Malabsorption; Diarrhea; Microscopic Colitis;* **Hospital:** Baylor Univ Medical Ctr; **Address:** Baylor Univ Med Ctr, Dept Med, 3500 Gaston Ave, Dallas, TX 75246; **Phone:** (214) 820-2672; **Med School:** Tulane Univ 1956; **Resid:** Internal Medicine, Parkland Hosp, Dallas, TX 1956-1958; **Fellow:** Gastroenterology, Mass Meml Hosp, Boston, MA 1960-1962

Galati, Joseph Steven MD (Ge) - *Spec Exp:* *Liver Disease; Transplant Medicine-Liver; Hepatitis C;* **Hospital:** St Luke's Episcopal Hosp - Houston; **Address:** 6624 Fannin, Ste 1990, Houston, TX 77030; **Phone:** (713) 794-0700; **Board Cert:** Internal Medicine 1990, Gastroenterology 1995; **Med School:** Grenada 1987; **Resid:** Internal Medicine, SUNY Hlth Sci Ctr-Kings Co Hosp, Brooklyn, NY 1988-1991; **Fellow:** Gastroenterology, Univ Nebraska, Omaha, NE 1991-1994; **Fac Appt:** Asst Prof Medicine, Univ Tex, Houston

Glombicki, Alan Paul MD (Ge) - *Spec Exp:* *Hepatitis-Antiviral Therapy; Transplant Medicine-Liver;* **Hospital:** St Luke's Episcopal Hosp - Houston; **Address:** 7737 SW Freeway, Ste 840, Houston, TX 77074; **Phone:** (713) 777-2555; **Board Cert:** Internal Medicine 1986, Gastroenterology 1987; **Med School:** Univ IL Coll Med 1981; **Resid:** Internal Medicine, Baylor Coll Med, Houston, TX 1982-1984; Hepatology, Baylor Coll Med, Houston, TX 1986-1987; **Fellow:** Gastroenterology, Baylor Coll Med, Houston, TX 1984-1986; **Fac Appt:** Asst Clin Prof Medicine, Univ Tex, Houston

Hodges, David S MD (Ge) - *Spec Exp:* *Inflammatory Bowel Disease/Crohn's;* **Hospital:** Univ Med Ctr - Lubbock; **Address:** Med Office Plaza, 3502 9th St, Ste 280, Lubbock, TX 79415; **Phone:** (806) 743-3085; **Board Cert:** Internal Medicine 1986, Gastroenterology 1989; **Med School:** Texas Tech Univ 1983; **Resid:** Internal Medicine, Lubbock Genl Hosp, Lubbock, TX 1983-1986; **Fellow:** Gastroenterology, Lubbock Genl Hosp, Lubbock, TX 1987-1989; **Fac Appt:** Assoc Prof Medicine, Texas Tech Univ

Levin, Bernard MD (Ge) - *Spec Exp:* *Gastrointestinal Cancer; Colon & Rectal Cancer;* **Hospital:** Univ of TX MD Anderson Cancer Ctr, The; **Address:** UT MD Anderson Cancer Ctr, 1515 Holcombe Blvd, Box 203, Houston, TX 77030-4095; **Phone:** (713) 792-3900; **Board Cert:** Internal Medicine 1972, Gastroenterology 1972; **Med School:** South Africa 1964; **Resid:** Internal Medicine, Rush Presby-St Lukes Hosp, Chicago, IL 1966-1968; **Fellow:** Pathology, Univ Chicago, Chicago, IL 1968-1970; Gastroenterology, Univ Chicago, Chicago, IL 1970-1972; **Fac Appt:** Prof Emeritus Medicine, Univ Tex, Houston

GASTROENTEROLOGY *Southwest*

Maddrey, Willis Crocker MD (Ge) - *Spec Exp:* Hepatitis C & B; Liver Disease-Drug Induced; Liver Disease-Alcohol Related; **Hospital:** Zale Lipshy Univ Hosp; **Address:** Univ Tex SW Med Ctr, 5323 Harry Hines Blvd, Dallas, TX 75390-8570; **Phone:** (214) 648-2024; **Board Cert:** Internal Medicine 1971; **Med School:** Johns Hopkins Univ 1964; **Resid:** Internal Medicine, Johns Hopkins Hosp, Baltimore, MD 1968-1970; Internal Medicine, Johns Hopkins Hosp, Baltimore, MD 1965-1966; **Fellow:** Hepatology, Yale, New Haven, CT 1970-1971; **Fac Appt:** Prof Medicine, Univ Tex SW, Dallas

Speeg, Kermit Vincent MD/PhD (Ge) - *Spec Exp:* Transplant Medicine-Liver; **Hospital:** Univ of Texas Hlth & Sci Ctr; **Address:** Univ Texas HSC, San Antonio, Med/GI, 7703 Floyd Curl, MC 7878, San Antonio, TX 78229-3900; **Phone:** (210) 567-4882; **Board Cert:** Internal Medicine 1976; **Med School:** Univ Tex SW, Dallas 1972; **Resid:** Internal Medicine, Vanderbilt Univ Hosp, Nashville, TN 1973-1974; **Fellow:** Gastroenterology, Vanderbilt Univ Hosp, Nashville, TN 1976-1977; **Fac Appt:** Prof Medicine, Univ Tex, San Antonio

West Coast and Pacific

Cello, John Patrick MD (Ge) - *Spec Exp:* Therapeutic Endoscopy; **Hospital:** UCSF Med Ctr; **Address:** San Francisco Genl Hosp, Div GI, 1001 Potrero Ave, San Francisco, CA 94110; **Phone:** (415) 206-4767; **Board Cert:** Internal Medicine 1972, Gastroenterology 1977; **Med School:** Harvard Med Sch 1969; **Resid:** Internal Medicine, Peter Bent Brigham Hosp, Boston, MA 1970-1972; **Fellow:** Gastroenterology, UCSF, San Francisco, CA 1975-1977; **Fac Appt:** Prof Medicine, UCSF

Ellis, Jonathan C MD (Ge) - *Spec Exp:* Colonoscopy; **Hospital:** Cedars-Sinai Med Ctr; **Address:** 8631 W Third St, Ste 540-E, Los Angeles, CA 90048-5901; **Phone:** (310) 659-9600; **Board Cert:** Internal Medicine 1985, Gastroenterology 1989; **Med School:** Stanford Univ 1982; **Resid:** Internal Medicine, Cedars Sinai Med Ctr, Los Angeles, CA 1983-1985; Internal Medicine, Cedars Sinai Med Ctr, Los Angeles, CA 1985-1986; **Fellow:** Gastroenterology, UCLA, Torrance, CA 1986-1988; **Fac Appt:** Assoc Prof Medicine, UCLA

Keeffe, Emmet B MD (Ge) - *Spec Exp:* Hepatitis-Antiviral Therapy; Liver Disease; **Hospital:** Stanford Med Ctr; **Address:** 750 Welch Rd, Ste 210, Palo Alto, CA 94304; **Phone:** (650) 498-5691; **Board Cert:** Gastroenterology 1975, Internal Medicine 1972; **Med School:** Creighton Univ 1969; **Resid:** Internal Medicine, Oreg Hlth Sci Univ, Portland, OR 1970-1973; Gastroenterology, Oreg Hlth Sci Univ, Portland, OR 1973-1974; **Fellow:** Gastroenterology, UCSF, Sanfrancisco, CA 1977-1979; **Fac Appt:** Prof Medicine, Stanford Univ

Kimmey, Michael Bryant MD (Ge) - *Spec Exp:* Pancreatic/Biliary Endoscopy (ERCP); Endoscopy; Endoscopic Ultrasound (EUS); **Hospital:** Univ WA Med Ctr; **Address:** Univ Washington, Div Gastroenterology, Box 356424, Seattle, WA 98195-0001; **Phone:** (206) 543-4404; **Board Cert:** Internal Medicine 1982, Gastroenterology 1987; **Med School:** Washington Univ, St Louis 1979; **Resid:** Internal Medicine, Univ Wash Med Ctr, Seattle, WA 1980-1982; **Fellow:** Gastroenterology, Univ Wash, Seattle, WA 1984-1987; **Fac Appt:** Prof Medicine, Univ Wash

Kozarek, Richard MD (Ge) - *Spec Exp:* Endoscopy; Inflammatory Bowel Disorders; **Hospital:** Virginia Mason Med Ctr; **Address:** 1100 9th Ave, Seattle, WA 98101-2756; **Phone:** (206) 223-6939; **Board Cert:** Internal Medicine 1977, Gastroenterology 1979; **Med School:** Univ Wisc 1973; **Resid:** Internal Medicine, Good Samaritan Hosp, Phoenix, AZ 1974-1976; **Fellow:** Gastroenterology, Univ Arizona/ VA Hosp, Phoenix, AZ 1976-1978; **Fac Appt:** Clin Prof Medicine, Univ Wash

Martin, Paul MD (Ge) - *Spec Exp: Liver Disease; Hepatitis; Transplant Medicine-Liver;* **Hospital:** Cedars-Sinai Med Ctr; **Address:** 8635 W Third St, Ste 590 West, Los Angeles, CA 90048-6110; **Phone:** (310) 423-2641; **Board Cert:** Internal Medicine 1984, Gastroenterology 1987; **Med School:** Ireland 1978; **Resid:** Internal Medicine, St Vincent's Hosp, Dublin, Ireland 1979-1982; Internal Medicine, Univ Alberta, Edmonton Alberta, Canada 1982-1984; **Fellow:** Gastroenterology, Queen Univ, Ontario, Canada 1984-1986; Hepatology, Natl Inst Hlth, Bethesda, MD 1987-1989; **Fac Appt:** Prof Medicine, UCLA

Ostroff, James Warren MD (Ge) - *Spec Exp: Pancreatic/Biliary Endoscopy(ERCP); Colonoscopy;* **Hospital:** UCSF Med Ctr; **Address:** 350 Parnassus Ave, Ste 410, San Francisco, CA 94117-3608; **Phone:** (415) 502-2112; **Board Cert:** Internal Medicine 1980, Gastroenterology 1983; **Med School:** Cornell Univ-Weill Med Coll 1977; **Resid:** Internal Medicine, New York Hosp-Cornell Med Ctr, New York, NY 1978-1980; **Fellow:** Gastroenterology, UCSF Hosps, San Francisco, CA 1980-1982; **Fac Appt:** Clin Prof Medicine, UCSF

Pimstone, Neville R MD (Ge) - *Spec Exp: Porphyria; Hepatitis C;* **Hospital:** Univ CA - Davis Med Ctr; **Address:** 4150 V St, Ste 3500, Sacramento, CA 95817; **Phone:** (916) 734-3751; **Med School:** South Africa 1960; **Resid:** Gastroenterology, Moffit Hosp- Univ Ca, San Francisco, CA; **Fac Appt:** Prof Medicine, UC Davis

Surawicz, Christina MD (Ge) - *Spec Exp: Clostridium Difficile Disease; Infectious Diarrhea;* **Hospital:** Univ WA Med Ctr; **Address:** 325 9th Ave, Box 359773, Seattle, WA 98104; **Phone:** (206) 341-4634; **Board Cert:** Internal Medicine 1976, Gastroenterology 1979; **Med School:** Univ KY Coll Med 1973; **Resid:** Internal Medicine, U Washington Med Ctr, Seattle, WA 1973-1976; **Fellow:** Gastroenterology, U Washington Med Ctr, Seattle, WA 1976-1979; **Fac Appt:** Prof Medicine, Univ Wash

Targan, Stephan Raoul MD (Ge) - *Spec Exp: Inflammatory Bowel Disease/Crohn's;* **Hospital:** Cedars-Sinai Med Ctr; **Address:** Cedars-Sinai IBD Center, 8631 W Third St, Ste 430E, Los Angeles, CA 90048; **Phone:** (310) 423-4100; **Board Cert:** Infectious Disease 1976, Gastroenterology 1979; **Med School:** Johns Hopkins Univ 1971; **Resid:** Internal Medicine, Harbor-UCLA Med Ctr, Torrance, CA 1971-1976; **Fellow:** Infectious Disease, Harbor-UCLA Med Ctr, Torrance, CA 1975-1976; Gastroenterology, UCLA Med Ctr, Los Angeles, CA 1976-1978; **Fac Appt:** Prof Gastroenterology, UCLA

Vierling, John Moore MD (Ge) - *Spec Exp: Liver Disease; Transplant Medicine-Liver;* **Hospital:** Cedars-Sinai Med Ctr; **Address:** 8635 W 3rd St #590W, Los Angeles, CA 90048-6101; **Phone:** (310) 423-6140; **Board Cert:** Internal Medicine 1975, Gastroenterology 1979; **Med School:** Stanford Univ 1972; **Resid:** Internal Medicine, Strong Meml Hosp, Rochester, NY 1973-1974; Hepatology, NIH-Liver Unit, Bethesda, MD 1974-1977; **Fellow:** Gastroenterology, UCSF Med Ctr, San Francisco, CA 1977-1978; **Fac Appt:** Prof Medicine, UCLA

GERIATRIC MEDICINE

(a subspecialty of INTERNAL MEDICINE or FAMILY PRACTICE)

An internist with special knowledge of the aging process and special skills in the diagnostic, therapeutic, preventive and rehabilitative aspects of illness in the elderly. This specialist cares for geriatric patients in the patient's home, the office, long-term care settings such as nursing homes and the hospital.

INTERNAL MEDICINE

An internist is a personal physician who provides long-term, comprehensive care in the office and the hospital, managing both common and complex illness of adolescents, adults and the elderly. Internists are trained in the diagnosis and treatment of cancer, infections and diseases affecting the heart, blood, kidneys, joints and digestive, respiratory and vascular systems. They are also trained in the essentials of primary care internal medicine which incorporates an understanding of disease prevention, wellness, substance abuse, mental health and effective treatment of common problems of the eyes, ears, skin, nervous system and reproductive organs.

FAMILY PRACTICE

A family physician is concerned with the total healthcare of the individual and the family, and is trained to diagnose and treat a wide variety of ailments in patients of all ages. The family physician receives a broad range of training that includes internal medicine, pediatrics, obstetrics and gynecology, psychiatry and geriatrics. Special emphasis is placed on prevention and the primary care of entire families, utilizing consultations and community resources when appropriate.

Training required: Three years in internal medicine or family pratice *plus* additional training and examination for certification in geriatric medicine.

THE MOUNT SINAI HOSPITAL
GERIATRICS AND ADULT DEVELOPMENT

One Gustave L. Levy Place (Fifth Avenue and 98th Street)
New York, NY 10029-6574   Phone: (212) 241-5561
Physician Referral: 1-800-MD-SINAI (637-4624)
www.mountsinai.org

The Mount Sinai Hospital is a pioneer in geriatric medicine. In 1909, a Mount Sinai physician coined the term "geriatrics," and in 1914, he wrote the first textbook on medical care for older adults.

Today, the Department continues to break new ground, offering comprehensive care, disease prevention, and the promotion of healthy and productive aging. The Department's enhanced expertise in assessing and managing patients with dementia greatly complements its established, interdisciplinary approach to patient care, in which the medical staff social workers and behavioral therapists address patients' needs as a team.

The Best in Clinical Care
We offer a full spectrum of patient care – including a specialized care unit for the elderly (to minimize complications sometimes associated with an older person's hospital stay); a primary care geriatrics practice for older adults living in the community; a hospital-based consultation service for patients throughout Mount Sinai; a number of community-linked programs and partnerships; and a Palliative Care team dedicated to assuring quality care and support for patients and families facing serious illness.

Groundbreaking Research
In addition, Mount Sinai's researchers continue to advance the understanding, prevention and treatment of age-related disorders.

The extensive research on aging conducted by the Department includes studies on health services research, medical decision-making and ethical dilemmas, palliative care, neurobiology of aging, and clinical interventions to promote independence in old age. And the Department's expertise is meant to be shared. It serves as a renowned educational resource for the Mount Sinai Health System and other institutions in teaching geriatrics and gerontology to medical students, medical residents, geriatrics fellows, established physicians and health professional trainees in other disciplines.

THE MOUNT SINAI MEDICAL CENTER

In recognition of the care offered to older patients, Mount Sinai specialists are cited time and time again as the finest in the nation. *U.S. News & World Reports* has consistently ranked The Mount Sinai Hospital as *number one in* New York for geriatric care.

We were the first freestanding department of geriatrics established by a U.S. medical school, and it continues to be one of the very best.

The **Brookdale Department of Geriatric and Adult Development** offers unparalleled inpatient and outpatient care and numerous treatment programs designed to meet the unique needs of older adults. And the hospital is home to world-class researchers dedicated to advancing our understanding of Alzheimer's disease and other common geriatric problems.

At the Department's heart are the patients, and the geriatricians of The Mount Sinai Hospital work hard to improve life and longevity for New York's elderly.

NYU Medical Center

550 First Avenue (at 31st Street)
New York, NY 10016
Physician Referral: (888) 7-NYU-MED
(888-769-8633)   www.nyumedicalcenter.org

NEW YORK UNIVERSITY

CARING FOR THE ELDERLY

Geriatrics, like Pediatrics, is by its nature a multi-disciplinary endeavor. All geriatricians are experts in spotting and treating the unique ways that common medical problems manifest themselves in the elderly. But the elderly also have problems and issues that other groups do not face, such as loss of bone density, changes in skin health and appearance, memory disorders, incontinence, partial or complete loss of vision, and many others. Our geriatricians are also expert in these.

Some of these disorders are still incurable and the guidelines for treating patients with them are unclear. When that is the case, as it is with Alzheimer's disease, NYU Medical Center geriatricians have first-hand access to the basic laboratories where studies of the disease and its manifestations have been carried out since 1973. In fact, **The William and Sylvia Silberstein Aging and Dementia Research Center** at NYU Medical Center is one of the oldest and largest centers of its kind in the nation. It is a National-Institute-on-Aging-designated Center of Excellence devoted to the diagnosis and treatment of Alzheimer's disease.

Bone health is another serious issue for the elderly. Weak bones pose a threat to mobility, and with it, independent life. That's why the **Geriatric Falls Prevention Program at the Hospital for Joint Diseases** is dedicated to the prevention, diagnosis, and treatment of falls in the elderly. The primary goal is to help older adults maintain a safe and independent lifestyle. Any older adults who have trouble with falls, loss of balance or fear of falling may benefit from this program.

A geriatrician and geriatric nurse practitioner evaluate each client. An in-depth history and physical exam are done to help determine the cause of the problem. Recommendations may include referrals to specialists such as a neurologist, othopaedist, physical or occupational therapist, or for tests or blood work. Other recommendations may include the use of a can or walker, more appropriate footwear or home safety improvements.

NYU MEDICAL CENTER

The William and Sylvia Silberstein Aging and Dementia Research Center provides:

- comprehensive diagnostic evaluations to determine if memory loss is "normal" or more serious

- a memory enhancement program for age-related memory decline

- pharmaceutical clinical trials for mild memory loss and for Alzheimer's treatment

- state-of-the-art brain imaging techniques

- methods to prevent excess disability in Alzheimer's disease patients

- and comprehensive, on-going counseling and support groups for patients, caregivers and family members.

Its longitudinal study of Alzheimer's patients is the most comprehensive ongoing study of its kind in the world.

PHYSICIAN LISTINGS

Geriatric Medicine

New England

Cooney, Leo MD (Ger) - *Spec Exp:* Geriatric Medicine - General; **Hospital:** Yale - New Haven Hosp; **Address:** 20 York St, Ste TMP17, New Haven, CT 06504-8900; **Phone:** (203) 785-2204; **Board Cert:** Internal Medicine 1974, Rheumatology 1978, Geriatric Medicine 2000; **Med School:** Yale Univ 1969; **Resid:** Internal Medicine, Boston City Hosp, Boston, MA 1970-1971; Internal Medicine, Boston City Hosp, Boston, MA 1973-1974; **Fellow:** Rheumatology, Boston Med Ctr, Boston, MA 1974-1975; **Fac Appt:** Prof Medicine, Yale Univ

Lipsitz, Lewis Arnold MD (Ger) - *Spec Exp:* Falls; Fainting; **Hospital:** Hebrew Rehab Ctr for the Aged; **Address:** 1200 Center St, Roslindale, MA 02131; **Phone:** (617) 363-8293; **Board Cert:** Internal Medicine 1980, Geriatric Medicine 2009; **Med School:** Univ Penn 1977; **Resid:** Internal Medicine, Beth Israel Hosp, Boston, MA 1978-1980; **Fellow:** Geriatric Medicine, Harvard, New Haven, CT 1980-1983; **Fac Appt:** Prof Medicine, Harvard Med Sch

Minaker, Kenneth MD (Ger) - *Spec Exp:* Aging; Neuroendocrine Disease; Cardiovascular Disease; **Hospital:** MA Genl Hosp; **Address:** Beacon Hill Senior Health, 100 Charles River Plaza, Boston, MA 02114; **Phone:** (617) 726-4600; **Board Cert:** Internal Medicine 1979, Geriatric Medicine 1985; **Med School:** Univ Toronto 1972; **Resid:** Internal Medicine, Univ Toronto, Canada 1979; **Fellow:** Geriatric Medicine, Mass Gen Hosp-Harvard, Boston, MA 1982

Tinetti, Mary MD (Ger) - *Spec Exp:* Fall Injuries; **Hospital:** Yale - New Haven Hosp; **Address:** 789 Howard St, Tompkins Basement, New Haven, CT 06519; **Phone:** (203) 688-6361; **Board Cert:** Geriatric Medicine 1988, Internal Medicine 1981; **Med School:** Univ Mich Med Sch 1978; **Resid:** Internal Medicine, Univ Minnesota, Minneapolis, MN 1978-1981; **Fellow:** Geriatric Medicine, Univ Rochester, Rochester, NY 1981-1984; **Fac Appt:** Prof Medicine, Yale Univ

Mid Atlantic

Bennett, Richard G MD (Ger) - *Spec Exp:* Geriatric Medicine - General; **Hospital:** Johns Hopkins Hosp - Baltimore; **Address:** 5505 Hopkins Bayview Rd, Baltimore, MD 21224; **Phone:** (410) 550-0781; **Board Cert:** Internal Medicine 1985, Geriatric Medicine 1998; **Med School:** Johns Hopkins Univ 1982; **Resid:** Internal Medicine, Johns Hopkins Hosp, Baltimore, MD 1983-1985; **Fellow:** Geriatric Medicine, Johns Hopkins Hosp, Baltimore, MD 1985-1987; **Fac Appt:** Assoc Prof Medicine, Johns Hopkins Univ

Blass, John MD/PhD (Ger) - *Spec Exp:* Alzheimer's Disease; Dementia; **Hospital:** Burke Rehab Hosp; **Address:** 785 Mamaroneck Ave, White Plains, NY 10605-2523; **Phone:** (914) 597-2359; **Med School:** Colombia 1965; **Resid:** Internal Medicine, Mass Genl Hosp, Boston, MA 1965-1967; Nat Heart Inst-NIH, Bethesda, MD 1967-1970; **Fac Appt:** Prof Neurology, Cornell Univ-Weill Med Coll

Bloom, Patricia MD (Ger) - *Spec Exp:* Dementia; **Hospital:** Mount Sinai Hosp (page 68); **Address:** 1470 Madison Ave, New York, NY 10029; **Phone:** (212) 824-7646; **Board Cert:** Internal Medicine 1978, Geriatric Medicine 1998; **Med School:** Univ Minn 1975; **Resid:** Internal Medicine, Montefiore Hosp, Bronx, NY 1975-1978; **Fac Appt:** Assoc Clin Prof Medicine, Mount Sinai Sch Med

Burton, John Russell MD (Ger) - *Spec Exp:* Geriatric Medicine - General; **Hospital:** Johns Hopkins Hosp - Baltimore; **Address:** 5505 Hopkins Bayview Cir, Baltimore, MD 21224-6821; **Phone:** (410) 550-0520; **Board Cert:** Internal Medicine 1980, Geriatric Medicine 1990; **Med School:** McGill Univ 1965; **Resid:** Internal Medicine, Baltimore City Hosp, Baltimore, MD 1969-1970; Internal Medicine, Baltimore City Hosp, Baltimore, MD 1970-1971; **Fellow:** Nephrology, Mass Genl Hosp, Boston, MA 1971-1972; **Fac Appt:** Prof Medicine, Johns Hopkins Univ

Freedman, Michael L MD (Ger) - *Spec Exp:* Alzheimer's Disease; Anemia; Nutrition; **Hospital:** NYU Med Ctr (page 71); **Address:** 530 First Ave, Ste 4J, New York, NY 10016-6402; **Phone:** (212) 263-7043; **Board Cert:** Internal Medicine 1971, Hematology 1974, Geriatric Medicine 1998; **Med School:** Tufts Univ 1963; **Resid:** Internal Medicine, Bellevue Hosp, New York, NY 1964-1965; Internal Medicine, Bellevue Hosp, New York, NY 1968-1969; **Fellow:** Hematology, Natl Inst Hlth-NCI, Bethesda, MD 1965-1968; **Fac Appt:** Prof Medicine, NYU Sch Med

Gambert, Steven MD (Ger) - *Spec Exp:* Endocrinology; Osteoporosis; Aging; **Hospital:** Sinai Hosp - Baltimore; **Address:** Sinai Hosp Baltimore, Hoffberger Bldg, 2401 W Belvedere Ave, Ste 56, Baltimore, MD 21215; **Phone:** (410) 601-6340; **Board Cert:** Internal Medicine 1978, Geriatric Medicine 1988; **Med School:** Columbia P&S 1975; **Resid:** Internal Medicine, Dartmouth Affl Hosp, Lebanon, NH 1975-1977; **Fellow:** Geriatric Medicine, Beth Israel Med Ctr, Boston, MA 1977-1979; **Fac Appt:** Prof Medicine, Johns Hopkins Univ

Libow, Leslie MD (Ger) - *Spec Exp:* Diagnostic Problems; **Hospital:** Mount Sinai Hosp (page 68); **Address:** 1 Gustave Levy Pl, Box 1070, New York, NY 10029; **Phone:** (212) 824-7646; **Board Cert:** Internal Medicine 1977, Geriatric Medicine 1988; **Med School:** Univ Hlth Sci/Chicago Med Sch 1958; **Resid:** Internal Medicine, Bronx VA Hosp, Bronx, NY 1959-1960; Internal Medicine, Mt Sinai Hosp, New York, NY 1963-1964; **Fac Appt:** Prof Geriatric Medicine, Mount Sinai Sch Med

Meier, Diane MD (Ger) - *Spec Exp:* Palliative Care; **Hospital:** Mount Sinai Hosp (page 68); **Address:** 101 Street at Madison Ave, Mount Sinai School of Medicine, New York, NY 10029-6501; **Phone:** (212) 824-7646; **Board Cert:** Internal Medicine 1981, Geriatric Medicine 1999; **Med School:** Northwestern Univ 1977; **Resid:** Internal Medicine, Oregon Hlth Sci Univ, Portland, OR 1981; **Fellow:** Geriatric Medicine, VA Med Ctr, Portland, OR 1983; **Fac Appt:** Prof Geriatric Medicine, Mount Sinai Sch Med

Paris, Barbara MD (Ger) - *Spec Exp:* Geriatric Medicine - General; **Hospital:** Mount Sinai Hosp (page 68); **Address:** One Gustave Levy Pl, Box 1070, New York, NY 10029; **Phone:** (212) 241-1305; **Board Cert:** Geriatric Medicine 1998, Internal Medicine 1982; **Med School:** SUNY Downstate 1977; **Resid:** Internal Medicine, St Vincents Hosp, New York, NY 1978-1981; **Fellow:** Geriatric Medicine, Mount Sinai Hosp, New York, NY 1983-1986; **Fac Appt:** Assoc Clin Prof Geriatric Medicine, Mount Sinai Sch Med

Resnick, Neil M. MD (Ger) - *Spec Exp:* Voiding Dysfunction; **Hospital:** UPMC - Presbyterian Univ Hosp; **Address:** Univ Pittsburgh, Div Geriatrics, 3520 Fifth Ave, Ste 300, Pittsburgh, PA 15213; **Phone:** (412) 383-1204; **Board Cert:** Internal Medicine 1980, Geriatric Medicine 1998; **Med School:** Stanford Univ 1977; **Resid:** Internal Medicine, Beth Israel Hosp, Boston, MA 1978-1980; **Fellow:** Geriatric Medicine, Harvard Univ, Boston, MA 1980-1982; Urology, Harvard Univ, Boston, MA 1982-1984; **Fac Appt:** Prof Medicine, Univ Pittsburgh

Southeast

Applegate, William MD (Ger) - *Spec Exp:* Hypertension; **Hospital:** Wake Forest Univ Baptist Med Ctr (page 81); **Address:** Wake Forest Univ Baptist Med Ctr, Internal Medicine, Medical Center Blvd, Winston-Salem, NC 27157; **Phone:** (336) 716-2020; **Board Cert:** Geriatric Medicine 1988, Internal Medicine 1976; **Med School:** Univ Louisville Sch Med 1972; **Resid:** Internal Medicine, Boston City, Boston, MA 1973-1975; Internal Medicine, NC Meml Hosp, Chapel Hill, NC 1975-1977; **Fac Appt:** Prof Medicine, Wake Forest Univ Sch Med

Ciocon, Jerry MD (Ger) - *Spec Exp:* Chronic Fatigue-Elderly; Pain-Musculoskeletal; Memory Disorders; **Hospital:** Cleveland Clin FL; **Address:** Cleveland Clinic Florida, 2950 Cleveland Clinic Blvd, Fort Lauderdale, FL 33331; **Phone:** (954) 659-5353; **Board Cert:** Internal Medicine 1985, Geriatric Medicine 1990; **Med School:** Philippines 1980; **Resid:** Internal Medicine, Mercy Hosp, Buffalo, NY 1983-1985; **Fellow:** Geriatric Medicine, LI Jewish Med Ctr, New Hyde Park, NY 1985-1987; **Fac Appt:** Asst Clin Prof Medicine, Ohio State Univ

Greganti, Mac Andrew MD (Ger) - *Spec Exp:* Geriatric Medicine; Diagnostic Problems; **Hospital:** Univ of NC Hosp (page 77); **Address:** Univ North Carolina Hosp, 5039 Old Clinic Bldg, Box 7005, Chapel Hill, NC 27599-7005; **Phone:** (919) 966-3063; **Board Cert:** Internal Medicine 1987, Geriatric Medicine 1988; **Med School:** Univ Miss 1972; **Resid:** Internal Medicine, Strong Meml Hosp, Rochester, NY 1972-1975; **Fac Appt:** Prof Medicine, Univ NC Sch Med

Groene, Linda A MD (Ger) - *Spec Exp:* Vitamin B-12 Metabolism; Sleep Disorders/Apnea; **Hospital:** Cleveland Clin FL; **Address:** 6405 N Federal Hwy, Ste 102, Ft Lauderdale, FL 33308; **Phone:** (954) 772-0062; **Board Cert:** Internal Medicine 1986, Geriatric Medicine 1990; **Med School:** Louisiana State Univ 1981; **Resid:** Pathology, Jackson Meml Hosp- Univ Miami, Miami, FL 1982-1983; Internal Medicine, Mt Sinai Med Ctr, Miami Beach, FL 1984-1986

Hanson, Laura Catherine MD (Ger) - *Spec Exp:* Frail Elderly; Palliative Care; **Hospital:** Univ of NC Hosp (page 77); **Address:** Univ North Carolina, 5039 Old Clinic Building, Box 7110, Chapel Hill, NC 27599-7110; **Phone:** (919) 966-2276; **Board Cert:** Internal Medicine 1989, Geriatric Medicine 1992; **Med School:** Harvard Med Sch 1986; **Resid:** Internal Medicine, Brigham & Women's Hosp, Boston, MA 1986-1988; Internal Medicine, UNC Hosp, Chapel Hill, NC 1988-1989; **Fellow:** Geriatric Medicine, UNC Hosp, Chapel Hill, NC 1989-1991; **Fac Appt:** Assoc Prof Medicine, Univ NC Sch Med

Lyles, Kenneth W MD (Ger) - *Spec Exp:* Bone Disorders-Metabolic; Tumoral Calcinosis; Parathyroid Disease; **Hospital:** Duke Univ Med Ctr (page 60); **Address:** Duke Univ Med Center, Box 3881, Durham, NC 27710; **Phone:** (919) 668-7630; **Board Cert:** Endocrinology, Diabetes & Metabolism 1979, Internal Medicine 1977; **Med School:** Med Coll VA 1974; **Resid:** Internal Medicine, Med Coll VA, Richmond, VA 1975-1977; **Fellow:** Endocrinology, Diabetes & Metabolism, Duke Univ Med Ctr, Durham, NC 1977-1979; Geriatric Medicine, VA Med Ctr, Durham, NC 1979-1981; **Fac Appt:** Prof Medicine, Duke Univ

Ouslander, Joseph MD (Ger) - *Spec Exp:* Incontinence; **Hospital:** Emory Univ Hosp; **Address:** 1841 Clifton Rd NE, Atlanta, GA 30329; **Phone:** (404) 728-6363; **Board Cert:** Geriatric Medicine 1998, Internal Medicine 1980; **Med School:** Case West Res Univ 1977; **Resid:** Internal Medicine, Univ Hosp, Cleveland, OH 1978-1979; Internal Medicine, Sepulveda Med Ctr, Sepulveda, CA 1979-1980; **Fellow:** Geriatric Medicine, UCLA Med Ctr, Los Angeles, CA 1980-1982

Snustad, Diane Gail MD (Ger) - *Spec Exp:* Osteoporosis; Dementia; **Hospital:** Univ of VA Hlth Sys (page 79); **Address:** Colonnades Medical Associates, 2610 Barracks Rd, Charlottesville, VA 22901; **Phone:** (434) 924-1212; **Board Cert:** Internal Medicine 1982, Geriatric Medicine 1998; **Med School:** Univ Minn 1979; **Resid:** Internal Medicine, West VA Univ, Morgantown, WV 1980-1982; **Fac Appt:** Assoc Prof Geriatric Medicine, Univ VA Sch Med

Tenover, Joyce Sander MD/PhD (Ger) - *Spec Exp:* Hormonal Disorders; **Hospital:** Wesley Woods Ger Hosp; **Address:** 1841 Clifton Rd NE, Atlanta, GA 30329; **Phone:** (404) 728-6331; **Board Cert:** Geriatric Medicine 1997, Internal Medicine 1983; **Med School:** Geo Wash Univ 1980; **Resid:** Internal Medicine, Univ Wash Alffil Hosp, Seattle, WA 1981-1983; Internal Medicine, VA Med Ctr, Seattle, WA 1983-1984; **Fellow:** Geriatric Medicine, VA Med Ctr, Seattle, WA 1984-1987; **Fac Appt:** Assoc Prof Medicine, Emory Univ

Weinberg, Andrew David MD (Ger) - *Spec Exp:* Elderly Long Term Care; **Hospital:** Wesley Woods Ger Hosp; **Address:** Wesley Woods Ctr for Geriatrics, 1841 Clifton Rd NE, Atlanta, GA 30329; **Phone:** (404) 728-6901; **Board Cert:** Geriatric Medicine 1992, Internal Medicine 1981; **Med School:** SUNY Syracuse 1978; **Resid:** Internal Medicine, Mayo Clin, Rochester, MN 1979-1981; **Fellow:** Endocrinology, Diabetes & Metabolism, Yale Sch Med, New Haven, CT 1981-1982; **Fac Appt:** Prof Medicine, Emory Univ

Midwest

Barnhart, William MD (Ger) - *Spec Exp:* Preventive Medicine; Geriatric Medicine; **Hospital:** Louis A Weiss Mem Hosp; **Address:** Medical Education, 4646 N Marine St N, Fl 7th, Chicago, IL 60640; **Phone:** (773) 564-5446; **Board Cert:** Geriatric Medicine 1994, Internal Medicine 1974; **Med School:** Northwestern Univ 1971; **Resid:** Internal Medicine, Wesley Hospital, Chicago, IL 1971-1972; Internal Medicine, Emory University, Atlanta, GA 1972-1974; **Fac Appt:** Assoc Clin Prof Geriatric Medicine, Univ Chicago-Pritzker Sch Med

Bentley, David Warren MD (Ger) - *Spec Exp:* Infectious Disease in Elderly; Infectious Disease-Hospital Acquired; **Hospital:** St Louis Univ Hospital; **Address:** St Louis Univ Hlth Sci Ctr, Div Geriatric Med, 1402 S Grand Blvd, rm M238, St Louis, MO 63104; **Phone:** (314) 894-6510; **Board Cert:** Internal Medicine 1969, Geriatric Medicine 1998; **Med School:** Univ Rochester 1963; **Resid:** Internal Medicine, Vanderbilt Univ Hosp, Nashville, TN 1964-1966; **Fellow:** Infectious Disease, Univ IL, Chicago, IL 1966-1968; **Fac Appt:** Prof Medicine, St Louis Univ

Carr, David Brian MD (Ger) - *Spec Exp:* Geriatric Medicine - General; **Hospital:** Barnes-Jewish Hosp (page 55); **Address:** Div Geriatric Medicine, 4488 Forest Park Ave, St Louis, MO 63108; **Phone:** (314) 286-2700; **Board Cert:** Geriatric Medicine 2000, Internal Medicine 1989; **Med School:** Univ MO-Columbia Sch Med 1985; **Resid:** Internal Medicine, Mich State Assoc Hosp, Lansing, MI 1986-1988; **Fellow:** Geriatric Medicine, Duke Univ, Durham, NC 1988-1990; **Fac Appt:** Prof Geriatric Medicine, Washington Univ, St Louis

Couch, Nancy MD (Ger) - *Spec Exp:* Geriatric Medicine - General; **Hospital:** Henry Ford Hosp; **Address:** 2799 W Grand Blvd, Ste K15, Detroit, MI 48202; **Phone:** (313) 916-1313; **Board Cert:** Internal Medicine 1986, Geriatric Medicine 1998; **Med School:** Wayne State Univ 1982; **Resid:** Internal Medicine, Wayne State Univ Affil Hosps, Detroit, MI 1982-1984; Internal Medicine, Henry Ford Hosp, Detroit, MI 1984-1985; **Fellow:** Geriatric Medicine, Univ of Mich/VA Medical Ctr, Ann Arbor, MI 1985-1987

Dale, Lowell C MD (Ger) - *Spec Exp:* Tobacco Abuse; Nutrition; Long Term Care; **Hospital:** Mayo Med Ctr & Clin - Rochester, MN; **Address:** Div of Cmnty Internal Med, 200 1st St SW, Rochester, MN 55902; **Phone:** (507) 266-5032; **Board Cert:** Internal Medicine 1984, Geriatric Medicine 1992; **Med School:** Univ Minn 1981; **Resid:** Internal Medicine, Mayo Clinic, Rochester, MN 1981-1984; **Fellow:** Internal Medicine, Mayo Clinic, Rochester, MN 1984-1985; **Fac Appt:** Asst Prof Medicine, Mayo Med Sch

Duthie, Edmund H MD (Ger) - *Spec Exp:* Geriatric Assessment; **Hospital:** Froedtert Meml Lutheran Hosp; **Address:** 9200 W Watertown Plank Rd, Milwaukee, WI 53295; **Phone:** (414) 259-2000; **Board Cert:** Internal Medicine 1979, Geriatric Medicine 1998; **Med School:** Georgetown Univ 1976; **Resid:** Internal Medicine, Med Coll Wisc Hosps, Milwaukee, WI 1977-1979; **Fellow:** Geriatric Medicine, Jewish Inst Geri Care-SUNY, NY 1979-1980; **Fac Appt:** Prof Nephrology, Med Coll Wisc

Gorbien, Martin MD (Ger) - *Spec Exp:* Depression; Alzheimer's Disease; Dementia; **Hospital:** Rush-Presby - St Luke's Med Ctr (page 72); **Address:** 1725 W Harrison St, Ste 319, Chicago, IL 60612; **Phone:** (312) 942-7030; **Board Cert:** Internal Medicine 1996, Geriatric Medicine 1998; **Med School:** Mexico 1983; **Resid:** Internal Medicine, Mercy Hosp & Med Ctr, Chicago, IL 1984-1987; **Fellow:** Geriatric Medicine, UCLA Med Ctr, Los Angeles, CA 1987-1989; **Fac Appt:** Assoc Prof Medicine, Rush Med Coll

Halter, Jeffrey Brian MD (Ger) - *Spec Exp:* Endocrinology; Diabetes; **Hospital:** Univ of MI Hlth Ctr; **Address:** Univ Michigan - CCGCB Room 1111, 1500 E Medical Center, Ann Arbor, MI 48109-0926; **Phone:** (734) 763-4002; **Board Cert:** Internal Medicine 1974, Endocrinology 1977; **Med School:** Univ Minn 1969; **Resid:** Internal Medicine, LA Co Harbor Gen Hosp, Torrance, CA 1970-1971; Internal Medicine, Univ Wash Affil Hosp, Seattle, WA 1973-1974; **Fellow:** Seattle VA Hospital, Seattle, WA 1975-1977; **Fac Appt:** Prof Medicine, Univ Mich Med Sch

Miller, Douglas Kent MD (Ger) - *Spec Exp:* Geriatric Medicine - General; **Hospital:** St Louis Univ Hospital; **Address:** 1402 S Grand Blvd, Ste M238, St Louis, MO 63104; **Phone:** (314) 577-6055; **Board Cert:** Internal Medicine 1978, Geriatric Medicine 1998; **Med School:** Washington Univ, St Louis 1972; **Resid:** Internal Medicine, Jewish Hosp, St Louis, MO 1972-1973; Internal Medicine, Hosp Univ Pa, Philadelphia, PA 1977-1978; **Fellow:** Geriatric Medicine, UCLA, Los Angeles, CA 1987-1988; **Fac Appt:** Prof Medicine, St Louis Univ

Morley, John MD (Ger) - *Spec Exp:* Nutrition; Endocrinology; Menopause-Male; **Hospital:** St Louis Univ Hospital; **Address:** St Louis Univ Hlth Sci Ctr, Div Ger Med, 1402 S Grand Blvd, rm M 238, St Louis, MO 63104; **Phone:** (314) 577-6055; **Board Cert:** Internal Medicine 1978, Geriatric Medicine 1998, Endocrinology 1981; **Med School:** South Africa 1972; **Resid:** Internal Medicine, Johannesburg Genl Hosp, Johannesburg, South Africa 1974; Internal Medicine, Baragwanath Hosp, Johannesburg, South Africa 1975-1976; **Fellow:** Endocrinology, Diabetes & Metabolism, Wadsworth VA Hosp UCLA, Los Angeles, CA 1977-1979; **Fac Appt:** Prof Geriatric Medicine, St Louis Univ

Olson, Jack Conrad MD (Ger) - *Spec Exp:* Geriatric Medicine - General; **Hospital:** Rush-Presby - St Luke's Med Ctr (page 72); **Address:** 1725 W Harrison St, Ste 319, Chicago, IL 60612; **Phone:** (312) 942-7030; **Board Cert:** Geriatric Medicine 1990, Internal Medicine 1987; **Med School:** Univ Mich Med Sch 1984; **Resid:** Internal Medicine, Univ Wisc Med Sch, Madison, WI 1985-1987; **Fellow:** Geriatric Medicine, Univ Wisc Med Sch, Madison, WI 1987-1989; **Fac Appt:** Assoc Prof Medicine, Univ Chicago-Pritzker Sch Med

Palmer, Robert MD (Ger) - *Spec Exp:* Geriatric Assessment; **Hospital:** Cleveland Clin Fdn (page 57); **Address:** 9500 Euclid Ave, MC A-91, Cleveland, OH 44195; **Phone:** (216) 444-8091; **Board Cert:** Internal Medicine 1975, Geriatric Medicine 1998; **Med School:** Univ Mich Med Sch 1971; **Resid:** Internal Medicine, LA Co Med Ctr, Los Angeles, CA 1972-1975; **Fellow:** Geriatric Medicine, UCLA, Los Angeles, CA 1985-1986; **Fac Appt:** Assoc Prof Medicine, Ohio State Univ

Sachs, Greg MD (Ger) - *Spec Exp:* Memory Disorders/Alzheimer's; **Hospital:** Univ of Chicago Hosps (page 76); **Address:** Dept Medicine, Sect Geriatrics, 5841 S Maryland Ave, MC-6098, Chicago, IL 60637; **Phone:** (773) 702-8840; **Board Cert:** Geriatric Medicine 1990, Internal Medicine 1988; **Med School:** Yale Univ 1985; **Resid:** Internal Medicine, Univ Chicago Hosps, Chicago, IL 1985-1987; **Fellow:** Geriatric Medicine, Univ Chicago Hosps, Chicago, IL 1987-1990; **Fac Appt:** Assoc Prof Medicine, Univ Chicago-Pritzker Sch Med

Sheehan, Myles MD (Ger) - *Spec Exp:* Dementia; Functional Assessment; **Hospital:** Loyola Univ Med Ctr; **Address:** Loyola Univ Med Ctr, 2160 S 1st Ave , Bldg 120 - rm 310, Maywood, IL 60153; **Phone:** (708) 216-8887; **Board Cert:** Internal Medicine 1984, Geriatric Medicine 1992; **Med School:** Dartmouth Med Sch 1981; **Resid:** Internal Medicine, Beth Israel Deaconcess Med Ctr, Boston, MA 1981-1984; **Fellow:** Geriatric Medicine, Beth Israel Deaconess Med Ctr, Boston, MA 1989-1991; **Fac Appt:** Assoc Prof Medicine, Loyola Univ-Stritch Sch Med

Supiano, Mark A. MD (Ger) - *Spec Exp:* Blood Pressure Regulation; Hypertension; Geriatric Assessment; **Hospital:** Univ of MI Hlth Ctr; **Address:** U-M Comp. Cancer and Ger Ctr. Turner Ger Clinic Lvl 1, 1500 E Med Ctr Dr, Ann Arbor, MI 48109-0926; **Phone:** (734) 764-6831; **Board Cert:** Geriatric Medicine 1998, Internal Medicine 1985; **Med School:** Univ Wisc 1982; **Resid:** Internal Medicine, U Mich., Ann Arbor, MI 1982-1985; **Fellow:** Geriatric Medicine, U Mich., Ann Arbor, MI 1985-1986; **Fac Appt:** Assoc Prof Medicine, Univ Mich Med Sch

Von Sternberg, Thomas MD (Ger) - *Spec Exp:* Dementia; **Hospital:** Fairview-Univ Med Ctr - Univ Campus; **Address:** Hlth Partners Riverside Clin, Adult Med, 2220 Riverside Ave S, Fl 1st, Minneapolis, MN 55454; **Phone:** (612) 371-1610; **Board Cert:** Family Practice 1997, Geriatric Medicine 1998; **Med School:** Ohio State Univ 1980; **Resid:** Family Practice, Fairview-Univ Med Ctr, Minneapolis, MN 1980-1983; **Fellow:** Geriatric Medicine, Westminster Med Sch, London 1983

Williamson, Wayne MD (Ger) - *Spec Exp:* Hypertension; Asthma; **Hospital:** Northwestern Meml Hosp; **Address:** 201 E Huron Fl 11 - Ste 105, Chicago, IL 60611; **Phone:** (312) 642-7493; **Board Cert:** Geriatric Medicine 1992, Internal Medicine 1984; **Med School:** Univ Cincinnati 1978; **Resid:** Internal Medicine, Rush Presby St Lukes Med Ctr, Chicago, IL 1979-1981; **Fac Appt:** Asst Prof Geriatric Medicine, Rush Med Coll

Great Plains and Mountains

Schwartz, Robert S MD (Ger) - *Spec Exp:* Diabetes; Eating Disorders-Obesity; Exercise Therapy; **Hospital:** Univ Colo HSC - Denver; **Address:** Univ Colo Hlth Scis Ctr, 4200 E Ninth Ave, Box B179, Denver, CO 80262; **Phone:** (303) 315-8668; **Board Cert:** Internal Medicine 1977, Endocrinology 1981, Geriatric Medicine 2000; **Med School:** Ohio State Univ 1974; **Resid:** Internal Medicine, Univ Wash, Seattle, WA 1975-1977; **Fellow:** Endocrinology, Diabetes & Metabolism, Univ Wash, Seattle, WA 1977-1980; **Fac Appt:** Prof Medicine, Univ Wash

Southwest

Bernard, Marie A MD (Ger) - *Spec Exp:* Osteoporosis in the Aged; **Hospital:** Univ OK Hlth Sci Ctr; **Address:** 921 NE 13th St, VAMC-11G, Oklahoma, OK 73104; **Phone:** (405) 271-8558; **Board Cert:** Internal Medicine 1979, Geriatric Medicine 1999; **Med School:** Univ Penn 1976; **Resid:** Internal Medicine, Temple Univ Med Ctr, Philadelphia, PA 1976-1979; **Fac Appt:** Prof Medicine, Univ Okla Coll Med

Carter, William Jerry MD (Ger) - *Spec Exp:* Geriatric Endocrinology; **Hospital:** VA Med Ctr; **Address:** Geriatrics Clinic, 3B, 2200 Fort Roots Drive, North Little Rock, AR 72114; **Phone:** (501) 257-2061; **Board Cert:** Geriatric Medicine 1994, Endocrinology, Diabetes & Metabolism 1975; **Med School:** Univ Ark 1963; **Resid:** Internal Medicine, University Ark, Little Rock, AR 1964-1967; **Fellow:** Endocrinology, Diabetes & Metabolism, University Ark, Little Rock, AR 1969-1971; **Fac Appt:** Prof Medicine, Univ Ark

Garb, Leslie Julian MD (Ger) - *Spec Exp:* Sigmoidoscopy; **Hospital:** Methodist Hosp - Houston; **Address:** 5420 Dashwood Dr, Ste 100, Houston, TX 77081; **Phone:** (713) 664-0719; **Board Cert:** Family Practice 1997, Geriatric Medicine 1997; **Med School:** South Africa 1963; **Resid:** Internal Medicine, Johnnesberg Genl Hosp, Johannesberg, S. Africa 1963-1968

Lichtenstein, Michael Joseph MD (Ger) - *Spec Exp:* Alzheimer's Disease; **Hospital:** Univ of Texas Hlth & Sci Ctr; **Address:** Univ TX Hlth Sci Ctr, Dept Med, 7703 Floyd Curl Dr, San Antonio, TX 78229-3900; **Phone:** (210) 592-0400; **Board Cert:** Geriatric Medicine 1999, Internal Medicine 1982; **Med School:** Baylor Coll Med 1978; **Fac Appt:** Prof Medicine, Univ Tex, San Antonio

Liem, Pham MD (Ger) - *Spec Exp:* Dementia; Alzheimer's Disease; **Hospital:** UAMS; **Address:** Univ Hosp Arkansas Med Sci, 4301 W Markham #748, Little Rock, AR 72205; **Phone:** (501) 686-8948; **Board Cert:** Family Practice 1999, Geriatric Medicine 1998; **Med School:** Vietnam 1973; **Resid:** Family Practice, Univ Ark Med Sch, Little Rock, AR 1977-1980; **Fellow:** Geriatric Medicine, Univ Ark Med Sch, Little Rock, AR 1980-1982; **Fac Appt:** Assoc Prof Geriatric Medicine, Univ Ark

Lipschitz, David Arnold MD/PhD (Ger) - *Spec Exp:* Nutrition; **Hospital:** UAMS; **Address:** Univ Arkansas Med Sci, 4301 W Markham St, MS 748, Little Rock, AR 72205-7101; **Phone:** (501) 686-5944; **Board Cert:** Internal Medicine 1975, Hematology 1976; **Med School:** Africa 1966; **Resid:** Internal Medicine, Johannesburg Genl Hosp, Johannesburg 1966-1972; **Fellow:** Hematology, Univ Washington, Seattle, WA 1972-1974; Internal Medicine, Montefiore Hosp, New York, NY 1974-1975; **Fac Appt:** Prof Geriatric Medicine, Univ Ark

Vicioso, Belinda Angelica MD (Ger) - *Spec Exp:* Geriatric Medicine - General; **Hospital:** Parkland Mem Hosp; **Address:** 5323 Harry Hines Blvd, Dallas, TX 75390-8889; **Phone:** (214) 648-9012; **Board Cert:** Internal Medicine 1989, Geriatric Medicine 1990; **Med School:** Dominican Republic 1979; **Resid:** Internal Medicine, St Francis Med Ctr, Trenton, NJ 1981-1983; **Fellow:** Geriatric Medicine, Univ Penn Med Sch, Philadelphia, PA 1984-1986; **Fac Appt:** Asst Prof Medicine, Univ Tex SW, Dallas

West Coast and Pacific

Abrass, Itamar MD (Ger) - *Spec Exp:* Endocrinology; Diabetes; **Hospital:** Univ WA Med Ctr; **Address:** Harborview Med Ctr, 325 9th Ave, Box 359755, Seattle, WA 98104-2499; **Phone:** (206) 731-4191; **Board Cert:** Geriatric Medicine 1988, Endocrinology, Diabetes & Metabolism 1975, Internal Medicine 1974; **Med School:** UCSF 1966; **Resid:** Internal Medicine, Columbia-Pesby Med Ctr, New York, NY 1966-1968; **Fellow:** Endocrinology, Diabetes & Metabolism, UC SanDiego Med Ctr, SanDiego, CA 1970-1971; **Fac Appt:** Prof Medicine, Univ Wash

Davis Jr, James William MD (Ger) - *Spec Exp:* Geriatric Medicine - General; **Hospital:** UCLA Med Ctr; **Address:** Dept Geriatrics, 200 UCLA Medical Plaza, Ste 420, Los Angeles, CA 90095; **Phone:** (310) 206-8272; **Board Cert:** Geriatric Medicine 2000, Internal Medicine 1979; **Med School:** Med Univ SC 1975; **Resid:** Internal Medicine, Mount Zion Med Ctr, San Fransisco, CA; Geriatric Medicine, Mount Zion Med Ctr, San Francisco, CA

Landefeld, Charles Seth MD (Ger) - *Spec Exp:* Cardiology-Geriatric; **Hospital:** UCSF Med Ctr; **Address:** 3333 California St, Ste 380, San Francisco, CA 94118; **Phone:** (415) 750-6625; **Board Cert:** Internal Medicine 1982, Geriatric Medicine 1990; **Med School:** Yale Univ 1979; **Resid:** Internal Medicine, UCSF Med Ctr, San Francisco, CA 1980-1983; **Fellow:** Geriatric Medicine, Brigham-Womens Hosp, Boston, MA 1983-1985; **Fac Appt:** Prof Medicine, UCSF

McCormick, Wayne MD (Ger) - *Spec Exp:* Dementia; AIDS/HIV; Elderly Long Term Care; **Hospital:** Univ WA Med Ctr; **Address:** 325 9th Ave, Box 359860, Seattle, WA 98104; **Phone:** (206) 731-4191; **Board Cert:** Internal Medicine 1986, Geriatric Medicine 1992; **Med School:** Washington Univ, St Louis 1983; **Resid:** Internal Medicine, Michael Reese Hosp, Chicago, IL 1984-1986; Internal Medicine, Michael Reese Hosp, Chicago, IL 1986-1987; **Fellow:** Geriatric Medicine, Univ Wash Med Ctr, Seattle, WA 1987-1990; **Fac Appt:** Asst Prof Medicine, Univ Wash

Reuben, David MD (Ger) - *Spec Exp:* Aging; **Hospital:** UCLA Med Ctr; **Address:** UCLA Dept Med, Div Geriatrics, 10945 Le Conte Ave, Ste 2339, Los Angeles, CA 90095; **Phone:** (310) 825-8253; **Board Cert:** Internal Medicine 1980, Geriatric Medicine 1988; **Med School:** Emory Univ 1977; **Resid:** Internal Medicine, Rhode Island Hosp, Providence, RI 1977-1980; **Fellow:** Geriatric Medicine, UCLA Med Ctr, Los Angeles, CA 1987; **Fac Appt:** Prof Medicine, UCLA

GYNECOLOGIC ONCOLOGY

(a subspecialty of OBSTETRICS AND GYNECOLOGY)

An obstetrician/gynecologist possesses special knowledge, skills and professional capability in the medical and surgical care of the female reproductive system and associated disorders. This physician serves as a consultant to other physicians and as a primary physician for women.

OBSTETRICS/GYNECOLOGY

An obstetrician/gynecologist who provides consultation and comprehensive management of patients with gynecologic cancer, including those diagnostic and therapeutic procedures necessary for the total care of the patient with gynecologic cancer and resulting complications.

Training required: Four years plus two years in clinical practice before certification in obstetrics and gynecology is complete *plus* additional training and examination in gynecologic oncology

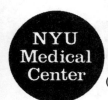

NYU Medical Center

550 First Avenue (at 31st Street)
New York, NY 10016
Physician Referral: (888) 7-NYU-MED
(888-769-8633) www.nyumedicalcenter.org

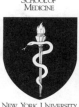

GYNECOLOGIC ONCOLOGY

The Division of Gynecologic Oncology is now one of the largest academic divisions of its kind in the United States. Working in concert with the Department of Medical Oncology, Radiation Oncology, Gynecological Pathology and Radiology, physicians within the Gynecologic Oncology program hold interdisciplinary meetings with doctors from each of these specialties to discuss patients at frequent and regular intervals.

The Division enjoys a close relationship with the NCI-designated Rita J. and Stanley H. Kaplan Comprehensive Cancer Center, also located on the NYU Medical Center campus, and it has established the Kaplan Cancer Center/Gynecological Cancer research Fund to support crucial research initiatives. Among these are: evaluation of combined teletherapy and brachytherapy with chemotherapy in the management of cervical carcinoma with established spread to the para-aortic lymph nodes; prospective evaluation of ultrasound and serum markers as screen for ovarian cancer; effects of topotecan, a topoisomerase inhibitor, and the preservation of fertility in cervical cancer patients.

Patient care at NYU Medical Center takes a circumspect approach when it comes to cancer, and our doctors emphasize the crucial importance of choosing the correct course of treatment right at the outset, within a very short time-frame. At the same time, NYU physicians know that patient comfort is paramount and that, especially with gynecologic cancers, good patient care is only half the story. Most patients have a strong psychological reaction to their diagnosis, and, at NYU Medical Center, doctors, social workers and therapists team up to help patients through this difficult period.

NYU MEDICAL CENTER

Women's Health at NYU Medical Center

- Obstetrics
- Gynecology
- Maternal-Fetal Medicine
- Gynecologic Oncology
- Reproductive Endocrinology and Infertility
- Reconstructive Pelvic Surgery and Urogynecology
- Endoscopic Pelvic Surgery and Family Planning
- Ultrasound Imaging
- Gynecological Pathology

PHYSICIAN LISTINGS

Gynecologic Oncology

New England

Currie, John L. MD (GO) - *Spec Exp:* Gynecologic Cancers; Pelvic Reconstruction; **Hospital:** Dartmouth - Hitchcock Med Ctr; , Lebanon, NH 03756; **Phone:** (603) 650-7625; **Board Cert:** Gynecologic Oncology 1982, Obstetrics & Gynecology 1991; **Med School:** Univ NC Sch Med 1967; **Resid:** Obstetrics & Gynecology, Hosp of the Univ of Pennsylvania, Philadelphia, PA 1968-1972; Surgery, Hosp of the Univ of Pennsylvania, Philadelphia, PA 1967; **Fellow:** Gynecologic Oncology, Duke Univ Med Ctr, Durham, NC 1978-1980

Fuller, Arlan F. MD (GO) - *Spec Exp:* Ovarian Cancer; Cervical Cancer; **Hospital:** MA Genl Hosp; **Address:** 100 Blossom St, Bldg Cox5, Boston, MA 02114; **Phone:** (617) 724-6880; **Board Cert:** Obstetrics & Gynecology 1979, Gynecologic Oncology 1982; **Med School:** Harvard Med Sch 1971; **Resid:** Surgery, Mass Genl Hosp, Boston, MA 1971-1974; Obstetrics & Gynecology, Brigham and Womens Hosp, Boston, MA 1974-1977; **Fellow:** Gynecologic Oncology, Memorial Sloan Kettering Cancer Ctr, New York, NY 1977-1979; **Fac Appt:** Assoc Prof Obstetrics & Gynecology, Harvard Med Sch

Goodman, Annekathryn MD (GO) - *Spec Exp:* Cervical Cancer; AIDS/HIV; **Hospital:** MA Genl Hosp; **Address:** 100 Blossom St, Bldg Cox5, Boston, MA 02114; **Phone:** (617) 726-2429; **Board Cert:** Obstetrics & Gynecology 1991, Gynecologic Oncology 1994; **Med School:** Tufts Univ 1983; **Resid:** Obstetrics & Gynecology, Tufts, Boston, MA 1983-1987; **Fellow:** Gynecologic Oncology, Mass Genl Hosp., Boston, MA 1987-1990; **Fac Appt:** Asst Prof Obstetrics & Gynecology, Harvard Med Sch

Niloff, Jonathan Mitchell MD (GO) - *Spec Exp:* Ovarian Cancer; Gynecologic Surgery-Complex; Endometrial Cancer; **Hospital:** Beth Israel Deaconess Med Ctr - Boston; **Address:** 330 Brookline Ave, rm KS-330, Boston, MA 02215-5400; **Phone:** (617) 667-4040; **Board Cert:** Obstetrics & Gynecology 1987, Gynecologic Oncology 1987; **Med School:** McGill Univ 1978; **Resid:** Obstetrics & Gynecology, Brigham & Women's Hosp, Boston, MA 1979-1982; **Fellow:** Gynecologic Oncology, Brigham & Women's Hosp, Boston, MA 1982-1984; **Fac Appt:** Assoc Prof Obstetrics & Gynecology, Harvard Med Sch

Schwartz, Peter MD (GO) - *Spec Exp:* Ovarian Cancer; Uterine Cancer; Gynecologic Surgery; **Hospital:** Yale - New Haven Hosp; **Address:** 333 Cedar St, Ste FM13316, New Haven, CT 06510-3289; **Phone:** (203) 785-4135; **Board Cert:** Obstetrics & Gynecology 1973, Gynecologic Oncology 1979; **Med School:** Albert Einstein Coll Med 1966; **Resid:** Obstetrics & Gynecology, Yale-New Haven Hosp, New Haven, CT 1967-1970; **Fellow:** Gynecologic Oncology, MD Anderson Cancer Ctr, Houston, TX 1973-1975; **Fac Appt:** Prof Obstetrics & Gynecology, Yale Univ

Tarraza, Hector MD (GO) - *Spec Exp:* Gynecologic Oncology; **Hospital:** Maine Med Ctr; **Address:** 34 Broad Cove Rd, Cape Elizabeth, ME; **Phone:** (207) 771-5549; **Board Cert:** Gynecologic Oncology 1998, Obstetrics & Gynecology 1998; **Med School:** Harvard Med Sch 1981; **Resid:** Obstetrics & Gynecology, Mass General Hospital, Boston, MA 1981-1985; **Fellow:** Gynecologic Oncology, Mass General Hospital, Boston, MA 1985-1987; **Fac Appt:** Asst Prof Univ VT Coll Med

Mid Atlantic

Barakat, Richard MD (GO) - *Spec Exp:* Laparoscopic Surgery; Ovarian Cancer; Uterine Cancer; **Hospital:** Mem Sloan Kettering Cancer Ctr; **Address:** Memorial Sloan Kettering Cancer Center, 1275 York Ave, rm C1096, New York, NY 10021; **Phone:** (212) 639-2453; **Board Cert:** Obstetrics & Gynecology 1992, Gynecologic Oncology 1994; **Med School:** SUNY Hlth Sci Ctr 1985; **Resid:** Obstetrics & Gynecology, Bellevue Hosp, New York, NY 1985-1989; **Fellow:** Gynecologic Oncology, Mem Sloan Kettering Cancer Ctr, New York, NY 1989-1991; **Fac Appt:** Assoc Prof Obstetrics & Gynecology, Cornell Univ-Weill Med Coll

Barnes, Willard MD (GO) - *Spec Exp:* Pelvic Tumors; **Hospital:** Georgetown Univ Hosp; **Address:** GUMC - Lombardi Cancer Center Dept OB/GYN, 3800 Reservoir Rd NW Fl 2, Washington, DC 20007-2194; **Phone:** (202) 687-2114; **Board Cert:** Obstetrics & Gynecology 1997, Gynecologic Oncology 1997; **Med School:** Univ Miss 1979; **Resid:** Obstetrics & Gynecology, Univ Miss Med Ctr, Jackson, MS 1979-1983; **Fellow:** Gynecologic Oncology, Georgetown Univ Med Ctr, Washington, DC 1983-1985; **Fac Appt:** Assoc Prof Obstetrics & Gynecology, Georgetown Univ

Barter, James MD (GO) - *Spec Exp:* Laparoscopic Surgery; **Hospital:** Georgetown Univ Hosp; **Address:** Georgetown Univ Hosp, Lombardi Cancer Ctr, 3800 Reservoir Rd NW, Washington, DC 20007; **Phone:** (202) 687-2114; **Board Cert:** Obstetrics & Gynecology 1997, Gynecologic Oncology 1997; **Med School:** Univ VA Sch Med 1977; **Resid:** Internal Medicine, Univ of KY, Lexington, KY 1978-1979; Obstetrics & Gynecology, Duke Univ, Durham, NC 1980-1983; **Fellow:** Gynecologic Oncology, Univ of Alabama, Birmingham, AL 1983-1986; **Fac Appt:** Assoc Prof Obstetrics & Gynecology, Georgetown Univ

Caputo, Thomas A MD (GO) - *Spec Exp:* Cervical Cancer; Ovarian Cancer; Uterine Cancer; **Hospital:** NY Presby Hosp - NY Weill Cornell Med Ctr (page 70); **Address:** 525 E 68th St, Ste J130, New York, NY 10021; **Phone:** (212) 746-3179; **Board Cert:** Obstetrics & Gynecology 1993, Gynecologic Oncology 1977; **Med School:** UMDNJ-NJ Med Sch, Newark 1965; **Resid:** Obstetrics & Gynecology, Martland Hosp-NJ Coll, Newark, NJ 1966-1969; **Fellow:** Gynecologic Oncology, Emory Univ Hosp, Atlanta, GA 1972-1974; **Fac Appt:** Clin Prof Obstetrics & Gynecology, Cornell Univ-Weill Med Coll

Carlson, John MD (GO) - *Spec Exp:* Gynecologic Cancer; Ovarian Cancer; **Hospital:** Thomas Jefferson Univ Hosp; **Address:** Thomas Jefferson Univ. Hosp., 111 S 11th St, Bldg Gibbons - rm 6200, Philadelphia, PA 19107; **Phone:** (215) 955-6200; **Board Cert:** Gynecologic Oncology 1982, Obstetrics & Gynecology 1981; **Med School:** Georgetown Univ 1974; **Resid:** Obstetrics & Gynecology, Hartford Hosp, Hartford, CT 1974-1975; Obstetrics & Gynecology, Hosp Univ Penn, Philadelphia, PA 1975-1978; **Fellow:** Gynecologic Oncology, MD Anderson Hosp, Houston, TX 1978-1980; **Fac Appt:** Prof Obstetrics & Gynecology, Jefferson Med Coll

Chalas, Eva MD (GO) - *Spec Exp:* Gynecologic Cancer; **Hospital:** Stony Brook Univ Hosp; **Address:** 994 W Jericho Tpke, Smithtown, NY 11787; **Phone:** (631) 864-5440; **Board Cert:** Obstetrics & Gynecology 1998, Gynecologic Oncology 1998; **Med School:** SUNY Stony Brook 1981; **Resid:** Obstetrics & Gynecology, Univ Hosp, Stony Brook, NY 1981-1985; **Fellow:** Gynecologic Oncology, Meml Sloan Kettering Cancer Ctr, New York, NY 1985-1987

Cohen, Carmel MD (GO) - *Spec Exp:* Ovarian Cancer; Cervical Cancer; Pelvic Surgery; **Hospital:** Mount Sinai Hosp (page 68); **Address:** Mt Sinai Hosp, 5 E 98th St, Fl 2, New York, NY 10029; **Phone:** (212) 427-9898; **Board Cert:** Obstetrics & Gynecology 1967, Gynecologic Oncology 1974; **Med School:** Tulane Univ 1958; **Resid:** Obstetrics & Gynecology, Mount Sinai, New York, NY 1959-1964; **Fellow:** Gynecologic Oncology, Mount Sinai Hosp, New York, NY 1964-1965; **Fac Appt:** Prof Obstetrics & Gynecology, Mount Sinai Sch Med

Curtin, John P MD (GO) - *Spec Exp:* *Uterine Cancer; Ovarian Cancer; Laparoscopic Surgery;* **Hospital:** NYU Med Ctr (page 71); **Address:** NYU Sch Med, Dept Gyn/Onc, 530 First Ave, Ste 9R, New York, NY 10016; **Phone:** (212) 263-2353; **Board Cert:** Gynecologic Oncology 1990, Obstetrics & Gynecology 1996; **Med School:** Creighton Univ 1979; **Resid:** Obstetrics & Gynecology, Univ Minn Med Ctr, Minneapolis, MN 1979-1984; **Fellow:** Gynecologic Oncology, Meml Sloan-Kettering Cancer Ctr, New York, NY 1986-1988; **Fac Appt:** Prof Gynecologic Oncology, NYU Sch Med

Kwon, Tae MD (GO) - *Spec Exp:* *Uterine Cancer; Cervical Cancer; Ovarian Cancer;* **Hospital:** Our Lady of Mercy Med Ctr; **Address:** 305 North St, White Plains, NY 10605; **Phone:** (914) 681-7171; **Board Cert:** Obstetrics & Gynecology 1978, Gynecologic Oncology 1981; **Med School:** South Korea 1965; **Resid:** Obstetrics & Gynecology, Lenox Hill Hosp, New York, NY 1970-1974; Gynecologic Oncology, Lenox Hill Hosp, New York, NY 1974-1976; **Fellow:** Gynecologic Oncology, Univ Mississippi Hosp, Jackson, MS 1976-1978; **Fac Appt:** Assoc Clin Prof Obstetrics & Gynecology, NY Med Coll

Montz, Fredrick John MD (GO) - *Spec Exp:* *Gynecologic Oncology - General;* **Hospital:** Johns Hopkins Hosp - Baltimore; **Address:** Johns Hopkins Med Inst., 600 N Wolfe St Bldg Phipps - rm 284, Baltimore, MD 21287; **Phone:** (410) 955-8240; **Board Cert:** Obstetrics & Gynecology 1999, Gynecologic Oncology 1997; **Med School:** Baylor Coll Med 1980; **Resid:** Obstetrics & Gynecology, LA Co-USC Med Ctr., Los Angeles, CA 1980-1984; **Fellow:** Gynecologic Oncology, LA Co-USC Med. Ctr., Los Angeles, CA 1985-1987; **Fac Appt:** Prof Obstetrics & Gynecology, Johns Hopkins Univ

Smith, Daniel MD (GO) - *Spec Exp:* *Gynecologic Oncology - General;* **Hospital:** NY Presby Hosp - Columbia Presby Med Ctr (page 70); **Address:** 161 Ft Washington Ave Bldg Herbert Irving - Ste 837, New York, NY 10032; **Phone:** (212) 305-3410; **Board Cert:** Obstetrics & Gynecology 1994, Gynecologic Oncology 1983; **Med School:** Harvard Med Sch 1972; **Resid:** Surgery, Mass Genl Hosp, Boston, MA 1978-1979; Obstetrics & Gynecology, LA Co USC Med Ctr, Los Angeles, CA 1975-1978; **Fellow:** Gynecologic Oncology, Mem Sloan Kettering Cancer Ctr, New York, NY 1979-1981; **Fac Appt:** Assoc Prof Obstetrics & Gynecology, Columbia P&S

Soisson, Andrew MD (GO) - *Spec Exp:* *Cervical Cancer;* **Hospital:** WV Univ Hosp - Ruby Memorial; **Address:** 4601 HSN, Morgantown, WV 26505; **Phone:** (304) 293-3141; **Board Cert:** Gynecologic Oncology 1999, Obstetrics & Gynecology 1997; **Med School:** Georgetown Univ 1981; **Resid:** Gynecologic Oncology, Duke Univ Med Ctr, Durham, NC 1987-1990; Obstetrics & Gynecology, Madigan AMC, Tacoma, WA 1981-1985; **Fac Appt:** Assoc Prof W VA Univ

Wallach, Robert C MD (GO) - *Spec Exp:* *Gynecologic Oncology - General;* **Hospital:** NYU Med Ctr (page 71); **Address:** 700 Park Ave, New York, NY 10021-4930; **Phone:** (212) 666-5566; **Board Cert:** Obstetrics & Gynecology 1967, Gynecologic Oncology 1974; **Med School:** Yale Univ 1969; **Resid:** Obstetrics & Gynecology, Beth Israel Med Ctr, New York, NY 1961-1965; **Fellow:** Gynecologic Oncology, SUNY Brooklyn Med Ctr, Brooklyn, NY 1965-1966; **Fac Appt:** Clin Prof Obstetrics & Gynecology, NYU Sch Med

Southeast

Alleyn, James MD (GO) - *Spec Exp:* *Gynecologic Oncology - General;* **Hospital:** Baptist Hosp - Miami; **Address:** 3661 S Miami Ave, Ste 308, Miami, FL 33133-4206; **Phone:** (305) 854-3603; **Board Cert:** Obstetrics & Gynecology 1978; **Med School:** Indiana Univ 1972; **Resid:** Obstetrics & Gynecology, Miami-Jackson Meml Hosp, Miami, FL 1973-1976; **Fellow:** Gynecologic Oncology, Miami-Jackson Meml Hosp, Miami, FL 1976-1978

GYNECOLOGIC ONCOLOGY

Berchuck, Andrew MD (GO) - *Spec Exp:* Ovarian Cancer-Hereditary; Uterine Cancer; **Hospital:** Duke Univ Med Ctr (page 60); **Address:** Duke Univ Med Center, Box 3079, Durham, NC 27710; **Phone:** (919) 684-3765; **Board Cert:** Obstetrics & Gynecology 1998, Gynecologic Oncology 1998; **Med School:** Case West Res Univ 1980; **Resid:** Obstetrics & Gynecology, Case Western Resrv, Cleveland, OH 1980-1984; **Fellow:** Gynecology, UT Southwestern, Dallas, TX 1984-1985; Gynecology, Meml Sloan-Kettering, New York, NY 1985-1987; **Fac Appt:** Prof Obstetrics & Gynecology, Duke Univ

Clarke-Pearson, Daniel L MD (GO) - *Spec Exp:* Pelvic Reconstruction; Gynecologic Surgery-Complex; **Hospital:** Duke Univ Med Ctr (page 60); **Address:** Duke Univ Med Ctr, Box 3079, Durham, NC 27710; **Phone:** (919) 684-3765; **Board Cert:** Obstetrics & Gynecology 1982, Gynecologic Oncology 1983; **Med School:** Case West Res Univ 1975; **Resid:** Obstetrics & Gynecology, Duke Med Ctr, NC 1975-1979; **Fellow:** Gynecologic Oncology, Duke Med Ctr 1979-1981; **Fac Appt:** Prof Obstetrics & Gynecology, Duke Univ

Fiorica, James Vincent MD (GO) - *Spec Exp:* Gynecologic Cancer; Breast Cancer; **Hospital:** H Lee Moffitt Cancer Ctr & Research Inst; **Address:** 12902 Magnolia Drive, Tampa, FL 33612; **Phone:** (813) 972-8450; **Board Cert:** Obstetrics & Gynecology 1999, Gynecologic Oncology 1999; **Med School:** Tufts Univ 1982; **Resid:** Obstetrics & Gynecology, Univ of S Fla Affil Hosp, Tampa, FL 1982-1986; **Fellow:** Gynecologic Oncology, Univ of S Fla Affil Hosp, Tampa, FL 1986-1989; Breast Disease, Tufts Univ, Boston, MA 1990; **Fac Appt:** Prof Obstetrics & Gynecology, Univ S Fla Coll Med

Fowler Jr, Wesley C MD (GO) - *Spec Exp:* Vulva Disease/Neoplasia; DES-Exposed Females; **Hospital:** Univ of NC Hosp (page 77); **Address:** U NC Chapel Hill, Div of Ob/Gyn, MacNider - CB 7570, Chapel Hill, NC 27599-7570; **Phone:** (919) 966-1196; **Board Cert:** Obstetrics & Gynecology 1991, Gynecologic Oncology 1979; **Med School:** Univ NC Sch Med 1966; **Resid:** Obstetrics & Gynecology, NC Meml Hosp, Chapel Hill, NC 1967-1971; **Fac Appt:** Prof Obstetrics & Gynecology, Univ NC Sch Med

Hoskins, William MD (GO) - *Spec Exp:* Ovarian Cancer; **Hospital:** Meml Med Ctr - Savannah; **Address:** Anderson Cancer Inst, Meml Hlth Univ Med Ctr, 4700 Waters Ave, Savannah, GA 31404; **Phone:** (912) 350-3071; **Board Cert:** Obstetrics & Gynecology 1993, Gynecologic Oncology 1979; **Med School:** Univ Tenn Coll Med, Memphis 1965; **Resid:** Obstetrics & Gynecology, Naval Med Ctr, New York, NY 1968-1971; **Fellow:** Gynecologic Oncology, Univ Miami Hosp, Miami, FL 1974-1975

Jones III, Howard Wilbur MD (GO) - *Spec Exp:* Gynecologic Oncology - General; **Hospital:** Vanderbilt Univ Med Ctr (page 80); **Address:** Vanderbilt Univ Med Ctr, Medical Center North, Box 1100, Nashville, TN 37232-2519; **Phone:** (615) 322-2114; **Board Cert:** Obstetrics & Gynecology 1999, Gynecologic Oncology 1999; **Med School:** Duke Univ 1968; **Resid:** Obstetrics & Gynecology, Univ Colo Med Ctr, Denver, CO 1969-1972; **Fellow:** Gynecologic Oncology, Univ Tex-MD Anderson Hosp, Houston, TX 1972-1974; **Fac Appt:** Prof Obstetrics & Gynecology, Vanderbilt Univ

Kohler, Matthew MD (GO) - *Spec Exp:* Surgery; Chemotherapy; **Hospital:** Med Univ Hosp Authority; **Address:** 96 Jonathan Lucas St, MUSC Medical Center, P.O.Box 29425, Charleston, SC 29425; **Phone:** (843) 792-8176; **Board Cert:** Obstetrics & Gynecology 1995, Gynecologic Oncology 1997; **Med School:** Duke Univ 1987; **Resid:** Obstetrics & Gynecology, Duke University Medical Center, Durham, NC 1987-1991; **Fellow:** Gynecologic Oncology, Duke University Medical Center, Durham, NC 1991-1994; **Fac Appt:** Assoc Prof Obstetrics & Gynecology, Med Univ SC

Parham, Groesbeck Preer MD (GO) - *Spec Exp:* *Cervical Cancer;* **Hospital:** Univ of Ala Hosp at Birmingham; **Address:** Univ Alabama at Birmingham, 619 19th St S, OHB 538, Birmingham, AL 35249-7337; **Phone:** (205) 934-4986; **Board Cert:** Obstetrics & Gynecology 1999, Gynecologic Oncology 1999; **Med School:** Univ Ala 1981; **Resid:** Obstetrics & Gynecology, Univ Ala Hosp, Birmingham, AL 1981-1985; **Fellow:** Gynecologic Oncology, UC Irvine Med Ctr, Orange, CA 1986-1988; **Fac Appt:** Prof Obstetrics & Gynecology, Univ Ala

Partridge, Edward E MD (GO) - *Spec Exp:* *Ovarian Cancer;* **Hospital:** Univ of Ala Hosp at Birmingham; **Address:** UAB, Div Gyn Onc, 619 19th St S Bldg Old Hillman - rm 538, Birmingham, AL 35249-7333; **Phone:** (205) 934-4986; **Board Cert:** Obstetrics & Gynecology 1980, Gynecologic Oncology 1981; **Med School:** Univ Ala 1973; **Resid:** Obstetrics & Gynecology, Univ Ala Sch Med, Birmingham, AL 1974-1977; **Fellow:** Gynecologic Oncology, Univ Ala Sch Med, Brimingham, AL 1978-1979; **Fac Appt:** Prof Obstetrics & Gynecology, Univ Ala

Poliakoff, Steven MD (GO) - *Spec Exp:* *Ovarian Cancer; Minimally Invasive Surgery; Genetic Testing;* **Hospital:** Mount Sinai Med Ctr; **Address:** 6280 Sunset Dr, Ste 502, South Miami, FL 33143-4870; **Phone:** (305) 596-0870; **Board Cert:** Obstetrics & Gynecology 1983; **Med School:** Univ NC Sch Med 1975; **Resid:** Obstetrics & Gynecology, Johns Hopkins Hosp, Baltimore, MD 1976-1979; Gynecologic Oncology, Jackson Meml Hosp/Univ Miami, Miami, FL 1979-1981

Taylor Jr., Peyton T. MD (GO) - *Spec Exp:* *Gynecologic Surgery-Complex; Gynecologic Cancer;* **Hospital:** Univ of VA Hlth Sys (page 79); **Address:** UVA Health Systems, Dept OB/GYN, PO Box 800712, Charlottesville, VA 22908; **Phone:** (804) 924-9933; **Board Cert:** Obstetrics & Gynecology 1994, Gynecologic Oncology 1981; **Med School:** Univ Ala 1968; **Resid:** Obstetrics & Gynecology, Univ VA Hosp, Charlottesville, VA 1969-1970; Obstetrics & Gynecology, Univ VA Hosp, Charlottesville, VA 1972-1975; **Fellow:** Gynecologic Oncology, Univ Va Hosp, Charlottesville, VA 1975-1977; Surgical Oncology, Natl Cancer Inst, Bethesda, MD 1970-1972; **Fac Appt:** Prof Obstetrics & Gynecology, Univ VA Sch Med

Van Nagell Jr., John R. MD (GO) - *Spec Exp:* *Ovarian Cancer; Cervical Cancer;* **Hospital:** Univ Kentucky Med Ctr; **Address:** Dept Ob/Gyn, 800 Rose St, rm MN-308, Lexington, KY 40536; **Phone:** (859) 323-5553; **Board Cert:** Gynecologic Oncology 1976, Obstetrics & Gynecology 1973; **Med School:** Univ Penn 1967; **Resid:** Obstetrics & Gynecology, Kentucky Med Ctr, Lexington, KY 1968-1971; **Fac Appt:** Prof Obstetrics & Gynecology, Univ KY Coll Med

Midwest

Belinson, Jerome Leslie MD (GO) - *Spec Exp:* *Ovarian Cancer; Cervical Cancer; Cervical Dysplasia;* **Hospital:** Cleveland Clin Fdn (page 57); **Address:** Cleveland Clinic Foundation-OB/Gyn, Euclid Ave, Bldg A - Ste 8, Cleveland, OH 44195; **Phone:** (216) 444-7933; **Board Cert:** Obstetrics & Gynecology 1998, Gynecologic Oncology 1980; **Med School:** Univ MO-Columbia Sch Med 1968; **Resid:** Obstetrics & Gynecology, Columbia Presby Med Ctr, New York, NY 1969-1973; **Fellow:** Gynecologic Oncology, Jackson Meml Hosp, Miami, Florida, FL 1975-1977; **Fac Appt:** Prof Obstetrics & Gynecology, Ohio State Univ

Copeland, Larry James MD (GO) - *Spec Exp:* *Ovarian Cancer; Pelvic Surgery;* **Hospital:** Arthur G James Cancer Hosp & Research Inst; **Address:** 1654 Upham Drive, Ste 505, Columbus, OH 43210-1250; **Phone:** (614) 293-8697; **Board Cert:** Obstetrics & Gynecology 1991, Gynecologic Oncology 1981; **Med School:** Canada 1973; **Resid:** Obstetrics & Gynecology, McMaster Univ Affiliated Hosp, Hamilton, CN 1973-1977; **Fellow:** Gynecologic Oncology, Univ Texas M.D. Anderson Cancer Center, Houston, TX 1977-1979; **Fac Appt:** Prof Obstetrics & Gynecology, Ohio State Univ

De Geest, Koen MD (GO) - *Spec Exp:* *Ovarian Cancer; Cervical Cancer; Clinical Trials;* **Hospital:** Rush-Presby - St Luke's Med Ctr (page 72); **Address:** 1725 W Harrison St, Ste 863, Chicago, IL 60612; **Phone:** (312) 942-6723; **Board Cert:** Gynecologic Oncology 1997, Obstetrics & Gynecology 1997; **Med School:** Belgium 1977; **Resid:** Obstetrics & Gynecology, Univ Ghent, Ghent, Belgium 1977-1982; **Fellow:** Gynecologic Oncology, Penn State/Hershey Med Ctr, Hershey, PA 1987-1990; **Fac Appt:** Assoc Prof Obstetrics & Gynecology, Rush Med Coll

Herbst, Arthur MD (GO) - *Spec Exp:* *Ovarian Cancer;* **Hospital:** Univ of Chicago Hosps (page 76); **Address:** 5841 S Maryland Ave, MS 2050, Chicago, IL 60637; **Phone:** (773) 702-6127; **Board Cert:** Obstetrics & Gynecology 1983, Gynecologic Oncology 1974; **Med School:** Harvard Med Sch 1959; **Resid:** Surgery, Mass Genl Hosp, Boston, MA 1960-1962; Obstetrics & Gynecology, Women's Hosp, Boston, MA 1962-1965; **Fac Appt:** Prof Obstetrics & Gynecology, Univ Chicago-Pritzker Sch Med

Johnston, Carolyn Marie MD (GO) - *Spec Exp:* *Gynecologic Cancer; Gynecologic Surgery-Complex;* **Hospital:** Univ of MI Hlth Ctr; **Address:** Womens Hosp, rm L4606, 1500 E Medical Center Dr, Ann Arbor, MI 48109-0276; **Phone:** (734) 647-8906; **Board Cert:** Gynecologic Oncology 2005, Obstetrics & Gynecology 2001; **Med School:** Yale Univ 1984; **Resid:** Obstetrics & Gynecology, Univ Chicago Hosp, Chicago, IL 1985-1988; **Fellow:** Gynecologic Oncology, Mt Sinai Hosp, New York, NY 1988-1990; **Fac Appt:** Asst Clin Prof Gynecologic Oncology, Univ Mich Med Sch

Kim, Woo Shin MD (GO) - *Spec Exp:* *Ovarian Cancer; Cervical Cancer;* **Hospital:** Henry Ford Hosp; **Address:** 2799 W Grand Blvd, Detroit, MI 48202-2608; **Phone:** (313) 916-2465; **Board Cert:** Obstetrics & Gynecology 1977, Gynecologic Oncology 1979; **Med School:** South Korea 1966; **Resid:** Obstetrics & Gynecology, Boston City Hosp, Boston, MA 1970-1973; **Fellow:** Gynecologic Oncology, Meml Sloan-Kettering Cancer Ctr, New York, NY 1973-1976; **Fac Appt:** Assoc Clin Prof Obstetrics & Gynecology, Wayne State Univ

Look, Katherine MD (GO) - *Spec Exp:* *Ovarian Cancer;* **Hospital:** IN Univ Hosp (page 63); **Address:** 535 Barnhill Drive, Ste 434, Indianapolis, IN 46202; **Phone:** (317) 274-8987; **Board Cert:** Obstetrics & Gynecology 1996, Gynecologic Oncology 1996; **Med School:** Univ Mich Med Sch 1979; **Resid:** Obstetrics & Gynecology, Univ Illinois, Chicago, IL 1979-1983; **Fellow:** Gynecologic Oncology, Meml Sloan Kettering Cancer Ctr, New York, NY 1984-1986; **Fac Appt:** Prof Obstetrics & Gynecology, Indiana Univ

Lurain, John R MD (GO) - *Spec Exp:* *Trophoblastic Disease; Uterine Cancer; Ovarian Cancer;* **Hospital:** Northwestern Meml Hosp; **Address:** Northwestern Meml Hosp, 333 E Superior St, Chicago, IL 60611-3056; **Phone:** (312) 926-7365; **Board Cert:** Obstetrics & Gynecology 1977, Gynecologic Oncology 1981; **Med School:** Univ NC Sch Med 1972; **Resid:** Obstetrics & Gynecology, Univ Pittsburgh, Pittsburgh, PA 1972-1975; **Fellow:** Gynecologic Oncology, Roswell Park Cancer Ctr, Buffalo, NY 1977-1979; **Fac Appt:** Prof Obstetrics & Gynecology, Northwestern Univ

Moore, David H MD (GO) - *Spec Exp:* *Cervical Cancer; Ovarian Cancer;* **Hospital:** IN Univ Hosp (page 63); **Address:** 535 Barnhill Drive, Ste 433, Indianapolis, IN 46202; **Phone:** (317) 274-2422; **Board Cert:** Obstetrics & Gynecology 1989, Gynecologic Oncology 1990; **Med School:** Indiana Univ 1982; **Resid:** Obstetrics & Gynecology, Indiana Univ, Indianapolis, IN 1982-1986; **Fellow:** Gynecologic Oncology, Univ North Carolina, Chapel Hill, NC 1986-1988; **Fac Appt:** Assoc Prof Gynecologic Oncology, Indiana Univ

Mutch, David MD (GO) - *Spec Exp:* Pelvic Reconstruction; **Hospital:** Barnes-Jewish Hosp (page 55); **Address:** 4911 Barnes Hospital Plaza, St. Louis, MO 63110; **Phone:** (314) 362-3181; **Board Cert:** Obstetrics & Gynecology 1999, Gynecologic Oncology 1996; **Med School:** Washington Univ, St Louis 1980; **Resid:** Obstetrics & Gynecology, Barnes Hosp/Wash Univ of St Louis, St Louis, MO 1981-1984; **Fellow:** Gynecologic Oncology, Duke Univ Med Ctr, Durham, NC 1984-1987; **Fac Appt:** Assoc Prof Obstetrics & Gynecology, Washington Univ, St Louis

Podratz, Karl C MD/PhD (GO) - *Spec Exp:* Pelvic Reconstruction; **Hospital:** Mayo Med Ctr & Clin - Rochester, MN; **Address:** 200 1st St SW, Rochester, MN 55905; **Phone:** (507) 266-7712; **Board Cert:** Obstetrics & Gynecology 1993, Gynecologic Oncology 1982; **Med School:** St Louis Univ 1974; **Resid:** Obstetrics & Gynecology, Univ Chicago Hosp, Chicago, IL 1974-1977; **Fellow:** Gynecologic Oncology, Mayo Clinic, Rochester, MN 1977-1979; **Fac Appt:** Prof Obstetrics & Gynecology, Mayo Med Sch

Potkul, Ronald MD (GO) - *Spec Exp:* Ovarian Cancer; Cervical Cancer; **Hospital:** Loyola Univ Med Ctr; **Address:** 2160 S First Ave, Bldg 112 - rm 267, Maywood, IL 60153; **Phone:** (708) 327-3314; **Board Cert:** Gynecologic Oncology 1990, Obstetrics & Gynecology 1989; **Med School:** Univ Chicago-Pritzker Sch Med 1981; **Resid:** Obstetrics & Gynecology, Univ Chicago Hosp, Chicago, IL 1981-1985; **Fellow:** Gynecologic Oncology, Georgetown Univ, Washington, DC 1985-1988; **Fac Appt:** Prof Obstetrics & Gynecology, Loyola Univ-Stritch Sch Med

Reynolds, R Kevin MD (GO) - *Spec Exp:* Gynecologic Oncology - General; **Hospital:** Univ of MI Hlth Ctr; **Address:** L4510 Women's Hosp, 1500 E Med Ctr Drive, Box 0276, Ann Arbor, MI 48109-0276; **Phone:** (734) 764-9106; **Board Cert:** Gynecologic Oncology 1998, Obstetrics & Gynecology 1998; **Med School:** Univ New Mexico 1982; **Resid:** Obstetrics & Gynecology, Univ Vt Hosp, Burlington, VT 1983-1986; **Fellow:** Gynecologic Oncology, Univ Michigan Med Ctr, Ann Arbor, MI 1988-1991; **Fac Appt:** Asst Prof Obstetrics & Gynecology, Univ Mich Med Sch

Rose, Peter G MD (GO) - *Spec Exp:* Cervical Cancer; **Hospital:** MetroHealth Medical Center; **Address:** MacDonald Women's Hosp, Univ Hosp-Cleveland, 11100 Euclid Ave Fl 7 - rm 7218, Cleveland, OH 44106; **Phone:** (216) 844-3340; **Board Cert:** Obstetrics & Gynecology 1999, Gynecologic Oncology 1990; **Med School:** Boston Univ 1981; **Resid:** Surgery, Vanderbilt Med Ctr, Nashville, TN 1981-1983; Obstetrics & Gynecology, Ohio State Univ Med Ctr, ColumbusBuffalo, NY 1983-1986; **Fellow:** Gynecologic Oncology, Roswell Park Med Ctr, Buffalo, NY 1986-1988; **Fac Appt:** Assoc Prof Case West Res Univ

Schink, Julian C MD (GO) - *Spec Exp:* Gynecologic Oncology - General; **Hospital:** Univ WI Hosp & Clins; **Address:** 600 Highland Ave, rm H4/636, Madison, WI 53792; **Phone:** (608) 263-1209; **Board Cert:** Gynecologic Oncology 1990, Obstetrics & Gynecology 1989; **Med School:** Univ Tex, San Antonio 1982; **Resid:** Obstetrics & Gynecology, Northwestern Univ Med Sch, Chicago, IL 1982-1986; **Fellow:** Gynecologic Oncology, UCLA Med Ctr, Los Angeles, CA 1986-1988; **Fac Appt:** Prof Gynecologic Oncology, Univ Wisc

Smith, Donna Marie MD (GO) - *Spec Exp:* Cervical Cancer; Ovarian Cancer; **Hospital:** Loyola Univ Med Ctr; **Address:** 2160 S First Ave, Bldg 112 - rm 340, Maywood, IL 60153; **Phone:** (708) 327-3314; **Board Cert:** Obstetrics & Gynecology 1997, Gynecologic Oncology 1997; **Med School:** Univ MO-Kansas City 1980; **Resid:** Obstetrics & Gynecology, Emory Univ Hosp, Atlanta, GA 1981-1984; **Fellow:** Gynecologic Oncology, Georgetown Univ Med Ctr, Washington, DC 1984-1987; **Fac Appt:** Assoc Prof Obstetrics & Gynecology, Loyola Univ-Stritch Sch Med

Waggoner, Steven MD (GO) - *Spec Exp: Ovarian Cancer; Cervical Cancer;* **Hospital:** Univ of Chicago Hosps (page 76); **Address:** Dept OB/GYN, 5841 S Maryland Ave, MS 2050, Chicago, IL 60637; **Phone:** (773) 702-6722; **Board Cert:** Gynecologic Oncology 1994, Obstetrics & Gynecology 1992; **Med School:** Univ Wash 1984; **Resid:** Obstetrics & Gynecology, Univ Chicago, Chicago, IL 1984-1988; **Fellow:** Gynecologic Oncology, Georgetown Univ, Washington, DC 1988-1991; **Fac Appt:** Prof Gynecologic Oncology, Univ Chicago-Pritzker Sch Med

Webb, Maurice James MD (GO) - *Spec Exp: Gynecologic Cancer; Pelvic Reconstruction;* **Hospital:** Mayo Med Ctr & Clin - Rochester, MN; **Address:** Mayo Clinic, 200 1st St SW, Rochester, MN 55905; **Phone:** (507) 266-8683; **Board Cert:** Obstetrics & Gynecology 1974, Gynecologic Oncology 1976; **Med School:** Australia 1965; **Resid:** Obstetrics & Gynecology, Univ Queensland-Royal Hosp, England, UK 1968-1969; Obstetrics & Gynecology, St Marys Hosp, Portsmouth, UK 1970-1971; **Fellow:** Gynecologic Oncology, Mayo Clinic, Rochester, MN 1971-1972; **Fac Appt:** Prof Obstetrics & Gynecology, Mayo Med Sch

Southwest

Finan, Michael A MD (GO) - *Spec Exp: Pelvic Cancer;* **Hospital:** Ochsner Found Hosp; **Address:** Ochsner Clin, Div Gyn Oncology, 1514 Jefferson Hwy, New Orleans, LA 70121-2429; **Phone:** (504) 842-4165; **Board Cert:** Obstetrics & Gynecology 1993, Gynecologic Oncology 1997; **Med School:** Louisiana State Univ 1986; **Resid:** Obstetrics & Gynecology, Univ South Fla Affiliated Hosps, Tampa, FL 1986-1990; **Fellow:** Gynecologic Oncology, Univ Soutt Fla Coll Med, Tampa, FL 1990-1992

Freedman, Ralph MD (GO) - *Spec Exp: Immune Deficiency; Ovarian Cancer;* **Hospital:** Univ of TX MD Anderson Cancer Ctr, The; **Address:** Univ Texas MD Anderson Canc Ctr, Dept Gyn Onc, 1515 Holcombe Blvd, Box 440, Houston, TX 77030; **Phone:** (713) 792-2764; **Board Cert:** Obstetrics & Gynecology 1980; **Med School:** South Africa 1965; **Resid:** Obstetrics & Gynecology, Queen Victoria-Johannesburg-Baragwanath Hosps, Johannesburg, S Africa 1968-1971; **Fellow:** Gynecologic Oncology, Univ Texas MD Anderson Canc Ctr, Houston, TX 1976; **Fac Appt:** Prof Gynecologic Oncology, Univ Tex, Houston

Fromm, Geri Lynn MD (GO) - *Spec Exp: Gynecologic Oncology - General;* **Hospital:** St Luke's Episcopal Hosp - Houston; **Address:** 2223 Dorrington St, Houston, TX 77030; **Phone:** (713) 665-0404; **Board Cert:** Obstetrics & Gynecology 1998, Gynecologic Oncology 1991; **Med School:** Northwestern Univ 1981; **Resid:** Obstetrics & Gynecology, Magee Womens-Univ Pittsburgh, Pittsburgh, PA 1981-1985; **Fellow:** Gynecologic Oncology, MD Anderson-Univ Texas, Houston, TX 1985-1987

Gershenson, David Marc MD (GO) - *Spec Exp: Ovarian Cancer; Uterine Cancer;* **Hospital:** Univ of TX MD Anderson Cancer Ctr, The; **Address:** Univ Tex-MD Anderson Cancer Ctr, 1515 Holcombe Blvd, Box 440, Houston, TX 77030; **Phone:** (713) 745-2565; **Board Cert:** Obstetrics & Gynecology 1991, Gynecologic Oncology 1981; **Med School:** Vanderbilt Univ 1971; **Resid:** Obstetrics & Gynecology, Yale-New Haven Hosp, New Haven, CT 1972-1975; **Fellow:** Gynecologic Oncology, MD Anderson Hosp, Houston, TX 1977-1979; **Fac Appt:** Clin Prof Obstetrics & Gynecology, Univ Tex, Houston

Roman-Lopez, Juan J MD (GO) - *Spec Exp: Vulva Disease/Neoplasia; Bladder Problems Post-Hysterectomy; Gynecologic Oncology;* **Hospital:** UAMS; **Address:** 4301 W Markham St, Ste 518, Little Rock, AR 72205-7199; **Phone:** (501) 296-1099; **Board Cert:** Obstetrics & Gynecology 1971; **Med School:** Univ Puerto Rico 1963; **Resid:** Obstetrics & Gynecology, San Juan City Hosp, Puerto Rico 1966-1967; Obstetrics & Gynecology, Tulane-Charity Hosp, New Orleans, LA 1967-1969; **Fellow:** Gynecologic Oncology, Tulane-LSU Med Ctr, New Orleans, LA 1969-1970; **Fac Appt:** Assoc Clin Prof Obstetrics & Gynecology, Univ Ark

West Coast and Pacific

Berek, Jonathan S MD (GO) - *Spec Exp:* Ovarian Cancer; **Hospital:** UCLA Med Ctr; **Address:** 200 UCLA Med Plaza, Ste 430, Los Angeles, CA 90095-6928; **Phone:** (310) 794-7274; **Board Cert:** Gynecologic Oncology 1983, Obstetrics & Gynecology 1991; **Med School:** Johns Hopkins Univ 1975; **Resid:** Obstetrics & Gynecology, Harvard Med Sch-Brigham & Woman's Hosp, Boston, MA 1976-1979; **Fellow:** Gynecologic Oncology, UCLA Sch Med, Los Angeles, CA 1979-1981; **Fac Appt:** Prof Obstetrics & Gynecology, UCLA

Berman, Michael Leonard MD (GO) - *Spec Exp:* Gynecologic Cancer; **Hospital:** UCI Med Ctr; **Address:** UCI Med Ctr, Div Gyn/Onc, 101 The City Drive S, Bldg 23 - rm 107, Orange, CA 92868-3298; **Phone:** (714) 456-6570; **Board Cert:** Obstetrics & Gynecology 1999, Gynecologic Oncology 1999; **Med School:** Geo Wash Univ 1967; **Resid:** Obstetrics & Gynecology, GW Univ Hosp, Washington, DC 1968-1969; Obstetrics & Gynecology, Los Angeles Co-Harbor, Torrence, CA 1971-1974; **Fellow:** Gynecologic Oncology, UCLA Med Ctr, Los Angeles, CA 1974-1976; **Fac Appt:** Prof Obstetrics & Gynecology, UC Irvine

Greer, Benjamin MD (GO) - *Spec Exp:* Gynecologic Oncology - General; **Hospital:** Univ WA Med Ctr; **Address:** Dept OB/GYN, Box 356460, 1959 NE Pacific St, Seattle, WA 98195; **Phone:** (206) 685-2463; **Board Cert:** Obstetrics & Gynecology 1989, Gynecologic Oncology 1983; **Med School:** Univ Penn 1966; **Resid:** Obstetrics & Gynecology, Univ Colorado Med Ctr, Denver, CO 1967-1970; **Fac Appt:** Prof Obstetrics & Gynecology, Univ Wash

Lagasse, Leo D MD (GO) - *Spec Exp:* Ovarian Cancer; **Hospital:** Cedars-Sinai Med Ctr; **Address:** Cedars-Sinai Med Ctr, 8700 Beverly Blvd Ste 160W, Los Angeles, CA 90048-1804; **Phone:** (310) 423-3373; **Board Cert:** Obstetrics & Gynecology 1967, Gynecologic Oncology 1974; **Med School:** Univ VA Sch Med 1959; **Resid:** Obstetrics & Gynecology, UCLA Med Ctr, Los Angeles, CA 1960-1964; **Fac Appt:** Prof Obstetrics & Gynecology, UCLA

Morrow, Charles Paul MD (GO) - *Spec Exp:* Gynecologic Oncology - General; **Hospital:** USC Norris Cancer Comp Ctr; **Address:** USC K Norris Jr Cancer Hosp, 1441 Eastlake Ave, Ste 7419, Los Angeles, CA 90033; **Phone:** (323) 865-3922; **Board Cert:** Obstetrics & Gynecology 1970, Gynecologic Oncology 1974; **Med School:** Loyola Univ-Stritch Sch Med 1962; **Resid:** Obstetrics & Gynecology, Little Co Mary Hosp, Evergreen, IL 1965-1966; Obstetrics & Gynecology, Chicago Mercy Hosp, Chicago, IL 1966-1968; **Fellow:** Gynecologic Oncology, MD Anderson Hosp Houston, Houston, TX 1968-1970; **Fac Appt:** Prof Obstetrics & Gynecology, UCLA

Stern, Jeffrey L MD (GO) - *Spec Exp:* Gynecologic Oncology - General; **Hospital:** Alta Bates Summit Med Ctr - Ashby Campus; **Address:** Womens Cancer Ctr Northern Calif, 2100 Webster St, Ste 319, San Francisco, CA 94115; **Phone:** (415) 202-1570; **Board Cert:** Obstetrics & Gynecology 1983, Gynecologic Oncology 1984; **Med School:** SUNY Syracuse 1976; **Resid:** Obstetrics & Gynecology, Johns Hopkins Hosp, Baltimore, MD 1977-1980; **Fellow:** Gynecologic Oncology, USC Med Ctr, Los Angeles, CA 1980-1982; **Fac Appt:** Assoc Prof Obstetrics & Gynecology, UCSF

Teng, Nelson NH MD/PhD (GO) - *Spec Exp:* Gynecologic Cancer; **Hospital:** Stanford Med Ctr; **Address:** Stanford Univ Sch Med, Dept Gyn Onc, 300 Pasteur Drive, rm HH333, Stanford, CA 94305-5317; **Phone:** (650) 498-8080; **Board Cert:** Obstetrics & Gynecology 1985, Gynecologic Oncology 1987; **Med School:** Univ Miami Sch Med 1977; **Resid:** Obstetrics & Gynecology, UCLA Med Ctr, Los Angeles, CA 1978-1981; **Fellow:** Gynecologic Oncology, Stanford Univ Sch Med, Stanford, CA 1984; **Fac Appt:** Assoc Prof Obstetrics & Gynecology, Stanford Univ

HAND SURGERY

(a subspecialty of ORTHOPAEDICS, SURGERY or PLASTIC SURGERY)

A specialist trained in the investigation, preservation and restoration by medical, surgical and rehabilitative means of all structures of the upper extremity directly affecting the form and function of the hand and wrist.

ORTHOPAEDICS

An orthopaedic surgeon is involved with the care of patients whose musculoskeletal problems include congenital deformities, trauma, infections, tumors, metabolic disturbances of the musculoskeletal system, deformities, injuries and degenerative diseases of the spine, hands, feet, knee, hip, shoulder and elbow in children and adults. An orthopaedic surgeon is also concerned with primary and secondary muscular problems and the effects of central or peripheral nervous system lesions of the musculoskeletal system.

SURGERY

A surgeon manages a broad spectrum of surgical conditions affecting almost any area of the body. The surgeon establishes the diagnosis and provides the preoperative, operative and postoperative care to surgical patients and is usually responsible for the comprehensive management of the trauma victim and the critically ill surgical patient. The surgeon uses a variety of diagnostic techniques, including endoscopy, for observing internal structures, and may use specialized instruments during operative procedures. A general surgeon is expected to be familiar with the salient features of other surgical specialties in order to recognize problems in those areas and to know when to refer a patient to another specialist.

PLASTIC SURGERY

A plastic surgeon deals with the repair, reconstruction or replacement of physical defects of form or function involving the skin, musculoskeletal system, craniomaxillofacial structures, hand, extremities, breast and trunk and external genitalia. He/she uses aesthetic surgical principles not only to improve undesirable qualities of normal structures but in all reconstructive procedures as well.

Training required: Five years (including general surgery) in orthopaedics *plus* two years in clinical practice before final certification is achieved *plus* additional training and examination in hand surgery OR five to seven years in plastic surgery *plus* additional training and examination in hand surgery

273

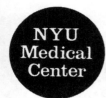

550 First Avenue (at 31st Street)
New York, NY 10016
Physician Referral: (888) 7-NYU-MED
(888-769-8633) www.nyumedicalcenter.org

HAND SURGERY

The **NYU-HJD Hand Service** (a joint division of NYU Medical Center and The Hospital for Joint Diseases Orthopedic Institute) provides comprehensive care of patients with hand and wrist disorders, including:

- Fractures
- Congenital anomalies
- Soft tissue and skeletal trauma
- Degenerative and rheumatoid arthritis
- Sports-related injuries of the hand and wrist
- Vascular disorders
- Tumors

Specific emphases include fractures of the wrist and distal radius and reconstructive aspects of hand surgery, as reflected by the large volume of cases involving posttraumatic, arthritis, congenital, neuromuscular, and neoplastic conditions.

The research focus of the **NYU-HJD Hand Service** is on a variety of clinical problems, including non-unions of the scaphoid, avascular necrosis of the lunate (Kienböck's disease), intercarpal subluxations, and neuropathies of the upper extremity. Basic research projects are also frequently conducted; one current study seeks to determine the efficacy of utilizing a cold laser for tendon healing.

After surgery, the **Rusk Institute of Rehabilitation Medicine's Hand Therapy Unit** helps surgical patients recover full or partial use of their hands, providing comprehensive rehabilitation for a variety of ailments associated with the hand and upper body. The Hand Therapy Unit specializes in fractures, traumatic injuries, tendonitis, sports injuries, work-related injuries, repetitive stress injuries, carpal tunnel syndrome, tendon and nerve repairs, and arthritis. It is staffed by licensed occupational therapists who specialize in the treatment of the hand and upper extremities.

NYU MEDICAL CENTER

Optimal care of hands requires a hand surgeon, a regional specialist who has extracted and mastered the appropriate aspects of traditional general, plastic, orthopedic, and neurological surgical specialities, along with post-operative rehabilitation techniques.

At NYU Medical Center, world-class hand surgery and rehabilitation are brought together, ensuring patients and their families have a positive outcome.

Physician Referral
(888) 7-NYU-MED
(888-769-8633)
www.nyumedicalcenter.org

PHYSICIAN LISTINGS

Hand Surgery

New England

Belsky, Mark R MD (HS) - *Spec Exp:* *Hand Surgery - General;* **Hospital:** Newton - Wellesley Hosp; **Address:** Bldg Green - Ste 563, 2000 Washington St, Newton, MA 02462; **Phone:** (617) 965-4263; **Board Cert:** Hand Surgery 1990, Orthopaedic Surgery 1982; **Med School:** Tufts Univ 1974; **Resid:** Surgery, Peter Bent Brigham Hosp, Boston, MA 1975-1976; Orthopaedic Surgery, Tufts-New Eng Med Ctr, Boston, MA 1976-1979; **Fellow:** Hand Surgery, Roosevelt Hosp, New York, NY 1980; **Fac Appt:** Assoc Clin Prof Orthopaedic Surgery, Tufts Univ

Upton, Joseph MD (HS) - *Spec Exp:* *Hand-Congenital Anomaly; Hand Microsurgical Reconstruction;* **Hospital:** Children's Hospital - Boston; **Address:** 830 Boylston St, Ste 212, Chestnut Hill, MA 02467; **Phone:** (617) 739-1972; **Board Cert:** Plastic Surgery 1981, Hand Surgery 1992; **Med School:** Baylor Coll Med 1970; **Resid:** Orthopaedic Surgery, Eisenhower Med Ctr, Augusta, GA 1972-1974; Surgery, St Joseph Hosp, Houston, TX 1974-1976; **Fellow:** Hand Surgery, Roosevelt Hosp, New York, NY 1976-1977; **Fac Appt:** Assoc Prof Surgery, Harvard Med Sch

Waters, Peter Michael MD (HS) - *Spec Exp:* *Brachial Plexus; Hand-Congenital Anomaly;* **Hospital:** Children's Hospital - Boston; **Address:** Chldrns Hosp, Dept Ortho Surg, 300 Longwood Ave, Boston, MA 02115-5724; **Phone:** (617) 355-6021; **Board Cert:** Orthopaedic Surgery 1991, Hand Surgery 1992; **Med School:** Tufts Univ 1981; **Resid:** Pediatrics, Mass Genl Hosp, Boston, MA 1981-1983; Orthopaedic Surgery, Harvard Combined Prog, Boston, MA 1984-1988; **Fellow:** Hand Surgery, Brigham/Childrens Hosp, Boston, MA 1988-1989; **Fac Appt:** Assoc Prof Orthopaedic Surgery, Harvard Med Sch

Weiss, Arnold Peter MD (HS) - *Spec Exp:* *Carpal Tunnel Syndrome; Wrist Surgery; Elbow Replacement;* **Hospital:** Rhode Island Hosp; **Address:** Univ Orth Inc, 2 Dudley St, Ste 200, Providence, RI 02905-3248; **Phone:** (401) 457-1520; **Board Cert:** Orthopaedic Surgery 1993, Hand Surgery 1994; **Med School:** Johns Hopkins Univ 1985; **Resid:** Orthopaedic Surgery, Johns Hopkins Hosp, Baltimore, MD 1986-1990; **Fellow:** Hand Surgery, Ind Hand Ctr, Indianapolis, IN 1990-1991; **Fac Appt:** Prof Orthopaedic Surgery, Brown Univ

Mid Atlantic

Beasley, Robert MD (HS) - *Spec Exp:* *Plastic Surgery of Hand; Paralytic Disorders; Arthritis Hand Surgery;* **Hospital:** NYU Med Ctr (page 71); **Address:** 345 E 37th St, Ste 306, New York, NY 10016-3256; **Phone:** (212) 986-9494; **Board Cert:** Plastic Surgery 1968; **Med School:** Univ Tenn Coll Med, Memphis 1953; **Resid:** Hand Surgery, St Luke's Roosevelt Hosp, New York, NY 1960-1961; Plastic Surgery, Clumbia-Presbyterian Med Ctr, New York, NY 1962-1963; **Fac Appt:** Prof Surgery, NYU Sch Med

Chiu, David MD (HS) - *Spec Exp:* *Hand & Microvascular Surgery; Cosmetic Surgery;* **Hospital:** NYU Med Ctr (page 71); **Address:** 900 Park Ave at 79th St, New York, NY 10021; **Phone:** (212) 879-8880; **Board Cert:** Plastic Surgery 1982, Hand Surgery 1990; **Med School:** Columbia P&S 1973; **Resid:** Surgery, Columbia-Presby Med Ctr, New York, NY 1973-1977; Plastic Surgery, Barnes Hosp-Washington Univ, St Louis, MO 1977-1979; **Fellow:** Hand Surgery, NYU Med Ctr, New York, NY 1980; **Fac Appt:** Prof Surgery, Columbia P&S

Culp, Randall MD (HS) - *Spec Exp:* *Microsurgery;* **Hospital:** Thomas Jefferson Univ Hosp; **Address:** 700 S Henderson Rd, Ste 200, King of Prussia, PA 19406; **Phone:** (610) 768-4474; **Board Cert:** Orthopaedic Surgery 1990, Hand Surgery 1992; **Med School:** Penn State Univ-Hershey Med Ctr 1982; **Resid:** Orthopaedic Surgery, Hosp Univ Penn, Philadelphia, PA 1983-1987; **Fellow:** Hand Surgery, Hosp Univ Penn, Philadelphia, PA 1987-1988; **Fac Appt:** Assoc Prof Orthopaedic Surgery, Jefferson Med Coll

Glickel, Steven MD (HS) - *Spec Exp:* Hand & Wrist Surgery; Elbow Disorders/Surgery; **Hospital:** St Luke's - Roosevelt Hosp Ctr - Roosevelt Div (page 58); **Address:** 1000 10th Ave Fl 3, New York, NY 10019; **Phone:** (212) 523-7590; **Board Cert:** Orthopaedic Surgery 1985, Hand Surgery 1998; **Med School:** Harvard Med Sch 1976; **Resid:** Surgery, Columbia Presby Hosp, New York, NY 1976-1978; Orthopaedic Surgery, Harvard Comb Ortho, Boston, MA 1978-1981; **Fellow:** Hand Surgery, St Luke's-Roosevelt Hosp Ctr, New York, NY 1982-1983; **Fac Appt:** Assoc Clin Prof Orthopaedic Surgery, Columbia P&S

Lubahn, John D MD (HS) - *Spec Exp:* Microsurgery; **Hospital:** Hamot Med Ctr; **Address:** 300 State St, Ste 205, Hamot Med Ctr, Erie, PA 16507-1429; **Phone:** (814) 456-6022; **Board Cert:** Orthopaedic Surgery 1992, Hand Surgery 1998; **Med School:** Case West Res Univ 1975; **Resid:** Surgery, Univ Rochester Med Ctr, Rochester, MN 1976-1977; Orthopaedic Surgery, Univ Rochester Med Ctr, Rochester, MN 1977-1980; **Fellow:** Hand Surgery, Univ Louisville Hosp, Louisville, KY 1980-1981

McCormack Jr, Richard R MD (HS) - *Spec Exp:* Dupuytren's Contracture; Arthritis Hand Surgery; Hand & Wrist Fractures; **Hospital:** Hosp For Special Surgery (page 62); **Address:** 535 E 70th St, New York, NY 10021; **Phone:** (212) 606-1230; **Board Cert:** Orthopaedic Surgery 1983, Hand Surgery 1992; **Med School:** Cornell Univ-Weill Med Coll 1975; **Resid:** Surgery, Roosevelt Hosp, New York, NY 1976-1977; Orthopaedic Surgery, Hosp For Special Surg, New York, NY 1977-1980; **Fellow:** Hand Surgery, Roosevelt Hosp, New York, NY 1980-1981; **Fac Appt:** Assoc Clin Prof Orthopaedic Surgery, Cornell Univ-Weill Med Coll

Melone Jr, Charles P MD (HS) - *Spec Exp:* Arthritis Hand Surgery; Wrist Surgery; **Hospital:** Beth Israel Med Ctr - Petrie Division (page 58); **Address:** 321 E 34th St, New York, NY 10016; **Phone:** (212) 340-0000; **Board Cert:** Orthopaedic Surgery 1976, Hand Surgery 1993; **Med School:** Georgetown Univ 1969; **Resid:** Surgery, Nassau County Med Ctr, East Meadow, NY 1970-1971; Orthopaedic Surgery, Nassau County Med Ctr, East Meadow, NY 1971-1974; **Fellow:** Hand Surgery, NYU Med Ctr, New York, NY 1974-1975; **Fac Appt:** Clin Prof Orthopaedic Surgery, Albert Einstein Coll Med

Patel, Mukund MD (HS) - *Spec Exp:* Arthritis; Carpal Tunnel Syndrome; **Hospital:** Maimonides Med Ctr (page 65); **Address:** Orthopedic Surg Assocs, 4901 Fort Hamilton Pkwy, Brooklyn, NY 11219; **Phone:** (718) 435-4944; **Board Cert:** Orthopaedic Surgery 1972, Hand Surgery 2000; **Med School:** India 1966; **Resid:** Orthopaedic Surgery, Maimonides Med Ctr, Brooklyn, NY 1968-1970; **Fellow:** Hand Surgery, Mass Genl Hosp, Boston, MA 1970-1971; **Fac Appt:** Asst Clin Prof Surgery, SUNY Hlth Sci Ctr

Peimer, Clayton Austin MD (HS) - *Spec Exp:* Hand Surgery - General; **Hospital:** Millard Fillmore Hosp; **Address:** Hand Center of Western New York, 3 Gates Cir, Buffalo, NY 14209-1120; **Phone:** (716) 887-4599; **Board Cert:** Orthopaedic Surgery 1978, Hand Surgery 2000; **Med School:** SUNY Syracuse 1971; **Resid:** Surgery, Beth Israel Med Ctr, New York, NY 1972-1973; Orthopaedic Surgery, SUNY Upstate Med tr, Syracuse, NY 1973-1976; **Fellow:** Hand Surgery, Mass Genl Hosp, Boston, MA 1976-1977; **Fac Appt:** Assoc Prof Orthopaedic Surgery, SUNY Buffalo

Strauch, Robert MD (HS) - *Spec Exp:* Hand-Congenital Anomaly; Hand & Elbow Nerve Disorders; Hand & Wrist Fractures; **Hospital:** NY Presby Hosp - Columbia Presby Med Ctr (page 70); **Address:** 161 Fort Washington Ave, New York, NY 10032-3713; **Phone:** (212) 305-4272; **Board Cert:** Orthopaedic Surgery 1994, Hand Surgery 1995; **Med School:** Columbia P&S 1986; **Resid:** Orthopaedic Surgery, Columbia-Presby Hosp, New York, NY 1988-1991; **Fellow:** Hand Surgery, Indiana Hand Center, Indianapolis, IN 1991-1992; **Fac Appt:** Asst Prof Orthopaedic Surgery, Columbia P&S

Weiland, Andrew J MD (HS) - *Spec Exp:* Wrist/Hand Injuries; **Hospital:** Hosp For Special Surgery (page 62); **Address:** 535 E 70th St, New York, NY 10021-4872; **Phone:** (212) 606-1575; **Board Cert:** Hand Surgery 1989, Orthopaedic Surgery 1992; **Med School:** Wake Forest Univ Sch Med 1968; **Resid:** Surgery, Univ Michigan Med Ctr, Ann Arbor, MI 1969-1970; Orthopaedic Surgery, Johns Hopkins Hosp, Baltimore, MD 1972-1975; **Fellow:** Hand Surgery, Kleinert Hosp, Louisville, KY 1975; **Fac Appt:** Prof Orthopaedic Surgery, Cornell Univ-Weill Med Coll

Wolfe, Scott W MD (HS) - *Spec Exp:* Wrist Surgery; Nerve Reconstruction; **Hospital:** Hosp For Special Surgery (page 62); **Address:** 535 E 70th St, New York, NY 10021; **Phone:** (212) 606-1529; **Board Cert:** Orthopaedic Surgery 1992, Hand Surgery 1993; **Med School:** Cornell Univ-Weill Med Coll 1984; **Resid:** Orthopaedic Surgery, Hosp Special Surg, New York, NY 1986-1989; **Fellow:** Hand Surgery, Columbia Presby Med Ctr, New York, NY 1989-1990; **Fac Appt:** Prof Orthopaedic Surgery, Cornell Univ-Weill Med Coll

Southeast

Breidenbach, Warren C MD (HS) - *Spec Exp:* Transplant-Hand; **Hospital:** Jewish Hosp HlthCre Svcs Inc; **Address:** 225 Abraham Flexner Way, Ste 700, Louisville, KY 40202; **Phone:** (502) 561-4263; **Board Cert:** Plastic Surgery 1988, Hand Surgery 1992; **Med School:** Univ Calgary 1975; **Resid:** Plastic Surgery, McGill Univ, Montreal, Quebec,Canada 1976-1982; **Fellow:** Microsurgery, Eastern Va Med Sch, Norfolk, VA 1982; Hand Surgery, Louisville, KY 1983; **Fac Appt:** Asst Clin Prof Plastic Surgery, Univ Louisville Sch Med

Carneiro, Ronaldo Dos Santos MD (HS) - *Spec Exp:* Hand Surgery - General; **Hospital:** Citrus Memorial Hosp; **Address:** Cleveland Clinic-Florida, 6101 Pine Ridge Rd, Naples, FL 34119; **Phone:** (941) 348-4000; **Board Cert:** Plastic Surgery 1990, Hand Surgery 1994; **Med School:** Brazil 1970; **Resid:** Surgery, Union Meml Hosp, Baltimore, MD 1971-1975; Plastic Surgery, Allentown & Sacred Heart Hosp Ctr, Allentown, PA 1975-1977; **Fellow:** Hand Surgery, Jackson Meml Hosp-Univ Miami Hosp, Miami, FL 1977; Plastic Surgery, Univ Miami Sch Med, Miami, FL 1978; **Fac Appt:** Assoc Clin Prof Plastic Surgery, Univ S Fla Coll Med

Freeland, Alan Edward MD (HS) - *Spec Exp:* Hand & Wrist Fractures; Joint Replacement-Hand & Wrist; **Hospital:** Univ Hosps & Clins - Mississippi; **Address:** Univ Mississippi Med Ctr, Orthopaedic Assocs, 2500 N State St, Jackson, MS 39216-4505; **Phone:** (601) 815-1220; **Board Cert:** Orthopaedic Surgery 1977, Hand Surgery 2000; **Med School:** Geo Wash Univ 1965; **Resid:** Orthopaedic Surgery, Letterman AMC, San Francisco, CA 1973-1975; Orthopaedic Surgery, Johns Hopkins Hosp, Baltimore, MD 1967-1970; **Fellow:** Hand Surgery, Jackson Meml Hosp-Univ Miami Med Ctr, Miami, FL 1975; **Fac Appt:** Prof Orthopaedic Surgery, Univ Miss

Freshwater, M Felix MD (HS) - *Spec Exp:* Plastic Surgery of Hand; **Hospital:** Baptist Hosp - Miami; **Address:** Miami Inst of Hand & Microsurgery, 9100 S Dadeland Blvd, Ste 502, Miami, FL 33156-7815; **Phone:** (305) 670-9988; **Board Cert:** Plastic Surgery 1980, Hand Surgery 1997; **Med School:** Yale Univ 1972; **Resid:** Surgery, Yale-New Haven Hosp, New Haven, CT 1972-1974; Plastic Surgery, Jackson Meml Hosp, Miami, FL 1977-1978; **Fellow:** Hand Surgery, Johns Hopkins Univ, Baltimore, MD 1974-1977; Hand Surgery, Univ Louisville, Louisville, KY 1979; **Fac Appt:** Asst Clin Prof Surgery, Univ Miami Sch Med

Greene, Thomas MD (HS) - *Spec Exp:* Microvascular Surgery; Nerve Surgery; **Hospital:** Tampa Genl Hosp; **Address:** 2727 W Dr Martin Luther King Jr Blvd, Ste 560, Tampa, FL 33607-6009; **Phone:** (813) 873-0337; **Board Cert:** Orthopaedic Surgery 1983, Hand Surgery 2000; **Med School:** Ohio State Univ 1975; **Resid:** Surgery, Univ Michigan, Ann Arbor, MI 1976-1977; Orthopaedic Surgery, Univ Michigan, Ann Arbor, MI 1977-1980; **Fellow:** Hand Surgery, St Vincent's Hosp, Indianapolis, IN 1980-1981; **Fac Appt:** Assoc Clin Prof Orthopaedic Surgery, Univ S Fla Coll Med

Koman, L Andrew MD (HS) - *Spec Exp:* Congenital Hand Deformities; Vascular Disorders-Upper Extremity; Pain-Nerve Injury; **Hospital:** Wake Forest Univ Baptist Med Ctr (page 81); **Address:** Wake Forest University Baptist Medical Center, Medical Center Blvd, Winston-Salem, NC 27157; **Phone:** (336) 716-2878; **Board Cert:** Orthopaedic Surgery 1981, Hand Surgery 2000; **Med School:** Duke Univ 1974; **Resid:** Surgery, Duke Univ Med Ctr., Durham, NC 1974-1975; Orthopaedic Surgery, Duke Univ Med Ctr., Durham, NC 1975-1979; **Fellow:** Hand Surgery, Duke Univ Med Ctr, Durham, NC 1979-1980; **Fac Appt:** Prof Orthopaedic Surgery, Wake Forest Univ Sch Med

McAuliffe, John A MD (HS) - *Spec Exp:* Elbow Surgery; Wrist/Hand Injuries; Nerve Compression; **Hospital:** Cleveland Clin FL; **Address:** 2950 Cleveland Clinic Blvd, Weston, FL 33331; **Phone:** (954) 659-5594; **Board Cert:** Orthopaedic Surgery 1999, Hand Surgery 1999; **Med School:** Univ Fla Coll Med 1982; **Resid:** Orthopaedic Surgery, Univ Fla Affil Hosp, Gainsville, FL 1983-1988; **Fellow:** Hand Surgery, Univ Miami, Miami, FL 1988-1989

Nunley, James MD (HS) - *Spec Exp:* Arthritis Hand Surgery; Ankle Joint Replacement; **Hospital:** Duke Univ Med Ctr (page 60); **Address:** Duke Univ Med Ctr, Box 2923, Durham, NC 27710-0001; **Phone:** (919) 684-4033; **Board Cert:** Orthopaedic Surgery 1981, Hand Surgery 1989; **Med School:** Tulane Univ 1973; **Resid:** Orthopaedic Surgery, Duke Univ Med Ctr, Durham, NC 1975-1979; **Fellow:** Hand Surgery, Duke Univ Med Ctr, Durham, NC 1979-1980; **Fac Appt:** Prof Orthopaedic Surgery, Duke Univ

Ouellette, Elizabeth Anne MD (HS) - *Spec Exp:* Hand Surgery - General; **Hospital:** Univ of Miami - Jackson Meml Hosp; **Address:** Dept Orthopaedics, 900 NW 17th St, Ste 549, Miami, FL 33136; **Phone:** (305) 326-6590; **Board Cert:** Orthopaedic Surgery 2000, Hand Surgery 2000; **Med School:** Univ Tex, San Antonio 1978; **Resid:** Orthopaedic Surgery, Univ Wash Hosp, Seattle, WA 1978-1983; **Fellow:** Hand Surgery, Jackson Meml Hosp, Miami, FL 1984-1985; **Fac Appt:** Assoc Prof Orthopaedic Surgery, Univ Miami Sch Med

Tsai, Tsu-Min MD (HS) - *Spec Exp:* Microsurgery; **Hospital:** Jewish Hosp HlthCre Svcs Inc; **Address:** 225 Abraham Flexner Way, Ste 700, Louisville, KY 40202; **Phone:** (502) 561-4263; **Board Cert:** Hand Surgery 1990, Orthopaedic Surgery 1984; **Med School:** Taiwan 1961; **Resid:** Surgery, Natl Taiwan Univ Hosp, Taipei, Taiwan 1964-1970; Orthopaedic Surgery, Univ Louisville Hosp, Louisville, KY 1976-1979; **Fellow:** Hand Surgery, Univ Louisville Hosp, Louisville, KY 1976; **Fac Appt:** Clin Prof Orthopaedic Surgery, Univ Louisville Sch Med

Urbaniak, James R MD (HS) - *Spec Exp:* Hand, Wrist, Elbow Microsurgery; Peripheral Nerve Surgery; **Hospital:** Duke Univ Med Ctr (page 60); **Address:** Duke Univ Med Ctr, Box 2912, Durham, NC 27710; **Phone:** (919) 684-5388; **Board Cert:** Orthopaedic Surgery 1992; **Med School:** Duke Univ 1962; **Resid:** Orthopaedic Surgery, Duke Univ Affl Hosps, Durham, NC 1965-1969; **Fac Appt:** Prof Orthopaedic Surgery, Duke Univ

Midwest

Bishop, Allen Thorp MD (HS) - *Spec Exp:* Microsurgery; Brachial Plexus; **Hospital:** Mayo Med Ctr & Clin - Rochester, MN; **Address:** Div of Hand Surgery, 200 1st St SW, Rochester, MN 55905; **Phone:** (507) 284-4149; **Board Cert:** Orthopaedic Surgery 2000, Hand Surgery 2000; **Med School:** Mayo Med Sch 1981; **Resid:** Orthopaedic Surgery, Mayo Clinic, Rochester, MN 1981-1986; **Fellow:** Hand Surgery, St Vincent Hosp, Indianapolis, IN 1986-1987; **Fac Appt:** Prof Orthopaedic Surgery, Mayo Med Sch

Carroll, Charles MD (HS) - *Spec Exp:* Carpal Tunnel Syndrome/ Hand Surgery; Upper Extremity Surgery; Shoulder & Elbow Surgery; **Hospital:** Northwestern Meml Hosp; **Address:** 676 N St. Clair, Ste 450, Chicago, IL 60611-2983; **Phone:** (312) 943-7850; **Board Cert:** Orthopaedic Surgery 2000, Hand Surgery 2000; **Med School:** Univ MD Sch Med 1982; **Resid:** Surgery, Johns Hopkins Hosp, Baltimore, MD 1983-1984; Orthopaedic Surgery, Johns Hopkins Hosp, Baltimore, MD 1984-1987; **Fellow:** Hand Surgery, Indiana Univ Med Ctr, Indianapolis, IN 1987-1988; Shoulder Surgery, Univ. of Western Ontario, London, Ontario 1988-1988; **Fac Appt:** Asst Clin Prof Orthopaedic Surgery, Northwestern Univ

Chung, Kevin MD (HS) - *Spec Exp:* Hand-Congenital Anomaly; Hand & Microvascular Surgery; Upper Extremity Trauma; **Hospital:** Univ of MI Hlth Ctr; **Address:** 24 Frank Lloyd Wright Drive, Box 441, Ann Arbor, MI 48106; **Phone:** (734) 998-6022; **Board Cert:** Plastic Surgery 1997, Hand Surgery 1997; **Med School:** Emory Univ 1987; **Resid:** Plastic Surgery, Univ Michigan Hosp & Hlth Ctr, Ann Arbor, MI 1992-1994; Hand Surgery, Union Meml Hosp, Baltimore, MD 1994-1995

Cooney, William MD (HS) - *Spec Exp:* Wrist/Hand Injuries; **Hospital:** Mayo Med Ctr & Clin - Rochester, MN; **Address:** Dept of Orthopedic Surgery, 200 1st St SW, Rochester, MN 55905; **Phone:** (507) 284-2994; **Board Cert:** Orthopaedic Surgery 1978, Hand Surgery 1989; **Med School:** St Louis Univ 1969; **Resid:** Surgery, Michigan Hosp 1969-1970; Orthopaedic Surgery, Mayo Clinic, Rochester, MN 1971-1975; **Fellow:** Hand Surgery, Mayo Clinic, Rochester, MN 1975-1976; **Fac Appt:** Prof Orthopaedic Surgery, Mayo Med Sch

Derman, Gordon Harris MD (HS) - *Spec Exp:* Carpal Tunnel Syndrome; Tendon Repair/ Reattachment; Repetitive Motion Injuries; **Hospital:** Rush-Presby - St Luke's Med Ctr (page 72); **Address:** 800 S Wells St, Ste 105, Chicago, IL 60607; **Phone:** (312) 408-0800; **Board Cert:** Plastic Surgery 1984, Hand Surgery 1999; **Med School:** Rush Med Coll 1975; **Resid:** Surgery, Loyola Univ Med Ctr, Maywood, IL 1977-1981; Plastic Surgery, Univ Mich Hosp, Ann Arbor, IL 1981-1983; **Fellow:** Microsurgery, Rush/Presby St Luke's, Chicago, IL 1976; **Fac Appt:** Asst Prof Surgery, Rush Med Coll

Failla, Joseph M MD (HS) - *Spec Exp:* Hand Surgery; Hand Reconstruction; **Hospital:** Henry Ford Hosp; **Address:** 6525 Second Ave, Detroit, MI 48202; **Phone:** (313) 876-2181; **Board Cert:** Orthopaedic Surgery 2001, Hand Surgery 2001; **Med School:** SUNY Buffalo 1982; **Resid:** Orthopaedic Surgery, SUNY-Buffalo, Buffalo, NY 1983-1987; **Fellow:** Hand Surgery, Mayo Clinic, Rochester, NY 1987-1988

Fischer, Thomas James MD (HS) - *Spec Exp:* Hand Surgery - General; **Hospital:** St Vincent's Hosp and Hlth Ctr - Indianapolis; **Address:** 8501 Harcourt Rd, Box 80434, indianapolis, IN 46280-0434; **Phone:** (315) 875-9105; **Board Cert:** Orthopaedic Surgery 2000, Hand Surgery 2000; **Med School:** Indiana Univ 1979; **Resid:** Orthopaedic Surgery, Univ Wash Affil Hosp, Seattle, WA 1980-1984; Hand Surgery, Duke Univ Med Ctr, Durham, NC 1986; **Fellow:** Hand Surgery, Hand Surg Assoc, Indianapolis, IN 1984-1985; Hand Surgery, Duke Univ Med Ctr, Durham, NC 1986; **Fac Appt:** Asst Clin Prof Orthopaedic Surgery, Indiana Univ

Gelberman, Richard MD (HS) - *Spec Exp:* Flexor Tendon Surgery; Peripheral Nerve Surgery; **Hospital:** Barnes-Jewish Hosp (page 55); **Address:** 1 Barnes Hospital Plaza, Ste 11300, St Louis, MO 63110; **Phone:** (314) 747-2531; **Board Cert:** Orthopaedic Surgery 1997, Hand Surgery 1996; **Med School:** Univ Tenn Coll Med, Memphis 1969; **Resid:** Surgery, Univ Wisc Med Ctr, Madison, WI 1971-1975; **Fellow:** Hand Surgery, Duke Univ Med Ctr, Durham, NC 1976-1977; Pediatric Orthopedic Surgery, Harvard Univ/Children's Hosp, Boston, MA 1985-1986; **Fac Appt:** Prof Orthopaedic Surgery, Washington Univ, St Louis

Hastings II, Hill MD (HS) - *Spec Exp:* Hand Surgery - General; **Hospital:** St Vincent's Hosp and Hlth Ctr - Indianapolis; **Address:** 8501 Harcourt Rd, Indianapolis, IN 46260; **Phone:** (317) 471-4338; **Board Cert:** Orthopaedic Surgery 1982, Hand Surgery 2000; **Med School:** USC Sch Med 1974; **Resid:** Surgery, Univ Colorado Med Ctr, Denver, CO 1975-1976; Orthopaedic Surgery, Mass Genl Hosp, Boston, MA 1977-1980; **Fellow:** Hand Surgery, St Vincent Hosp, Indianapolis, IN 1980-1981; **Fac Appt:** Assoc Clin Prof Orthopaedic Surgery, Indiana Univ

Hunt III, Thomas MD (HS) - *Spec Exp:* Hand Surgery; Wrist Surgery; **Hospital:** Cleveland Clin Fdn (page 57); **Address:** 9500 Euclid Ave, MC A40, Cleveland, OH 44195; **Phone:** (216) 445-6426; **Board Cert:** Orthopaedic Surgery 1995, Hand Surgery 1996; **Med School:** Vanderbilt Univ 1986; **Resid:** Orthopaedic Surgery, Univ Kansas Med Ctr, Kansas City, KS 1987-1992; **Fellow:** Hand Surgery, Hospital of the Univ. of Pennsylvania, Philadelphia, PA 1992-1993

Idler, Richard S. MD (HS) - *Spec Exp:* Hand Surgery; **Hospital:** IN Univ Hosp (page 63); **Address:** 8501 Harcourt Rd, Indianapolis, IN 46260; **Phone:** (317) 471-4334; **Board Cert:** Orthopaedic Surgery 1985, Hand Surgery 1989; **Med School:** Dartmouth Med Sch 1975; **Resid:** Surgery, UCLA Med Ctr, Los Angeles, CA 1976-1977; Plastic Surgery, UCLA Med Ctr, Los Angeles, CA 1977-1978; **Fellow:** Hand Surgery, St Vincent Hosp, Indianapolis, IN 1981-1982; **Fac Appt:** Asst Clin Prof Orthopaedic Surgery, Indiana Univ

Light, Terry MD (HS) - *Spec Exp:* Hand-Congenital Anomaly; Hand Trauma-Pediatric; Arthritis Hand Surgery; **Hospital:** Loyola Univ Med Ctr; **Address:** Loyola Univ Med Ctr, Dept Ortho, 2160 S First Ave, Maywood, IL 60153-5590; **Phone:** (708) 216-4570; **Board Cert:** Orthopaedic Surgery 1979, Hand Surgery 2000; **Med School:** Univ Hlth Sci/Chicago Med Sch 1973; **Resid:** Orthopaedic Surgery, Yale-New Haven Hosp, New Haven, CT 1974-1977; **Fellow:** Hand Surgery, Hartford Combined Prog., Hartford, CT 1977; **Fac Appt:** Prof Orthopaedic Surgery, Loyola Univ-Stritch Sch Med

Louis, Dean MD (HS) - *Spec Exp:* Hand-Congenital Anomaly; Wrist Sugergy; Arthritis Hand Surgery; **Hospital:** Univ of MI Hlth Ctr; **Address:** A Alfred Taubman Hlth Care Ctr, 1500 E Medical Center Drive, 2nd FL, Reception Area C, Rm 2912, Ann Arbor, MI 48109-0328; **Phone:** (734) 936-5200; **Board Cert:** Orthopaedic Surgery 1998, Hand Surgery 1998; **Med School:** Univ VT Coll Med 1962; **Resid:** Orthopaedic Surgery, Univ Michigan Med Ctr, Ann Arbor, MI 1967-1970; **Fellow:** Hand Surgery, Columbia Presby Hosp, New York, NY 1970-1971; **Fac Appt:** Prof Surgery, Univ Mich Med Sch

Manske, Paul MD (HS) - *Spec Exp:* Hand Surgery - General; **Hospital:** Barnes-Jewish Hosp (page 55); **Address:** One Barnes Hosp Plaza, West Pavilion, Ste 11300, St. Louis, MO 63110; **Phone:** (314) 747-2500; **Board Cert:** Orthopaedic Surgery 1974, Hand Surgery 2000; **Med School:** Washington Univ, St Louis 1964; **Resid:** Surgery, Univ Wash Med Ctr, Seattle, WA 1965-1966; Orthopaedic Surgery, Wash Univ/Barnes Hosp, St Louis, MO 1969-1972; **Fellow:** Hand Surgery, Univ Louisville Hosp, Louisville, KY 1971; **Fac Appt:** Prof Orthopaedic Surgery, Washington Univ, St Louis

Mass, Daniel MD (HS) - *Spec Exp:* Tendon/nerve injuries; Arthritis Hand Surgery; **Hospital:** Univ of Chicago Hosps (page 76); **Address:** 5841 S Maryland Ave, MS 3079, Chicago, IL 60637; **Phone:** (773) 834-3531; **Board Cert:** Orthopaedic Surgery 1994, Hand Surgery 2000; **Med School:** Univ Chicago-Pritzker Sch Med 1975; **Resid:** Orthopaedic Surgery, Univ Chicago Hosp, Chicago, IL 1976-1979; **Fellow:** Hand Surgery, St Francis Hosp, San Francisco, CA 1980; **Fac Appt:** Clin Prof Surgery, Univ Chicago-Pritzker Sch Med

Mih, Alexander MD (HS) - *Spec Exp:* *Microsurgery;* **Hospital:** IN Univ Hosp (page 63); **Address:** Clinical Bldg 600, 541 Clinical Dr, Indianapolis, IN 46202-5111; **Phone:** (317) 274-5648; **Board Cert:** Orthopaedic Surgery 1992, Hand Surgery 1993; **Med School:** Johns Hopkins Univ 1984; **Resid:** Orthopaedic Surgery, Mayo Clinic, Rochester, MN 1984-1989; **Fellow:** Hand Surgery, Indiana Ctr for Hand Surg, Indianapolis, IA 1989-1990; **Fac Appt:** Assoc Prof Orthopaedic Surgery, Indiana Univ

Nagle, Daniel J MD (HS) - *Spec Exp:* *Hand Surgery; Carpal Tunnel Syndrome; Wrist Problems;* **Hospital:** Northwestern Meml Hosp; **Address:** 448 E Ontario St, Ste 500, Chicago, IL 60611-7108; **Phone:** (312) 908-3366; **Board Cert:** Orthopaedic Surgery 1986, Hand Surgery 1989; **Med School:** Belgium 1978; **Resid:** Orthopaedic Surgery, Northwestern Univ Med Sch, Chicago, IL 1979-1983; **Fellow:** Hand Surgery, Christine Kleinert, Louisville, KY 1983-1984; **Fac Appt:** Assoc Prof Orthopaedic Surgery, Northwestern Univ

Putnam, Matthew Douglas MD (HS) - *Spec Exp:* *Hand Surgery - General;* **Hospital:** Fairview-Univ Med Ctr - Univ Campus; **Address:** Dept Orthopedic Surgery, 401 E River Rd, Minneapolis, MN 55455; **Phone:** (612) 625-1192; **Board Cert:** Hand Surgery 1990, Orthopaedic Surgery 1998; **Med School:** Dartmouth Med Sch 1977; **Resid:** Surgery, Roosevelt Hosp, New York, NY 1978-1979; Orthopaedic Surgery, Univ Pittsburgh, Pittsburgh, PA 1981-1984; **Fellow:** Hand Surgery, NVOH, New York, NY 1984-1985; **Fac Appt:** Asst Prof Orthopaedic Surgery, Univ Minn

Schenck, Robert Roy MD (HS) - *Spec Exp:* *Carpal Tunnel Syndrome; Trigger Finger; Finger Fractures;* **Hospital:** Rush-Presby - St Luke's Med Ctr (page 72); **Address:** 1725 W Harrison St, rm 263, Chicago, IL 60612; **Phone:** (312) 738-3426; **Board Cert:** Plastic Surgery 1973, Hand Surgery 1998; **Med School:** Univ IL Coll Med 1955; **Resid:** Surgery, Western Penn Hosp, Pittsburgh, PA 1967-1969; Plastic Surgery, Columbia-Presby Hosp, New York, NY 1969-1971; **Fellow:** Hand Surgery, Roosevelt Hosp, New York, NY 1971-1972; **Fac Appt:** Assoc Prof Surgery, Rush Med Coll

Stern, Peter MD (HS) - *Spec Exp:* *Hand Injuries; Microsurgery;* **Hospital:** Good Samaritan Hosp - Cincinnati; **Address:** 2800 Winslow Ave, Ste 401, Cincinnati, OH 45206-1174; **Phone:** (513) 961-4263; **Board Cert:** Orthopaedic Surgery 1993, Hand Surgery 2000; **Med School:** Washington Univ, St Louis 1970; **Resid:** Surgery, Beth Israel Hosp, Boston, MA 1970-1972; Orthopaedic Surgery, Harvard Combined Pgrm., Boston, MA 1975-1977; **Fellow:** Hand Surgery, Univ Louisville Hosp, Loisville, KY 1978; **Fac Appt:** Prof Orthopaedic Surgery, Univ Cincinnati

Great Plains and Mountains

Ferlic, Donald C. MD (HS) - *Spec Exp:* *Hand Surgery - General;* **Hospital:** Presby - St Luke's Med Ctr; **Address:** Denver Orthopedic Clinic, 1601 E 19th Avenue #5000, Denver, CO 80218; **Phone:** (303) 839-5383; **Board Cert:** Orthopaedic Surgery 1992, Hand Surgery 1989; **Med School:** Johns Hopkins Univ 1961; **Resid:** Orthopaedic Surgery, Duke Univ Med Ctr, Durham, NC 1962-1968; Pediatric Orthopedic Surgery, NC Ortho Hosp, NC 1966-1967; **Fac Appt:** Assoc Clin Prof Orthopaedic Surgery, Univ Colo

Southwest

Ezaki, Marybeth MD (HS) - *Spec Exp:* *Hand-Congenital Anomaly; Hand Reconstruction-Pediatric;* **Hospital:** Texas Scottish Rite Hosp for Children - Dallas; **Address:** 2222 Welborn St, Ste 131, Dallas, TX 75219; **Phone:** (214) 559-7842; **Board Cert:** Orthopaedic Surgery 1993, Hand Surgery 2000; **Med School:** Yale Univ 1977; **Resid:** Orthopaedic Surgery, U Tex SW Affil Hosp, Dallas, TX 1978-1982; **Fellow:** Hand Surgery, Weyham Pk Hosp, Slough, England 1982; **Fac Appt:** Assoc Prof Orthopaedic Surgery, Univ Tex SW, Dallas

Moneim, Moheb S.A. MD (HS) - *Spec Exp:* Hand Surgery; **Hospital:** Univ NM Hosp; **Address:** Univ. New Mexico Hlth Scis Ctr, Dept. Orthopaedics, Albuquerque, NM 87131-5296; **Phone:** (505) 272-4107; **Board Cert:** Orthopaedic Surgery 1998, Hand Surgery 1998; **Med School:** Egypt 1963; **Resid:** Orthopaedic Surgery, Duke Univ Med ctr, Durham, NC 1972-1975; **Fellow:** Hand Surgery, Hosp for Spec Surg/Cornell, NYC, NY 1975-1976; **Fac Appt:** Prof Orthopaedic Surgery, Univ New Mexico

Rayan, Ghazi M. MD (HS) - *Spec Exp:* Microsurgery; Congenital Limb Abnormalities; Arthritis Reconstructive Surgery; **Hospital:** Intergris Baptist Med Ctr - OK; **Address:** Physicians Building D, 3366 NW Expressway #700, Oklahoma City, OK 73112-4439; **Phone:** (405) 945-4888; **Board Cert:** Orthopaedic Surgery 1983; **Med School:** Egypt 1973; **Resid:** Surgery, S Baltimore Genl Hosp-Univ Md Sch Med, Baltimore, MD 1976-1977; Orthopaedic Surgery, Union Meml Hosp-Johns Hopkins, Baltimore, MD 1977-1980; **Fellow:** Hand Surgery, Union Meml Hosp, Baltimore, MD 1980; **Fac Appt:** Clin Prof Orthopaedic Surgery, Univ Okla Coll Med

West Coast and Pacific

Diao, Edward MD (HS) - *Spec Exp:* Microvascular Surgery; **Hospital:** UCSF Med Ctr; **Address:** 1701 Divisadero Ave Fl 2 - Ste 280, San Francisco, CA 94115; **Phone:** (415) 353-2808; **Board Cert:** Hand Surgery 1993, Orthopaedic Surgery 1992; **Med School:** Columbia P&S 1981; **Resid:** Surgery, Beth Israel Hosp, Boston, MA 1982-1983; Orthopaedic Surgery, Mass Gen Hosp-Harvard, Boston, MA 1983-1987; **Fellow:** Hand Surgery, Roosevelt Hosp, New York, NY 1988; **Fac Appt:** Assoc Prof Orthopaedic Surgery, UCSF

Godzik, Cathleen MD (HS) - *Spec Exp:* Hand Surgery - General; **Hospital:** Orthopaedic Hosp; **Address:** 2300 S Hope St, Ste 300, Los Angeles, CA 90007; **Phone:** (213) 742-9708; **Board Cert:** Hand Surgery 1992, Orthopaedic Surgery 1990; **Med School:** NY Med Coll 1981; **Resid:** Surgery, Brown Univ Sch Med, Providence, RI 1982-1983; Orthopaedic Surgery, Univ Conn Sch Med, Farmington, CT 1983-1984; **Fellow:** Hand Surgery, Joseph Boyes Hand Fell-USC, Los Angeles, CA 1986-1987

Hanel, Douglas MD (HS) - *Spec Exp:* Reconstructive Microvascular Surgery; Hand-Congenital Anomaly; **Hospital:** Univ WA Med Ctr; **Address:** 325 9th Ave, Seattle, WA 98104-2420; **Phone:** (206) 731-3462; **Board Cert:** Orthopaedic Surgery 1997, Hand Surgery 1997; **Med School:** St Louis Univ 1977; **Resid:** Orthopaedic Surgery, St Louis Univ Hosp, St Louis, MO 1978-1982; Hand Surgery, Univ Louisville Hosp, Louisville, KY 1982-1983; **Fellow:** Microsurgery, Univ Louisville Hosp, Louisville, KY 1983; **Fac Appt:** Prof Orthopaedic Surgery, Univ Wash

Hentz, Vincent R MD (HS) - *Spec Exp:* Plastic Surgery; **Hospital:** Stanford Med Ctr; **Address:** 900 Blake Wilbur Drive, Ste W1083, Stanford, CA 94305; **Phone:** (650) 723-5256; **Board Cert:** Plastic Surgery 1977; **Med School:** Univ Fla Coll Med 1968; **Resid:** Plastic Surgery, Stanford Univ Hosp, Stanford, CA 1969-1974; **Fellow:** Hand Surgery, Roosevelt Hosp, New York, NY 1974-1975; **Fac Appt:** Prof Surgery, Stanford Univ

Jones, Neil MD (HS) - *Spec Exp:* Hand Surgery - General; **Hospital:** UCLA Med Ctr; **Address:** 200 UCLA Med Plz , Ste 140, Los Angeles, CA 90095; **Phone:** (310) 794-7784; **Board Cert:** Plastic Surgery 1985, Hand Surgery 1990; **Med School:** England 1974; **Resid:** Surgery, Nat Inst Health, Bethesda, MD 1976-1979; Plastic Surgery, Univ Mich Med Ctr, Ann Arbor, MI 1979-1981; **Fellow:** Plastic Surgery, St Bartholomew's, London, England 1982; Hand Surgery, Mass Gen Hosp/Harvard, Boston, MA 1983; **Fac Appt:** Prof Plastic Surgery, UCLA

Meals, Roy Allen MD (HS) - *Spec Exp:* Hand Surgery - General; **Hospital:** UCLA Med Ctr; **Address:** 100 UCLA Medical Plaza, Ste 305, Los Angeles, CA 90024-6970; **Phone:** (310) 206-6337; **Board Cert:** Orthopaedic Surgery 1980, Hand Surgery 2000; **Med School:** Vanderbilt Univ 1971; **Resid:** Surgery, Johns Hopkins Hosp, Baltimore, MD 1972-1973; Orthopaedic Surgery, Johns Hopkins Hosp, Baltimore, MD 1974-1978; **Fellow:** Hand Surgery, Mass General Hosp, Boston, MA 1978-1979; **Fac Appt:** Assoc Prof Surgery, UCLA

Szabo, Robert MD (HS) - *Spec Exp:* Peripheral Nerve Surgery; Hand Injuries; Upper Extremity Tumors; **Hospital:** Univ CA - Davis Med Ctr; **Address:** UC Davis, Dept Ortho, 4860 Y St, Ste 3800, Sacramento, CA 95817-2307; **Phone:** (916) 734-3678; **Board Cert:** Orthopaedic Surgery 1998, Hand Surgery 1998; **Med School:** SUNY Buffalo 1977; **Resid:** Surgery, Mt Sinai Med Ctr, New York, NY 1978-1979; Orthopaedic Surgery, Mt Sinai Med Ctr, New York, NY 1978-1982; **Fellow:** Hand Surgery, UCSD, San Diego, CA 1982-1983; Epidemiology, UC Berkeley, Berkeley, CA 1994-1995; **Fac Appt:** Prof Orthopaedic Surgery, UC Davis

Taleisnik, Julio MD (HS) - *Spec Exp:* Wrist/Hand Injuries; Arthritis Hand Surgery; **Hospital:** St Joseph's Hosp - Orange; **Address:** 1140 W La Veta Ave, Ste 860, Orange, CA 92868-4218; **Phone:** (714) 835-6500; **Board Cert:** Orthopaedic Surgery 1968; **Med School:** Argentina 1957; **Resid:** Orthopaedic Surgery, Mayo Clinic, Rochester, MN 1961-1966; **Fac Appt:** Clin Prof Orthopaedic Surgery, UC Irvine

Trumble, Thomas MD (HS) - *Spec Exp:* Nerve Regeneration; Upper Extremity Trauma; Biomechanics-Arms; **Hospital:** Univ WA Med Ctr; **Address:** Bone and Joint Center, 4245 Roosevelt Way NE, Seattle, WA 98105; **Phone:** (206) 598-4288; **Board Cert:** Orthopaedic Surgery 1999, Hand Surgery 1999; **Med School:** Yale Univ 1979; **Resid:** Orthopaedic Surgery, Yale-New Haven Hosp, New Haven, CT 1980-1984; **Fellow:** Microvascular Surgery, Duke Univ Med Ctr, Durham, NC 1984; Hand Surgery, Mass Genl Hosp, Boston, MA 1985; **Fac Appt:** Assoc Prof Surgery, Univ Wash

HEMATOLOGY &
MEDICALONCOLOGY

(a subspecialty of INTERNAL MEDICINE)

Hematology: An internist with additional training who specializes in diseases of the blood, spleen and lymph glands. This specialist treats conditions such as anemia, clotting disorders, sickle cell disease, hemophilia, leukemia and lymphoma.

Medical Oncology: An internist who specializes in the diagnosis and treatment of all types of cancer and other benign and malignant tumors. This specialist decides on and administers chemotherapy for malignancy, as well as consulting with surgeons and radiotherapists on other treatments for cancer.

INTERNAL MEDICINE

An internist is a personal physician who provides long-term, comprehensive care in the office and the hospital, managing both common and complex illness of adolescents, adults and the elderly. Internists are trained in the diagnosis and treatment of cancer, infections and diseases affecting the heart, blood, kidneys, joints and digestive, respiratory and vascular systems. They are also trained in the essentials of primary care internal medicine which incorporates an understanding of disease prevention, wellness, substance abuse, mental health and effective treatment of common problems of the eyes, ears, skin, nervous system and reproductive organs.

Training required: Three years in internal medicine *plus* additional training and examination for certification in hematology or medical oncology

SITEMAN CANCER CENTER
BARNES-JEWISH HOSPITAL • WASHINGTON UNIVERSITY SCHOOL OF MEDICINE

A National Cancer Institute-Designated Cancer Center

Barnes-Jewish Hospital • Washington University School of Medicine

660 S. Euclid Avenue
Campus Box 8100
St. Louis, MO 63110

Toll free: 800-600-3606
www.siteman.wustl.edu

one of the world's elite in the battle against cancer

For more than 100 years, Barnes-Jewish Hospital and Washington University School of Medicine have provided the finest cancer care anywhere. These two premier institutions and St. Louis Children's Hospital, a leader in pediatric oncology, have joined to create the Alvin J. Siteman Cancer Center. This dedicated cancer care facility:

- is the only National Cancer Institute-designated cancer center in Missouri and the surrounding five-state region

- treats more than 5,000 newly diagnosed patients and over 24,000 follow-up patients annually. Additionally, more than 30,000 people are reached annually through cancer screening and education programs. Combined, these numbers make the program the largest in the Midwest

- recently opened a state-of-the-art outpatient cancer center, which offers integrated evaluation services and treatment for patients and their families. Created with a patient-centered design, this single-site facility highlights patient and family convenience

offering the latest research and treatment

Future advances in cancer research and treatment will come from many fronts, in part based on the knowledge scientists will gain from endeavors such as Washington University's Human Genome Project, which will help us better understand the genetics of cancer development. The Siteman Cancer Center:

- remains one of the country's research leaders, devoting more than $80 million each year to cancer research that involves more than 250 clinical trials and over 1,200 patients

- offers a multidisciplinary team of more than 300 eminent clinicians and medical researchers. This approach to cancer care includes medical oncology, radiation oncology, surgery and psychosocial support

- provides specialists who lead research and clinical care teams in: Breast · GI (esophagus, stomach, colon, pancreatic, liver) · Gynecological (cervical, endometrial, uterine, ovarian) · Pediatric · Lung · Skin · Musculoskeletal · Urological (prostate, bladder, kidney, testicular) · Thyroid · Brain · Head and Neck · Hematology/Leukemia/Lymphoma · Bone marrow transplant

looking ahead to put cancer behind us

"Our physicians work side by side to rapidly share new knowledge that ultimately will mean better care for our patients."

— Timothy J. Eberlein, MD
Director, Alvin J. Siteman
Cancer Center

If you need a cancer specialist, call toll free:
800-600-3606
www.siteman.wustl.edu

CONTINUUM HEALTH PARTNERS, INC.
THE CONTINUUM CANCER CENTERS OF NEW YORK

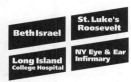

Phone (212) 420-4004

Continuum Health Partners, Inc.

The hospitals of Continuum — Beth Israel Medical Center, St. Luke's-Roosevelt Hospital Center, Long Island College Hospital and the New York Eye and Ear Infirmary — are leading providers of cancer care through the Continuum Cancer Centers of New York. Our integrated system allows us to build on the clinical strengths found at our four partner hospitals.

The goal — and result — is delivery of care in ways that are more efficient, more attractive and more convenient for patients. Specifically, it means that cancer patients at any Continuum hospital can benefit from system-wide cancer expertise, facilities and resources. The Cancer Centers feature world-renowned cancer specialists, including top-rated surgeons, medical oncologists, physicians, radiation oncologists, radiologists, and oncology nurses.

Comprehensive diagnostic and treatment services are available for breast cancer, prostate cancers, head and neck cancers, skin cancer, lung cancer, colorectal and other gastrointestinal cancers, Lymphoma/Hodgkin's Disease, gynecological cancers, and cancers of the brain and central nervous system. Delivered efficiently in a friendly and supportive environment, services include prevention programs—such as community education, screenings and early detection—expert diagnosis, outpatient treatment, inpatient services, home care and, when necessary, hospice care. In addition, the Cancer Centers Research Program offers patients access to investigational protocols through a wide number of clinical trials.

Support services play an important role at The Cancer Centers. Nurses, social workers, psychiatrists, chaplains, pharmacists, rehabilitation therapists and nutritionists—each with specialized knowledge and expertise in the field of oncology—work together to ensure that patients' medical, emotional and family needs are addressed appropriately and in a timely manner.

COMPREHENSIVE BREAST CENTER

The Comprehensive Breast Center at St. Luke's-Roosevelt combines state-of-the-art diagnosis and treatment of breast cancer with a supportive approach to health care that addresses emotional as well as physical needs. With radiology, pathology and consultation services available on site, a suspected malignancy can be confirmed or ruled out quickly and treatment options—including plastic surgery—can be outlined in a single visit. Services also include genetic testing, gynecologic cancer screening, referral to complementary therapies, psychiatric care and support groups.

BARBARA ANN KARMANOS CANCER INSTITUTE

4100 John R • Detroit, Michigan 48201
1-800-KARMANOS • www.karmanos.org

FIGHTING CANCER. IT'S ALL WE DO.

The Barbara Ann Karmanos Cancer Institute fights cancer on three fronts: state-of-the-science research; compassionate, advanced treatment; and education of health care professionals, cancer patients, and the public at large. It is Michigan's first National Cancer Institute-designated Comprehensive Cancer Center and one of only two in the state. Only 40 centers hold the prestigious distinction in the United States.

A LEADER IN RESEARCH

The Meyer L. Prentis Cancer Center is the Institute's primary laboratory research facility. Programs include breast cancer, developmental therapeutics, cancer genetics, immunotherapy and a cancer registry to help document and understand cancer among Detroit's diverse population. Members of the Institute's faculty create and participate in 300 clinical research studies, widely believed to be the best treatment option for many patients. Meanwhile, Karmanos scientists are aggressively developing new diagnostic tools to detect tumors at their earliest, and most-curable stages.

SPECIALIZED CARE

The Institute is sustained by more than 5,000 researchers, physicians, educators, support staff and volunteers. It is broken into 12 multispecialty teams — groups of cancer experts from various disciplines who review cases and determine the best treatment options for the patient. Teams include surgeons, radiation and medical oncologists, immunotherapists and veteran nurses focusing on each major type of cancer. This process eliminates unnecessary duplication of tests and procedures reducing anxiety, discomfort and appointment time, all critical factors for cancer patients.

THE HUMAN TOUCH

Karmanos Cancer Institute stands apart for its ability to understand the unique needs of cancer patients and offers a wide array of specialized programs including hospice, counseling, guest housing, transportation and family support services. AARP's *Modern Maturity* magazine recently honored the Institute as one of the 15 hospitals "with heart" for its caring compassionate care.

THE KARMANOS CANCER INSTITUTE OFFERS TREATMENT AVAILABLE AT FEW OTHER PLACES:

- Neutron radiation therapy — one of only two U.S. sites to offer this treatment.

- Cryotherapy to freeze tumor cells as an alternative or supplement to conventional surgery.

- Radiosurgery, form of brain surgery "without a knife."

- Immunotherapy, harnessing the body's immune system to destroy cancer cells.

- Photodynamic therapy, utilizing lasers and light-sensitive drugs.

BARBARA ANN
KARMANOS
CANCER INSTITUTE
Detroit Medical Center
Wayne State University

**Fighting Cancer.
It's all we do.**

Duke Comprehensive Cancer Center
DUKE UNIVERSITY HEALTH SYSTEM

Durham, North Carolina
1-888-ASK-DUKE • *Online at* cancer.duke.edu

One of the nation's first comprehensive cancer centers, the Duke Comprehensive Cancer Center has made many breakthroughs in understanding and treating cancer that are quickly translated to help patients. Duke also offers extensive support programs to help patients and families cope with cancer.

PROGRAM HIGHLIGHTS

Duke Breast Program faculty include leaders in breast conservation therapy and in development of early breast cancer detection technologies. Duke researchers were part of the team that discovered the breast cancer genes BRCA1 and BRCA2.

Neuro-Oncology Program. Duke's Brain Tumor Center is the largest and most successful in the nation, according to the NCI. Duke houses one of three NIH-recognized brain tumor research programs, and offers more active clinical trials than any other known treatment center.

The Adult Bone Marrow and Stem Cell Transplant Program has pioneered efforts in treating breast cancer with autologous bone marrow transplantation and in treating leukemia, lymphoma and myeloma.

The largest dedicated pediatric transplant program in the nation, Duke's **Pediatric Bone Marrow and Stem Cell Transplant Program** is a leader in developing allogeneic stem-cell transplants using umbilical cord blood and in performing haplo-identical transplants and transplants for patients with immunodeficiency diseases.

Duke's **Lung Cancer Program** is known for use of leading-edge imaging technologies as well as for new drug development.

Leukemias and Lymphomas. Duke offers bone marrow transplants, biological therapies, and access to new techniques, such as the use of growth factors to stimulate platelet recovery and aid in recovery from chemotherapy.

The Melanoma Clinic is rated as one of the nation's leading specialty clinics by the NCI. Duke pioneered the use of CD-ROM technology for early melanoma detection and is perfecting techniques to enhance the safety and efficacy of treatment.

Prostate Cancer Program. Duke offers patients the latest treatment options as well as techniques to help maintain or restore as much sexual functioning as possible.

Surgical Oncology. Duke is home to the American College of Surgeons Oncology Group, which oversees the nation's largest number of clinical trials of surgical approaches to cancer.

The Hereditary Cancer Clinic offers comprehensive cancer risk assessment, counseling, and education.

DCCC FACTS

U.S. News & World Report has consistently ranked Duke among the nation's top ten centers for cancer care.

≈

Since its founding in 1972, DCCC has maintained its status as a "comprehensive cancer center"—a recognition from the National Cancer Institute (NCI) requiring rigorous peer review, strong basic laboratory and clinical research programs, and an ability to translate research findings into clinical practice.

≈

In 1998, DCCC received an "outstanding" score—the highest ranking given to any research institution—from the NCI on its core grant renewal application and site visit.

MONTEFIORE-EINSTEIN CANCER CENTER
MONTEFIORE MEDICAL CENTER
The University Hospital for the Albert Einstein College of Medicine

Montefiore Medical Center
111 East 210th Street
Bronx, New York 10467

Albert Einstein College of Medicine
1825 Eastchester Road
Bronx, New York 10461

CUTTING-EDGE RESEARCH

Recognized internationally for their research, Montefiore's physicians continue to make major contributions to the advancement of patient care. Known throughout the tri-state region as research innovators, patients seek solutions from multidisciplinary teams of specialists who accomplish groundbreaking treatment techniques. Specialists in medical oncology, surgical oncology, gynecologic oncology and radiation oncology offer a comprehensive approach to cancer treatment that allows patients to receive integrated care in one location. The team's innovative approach emphasizes caring for each patient as a whole with a focus on their individual needs.

LUNG CANCER PROGRAM: EARLY INTERVENTION AND DETECTION

Lung cancer is the leading cause of death for men and women in America. Smokers and former smokers represent 85% of lung cancer cases. The Lung Cancer Program is a multi-disciplinary team of experts who dedicate themselves to the latest patient care and revolutionary research focusing on early detection, early intervention and prevention.

TUMOR VACCINE PROGRAM: RESEARCH & DEVELOP NEW CANCER VACCINES

The program, unique in the Metropolitan New York area, is dedicated to finding ways of using a patient's immune system to fight cancer. The program includes doctors and nurses with specialized training in biologic therapy and vaccines who are actively conducting clinical studies of tumor vaccines. Scientists are also working in the research laboratory within the Montefiore-Einstein Cancer Center to develop new vaccines and perform research to further understanding of how vaccines work in cancer patients.

COLORECTAL CANCER PROGRAM: DEDICATED TO PREVENTION & EARLY DIAGNOSIS

Montefiore Medical Center's team of experts within the Colorectal Cancer Program dedicate themselves to minimizing their patients risk of developing colorectal cancer with state-of-the-art technology. Montefiore created The New York Metropolitan Familial Colorectal Cancer Registry to help individuals and families clarify their risk of developing colorectal cancer based on personal and family history. The registry's program initiatives include *Hereditary Nonpolyposis Colorectal Cancer (HNPCC) and Familial Adenomatous Polyposis (FAP) Surveillance, Treatment and Support, Individual and Family Colorectal Cancer Risk Assessment, Women's Program, Patient and Provider Education Programs.*

AN ELITE CANCER CENTER

The Albert Einstein College of Medicine's designation as a National Cancer Institute (NCI) Comprehensive Cancer Center – one of a few in this nation – supports Montefiore's full range of cancer prevention, diagnosis and treatment options with cutting-edge research. Montefiore's physicians are internationally recognized for their cancer research, which contributes to improved patient care. Multi-disciplinary teams care for all of the patient's needs from detection through effective treatment of all cancers, including breast, colon, prostate, lung and ovarian.

1-800-MD-MONTE   **www.montefiore.org/cancer**

THE MOUNT SINAI HOSPITAL
ONCOLOGY / CANCER CARE

One Gustave L. Levy Place (Fifth Avenue and 98th Street)
New York, NY 10029-6574   Phone: (212) 241-6500
Physician Referral: 1-800-MD-SINAI (637-4624)
www.mountsinai.org

A Tradition of Commitment and Dedication

Mount Sinai has dedicated itself to one of the most wide-spread life-threatening diseases.

Superb Care

In an atmosphere of learning, clinical excellence, and superb patient care, The Hospital coordinates a full service diagnostic and treatment program for the cancer patient.

A Wide Range of Programs

Programs include medical chemotherapy, radiation, surgery, bone marrow and stem cell transplants, clinical trials for adults and children, and palliative care.

Advance Techniques

Mount Sinai specialists use the most recent advances in the diagnosis and treatment of all cancers and especially, breast, colorectal, liver, lung, prostate, head and neck, gynecological and genitourinary cancers, and cancers of the blood and lymph systems.

Teamwork

Using a multi-disciplinary approach, The Hospital's cancer specialists work with their colleagues in Medical Oncology, Radiation Oncology, Radiology, Surgery, and Pathology to treat the wide types and locations of cancer.

Innovation

In addition, The Hospital takes innovative approaches to the treatment of cancer patients: minimal access, local therapy for endocrine tumors, high risk screening, genetics of breast cancer, women's breast cancer center, multi-modality therapy for gastrointestinal cancer, melanoma screening, vaccine program, and minimal access surgery for cancer in elderly. And with the knowledge gained through the Human Genome Project, Mount Sinai researchers are working on a gene therapy program for colon, pancreas, and breast cancer.

THE MOUNT SINAI HOSPITAL

The mission of the **Derald H. Ruttenberg Cancer Center** at the Mount Sinai School of Medicine is to reduce the burden of human cancer through its outstanding interdisciplinary programs in research and patient care, including cancer prevention, treatment, early detection, and education.

The members of the Cancer Center, scientists and medical professionals, are working together to develop cancer therapies and prevention strategies to improve cancer care. New translational cancer research initiatives, from "bench to bedside" are being developed in a number of research laboratories with funding from the National Cancer Institute.

NewYork-Presbyterian
The University Hospitals of Columbia and Cornell

Columbia Weill Cornell Cancer Centers

Herbert Irving Comprehensive Cancer Center
At Columbia Presbyterian Medical Center
161 Fort Washington Avenue
New York, NY 10032

NewYork Weill Cornell Cancer Center
At NewYork Weill Cornell Medical Center
525 East 68th Street
New York, NY 10021

OVERVIEW:

Columbia Weill Cornell Cancer Centers are dedicated to reducing cancer morbidity and mortality by providing

- a full continuum of multidisciplinary, state-of-the-art screening, diagnostic, treatment and support services for all phases of the disease process;

- cutting-edge basic, clinical, and public health research;

- full range of cancer-related educational programs and resources to clinicians, scientists, patients and survivors, families, and the cancer prevention community.

The Cancer Centers, which treat over 6,000 new patients annually, draw on the innovation and excellence of the NCI- designated Herbert Irving Comprehensive Cancer Center at Columbia Presbyterian Medical Center and oncology services at NewYork Weill Cornell Medical Center. Programs include:

- AIDS-related Malignancies
- Bone Marrow Transplant
- Breast Cancer
- Dermatologic/Skin Cancer
- Gastrointestinal Cancers
- Genitourinary Cancers
- Gynecologic Cancers
- Head and Neck Cancers
- Hematologic Malignancies, such as lymphoma, myeloma and leukemias
- Lung Cancer
- Neurologic Cancer
- Ophthalmic Cancer
- Pediatric Hematology/Oncology
- Urologic Cancers, including bladder, kidney and prostate cancer
- Sarcomas and Mesotheiliomas

The Centers are frequent recipients of major grants and gifts to support research programs. Recent highlights include:
- Avon Products Foundation $10 million award to Columbia Presbyterian Medical Center and Columbia University for establishment of the Avon Products Breast Center to support basic, clinical and public health research in breast cancer;

- The Leukemia and Lymphoma Society five-year $7.5 million grant to NewYork Weill Cornell Medical Center to study fundamental causes of multiple myeloma

Physician Referral: For a physician referral call toll free **1-877-NYP-WELL** (1-877-697-9355) to learn more about the Columbia Weill Cornell Cancer Centers visit our Web site at **www.nypcancer.com**.

COMPREHENSIVE SERVICES INCLUDE:

- Access to over 400 clinical trials supported by the National Institutes of Health and many prominent pharmaceutical companies.

- Bone marrow and blood stem cell transplant, including New York State approval to perform transplants using unrelated donors for patients with hematologic malignancies

- CT screening for early lung cancer detection

- Sentinel node biopsy to assess spread of breast cancer

- Skin-sparing mastectomy and reconstruction

- Laparoscopic surgery for colon cancer

- Intraoperative brachytherapy for GI, prostate and other cancers

- Stereotactic biopsies for breast cancer and brain cancer

- Stereotactic gamma radiation for brain tumors

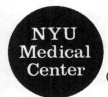

NYU Medical Center

SCHOOL OF MEDICINE

550 First Avenue (at 31st Street)
New York, NY 10016
Physician Referral: (888) 7-NYU-MED
(888-769-8633) www.nyumedicalcenter.org

NEW YORK UNIVERSITY

HEMATOLOGY/ONCOLOGY

The Division of Hematology in NYU Medical Center's Department of Medicine is one of the few centers in the United States to have a National Institutes of Health-funded training program in hematology – a specialty that focuses on the study, diagnosis, and treatment of diseases of the blood. Future hematologists are trained in close coordination with the NYU Cancer Institute and the Division of Medical Oncology, allowing them to become board-eligible in either or both specialties.

Patients with a wide range of benign and malignant hematological problems seek – and find – superior care at Tisch Hospital and affiliated hospital campuses, including Bellevue Hospital and the New York Department of Veterans Affairs Medical Center. NYU's hematologists bring outstanding expertise to treating patients with the following conditions:

- Anemia
- White blood cell and platelet disorders
- Enlargement of the lymph nodes or spleen
- Bleeding and clotting disorders
- Leukemia
- Lymphoma
- Lymphoproliferative and myeloproliferative disorders

At NYU, the Divisions of Hematology and Immunopathology enjoy a close working relationship. Together, physicians and researchers in each specialty participate in the laboratory evaluation of blood, bone marrow, and lymph node specimens using flow cytometric, immunocytochemical, and molecular biologic techniques. The NYU Medical Center Blood Bank also performs serologic techniques, evaluation of transfusion complications, and apheresis – infusion of a patient's own blood, from which certain elements have been removed.

BONE MARROW TRANSPLANTATION

The newly established bone marrow transplant facility at Tisch Hospital conducts bone marrow and peripheral blood stem cell harvesting, marrow ablation via treatment with high-dose chemotherapy, and management of patients during the post-transplant period.

NYU MEDICAL CENTER

Working closely with the Division of Hematology, Medical Oncology is a major component of the NYU Cancer Center, offering diagnosis and treatment of both hematological and solid tumors. Its research focus is on the development and testing of new cytotoxic agents used in chemotherapy – both biologic and synthetic – and on multi-modality treatment. Close collaboration with Radiation Oncology and the various surgical subspecialties in Oncology is actively pursued.

Most recently, the Division of Medical Oncology has engaged in the quest for cancer prevention strategies, including the study of biomarkers that may suggest early cancer development or may be used as diagnostic and prognostic tools.

UNIVERSITY OF FLORIDA SHANDS CANCER CENTER
SHANDS AT THE UNIVERSITY OF FLORIDA

1600 SW Archer Road, Gainesville, FL 32610
Patient referral: 800.749.7424
Physician-to-physician referral: 800.633.2122
www.shands.org

SPECIALIZED SERVICES

The UFSCC was among the first in the nation to perform many of the newest medical procedures, some of which were developed by UF physicians. The center combines personalized cancer treatment with access to advanced procedures and innovative research alternatives.

The UF faculty cancer specialists and their teams provide many services, including:

- Surgical procedures
- Chemotherapy
- Hematology/oncology
- Bone marrow transplantation
- Radiation oncology, with three high-energy linear accelerators and advanced computer simulation
- Lymphography and sophisticated nuclear medicine studies
- Sentinel lymph node biopsy for breast cancer patients
- Gene therapy to attack tumors at a molecular level without destroying normal tissue
- Minimally invasive techniques to remove tumors

CLINICAL TRIALS AND RESEARCH

The UFSCC's research mission is to provide a multidisciplinary approach to the study of cancer that will result in improved outcomes for prevention, diagnosis and treatment. Enhancing translational research is the key to making progress toward improved outcomes, and linking basic and clinical scientists brings a new dimension to cancer research at UF. A variety of clinical trials, including numerous national clinical trials, are available to further advance understanding of cancer biology and create improved treatment options for patients.

PHYSICIAN REFERRAL

The Shands Consultation Center is your link to UF physicians at the UFSCC. For more information or to schedule an appointment, please call 800.749.7424 or visit our Web site at shands.org.

WORLD-CLASS-CANCER CARE

The University of Florida Shands Cancer Center (UFSCC) is an interdisciplinary initiative at the UF Health Science Center's Gainesville and Jacksonville campuses, Shands at UF in Gainesville, and Shands Jacksonville. Clinicians and scientists affiliated with the UFSCC perform original scientific research and enhance clinical strategies for the diagnosis, treatment and prevention of cancer. Multidisciplinary teams work together to utilize the latest diagnostic and therapeutic innovations to optimize treatment outcomes. UFSCC cancer care services consistently are ranked among the nation's best by *U.S. News & World Report*.

The University of Chicago Hospitals
Cancer Program

5841 S. Maryland Avenue
Chicago, Illinois 60637-1470
For help finding a physician: 1-888-UCH-0200

AT THE FOREFRONT OF CANCER CARE

The University of Chicago Hospitals' cancer program ranks seventh in the nation and first in Illinois, according to *U.S. News & World Report*. More than 500 scientists, physicians, and other professionals from 20 different academic and clinical departments fight cancer here. Their work encompasses all aspects of the disease: prevention, detection, diagnosis, and treatment.

Designated by the National Cancer Institute (NCI) as a Comprehensive Cancer Center, the University of Chicago Hospitals is currently working with more than $30 million in cancer research grants -- more funding than any other hospital in Illinois. We are one of only a few centers in the United States selected by the NCI for Phase I and II clinical trials on new cancer-fighting drugs. Our cancer experts -- among the most renowned in the world – can quickly translate new knowledge from the scientific lab to the patient's bedside, providing innovative treatments long before they are available at most other hospitals.

NEW, EFFECTIVE TREATMENTS AND CLINICAL TRIALS

- Sophisticated diagnostics, including a computerized system that combines an MRI, PET scan and CT scan to produce a three-dimensional image of the brain. This detailed image allows doctors to pinpoint tumor location before radiation therapy or surgery.

- Advanced techniques that preserve organ function and healthy tissue whenever possible, so patients with colon, rectal, head and neck, and other cancers can maintain normal body functioning and appearance.

- Bone marrow transplants for treatment of Hodgkin's and non-Hodgkin's lymphomas, and all types of leukemia in children and adults. Bone marrow transplants are also used to treat solid tumors in the breasts, testicles, and other areas. Stem-cell transplants are provided as well.

**To Find a University of Chicago
Cancer Specialist,
Call 1-888-UCH-0200
Visit our web site at www.uchospitals.edu**

SERVING PATIENTS FROM AROUND THE WORLD

According to *U.S. News & World Report*, the University of Chicago's cancer program ranks 6th in the nation.

Our cancer program draws patients from throughout the Chicago area, the Midwest, the nation, and even the world. Our patients' problems are diverse, yet they reach for a common goal: to find the most effective solutions to meet their unique needs.

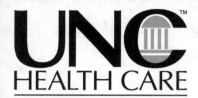

UNC Lineberger Comprehensive Cancer Center
The University of North Carolina Health Care System
101 Manning Drive Chapel Hill, NC 27514

www.unchealthcare.org

UNC LINEBERGER COMPREHENSIVE CANCER CENTER

The UNC Lineberger Comprehensive Cancer Center is one of 41 comprehensive cancer centers designated by the National Cancer Institute as a research and clinical care leader. A component of the University of North Carolina at Chapel Hill School of Medicine and working as the cancer care program of UNC Hospitals, the Lineberger Center is a national leader in research and care innovation. The center also has a Specialized Program of Research Excellence (SPORE) in breast cancer, one of eight programs in the country designated by the National Cancer Institute. The mission of the center and its Breast Cancer SPORE is to provide leading-edge care and developing novel therapies for cancer.

PATIENT CARE

■ Multidisciplinary approach means that a team of cancer specialists provide individualized treatment plans and care for each patient. Programs include: Bone Marrow and Stem Cell Transplantation, Breast Cancer, Cancer Genetics, Gastrointestinal Cancer, Gynecologic Oncology, Head and Neck Cancer, Lung and Thoracic Cancer, Lymphoma/Leukemia and Myelomas, Melanoma, Neuro-Oncology, Pediatric Oncology, Sarcomas, and Urologic Cancers.
■ Leading-edge technology – from early breast cancer detection, using digital mammography, to innovative clinical trials for late-stage cancers with molecular gene profiling of patients' tumors to analyze the best therapy.
■ Genetic counseling for patients and families at increased risk for cancer.
■ Patient programs including a Patient/Family Resource Center, support groups, wig/scarves loan program, patient and family counseling, and free massages offered weekly.

RESEARCH

■ Clinical trials for virtually all cancer types and stages, from innovative studies developed at UNC to national trials offered through clinical cooperative groups.
■ UNC is ranked in the top 15 institutions nationally in cancer research funding.
■ Regional population studies to seek environmental causes of cancers.

PREVENTION

■ Trials to prevent cancer in people at high risk.
■ Projects that work in communities with citizens and practitioners to reduce cancer risk by promoting early detection, screening, and healthy lifestyles.

UNC patients receive individualized care from a multidisciplinary team. A broad cancer genetics program extends from patient and family counseling and risk assessment to the use of leading-edge technologies to plan therapy and evaluate the extent of the cancer. Innovative clinical trials are available for those with advanced cancer. For more information about UNC Lineberger's cancer programs, please visit: http://cancer.med.unc.edu. To make an appointment, please call toll-free 1-866-828-0270.

PENN CANCER SERVICES
UNIVERSITY OF PENNSYLVANIA HEALTH SYSTEM

1-800-789-PENN
Philadelphia, PA
www.pennhealth.com

LEADERS IN CANCER

The University of Pennsylvania Cancer Center is one of a select group of cancer centers approved and awarded the prestigious designation of Comprehensive Cancer Center by the National Cancer Institute. It was among the first cancer centers to receive this designation and has maintained the status continuously since the early 1970s. With more than 330 faculty actively involved in the diagnosis and treatment of cancer patients, the Cancer Center offers a team of experts who provide coordinated patient care.

As one of the nation's foremost cancer centers, the University of Pennsylvania Cancer Center offers tremendous medical services and technological resources to meet any need throughout the course of treatment and follow-up care.

The University of Pennsylvania Cancer Network, established in 1991, is a select group of community hospitals throughout Pennsylvania and New Jersey collaborating with the University of Pennsylvania Cancer Center to provide excellence in patient care throughout the region. Penn's Cancer Network includes more than 25 hospitals that are recognized for excellence in patient care and commitment to improving the health and well-being of the community.

Pennsylvania Hospital, founded in 1751, offers a wide-ranging program that combines leading-edge technology and broad-based expertise with the intimacy of a personalized medical practice. At the Joan Karnell Cancer Center at Pennsylvania Hospital, patients have access to the latest cancer treatments, clinical trials and education programs through Penn's Cancer Network. A closely integrated team of medical, surgical, radiation and related cancer specialists use their knowledge and experience to bring patients a level of care that reflects the most current approaches to physical, emotional, family and social needs.

The Cancer Center at Phoenixville Hospital provides comprehensive care for patients close to home. The center provides a multi-disciplinary approach to cancer care and offers state-of-the-art radiation therapy, chemotherapy services in two locations, immunotherapy and supportive care management. A team of physicians, nurses, nutritionists and technicians create a synergy unique to Phoenixville Hospital. Through its membership in the University of Pennsylvania Cancer Network, patients have access to the latest cancer treatments, clinical trials and education programs.

For direct connection to one of our Penn physicians, call PennLine **1-800-635-7780**.

OVERVIEW

The University of Pennsylvania Health System is one of the leading health care providers in the country, known for its innovative approaches to cancer diagnosis and treatment as well as the care and compassion of its staff. United in a commitment to science and patient care, the University of Pennsylvania Health System has made enormous strides in understanding cancer's underlying causes. Each new advance improves the chances for recovery and enhances the quality of life for patients.

LOCATIONS

- University of Pennsylvania Medical Center
- Phoenixville Hospital
- Pennsylvania Hospital
- Presbyterian Medical Center
- Penn Medicine at Radnor
- Penn Medicine at Limerick

THE CANCER CENTER *AT THE*
UNIVERSITY OF VIRGINIA HEALTH SYSTEM

CHANGING THE FACE OF MEDICINE

The nationally recognized Cancer Center at the University of Virginia Health System is dedicated to providing exceptional care and comfort to cancer patients and their families. Our comprehensive services combine advanced medical care and research with extensive education and support.

Breadth of care sets us apart

Our cancer researchers are among the most highly respected in the world, searching for better treatments by teasing out the molecular and cellular processes that lead to cancer. Our clinical trials offer vast alternatives to patients who have exhausted traditional measures and accelerate the introduction of potentially lifesaving drugs. UVa is an international leader in the development of cancer vaccines for melanoma and ovarian cancer and in gene therapy for prostate cancer.

The UVa Cancer Center was one of the first centers in the nation to establish multidisciplinary teams of experts who collaborate on treating a specific cancer site, including lung, breast and prostate. This approach gives patients the most effective care by bringing together the expertise of medical oncologists, surgeons, radiologists, radiation oncologists, social workers, educators, psychologists and nurses. Our more than 30 nurses certified by the Oncology Nursing Society serve a vital role by guiding our patients through the complex process of cancer care.

Connected to our extraordinary clinical care and research is an extensive network of patient education and support: educational counseling, cancer genetics counseling, social work services, psychological counseling, nutrition, chaplaincy and a host of educational and support groups as well as yoga, meditation and exercise classes.

Changing the future of cancer care

The UVa Cancer Center has been judged consistently as one of the top 25 Cancer Centers by *US News & World Report* and is among a handful of clinical cancer centers designated by the National Cancer Institute. We have also received the highest designation by The American College of Surgeons.

Combining our world-class research, our innovative clinical trials, our exceptional patient care and our broad range of support services, the Cancer Center has created a unique tapestry where science and medicine merge and where excellent care is blended with compassion.

UVA HEALTH SYSTEM: HEADING THE CHARGE AGAINST PROSTATE CANCER

With a $20 million gift from a patient, the University of Virginia Health System has established the Mellon Prostate Cancer Research Institute to wage an all-out assault on a cancer that accounts for one of every three cancers among American men.

Through the institute, UVa is leading the way in understanding the causes of prostate cancer, which can be effectively treated when detected early. The Mellon Prostate Cancer Research Institute was established by a bequest from the estate of the late Paul Mellon, a noted philanthropist who died of prostate cancer in 1999. Mellon's generosity was motivated by the excellent care he received from a UVa urologist.

For more information, please visit www.med.virginia.edu/cancer or call 434 924-9333 or 800 251-3627.

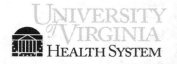

Vanderbilt-Ingram Cancer Center

Vanderbilt University Medical Center
691 Frances Williams Preston Building
Nashville, Tennessee 37232-6838
Tel. 615.936.5855 Fax. 615.936.5879 www.vicc.org

A Comprehensive Cancer Center

The Vanderbilt-Ingram Cancer Center is the only Comprehensive Cancer Center designated by the National Cancer Institute in Tennessee and one of only 41 nationwide. The designation, the highest distinction awarded to cancer centers, recognizes research excellence in cancer causes, development, treatment and prevention, as well as a demonstrated commitment to community education, information and outreach.

Clinical Trials and Research

Vanderbilt-Ingram conducts a full spectrum of research, from basic science to population-based studies that seek out cancer causes, to development of innovative treatment and prevention strategies. At any one time, the center offers more than 120 investigational therapies. Many of these studies are available to patients through Vanderbilt-Ingram's Affiliate Network, which includes more than a dozen hospitals throughout Tennessee, Alabama, Kentucky and Georgia.

Care and Support for Patients and Families

In addition to providing the latest in cancer treatment and conducting world-class research, Vanderbilt-Ingram offers programs to care for patients and families facing emotional, symptomatic, psychological, and social issues related to cancer and cancer treatment. These include Patient and Family Care, which offers in-clinic refreshments, music and pet therapy, free wigs and other support; Pain and Symptom Management; Strength for Life, which assists patients who have recently completed treatment make the transition back to "normalcy," and the Family Cancer Risk Service, which consults with individuals and families concerned about inherited risks of cancer and genetic testing.

Vanderbilt-Ingram Team

Vanderbilt-Ingram includes more than 1,000 doctors, researchers, nurses, technicians and other staff, all dedicated to the vision of preventing most cancers and curing the rest with innovative therapies and few, if any, side effects. The center includes more than 100 laboratories throughout Vanderbilt University and Medical Center, as well as the Henry-Joyce Cancer Clinic and Clinical Research Center and inpatient units in the Vanderbilt Hospital and Children's Hospital.

Since its inception in 1993, the center has been led by Dr. Harold Moses, Benjamin F. Byrd Professor of Oncology and director of the Frances Williams Preston Laboratories of the T.J. Martell Foundation. Moses, nationally known for his research in growth factors and cancer, is currently vice president and president-elect of the American Association of Cancer Institutes and a member of the National Dialogue on Cancer.

WESTCHESTER MEDICAL CENTER
WORLD-CLASS MEDICINE THAT'S NOT A WORLD AWAY.®

Valhalla Campus • Valhalla, NY 10595 • (914) 4-CANCER

Website: www.worldclassmedicine.com

OVERVIEW

Groundbreaking research, state-of-the-art treatment, internationally renowned doctors and the highest level of compassionate care make the Arlin Cancer Institute at Westchester Medical Center the choice for people from throughout the region and beyond who are facing cancer. The Cancer Institute's team strives to involve patients in their treatment and recovery by making them partners in care, and assists patients and their families in living with and fighting cancer.

The Cancer Institute is home to one of the world's most active bone marrow transplant programs, and one of the few programs in New York State approved by the National Marrow Donor program as an unrelated bone marrow transplant and collection center. As part of the Medical Center's affiliation with New York Medical College, the Cancer Institute collaborates with key national study groups and universities in dozens of cutting-edge research projects for such cancers as leukemia, lymphoma, myeloma and prostate, brain, breast, lung and an array of gynecologic cancers. Patients are able to participate in and benefit from scientific advances in oncologic medicine and technology years before they are available to the general public.

The Arlin Cancer Institute continues to break ground in therapeutic anticancer approaches, including matched unrelated marrow and cord blood transplantation, stereotactic radiosurgery, high-dose-rate brachytherapy, hyperthermia and cryosurgical procedures. A gene screening and therapy program and expansion of molecular biology services are among the many innovations on the horizon at Westchester Medical Center.

At the forefront of medical technology, Westchester Medical Center recently became one of just five hospitals in the nation to offer Novalis® Shaped Beam Surgery—the least invasive and most precise treatment option available to patients diagnosed with cancer, brain tumors, and neurologic and vascular disorders.

Each year more than 25,000 radiation therapy procedures performed at the Medical Center help Cancer Institute patients battle cancer. Fifty years ago only one cancer patient in five survived. Today nearly half of all cancer patients win their fight against cancer. Research at Westchester Medical Center has made significant contributions to the enhanced survival of cancer patients in the U.S. and abroad.

ARLIN CANCER INSTITUTE

At the forefront of medical technology, Westchester Medical Center recently became one of just five hospitals in the nation to offer Novalis® Shaped Beam Surgery — the least invasive and most precise treatment option available to patients diagnosed with cancer, brain tumors, and neurologic and vascular disorders. This revolutionary system, comprised of four state-of-the-art radiosurgery and radiotherapy applications, custom shapes the treatment beam to better target affected tissue while protecting healthy tissue.

For more information on Novalis® Shaped Beam Surgery:
Call 1-866-BEAM CENTER

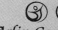

Arlin Cancer Institute

Physician Listings

New England

Benz, Edward MD (Hem) - *Spec Exp:* Anemias & Red Cell Disorders; Bone Marrow Transplant; **Hospital:** Dana Farber Cancer Inst; **Address:** 44 Binney St, Ste 1628, Boston, MA 02115; **Phone:** (617) 632-2159; **Board Cert:** Hematology 1982, Internal Medicine 1979; **Med School:** Harvard Med Sch 1973; **Resid:** Internal Medicine, Peter Bent Brigham Hosp, Boston, MA 1973-1975; Hematology, Yale New Haven Hosp, New Haven, CT 1978-1980; **Fellow:** Hematology, Natl Inst of Hlth, Bethesda, MD 1975-1978; **Fac Appt:** Prof Medicine, Harvard Med Sch

Duffy, Thomas MD (Hem) - *Spec Exp:* Mast Cell Diseases; **Hospital:** Yale - New Haven Hosp; **Address:** Yale Univ, Hematology Sect, Rm 403-WWW, 333 Cedar St, New Haven, CT 06510; **Phone:** (203) 785-4744; **Board Cert:** Hematology 1974, Internal Medicine 1972; **Med School:** Johns Hopkins Univ 1962; **Resid:** Internal Medicine, Johns Hopkins Hosp, Baltimore, MD 1963-1965; **Fellow:** Hematology, Johns Hopkins Hosp, Baltimore, MD 1968-1970; **Fac Appt:** Prof Medicine, Yale Univ

Groopman, Jerome E. MD (Hem) - *Spec Exp:* AIDS/HIV; AIDS Related Cancers; **Hospital:** Beth Israel Deaconess Med Ctr - Boston; **Address:** 330 Brookline Ave, Boston, MA 02215; **Phone:** (617) 667-0070; **Board Cert:** Hematology 1984, Medical Oncology 1981; **Med School:** Columbia P&S 1976; **Resid:** Internal Medicine, Mass Genl Hosp., Boston, MA 1978

Miller, Kenneth B. MD (Hem) - *Spec Exp:* Bone Marrow Transplant; Leukemia; **Hospital:** New England Med Ctr - Boston; **Address:** New England Medical Center, 860 Washington St, Box 542, Boston, MA 02111; **Phone:** (617) 636-5144; **Board Cert:** Internal Medicine 1976, Hematology 1980; **Med School:** NY Med Coll 1972; **Resid:** Internal Medicine, NYU Med Ctr/VA Hosp, New York, NY 1973-1976; Internal Medicine, NYU Med Ctr, New York, NY 1975-1976; **Fellow:** Hematology, New England Med Ctr., Boston, MA 1976-1979; **Fac Appt:** Assoc Prof Medicine, Tufts Univ

Spitzer, Thomas R MD (Hem) - *Spec Exp:* Bone Marrow Transplant; **Hospital:** MA Genl Hosp; **Address:** Mass Genl Hosp-Bone Marrow Tranplant Program, 100 Blossom St Bldg Cox 640, Boston, MA 02114; **Phone:** (617) 724-1124; **Board Cert:** Internal Medicine 1977, Medical Oncology 1983, Hand Surgery 1984; **Med School:** Univ Rochester 1974; **Resid:** Internal Medicine, New York Hosp-Cornell, New York, NY 1975-1977; **Fellow:** Hematology and Oncology, Case West Res Univ, Cleveland, OH 1981-1983; **Fac Appt:** Assoc Prof Medicine, Harvard Med Sch

Stone, Richard Maury MD (Hem) - *Spec Exp:* Leukemia-Adult; **Hospital:** MA Genl Hosp; **Address:** 44 Binney St, rm D-840B, Boston, MA 02115-6013; **Phone:** (617) 632-2214; **Board Cert:** Medical Oncology 1987, Hematology 1988; **Med School:** Harvard Med Sch 1981; **Resid:** Internal Medicine, Brigham & Womens Hosp, Boston, MA 1982-1984; **Fellow:** Medical Oncology, Dana Farber Cancer Inst, Boston, MA 1984-1987; **Fac Appt:** Assoc Prof Medicine, Harvard Med Sch

Mid Atlantic

Coller, Barry MD (Hem) - *Spec Exp:* Bleeding/Coagulation Disorders; Thrombotic Disorders; Glanzmann's Thrombasthenia; **Hospital:** Rockefeller Univ; **Address:** Rockefeller Univ, 1230 York Ave, New York, NY 10021; **Phone:** (212) 327-7494; **Board Cert:** Internal Medicine 1973, Hematology 1975; **Med School:** NYU Sch Med 1970; **Resid:** Internal Medicine, Bellevue Hosp, New York, NY 1970-1974

Diuguid, David Lincoln MD (Hem) - *Spec Exp:* Bleeding/Coagulation Disorders; **Hospital:** NY Presby Hosp - Columbia Presby Med Ctr (page 70); **Address:** 161 Ft Washington Ave, Rm 862, New York, NY 10032; **Phone:** (212) 305-0527; **Board Cert:** Hematology 1986, Medical Oncology 1985; **Med School:** Cornell Univ-Weill Med Coll 1979; **Resid:** Internal Medicine, Boston Univ Med Ctr, Boston, MA 1980-1983; **Fellow:** Hematology, New England Med Ctr, Boston, MA 1983-1986; **Fac Appt:** Asst Prof Clinical Pathology, Columbia P&S

Fruchtman, Steven MD (Hem) - *Spec Exp:* Bone Marrow Transplant; Stem Cell Transplant; Polycythemia Rubra Vera; **Hospital:** Mount Sinai Hosp (page 68); **Address:** 5 E 98th St, Box 1410, New York, NY 10029; **Phone:** (212) 241-6021; **Board Cert:** Internal Medicine 1980, Hematology 1984; **Med School:** NY Med Coll 1977; **Resid:** Internal Medicine, Univ Hosp/SUNY, Brooklyn, NY 1977-1981; **Fellow:** Hematology, Mount Sinai Med Ctr, New York, NY 1981-1984; Hematology, Meml SloanKettering Cancar Ctr, New York, NY 1984-1985; **Fac Appt:** Assoc Prof Hematology, NY Med Coll

Kempin, Sanford Jay MD (Hem) - *Spec Exp:* Leukemia; Lymphoma; **Hospital:** St Vincent Cath Med Ctrs - Manhattan (page 75); **Address:** St Vincents Cancer Ctr, 325 W 15th St, Ground Fl, New York, NY 10011; **Phone:** (212) 604-6010; **Board Cert:** Internal Medicine 1979, Medical Oncology 1977, Hematology 1978; **Med School:** Belgium 1971; **Resid:** Internal Medicine, Lemuel Shattuck Hosp, Boston, MA 1971-1972; **Fellow:** Hematology, St Jude Chldns Hosp, Memphis, TN 1973-1975; **Fac Appt:** Assoc Clin Prof Medicine, NY Med Coll

Schuster, Michael MD (Hem) - *Spec Exp:* Bone Marrow Transplant; **Hospital:** NY Presby Hosp - NY Weill Cornell Med Ctr (page 70); **Address:** 525 E 68th St, New York, NY 10044; **Phone:** (212) 746-2119; **Board Cert:** Internal Medicine 1984, Hematology 1986; **Med School:** Dartmouth Med Sch 1980; **Resid:** Internal Medicine, New England Deaconess Hosp, Boston, MA 1980-1983; **Fellow:** Hematology and Oncology, Beth Israel Hosp-Harvard, Boston, MA 1983-1987; **Fac Appt:** Assoc Prof Medicine, Cornell Univ-Weill Med Coll

Silverstein, Roy MD (Hem) - *Spec Exp:* Aplastic Anemia; Thrombotic Disorders; **Hospital:** NY Presby Hosp - NY Weill Cornell Med Ctr (page 70); **Address:** 525 E 68th St Bldg Payson 3, New York, NY 10021; **Phone:** (212) 746-2075; **Board Cert:** Hematology 1984, Medical Oncology 1985; **Med School:** Emory Univ 1979; **Resid:** Internal Medicine, New York Hosp-Cornell Med Ctr, New York, NY 1979-1982; Hematology, New York Hosp-Cornell Med Ctr, New York, NY 1982-1984; **Fac Appt:** Prof Hematology, Cornell Univ-Weill Med Coll

Spivak, Jerry L. MD (Hem) - *Spec Exp:* Myeloproliferative Disorders; Polycythemia Vera; **Hospital:** Johns Hopkins Hosp - Baltimore; **Address:** Traylor, Rm 924, 720 Rutland Ave, Baltimore, MD 21205; **Phone:** (410) 955-5454; **Board Cert:** Hematology 1974, Internal Medicine 1971; **Med School:** Cornell Univ-Weill Med Coll 1964; **Resid:** Internal Medicine, New York Hosp, New York, NY 1968-1969; Internal Medicine, Johns Hopkins Hosp., Baltimore, MD 1965-1966; **Fellow:** Hematology, Johns Hopkins Hosp., Baltimore, MD 1969-1971; **Fac Appt:** Prof Hematology, Johns Hopkins Univ

Wisch, Nathaniel MD (Hem) - *Spec Exp:* Lymphoma; Breast Cancer; Leukemia; **Hospital:** Lenox Hill Hosp (page 64); **Address:** 12 E 86th St, New York, NY 10028-0506; **Phone:** (212) 861-6660; **Board Cert:** Internal Medicine 1965, Hematology 1972, Medical Oncology 1977; **Med School:** Northwestern Univ 1958; **Resid:** Internal Medicine, VA Hosp, Brooklyn, NY 1959-1960; Internal Medicine, Montefiore Hosp, Bronx, NY 1960-1961; **Fellow:** Hematology, Mount Sinai Hosp, New York, NY 1961-1962; **Fac Appt:** Assoc Prof Medicine, Mount Sinai Sch Med

Zalusky, Ralph MD (Hem) - *Spec Exp:* Anemia; Leukemia; **Hospital:** Beth Israel Med Ctr - Petrie Division (page 58); **Address:** 1st Ave & 16th St Fl 19, New York, NY 10003; **Phone:** (212) 420-4185; **Board Cert:** Internal Medicine 1964, Hematology 1972; **Med School:** Boston Univ 1957; **Resid:** Internal Medicine, Duke Univ Med, Durham, NC 1957-1959; Internal Medicine, Duke Univ Med, Durham, NC 1961-1962; **Fellow:** Hematology, Boston Med Ctr, Boston, MA 1959-1961; **Fac Appt:** Prof Medicine, Albert Einstein Coll Med

Southeast

De Simone, Philip A MD (Hem) - *Spec Exp:* Hematology - General; **Hospital:** Univ Kentucky Med Ctr; **Address:** Markey Cancer Ctr, CC-454, 800 Rose St, Lexington, KY 40536; **Phone:** (859) 323-6562; **Board Cert:** Hematology 1974, Internal Medicine 1972; **Med School:** Univ VT Coll Med 1967; **Resid:** Internal Medicine, Univ Kentucky Hosp, Lexington, KY 1968-1974; **Fac Appt:** Prof Medicine, Univ KY Coll Med

Lutcher, Charles MD (Hem) - *Spec Exp:* Hemophilia-Adult; **Hospital:** Med Coll of GA Hosp and Clin; **Address:** Dept Hematology-Oncology, 1120 15th St, rm BAA-5407, Augusta, GA 30912; **Phone:** (706) 721-2505; **Board Cert:** Internal Medicine 1987, Hematology 1974; **Med School:** Washington Univ, St Louis 1961; **Resid:** Hematology, Univ Oregon Hosp, Eugene, OR 1963-1964; Internal Medicine, Univ Wash City Hosp, St Louis, MO 1962-1963; **Fellow:** Hematology, Univ Oregon Hosp, Eugene, OR 1964-1966; **Fac Appt:** Prof Medicine, Med Coll GA

Solberg, Lawrence MD (Hem) - *Spec Exp:* Bone Marrow Transplant; **Hospital:** St Luke's Hosp; **Address:** Mayo Clinic - Jacksonville, 4500 San Pablo Rd, Jacksonville, FL 32224; **Phone:** (904) 953-7292; **Board Cert:** Internal Medicine 1978, Hematology 1980; **Med School:** St Louis Univ 1975; **Resid:** Internal Medicine, Mayo Grad Sch, Rochester, MN 1976-1978; **Fellow:** Hematology, Mayo Grad Sch, Rochester, MN 1978-1980

Telen, Marilyn J MD (Hem) - *Spec Exp:* Transfusion Medicine; Hemolytic Anemia; **Hospital:** Duke Univ Med Ctr (page 60); **Address:** Duke Univ Med Ctr, Box 2615, Durham, NC 27710; **Phone:** (919) 684-5426; **Board Cert:** Internal Medicine 1980, Hematology 1984; **Med School:** NYU Sch Med 1977; **Resid:** Internal Medicine, Erie Co Med Cr-SUNY-Buffalo, Buffalo, NY 1978-1980; **Fellow:** Hematology, Duke Univ Med Ctr, Durham, NC 1980-1982; **Fac Appt:** Prof Medicine, Duke Univ

Zuckerman, Kenneth MD (Hem) - *Spec Exp:* Leukemia; Myeloproliferative Disorders; **Hospital:** H Lee Moffitt Cancer Ctr & Research Inst; **Address:** H Lee Moffitt Cancer Ctr, 12902 Magnolia Drive, Ste 3157, Tampa, FL 33612-9416; **Phone:** (813) 972-8400; **Board Cert:** Internal Medicine 1975, Hematology 1978; **Med School:** Ohio State Univ 1972; **Resid:** Internal Medicine, Ohio State Univ Hosp, Columbus, OH 1973-1975; **Fellow:** Hematology, Peter Bent Brigham Hosp, Boston, MA 1975-1978; **Fac Appt:** Prof Medical Oncology, Univ S Fla Coll Med

Midwest

Adler, Solomon Stanley MD (Hem) - *Spec Exp:* Lymphoma; Leukemia; Myelodysplastic Syndromes; **Hospital:** Rush-Presby - St Luke's Med Ctr (page 72); **Address:** 1725 W Harrison St, Ste 862, Chicago, IL 60612; **Phone:** (312) 563-2320; **Board Cert:** Hematology 1973, Medical Oncology 1975; **Med School:** Albert Einstein Coll Med 1970; **Resid:** Internal Medicine, Brookdale Hosp Med Ctr, Brooklyn, NY 1971-1972; Hematology, Brookdale Hosp Med Ctr, Brooklyn, NY 1972-1973; **Fellow:** Hematology, Rush/Presby-St Lukes Hosp, Chicago, IL 1973-1975; **Fac Appt:** Prof Medicine, Rush Med Coll

Baron, Joseph M MD (Hem) - *Spec Exp:* Bleeding/Coagulation Disorders; Lymphoma; Myeloproliferative Disorders; **Hospital:** Univ of Chicago Hosps (page 76); **Address:** 5758 S Maryland Ave, MC 9015, Chicago, IL 60637; **Phone:** (773) 702-6149; **Board Cert:** Hematology 1972, Medical Oncology 1975; **Med School:** Univ Chicago-Pritzker Sch Med 1962; **Resid:** Internal Medicine, Univ Chicago, Chicago, IL 1962-1964; **Fellow:** Hematology, Univ Chicago, Chicago, IL 1967-1968; **Fac Appt:** Assoc Prof Medicine, Univ Chicago-Pritzker Sch Med

Blinder, Morey MD (Hem) - *Spec Exp:* Bleeding/Coagulation Disorders; Anemia; Sickle Cell Disease; **Hospital:** Barnes-Jewish Hosp (page 55); **Address:** 4960 Children's Pl Fl 4, MC 8125, St. Louis, MO 63110; **Phone:** (314) 362-8808; **Board Cert:** Internal Medicine 1984, Hematology 1988, Hematology 1987; **Med School:** St Louis Univ 1981; **Resid:** Internal Medicine, Univ Illinois Hosp, Chicago, IL 1981-1984; **Fac Appt:** Assoc Prof Medicine, Washington Univ, St Louis

Bockenstedt, Paula MD (Hem) - *Spec Exp:* Bleeding/Coagulation Disorders; Leukemia/Hematopoietic Malignancy; Von Willebrand's Disease; **Hospital:** Univ of MI Hlth Ctr; **Address:** 1500 E Med Center Drive, Ste 3588 Reception B, Ann Arbor, MI 48109-0640; **Phone:** (734) 647-8901; **Board Cert:** Internal Medicine 1981, Hematology 1984; **Med School:** Harvard Med Sch 1978; **Resid:** Internal Medicine, Brigham-Womens Hosp, Boston, MA 1979-1981; **Fellow:** Hematology, Brigham-Womens Hosp, Boston, MA 1981-1984; **Fac Appt:** Asst Clin Prof Hematology, Univ Mich Med Sch

Bricker, Leslie J MD (Hem) - *Spec Exp:* Hospice Care; Palliative Care; **Hospital:** Henry Ford Hosp; **Address:** 2799 W Grand Blvd, Detroit, MI 48202; **Phone:** (313) 916-1859; **Board Cert:** Hematology 1982, Medical Oncology 1983; **Med School:** Wayne State Univ 1977; **Resid:** Internal Medicine, Sinai Hosp, Detroit, MI 1978-1980; **Fellow:** Hematology, Univ Mich Hosp, Ann Arbor, MI 1980

Bukowski, Ronald Mathew MD (Hem) - *Spec Exp:* Kidney Cancer; **Hospital:** Cleveland Clin Fdn (page 57); **Address:** 9500 Euclid Ave, Cleveland, OH 44195-0001; **Phone:** (216) 444-6825; **Board Cert:** Infectious Disease 1974, Medical Oncology 1975, Hematology 1976; **Med School:** Northwestern Univ 1967; **Resid:** Internal Medicine, Cleveland Clinic, Cleveland, OH 1968-1969; Internal Medicine, Cleveland Clinic, Cleveland, OH 1972-1973; **Fellow:** Hematology, Cleveland Clinic, Cleveland, OH 1973

Gaynor, Ellen MD (Hem) - *Spec Exp:* Lymphoma; **Hospital:** Loyola Univ Med Ctr; **Address:** Loyola Univ Med Ctr, Dept Hematology, 2160 S First Ave, Maywood, IL 60153; **Phone:** (708) 327-3214; **Board Cert:** Medical Oncology 1985, Hematology 1986; **Med School:** Univ Wisc 1978; **Resid:** Internal Medicine, Loyola Univ Med Ctr, Maywood, IL 1979-1982; **Fellow:** Medical Oncology, Loyola Univ Med Ctr, Maywood, IL 1980-1981; Hematology and Oncology, Univ Chicago Hosp, Chicago, IL 1982-1984; **Fac Appt:** Assoc Prof Medicine, Loyola Univ-Stritch Sch Med

Godwin, John MD (Hem) - *Spec Exp:* Hematology - General; **Hospital:** Loyola Univ Med Ctr; **Address:** Loyola Univ Med Ctr, Dept Hematology, 2160 S 1st Ave Bldg 112 - rm 342, Maywood, IL 60153; **Phone:** (708) 327-3180; **Board Cert:** Hematology 1986, Internal Medicine 1981; **Med School:** Univ Ala 1978; **Resid:** Internal Medicine, Baylor Coll Med, Houston, TX 1979-1981; Hematology, Baylor Coll Med, Houston, TX 1981-1983; **Fellow:** Hematology, NC Meml Hosp-U NC, Chapel Hill, NC 1983-1985; **Fac Appt:** Assoc Prof Medicine, Loyola Univ-Stritch Sch Med

Gordon, Leo I MD (Hem) - *Spec Exp:* Non-Hodgkins Lymphoma/Leukemia; Hodgkin's Disease; Bone Marrow Transplant; **Hospital:** Northwestern Meml Hosp; **Address:** 676 N St Clair St, Ste 850, Chicago, IL 60611-3124; **Phone:** (312) 695-4546; **Board Cert:** Hematology 1978, Medical Oncology 1979; **Med School:** Univ Cincinnati 1973; **Resid:** Internal Medicine, Univ Chicago Hosps, Chicago, IL 1974-1976; **Fellow:** Hematology, Univ Minn Hosps, Minneapolis, MN 1976-1978; Hematology and Oncology, Univ Chicago Hosps, Chicago, IL 1978-1979; **Fac Appt:** Prof Medicine, Northwestern Univ

Green, David MD (Hem) - *Spec Exp:* Bleeding/Coagulation Disorders; **Hospital:** Northwestern Meml Hosp; **Address:** 345 E Superior St, Ste 1407, Chicago, IL 60611-4496; **Phone:** (312) 238-4701; **Board Cert:** Internal Medicine 1987, Hematology 1972; **Med School:** Jefferson Med Coll 1960; **Resid:** Internal Medicine, Jefferson Hosp, Philadelphia, PA 1961-1963; **Fellow:** Hematology, Jefferson Hosp, Philadelphia, PA 1963-1964; **Fac Appt:** Prof Medicine, Northwestern Univ

Gregory, Stephanie A MD (Hem) - *Spec Exp:* Lymphoma; Leukemia; Plasma Cell Disorders; **Hospital:** Rush-Presby - St Luke's Med Ctr (page 72); **Address:** 1725 W Harrison St, Ste 809, Chicago, IL 60612-3861; **Phone:** (312) 563-2320; **Board Cert:** Internal Medicine 1972, Hematology 1972; **Med School:** Med Coll PA Hahnemann 1965; **Resid:** Internal Medicine, Rush/Presby-St Luke's Med Ctr, Chicago, IL 1966-1969; **Fellow:** Hematology, Rush/Presby-St Luke's Med Ctr, Chicago, IL 1969-1972; **Fac Appt:** Prof Medicine, Rush Med Coll

Greipp, Philip R MD (Hem) - *Spec Exp:* Multiple Myeloma; **Hospital:** Mayo Med Ctr & Clin - Rochester, MN; **Address:** Div Hematology, 200 1st St SW, Rochester, MN 55905; **Phone:** (507) 284-3159; **Board Cert:** Internal Medicine 1974, Hematology 1994; **Med School:** Georgetown Univ 1968; **Resid:** Internal Medicine, Mayo Clinic, Rochester, MN 1971-1973; **Fellow:** Hematology, Mayo Clinic, Rochester, MN 1973-1975; **Fac Appt:** Prof Medicine, Mayo Med Sch

Lazarus, Hillard M MD (Hem) - *Spec Exp:* Bone Marrow Transplant; Stem Cell Transplant; **Hospital:** Univ Hosp of Cleveland; **Address:** Univ Hosp of Cleveland, 11100 Euclid Ave Bldg Wearn - rm 341, Cleveland, OH 44106-5065; **Phone:** (216) 844-3629; **Board Cert:** Internal Medicine 1977, Medical Oncology 1979, Hematology 1980; **Med School:** Univ Rochester 1974; **Resid:** Internal Medicine, Univ Hosp, Cleveland, OH 1975-1977; **Fellow:** Hematology and Oncology, Univ Hosp, Cleveland, OH 1977-1979; **Fac Appt:** Prof Medicine, Case West Res Univ

Litzow, Mark Robert MD (Hem) - *Spec Exp:* Bone Marrow Transplant; Leukemia; **Hospital:** Mayo Med Ctr & Clin - Rochester, MN; **Address:** Div Hematology, 200 1st St SW, Rochester, MN 55905; **Phone:** (507) 284-5302; **Board Cert:** Medical Oncology 1989, Hematology 1988; **Med School:** Univ Chicago-Pritzker Sch Med 1980; **Resid:** Internal Medicine, Mayo Clinic, Rochester, MN 1980-1984; **Fellow:** Medical Oncology, Mayo Clinic, Rochester, MN 1985-1990; **Fac Appt:** Asst Prof Medicine, Mayo Med Sch

Mosher, Deane F MD (Hem) - *Spec Exp:* Hematology - General; **Hospital:** Univ WI Hosp & Clins; **Address:** Univ Wisc Hosp, Dept Hematology, 600 Highland Avenue, Madison, WI 53792; **Phone:** (608) 263-7022; **Board Cert:** Hematology 1980, Internal Medicine 1973; **Med School:** Harvard Med Sch 1968; **Resid:** Internal Medicine, Beth Israel Hosp, Boston, MA 1969-1970; **Fellow:** Hematology, Harvard, Boston, MA 1970-1972; **Fac Appt:** Prof Medicine, Univ Wisc

Nand, Sucha MD (Hem) - *Spec Exp:* Myelodysplastic Syndromes; Myeloproliferative Disorders; **Hospital:** Loyola Univ Med Ctr; **Address:** Cardinal Bernardin Cancer Ctr, 2160 S First Ave, Maywood, IL 60153-3304; **Phone:** (708) 327-3217; **Board Cert:** Internal Medicine 1979, Medical Oncology 1981, Hematology 1982; **Med School:** India 1971; **Resid:** Physical Medicine & Rehabilitation, Northwestern Meml Hosp, Chicago, IL 1975-1976; Internal Medicine, North Chicago VA Hospital, Chicago, IL 1977-1978; **Fellow:** Medical Oncology, Northwestern Meml Hosp, Chicago, IL 1979-1981; **Fac Appt:** Prof Medicine, Loyola Univ-Stritch Sch Med

Palascak, Joseph E MD (Hem) - *Spec Exp:* Hemophilia; Bleeding/Coagulation Disorders; **Hospital:** Univ Hosp - Cincinnati; **Address:** Univ Hosp, Cincinatti, 231 Albert Sabin Way, rm 6367, Cincinnati, OH 45267-0562; **Phone:** (513) 558-4233; **Board Cert:** Internal Medicine 1975, Hematology 1978; **Med School:** Jefferson Med Coll 1968; **Resid:** Internal Medicine, Thomas Jefferson Univ Hosp, Philadelphia, PA 1969-1971; **Fellow:** Hematology, Thomas Jefferson Univ Hosp, Philadelphia, PA 1971-1974; **Fac Appt:** Assoc Prof Medicine, Univ Cincinnati

Preisler, Harvey D MD (Hem) - *Spec Exp:* Lymphoma; **Hospital:** Rush-Presby - St Luke's Med Ctr (page 72); **Address:** 1725 W Harrison St, Ste 809, Chicago, IL 60612-3728; **Phone:** (312) 563-2190; **Board Cert:** Medical Oncology 1975, Internal Medicine 1972; **Med School:** Univ Rochester 1965; **Resid:** Internal Medicine, Buffalo Genl Hosp, Buffalo, NY 1966-1967; Internal Medicine, Roswell Cancer Ctr, Buffalo, NY 1966-1967; **Fellow:** Hematology, Columbia-Presby Hosp, New York, NY 1969-1971; **Fac Appt:** Prof Medicine, Univ Chicago-Pritzker Sch Med

Stiff, Patrick J MD (Hem) - *Spec Exp:* Bone Marrow Transplant; Non-Hodgkin's Lymphoma; Leukemia; **Hospital:** Loyola Univ Med Ctr; **Address:** 2160 S First Ave, Maywood, IL 60153; **Phone:** (708) 169-9000; **Board Cert:** Medical Oncology 1981, Hematology 1982; **Med School:** Loyola Univ-Stritch Sch Med 1975; **Resid:** Internal Medicine, Cleveland Clinic, Cleveland, OH 1976-1978; **Fellow:** Hematology and Oncology, Meml Sloan Kettering Cancer Ctr, New York, NY 1978-1981; **Fac Appt:** Prof Medicine, Loyola Univ-Stritch Sch Med

Tallman, Martin S MD (Hem) - *Spec Exp:* Bone Marrow Transplant; Leukemia; **Hospital:** Northwestern Meml Hosp; **Address:** 675 N St Clair St Fl 14 - Ste 100, Chicago, IL 60611; **Phone:** (312) 695-8697; **Board Cert:** Internal Medicine 1983, Medical Oncology 1987, Hematology 1988; **Med School:** Univ Hlth Sci/Chicago Med Sch 1980; **Resid:** Internal Medicine, Evanston Hosp/Northwestern 1981-1983; **Fellow:** Medical Oncology, U. Wash, Seattle, WA 1984-1987

White, Peter MD (Hem) - *Spec Exp:* Porphyria; **Hospital:** Med Coll of Ohio Hosps; **Address:** Ruppert Health Ctr, 3120 Glendale Ave, rm 1100, Toledo, OH 43614; **Phone:** (419) 383-3747; **Board Cert:** Internal Medicine 1974, Hematology 1974; **Med School:** Univ Penn 1955; **Resid:** Internal Medicine, Hosp Univ Penn, Philadelphia, PA 1956-1960; **Fellow:** Hematology, Hosp Univ Penn, Philadelphia, PA 1963-1965; **Fac Appt:** Prof Medicine, Med Coll OH

Winter, Jane N MD (Hem) - *Spec Exp:* Hodgkin's Disease; Bone Marrow Transplant; Non-Hodgkin's Lymphoma; **Hospital:** Northwestern Meml Hosp; **Address:** 675 N St Claire St, Fl 14 - Ste 100, Chicago, IL 60611; **Phone:** (312) 695-8697; **Board Cert:** Internal Medicine 1980, Hematology 1982, Medical Oncology 1983; **Med School:** Univ Penn 1977; **Resid:** Internal Medicine, Univ Chicago Hosp, Chcago, IL 1978-1980; **Fellow:** Hematology and Oncology, Columbia Presby Hosp, New York, NY 1980-1981; Hematology, Northwestern Univ Hosp, Chicago, IL 1981-1983; **Fac Appt:** Prof Medicine, Northwestern Univ

Southwest

Barlogie, Bartholomew MD/PhD (Hem) - *Spec Exp:* Bone Marrow Transplant; Plasma Cell Disorders; Myeloma; **Hospital:** UAMS; **Address:** Univ Hosp Arkansas Med Sci, Bone Marrow Clinic, 4301 West Markham St - Slot 623, Little Rock, AR 72205; **Phone:** (501) 686-6000; **Med School:** Germany 1969; **Fellow:** Medical Oncology, MD Anderson Cancer Ctr, Houston, TX 1974-1976; **Fac Appt:** Prof Medicine, Univ Ark

Cobos, Everardo MD (Hem) - ***Spec Exp:*** *Bone Marrow Transplant; Bleeding/Coagulation Disorders;* **Hospital:** Univ Med Ctr - Lubbock; **Address:** Texas Tech Univ Med Sch, Dept Med, 3601 4th St, Lubbock, TX 79430; **Phone:** (806) 743-3155; **Board Cert:** Hematology 1988, Medical Oncology 1987; **Med School:** Univ Tex, San Antonio 1981; **Resid:** Internal Medicine, Letterman Army Med Ctr, San Francisco, CA 1983-1985; **Fellow:** Hematology and Oncology, Letterman Army Med Ctr, San Francisco, CA 1985-1988; **Fac Appt:** Assoc Prof Medicine, Texas Tech Univ

Kantarjian, Hagop M MD (Hem) - ***Spec Exp:*** *Leukemia;* **Hospital:** Univ of TX MD Anderson Cancer Ctr, The; **Address:** 1515 Holcombe Blvd, Box 428, Houston, TX 77030-4009; **Phone:** (713) 792-7026; **Board Cert:** Medical Oncology 1985, Hematology 1990; **Med School:** Lebanon 1979; **Resid:** Internal Medicine, Univ Tex MD Anderson, Houston, TX 1981-1983; **Fellow:** Univ Texas MD Anderson Cancer Ctr, Houston, TX 1981-1983; **Fac Appt:** Prof Medicine, Univ Tex, Houston

List, Alan F MD (Hem) - ***Spec Exp:*** *Bone Marrow Transplant; Leukemia;* **Hospital:** Univ Med Ctr; **Address:** Univ Arizona Hlth Scis, 1515 N Campbell Ave, rm 3945, Tucson, AZ 85724; **Phone:** (520) 626-2340; **Board Cert:** Internal Medicine 1983, Medical Oncology 1985, Hematology 1986; **Med School:** Univ Penn 1980; **Resid:** Internal Medicine, Good Samaritan Hosp, Phoenix, AZ 1980-1983; Oncology, Vanderbilt Univ Med Ctr, Nashville, TN 1983-1985; **Fellow:** Hematology, Vanderbilt Univ Med Ctr, Nashville, TN 1985-1986; **Fac Appt:** Assoc Prof Medicine, Univ Ariz Coll Med

Miro-Quesada, Miguel MD (Hem) - ***Spec Exp:*** *Hematology - General;* **Hospital:** St Luke's Episcopal Hosp - Houston; **Address:** 920 Frostwood, Ste 780, Houston, TX 77030; **Phone:** (713) 827-9525; **Board Cert:** Internal Medicine 1972, Hematology 1974; **Med School:** Johns Hopkins Univ 1969; **Resid:** Internal Medicine, Northwestern Univ Hosp, Chicago, IL 1970-1971; Internal Medicine, Rush-Presby-St Luke's Med Ctr, Chicago, IL 1971-1972; **Fellow:** Hematology, Montefiore Hosp, New York, NY 1973-1974

West Coast and Pacific

Feinstein, Donald I MD (Hem) - ***Spec Exp:*** *Bleeding/Coagulation Disorders;* **Hospital:** USC Norris Cancer Comp Ctr; **Address:** USC Keck Sch Med, Topping Tower, 1441 Eastlake Ave, Ste 3436, Los Angeles, CA 90033-9172; **Phone:** (323) 865-3964; **Board Cert:** Hematology 1974, Internal Medicine 1965; **Med School:** Stanford Univ 1958; **Resid:** Internal Medicine, LAC-USC Med Ctr, Los Angeles, CA 1959-1962; **Fellow:** Hematology, NYU Med Ctr, New York, NY 1964-1966; **Fac Appt:** Prof Medicine, USC Sch Med

Kaushansky, Kenneth MD (Hem) - ***Spec Exp:*** *Hematology - General;* **Hospital:** Univ WA Med Ctr; **Address:** 1959 NE Pacific St, HSB K-260, Box 357710, Seattle, WA 98195-7710; **Phone:** (206) 685-7868; **Board Cert:** Internal Medicine 1982, Hematology 1984; **Med School:** UCLA 1979; **Resid:** Internal Medicine, Univ Wash Med Ctr, Seattle, WA 1979-1982; **Fellow:** Hematology, Univ Wash Med Ctr, Seattle, WA 1982-1986; **Fac Appt:** Prof Medicine, Univ Wash

Leung, Lawrence L MD (Hem) - ***Spec Exp:*** *Thrombotic Disorders;* **Hospital:** Stanford Med Ctr; **Address:** Stanford Univ Med Ctr, Dept Hem, 269 Tempest Dr CCSR Bldg Rm 1155, Stanford, CA 94305-5156; **Phone:** (650) 723-5007; **Board Cert:** Hematology 1980, Medical Oncology 1981; **Med School:** Columbia P&S 1975; **Resid:** Internal Medicine, NY Hosp/Cornell Med Ctr, New York, NY 1976-1978; **Fellow:** Hematology, NY Hosp/Cornell Med Ctr, New York, NY 1978-1981; **Fac Appt:** Assoc Prof Medicine, Stanford Univ

Levine, Alexandra Mary MD (Hem) - *Spec Exp:* Leukemia; Acute Promyelocytic Leukemia((APL); Tranfusion Free Medicine; **Hospital:** USC Norris Cancer Comp Ctr; **Address:** USC Kenneth Norris Jr Cancer Hosp, 1441 Eastlake Ave, rm 3468, Los Angeles, CA 90033; **Phone:** (323) 865-3913; **Med School:** USC Sch Med 1971; **Resid:** Internal Medicine, LA Cc-USC Med Ctr, Los Angeles, CA 1972-1974; **Fellow:** Hematology, Grady Meml Hosp-Emory Univ, Atlanta, GA 1974-1975; Hematology, LA Co-USC Med Ctr, Los Angeles, CA 1975-1976; **Fac Appt:** Prof Medicine, USC Sch Med

Linenberger, Michael MD (Hem) - *Spec Exp:* Hematology - General; **Hospital:** Univ WA Med Ctr; **Address:** 825 Eastlake Ave E, Box 19023, Seattle, WA 98109; **Phone:** (206) 288-2038; **Board Cert:** Internal Medicine 1985, Hematology 1988; **Med School:** Univ Kans 1982; **Resid:** Internal Medicine, Rhode Island Hosp, Providence, RI 1983-1985; **Fellow:** Hematology, Univ Wash Med Ctr, Seattle, WA 1986-1989; **Fac Appt:** Assoc Prof Medicine, Univ Wash

Schiller, Gary John MD (Hem) - *Spec Exp:* Leukemia; **Hospital:** UCLA Med Ctr; **Address:** UCLA Med Ctr, CHS, 10833 Le Conte Ave, rm 42-121, Los Angeles, CA 90095; **Phone:** (310) 825-5513; **Board Cert:** Internal Medicine 1987, Medical Oncology 1989, Hematology 2000; **Med School:** USC Sch Med 1984; **Resid:** Internal Medicine, UCLA Med Ctr, Los Angeles, CA 1984-1987; **Fellow:** Hematology and Oncology, UCLA Med Ctr, Los Angeles, CA 1987-1990; **Fac Appt:** Assoc Prof Medicine, UCLA

New England

Antin, Joseph Harry MD (Onc) - *Spec Exp:* Bone Marrow Transplant; **Hospital:** Brigham & Women's Hosp; **Address:** 44 Binney St, Quarterdeck, Boston, MA 02115; **Phone:** (617) 632-2525; **Board Cert:** Hematology 1984, Medical Oncology 1983; **Med School:** Cornell Univ-Weill Med Coll 1978; **Resid:** Internal Medicine, Peter Bent Brigham Hosp., Boston, MA 1979-1981; **Fellow:** Medical Oncology, Brigham-Womens, Boston, MA 1981-1984; **Fac Appt:** Assoc Prof Medicine, Harvard Med Sch

Canellos, George Peter MD (Onc) - *Spec Exp:* Lymphoma; Leukemia; Breast Cancer; **Hospital:** Dana Farber Cancer Inst; **Address:** 44 Binney St, Boston, MA 02115; **Phone:** (617) 632-3470; **Board Cert:** Medical Oncology 1973, Hematology 1972; **Med School:** Columbia P&S 1960; **Resid:** Internal Medicine, Mass Genl Hosp, Boston, MA 1962-1963; Internal Medicine, Mass Genl Hosp, Boston, MA 1965-1966; **Fellow:** Medical Oncology, Natl Cancer Inst, Bethesda, MD 1963-1965; Hematology, Hammersmith Hosp, London, England 1966-1967; **Fac Appt:** Prof Medicine, Harvard Med Sch

Come, Steven Eliot MD (Onc) - *Spec Exp:* Breast Cancer; Hodgkin's Disease; **Hospital:** Beth Israel Deaconess Med Ctr - Boston; **Address:** 330 Brookline Ave, Boston, MA 02215-5491; **Phone:** (617) 667-4599; **Board Cert:** Medical Oncology 1979, Internal Medicine 1975; **Med School:** Harvard Med Sch 1972; **Resid:** Internal Medicine, Beth Israel Hosp, Boston, MA 1973-1977; **Fellow:** Medical Oncology, Natl Cancer Inst, Bethesda, MD 1974-1976; **Fac Appt:** Assoc Prof Medicine, Harvard Med Sch

De Fusco, Patricia A MD (Onc) - *Spec Exp:* Breast Cancer; **Hospital:** Hartford Hosp; **Address:** 100 Retreat Ave, Hartford, CT 06106-2528; **Phone:** (860) 246-6647; **Board Cert:** Internal Medicine 1983, Medical Oncology 1987; **Med School:** Boston Univ 1980; **Resid:** Internal Medicine, Hartford, Hartford, CT 1981-1984; **Fellow:** Medical Oncology, Mayo Clinic, Rochester, MN 1984-1986

De Vita Jr, Vincent T MD (Onc) - *Spec Exp:* Lymphoma; Hodgkin's Disease; **Hospital:** Yale - New Haven Hosp; **Address:** 333 Cedar St, rm WWW-205, Box 208028, New Haven, CT 06520-8028; **Phone:** (203) 785-4371; **Board Cert:** Medical Oncology 1973, Hematology 1972; **Med School:** Geo Wash Univ 1961; **Resid:** Internal Medicine, Geo Wash Hosp, Washington, DC 1962-1963; Internal Medicine, Yale-New Haven Hosp, New Haven, CT 1965-1966; **Fellow:** Medical Oncology, Natl Cancer Inst, Bethesda, MD 1963-1965; **Fac Appt:** Prof Medicine, Yale Univ

Garber, Judy E MD (Onc) - *Spec Exp:* Breast Cancer; **Hospital:** Dana Farber Cancer Inst; **Address:** 44 Binney St, Boston, MA 02115; **Phone:** (617) 632-2282; **Board Cert:** Hematology 1988, Medical Oncology 1987, Internal Medicine 1984; **Med School:** Yale Univ 1981; **Resid:** Internal Medicine, Brigham & Women's Hosp, Boston, MA 1982-1984; **Fellow:** Medical Oncology, Dana Farber Canc Inst, Boston, MA 1985-1988; Epidemiology, Dana Farber Canc Inst, Boston, MA 1986-1990; **Fac Appt:** Asst Prof Medicine, Harvard Med Sch

Garnick, Marc Bennett MD (Onc) - *Spec Exp:* Prostate Cancer; Biotechnology; **Hospital:** Beth Israel Deaconess Med Ctr - Boston; **Address:** 330 Brookline Ave, Boston, MA 02215; **Phone:** (617) 667-5288; **Board Cert:** Internal Medicine 1976, Medical Oncology 1979; **Med School:** Univ Penn 1972; **Resid:** Internal Medicine, Univ Penn Hosp, Philadelphia, PA 1973-1974; **Fellow:** Research, Natl Inst Hlth, Boston, MA 1974-1976; Medical Oncology, Dana-Farber Cancer Inst, Boston, MA 1976-1978; **Fac Appt:** Assoc Prof Medicine, Harvard Med Sch

Johnson, Bruce Evan MD (Onc) - *Spec Exp:* Lung Cancer; **Hospital:** Dana Farber Cancer Inst; **Address:** Lowe Ctr. Thoracic Onc-Dana Farber Cancer Inst., 44 Binney St, Ste 1234, Boston, MA 02115; **Phone:** (617) 632-4790; **Board Cert:** Medical Oncology 1985, Internal Medicine 1982; **Med School:** Univ Minn 1979; **Resid:** Internal Medicine, Univ Chicago, Chicago, IL 1980-1982; **Fellow:** Medical Oncology, Natl Cancer Inst., Bethesda, MD 1982-1985; **Fac Appt:** Assoc Prof Medical Oncology, Harvard Med Sch

Kaelin, William G MD (Onc) - *Spec Exp:* Medical Oncology - General; **Hospital:** Dana Farber Cancer Inst; **Address:** Dana Farber Cancer Inst, 44 Binney St, rm M-457, Boston, MA 02115; **Phone:** (617) 632-3975; **Board Cert:** Internal Medicine 1987, Medical Oncology 1989; **Med School:** Duke Univ 1982; **Resid:** Internal Medicine, Johns Hopkins Hosp, Baltimore, MD 1983-1986; **Fellow:** Medical Oncology, Dana Farber Cancer Inst, Boston, MA 1987-1989; **Fac Appt:** Assoc Prof Medicine, Harvard Med Sch

Karp, Daniel David MD (Onc) - *Spec Exp:* Lung Cancer; **Hospital:** Beth Israel Deaconess Med Ctr - Boston; **Address:** 330 Brookline Ave, Ste E/KS-158, Boston, MA 02111; **Phone:** (617) 667-1910; **Board Cert:** Internal Medicine 1976, Hematology 1980, Medical Oncology 1981; **Med School:** Duke Univ **Resid:** Internal Medicine, Dartmouth-Hitchcock Med Ctr., Hanover, NH 1974-1976; **Fellow:** Hematology, Dartmouth-Hitchcock Med Ctr., Hanover, NH 1976-1978; Medical Oncology, Dana Farber Inst., Boston, MA 1978-1979; **Fac Appt:** Assoc Prof Medicine, Harvard Med Sch

Kaufman, Peter A. MD (Onc) - *Spec Exp:* Breast Cancer; **Hospital:** Dartmouth - Hitchcock Med Ctr; **Address:** One Medical Center Drive, Lebanon, NH 03756; **Phone:** (603) 650-5000; **Board Cert:** Medical Oncology 1989, Hematology 1990; **Med School:** NYU Sch Med 1983; **Resid:** Internal Medicine, Duke Univ Med Ctr, Durham, NC 1984-1986; **Fellow:** Hematology and Oncology, Duke Univ Med Ctr, Durham, NC 1986

Lynch, Thomas MD (Onc) - *Spec Exp:* Lung Cancer; **Hospital:** MA Genl Hosp; **Address:** Mass Genl Hosp, Dept Hem/Onc, 55 Fruit Street, Boston, MA 02114; **Phone:** (617) 724-1136; **Board Cert:** Internal Medicine 1989, Medical Oncology 1991; **Med School:** Yale Univ 1986; **Resid:** Internal Medicine, Mass Genl Hosp, Boston, MA 1987-1989; **Fellow:** Medical Oncology, Dana-Farber Cancer Inst, Boston, MA 1989-1991; **Fac Appt:** Asst Prof Medicine, Harvard Med Sch

Mayer, Robert James MD (Onc) - *Spec Exp:* Colon & Rectal Cancer; **Hospital:** Dana Farber Cancer Inst; **Address:** Dana Farber Cancer Inst., 44 Binney St., rm D1608, Boston, MA 02115-6084; **Phone:** (617) 632-3474; **Board Cert:** Internal Medicine 1973, Medical Oncology 1975, Hematology 1976; **Med School:** Harvard Med Sch 1969; **Resid:** Internal Medicine, Mt Sinai Hosp, New York, NY 1979-1971; Hematology and Oncology, Natl Cancer Inst, Bethesda, MD 1971-1974; **Fellow:** Sidney Farber Cancer Inst., Boston, MA 1974-1976; **Fac Appt:** Prof Medicine, Harvard Med Sch

Muss, Hyman MD (Onc) - *Spec Exp:* Breast Cancer; **Hospital:** Fletcher Allen Hlth Care Med Ctr - Campus; **Address:** 1 S Prospect St Bldg Arnold 2, Burlington, VT 05401-1429; **Phone:** (802) 847-8400; **Board Cert:** Hematology 1974, Medical Oncology 1975; **Med School:** SUNY Downstate 1968; **Resid:** Internal Medicine, Peter Bent Brigham Hosp, Boston, MA 1968-1970; **Fellow:** Medical Oncology, Peter Bent Brigham Hosp, Boston, MA 1972-1974; **Fac Appt:** Prof Medicine, Univ VT Coll Med

Nadler, Lee Marshall MD (Onc) - *Spec Exp:* Lymphoma; **Hospital:** Dana Farber Cancer Inst; **Address:** Dana-Farber Cancer Inst, 44 Binney St, Boston, MA 02115; **Phone:** (617) 632-3331; **Board Cert:** Internal Medicine 1976; **Med School:** Harvard Med Sch 1973; **Resid:** Internal Medicine, Columbia-Presby Hosp, New York, NY 1973-1975; **Fellow:** Medical Oncology, Dana-Farber Cancer Inst, Boston, MA 1977-1978; Medical Oncology, Natl Cancer Inst, Bethesda, MD 1975-1977; **Fac Appt:** Prof Medicine, Harvard Med Sch

Weisberg, Tracey MD (Onc) - *Spec Exp:* Breast Cancer; **Hospital:** Maine Med Ctr; **Address:** 100 US Route One, Scarborough, ME 04074; **Phone:** (207) 885-7600; **Board Cert:** Internal Medicine 1987, Medical Oncology 1989; **Med School:** SUNY Stony Brook 1983; **Resid:** Internal Medicine, Mount Sinai Hospital, New York, NY 1984-1985; Internal Medicine, Hartford Hospital, Hartford, CT 1985-1986; **Fellow:** Medical Oncology, Yale University Hospital, New Haven, CT; **Fac Appt:** Clin Inst Univ VT Coll Med

Winer, Eric P MD (Onc) - *Spec Exp:* Breast Cancer; **Hospital:** Dana Farber Cancer Inst; **Address:** 44 Binney St, Ste 1210, Boston, MA 02115; **Phone:** (617) 632-3800; **Board Cert:** Internal Medicine 1987, Medical Oncology 1989; **Med School:** Yale Univ 1983; **Resid:** Internal Medicine, Yale-New Haven Hosp, New Haven, CT 1983-1987; **Fellow:** Hematology and Oncology, Duke Univ, Durham, NC 1987-1989; **Fac Appt:** Assoc Clin Prof Medicine, Harvard Med Sch

Mid Atlantic

Abeloff, Martin MD (Onc) - *Spec Exp:* Breast Cancer; **Hospital:** Johns Hopkins Hosp - Baltimore; **Address:** 401 N Broadway, Baltimore, MD 21231; **Phone:** (410) 955-8822; **Board Cert:** Medical Oncology 1973, Internal Medicine 1973; **Med School:** Johns Hopkins Univ 1966; **Resid:** Internal Medicine, Beth Israel Hosp, Boston, MA 1969-1970; **Fellow:** Hematology, New England Med Ctr, Boston, MA 1970-1971; **Fac Appt:** Prof Medicine, Johns Hopkins Univ

Ahlgren, James David MD (Onc) - *Spec Exp:* Gastrointestinal Cancer; **Hospital:** G Washington Univ Hosp; **Address:** Geo Wash Univ Med Ctr, Dept Hem & Onc, 2150 Pennsylvania Ave NW, Ste 3-428, Washington, DC 20037-3201; **Phone:** (202) 994-2746; **Board Cert:** Internal Medicine 1980, Medical Oncology 1989; **Med School:** Georgetown Univ 1977; **Resid:** Internal Medicine, Georgetown Univ Hosp, Washington, DC 1978-1979; **Fellow:** Medical Oncology, Georgetown Univ Hosp, Washington, DC 1979-1981; **Fac Appt:** Prof Medicine, Geo Wash Univ

Aisner, Joseph MD (Onc) - *Spec Exp:* Lung Cancer; **Hospital:** Cancer Inst of NJ, The; **Address:** 195 Little Albany St, Ste 2005, New Brunswick, NJ 08901; **Phone:** (732) 235-2465; **Board Cert:** Medical Oncology 1975, Internal Medicine 1973; **Med School:** Wayne State Univ 1970; **Resid:** Internal Medicine, Georgetown Univ Hosp, Washington, DC 1971-1972; **Fellow:** Medical Oncology, Natl Cancer Inst, Bethesda, MD 1972-1975

Algazy, Kenneth M MD (Onc) - *Spec Exp:* Lung Cancer; Mesothelioma; **Hospital:** Hosp Univ Penn (page 78); **Address:** 51 N 39th St, Medical Arts Building, Ste 103, Philadelphia, PA 19104; **Phone:** (215) 662-8947; **Board Cert:** Internal Medicine 1972, Hematology 1974, Medical Oncology 1979; **Med School:** Temple Univ 1969; **Resid:** Internal Medicine, Univ Rocheste-Strong Meml Hospr, Rochester, NY 1970-1972; **Fellow:** Hematology and Oncology, Johns Hopkins Med Ctr, Baltimore, MD 1972-1974

Antman, Karen MD (Onc) - *Spec Exp:* Breast Cancer; Sarcoma; **Hospital:** NY Presby Hosp - Columbia Presby Med Ctr (page 70); **Address:** 177 Fort Washington Ave, New York, NY 10032-3713; **Phone:** (212) 305-8602; **Board Cert:** Internal Medicine 1977, Medical Oncology 1979; **Med School:** Columbia P&S 1974; **Resid:** Internal Medicine, Columbia-Presby Med Ctr, New York, NY 1974-1977; **Fellow:** Medical Oncology, Dana-Farber Cancer Institute, Boston, MA 1977-1979; **Fac Appt:** Prof Medicine, Columbia P&S

Belani, Chandra MD (Onc) - *Spec Exp:* Lung Cancer; **Hospital:** UPMC - Presbyterian Univ Hosp; **Address:** Univ Pittsburgh Med Ctr - Montefiore, 3459 Fifth Ave, 7 Main, Pittsburgh, PA 15213; **Phone:** (412) 648-6619; **Board Cert:** Internal Medicine 1986, Medical Oncology 1987; **Med School:** India 1978; **Resid:** Internal Medicine, SMS Med Hosp, Jaipur, India 1978-1981; Internal Medicine, Good Samaritan/Univ MD Hosp, Baltimore, MD 1983-1984; **Fellow:** Hematology and Oncology, Univ MD Hosp, Baltimore, MD 1985; **Fac Appt:** Prof Medicine, Univ Pittsburgh

Bosl, George MD (Onc) - *Spec Exp:* Testicular Cancer; Head & Neck Cancer; **Hospital:** Mem Sloan Kettering Cancer Ctr; **Address:** 1275 York Ave, New York, NY 10021-6094; **Phone:** (212) 639-8473; **Board Cert:** Internal Medicine 1976, Medical Oncology 1979; **Med School:** Creighton Univ 1973; **Resid:** Internal Medicine, NY Hosp, New York, NY 1974-1975; Internal Medicine, Memorial Sloan-Kettering Cancer Ctr, New York, NY 1974-1977; **Fellow:** Medical Oncology, Univ Minn, Minneapolis, MN 1977-1979; **Fac Appt:** Prof Medicine, Cornell Univ-Weill Med Coll

Chapman, Paul MD (Onc) - *Spec Exp:* Melanoma; Immunology; **Hospital:** Mem Sloan Kettering Cancer Ctr; **Address:** 1275 York Ave, New York, NY 10021-6007; **Phone:** (212) 639-5015; **Board Cert:** Internal Medicine 1984, Medical Oncology 1987; **Med School:** Cornell Univ-Weill Med Coll 1981; **Resid:** Internal Medicine, Univ Chicago, Chicago, IL 1982-1984; **Fellow:** Medical Oncology, Meml Sloan-Kettering Cancer Ctr, New York, NY 1984; **Fac Appt:** Assoc Prof Medicine, Cornell Univ-Weill Med Coll

Cohen, Philip MD (Onc) - *Spec Exp:* Breast Cancer; **Hospital:** Georgetown Univ Hosp; **Address:** Georgetown Univ Hosp, Lombardi Cancer Ctr, 3800 Reservoir Rd NW, Washington, DC 20007; **Phone:** (202) 687-2198; **Board Cert:** Internal Medicine 1973, Medical Oncology 1975, Hematology 1976; **Med School:** Harvard Med Sch 1970; **Resid:** Infectious Disease, Mass Genl Hosp, Boston, MA 1971-1972; **Fellow:** Medical Oncology, Natl Cancer Inst, Bethesda, MD 1972-1974; **Fac Appt:** Assoc Clin Prof Medicine, Geo Wash Univ

Cohen, Seymour MD (Onc) - *Spec Exp:* Melanoma; Breast Cancer; Lung Cancer; **Hospital:** Mount Sinai Hosp (page 68); **Address:** 1045 5th Ave, New York, NY 10028-0138; **Phone:** (212) 249-9141; **Board Cert:** Internal Medicine 1971, Medical Oncology 1973; **Med School:** Univ Pittsburgh 1962; **Resid:** Internal Medicine, Montefiore Med Ctr, Bronx, NY 1963-1964; Internal Medicine, Mount Sinai Med Ctr, New York, NY 1964-1965; **Fellow:** Hematology, Mount Sinai Med Ctr, New York, NY 1965-1967; Hematology and Oncology, LI Jewish Hosp, New Hyde Park, NY 1968-1969; **Fac Appt:** Assoc Clin Prof Medicine, Mount Sinai Sch Med

Coleman, Morton MD (Onc) - *Spec Exp:* Lymphoma-Hodgkins & Non-Hodgkins; Myeloma; Leukemia; **Hospital:** NY Presby Hosp - NY Weill Cornell Med Ctr (page 70); **Address:** 407 E 70th St, FL 3, New York, NY 10021; **Phone:** (212) 517-5900; **Board Cert:** Medical Oncology 1973, Hematology 1972; **Med School:** Med Coll VA 1963; **Resid:** Internal Medicine, NY Hosp, New York, NY 1967-1968; Internal Medicine, Grady Mem, Atlanta, GA 1963-1965; **Fellow:** Hematology and Oncology, NY Hosp, New York, NY 1968-1970; **Fac Appt:** Clin Prof Medicine, Cornell Univ-Weill Med Coll

Comis, Robert L MD (Onc) - *Spec Exp:* Lung Cancer; Oncology; **Hospital:** Hahnemann Univ Hosp; **Address:** 1818 Market St, Ste 1100, Philadelphia, PA 19103; **Phone:** (215) 789-3645; **Board Cert:** Internal Medicine 1975, Medical Oncology 1977; **Med School:** SUNY Syracuse 1971; **Resid:** Internal Medicine, SUNY Hlth Sci Ctr, Syracuse, NY 1971-1975

Cullen, Kevin MD (Onc) - *Spec Exp:* Head & Neck Cancer; **Hospital:** Georgetown Univ Hosp; **Address:** Georgetown Univ Hosp, Lombardi Cancer Ctr, 3800 Reservoir Rd NW, Washington, DC 20007; **Phone:** (202) 687-3013; **Board Cert:** Infectious Disease 1986, Medical Oncology 1989; **Med School:** Harvard Med Sch 1983; **Resid:** Infectious Disease, Beth Israel Hosp, Boston, MA 1984-1986; **Fellow:** Medical Oncology, Natl Cancer Inst, Bethesda, MD 1986-1987; **Fac Appt:** Assoc Prof Medicine, Georgetown Univ

Davidson, Nancy E MD (Onc) - *Spec Exp:* Breast Cancer; Bone Marrow Transplant; **Hospital:** Johns Hopkins Hosp - Baltimore; **Address:** Johns Hopkins Oncology Center, 1650 Orleans St, Bldg CRB - rm 409, Baltimore, MD 21231-1000; **Phone:** (410) 955-8964; **Board Cert:** Internal Medicine 1982, Medical Oncology 1985; **Med School:** Harvard Med Sch 1979; **Resid:** Internal Medicine, Johns Hopkins Hosp, Baltimore, MD 1980-1982; **Fellow:** Medical Oncology, Natl Cancer Inst, Bethesda, MD 1982-1986; **Fac Appt:** Prof Medical Oncology, Johns Hopkins Univ

Donehower, Ross Carl MD (Onc) - *Spec Exp:* Pancreatic Cancer; Colon Cancer; Prostate Cancer; **Hospital:** Johns Hopkins Hosp - Baltimore; **Address:** 1650 Orleans St, Ste 187, Baltimore, MD 21231; **Phone:** (410) 955-8838; **Board Cert:** Internal Medicine 1977, Medical Oncology 1979; **Med School:** Univ Minn 1974; **Resid:** Internal Medicine, Johns Hopkins Hosp, Baltimore, MD 1975-1976; **Fellow:** Medical Oncology, Natl Inst Hlth, Bethesda, MD 1976-1980; **Fac Appt:** Prof Medicine, Johns Hopkins Univ

Eisenberger, Mario MD (Onc) - *Spec Exp:* Prostate Cancer; **Hospital:** Johns Hopkins Hosp - Baltimore; **Address:** Johns Hopkins Univ, 1650 Orleans St, rm 1M51, Baltimore, MD 21231; **Phone:** (410) 614-3511; **Board Cert:** Internal Medicine 1976, Medical Oncology 1979; **Med School:** Brazil 1972

Ettinger, David Seymour MD (Onc) - *Spec Exp:* Lung Cancer; **Hospital:** Johns Hopkins Hosp - Baltimore; **Address:** Bunting Blaustein Cancer Rsrch Bldg, 1650 Orleans St, Baltimore, MD 21231-1000; **Phone:** (410) 955-8847; **Board Cert:** Internal Medicine 1976, Medical Oncology 1977; **Med School:** Univ Louisville Sch Med 1967; **Resid:** Internal Medicine, Mayo Grad Schl, Rochester, MN 1968-1971; **Fellow:** Medical Oncology, Johns Hopkins Hosp, Baltimore, MD 1973-1975; **Fac Appt:** Prof Medical Oncology, Johns Hopkins Univ

Fisher, Richard I MD (Onc) - *Spec Exp:* Lymphoma; Hodgkin's Disease; **Hospital:** Strong Memorial Hosp - URMC; **Address:** James P. Wilmot Cancer Ctr, 601 Elmwood Ave, Box 704, Rochester, NY 14642; **Phone:** (585) 275-0842; **Board Cert:** Internal Medicine 1973, Medical Oncology 1977; **Med School:** Harvard Med Sch 1970; **Resid:** Internal Medicine, Mass Genl Hosp, Boston, MA 1971-1972; **Fac Appt:** Prof Medical Oncology, Univ Rochester

Gabrilove, Janice MD (Onc) - *Spec Exp:* Myelodysplastic Syndromes; Leukemia; **Hospital:** Mount Sinai Hosp (page 68); **Address:** 5 E 98th St, Fl 14, Box 1129, New York, NY 10029; **Phone:** (212) 241-9650; **Board Cert:** Internal Medicine 1980, Medical Oncology 1983; **Med School:** Mount Sinai Sch Med 1977; **Resid:** Internal Medicine, Columbia-Presby Med Ctr, New York, NY 1978-1980; **Fellow:** Hematology and Oncology, Meml Sloan-Kettering Cancer Ctr, New York, NY 1984; **Fac Appt:** Prof Medicine, Mount Sinai Sch Med

Glick, John H MD (Onc) - *Spec Exp:* Breast Cancer; Hodgkin's Disease; Non-Hodgkins Lymphoma; **Hospital:** Hosp Univ Penn (page 78); **Address:** Univ Penn Cancer Ctr, 3400 Spruce St, Fl 16, Philadelphia, PA 19104-4206; **Phone:** (215) 662-6334; **Board Cert:** Internal Medicine 1973, Medical Oncology 1975; **Med School:** Columbia P&S 1969; **Resid:** Internal Medicine, Presbyterian Hosp, New York, NY 1969-1971; **Fellow:** Medical Oncology, Natl Cancer Inst, Bethesda, MD 1971-1973; Medical Oncology, Stanford Univ, Stanford, CA 1973-1974; **Fac Appt:** Prof Medicine, Univ Penn

Goldstein, Lori J MD (Onc) - *Spec Exp:* Breast Cancer; **Hospital:** Fox Chase Cancer Ctr; **Address:** Fox Chase Cancer Ctr, Dept Med Oncology, 7701 Burholme Ave, Philadelphia, PA 19111; **Phone:** (215) 728-2689; **Board Cert:** Medical Oncology 1991, Internal Medicine 1985; **Med School:** SUNY Syracuse 1982; **Resid:** Internal Medicine, Presby U Hosp, Pittsburgh, PA 1983-1985; **Fellow:** Medical Oncology, NCI/NIH, Bethesda, MD 1986; **Fac Appt:** Assoc Prof Medical Oncology, Temple Univ

Grossbard, Michael Laurence MD (Onc) - *Spec Exp:* Lymphoma; Gastrointestinal Cancer; **Hospital:** St Luke's - Roosevelt Hosp Ctr - Roosevelt Div (page 58); **Address:** 425 W 59th St, Ste 1A, New York, NY 10019; **Phone:** (212) 523-5419; **Board Cert:** Internal Medicine 1989, Medical Oncology 1991; **Med School:** Yale Univ 1986; **Resid:** Internal Medicine, Mass Genl Hosp, Boston, MA 1986-1989; **Fellow:** Medical Oncology, Dana Farber Cancer Inst, Boston, MA 1989; **Fac Appt:** Asst Clin Prof Medicine, Columbia P&S

Hait, William MD/PhD (Onc) - *Spec Exp:* Breast Cancer; **Hospital:** Robert Wood Johnson Univ Hosp @ New Brunswick; **Address:** Cancer Inst of NJ, 195 Little Albany St, New Brunswick, NJ 08901-1914; **Phone:** (732) 235-8064; **Board Cert:** Internal Medicine 1982, Medical Oncology 1987; **Med School:** Univ Penn 1978; **Resid:** Internal Medicine, Yale Univ Sch Med, New Haven, CT 1979-1982; **Fellow:** Medical Oncology, Yale Univ Sch Med, New Haven, CT 1982-1983; **Fac Appt:** Prof Medicine, UMDNJ-RW Johnson Med Sch

Haller, Daniel MD (Onc) - *Spec Exp:* Gastrointestinal Cancer; Colon & Rectal Cancer; **Hospital:** Hosp Univ Penn (page 78); **Address:** Hosp of the Univ PA, Dept Hem Onc, 3400 Spruce St, Penn Tower Bldg, Fl 16, Philadelphia, PA 19104; **Phone:** (215) 662-7666; **Board Cert:** Internal Medicine 1976, Medical Oncology 1979; **Med School:** Univ Pittsburgh 1973; **Resid:** Internal Medicine, Georgetown Univ Hosp, Washington, DC 1974-1976; **Fellow:** Medical Oncology, Georgetown Univ Hosp, Washington, DC 1976-1978

Holland, James F MD (Onc) - *Spec Exp:* Breast Cancer; **Hospital:** Mount Sinai Hosp (page 68); **Address:** 5 E 98th St Fl 14, New York, NY 10029; **Phone:** (212) 241-4495; **Board Cert:** Internal Medicine 1955; **Med School:** Columbia P&S 1947; **Resid:** Internal Medicine, Columbia-Presby, New York, NY 1947-1949; **Fellow:** Internal Medicine, Francis Delafield Hosp, New York, NY 1951-1953; **Fac Appt:** Prof Medicine, Mount Sinai Sch Med

Hudes, Gary Robert MD (Onc) - *Spec Exp:* Prostate Cancer; Genitourinary Cancer; **Hospital:** Fox Chase Cancer Ctr; **Address:** Fox Chase Cancer Ctr, 7701 Burholme Ave, rm W250, Philadelphia, PA 19111; **Phone:** (215) 728-3889; **Board Cert:** Hematology 1984, Medical Oncology 1985; **Med School:** SUNY Downstate 1979; **Resid:** Internal Medicine, Graduate Hosp-Tenet Hlth Sys, Philadelphia, PA 1979-1982; **Fellow:** Hematology and Oncology, Presby-Univ Penn Med Ctr, Philadelphia, PA 1982-1985

Kelsen, David MD (Onc) - *Spec Exp:* Gastrointestinal Cancer; Neuroendocrine Tumors; **Hospital:** Mem Sloan Kettering Cancer Ctr; **Address:** Gastrointestinal Oncology Service, 1275 York Ave Bldg Howard Fl 9 - rm 918, New York, NY 10021; **Phone:** (212) 639-8470; **Board Cert:** Internal Medicine 1976, Medical Oncology 1979; **Med School:** Hahnemann Univ 1972; **Resid:** Internal Medicine, Temple U Hosp, Philadelphia, PA 1972-1976; **Fellow:** Medical Oncology, Meml Sloan Kettering Cancer Ctr, New York, NY 1976-1978; **Fac Appt:** Prof Medicine, Cornell Univ-Weill Med Coll

Kemeny, Nancy MD (Onc) - *Spec Exp:* Colon Cancer; Rectal Cancer; **Hospital:** Mem Sloan Kettering Cancer Ctr; **Address:** Meml Sloan Kettering Cancer Ctr, Howard 916, 1275 York Ave, New York, NY 10021; **Phone:** (212) 639-8068; **Board Cert:** Internal Medicine 1974, Medical Oncology 1981; **Med School:** UMDNJ-NJ Med Sch, Newark 1971; **Resid:** Internal Medicine, St Luke's Roosevelt Hosp Ctr, New York, NY 1972-1974; **Fellow:** Medical Oncology, Mem Sloan Kettering Cancer Ctr, New York, NY 1974-1976; **Fac Appt:** Prof Medicine, Cornell Univ-Weill Med Coll

Kirkwood, John Munn MD (Onc) - *Spec Exp:* Melanoma; Sentinel Node Assessment/Adjuvant Therap; **Hospital:** UPMC - Presbyterian Univ Hosp; **Address:** Presbyterian University Hosp, North Wing, 200 Lothrop St, rm N758, Pittsburgh, PA 15413; **Phone:** (412) 648-6570; **Board Cert:** Medical Oncology 1981, Internal Medicine 1976; **Med School:** Yale Univ 1973; **Resid:** Yale Univ. Hosp., CT; **Fellow:** Dana Farber Cancer Inst., Boston, MA; Harvard Medical School, Boston, MA

Kris, Mark MD (Onc) - *Spec Exp:* Lung Cancer; Antiemetic Therapy; Mediastinal Tumors; **Hospital:** Mem Sloan Kettering Cancer Ctr; **Address:** 1275 York Ave Bldg Howard Fl 10, New York, NY 10021-6094; **Phone:** (212) 639-7590; **Board Cert:** Internal Medicine 1980, Medical Oncology 1983; **Med School:** Cornell Univ-Weill Med Coll 1977; **Resid:** Internal Medicine, New York Hosp, New York, NY 1977-1980; **Fellow:** Medical Oncology, Meml Sloan Kettering Cancer Ctr, New York, NY 1980-1983; **Fac Appt:** Prof Medicine, Cornell Univ-Weill Med Coll

Kwak, Larry Wonshin MD (Onc) - *Spec Exp:* Lymphoma; **Hospital:** Natl Inst of Hlth - Clin Ctr; **Address:** National Cancer Institute, Bldg 567 - rm 205, Fredrick, MD 21702; **Phone:** (301) 846-1607; **Board Cert:** Internal Medicine 1987, Medical Oncology 1989; **Med School:** Northwestern Univ 1982; **Resid:** Internal Medicine, Stanford Univ Hosp, Stanford, CA 1984-1987; **Fellow:** Oncology, Stanford Univ Hosp, Stanford, CA 1987-1989

Langer, Corey Jay MD (Onc) - *Spec Exp:* Lung Cancer; Head & Neck Cancer; **Hospital:** Fox Chase Cancer Ctr; **Address:** Fox Chase Cancer Center, 7701 Burholme Ave, rm C307, Philadelphia, PA 19111; **Phone:** (215) 728-2985; **Board Cert:** Medical Oncology 1986, Hematology 1986; **Med School:** Boston Univ 1981; **Resid:** Internal Medicine, Grad Hosp U Penn, Philadelphia, PA 1982-1984; Hematology and Oncology, Presby-Hosp U Penn, Philadelphia, PA 1984-1986; **Fellow:** Medical Oncology, Fox Chase Cancer Ctr, Philadelphia, PA 1986-1987

Leichman, Lawrence Peter MD (Onc) - *Spec Exp:* Esophageal Cancer; Gastrointestinal Cancer; **Hospital:** Albany Medical Center; **Address:** Cancer Center of Albany Med, 47 New Scotland Ave, MC 173, Albany, NY 12208; **Phone:** (518) 262-3829; **Board Cert:** Internal Medicine 1977, Medical Oncology 1983; **Med School:** Wayne State Univ 1973; **Resid:** Internal Medicine, Detroit Genl Hosp, Detroit, MI 1974-1977; **Fellow:** Medical Oncology, Wayne Hospital, Wayne, MI 1977-1979; **Fac Appt:** Prof Medicine, Albany Med Coll

Levine, Ellis MD (Onc) - *Spec Exp:* Breast Cancer; Urologic Cancer; **Hospital:** Roswell Park Cancer Inst; **Address:** Roswell Park Cancer Institute, Elm & Carlton Sts, Buffalo, NY 14263; **Phone:** (716) 845-8547; **Board Cert:** Medical Oncology 1985, Internal Medicine 1982; **Med School:** Univ Pittsburgh 1979; **Resid:** Internal Medicine, U Minn Hosps., MN 1980-1982; **Fellow:** Medical Oncology, U Minn., MN 1982-1984

Livingston, Philip MD (Onc) - *Spec Exp:* Breast Cancer; **Hospital:** Mem Sloan Kettering Cancer Ctr; **Address:** 1275 York Ave, New York, NY 10021; **Phone:** (212) 639-7425; **Board Cert:** Allergy & Immunology 1974, Medical Oncology 1981; **Med School:** Harvard Med Sch 1969; **Resid:** Internal Medicine, N Shore Hosp-Cornell Med Ctr, New York, NY 1969-1970; **Fellow:** Immunology, NYU Med Ctr, New York, NY 1971-1973; **Fac Appt:** Prof Medical Oncology, Cornell Univ-Weill Med Coll

Macdonald, John MD (Onc) - *Spec Exp:* Colon Cancer; **Hospital:** St Vincent Cath Med Ctrs - Manhattan (page 75); **Address:** 325 W 15th St, New York, NY 10011; **Phone:** (212) 604-6011; **Board Cert:** Internal Medicine 1973, Medical Oncology 1975; **Med School:** Harvard Med Sch 1969; **Resid:** Internal Medicine, Beth Israel Hosp, Boston, MA 1969-1971; **Fellow:** Hematology and Oncology, Natl Cancer Inst, Bethesda, MD 1971-1974; **Fac Appt:** Prof Medicine, NY Med Coll

Marks, Stanley M MD (Onc) - *Spec Exp:* Medical Oncology - General; **Hospital:** Shadyside Hosp - Pittsburgh; **Address:** Shadyside Place, 580 S Aiken Ave, Ste 430, Pittsburg, PA 15232; **Phone:** (412) 235-1020; **Board Cert:** Internal Medicine 1976, Hematology 1978; **Med School:** Univ Pittsburgh 1973; **Resid:** Internal Medicine, Presby Univ Hosp, Pittsburgh, PA 1974-1976; **Fellow:** Hematology, Peter Bent Brigham Hosp, Boston, MA 1976-1978; **Fac Appt:** Assoc Prof Medicine, Hahnemann Univ

Moore, Anne MD (Onc) - *Spec Exp:* Breast Cancer; **Hospital:** NY Presby Hosp - NY Weill Cornell Med Ctr (page 70); **Address:** New York Presbyterian Hospital, 428 E 72nd St, Ste 300, New York, NY 10021-4873; **Phone:** (212) 746-2085; **Board Cert:** Internal Medicine 1973, Medical Oncology 1977; **Med School:** Columbia P&S 1969; **Resid:** Internal Medicine, Cornell Univ Med Ctr, New York, NY 1970-1973; **Fellow:** Medical Oncology, Rockefeller Univ, New York, NY 1972-1973; **Fac Appt:** Prof Medical Oncology, Cornell Univ-Weill Med Coll

Motzer, Robert J MD (Onc) - *Spec Exp:* Kidney Cancer; Testicular Cancer; **Hospital:** Mem Sloan Kettering Cancer Ctr; **Address:** 1275 York Ave, Box 239, New York, NY 10021; **Phone:** (646) 422-4312; **Board Cert:** Internal Medicine 1984, Medical Oncology 1987; **Med School:** Univ Mich Med Sch 1981; **Resid:** Internal Medicine, Meml Sloan Kettering, New York, NY 1982-1984; **Fellow:** Medical Oncology, Meml Sloan Kettering, New York, NY 1984-1987; **Fac Appt:** Assoc Prof Medicine, Cornell Univ-Weill Med Coll

Nissenblatt, Michael MD (Onc) - *Spec Exp:* Breast & Lung Cancer; Lymphoma; Hereditary & Familial Cancers; **Hospital:** Robert Wood Johnson Univ Hosp @ New Brunswick; **Address:** 205 Easton Ave, New Brunswick, NJ 08901-1722; **Phone:** (732) 828-9570; **Board Cert:** Internal Medicine 1976, Medical Oncology 1979; **Med School:** Columbia P&S 1973; **Resid:** Internal Medicine, Johns Hopkins Hosp, Baltimore, MD 1973-1976; **Fellow:** Medical Oncology, Johns Hopkins Hosp, Baltimore, MD 1976-1978; **Fac Appt:** Clin Prof Medicine, Robert W Johnson Med Sch

Norton, Larry MD (Onc) - *Spec Exp:* Breast Cancer; **Hospital:** Mem Sloan Kettering Cancer Ctr; **Address:** 205 E 64th St, Concourse Level, New York, NY 10021; **Phone:** (212) 639-5438; **Board Cert:** Internal Medicine 1972, Medical Oncology 1977; **Med School:** Columbia P&S 1972; **Resid:** Internal Medicine, Bronx Municipal Hosp Ctr-Albert Einstein Coll Med, Bronx, NY 1973-1974; **Fac Appt:** Prof Medicine, Cornell Univ-Weill Med Coll

Offit, Kenneth MD (Onc) - *Spec Exp:* Cancer Genetics; Breast Cancer; Lymphoma; **Hospital:** Mem Sloan Kettering Cancer Ctr; **Address:** 1275 York Ave, Box 192, New York, NY 10021-6094; **Phone:** (212) 434-5166; **Board Cert:** Internal Medicine 1985, Medical Oncology 1987; **Med School:** Harvard Med Sch 1982; **Resid:** Internal Medicine, Lenox Hill Hosp, New York, NY; **Fellow:** Hematology and Oncology, Mem Sloan Kettering Cancer Ctr, New York, NY 1985-1987; Cancer Genetics, Mem Sloan Kettering Cancer Ctr, New York, NY 1987-1988; **Fac Appt:** Assoc Prof Medical Oncology, Cornell Univ-Weill Med Coll

Oster, Martin MD (Onc) - **Spec Exp:** *Breast Cancer; Lung Cancer; Prostate Cancer;* **Hospital:** NY Presby Hosp - Columbia Presby Med Ctr (page 70); **Address:** 161 Fort Washington Ave, New York, NY 10032-3713; **Phone:** (212) 305-8231; **Board Cert:** Internal Medicine 1974, Medical Oncology 1975; **Med School:** Columbia P&S 1971; **Resid:** Internal Medicine, Mass Genl Hosp, Boston, MA 1971-1973; **Fellow:** Medical Oncology, Natl Cancer Inst/Natl Inst Hlth, Bethesda, MD 1973-1976; **Fac Appt:** Assoc Clin Prof Medical Oncology, Columbia P&S

Ozols, Robert F MD/PhD (Onc) - **Spec Exp:** *Ovarian Cancer;* **Hospital:** Fox Chase Cancer Ctr; **Address:** Fox Chase Cancer Ctr, 7701 Burholme Ave, rm P 2050, Philadelphia, PA 19111; **Phone:** (215) 728-2673; **Board Cert:** Internal Medicine 1977, Medical Oncology 1979; **Med School:** Univ Rochester 1974; **Resid:** Internal Medicine, Dartmouth-Hitchcock Hosp, Lebanon, NH 1975-1976; **Fellow:** Medical Oncology, Natl Cancer Inst, Bethesda, MD 1976-1979; **Fac Appt:** Assoc Prof Medicine, Temple Univ

Scheinberg, David MD/PhD (Onc) - **Spec Exp:** *Leukemia; Immunotherapy; Cancer Vaccines;* **Hospital:** Mem Sloan Kettering Cancer Ctr; **Address:** 1275 York Ave, New York, NY 10021-6094; **Phone:** (212) 639-5010; **Board Cert:** Internal Medicine 1986, Medical Oncology 1995; **Med School:** Johns Hopkins Univ 1983; **Resid:** Internal Medicine, NY Hosp Cornell, New York, NY 1984-1985; **Fellow:** Medical Oncology, Meml Sloan Kettering Med Ctr, New York, NY 1985-1987; **Fac Appt:** Prof Medicine, Cornell Univ-Weill Med Coll

Scher, Howard MD (Onc) - **Spec Exp:** *Genitourinary Cancer; Prostate Cancer; Bladder Cancer;* **Hospital:** Mem Sloan Kettering Cancer Ctr; **Address:** 1275 York Ave, New York, NY 10021; **Phone:** (646) 422-4330; **Board Cert:** Internal Medicine 1979, Medical Oncology 1985; **Med School:** NYU Sch Med 1976; **Resid:** Internal Medicine, Bellevue Hosp, New York, NY 1977-1980; **Fellow:** Medical Oncology, Meml Sloan Kettering, New York, NY 1980-1983

Speyer, James MD (Onc) - **Spec Exp:** *Ovarian Cancer; Breast Cancer;* **Hospital:** NYU Med Ctr (page 71); **Address:** 160 E 32nd St, Fl 2, New York, NY 10016-6004; **Phone:** (212) 652-1918; **Board Cert:** Medical Oncology 1979, Hematology 1978, Internal Medicine 1977; **Med School:** Johns Hopkins Univ 1974; **Resid:** Internal Medicine, Columbia-Presby Med Ctr, New York, NY 1975-1976; Hematology, Columbia-Presby Med Ctr, NY, NY 1976-1977; **Fellow:** Medical Oncology, Natl Cancer Inst, Bethesda, MD 1977-1979; **Fac Appt:** Clin Prof Medicine, NYU Sch Med

Treat, Joseph MD (Onc) - **Spec Exp:** *Lung Cancer;* **Hospital:** Fox Chase Cancer Ctr; **Address:** 3322 N Broad St, Philadelphia, PA 19140; **Phone:** (215) 707-8030; **Board Cert:** Medical Oncology 1985, Internal Medicine 1982; **Med School:** Temple Univ 1979; **Resid:** Internal Medicine, Georgetown Univ Hosp, Washington, DC 1980-1982; **Fellow:** Medical Oncology, Georgetown Univ Hosp, Washington, DC 1982-1984; **Fac Appt:** Prof Medical Oncology, Temple Univ

Weber, Barbara L MD (Onc) - **Spec Exp:** *Breast Cancer;* **Hospital:** Hosp Univ Penn (page 78); **Address:** Univ Penn Cancer Ctr, 3400 Spruce St, Bldg Penn Tower - Fl 14, Philadelphia, PA 19104; **Phone:** (215) 898-0247; **Board Cert:** Internal Medicine 1985, Medical Oncology 1987; **Med School:** Univ Wash 1982; **Resid:** Internal Medicine, Yale Univ, New Haven, CT 1983-1985; **Fellow:** Medical Oncology, Dana-Farber Cancer Inst, Boston, MA 1985; **Fac Appt:** Prof Medical Oncology, Univ Penn

Weiner, Louis M MD (Onc) - **Spec Exp:** *Gastrointestinal Cancer; Immunotherapy;* **Hospital:** Fox Chase Cancer Ctr; **Address:** Fox Chase Cancer Ctr, 7701 Burholme Ave, Philadelphia, PA 19111; **Phone:** (215) 728-2480; **Board Cert:** Medical Oncology 1985, Internal Medicine 1980; **Med School:** Mount Sinai Sch Med 1977; **Resid:** Internal Medicine, Med Ctr Hosp of VT, Burlington, VT; **Fellow:** Hematology and Oncology, New England Med Ctr - Tufts Univ Sch Med, Boston, MA

MEDICAL ONCOLOGY

Zelenetz, Andrew D MD/PhD (Onc) - *Spec Exp:* Lymphoma; **Hospital:** Mem Sloan Kettering Cancer Ctr; **Address:** Meml Sloan-Kettering Cancer Ctr, 1275 York Ave, Box 330, New York, NY 10021; **Phone:** (212) 639-2656; **Board Cert:** Internal Medicine 1992, Medical Oncology 1993; **Med School:** Harvard Med Sch 1984; **Resid:** Internal Medicine, Stanford Univ Med Ctr, Stanford, CA 1985-1986; **Fellow:** Medical Oncology, Stanford Univ Med Ctr, Stanford, CA 1986-1989; **Fac Appt:** Asst Prof Medicine, Cornell Univ-Weill Med Coll

Southeast

Balducci, Lodovico MD (Onc) - *Spec Exp:* Genitourinary Cancer; Breast Cancer; **Hospital:** H Lee Moffitt Cancer Ctr & Research Inst; **Address:** 12902 Magnolia Dr, rm 3157, Tampa, FL 33612; **Phone:** (813) 979-3822; **Board Cert:** Medical Oncology 1979, Internal Medicine 1976; **Med School:** Italy 1968; **Resid:** Internal Medicine, Univ Miss Med Ctr, Jackson, MS 1973-1976; Hematology and Oncology, Univ Miss Med Ctr, Jackson, MS 1976-1979; **Fellow:** Internal Medicine, A Gemelli Genl Hosp, Rome, Italy 1968-1970; **Fac Appt:** Prof Medicine, Univ S Fla Coll Med

Crawford, Jeffrey MD (Onc) - *Spec Exp:* Lung Cancer; **Hospital:** Duke Univ Med Ctr (page 60); **Address:** Duke Univ Med Ctr, Box 3198, Durham, NC 27710; **Phone:** (919) 684-5621; **Board Cert:** Hematology 1980, Medical Oncology 1981; **Med School:** Ohio State Univ 1974; **Resid:** Internal Medicine, Duke Med Ctr, Durham, NC 1975-1977; Internal Medicine, Duke Med Ctr, Durham, NC 1978-1979; **Fellow:** Medical Oncology, Duke Med Ctr, Durham, NC 1977-1978; Hematology, Duke Med Ctr, Durham, NC 1979-1981; **Fac Appt:** Prof Medicine, Duke Univ

Gockerman, Jon Paul MD (Onc) - *Spec Exp:* Leukemia; Lymphoma; **Hospital:** Duke Univ Med Ctr (page 60); **Address:** Duke Univ Med Ctr, Box 3872, Durham, NC 27710; **Phone:** (919) 684-8964; **Board Cert:** Medical Oncology 1973, Hematology 1974; **Med School:** Univ Chicago-Pritzker Sch Med 1967; **Resid:** Internal Medicine, Duke Univ Med Ctr, Durham, NC 1968-1969; **Fellow:** Hematology and Oncology, Duke Univ Med Ctr, Durham, NC 1969-1971

Graham, Mark MD (Onc) - *Spec Exp:* Breast Cancer; Breast Cancer Genetics; **Hospital:** Western Wake Med Ctr; **Address:** Univ NC Hlthcare - Cary Oncology, 300 Ashville Ave, Ste 180, Cary, NC 27511; **Phone:** (919) 859-6631; **Board Cert:** Internal Medicine 1989; **Med School:** Mayo Med Sch 1982; **Resid:** Internal Medicine, Duke Univ Med Ctr, Durham, NC 1983-1985; **Fellow:** Medical Oncology, Univ CO Hlth Sci Ctr, Denver, CO 1986-1990; **Fac Appt:** Assoc Clin Prof Medicine, Univ NC Sch Med

Greco, F Anthony MD (Onc) - *Spec Exp:* Lung Cancer; **Hospital:** Centennial Med Ctr; **Address:** Sarah Cannon - Minnie Pearl Cancer Center, 250 25th Ave N, Ste 110, Nashville, TN 37203; **Phone:** (615) 342-1725; **Board Cert:** Internal Medicine 1975, Medical Oncology 1977; **Med School:** W VA Univ 1972; **Resid:** Internal Medicine, Univ West Virginia Hosp, Morgantown, WV 1973-1974; **Fellow:** Medical Oncology, Natl Canc Inst, Bethesda, MD 1974-1976

Green, Mark MD (Onc) - *Spec Exp:* Lung Cancer; **Hospital:** Med Univ Hosp Authority; **Address:** Med Univ South Carolina, 96 Jonathan Lucas St, 903 Clin Sciences Bldg, Charleston, SC 29425; **Phone:** (843) 792-4271; **Board Cert:** Internal Medicine 1973, Medical Oncology 1975; **Med School:** Harvard Med Sch 1970; **Resid:** Internal Medicine, Beth Israel Hosp, Boston, MA 1971-1972; Internal Medicine, Stanford Univ Hosp, Stanford, CA 1974-1975; **Fellow:** Medical Oncology, Natl Canc Inst, Bethesda, MD 1972-1974; Medical Oncology, Stanford Univ Hosp, Stanford, CA 1975-1976; **Fac Appt:** Prof Medicine, Univ SC Sch Med

Grosh, William W MD (Onc) - *Spec Exp:* Melanoma & Sarcoma; Liver Cancer; Carcinoid Tumors; **Hospital:** Univ of VA Hlth Sys (page 79); **Address:** PO Box 800716, Charlottesville, VA 22908; **Phone:** (804) 924-1904; **Board Cert:** Medical Oncology 1985, Internal Medicine 1978; **Med School:** Columbia P&S 1974; **Resid:** Internal Medicine, Vanderbilt Univ Med Ctr, Nashville, TN 1975-1977; **Fellow:** Medical Oncology, Vanderbilt Univ Med Ctr, Nashville, TN 1980-1983

Hande, Kenneth MD (Onc) - *Spec Exp:* Breast Cancer; Sarcoma; Carcinoid Tumors; **Hospital:** Vanderbilt Univ Med Ctr (page 80); **Address:** Vanderbilt Univ Med Ctr, 1956 The Vanderbilt Clinic, Nashville, TN 37232-5536; **Phone:** (615) 322-4967; **Board Cert:** Internal Medicine 1975, Medical Oncology 1977; **Med School:** Johns Hopkins Univ 1972; **Resid:** Internal Medicine, Barnes Hosp, St Louis, MO 1973-1974; **Fellow:** Medical Oncology, Natl Cancer Inst, Bethesda, MD 1974-1977; **Fac Appt:** Prof Medicine, Vanderbilt Univ

Horton, John MD (Onc) - *Spec Exp:* Breast Cancer; **Hospital:** H Lee Moffitt Cancer Ctr & Research Inst; **Address:** 12902 Magnolia Dr, Ste 4035, Tampa, FL 33612-9416; **Phone:** (813) 972-8470; **Board Cert:** Internal Medicine 1968, Medical Oncology 1973; **Med School:** England 1957; **Resid:** Internal Medicine, Albany Med Ctr Hosp, Albany, NY 1957-1962; **Fellow:** Medical Oncology, Albany Med Ctr Hosp, Albany, NY 1962-1963; **Fac Appt:** Prof Medical Oncology, Univ S Fla Coll Med

Jillella, Anand MD (Onc) - *Spec Exp:* Bone Marrow Transplant; Stem Cell Transplantation; **Hospital:** Med Coll of GA Hosp and Clin; **Address:** Med Coll of GA, Comprehensive Cancer Ctr, 1120 15th St, Augusta, GA 30912; **Phone:** (706) 721-2505; **Board Cert:** Internal Medicine 1992, Medical Oncology 1997; **Med School:** India 1985; **Resid:** Internal Medicine, Med Coll of GA, Augusta, GA; Medical Oncology, Yale University, New Haven, CT; **Fac Appt:** Assoc Prof Medicine, Med Coll GA

Johnson, David H MD (Onc) - *Spec Exp:* Lung Cancer; **Hospital:** Vanderbilt Univ Med Ctr (page 80); **Address:** Vanderbilt Univ Med Ctr, Div Med Onc, 2220 Pierce Ave, 777 PRB, Nashville, TN 37232; **Phone:** (615) 322-4967; **Board Cert:** Internal Medicine 1979, Medical Oncology 1983; **Med School:** Med Coll GA 1976; **Resid:** Internal Medicine, Univ South Alabama Med Ctr, Mobile, AL 1977-1979; Internal Medicine, Med Coll Georgia Hosps, Augusta, GA 1979-1980; **Fellow:** Medical Oncology, Vanderbilt Univ Med Ctr, Nashville, TN 1981-1983; **Fac Appt:** Prof Medicine, Vanderbilt Univ

Lyckholm, Laurel Jean MD (Onc) - *Spec Exp:* Neuro-Onocology; **Hospital:** Med Coll of VA Hosp; **Address:** PO Box 980230, Richmond, VA 23298; **Phone:** (804) 828-9723; **Board Cert:** Hematology 1994, Medical Oncology 1993, Internal Medicine 1989; **Med School:** Creighton Univ 1985; **Resid:** Creighton U., NE 1986-1989; **Fellow:** Medical Oncology, U IA Coll Med., IA 1989-1992; Hematology, Univ IA Coll Med, IA 1989-1992; **Fac Appt:** Asst Prof Medicine, Med Coll VA

McCarley, Dean L MD (Onc) - *Spec Exp:* Solid Tumors; Urologic Cancer; Lung Cancer; **Hospital:** Shands Hlthcre at Univ of FL (page 73); **Address:** Shands Healthcare-Univ Florida, 2000 SW Archer Road, Gainesville, FL 32608; **Phone:** (352) 265-0725; **Board Cert:** Internal Medicine 1978, Medical Oncology 1985; **Med School:** Duke Univ 1975; **Resid:** Internal Medicine, Univ Fla Affil. Hosp, Gainesville, FL 1976-1978; **Fellow:** Hematology and Oncology, Shands Tchg Hosp, Gainesville, FL 1978-1981; **Fac Appt:** Assoc Prof Medical Oncology, Univ Fla Coll Med

Mitchell, Beverly MD (Onc) - *Spec Exp:* Hematopoietic; Leukemia; Lymphoma; **Hospital:** Univ of NC Hosp (page 77); **Address:** Div Hematology, 3009 Old Clinic Bldg, Box 7305, Chapel Hill, NC 27599-7305; **Phone:** (919) 966-5720; **Board Cert:** Internal Medicine 1973, Hematology 1978; **Med School:** Harvard Med Sch 1969; **Resid:** Internal Medicine, Univ Washington, Seattle, WA 1969-1972; **Fellow:** Metabolism, Univ Zurich, Zurich, Switzerland 1973-1975; Hematology and Oncology, Univ Michigan, Ann Arbor, MI 1975-1977; **Fac Appt:** Prof Medicine, Univ NC Sch Med

Moores, Russell MD (Onc) - *Spec Exp:* Medical Oncology - General; **Hospital:** Med Coll of GA Hosp and Clin; **Address:** Hematology-Oncology Section, 1120 15th St, rm BAA-6407, Augusta, GA 30912; **Phone:** (706) 721-2505; **Board Cert:** Internal Medicine 1965; **Med School:** Univ Ark 1958; **Resid:** Internal Medicine, Strong Meml Hosp, Rochester, NY 1959-1960; Internal Medicine, Barnes Hosp, St. Louis, MO 1960-1961; **Fellow:** Hematology, Natl Inst Hlth, Bethesda, MD 1961-1963; **Fac Appt:** Prof Medical Oncology, Med Coll GA

Nixon, Daniel MD (Onc) - *Spec Exp:* Medical Oncology - General; **Hospital:** Mount Sinai Med Ctr; **Address:** Mount Sinai Comprehensive Ctr, 4306 Alton Rd, Fl 3, Miami, FL 33140-2840; **Phone:** (305) 535-3300; **Board Cert:** Internal Medicine 1967, Medical Oncology 1973; **Med School:** Univ Pittsburgh 1959; **Resid:** Internal Medicine, Univ Pittsburgh, Pittsburgh, PA 1960-1961; Internal Medicine, Mt Sinai Hosp, New York, NY 1961-1962; **Fellow:** Hematology, Mt Sinai Hosp, New York, NY 1962-1963; Medical Oncology, Delafield-Columbia Univ, New York, NY 1968-1969; **Fac Appt:** Assoc Clin Prof Medical Oncology, Univ Miami Sch Med

Powell, Bayard Lowery MD (Onc) - *Spec Exp:* Leukemia; Myelodysplastic Syndromes; **Hospital:** Wake Forest Univ Baptist Med Ctr (page 81); **Address:** Wake Forest Univ Baptist Med Ctr, Med Ctr Blvd-Cancer Center, Winston-Salem, NC 27157; **Phone:** (336) 716-2946; **Board Cert:** Medical Oncology 1985, Internal Medicine 1983; **Med School:** Univ NC Sch Med 1980; **Resid:** Internal Medicine, NC Baptist Hospital, Winston Salem, NC 1981-1983; **Fellow:** Medical Oncology, Wake Forest U Sch of Med, Winston Salem, NC 1983-1986; **Fac Appt:** Prof Hematology, Wake Forest Univ Sch Med

Robert, Nicholas J MD (Onc) - *Spec Exp:* Breast Cancer; Hematology; **Hospital:** Inova Fairfax Hosp; **Address:** 8503 Arlington Blvd, Ste 400, Fairfax, VA 22031; **Phone:** (703) 280-5390; **Board Cert:** Hematology 1984, Medical Oncology 1981; **Med School:** McGill Univ 1974; **Resid:** Internal Medicine, Royal Victoria Hosp, Montreal, Canada 1975-1976; Pathology, Mass Genl Hosp, Boston, MA 1976-1979; **Fellow:** Hematology, Peter Bent Brigham Hosp, Boston, MA 1979-1984

Ross, Maureen MD/PhD (Onc) - *Spec Exp:* adult bone marrow transpl.; breast cancer; **Hospital:** Univ of VA Hlth Sys (page 79); **Address:** Univ of VA Hospital, Box 800-130, Charlottesville, VA 22908; **Phone:** (434) 924-1693; **Board Cert:** Medical Oncology 1989, Hematology 1983; **Med School:** Univ Miami Sch Med 1984; **Resid:** Internal Medicine, Duke Univ. Med. Ctr., Durham, NC 1984-1987; **Fellow:** Hematology and Oncology, Duke Univ. Med. Ctr., Durham, NC 1987; Transplant/Immunology, Duke Univ. Med. Ctr., Durham, NC; **Fac Appt:** Prof Medical Oncology, Univ VA Sch Med

Roth, Bruce Joseph MD (Onc) - *Spec Exp:* Prostate Cancer; Bladder Cancer; Testicular Cancer; **Hospital:** Vanderbilt Univ Med Ctr (page 80); **Address:** Vanderbilt Ingram Cancer Center, 777 Preston Research Bldg, Nashville, TN 37232-6307; **Phone:** (615) 322-4967; **Board Cert:** Internal Medicine 1983, Medical Oncology 1985; **Med School:** St Louis Univ 1980; **Resid:** Internal Medicine, Ind Univ Med Ctr, Indianapolis, IN 1981-1983; **Fellow:** Medical Oncology, Ind Univ Med Ctr, Indianapolis, IN 1983-1986; **Fac Appt:** Prof Medicine, Vanderbilt Univ

Rothenberg, Mace MD (Onc) - *Spec Exp:* Pancreatic Cancer; Colon & Rectal Cancer; **Hospital:** Vanderbilt Univ Med Ctr (page 80); **Address:** Vanderbilt Ingram Cancer Center, 777 Preston Research Bldg, Nashville, TN 37232-6307; **Phone:** (615) 322-4967; **Board Cert:** Internal Medicine 1985, Medical Oncology 1987; **Med School:** NYU Sch Med 1982; **Resid:** Internal Medicine, Vanderbilt Univ Med Ctr, Nashville, TN 1982-1985; **Fellow:** Medical Oncology, Natl Cancer Inst, Bethesda, MD 1985-1988; **Fac Appt:** Assoc Prof Medical Oncology, Vanderbilt Univ

Ruckdeschel, John C MD (Onc) - *Spec Exp:* Lung Cancer; **Hospital:** H Lee Moffitt Cancer Ctr & Research Inst; **Address:** H Lee Moffitt Cancer Ctr, 12908 Magnolia Dr, Tampa, FL 33612-9497; **Phone:** (813) 979-7265; **Board Cert:** Internal Medicine 1976, Medical Oncology 1977; **Med School:** Albany Med Coll 1971; **Resid:** Internal Medicine, Johns Hopkins Hosp, Baltimore, MD 1971-1972; Internal Medicine, Beth Israel Hosp, Boston, MA 1972-1975; **Fellow:** Medical Oncology, Natl Cancer Inst, Baltimore, MD 1975-1977; **Fac Appt:** Prof Medical Oncology, Univ S Fla Coll Med

Schwartz, Michael MD (Onc) - *Spec Exp:* Breast Cancer; Lymphoma; **Hospital:** Mount Sinai Med Ctr; **Address:** 4306 Alton Rd, FL 3, Oncology Hematology Assoc, Miami Beach, FL 33140; **Phone:** (305) 535-3310; **Board Cert:** Medical Oncology 1991, Hematology 1992; **Med School:** UMDNJ-RW Johnson Med Sch 1986; **Resid:** Medical Oncology, Meml Sloan Kettering, New York, NY; Internal Medicine, Mt Sinai Med Ctr, New York, NY; **Fellow:** Meml Sloan Kettering, New York, NY 1989-1992; **Fac Appt:** Asst Clin Prof Medical Oncology, Univ Miami Sch Med

Shea, Thomas MD (Onc) - *Spec Exp:* Bone Marrow Transplant; Lymphoma; Leukemia; **Hospital:** Univ of NC Hosp (page 77); **Address:** Univ North Carolina-Chapel Hill, Dept Medicine, 3009 Old Clinic Bldg, Chapel Hill, NC 27599; **Phone:** (919) 966-7746; **Board Cert:** Clinical Genetics 1985, Hematology 1989; **Med School:** Univ NC Sch Med 1980; **Resid:** Internal Medicine, Univ North Carolina-Chapel Hill, Chapel Hill, NC 1980; Internal Medicine, Beth Israel Deaconess Med Ctr, Boston, MA 1981-1982; **Fellow:** Hematology and Oncology, Beth Israel Deaconess Med Ctr, Boston, MA 1982-1985; Bone Marrow Transplant, Dana Farber Cancer Inst, Boston, MA 1985-1988; **Fac Appt:** Prof Medicine, Univ NC Sch Med

Smith, Thomas Joseph MD (Onc) - *Spec Exp:* Breast Cancer; Palliative Care; **Hospital:** Med Coll of VA Hosp; **Address:** 1101 E Marshall St, rm 6030, Richmond, VA 23298; **Phone:** (804) 828-5116; **Board Cert:** Hematology 1990, Medical Oncology 1987; **Med School:** Yale Univ 1979; **Resid:** Internal Medicine, Hosp Univ Penn, Philadelphia, PA 1980-1982; Medical Oncology, Med Coll VA, Richmond, VA 1984-1987; **Fac Appt:** Prof Medicine, Med Coll VA

Socinski, Mark A MD (Onc) - *Spec Exp:* Lung Cancer; **Hospital:** Univ of NC Hosp (page 77); **Address:** 3009 Old Clinic Bldg, Box CB7305, Chapel Hill, NC 27599-7305; **Phone:** (919) 966-4431; **Board Cert:** Internal Medicine 1988, Medical Oncology 1991; **Med School:** Univ VT Coll Med 1984; **Resid:** Internal Medicine, Beth Israel Hosp, Boston, MA 1984-1986; **Fellow:** Medical Oncology, Dana-Farber Cancer Inst, Boston, MA 1986-1989; **Fac Appt:** Asst Prof Medicine, Univ NC Sch Med

Stone, Joel MD (Onc) - *Spec Exp:* Lung Cancer; Breast Cancer; **Hospital:** St Vincent's Med Ctr - Jacksonville; **Address:** 1801 Barrs St, Ste 800, Jacksonville, FL 32204-4751; **Phone:** (904) 388-2619; **Board Cert:** Internal Medicine 1977, Medical Oncology 1979; **Med School:** Univ VA Sch Med 1974; **Resid:** Internal Medicine, Univ KY Med Ctr, Lexington, KY 1975-1977; **Fellow:** Hematology and Oncology, Emory Univ, Atlanta, GA 1977-1979

Torti, Frank M MD (Onc) - *Spec Exp:* Prostate Cancer; Urologic Cancer; **Hospital:** Wake Forest Univ Baptist Med Ctr (page 81); **Address:** Wake Forest Baptist Med Ctr-Comprehensive Cancer Ctr, Med Center Blvd, Winston-Salem, NC 27157; **Phone:** (336) 716-7971; **Board Cert:** Internal Medicine 1978, Medical Oncology 1979; **Med School:** Harvard Med Sch 1974; **Resid:** Internal Medicine, Beth Israel Hosp, New York, NY 1975-1976; **Fellow:** Medical Oncology, Stanford Univ Med Ctr, Stanford, CA 1977-1979; **Fac Appt:** Prof Medicine, Wake Forest Univ Sch Med

Troner, Michael MD (Onc) - *Spec Exp:* Medical Oncology - General; **Hospital:** Baptist Hosp - Miami; **Address:** 8950 N Kendall Dr, Ste 503, Miami, FL 33176-2132; **Phone:** (305) 271-6467; **Board Cert:** Internal Medicine 1972, Medical Oncology 1973; **Med School:** SUNY Downstate 1968; **Resid:** Internal Medicine, Univ Maryland Hosp, Baltimore, MD 1969-1971; **Fellow:** Medical Oncology, Univ Miami Med Ctr, Miami, FL 1971-1973; **Fac Appt:** Assoc Clin Prof Medical Oncology, Univ Miami Sch Med

Williams, Michael MD (Onc) - *Spec Exp:* Lymphoma; Multiple Myeloma; Leukemia; **Hospital:** Univ of VA Hlth Sys (page 79); **Address:** UVA Health System, Dept Hematology, PO Box 800716, Charlottesville, VA 22908; **Phone:** (804) 924-9637; **Board Cert:** Hematology 1988, Medical Oncology 1987; **Med School:** Univ Cincinnati 1979; **Resid:** Internal Medicine, Univ Virginia Med Ctr, Charlottesville, VA 1980-1983; **Fellow:** Medical Oncology, Univ Virginia Med Ctr, Charlottesville, VA 1983-1986; **Fac Appt:** Prof Medicine, Univ VA Sch Med

Wingard, John R MD (Onc) - *Spec Exp:* Bone Marrow Transplant; Leukemia; Multiple Myeloma; **Hospital:** Shands Hlthcre at Univ of FL (page 73); **Address:** 1600 SW Archer Rd, rm 116, Box 27, MS 100277, Gainesville, FL 32610; **Phone:** (352) 846-2814; **Board Cert:** Internal Medicine 1977, Medical Oncology 1981; **Med School:** Johns Hopkins Univ 1973; **Resid:** Internal Medicine, Memphis City Hosps, Memphis, TN 1974-1976; Internal Medicine, VA Hosp, Memphis, TN 1976-1977; **Fellow:** Medical Oncology, Johns Hopkins Hosp, Baltimore, MD 1977-1979; **Fac Appt:** Prof Medicine, Univ Fla Coll Med

Midwest

Albain, Kathy MD (Onc) - *Spec Exp:* Breast Cancer; Lung Cancer; **Hospital:** Loyola Univ Med Ctr; **Address:** Loyola Univ Med Ctr, 2160 S First Ave, Bldg 112 - Ste 109, Maywood, IL 60153-5590; **Phone:** (708) 327-3102; **Board Cert:** Internal Medicine 1981, Medical Oncology 1983; **Med School:** Univ Mich Med Sch 1978; **Resid:** Internal Medicine, Univ Illinois Med Ctr, Chicago, IL 1979-1981; **Fellow:** Hematology and Oncology, Univ Chicago Med Ctr, Chicago, IL 1981-1984; **Fac Appt:** Prof Medicine, Loyola Univ-Stritch Sch Med

Anderson, Joseph MD (Onc) - *Spec Exp:* Breast Cancer; Palliative Care; **Hospital:** Henry Ford Hosp; **Address:** 2799 W Grand Blvd, Detroit, MI 48202; **Phone:** (313) 916-1854; **Board Cert:** Internal Medicine 1985, Medical Oncology 1989; **Med School:** Univ Mich Med Sch 1982; **Resid:** Internal Medicine, Henry Ford Hosp, Detroit, MI 1982-1986; **Fellow:** Medical Oncology, Henry Ford Hosp, Detroit, MI 1986-1988

Baker, Laurence H DO (Onc) - *Spec Exp:* Sarcoma-Soft Tissue & Bone; Breast Cancer; **Hospital:** Univ of MI Hlth Ctr; **Address:** 1500 E Med Center Drive, Ste 7216CCGC, Ann Arbor, MI 48109-0948; **Phone:** (734) 647-8902; **Med School:** Univ Hlth Sci, Coll Osteo Med 1966; **Resid:** Internal Medicine, Genesys Reg M C-W Flint Campus, Flint, MI 1966-1967; **Fellow:** Medical Oncology, Wayne State Univ Affil Hosp, Detroit, MI 1970-1972; **Fac Appt:** Prof Medicine, Univ Mich Med Sch

Benson III, Al B MD (Onc) - *Spec Exp:* Colon Cancer; Carcinoid Tumors; Gastrointestinal Cancer; **Hospital:** Northwestern Meml Hosp; **Address:** 676 N St Clair, Ste 850, Chicago, IL 60611; **Phone:** (312) 695-8697; **Board Cert:** Internal Medicine 1979, Medical Oncology 1983; **Med School:** SUNY Buffalo 1976; **Resid:** Internal Medicine, Univ Wisc Hosps, Madison, WI 1977-1979; **Fellow:** Medical Oncology, Univ Wisc Hosps, Madison, WI 1981-1984; **Fac Appt:** Prof Medicine, Northwestern Univ

Bitran, Jacob MD (Onc) - *Spec Exp:* Breast Cancer; Bone Marrow Transplant; Lung Cancer; **Hospital:** Advocate Lutheran Gen Hosp; **Address:** Advocate Medical Group, 1700 Luther Ln, Park Ridge, IL 60068-1270; **Phone:** (847) 723-2500; **Board Cert:** Hematology 1985, Medical Oncology 1977; **Med School:** Univ IL Coll Med 1971; **Resid:** Pathology, Rush Presby St Luke's Hosp, Chicago, IL 1972-1973; Internal Medicine, Michael Reese Hosp, Chicago, IL 1972-1973; **Fellow:** Hematology and Oncology, Univ Chicago Hosp, Chicago, IL 1975-1977

Bonomi, Philip MD (Onc) - *Spec Exp:* Mesothelioma; Thymoma; Lung Cancer; **Hospital:** Rush-Presby - St Luke's Med Ctr (page 72); **Address:** 1725 W Harrison St, Ste 821, Chicago, IL 60612; **Phone:** (312) 942-3312; **Board Cert:** Internal Medicine 1975, Medical Oncology 1977; **Med School:** Univ IL Coll Med 1970; **Resid:** Internal Medicine, Geisinger, Danville, PA 1971-1972; Internal Medicine, Geisinger, Danville, PA 1974-1975; **Fellow:** Medical Oncology, Rush Presby-St Luke's Med Ctr, Chicago, IL 1975-1977; **Fac Appt:** Prof Medicine, Rush Med Coll

Budd, George Thomas MD (Onc) - *Spec Exp:* Breast Cancer; **Hospital:** Cleveland Clin Fdn (page 57); **Address:** Cleveland Clinic, Taussig Cancer Ctr, 9500 Euclid Ave, MC R35, Cleveland, OH 44195-0001; **Phone:** (216) 444-6480; **Board Cert:** Medical Oncology 1983, Internal Medicine 1980; **Med School:** Univ Kans 1976; **Resid:** Internal Medicine, Cleveland Clin, Cleveland, OH 1978-1980; **Fellow:** Hematology and Oncology, Cleveland Clin, Cleveland, OH 1980-1982

Cobleigh, Melody MD (Onc) - *Spec Exp:* Breast Cancer; **Hospital:** Rush-Presby - St Luke's Med Ctr (page 72); **Address:** 1725 W Harrison St, Ste 821, Chicago, IL 60612-3828; **Phone:** (312) 942-3240; **Board Cert:** Internal Medicine 1979, Medical Oncology 1981; **Med School:** Rush Med Coll 1976; **Resid:** Internal Medicine, Rush Presby-St Lukes Med Ctr, Chicago, IL 1977-1979; **Fellow:** Medical Oncology, Indiana Univ, Indianapolis, IN 1979-1981; **Fac Appt:** Prof Medicine, Rush Med Coll

Di Persio, John MD/PhD (Onc) - *Spec Exp:* Bone Marrow Transplant; Hematology; **Hospital:** Barnes-Jewish Hosp (page 55); **Address:** Washington Univ, 660 S Euclid Ave, Box 8007, St Louis, MO 63110; **Phone:** (314) 454-8313; **Board Cert:** Medical Oncology 1987, Hematology 1988; **Med School:** Univ Rochester 1980; **Resid:** Internal Medicine, Parkland Meml Hosp, Dallas, TX 1981-1984; **Fellow:** Hematology and Oncology, UCLA Sch Med, Los Angeles, CA 1984-1987; **Fac Appt:** Prof Medicine, Washington Univ, St Louis

Dreicer, Robert MD (Onc) - *Spec Exp:* Breast Cancer; Prostate Cancer; **Hospital:** Cleveland Clin Fdn (page 57); **Address:** Cleveland Clinic, Taussig Cancer Ctr, 9500 Euclid Ave, MC R35, Cleveland, OH 44195-0001; **Phone:** (216) 445-4623; **Board Cert:** Medical Oncology 1989, Internal Medicine 1986; **Med School:** Univ Tex, Houston 1983; **Resid:** Internal Medicine, Ind Univ, Indianapolis, IN 1984-1986; **Fellow:** Medical Oncology, Univ Wisc, Madison, WI 1986-1989

Einhorn, Lawrence MD (Onc) - *Spec Exp:* Testicular Cancer; Lung Cancer; **Hospital:** IN Univ Hosp (page 63); **Address:** 535 Barnhill Drive, Ste 473, Indianapolis, IN 46202; **Phone:** (317) 274-0920; **Board Cert:** Internal Medicine 1972, Medical Oncology 1975; **Med School:** UCLA 1967; **Resid:** Internal Medicine, Indiana U Hosp, Indianapolis, IN 1968-1969; **Fellow:** Medical Oncology, Indiana U Hosp, Indianapolis, IN 1971-1972

Flynn, Patrick MD (Onc) - *Spec Exp:* Medical Oncology - General; **Hospital:** Fairview-Univ Med Ctr - Univ Campus; **Address:** Fairview Physicians Associates, 8006 28th St, Ste 405, Minneapolis, MN 55407; **Phone:** (612) 863-8585; **Board Cert:** Medical Oncology 1981, Hematology 1982; **Med School:** Univ Minn 1975; **Resid:** Internal Medicine, Hennepin Co Med Ctr-Univ Minn, Minneapolis, MN 1976-1978; **Fellow:** Hematology and Oncology, Univ Minnesota Hosp, Minneapolis, MN 1979-1981; **Fac Appt:** Asst Prof Medicine, Univ Minn

Hartmann, Lynn Carol MD (Onc) - *Spec Exp:* Breast Cancer; Ovarian Cancer; **Hospital:** Mayo Med Ctr & Clin - Rochester, MN; **Address:** 200 First St SW, Mayo Clinic, Div Medical Oncology, Rochester, MN 55905; **Phone:** (507) 284-3903; **Board Cert:** Internal Medicine 1986, Medical Oncology 1989; **Med School:** Northwestern Univ 1983; **Resid:** Internal Medicine, U Ia. Hosps/Clinics, Iowa City, IA 1984-1986; **Fellow:** Medical Oncology, Mayo Med Fdn., Rochester, MN 1987-1989

Hayes, Daniel Fleming MD (Onc) - *Spec Exp:* Breast Cancer; **Hospital:** Univ of MI Hlth Ctr; **Address:** 1500 E Medical Center Drive, 6312 Cancer Center, Ann Arbor, MI 48109; **Phone:** (734) 615-6725; **Board Cert:** Medical Oncology 1985, Internal Medicine 1982; **Med School:** Indiana Univ 1979; **Resid:** Internal Medicine, Parkland Meml Hosp, San Antonio, TX 1979-1982; **Fellow:** Medical Oncology, Dana Farber Cancer Inst., Boston, MA 1982-1985; **Fac Appt:** Prof Medicine, Univ Mich Med Sch

Hussein, Mohammed Ahmed MD (Onc) - *Spec Exp:* Multiple Myeloma; Amyloidosis; Plasmacytoma; **Hospital:** Cleveland Clin Fdn (page 57); **Address:** Cleveland Clinic,Dept Hematology/Oncology-Desk R35, 9500 Euclid Ave, Cleveland, OH 44195-5236; **Phone:** (216) 445-6830; **Board Cert:** Medical Oncology 1989, Internal Medicine 1986; **Med School:** Egypt 1981; **Resid:** Internal Medicine, Univ Miss Med Ctr, Jackson, MS 1983-1985; Internal Medicine, Cleveland Clin Fdn, Cleveland, OH 1985-1986; **Fellow:** Medical Oncology, U Md Canc Ctr, Baltimore, MD 1986-1989

Ingle, James N MD (Onc) - *Spec Exp:* Breast Cancer; **Hospital:** Rochester Meth Hosp; **Address:** Mayo Clinic, 200 First St SW Fl 12 East, Rochester, MN 55905; **Phone:** (507) 284-8432; **Board Cert:** Internal Medicine 1974, Medical Oncology 1975; **Med School:** Johns Hopkins Univ 1971; **Resid:** Internal Medicine, Johns Hopkins Hosp, Baltimore, MD 1972-1976; Medical Oncology, Natl Cancer Inst, Bethesda, MD 1973-1975; **Fac Appt:** Prof Medical Oncology, Mayo Med Sch

Kosova, Leonard MD (Onc) - *Spec Exp:* Breast Cancer; Lymphoma; Lung Cancer; **Hospital:** Advocate Lutheran Gen Hosp; **Address:** 8915 W Golf Rd, Ste 3, Niles, IL 60714; **Phone:** (847) 827-9060; **Board Cert:** Hematology 1972, Medical Oncology 1975; **Med School:** Univ IL Coll Med 1961; **Resid:** Internal Medicine, Hines VA Hosp, Hines, IL 1962-1964; **Fellow:** Hematology and Oncology, Hektoen Inst-Cook Cty Hosp, Chicago, IL 1964-1965

Lippman, Marc E MD (Onc) - *Spec Exp:* Breast Cancer; **Hospital:** Univ of MI Hlth Ctr; **Address:** Univ Mich Health Sci Ctr, 3101 Taubman Ctr, 1500 E Medical , Box 0368, Ann Arbor, MI 48109-0368; **Phone:** (734) 647-8916; **Board Cert:** Endocrinology, Diabetes & Metabolism 1975, Medical Oncology 1977; **Med School:** Yale Univ 1968; **Resid:** Internal Medicine, Johns Hopkins Hosp, Baltimore, MD 1969-1970; **Fellow:** Endocrinology, Diabetes & Metabolism, Yale, New Haven, CT 1973-1974; Medical Oncology, Natl Cancer Inst, Bethesda, MD 1970-1973; **Fac Appt:** Prof Medicine, Univ MD Sch Med

Loprinzi, Charles L MD (Onc) - *Spec Exp:* Melonoma; Breast Cancer; **Hospital:** Mayo Med Ctr & Clin - Rochester, MN; **Address:** Mayo Medical Center-Dept. Med. Onc., 200 First St SW, Rochester, MN 55905-0001; **Phone:** (507) 284-4137; **Board Cert:** Medical Oncology 1985, Internal Medicine 1982; **Med School:** Oregon Hlth Scis Univ 1979; **Resid:** Internal Medicine, Maricopa Co. Hosp., Phoenix, AZ 1980-1982; **Fellow:** Medical Oncology, U Wisc Med Ctr, Madison, WI 1982-1984; **Fac Appt:** Prof Medicine, Mayo Med Sch

Markman, Maurie MD (Onc) - *Spec Exp:* Ovarian Cancer; **Hospital:** Cleveland Clin Fdn (page 57); **Address:** Cleveland Clinic Foundation- Dept Hem/Onc, 9500 Euclid Ave, MC-Desk R35, Cleveland, OH 44195; **Phone:** (216) 445-6888; **Board Cert:** Medical Oncology 1981, Hematology 1982; **Med School:** NYU Sch Med 1974; **Resid:** Internal Medicine, Bellevue Hosp Ctr, New York, NY 1975-1978; **Fellow:** Medical Oncology, Johns Hopkins Hosp, Baltimore, MD 1980; **Fac Appt:** Prof Medicine, Ohio State Univ

Markowitz, Sanford D MD (Onc) - *Spec Exp:* Colon & Rectal Cancer; Familial Cancer; **Hospital:** Univ Hosp of Cleveland; **Address:** Howard Hughes Research Labs, 11001 Cedar Ave Bldg Samuel Gerber - Ste 200, Cleveland, OH 44106; **Phone:** (216) 844-8236; **Board Cert:** Internal Medicine 1984, Medical Oncology 1987; **Med School:** Yale Univ 1980; **Resid:** Internal Medicine, Univ Chicago Hosp, Chicago, IL 1982-1984; **Fellow:** Medical Oncology, Natl Cancer Inst, Bethesda, MD 1984-1986; **Fac Appt:** Prof Medicine, Case West Res Univ

Masters, Gregory MD (Onc) - *Spec Exp:* Lung Cancer; Esophageal Cancer; Thoracic Cancers; **Hospital:** Evanston Hosp; **Address:** 2650 Ridge Ave, Evanston, IL 60201; **Phone:** (847) 570-2110; **Board Cert:** Internal Medicine 1993, Medical Oncology 1996; **Med School:** Northwestern Univ 1990; **Resid:** Internal Medicine, Hosp Univ Penn, Philadelphia, PA 1991-1993; **Fellow:** Medical Oncology, Univ Chicago, Chicago, IL 1993; **Fac Appt:** Asst Prof Medicine, Northwestern Univ

Mortimer, Joanne MD (Onc) - *Spec Exp:* Breast Oncology; **Hospital:** Barnes-Jewish Hosp (page 55); **Address:** 660 S Euclid Ave, Box CB8056, St Louis, MO 63110; **Phone:** (314) 362-7502; **Board Cert:** Internal Medicine 1980, Medical Oncology 1983; **Med School:** Loyola Univ-Stritch Sch Med 1977; **Resid:** Internal Medicine, Cleveland Clin, Cleveland, OH 1978-1980; **Fellow:** Medical Oncology, Cleveland Clin, Cleveland, OH 1980-1982; **Fac Appt:** Prof Medical Oncology, Washington Univ, St Louis

Olopade, Olufunmilayo I F MD (Onc) - *Spec Exp:* Breast Cancer; Lymphoma; Cancer Genetic Testing; **Hospital:** Univ of Chicago Hosps (page 76); **Address:** 5758 S Maryland Ave, MC 9015, Chicago, IL 60637; **Phone:** (773) 702-6149; **Board Cert:** Medical Oncology 1989, Hematology 1990; **Med School:** Nigeria 1980; **Resid:** Internal Medicine, Cook Co Hosp, Chicago, IL 1984-1986; **Fellow:** Hematology and Oncology, Univ Chicago Med Ctr, Chicago, IL 1987-1991; **Fac Appt:** Assoc Prof Medicine, Univ Chicago-Pritzker Sch Med

Perry, Michael MD (Onc) - *Spec Exp:* Lung Cancer; Breast Cancer; **Hospital:** Univ of Missouri Hosp & Clinics; **Address:** Ellis Fischel Cancer Ctr., 115 Business Loop 70 W, rm 524, Columbia, MO 65203; **Phone:** (573) 882-4979; **Board Cert:** Medical Oncology 1975, Hematology 1974; **Med School:** Wayne State Univ 1970; **Resid:** Internal Medicine, Mayo Grad Sch, Rochester, MN 1971-1972; **Fellow:** Medical Oncology, Mayo Grad Sch, Rochester, MN 1974-1975; Hematology, Mayo Grad Sch, Rochester, MN 1972-1974; **Fac Appt:** Prof Medicine, Univ Hlth Sci Coll -Osteo Med

Peters, William P MD/PhD (Onc) - *Spec Exp:* Breast Cancer; **Hospital:** Barbara Ann Karmanos Cancer Inst; **Address:** Barbara Ann Karmanos Cancer Inst, 4100 John R St Bldg CETAID - rm 437, Detroit, MI 48201; **Phone:** (313) 993-7777; **Board Cert:** Internal Medicine 1981, Medical Oncology 1983; **Med School:** Columbia P&S 1978; **Resid:** Internal Medicine, Brigham & Women's Hosp, Boston, MA 1978-1981; **Fellow:** Medical Oncology, Dana-Farber Cancer Inst, Boston, MA 1981-1983

Piel, Ira MD (Onc) - *Spec Exp:* Breast Cancer; Colon Cancer; Lymphoma; **Hospital:** Lake Forest Hosp; **Address:** 900 N Westmoreland Road, Ste 105, Lake Forest, IL 60045; **Phone:** (847) 234-6155; **Board Cert:** Internal Medicine 1973, Medical Oncology 1975; **Med School:** Univ IL Coll Med 1967; **Resid:** Internal Medicine, St Lukes Hosp, Chicago, IL 1970-1972; **Fellow:** Medical Oncology, St Lukes Hosp, Chicago, IL 1972-1974; **Fac Appt:** Rush Med Coll

Ratain, Mark J MD (Onc) - *Spec Exp:* Solid Tumors; **Hospital:** Univ of Chicago Hosps (page 76); **Address:** 5758 S Maryland Ave, rm 6D, Chicago, IL 60637; **Phone:** (773) 702-4400; **Board Cert:** Hematology 1986, Medical Oncology 1985; **Med School:** Yale Univ 1980; **Resid:** Internal Medicine, Johns Hopkins Hosp, Baltimore, MD 1981-1983; **Fellow:** Hematology and Oncology, Univ Chicago, Chicago, IL 1983-1986; **Fac Appt:** Prof Medicine, Univ Chicago-Pritzker Sch Med

Richards, Jon MD/PhD (Onc) - *Spec Exp:* Testicular Cancer; Prostate Cancer; Melanoma; **Hospital:** Advocate Lutheran Gen Hosp; **Address:** 1700 Luther Ln, Park Ridge, IL 60068; **Phone:** (847) 723-2500; **Board Cert:** Internal Medicine 1998; **Med School:** Cornell Univ-Weill Med Coll 1983; **Resid:** Internal Medicine, Univ Chicago Hosp, Chicago, IL 1984-1985; **Fellow:** Hematology and Oncology, Univ Chicago Hosp, Chicago, IL 1985-1988; **Fac Appt:** Asst Prof Medicine, Univ IL Coll Med

Rosen, Steven T MD (Onc) - *Spec Exp:* Hemopoeitic Malignacies; Breast Cancer; **Hospital:** Northwestern Meml Hosp; **Address:** Northwestern Univ, 303 E Chicago Ave, Olsen Pavillion, Ste 8250, Chicago, IL 60611-3013; **Phone:** (312) 695-8697; **Board Cert:** Internal Medicine 1979, Medical Oncology 1981, Hematology 1984; **Med School:** Northwestern Univ 1976; **Resid:** Internal Medicine, Northwestern Univ Hosp, Chicago, IL 1977-1979; **Fellow:** Medical Oncology, Natl Cancer Instr, Bethesda, MD 1979-1981; **Fac Appt:** Prof Medicine, Northwestern Univ

Samuels, Brian Louis MD (Onc) - *Spec Exp:* Medical Oncology - General; **Hospital:** Advocate Lutheran Gen Hosp; **Address:** Cancer Care Ctr, Oncology Specialists, 1700 Luther Ln, Park Ridge, IL 60068; **Phone:** (847) 723-2500; **Board Cert:** Medical Oncology 1987, Internal Medicine 1984; **Med School:** Zimbabwe 1976; **Resid:** Internal Medicine, Albert Einstein Med Ctr, Philadelphia, PA 1979-1981; Internal Medicine, Albert Einstein Med Ctr, Philadelphia, PA 1983-1984; **Fellow:** Hematology and Oncology, Univ Chicago, Chicago, IL 1984-1988; **Fac Appt:** Assoc Prof Medicine, Univ IL Coll Med

Schiffer, Charles A MD (Onc) - *Spec Exp:* Leukemia; Lymphoma; **Hospital:** Harper Hosp (page 59); **Address:** Harper Hosp, Dept Hematology/Oncology, 3990 John R, 5 Hudson, Detroit, MI 48201; **Phone:** (313) 745-8910; **Board Cert:** Medical Oncology 1973, Internal Medicine 1972; **Med School:** NYU Sch Med 1968; **Resid:** Internal Medicine, NYU, Bellevue-New York VA Hosp., New York, NY 1968-1972; **Fac Appt:** Prof Medical Oncology, Wayne State Univ

Schiller, Joan H MD (Onc) - *Spec Exp:* Lung Cancer; **Hospital:** Univ WI Hosp & Clins; **Address:** 600 Highland Ave, rm K4/636, Madison, WI 53792; **Phone:** (608) 263-8090; **Board Cert:** Medical Oncology 1987, Internal Medicine 1983; **Med School:** Univ IL Coll Med 1980; **Resid:** Internal Medicine, Northwestern Meml Hosp, Chicago, IL 1981-1983; **Fellow:** Medical Oncology, U Wisc Hosp, Madison, WI 1984-1986; **Fac Appt:** Prof Medicine, Univ Wisc

Schwartz, Burton MD (Onc) - *Spec Exp:* Lymphoma; Breast Cancer; **Hospital:** Abbott - Northwestern Hosp; **Address:** Abott - Northwestern Hosp, 800 E 28th St, Minneapolis, MN 55417; **Phone:** (612) 863-8585; **Board Cert:** Internal Medicine 1972, Medical Oncology 1977, Hand Surgery 1976; **Med School:** Meharry Med Coll 1968; **Resid:** Internal Medicine, Michael Reese Hospital, Chicago, IL 1969-1971; **Fellow:** Hematology, U Minn Hosp, Minnesota, MN 1974-1976; **Fac Appt:** Clin Prof Hematology, Univ Minn

Shapiro, Charles L MD (Onc) - *Spec Exp:* Breast Cancer; **Hospital:** Arthur G James Cancer Hosp & Research Inst; **Address:** 320 W 10th Ave Bldg Starling Loving Hall - rm B405, Columbus, OH 43210-1240; **Phone:** (614) 293-7530; **Board Cert:** Internal Medicine 1987, Medical Oncology 1991; **Med School:** SUNY Buffalo 1984; **Resid:** Internal Medicine, Temple Univ, Philadelphia, PA 1984-1987

Sledge Jr, George W MD (Onc) - *Spec Exp:* Breast Cancer; **Hospital:** IN Univ Hosp (page 63); **Address:** 535 Barnhill Drive, Ste 473, Indianapolis, IN 46202; **Phone:** (317) 274-0920; **Board Cert:** Internal Medicine 1980, Medical Oncology 1983; **Med School:** Tulane Univ 1977; **Resid:** Internal Medicine, St Louis Univ, St Louis, MO 1977-1980; **Fellow:** Medical Oncology, Univ Texas, San Antonio, TX 1980-1983; **Fac Appt:** Prof Medicine, Indiana Univ

Todd III, Robert F MD/PhD (Onc) - *Spec Exp:* Gastrointestinal Cancer; Lung Cancer; **Hospital:** Univ of MI Hlth Ctr; **Address:** Univ Michigan Cancer Ctr, B1371 1500 E Med Ctr Dr, Box 0913, Ann Arbor, MI 48109-0948; **Phone:** (734) 647-8903; **Board Cert:** Internal Medicine 1979, Medical Oncology 1981; **Med School:** Duke Univ 1976; **Resid:** Internal Medicine, Peter Bent Brigham Hosp, Boston, MA 1977-1978; **Fellow:** Medical Oncology, Dana Farber Cancer Inst, Boston, MA 1978-1981; **Fac Appt:** Prof Medicine, Univ Mich Med Sch

Urba, Susan G MD (Onc) - *Spec Exp:* Head & Neck Cancer; **Hospital:** Univ of MI Hlth Ctr; **Address:** Univ Michigan Med Ctr, Div Hematology/Oncology, 1500 East Medical Center Drive, Ann Arbor, MI 48109-0374; **Phone:** (734) 936-5281; **Board Cert:** Internal Medicine 1986, Medical Oncology 1991; **Med School:** Univ Mich Med Sch 1983; **Resid:** Internal Medicine, Univ Michigan Med Ctr, Ann Arbor, MI 1984-1986; **Fellow:** Hematology and Oncology, Univ Michigan Med Ctr, Ann Arbor, MI 1986-1988

Vogelzang, Nicholas MD (Onc) - *Spec Exp:* Prostate Cancer; Mesothelioma; Kidney Cancer; **Hospital:** Univ of Chicago Hosps (page 76); **Address:** Cancer Research Ctr, 5841 S Maryland Ave, MS 1140, Chicago, IL 60637; **Phone:** (773) 702-6149; **Board Cert:** Internal Medicine 1978, Medical Oncology 1981; **Med School:** Univ IL Coll Med 1974; **Resid:** Internal Medicine, Rush-Presby St Luke's Med Ctr, Chicago, IL 1974-1978; **Fellow:** Medical Oncology, Univ Minn, Minneapolis, MN 1978-1981; **Fac Appt:** Prof Medicine, Univ Chicago-Pritzker Sch Med

Vokes, Everett Emmett MD (Onc) - *Spec Exp:* Lung Cancer; Head & Neck Cancer; **Hospital:** Univ of Chicago Hosps (page 76); **Address:** Univ Chicago Med Ctr, 5841 S Maryland Ave, MS 2115, Chicago, IL 60637-1470; **Phone:** (773) 834-3093; **Board Cert:** Internal Medicine 1983, Medical Oncology 1985; **Med School:** Germany 1980; **Resid:** Internal Medicine, Ravenswood Hosp-U IL, Chicago, IL 1981-1982; Internal Medicine, USC Med Ctr, Los Angeles, CA 1982-1983; **Fellow:** Medical Oncology, Univ Chicago, Chicago, IL 1983-1986; **Fac Appt:** Prof Medicine, Univ Chicago-Pritzker Sch Med

Wicha, Max S MD (Onc) - *Spec Exp:* Breast Cancer; **Hospital:** Univ of MI Hlth Ctr; **Address:** Cancer and Geriatric Ctr, 1500 E Med Ctr Dr, fl B1, rm 371, Box 0916, Ann Arbor, MI 48109; **Phone:** (734) 936-6000; **Board Cert:** Internal Medicine 1977, Medical Oncology 1983; **Med School:** Stanford Univ 1974; **Resid:** Internal Medicine, Univ Chicago Hosp, Chicago, IL 1976-1977; **Fellow:** Medical Oncology, Natl Inst Hlth, Bethesda, MD 1977-1980; **Fac Appt:** Prof Medicine, Univ Mich Med Sch

Great Plains and Mountains

Armitage, James MD (Onc) - *Spec Exp: Lymphoma; Bone Marrow Transplant;* **Hospital:** Nebraska Hlth Sys; **Address:** 986545 Nebraska Medical Center, Omaha, NE 68198; **Phone:** (402) 559-7290; **Board Cert:** Internal Medicine 1976, Medical Oncology 1977; **Med School:** Univ Nebr Coll Med 1973; **Resid:** Internal Medicine, Univ Nebr Med Ctr, Omaha, NE 1974-1975; **Fellow:** Hematology and Oncology, Univ Iowa Hosp, Iowa City, IA 1975-1977; **Fac Appt:** Prof Medicine, Univ Nebr Coll Med

Bunn Jr, Paul MD (Onc) - *Spec Exp: Lung Cancer; Lymphoma;* **Hospital:** Univ Colo HSC - Denver; **Address:** Univ Colorado Cancer Ctr, 4200 E Ninth Ave, Box B 188, Denver, CO 80262; **Phone:** (303) 315-3007; **Board Cert:** Internal Medicine 1974, Medical Oncology 1975; **Med School:** Cornell Univ-Weill Med Coll 1971; **Resid:** Internal Medicine, HC Moffitt/Univ California, San Francisco, CA 1972-1973; **Fellow:** Medical Oncology, Natl Cancer Inst, Bethesda, MD 1973-1976; **Fac Appt:** Prof Medicine, Univ Colo

Ebbert, Larry P. MD (Onc) - *Spec Exp: Medical Oncology - General;* **Hospital:** Rapid City Reg Hosp; **Address:** 353 Fairmont Blvd, Rapid City, SD 57701; **Phone:** (605) 719-2301; **Board Cert:** Medical Oncology 1975, Hematology 1974, Internal Medicine 1973; **Med School:** Ohio State Univ 1969; **Resid:** Internal Medicine, Univ of Missouri Med Ctr, Columbia, MO 1970-1971; **Fellow:** Hematology and Oncology, Duke Univ Med Ctr, Durham, NC 1971-1973; **Fac Appt:** Asst Clin Prof Univ SD Sch Med

Fabian, Carol J MD (Onc) - *Spec Exp: Breast Cancer;* **Hospital:** Univ Kansas Med Ctr; **Address:** Univ Kansas Med Ctr, Div Clin Onc, 3901 Rainbow Blvd, Ste 1347 Bell, Kansas City, KS 66160; **Phone:** (913) 588-7791; **Board Cert:** Internal Medicine 1976, Medical Oncology 1977; **Resid:** Internal Medicine, Wesley Med Ctr, Wichita, KS 1973-1975; **Fellow:** Medical Oncology, Univ Kansas Med Ctr, Kansas City, KS 1975-1977; **Fac Appt:** Prof Medicine, Univ Kans

Walters, Theodore MD (Onc) - *Spec Exp: Medical Oncology - General;* **Hospital:** St. Luke's Reg Med Ctr - Boise; **Address:** 901 N Curtis Rd, Ste 402, Boise, ID 83706; **Phone:** (208) 367-2878; **Board Cert:** Hematology 1976, Internal Medicine 1972; **Med School:** Oregon Hlth Scis Univ 1963; **Resid:** Internal Medicine, University of Oregon Med. Ctr., Portland, OR 1967-1970; **Fellow:** Hematology, University of Oregon Med. Ctr., Portland, OR 1970-1972; **Fac Appt:** Asst Clin Prof Univ Wash

Ward, John Harris MD (Onc) - *Spec Exp: Medical Oncology - General;* **Hospital:** Univ Utah Hosp and Clin; **Address:** Huntsman Cancer Inst, 2000 Circle of Hope, Ste 2100, Salt Lake City, UT 84112-5550; **Phone:** (801) 585-0255; **Board Cert:** Internal Medicine 1979, Medical Oncology 1981; **Med School:** Univ Utah 1976; **Resid:** Internal Medicine, Duke Univ, Durham, NC 1977-1979; **Fellow:** Hematology and Oncology, Univ Utah, Salt Lake City, UT 1979-1981; **Fac Appt:** Prof Medicine, Univ Utah

Southwest

Abbruzzese, James L MD (Onc) - *Spec Exp: Gastrointestinal Cancer; Pancreatic Cancer;* **Hospital:** Univ of TX MD Anderson Cancer Ctr, The; **Address:** Univ Texas MD Anderson Cancer Ctr, 1515 Holcombe Blvd, Box 426, Houston, TX 77030-4009; **Phone:** (713) 792-2828; **Board Cert:** Internal Medicine 1981, Medical Oncology 1983; **Med School:** Univ Chicago-Pritzker Sch Med 1978; **Resid:** Internal Medicine, Johns Hopkins Hosp, Baltimore, MD 1979-1981; **Fellow:** Medical Oncology, Dana-Farber Cancer Inst, Boston, MA 1981-1983; **Fac Appt:** Assoc Prof Medicine, Univ Tex, Houston

Benjamin, Robert S MD (Onc) - *Spec Exp:* Sarcoma-Soft Tissue; Sarcoma-Bone; **Hospital:** Univ of TX MD Anderson Cancer Ctr, The; **Address:** UT MD Anderson Cancer Ctr, 1515 Holcombe Blvd, Box 450, Houston, TX 77030; **Phone:** (713) 792-3626; **Board Cert:** Internal Medicine 1973, Medical Oncology 1973; **Med School:** NYU Sch Med 1968; **Resid:** Internal Medicine, Bellevue Hosp Ctr/NYU, New York, NY 1969-1970; **Fellow:** Medical Oncology, Baltimore Cancer Rsrch Ctr, Baltimore, MD 1970-1972; **Fac Appt:** Prof Medicine, Univ Tex, Houston

Buzdar, Aman U MD (Onc) - *Spec Exp:* Breast Cancer; **Hospital:** Univ of TX MD Anderson Cancer Ctr, The; **Address:** U Texas-MD Anderson Cancer Ctr, Dept Breast Med Oncology, 1515 Holcombe Blvd, Houston, TX 77030; **Phone:** (713) 792-2817; **Board Cert:** Internal Medicine 1975, Medical Oncology 1979; **Med School:** Pakistan 1967; **Resid:** Internal Medicine, Norwalk Hosp, Norwalk, CT 1972-1973; Internal Medicine, Lakewood Hosp 1970-1971; **Fellow:** Hematology, Norwalk Hosp, Norwalk, CT 1973-1974; **Fac Appt:** Prof Medicine, Univ Tex, Houston

Fossella, Frank V MD (Onc) - *Spec Exp:* Lung Cancer; **Hospital:** Univ of TX MD Anderson Cancer Ctr, The; **Address:** 1400 Holcombe Blvd, Box 432, Houston, TX 77030; **Phone:** (713) 792-6363; **Board Cert:** Internal Medicine 1985, Medical Oncology 1987; **Med School:** Baylor Coll Med 1982; **Resid:** Internal Medicine, Baylor Coll Med, Houston, TX 1983-1985; **Fellow:** Medical Oncology, Baylor Coll Med, Houston, TX 1985-1987; **Fac Appt:** Medical Oncology, Univ Tex, Houston

Glisson, Bonnie S MD (Onc) - *Spec Exp:* Head & Neck Cancer; Lung Cancer; **Hospital:** Univ of TX MD Anderson Cancer Ctr, The; **Address:** Univ Texas - MD Anderson Cancer Ctr, 1515 Holcombe Blvd, Box 432, Houston, TX 77030; **Phone:** (713) 792-6363; **Board Cert:** Medical Oncology 1985, Internal Medicine 1982; **Med School:** Ohio State Univ 1979; **Resid:** Internal Medicine, Univ Virginia Med Ctr, Charlottesville, VA 1979-1982; **Fellow:** Medical Oncology, Univ Florida Hosps, Gainesville, FL 1982-1985; **Fac Appt:** Prof Medical Oncology, Univ Tex, Houston

Hong, Waun Ki MD (Onc) - *Spec Exp:* Chemoprevention of Cancer; Lung Cancer; **Hospital:** Univ of TX MD Anderson Cancer Ctr, The; **Address:** 1515 Holcombe Blvd, Box 432, Houston, TX 77030; **Phone:** (713) 792-6363; **Board Cert:** Internal Medicine 1976, Medical Oncology 1979; **Med School:** South Korea 1967; **Resid:** Internal Medicine, Boston VA Hosp., Boston, MA 1971-1973; **Fellow:** Medical Oncology, Sloan-Kettering, New York, NY 1973-1975

Hortobagyi, Gabriel N MD (Onc) - *Spec Exp:* Breast Cancer; **Hospital:** Univ of TX MD Anderson Cancer Ctr, The; **Address:** U Texas-MD Anderson Cancer Ctr, Dept Breast Med Oncology, 1515 Holcombe Blvd, Houston, TX 77030; **Phone:** (713) 792-2817; **Board Cert:** Internal Medicine 1975, Medical Oncology 1977; **Med School:** Colombia 1970; **Resid:** Internal Medicine, St. Lukes Hosp, Cleveland, OH 1972-1974; **Fellow:** Medical Oncology, U Texas-MD Anderson Hosp, Houston, TX 1974-1976; **Fac Appt:** Prof Medicine, Univ Tex Med Br, Galveston

Hutchins, Laura MD (Onc) - *Spec Exp:* Breast Cancer; Melanoma; **Hospital:** UAMS; **Address:** Univ Arkansas Med Sci, Dept Hem/Onc, 4301 W Markham St, MS 508, Little Rock, AR 72205-7101; **Phone:** (501) 686-8511; **Board Cert:** Internal Medicine 1980, Hematology 1984, Medical Oncology 1987; **Med School:** Univ Ark 1977; **Resid:** Internal Medicine, Univ Ark Med Scis, Little Rock, AR 1977-1980; **Fellow:** Medical Oncology, Univ Ark Med Scis, Little Rock, AR 1980-1983; **Fac Appt:** Prof Medicine, Univ Ark

Jones, Stephen E MD (Onc) - *Spec Exp:* Breast Cancer; **Hospital:** Baylor Univ Medical Ctr; **Address:** Texas Oncology PA, 3535 Worth St, Ste 600, Dallas, TX 75246; **Phone:** (214) 370-1000; **Board Cert:** Internal Medicine 1972, Medical Oncology 1973; **Med School:** Case West Res Univ 1966; **Resid:** Internal Medicine, Stanford Univ, Stanford, CA 1967-1968; **Fellow:** Medical Oncology, Stanford Univ, Stanford, CA 1970-1972; **Fac Appt:** Prof Medical Oncology, Baylor Coll Med

Legha, Sewa Singh MD (Onc) - *Spec Exp:* *Melanoma; Breast Cancer; Thyroid & Adrenal Cancers;* **Hospital:** St Luke's Episcopal Hosp - Houston; **Address:** 6624 Fannin, Ste 1440, Houston, TX 77030; **Phone:** (713) 797-9711; **Board Cert:** Internal Medicine 1987, Medical Oncology 1977; **Med School:** India 1970; **Resid:** Internal Medicine, Milwaukee Co Genl Hosp/Med Coll Wisc, Milwaukee, WI 1972-1974; Medical Oncology, Natl Cancer Inst, Bethesda, MD 1974-1976; **Fellow:** Medical Oncology, MD Anderson Hosp, Houston, TX 1976-1977; **Fac Appt:** Clin Prof Medicine, Baylor Coll Med

Logothetis, Christopher John MD (Onc) - *Spec Exp:* *Prostate Cancer; Bladder Cancer;* **Hospital:** Univ of TX MD Anderson Cancer Ctr, The; **Address:** UT-MD Anderson MC, 1515 Holcombe Blvd, Box 0013, Houston, TX 77030-4009; **Phone:** (713) 792-2830; **Board Cert:** Internal Medicine 1978, Medical Oncology 1981; **Med School:** Greece 1975; **Fac Appt:** Assoc Prof Medical Oncology, Univ Tex, Houston

O'Brien, Susan M MD (Onc) - *Spec Exp:* *Leukemia; Lymphoma;* **Hospital:** Univ of TX MD Anderson Cancer Ctr, The; **Address:** Univ Texas MD Anderson Cancer Ctr, 1515 Holcombe Blvd, Box 428, Houston, TX 77030; **Phone:** (713) 792-7305; **Board Cert:** Internal Medicine 1983, Medical Oncology 1987; **Med School:** UMDNJ-NJ Med Sch, Newark 1980; **Resid:** Internal Medicine, UMDNJ Med Ctr, Newark, NJ 1981-1983; **Fellow:** Medical Oncology, Univ TX MD Anderson Med Ctr, Houston, TX 1985-1987; **Fac Appt:** Prof Medicine, Univ Tex, Houston

Osborne, Charles Kent MD (Onc) - *Spec Exp:* *Breast Cancer;* **Hospital:** Univ of Texas Hlth & Sci Ctr; **Address:** 1 Baylor Plaza, rm N-500, MC BCM-600, Houston, TX 77030; **Phone:** (713) 798-1600; **Board Cert:** Medical Oncology 1977, Internal Medicine 1975; **Med School:** Univ MO-Columbia Sch Med 1972; **Resid:** Internal Medicine, Johns Hopkins Hosp., Baltimore, MD 1973-1974; **Fellow:** Medical Oncology, Natl Cancer Inst., Bethesda, MD 1974-1977; **Fac Appt:** Prof Medicine, Baylor Coll Med

Patt, Yehuda Z MD (Onc) - *Spec Exp:* *Liver Cancer; Biliary Cancer;* **Hospital:** Univ of TX MD Anderson Cancer Ctr, The; **Address:** Univ Texas-MD Anderson Cancer Ctr, 1515 Holcombe Blvd, Box 426, Houston, TX 77030-4009; **Phone:** (713) 792-2828; **Board Cert:** Internal Medicine 1982, Medical Oncology 1987; **Med School:** Israel 1967; **Resid:** Internal Medicine, Tel Aviv-Sheba Med Ctr, Israel 1970-1974; **Fac Appt:** Assoc Prof Medicine, Univ Tex, Houston

Pisters, Katherine M W MD (Onc) - *Spec Exp:* *Lung Cancer;* **Hospital:** Univ of TX MD Anderson Cancer Ctr, The; **Address:** MD Anderson Cancer Ctr, 1515 Holcombe Blvd, Box 432, Houston, TX 77030; **Phone:** (713) 792-6363; **Board Cert:** Internal Medicine 1988, Medical Oncology 1991; **Med School:** Canada 1985; **Resid:** Internal Medicine, North Shore Univ Hosp, Manhasset, NY 1986-1988; **Fellow:** Medical Oncology, Meml Sloan Kettering Cancer Ctr, New York, NY 1988-1991

Saiki, John H. MD (Onc) - *Spec Exp:* *Hematology/Oncology;* **Hospital:** Univ NM Hosp; **Address:** 2211 NE Lomas, Albuquerque, NM 87106; **Phone:** (505) 272-4661; **Board Cert:** Internal Medicine 1970, Gynecologic Oncology 1973; **Med School:** McGill Univ 1961; **Resid:** Hematology, University of New Mexico, Albuquerque, NM 1968-1969; Internal Medicine, University of New Mexico, Albuquerque, NM 1966-1968; **Fellow:** Medical Oncology, M D Anderson Hospital, Houston, TX 1969-1970; **Fac Appt:** Prof Medicine, Univ New Mexico

Salem, Philip Adeeb MD (Onc) - *Spec Exp:* *Breast Cancer; Lymphoma;* **Hospital:** St Luke's Episcopal Hosp - Houston; **Address:** 6624 Fannin St, Ste 1630, Houston, TX 77030; **Phone:** (713) 796-1221; **Med School:** Lebanon 1965; **Resid:** Medical Oncology, Meml Sloan Kettering Cancer Ctr, New York, NY 1968-1970; **Fellow:** Oncology Research, MD Anderson Cancer Ctr, Houston, TX 1971-1972; **Fac Appt:** Clin Prof Medicine, Univ Tex, Houston

Valero, Vicente MD (Onc) - *Spec Exp:* Breast Cancer; **Hospital:** Univ of TX MD Anderson Cancer Ctr, The; **Address:** Univ Texas MD Anderson Cancer Ctr, 1515 Holcombe Blvd, Box 424, Houston, TX 77030; **Phone:** (713) 792-2817; **Board Cert:** Internal Medicine 1985, Hematology 1988, Medical Oncology 1987; **Med School:** Mexico 1980; **Resid:** Internal Medicine, Univ Cincinnati Coll Med, Cincinnati, OH 1982-1985; Hematology and Oncology, Univ Cincinnati Coll Med, Cincinnati, OH 1985-1987; **Fellow:** Hematology and Oncology, Univ Texas Med Br, Galveston, TX 1987-1988

West Coast and Pacific

Abrams, Donald Ira MD (Onc) - *Spec Exp:* AIDS/HIV; **Hospital:** San Francisco Gen Hosp; **Address:** Positive Hlth Program Bldg 80, Ward 84, 995 Potrero Ave, San Francisco, CA 94110; **Phone:** (415) 476-4082; **Board Cert:** Internal Medicine 1980, Medical Oncology 1983; **Med School:** Stanford Univ 1977; **Resid:** Internal Medicine, Kaiser Fdn Hosp, San Francisco, CA 1978-1980; **Fellow:** Medical Oncology, UCSF Cancer Rsch, San Francisco, CA 1980-1982; **Fac Appt:** Prof Medicine, UCSF

Ball, Edward David MD (Onc) - *Spec Exp:* Bone Marrow & Stem Cell Transplant; Leukemia/Lymphoma; Multiple Myeloma; **Hospital:** UCSD Healthcare; **Address:** 9500 Gilman Dr, Box 0960, La Jolla, CA 92093-0960; **Phone:** (858) 657-7053; **Board Cert:** Internal Medicine 1979, Medical Oncology 1983, Hematology 2000; **Med School:** Case West Res Univ 1976; **Resid:** Internal Medicine, Hartford Hosp, Hartford, CT 1977-1979; **Fellow:** Hematology, Univ Hosps Cleveland, Cleveland, OH 1979-1981; Hematology and Oncology, Dartmouth-Hitchcock Hosp, Hanover, NH 1981-1982; **Fac Appt:** Prof Medicine, UCSD

Carlson, Robert Wells MD (Onc) - *Spec Exp:* Breast Cancer; **Hospital:** Stanford Med Ctr; **Address:** 300 Pasteur Drive, rm H0274, Stanford, CA 94305; **Phone:** (650) 723-7621; **Board Cert:** Internal Medicine 1981, Medical Oncology 1983; **Med School:** Stanford Univ 1978; **Resid:** Internal Medicine, Barnes Hosp Group, St Louis, MO 1978-1980; Internal Medicine, Stanford Univ Hosp, Stanford, CA 1980-1981; **Fellow:** Medical Oncology, Stanford Univ Med Ctr, Stanford, CA 1981-1983; **Fac Appt:** Prof Medicine, Stanford Univ

Chap, Linnea MD (Onc) - *Spec Exp:* Breast Cancer; **Hospital:** UCLA Med Ctr; **Address:** UCLA Med Ctr, 0945 Le Conte Ave, Ste 2333, Los Angeles, CA 91436-3718; **Phone:** (310) 206-6144; **Board Cert:** Internal Medicine 1991, Hematology 1994, Maternal & Fetal Medicine 1995; **Med School:** Univ Chicago-Pritzker Sch Med 1988; **Resid:** Internal Medicine, Northwestern Meml Hosp, Chicago, IL 1988-1991; **Fellow:** Hematology and Oncology, UCLA Med Ctr, Los Angeles, CA 1991-1992

Chlebowski, Rowan Thomas MD/PhD (Onc) - *Spec Exp:* Breast Cancer; Women's Health; **Hospital:** LAC - Harbor - UCLA Med Ctr; **Address:** 1000 W Carson St Bldg J3, Torrance, CA 90509; **Phone:** (310) 222-2218; **Board Cert:** Internal Medicine 1980, Medical Oncology 1981; **Med School:** Case West Res Univ 1974; **Resid:** Internal Medicine, MetroHealth Med Ctr, Cleveland, OH 1974-1976; Medical Oncology, LAC-USC Med Ctr, Los Angeles, CA 1978-1979; **Fac Appt:** Prof Medical Oncology, UCLA

Gandara, David R MD (Onc) - *Spec Exp:* Lung Cancer; **Hospital:** Univ CA - Davis Med Ctr; **Address:** UC Davis Cancer Center, 4501 X St, Sacramento, CA 95817; **Phone:** (916) 734-5959; **Board Cert:** Medical Oncology 1979, Internal Medicine 1976; **Med School:** Univ Tex Med Br, Galveston 1973; **Resid:** Internal Medicine, Madigan Med Ctr, Tacoma, WA 1974-1976; **Fellow:** Medical Oncology, Letterman AMC, San Francisco, CA 1976-1978; **Fac Appt:** Asst Prof Medicine, UC Davis

MEDICAL ONCOLOGY

Ganz, Patricia Anne MD (Onc) - *Spec Exp:* Breast Cancer; **Hospital:** UCLA Med Ctr; **Address:** Div Cancer Prev & Control Research, 650 Charles Young Drive S, Box 956900, Los Angeles, CA 90095; **Phone:** (310) 206-1404; **Board Cert:** Medical Oncology 1979, Internal Medicine 1976; **Med School:** UCLA 1973; **Resid:** Internal Medicine, UCLA Med Ctr, Los Angeles, CA 1974-1976; **Fellow:** Hematology, UCLA Med Ctr, Los Angeles, CA 1976-1978; **Fac Appt:** Prof Medicine, UCLA

Jacobs, Charlotte DeCroes MD (Onc) - *Spec Exp:* Medical Oncology - General; **Hospital:** Stanford Med Ctr; **Address:** 1000 Welch Rd, Ste 202, Palo Alto, CA 94304; **Phone:** (650) 725-8738; **Board Cert:** Internal Medicine 1975, Medical Oncology 1977; **Med School:** Washington Univ, St Louis 1972; **Resid:** Internal Medicine, Barnes Hosp, St Louis, MO 1974; Internal Medicine, UCSF, San Francisco, CA 1975; **Fellow:** Medical Oncology, Stanford, Stanford, CA 1977; **Fac Appt:** Prof Medicine, Stanford Univ

Livingston, Robert B MD (Onc) - *Spec Exp:* Bone Marrow Transplant; Breast Cancer; Lung Cancer; **Hospital:** Univ WA Med Ctr; **Address:** 825 Eastlake Ave E, Seattle, WA 98109-1023; **Phone:** (206) 288-1085; **Board Cert:** Internal Medicine 1972, Medical Oncology 1973; **Med School:** Univ Okla Coll Med 1965; **Resid:** Internal Medicine, U Oklahoma Med Ctr, Oklahoma City, OK 1969-1971; **Fellow:** Medical Oncology, U Texas, Houston, TX 1971-1973; **Fac Appt:** Prof Medicine, Univ Wash

Natale, Ronald B MD (Onc) - *Spec Exp:* Lung Cancer; **Hospital:** Cedars-Sinai Med Ctr; **Address:** Cedars-Sinai Comprehensive Cancer Dtr, Area C2000, 8700 Beverly Blvd, Los Angeles, CA 90048; **Phone:** (310) 423-1101; **Board Cert:** Internal Medicine 1977, Medical Oncology 1979; **Med School:** Wayne State Univ 1974; **Resid:** Internal Medicine, Wayne State Univ. 1975-1977; **Fellow:** Medical Oncology, Meml Sloan Kettering, New York, NY 1977-1980; **Fac Appt:** Prof Medical Oncology, Univ Mich Med Sch

Press, Oliver William MD/PhD (Onc) - *Spec Exp:* Lymphoma; Bone Marrow Transplant; **Hospital:** Univ WA Med Ctr; **Address:** 1100 Fairview Ave N, MS D3-190, Seattle, WA 98109; **Phone:** (206) 667-1864; **Board Cert:** Medical Oncology 1985, Internal Medicine 1982; **Med School:** Univ Wash 1979; **Resid:** Internal Medicine, U Hosp., Seattle, WA 1982-1983; Internal Medicine, Mass Genl Hosp., Boston, MA 1980-1982; **Fellow:** Medical Oncology, U Wash., Seattle, WA 1983-1985; **Fac Appt:** Prof Medicine, Univ Wash

Rosen, Peter J MD (Onc) - *Spec Exp:* Lymphoma; Breast Cancer; **Hospital:** UCLA Med Ctr; **Address:** 10945 Le Conte Ave, Ste 2333, Los Angeles, CA 90095; **Phone:** (310) 794-1092; **Board Cert:** Hematology 1974, Medical Oncology 1975; **Med School:** USC Sch Med 1966; **Resid:** Internal Medicine, Johns Hopkins Hosp, Baltimore, MD 1966-1968; **Fellow:** Hematology, USC, Los Angeles, CA 1970-1972

Tempero, Margaret MD (Onc) - *Spec Exp:* Pancreatic Cancer; **Hospital:** UCSF Med Ctr; **Address:** UCSF-Comprehensive Cancer Ctr, 2356 Sutter St, Ste 711, San Francisco, CA 94115; **Phone:** (415) 885-3846; **Board Cert:** Medical Oncology 1983, Hematology 1984; **Med School:** Univ Nebr Coll Med 1977; **Resid:** Internal Medicine, Univ Nebraska, Omaha, NE 1978-1980; **Fellow:** Medical Oncology, Univ Nebraska, Omaha, NE 1982

Urba, Walter J MD (Onc) - *Spec Exp:* Breast Cancer; **Hospital:** Providence Portland Med Ctr; **Address:** Oregon Clinic, Div of Medical Oncology, 550 NE Hoyt St, Ste 611, Portland, OR 97213; **Phone:** (503) 215-5696; **Board Cert:** Internal Medicine 1985, Medical Oncology 1987; **Med School:** Univ Miami Sch Med 1981; **Resid:** Internal Medicine, Morristown Meml Hosp 1981-1983; **Fellow:** Medical Oncology, Natl Cancer Inst, Bethesda, MD 1983-1986; **Fac Appt:** Assoc Clin Prof Medicine, Oregon Hlth Scis Univ

Volberding, Paul Arthur MD (Onc) - *Spec Exp:* *AIDS/HIV;* **Hospital:** UCSF Med Ctr; **Address:** 4150 Clemens St, Ste BAMC 111, San Francisco, CA 94121; **Phone:** (415) 476-4082; **Board Cert:** Internal Medicine 1978, Medical Oncology 1981; **Med School:** Univ Minn 1975; **Resid:** Internal Medicine, Univ Utah, Salt Lake City, UT 1976-1978; **Fellow:** Medical Oncology, UCSF Med Ctr, San Francisco, CA 1978-1981; **Fac Appt:** Prof Medicine, UCSF

INFECTIOUS DISEASE

(a subspecialty of INTERNAL MEDICINE)

An internist who deals with infectious diseases of all types and in all organs. Conditions requiring selective use of antibiotics call for this special skill. This physician often diagnoses and treats AIDS patients and patients with fevers which have not been explained. Infectious disease specialists may also have expertise in preventive medicine and conditions associated with travel.

INTERNAL MEDICINE

An internist is a personal physician who provides long-term, comprehensive care in the office and the hospital, managing both common and complex illness of adolescents, adults and the elderly. Internists are trained in the diagnosis and treatment of cancer, infections and diseases affecting the heart, blood, kidneys, joints and digestive, respiratory and vascular systems. They are also trained in the essentials of primary care internal medicine which incorporates an understanding of disease prevention, wellness, substance abuse, mental health and effective treatment of common problems of the eyes, ears, skin, nervous system and reproductive organs.

Training required: Three years in internal medicine *plus* additional training and examination for certification in infectious disease

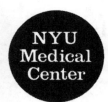

NYU Medical Center

550 First Avenue (at 31st Street)
New York, NY 10016
Physician Referral: (888) 7-NYU-MED
(888-769-8633) www.nyumedicalcenter.org

SCHOOL OF MEDICINE

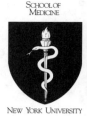

NEW YORK UNIVERSITY

INFECTIOUS DISEASES

Public Health officials estimate that, unless something is done to prevent the spread of AIDS, it will soon surpass the Black Plague as humankind's most deadly virus. Yet, researchers who face the daunting task of unraveling the medical mystery of AIDS must fight a battle on two fronts – developing treatments to prolong life for those already infected, and preventing infection among the healthy.

The history of AIDS research in the United States and the scientific contributions of NYU CFAR investigators are closely linked. The CFAR at NYU Medical Center was one of thirteen original Centers for AIDS research designated by the NIH to coordinate, enhance and expedite HIV/AIDS research efforts at selected institutions. NYU Faculty were among the first to document the immune deficiency associated with AIDS and the first to determine that immune abnormalisties could be found in asymptomatic members of the gay community. They were the first to identify Kaposi's sarcoma as a manifestation of the disease.

Drawing from NYU's pioneering contributions in the field of AIDS research, the NYU CFAR is committed to discovering treatments for people with HIV disease and ultimately, developing a vaccine for the virus. To accomplish this, the CFAR is organized into five different research programs, focusing on:

- development of new therapies and treatments for infected individuals

- understanding of the disease's transmission and prevention

- treatment of HIV-associated diseases like tuberculosis and hepatitis

- development of an AIDS vaccine

- viral pathogenesis

NYU MEDICAL CENTER

Maternal-Fetal Medicine at NYU Medical Center

- Specialized care to women with high-risk pregnancies by highly-trained Perinatologists

- Genetic counseling to provide education and genetic tests to evaluate family history

- Tests to help predict patients at risk for preterm labor and delivery, and medications for the mother

- Screening for complications, including preeclampsia, pregnancy-induced hypertension

- Nutritional counseling and education for gestational diabetes, diabetes disovered during pregnancy

---

Physician Referral
(888) 7-NYU-MED

(888-769-8633)

www.nyumedicalcenter.org

PHYSICIAN LISTINGS

Infectious Disease

New England

Craven, Donald Edward MD (Inf) - *Spec Exp:* AIDS/HIV; Hepatitis C; Pneumonia; **Hospital:** Lahey Cli.; **Address:** 41 Mall Rd, Burlington, MA -00003-4696; **Phone:** (781) 744-8608; **Board Cert:** Internal Medicine 1973, Infectious Disease 1982; **Med School:** Albany Med Coll 1970; **Resid:** Internal Medicine, Royal Victoria Hosp-McGill, Montreal, Canada 1971-1973; Infectious Disease, Boston Univ Hosp, Boston, MA 1974-1976; **Fellow:** Internal Medicine, Royal Victoria Hosp, Montreal, Canada 1973-1974; **Fac Appt:** Prof Medicine, Boston Univ

Hirsch, Martin Stanley MD (Inf) - *Spec Exp:* AIDS/HIV; Viral Infections; **Hospital:** MA Genl Hosp; **Address:** MA Genl Hosp - Inf Dis Unit, 55 Fruit St, Boston, MA 02114; **Phone:** (617) 726-3815; **Board Cert:** Internal Medicine 1972, Infectious Disease 1976; **Med School:** Johns Hopkins Univ 1964; **Resid:** Internal Medicine, Chicago Clins Hosps, Chicago, IL 1965-1966; **Fellow:** Infectious Disease, Mass Genl Hosp, Boston, MA 1969-1971; **Fac Appt:** Prof Medicine, Harvard Med Sch

Hopkins, Cyrus Clark MD (Inf) - *Spec Exp:* Infections-Hospital Acquired; **Hospital:** MA Genl Hosp; **Address:** 55 Fruit St, Clinic 131, Boston, MA 02114; **Phone:** (617) 726-2036; **Board Cert:** Internal Medicine 1972, Infectious Disease 1972; **Med School:** Harvard Med Sch 1964; **Resid:** Internal Medicine, Mass Genl Hosp, Boston, MA 1965-1966; Internal Medicine, Mass Genl Hosp, Boston, MA 1968-1970; **Fellow:** Infectious Disease, Mass Genl Hosp, Boston, MA 1969; **Fac Appt:** Assoc Prof Medicine, Harvard Med Sch

Karchmer, Adolph W MD (Inf) - *Spec Exp:* Infective Endocarditis; **Hospital:** Beth Israel Deaconess Med Ctr - Boston; **Address:** 1 Autumn St, Ste Kennedy 6, Boston, MA 02215; **Phone:** (617) 632-0760; **Board Cert:** Internal Medicine 1972; **Med School:** Harvard Med Sch 1964; **Resid:** Internal Medicine, Mass Genl Hosp, Boston, MA 1965-1966; Internal Medicine, Mass Genl Hosp, Boston, MA 1969-1970; **Fellow:** Infectious Disease, Mass Genl Hosp, Boston, MA 1970-1971; **Fac Appt:** Prof Medicine, Harvard Med Sch

Mid Atlantic

Auwaerter, Paul MD (Inf) - *Spec Exp:* Ehrlichiosis; Tick-borne Diseases; **Hospital:** Johns Hopkins Hosp - Baltimore; **Address:** 10755 Falls Rd, Ste 360, Lutherville, MD 21093; **Phone:** (410) 583-2774; **Board Cert:** Internal Medicine 1992, Infectious Disease 1994; **Med School:** Columbia P&S 1988; **Resid:** Internal Medicine, Johns Hopkins Med Ctr, Baltimore, MD 1989-1991; Infectious Disease, Johns Hopkins Med Ctr, Baltimore, MD 1991-1992; **Fellow:** Infectious Disease, Johns Hopkins Med Ctr, Baltimore, MD 1993-1996; **Fac Appt:** Asst Prof Medicine, Johns Hopkins Univ

Bartlett, John Gill MD (Inf) - *Spec Exp:* AIDS/HIV; Fevers-Unknown Origin; Pneumonia; **Hospital:** Johns Hopkins Hosp - Baltimore; **Address:** 1830 E Monument St, Ste 439, Baltimore, MD 21287-0003; **Phone:** (410) 955-7634; **Board Cert:** Internal Medicine 1972; **Med School:** SUNY Syracuse 1963; **Resid:** Internal Medicine, Univ Hosp Birmingham, Birmingham, AL 1967-1968; Internal Medicine, Peter B Brigham Hosp., Boston, MA 1964-1965; **Fellow:** Infectious Disease, Wadsworth VA Hosp., Los Angeles, CA 1968-1970

Berkowitz, Leonard B MD (Inf) - *Spec Exp:* AIDS/HIV; **Hospital:** Brooklyn Hosp Ctr-Downtown; **Address:** 121 DeKalb Ave, Brooklyn, NY 11201-5425; **Phone:** (718) 250-6141; **Board Cert:** Internal Medicine 1980, Infectious Disease 1984; **Med School:** SUNY Hlth Sci Ctr 1977; **Resid:** Internal Medicine, Univ Hosp, Kings Co Med Ctr, Brooklyn, NY 1977-1981; **Fellow:** Infectious Disease, Univ Hosp, Kings Co Med Ctr, Brooklyn, NY 1981-1983; **Fac Appt:** Asst Prof Medicine, SUNY Hlth Sci Ctr

Blaser, Martin Jack MD (Inf) - *Spec Exp:* Helicobacter Pylori; **Hospital:** NYU Med Ctr (page 71); **Address:** 550 1st Ave NVB 16 North 1, New York, NY 10016-6402; **Phone:** (212) 263-6394; **Board Cert:** Internal Medicine 1977, Infectious Disease 1980; **Med School:** NYU Sch Med 1973; **Resid:** Internal Medicine, U Colo Med Ctr, Denver, CO 1974-1977; **Fellow:** Infectious Disease, U Colo Med Ctr, Denver, CO 1977-1979; **Fac Appt:** Prof Medicine, NYU Sch Med

Brause, Barry MD (Inf) - *Spec Exp:* Bone/Joint Infections; Lyme Disease; **Hospital:** NY Presby Hosp - NY Weill Cornell Med Ctr (page 70); **Address:** 215 E 68th St, New York, NY 10021-5718; **Phone:** (212) 570-6122; **Board Cert:** Internal Medicine 1973, Infectious Disease 1976; **Med School:** Univ Pittsburgh 1970; **Resid:** Internal Medicine, New York Hosp, New York, NY 1971-1973; **Fellow:** Infectious Disease, New York Hosp, New York, NY 1973-1975; **Fac Appt:** Clin Prof Medicine, Cornell Univ-Weill Med Coll

Brennan, Patrick J MD (Inf) - *Spec Exp:* Tuberculosis; Infections in Immune Deficient; **Hospital:** Hosp Univ Penn (page 78); **Address:** U Penn Med Ctr-Infectious Dis, 3400 Spruce St Bldg 3 Silverstein - Ste D, Philadelphia, PA 19104; **Phone:** (215) 662-6932; **Board Cert:** Internal Medicine 1985, Infectious Disease 1990; **Med School:** Temple Univ 1982; **Resid:** Internal Medicine, Temple Univ Hosp, Philadelphia, PA 1983-1985; **Fellow:** Infectious Disease, Hosp Univ Penn, Philadelphia, PA 1985-1986; **Fac Appt:** Assoc Prof Medicine, Univ Penn

Chaisson, Richard Ernest MD (Inf) - *Spec Exp:* AIDS/HIV; Tuberculosis; **Hospital:** Johns Hopkins Hosp - Baltimore; **Address:** 424 N Bond St, Ste 114, Baltimore, MD 21231; **Phone:** (410) 955-1755; **Board Cert:** Internal Medicine 1985; **Med School:** Univ Mass Sch Med 1982; **Resid:** Internal Medicine, UCSF Med Ctr, San Francisco, CA 1983-1985; **Fellow:** Infectious Disease, UCSF Med Ctr, San Francisco, CA 1985-1987; **Fac Appt:** Assoc Prof Medicine, Johns Hopkins Univ

Cunha, Burke A MD (Inf) - *Spec Exp:* Infections in Compromised Host; Pneumonias; Fevers of Unknown Origin; **Hospital:** Winthrop - Univ Hosp; **Address:** 222 Station Plz N, Ste 432, Mineola, NY 11501; **Phone:** (516) 663-2507; **Board Cert:** Internal Medicine 1977, Infectious Disease 1978; **Med School:** Penn State Univ-Hershey Med Ctr 1972; **Resid:** Internal Medicine, Hartford Hosp, Hartford, CT 1972-1975; **Fellow:** Infectious Disease, Hartford Hosp/Univ Conn Sch Med, Hartford, CT 1975-1977; **Fac Appt:** Prof Medicine, SUNY Stony Brook

Ellner, Jerrold Jay MD (Inf) - *Spec Exp:* AIDS/HIV; Tuberculosis in AIDS/HIV; **Hospital:** UMDNJ-Univ Hosp-Newark; **Address:** UMDNJ-New Jersey Medical School, Dept Med, 185 S Orange Ave, Newark, NJ 07103; **Phone:** (973) 972-4595; **Board Cert:** Internal Medicine 1973, Infectious Disease 1978; **Med School:** Johns Hopkins Univ 1970; **Resid:** Internal Medicine, Johns Hopkins Hosp, Baltimore, MD 1970-1972

Fauci, Anthony Stephen MD (Inf) - *Spec Exp:* AIDS/HIV; **Hospital:** Natl Inst of Hlth - Clin Ctr; **Address:** NIAID , Bldg 31 - rm 7A03, 31 Center Drive MSC 2520, Bethesda, MD 20892-2520; **Phone:** (301) 496-2263; **Board Cert:** Allergy & Immunology 1974, Infectious Disease 1974; **Med School:** Cornell Univ-Weill Med Coll 1966; **Resid:** Internal Medicine, NY Hosp Cornell Med Ctr, New York, NY 1967-1968; Internal Medicine, NY Hosp Cornell Med Ctr, New York, NY 1971-1972; **Fellow:** Infectious Disease, Natl Inst Infectious Disease NIH, Bethesda, MD 1968-1971

Frank, Ian MD (Inf) - *Spec Exp:* AIDS/HIV; **Hospital:** Hosp Univ Penn (page 78); **Address:** Univ Penn Medical Center-Infectious Disease, 3400 Spruce St, Philadelphia, PA 19104-6073; **Phone:** (215) 662-6932; **Board Cert:** Internal Medicine 1983, Infectious Disease 1992; **Med School:** Dartmouth Med Sch 1980; **Resid:** Internal Medicine, Graduate Hosp, Philadelphia, PA 1981-1983; **Fellow:** Infectious Disease, Hosp Univ Penn, Philadelphia, PA 1983; **Fac Appt:** Assoc Prof Medicine, Univ Penn

Friedman, Harvey Michael MD (Inf) - *Spec Exp:* AIDS/HIV; Herpes Simplex; Viral Infections; **Hospital:** Hosp Univ Penn (page 78); **Address:** U Penn, 502 Johnson Pavillion, Philadelphia, PA 19104-6073; **Phone:** (215) 662-3557; **Board Cert:** Internal Medicine 1975, Infectious Disease 1976; **Med School:** McGill Univ 1969; **Resid:** Internal Medicine, Jewish Genl Hosp, Montreal, Canada 1970-1971; Virology, Wistar Inst, Philadelphia, PA 1971-1973; **Fellow:** Infectious Disease, Hosp Univ Penn, Philadelphia, PA 1973-1975; **Fac Appt:** Prof Medicine, Univ Penn

Garvey, Glenda Josephine MD (Inf) - *Spec Exp:* Infective Endocarditis; Septic Shock; **Hospital:** NY Presby Hosp - Columbia Presby Med Ctr (page 70); **Address:** Columbia-Presbyterian Med Ctr, Div Infectious Diseases, 622 W 168th St, PH8-876, New York, NY 10032; **Phone:** (212) 305-3272; **Board Cert:** Critical Care Medicine 1999, Infectious Disease 1976, Internal Medicine 1972; **Med School:** Columbia P&S 1969; **Resid:** Internal Medicine, Columbia Presby Med Ctr, New York, NY 1969-1972; **Fellow:** Infectious Disease, Columbia Presby Med Ctr, New York, NY 1972-1974; **Fac Appt:** Prof Medicine, Columbia P&S

Hammer, Glenn MD (Inf) - *Spec Exp:* AIDS/HIV; **Hospital:** Mount Sinai Hosp (page 68); **Address:** 1100 Park Ave, New York, NY 10128; **Phone:** (212) 427-9550; **Board Cert:** Infectious Disease 1974, Internal Medicine 1973; **Med School:** NYU Sch Med 1969; **Resid:** Internal Medicine, Mount Sinai Hosp, New York, NY 1970-1972; **Fellow:** Infectious Disease, Mount Sinai Hosp, New York, NY 1972-1974; **Fac Appt:** Asst Clin Prof Medicine, Mount Sinai Sch Med

Hartman, Barry Jay MD (Inf) - *Spec Exp:* Endocarditis; Infections-Surgical; Parasitic Infections; **Hospital:** NY Presby Hosp - NY Weill Cornell Med Ctr (page 70); **Address:** 407 E 70th St, Fl 4, New York, NY 10021-5302; **Phone:** (212) 744-4882; **Board Cert:** Internal Medicine 1976, Infectious Disease 1980; **Med School:** Penn State Univ-Hershey Med Ctr 1973; **Resid:** Internal Medicine, NY Hosp /Cornell Med Ctr, New York, NY 1974-1976; **Fellow:** Infectious Disease, NY Hosp/ Cornell Med Ctr, New York, NY 1978-1981; **Fac Appt:** Clin Prof Medicine, Cornell Univ-Weill Med Coll

Johnson, Warren MD (Inf) - *Spec Exp:* Travel Medicine; Parasitic Infections; Toxoplasmosis, Amebiasis; **Hospital:** NY Presby Hosp - NY Weill Cornell Med Ctr (page 70); **Address:** 1300 York Ave, Ste A-421, New York, NY 10021; **Phone:** (212) 746-6320; **Board Cert:** Infectious Disease 1974, Internal Medicine 1971; **Med School:** Columbia P&S 1962; **Resid:** Internal Medicine, NY Hosp-Cornell Med Ctr, New York, NY 1963-1964; Internal Medicine, NY Hosp-Cornell Med Ctr, New York, NY 1968-1969; **Fellow:** Infectious Disease, NY Hosp-Cornell Med Ctr, New York, NY 1966-1968; **Fac Appt:** Prof Medicine, Cornell Univ-Weill Med Coll

Kaplan, Mark H MD (Inf) - *Spec Exp:* AIDS/HIV; **Hospital:** N Shore Univ Hosp at Manhasset; **Address:** North Shore Univ Hosp, Div Infectious Disease, 300 Community Drive, Manhasset, NY 11030; **Phone:** (516) 562-4280; **Board Cert:** Infectious Disease 1974, Internal Medicine 1972; **Med School:** Cornell Univ-Weill Med Coll 1966; **Resid:** Internal Medicine, Bellevue Hosp Ctr, New York, NY 1967-1968; Internal Medicine, Mem Sloan Kettering Cancer Ctr, New York, NY 1970-1971; **Fellow:** Infectious Disease, Mem Sloan Kettering Cancer Ctr, New York, NY 1973-1974; **Fac Appt:** Clin Prof Medicine, NYU Sch Med

Masur, Henry MD (Inf) - *Spec Exp:* Critical Care; AIDS/HIV; **Hospital:** Natl Inst of Hlth - Clin Ctr; **Address:** National Institute of Health, 10 Center Drive Bldg Clinical Center 7D43, Bethesda, MD 20892; **Phone:** (301) 496-9320; **Board Cert:** Internal Medicine 1975, Infectious Disease 1978; **Med School:** Cornell Univ-Weill Med Coll 1972; **Resid:** Internal Medicine, New York Hosp, NewYork, NY 1973-1974; Internal Medicine, Johns Hopkins Hosp, Baltimore, MD 1974-1975; **Fellow:** Infectious Disease, New York Hosp-Cornell Med Ctr, New York, NY 1975-1977

Mildvan, Donna MD (Inf) - *Spec Exp:* AIDS/HIV; **Hospital:** Beth Israel Med Ctr - Petrie Division (page 58); **Address:** Div Infectious Disease, 1st Ave at 16th St, New York, NY 10003; **Phone:** (212) 420-4005; **Board Cert:** Internal Medicine 1972, Infectious Disease 1972; **Med School:** Johns Hopkins Univ 1967; **Resid:** Internal Medicine, Mount Sinai Hosp, New York, NY 1968-1970; **Fellow:** Infectious Disease, Mount Sinai Hosp, New York, NY 1970-1972; **Fac Appt:** Prof Medicine, Albert Einstein Coll Med

Perlman, David MD (Inf) - *Spec Exp:* AIDS/HIV; Lyme Disease; Travel Medicine; **Hospital:** Beth Israel Med Ctr - Petrie Division (page 58); **Address:** Beth Israel Med Ctr, 1st Ave at 16th St, New York, NY 10003; **Phone:** (212) 420-4470; **Board Cert:** Internal Medicine 1986, Infectious Disease 1988; **Med School:** Albert Einstein Coll Med 1983; **Resid:** Internal Medicine, NY Hosp/Meml Sloan Kettering, New York, NY 1984-1986; **Fellow:** Infectious Disease, Montefiore Hosp, Bronx, NY 1986-1988; **Fac Appt:** Prof Medicine, Albert Einstein Coll Med

Polsky, Bruce MD (Inf) - *Spec Exp:* AIDS/HIV; Viral Infections; Infectious Complications of Cancer; **Hospital:** St Luke's - Roosevelt Hosp Ctr - Roosevelt Div (page 58); **Address:** Univ Med Practice, 425 W 59th St, New York, NY 10019; **Phone:** (212) 523-2525; **Board Cert:** Internal Medicine 1983, Infectious Disease 1986; **Med School:** Wayne State Univ 1980; **Resid:** Internal Medicine, Montefiore Hosp, Bronx, NY 1981-1983; **Fellow:** Infectious Disease, Meml Sloan Kettering Hosp, New York, NY 1983-1986; **Fac Appt:** Prof Medicine, Columbia P&S

Rahal, James MD (Inf) - *Spec Exp:* West Nile Virus; **Hospital:** NY Hosp Med Ctr of Queens; **Address:** 56-45 Main St, Flushing, NY 11355-5095; **Phone:** (718) 670-1525; **Board Cert:** Internal Medicine 1967, Infectious Disease 1972; **Med School:** Tufts Univ 1959; **Resid:** Internal Medicine, New England Ctr Hosp, Boston, MA 1961-1964; **Fellow:** Infectious Disease, New England Ctr Hosp, Boston, MA 1962-1965; **Fac Appt:** Clin Prof Medicine, Cornell Univ-Weill Med Coll

Rao, Nalini MD (Inf) - *Spec Exp:* Orthopaedic Infectious Disease; Tropical Diseases; **Hospital:** UPMC - Presbyterian Univ Hosp; **Address:** Centre Commons, Suite 510, 5750 Centre Ave, Pittsburgh, PA 15206; **Phone:** (412) 661-1633; **Board Cert:** Infectious Disease 1980, Internal Medicine 1975; **Med School:** India 1970; **Resid:** Internal Medicine, Geo Wash Univ Hosp, Washington, DC 1973-1974; Infectious Disease, Baylor College Med, Houston, TX 1974-1975; **Fellow:** Infectious Disease, U Pittsburgh Sch Med, Pittsburgh, PA 1975-1977; **Fac Appt:** Assoc Clin Prof Medicine, Univ Pittsburgh

Sepkowitz, Kent MD (Inf) - *Spec Exp:* AIDS/HIV; Infections In Cancer Patients; **Hospital:** Mem Sloan Kettering Cancer Ctr; **Address:** 1275 York Ave, New York, NY 10021-0033; **Phone:** (212) 639-2441; **Board Cert:** Internal Medicine 1983, Infectious Disease 2000; **Med School:** Univ Okla Coll Med 1980; **Resid:** Internal Medicine, Roosevelt Hosp, New York, NY 1981-1984; **Fellow:** Infectious Disease, Meml Sloan Kettering Cancer Ctr, New York, NY 1988-1991; **Fac Appt:** Assoc Prof Medicine, Cornell Univ-Weill Med Coll

Smith, Leon G MD (Inf) - *Spec Exp:* AIDS/HIV; Bone/Joint Infections; Hepatitis; **Hospital:** Saint Michael's Med Ctr; **Address:** 268 Martin Luther King Jr Blvd, Newark, NJ 07102-2011; **Phone:** (973) 877-5481; **Board Cert:** Internal Medicine 1963, Infectious Disease 1974; **Med School:** Georgetown Univ 1956; **Resid:** Infectious Disease, Nat Inst Health, Bethesda, MD 1957-1959; Internal Medicine, Yale-New Haven Hosp, New Haven, CT 1960-1962; **Fellow:** Infectious Disease, Yale-New Haven Hosp, New Haven, CT 1959-1960; **Fac Appt:** Prof Medicine, UMDNJ-NJ Med Sch, Newark

Straus, Stephen MD (Inf) - *Spec Exp:* Chronic Fatigue Syndrome; **Hospital:** Natl Inst of Hlth - Clin Ctr; **Address:** NIH Bldg 10 - rm 11-N-228, 10 Center Drive, Bethesda, MD 20892; **Phone:** (301) 496-5807; **Board Cert:** Infectious Disease 1980, Internal Medicine 1977; **Med School:** Columbia P&S 1972; **Resid:** Internal Medicine, Barnes Hosp, St Louis, MO 1975-1976; **Fellow:** Infectious Disease, Barnes Hosp-Wash Univ, St Louis, MO 1976-1978

Welch, Peter MD (Inf) - *Spec Exp:* *Lyme Disease; Tick-Borne Diseases;* **Hospital:** Northern Westchester Hosp Ctr; **Address:** 16 Orchard Drive, Armonk, NY 10504; **Phone:** (914) 666-1308; **Board Cert:** Internal Medicine 1977, Infectious Disease 1980; **Med School:** SUNY Buffalo 1974; **Resid:** Internal Medicine, NY Hosp, Westchester, NY 1974-1977; **Fellow:** Infectious Disease, NY Hosp, New York, NY 1977-1979

Wormser, Gary MD (Inf) - *Spec Exp:* *Lyme Disease; AIDS/HIV;* **Hospital:** Westchester Med Ctr (page 82); **Address:** Westchester County Med Ctr, Munger Pavilion Fl 2, Valhalla, NY 10595; **Phone:** (914) 493-8865; **Board Cert:** Internal Medicine 1978, Infectious Disease 1982; **Med School:** Johns Hopkins Univ 1972; **Resid:** Internal Medicine, Mount Sinai Hosp, New York, NY 1973-1975; **Fellow:** Infectious Disease, Mount Sinai Hosp, New York, NY 1975-1977; **Fac Appt:** Prof Medicine, NY Med Coll

Yancovitz, Stanley MD (Inf) - *Spec Exp:* *Lyme Disease; AIDS/HIV;* **Hospital:** Beth Israel Med Ctr - Petrie Division (page 58); **Address:** 10 Union Square East, Ste 3-F, New York, NY 10003; **Phone:** (212) 420-2600; **Board Cert:** Internal Medicine 1973, Infectious Disease 1976; **Med School:** SUNY Downstate 1967; **Resid:** Internal Medicine, Metropolitan Hosp, New York, NY 1968-1969; Internal Medicine, Beth Israel Med Ctr, New York, NY 1971-1972; **Fellow:** Infectious Disease, Mount Sinai Hosp, New York, NY 1973-1975; **Fac Appt:** Assoc Prof Medicine, Albert Einstein Coll Med

Yu, Victor MD (Inf) - *Spec Exp:* *Legionnaire's Disease;* **Hospital:** VA Pittsburgh Hlth Care Sys; **Address:** Infectious Disease Sect, University Drive C, Rm 2-A-137, Pittsburgh, PA 15240; **Phone:** (412) 688-6179; **Board Cert:** Infectious Disease 1982, Internal Medicine 1978; **Med School:** Univ Minn 1970; **Resid:** Internal Medicine, Univ Colo Med Ctr, Denver, CO 1971-1972; Internal Medicine, Stanford Univ Med Ctr, Stanford, CA 1974-1975; **Fellow:** Infectious Disease, Stanford Univ Med Ctr, Stanford, CA 1975-1977; **Fac Appt:** Prof Medicine, Univ Pittsburgh

Southeast

Alvarez-Elcoro, Salvador MD (Inf) - *Spec Exp:* *Tuberculosis; Travel Medicine; Transplantation Medicine;* **Hospital:** St Luke's Hosp; **Address:** Mayo Clinic, Dept Infectious Disease, 4500 San Pablo Rd, Jacksonville, FL 32224; **Phone:** (904) 953-2419; **Board Cert:** Internal Medicine 1977, Infectious Disease 1982; **Med School:** Mexico 1972; **Resid:** Internal Medicine, Charity Hosp, New Orleans, LA 1974-1977; **Fellow:** Infectious Disease, Boston City Hosp, Boston, MA 1977-1979; **Fac Appt:** Prof Medicine, Univ Fla Coll Med

Archer, Gordon Lee MD (Inf) - *Spec Exp:* *Staphylococcal Infections;* **Hospital:** Med Coll of VA Hosp; **Address:** Med Coll VA, Box 980049, Richmond, VA 23298-0049; **Phone:** (804) 828-9711; **Board Cert:** Internal Medicine 1972, Infectious Disease 1976; **Med School:** Univ VA Sch Med 1969; **Resid:** Internal Medicine, Univ Mich Hosps, Ann Arbor, MI 1970-1972; **Fellow:** Infectious Disease, Univ Mich Hosps, Ann Arbor, MI 1972-1974; **Fac Appt:** Prof Medicine, Med Coll VA

Bartlett, John A MD (Inf) - *Spec Exp:* *AIDS/HIV;* **Hospital:** Duke Univ Med Ctr (page 60); **Address:** Duke Univ Med Ctr, Box 3238, Durham, NC 27710; **Phone:** (919) 684-6416; **Board Cert:** Internal Medicine 1984, Infectious Disease 1988; **Med School:** Univ VA Sch Med 1981; **Resid:** Internal Medicine, Duke Univ Med Ctr, Durham, NC 1982-1985; **Fellow:** Infectious Disease, Duke Univ Med Ctr, Durham, NC 1985; **Fac Appt:** Assoc Prof Medicine, Duke Univ

Cancio, Margarita MD (Inf) - *Spec Exp:* AIDS/HIV; **Hospital:** Tampa Genl Hosp; **Address:** 4 Columbia Dr, Ste 820, Tampa, FL 33606; **Phone:** (813) 251-8444; **Board Cert:** Infectious Disease 1988, Internal Medicine 1985; **Med School:** Univ S Fla Coll Med 1982; **Resid:** Internal Medicine, Univ S Fla Coll Med, Tampa, FL 1982-1983; Internal Medicine, Univ S Fla Coll Med, Tampa, FL 1983-1985; **Fellow:** Infectious Disease, Univ S Fla Coll Med, Tampa, FL 1986-1987; Infectious Disease, Univ S Fla Coll Med, Tampa, FL 1987-1988; **Fac Appt:** Assoc Prof Medicine, Univ S Fla Coll Med

Chan, Joseph MD (Inf) - *Spec Exp:* AIDS/HIV; **Hospital:** Mount Sinai Med Ctr; **Address:** Mt Sinai Medical Ctr, 4300 Alton Rd, Ste G-23, Miami, FL 33140-2849; **Phone:** (305) 674-2766; **Board Cert:** Internal Medicine 1980, Infectious Disease 1982; **Med School:** UCSF 1977; **Resid:** Internal Medicine, Univ Miami Affil Hosps, Miami, FL 1978-1980; **Fellow:** Infectious Disease, Univ Miami Affil Hosps, Miami, FL 1980-1982; **Fac Appt:** Assoc Prof Medicine, Univ Miami Sch Med

Cohen, Myron S MD (Inf) - *Spec Exp:* Infections in Immune Deficient; **Hospital:** Univ of NC Hosp (page 77); **Address:** Univ N Carolina Hosps, Div Infectious Disease, 547 Burnett-Womack Bldg, Box 7030, Chapel Hill, NC 27599-7030; **Phone:** (919) 966-2536; **Board Cert:** Internal Medicine 1977, Infectious Disease 1982; **Med School:** Rush Med Coll 1974; **Resid:** Internal Medicine, Univ Mich Hlth Ctr, Ann Arbor, MI 1975-1977; **Fellow:** Infectious Disease, Yale-New Haven Hosp, New Haven, CT 1977-1979; **Fac Appt:** Prof Infectious Disease, Univ NC Sch Med

Corey, G Ralph MD (Inf) - *Spec Exp:* Tropical Diseases; Travel Medicine; **Hospital:** Duke Univ Med Ctr (page 60); **Address:** Dept Inf Diseases, Box 3038, Durham, NC 27710; **Phone:** (919) 681-2458; **Board Cert:** Internal Medicine 1977, Infectious Disease 1980; **Med School:** Baylor Coll Med 1973; **Resid:** Internal Medicine, Duke Univ Med Ctr, Durham, NC 1975-1978; **Fellow:** Infectious Disease, Duke Univ Med Ctr, Durham, NC 1978-1980; **Fac Appt:** Assoc Prof Medicine, Duke Univ

Dismukes, William Ernest MD (Inf) - *Spec Exp:* Fungal Infections; **Hospital:** Univ of Ala Hosp at Birmingham; **Address:** 1900 Univ Blvd, rm 229THT, Brimingham, AL 35294-0006; **Phone:** (205) 934-5191; **Board Cert:** Internal Medicine 1977, Infectious Disease 1972; **Med School:** Univ Ala 1964; **Resid:** Internal Medicine, Peter Bent Brigham Hosp, Boston, MA 1965-1966; Internal Medicine, Peter Bent Brigham Hosp, Boston, MA 1968-1969; **Fellow:** Infectious Disease, Mass Genl Hosp, Boston, MA 1969-1971; **Fac Appt:** Prof Medicine, Univ Ala

Droller, David G MD (Inf) - *Spec Exp:* AIDS/HIV; Infections-Orthopedic; Infections-Post Operative; **Hospital:** Broward General Med Ctr; **Address:** 5333 N Dixie Hwy, Ste 208, Fort Lauderdale, FL 33334-3454; **Phone:** (954) 771-7988; **Board Cert:** Internal Medicine 1977, Infectious Disease 1980; **Med School:** NYU Sch Med 1974; **Resid:** Internal Medicine, Univ of Miami Affil Hosps, Miami, FL 1974-1977; **Fellow:** Infectious Disease, Univ of Miami Affil Hosps, Miami, FL 1977-1979; **Fac Appt:** Assoc Prof Medicine, Univ Miami Sch Med

Guerrant, Richard MD (Inf) - *Spec Exp:* Tropical Diseases; Infectious Diarrhea; Travel Medicine; **Hospital:** Univ of VA Hlth Sys (page 79); **Address:** Div Geographic & Int'l Medicine, PO Box 801379, Charlottesville, VA 22908-1379; **Phone:** (804) 924-5242; **Board Cert:** Infectious Disease 1976, Internal Medicine 1973; **Med School:** Univ VA Sch Med 1968; **Resid:** Internal Medicine, Boston City Hosp, Boston, MA 1969-1970; Internal Medicine, Univ Virginia Hosp, Charlottesville, VA 1972-1973; **Fellow:** Infectious Disease, Univ Virginia Hosp, Charlottesville, VA 1973-1974; **Fac Appt:** Prof Medicine, Univ VA Sch Med

Houston, Sally MD (Inf) - *Spec Exp:* Infections-Transplant; **Hospital:** Tampa Genl Hosp; **Address:** Tampa Genl Hosp, Inf Dis Ctr, PO Box 1289, Tampa, FL 33601-1289; **Phone:** (813) 251-7670; **Board Cert:** Internal Medicine 1990, Infectious Disease 1992; **Med School:** Vanderbilt Univ 1987; **Resid:** Internal Medicine, Univ South Fla, Tampa, FL 1990; **Fellow:** Infectious Disease, Univ South Fla, Tampa, FL 1992; **Fac Appt:** Assoc Prof Medicine, Univ S Fla Coll Med

Katner, Harold MD (Inf) - *Spec Exp:* AIDS/HIV; **Hospital:** Med Ctr of Central GA; **Address:** Dept Internal Medicine, 707 Pine St, Macon, GA 31207; **Phone:** (478) 301-5851; **Board Cert:** Infectious Disease 1986, Internal Medicine 1983; **Med School:** Louisiana State Univ 1980; **Resid:** Internal Medicine, Univ Med Ctr, Lafayette, LA 1981-1983; **Fellow:** Infectious Disease, Ochsner Fdn Hosp, New Orleans, LA 1983-1986; **Fac Appt:** Prof Medicine, Mercer Univ Sch Med

Maguire, James MD (Inf) - *Spec Exp:* Tropical Diseases; Parasitic Infections; **Hospital:** Emory Univ Hosp; **Address:** CDC, Div of Parasitic Disease, 4770 Buford Hwy NE, MS F22, Atlanta, GA 30341; **Phone:** (770) 488-7766; **Board Cert:** Infectious Disease 1978, Internal Medicine 1977; **Med School:** Harvard Med Sch 1974; **Resid:** Internal Medicine, Peter Bent Brigham Hosp, Boston, MA 1975-1977; **Fellow:** Infectious Disease, Peter Bent Brigham Hosp, Boston, MA 1976-1978; **Fac Appt:** Assoc Prof Medicine, Harvard Med Sch

Mandell, Gerald MD (Inf) - *Spec Exp:* White Cell Defects (Agranulocytosis); **Hospital:** Univ of VA Hlth Sys (page 79); **Address:** UVA Health System, Div Infectious Disease, Box 801341, Charlottesville, VA 22908; **Phone:** (804) 924-5942; **Board Cert:** Infectious Disease 1972, Internal Medicine 1968; **Med School:** Cornell Univ-Weill Med Coll 1962; **Resid:** Internal Medicine, NY Hosp-Cornell Ct, New York, NY 1965-1967; **Fellow:** Infectious Disease, Cornell Med Ctr, New York, NY 1967-1969; **Fac Appt:** Prof Medicine, Univ VA Sch Med

McGowan Jr, John E MD (Inf) - *Spec Exp:* Infections-Hospital Acquired; Tuberculosis; **Hospital:** Emory Univ Hosp; **Address:** 1634 Clinton Rd NE, Atlanta, GA 30302; **Phone:** (404) 727-9365; **Board Cert:** Infectious Disease 1978, Internal Medicine 1971; **Med School:** Harvard Med Sch 1967; **Resid:** Internal Medicine, Boston City Hosp, Boston, MA 1968-1969; **Fellow:** Infectious Disease, Boston City Hosp, Boston, MA 1971-1973; **Fac Appt:** Prof Medicine, Emory Univ

Pearson, Richard Dale MD (Inf) - *Spec Exp:* Tropical Diseases; Travel Medicine; Infectious Diseases; **Hospital:** Univ of VA Hlth Sys (page 79); **Address:** Dept of Internal Medicine, McKin Hall, Box 800739, Charlottesville, VA 22908-0739; **Phone:** (804) 924-5579; **Board Cert:** Internal Medicine 1976, Infectious Disease 1980; **Med School:** Univ Mich Med Sch 1973; **Resid:** Internal Medicine, Rochester/Strong Meml Hosp, Rochester, NY 1974-1976; **Fellow:** Infectious Disease, Rochester/Strong Meml Hosp, Rochester, NY 1978-1979; **Fac Appt:** Prof Medicine, Univ VA Sch Med

Pegram Jr., Paul Samuel MD (Inf) - *Spec Exp:* AIDS/HIV; **Hospital:** Wake Forest Univ Baptist Med Ctr (page 81); **Address:** Wake Forest Baptist Med Ctr, Med Ctr Blvd, Winston Salem, NC 27157-1042; **Phone:** (336) 716-2700; **Board Cert:** Infectious Disease 1978, Internal Medicine 1976; **Med School:** Wake Forest Univ Sch Med 1970; **Resid:** Internal Medicine, NC Baptist Hosp, Winston Salem, NC 1973-1975; **Fellow:** Infectious Disease, NC Baptist Hosp, Winston Salem, NC 1976-1978; **Fac Appt:** Prof Medicine, Wake Forest Univ Sch Med

Ratzan, Kenneth MD (Inf) - *Spec Exp:* AIDS/HIV; **Hospital:** Mount Sinai Med Ctr; **Address:** 4300 Alton Rd, rm G23, Miami Beach, FL 33140-2800; **Phone:** (305) 673-5490; **Board Cert:** Internal Medicine 1971, Infectious Disease 1974; **Med School:** Harvard Med Sch 1965; **Resid:** Internal Medicine, Columbia Presby Med Ctr, New York, NY 1966-1967; Infectious Disease, Tufts New Engl Med Ctr, Boston, MA 1971-1972; **Fellow:** Infectious Disease, Tufts New England Med Ctr, Boston, MA 1969-1971; **Fac Appt:** Prof Medicine, Univ Miami Sch Med

Saag, Michael S MD (Inf) - *Spec Exp:* AIDS/HIV; **Hospital:** Univ of Ala Hosp at Birmingham; **Address:** 908 20th St S, Bldg Community Care, Birmingham, AL 35205; **Phone:** (205) 934-1917; **Board Cert:** Internal Medicine 1985, Infectious Disease 1988; **Med School:** Univ Louisville Sch Med 1981; **Resid:** Internal Medicine, Univ Ala Hosp, Birmingham, AL 1981-1984; **Fellow:** Infectious Disease, Univ Ala Hosp, Birmingham, AL 1985-1987

INFECTIOUS DISEASE

Scheld, William Michael MD (Inf) - *Spec Exp:* Meningitis; **Hospital:** Univ of VA Hlth Sys (page 79); **Address:** Univ VA Hlth Sci Ctr, PO Box 801342, Charlottesville, VA 22908; **Phone:** (804) 924-5241; **Board Cert:** Internal Medicine 1976, Infectious Disease 1978; **Med School:** Cornell Univ-Weill Med Coll 1973; **Resid:** Internal Medicine, Univ VA Med Ctr, Charlottesville, VA 1974-1976; **Fellow:** Infectious Disease, Univ VA Med Ctr, Charlottesville, VA 1976-1979; **Fac Appt:** Prof Medicine, Univ VA Sch Med

Sexton, Daniel John MD (Inf) - *Spec Exp:* Rocky Mountain Spotted Fever; Infective Endocarditis; **Hospital:** Duke Univ Med Ctr (page 60); **Address:** PO Box 3065, Durham, NC 27702-3065; **Phone:** (919) 684-4596; **Board Cert:** Internal Medicine 1977, Infectious Disease 1978; **Med School:** Northwestern Univ 1971; **Resid:** Internal Medicine, Univ Missouri Med Ctr, Columbia, MO 1975-1977; **Fellow:** Infectious Disease, Duke Univ Med Ctr, Durham, NC 1974-1975; **Fac Appt:** Prof Medicine, Duke Univ

Sparling, Philip Frederick MD (Inf) - *Spec Exp:* Sexually Transmitted Diseases; **Hospital:** Univ of NC Hosp (page 77); **Address:** 547 Burnett-Womack Bldg, Box CB7030, Chapel Hill, NC 27599; **Phone:** (919) 966-2536; **Board Cert:** Internal Medicine 1970, Infectious Disease 1976; **Med School:** Harvard Med Sch 1962; **Resid:** Internal Medicine, Mass Genl Hosp, Boston, MA 1963-1964; **Fellow:** Infectious Disease, Mass Genl Hosp, Boston, MA 1968-1969; **Fac Appt:** Prof Medicine, Univ NC Sch Med

Van Der Horst, Charles MD (Inf) - *Spec Exp:* AIDS/HIV; Fungal Infections; Viral Infections; **Hospital:** Univ of NC Hosp (page 77); **Address:** Univ NC-Dept Med, Box CB7030, Chapel Hill, NC 27599-7030; **Phone:** (919) 966-2536; **Board Cert:** Internal Medicine 1982, Infectious Disease 1986; **Med School:** Harvard Med Sch 1979; **Resid:** Internal Medicine, Monteifore Hosp, Bronx, NY 1980-1982; **Fellow:** Infectious Disease, NC Meml Hosp, Chapel Hill, NC 1982-1985; **Fac Appt:** Prof Infectious Disease, Univ NC Sch Med

Midwest

Bakken, Johan Septimus MD (Inf) - *Spec Exp:* Ehrlichiosis; Tick-borne Diseases; **Hospital:** St Mary's Med Ctr - Duluth; **Address:** St Mary's-Duluth Clin Hlth Sys/ Sec Inf Dis, 400 E Third St, Duluth, MN 55805; **Phone:** (218) 786-3737; **Board Cert:** Internal Medicine 1999; **Med School:** Univ Wash 1972; **Resid:** Internal Medicine, Univ Wash Hosp, Seattle, WA 1975-1977; Internal Medicine, Lillehammer Fylkessykehus, Lillehammer,Norway 1978-1981; **Fellow:** Infectious Disease, Ulleval Hosp, Oslo,Norway 1981-1986; Microbiology, Creighton Univ, Omaha, NE 1986-1988; **Fac Appt:** Assoc Prof Family Practice, Univ Minn

Campbell, J William MD (Inf) - *Spec Exp:* AIDS/HIV; **Hospital:** Barnes-Jewish Hosp (page 55); **Address:** 114 N Taylor Ave, St Louis, MO 63108; **Phone:** (314) 534-8600; **Board Cert:** Infectious Disease 1982, Internal Medicine 1980; **Med School:** Washington Univ, St Louis 1977; **Resid:** Internal Medicine, Barnes Hosp-Wash U, St Louis, MO 1978-1980; **Fellow:** Infectious Disease, U Texas Hlth Sci Ctr, San Antonio, TX 1980-1981; Infectious Disease, Wash Univ St Louis, St Louis, MO 1981-1982; **Fac Appt:** Assoc Clin Prof Medicine, Washington Univ, St Louis

Kazanjian Jr, Powel H MD (Inf) - *Spec Exp:* AIDS/HIV; **Hospital:** Univ of MI Hlth Ctr; **Address:** Infectious Disease Clinic, TC Level 3, reception D, 1500 E Medical Center Drive, Ann Arbor, MI 48109-0378; **Phone:** (734) 647-5899; **Board Cert:** Internal Medicine 1982, Infectious Disease 1986; **Med School:** Tufts Univ 1979; **Resid:** Internal Medicine, Univ Chicago Hosp, Chicago, IL 1980-1982; **Fellow:** Infectious Disease, Brigham-Womens Hosp, Boston, MA 1982-1984; **Fac Appt:** Assoc Prof Medicine, Univ Mich Med Sch

Maki, Dennis G MD (Inf) - *Spec Exp:* Urinary Tract Infections; **Hospital:** Univ WI Hosp & Clins; **Address:** 600 Highland Ave, rm B6/242, Madison, WI 53792; **Phone:** (608) 263-0946; **Board Cert:** Critical Care Medicine 1987, Infectious Disease 1974; **Med School:** Univ Wisc 1967; **Resid:** Infectious Disease, Mass Genl Hosp, Boston, MA 1971-1972; Internal Medicine, Harvard-Boston City Hosp, Boston, MA 1972-1973; **Fellow:** Infectious Disease, Mass Genl Hosp, Boston, MA 1973-1974; **Fac Appt:** Prof Medicine, Univ Wisc

Paya, Carlos Vicente MD (Inf) - *Spec Exp:* AIDS/HIV; Cytomegalovirus PTLD; **Hospital:** Mayo Med Ctr & Clin - Rochester, MN; **Address:** Mayo Clinic, 200 1st St SW, Rochester, MN 55905-0002; **Phone:** (507) 284-3747; **Board Cert:** Internal Medicine 1986, Infectious Disease 1988; **Med School:** Spain 1981; **Resid:** Internal Medicine, Hennepin Co Med Ctr, Minneapolis, MN 1983-1984; Internal Medicine, Mayo Grad Sch, Rochester, MN 1984-1986; **Fellow:** Infectious Disease, Mayo Grad Sch, Rochester, MN 1986; **Fac Appt:** Prof Medicine, Mayo Med Sch

Powderly, William MD (Inf) - *Spec Exp:* AIDS/HIV; Fungal Infections; **Hospital:** Barnes-Jewish Hosp (page 55); **Address:** 660 S Euclid Ave, Ste 8051, St Louis, MO 63110; **Phone:** (314) 362-7601; **Med School:** Ireland 1979; **Fellow:** Infectious Disease, Barnes Jewish Hosp, St Louis, MO 1983-1987; **Fac Appt:** Prof Medicine, Washington Univ, St Louis

Slama, Thomas MD (Inf) - *Spec Exp:* Fungal Infections; Bone Infections; Infective Endocarditis; **Hospital:** St Vincent's Hosp and Hlth Ctr - Indianapolis; **Address:** 8240 Naab Rd, Ste 250, Indianapolis, IN 46260; **Phone:** (317) 870-1970; **Board Cert:** Internal Medicine 1976, Infectious Disease 1978; **Med School:** India 1973; **Resid:** Internal Medicine, Indianapolis Meth Hosp, Indianapolis, IN 1974-1976; **Fellow:** Infectious Disease, Univ Ohio Hosps, OH 1976-1978; **Fac Appt:** Clin Prof Medicine, Indiana Univ

Sobel, Jack MD (Inf) - *Spec Exp:* Sexually Transmitted Diseases; Vaginitis; **Hospital:** Harper Hosp (page 59); **Address:** Harper Hosp, 4 Brush Ctr, 3990 John R St, rm 4811, Detroit, MI 48201; **Phone:** (313) 745-7105; **Board Cert:** Internal Medicine 1978, Infectious Disease 1982; **Med School:** South Africa 1965; **Resid:** Internal Medicine, S Africa 1966-1970; **Fellow:** Infectious Disease, Univ Penn Hosps, Philadelphia, PA 1976-1977; Research, Natl Inst Hlth, Bethesda, MD 1977-1978; **Fac Appt:** Prof Medicine, Wayne State Univ

Wilson, Walter Ray MD (Inf) - *Spec Exp:* Musculoskeletal Infections; **Hospital:** Mayo Med Ctr & Clin - Rochester, MN; **Address:** Infectious Diseases Div, 200 1st St SW, Rochester, MN 55905; **Phone:** (507) 255-7761; **Board Cert:** Internal Medicine 1973, Infectious Disease 1974; **Med School:** Baylor Coll Med 1967; **Resid:** Internal Medicine, Methodist Hosp, Houston, TX 1967-1968; Internal Medicine, Mayo Clinic, Rochester, MN 1972-1973; **Fellow:** Infectious Disease, Mayo Clinic, Rochester, MN 1973-1974; Microbiology, Mayo Clinic, Rochester, MN 1974-1975; **Fac Appt:** Prof Medicine, Mayo Med Sch

Great Plains and Mountains

Cohn, David MD (Inf) - *Spec Exp:* Tuberculosis; AIDS/HIV; **Hospital:** Denver Health Med Ctr; **Address:** Denver Public Health, 605 Bannock Street, Denver, CO 80204-4507; **Phone:** (303) 436-7204; **Board Cert:** Internal Medicine 1978, Infectious Disease 1982; **Med School:** Univ IL Coll Med 1975; **Resid:** Internal Medicine, Univ Wisc Hosp, Madison, WI 1976-1978; **Fellow:** Infectious Disease, Univ Colo Hosp, Denver, CO 1979-1981; **Fac Appt:** Prof Medicine, Univ Colo

Southwest

DuPont, Herbert Lancashire MD (Inf) - *Spec Exp:* Tropical Diseases; Diarrhea; **Hospital:** St Luke's Episcopal Hosp - Houston; **Address:** 6720 Bertner Ave, MC 1-164, Houston, TX 77030-1602; **Phone:** (832) 355-4122; **Board Cert:** Internal Medicine 1972; **Med School:** Emory Univ 1965; **Resid:** Internal Medicine, Univ Minn Hosps, Minneapolis, MN 1966-1967; **Fellow:** Infectious Disease, Univ MD Hosp, Baltimore, MD 1968-1969; **Fac Appt:** Prof Medicine, Baylor Coll Med

Keiser, Philip MD (Inf) - *Spec Exp:* AIDS/HIV; **Hospital:** Zale Lipshy Univ Hosp; **Address:** Univ TX SW Med Ctr, 5323 Harry Hines Blvd, MC-9173, Dallas, TX 75390; **Phone:** (214) 648-8942; **Board Cert:** Internal Medicine 1989, Infectious Disease 1992; **Med School:** Univ MD Sch Med 1986; **Resid:** Internal Medicine, Francis Scott Key Med Ctr, Baltimore, MD 1986-1989; **Fellow:** Infectious Disease, Univ Maryland, Baltimore, MD 1989; **Fac Appt:** Assoc Prof Medicine, Univ Tex SW, Dallas

Kimbrough, Robert MD (Inf) - *Spec Exp:* Infectious Disease - General; **Hospital:** Univ Med Ctr - Lubbock; **Address:** Tex Tech U Hlth Scis Ctr, Dept IM Div Inf Dis- 3601 4th Street, Lubbock, TX 79430; **Phone:** (806) 743-3155; **Board Cert:** Internal Medicine 1977, Infectious Disease 1978; **Med School:** Univ Kans 1969; **Resid:** Internal Medicine, Baylor Affil Hosp, Houston, TX 1970-1973; **Fellow:** Infectious Disease, Baylor Univ, Houston, TX 1973-1974; Infectious Disease, Oreg Hlth Sci Univ, Portland, OR 1974-1975; **Fac Appt:** Prof Medicine, Texas Tech Univ

Luby, James P MD (Inf) - *Spec Exp:* Viral Infections; **Hospital:** Parkland Mem Hosp; **Address:** Univ Tex SW Med Ctr, 5323 Henry Hines Blvd, Dallas, TX 75239-9113; **Phone:** (214) 648-3480; **Board Cert:** Infectious Disease 1972, Internal Medicine 1968; **Med School:** Northwestern Univ 1961; **Resid:** Internal Medicine, Northwestern Univ, Chicago, IL 1962-1964; **Fac Appt:** Prof Infectious Disease, Univ Tex SW, Dallas

Patterson, Jan E Evans MD (Inf) - *Spec Exp:* Hospital Infection Control; **Hospital:** Univ of Texas Hlth & Sci Ctr; **Address:** Dept Medicine, Div Infectious Disease, 7703 Floyd Curl Drive, San Antonio, TX 78229-3900; **Phone:** (210) 567-4823; **Board Cert:** Internal Medicine 1985, Infectious Disease 1988; **Med School:** Univ Tex, Houston 1982; **Resid:** Internal Medicine, Vanderbilt Univ Hosp, Nashville, TN 1983-1985; **Fellow:** Infectious Disease, Yale-New Haven Hosp, New Haven, CT 1985-1988; **Fac Appt:** Assoc Prof Medicine, Univ Tex, San Antonio

Patterson, Thomas F. MD (Inf) - *Spec Exp:* AIDS/HIV; **Hospital:** Univ of Texas Hlth & Sci Ctr; **Address:** Dept Medicine, Div Infectious Dis, 7703 Floyd Curl Drive, San Antonio, TX 78229-3900; **Phone:** (210) 567-4823; **Board Cert:** Internal Medicine 1986, Infectious Disease 1988; **Med School:** Univ Tex, Houston 1983; **Resid:** Internal Medicine, Vanderbilt Univ Hosp, Nashville, TN 1984-1985; Internal Medicine, Yale-New Haven Hosp, New Haven, CT 1985-1986; **Fellow:** Infectious Disease, Yale-New Haven Hosp., New Haven, CT 1986-1989; **Fac Appt:** Assoc Prof Medicine, Univ Tex, San Antonio

Wallace Jr, Richard James MD (Inf) - *Spec Exp:* AIDS/HIV; Tuberculosis; **Hospital:** Univ of Texas Hlth & Sci Ctr; **Address:** Univ Tex Health Science Ctr, 119 37 US Hwy 271, Tyler, TX 75708; **Phone:** (903) 877-7680; **Board Cert:** Internal Medicine 1975, Infectious Disease 1976; **Med School:** Baylor Coll Med 1972; **Resid:** Internal Medicine, Boston City Hosp, Boston, MA 1973-1974; **Fellow:** Infectious Disease, Boston City Hosp, Boston, MA 1974-1975; Infectious Disease, Baylor Coll Med, Houston, TX 1975-1977

West Coast and Pacific

Ballon-Landa, Gonzalo MD (Inf) - *Spec Exp:* Nosocomial Infections; AIDS/HIV; **Hospital:** Mercy Hosp & Med Ctr - San Diego; **Address:** 4136 Bachman Pl, San Diego, CA 92103-2028; **Phone:** (619) 298-1443; **Board Cert:** Internal Medicine 1980, Infectious Disease 1984; **Med School:** Northwestern Univ 1977; **Resid:** Internal Medicine, Evanston Hosp, Evanston, IL 1978-1981; **Fellow:** Infectious Disease, UCSD Med Ctr, San Diego, CA 1981-1983

Bayer, Arnold Sander MD (Inf) - *Spec Exp:* Infective Endocarditis; Arthritis-Septic; Coccidioidomycosis; **Hospital:** LAC - Harbor - UCLA Med Ctr; **Address:** 1000 W Carson St, Bldg RB2 - Fl 2, Torrance, CA 90502; **Phone:** (310) 222-3813; **Board Cert:** Internal Medicine 1973, Infectious Disease 1978; **Med School:** Temple Univ 1970; **Resid:** Internal Medicine, Thomas Jefferson Univ Hosp, Philadelphia, PA 1971-1972; Internal Medicine, LAC-Harbor UCLA Med Ctr, Torrance, CA 1973-1974; **Fellow:** Infectious Disease, Veterans Affairs Med Ctr, Los Angeles, CA 1975-1976; Infectious Disease, LAC-Harbor UCLA Med Ctr, Torrance, CA 1974-1977; **Fac Appt:** Prof Medicine, UCLA

Edwards Jr., John Ellis MD (Inf) - *Spec Exp:* Fungal Infections; Infections in Immune Deficient; **Hospital:** LAC - Harbor - UCLA Med Ctr; **Address:** 1124 W Carson St, Ste RB-2, Torrance, CA 90509; **Phone:** (310) 222-3813; **Board Cert:** Internal Medicine 1980, Infectious Disease 1974; **Med School:** UC Irvine 1968; **Resid:** Internal Medicine, Harbor-UCLA Med Ctr, Los Angeles, CA 1969-1971; **Fellow:** Infectious Disease, Harbor-UCLA Med Ctr, Los Angeles, CA 1971-1973; **Fac Appt:** Prof Medicine, UCLA

Hollander, Harry MD (Inf) - *Spec Exp:* AIDS/HIV; **Hospital:** UCSF Med Ctr; **Address:** 400 Parnassus Ave, Box 378, San Francisco, CA 94143; **Phone:** (415) 353-2119; **Board Cert:** Internal Medicine 1983, Infectious Disease 1988; **Med School:** Univ Penn 1980; **Resid:** Internal Medicine, UCSF Med Ctr, San Francisco, CA 1981-1983; **Fac Appt:** Clin Prof Medicine, UCSF

Holmes, King K MD (Inf) - *Spec Exp:* AIDS/HIV; Sexually Transmitted Diseases; **Hospital:** Univ WA Med Ctr; **Address:** Box 359931, 325 Ninth Ave, Seattle, WA 98104; **Phone:** (206) 731-3000; **Board Cert:** Infectious Disease 1974, Internal Medicine 1971; **Med School:** Cornell Univ-Weill Med Coll 1963; **Resid:** Internal Medicine, Univ Wash Med Ctr, Seattle, WA 1967-1969; **Fellow:** Infectious Disease, Univ Wash Med Ctr, Seattle, WA 1969-1970; **Fac Appt:** Prof Medicine, Univ Wash

Richman, Douglas MD (Inf) - *Spec Exp:* AIDS/HIV; **Hospital:** UCSD Healthcare; **Address:** UCSD, Dept Path & Med, 9500 Gilman Dr, La Jolla, CA 92093-0679; **Phone:** (858) 552-7439; **Board Cert:** Internal Medicine 1973, Infectious Disease 1976; **Med School:** Stanford Univ 1970; **Resid:** Infectious Disease, Stanford Univ Hosp, Stanford, CA 1971-1972; **Fellow:** Infectious Disease, NIAID/NIH, Bethdesda, MD 1972-1975; Infectious Disease, Beth Israel Deaconess Med Ctr, Boston, MA 1975-1976; **Fac Appt:** Prof Medicine, UCSD

Wiviott, Lory David MD (Inf) - *Spec Exp:* AIDS/HIV; **Hospital:** CA Pacific Med Ctr - Pacific Campus; **Address:** 2100 Webster St, Ste 404, San Francisco, CA 94115; **Phone:** (415) 923-3883; **Board Cert:** Infectious Disease 1990, Internal Medicine 1986; **Med School:** Albert Einstein Coll Med 1982; **Resid:** Internal Medicine, Columbia Presby Med Ctr, New York, NY 1982-1985; **Fellow:** Infectious Disease, UCSF Med Ctr, San Francisco, CA 1986-1989; **Fac Appt:** Asst Clin Prof Medicine, UCSF

Yoshikawa, Thomas T MD (Inf) - *Spec Exp:* Infections in the Elderly; **Hospital:** LAC - King/Drew Med Ctr; **Address:** Dept Internal Medicine, 12021 S Wilmington Ave, rm 4015, Los Angeles, CA 90059; **Phone:** (310) 668-4574; **Board Cert:** Infectious Disease 1974, Internal Medicine 1971; **Med School:** Univ Mich Med Sch 1966; **Resid:** Internal Medicine, Harbor Genl Hosp, Torrance, CA 1967-1970; **Fellow:** Infectious Disease, Harbor Genl Hosp, Torrance, CA 1972; **Fac Appt:** Prof Medicine, Charles Drew Univ Med & Sci

INTERNAL MEDICINE

A personal physician who provides long-term, comprehensive care in the office and the hospital, managing both common and complex illness of adolescents, adults and the elderly. Internists are trained in the diagnosis and treatment of cancer, infections and diseases affecting the heart, blood, kidneys, joints and digestive, respiratory and vascular systems. They are also trained in the essentials of primary care internal medicine which incorporates an understanding of disease prevention, wellness, substance abuse, mental health and effective treatment of common problems of the eyes, ears, skin, nervous system and reproductive organs.

Training required: Three years

DUKE WELLNESS PROGRAMS

Durham, North Carolina • 1-888-ASK-DUKE • www.dukecenter.org

 # DUKE UNIVERSITY HEALTH SYSTEM

Part of the world-class Duke University Health System, the Duke Center for Living helps people achieve optimal health through a comprehensive, interdisciplinary approach to disease prevention and lifestyle management. The Center offers a variety of wellness programs, most located on its beautiful, private campus near Duke University.

DUKE EXECUTIVE HEALTH PROGRAM

The DEHP offers health management programs for busy professionals. Programs include a comprehensive one- to two-day physical where clients spend at least a full hour and a half with an internist, along with exercise, nutrition and stress management evaluations; a Women's Program offering one-, two-, and three-day programs designed to address women's special health needs; Executive Escapes, a three-day individualized lifestyle management program that includes a full-day physical exam and customized counseling, fitness, nutrition and stress management sessions; and the Executive Lifestyle Retreat, a three-day customized lifestyle management program for corporate management teams. The retreat includes a full-day comprehensive physical, along with wellness workshops suited to the needs of the corporate client.

DUKE DIET & FITNESS CENTER

Founded in 1969, the DFC, located near downtown Durham, is one of the country's most successful weight management centers. Staffed by physicians, physician assistants, exercise physiologists, physical therapists, registered dietitians, health psychologists, clinical social workers and massage therapists, the residential program follows a sensible approach incorporating weight loss, physical activity, and stress management. A study of participants showed that after two years, 55% maintained their weight loss; at three years, 47% maintained, and for four or more years, 42% maintained their weight loss—making this program one of the most effective in the field.

DUKE HEALTH & FITNESS CENTER

The DHFC is a total wellness program focusing on exercise, nutrition, stress management, and lifestyle change programs. New participants begin with a comprehensive health and fitness assessment, with medical monitoring available as needed. Specialized offerings include the Arthritis Program, Cancer Exercise Program, Cardiac and Pulmonary Rehabilitation, locally based Weight Management Programs, and a three-day customized lifestyle program, Healthy Escapes.

DUKE CENTER FOR INTEGRATIVE MEDICINE

Opened in 2000 on the Center for Living campus, the Duke Center for Integrative Medicine seeks to improve medical care by combining the best of conventional Western medicine with mind-body-spirit approaches to health.

Directed by nationally recognized leaders in integrative medicine, the Center collaborates with patients' primary care and specialist physicians to create individually tailored wellness plans. Services that may be recommended include the full scope of conventional treatment modalities, lifestyle interventions such as nutrition and exercise, and complementary therapies such as acupuncture, Chinese medicine, biofeedback sessions, massage, yoga, mindfulness-based stress reduction workshops, and other techniques that have proven efficacy.

The Center also offers week-long Healing Life Retreats and conferences that give participants new tools to maximize personal wellness.

www.dcim.org
1-866-313-0959 (toll-free)

THE MOUNT SINAI HOSPITAL
OCCUPATIONAL AND ENVIRONMENTAL MEDICINE

One Gustave L. Levy Place (Fifth Avenue and 98th Street)
New York, NY 10029-6574   Phone: (212) 987-6043
Physician Referral: 1-800-MD-SINAI (637-4624)
www.mountsinai.org

A Reputation for Excellence

The Irving J. Selikoff Clinical Center for Occupational and Environmental Medicine is an internationally respected diagnostic and treatment center.

The mission of Center is to prevent occupational disease in the workplace and reduce morbidity and mortality associated to work. To achieve this goal, we utilize a preventive medicine model that includes three integrated components:

Clinical Care – These services include the diagnosis, treatment, and management of occupational diseases and work-related musculoskeletal disorders for current and retired workers. We offer disability assessment and rehabilitation services to facilitate safe return to work and appropriate accommodations. Our social work services include counseling regarding the financial, social, and psychological aspects of occupational disease.

Disease Prevention Services – These services include the education of patients, health care providers, workers, unions, employers, and communities in the signs and symptoms of occupational disease. Comprehensive industrial hygiene and ergonomic services are available to evaluate exposures and recommend effective preventive measures. Technical assistance and consultation services are provided for employers, unions, and public health agencies.

Surveillance & Data Management – We study the pattern and prevalence of occupational disease and identify new associations between workplace exposure and disease.

***

To promote disease prevention, the Center treats each newly identified case of occupational disease as a potential sentinel health event, that is, as a signal that there may be other similar cases of disease in the patient's co-workers. This approach, coupled with our efforts to reduce workplace hazards, projects the Center's impact well beyond individual patient evaluations.

The Clinical Center has satellite sites in Westchester County and Queens, where staff physicians see patients several days a week.

To help achieve our goal of improving public health by preventing occupational and environmental disease, and by early detection of work-related illness when it has occurred, we work closely with labor unions, employers, government, and service organizations, health care providers, and community organizations.

THE MOUNT SINAI HOSPITAL

Some of the services available at the Irving J. Selikoff Center for Occupational and Environmental Medicine:

- Medical evaluation of groups or individuals with hazardous exposures.

- Assistance evaluating specific workplace environments and suggesting ways of eliminating dangerous conditions.

- Educational programs for unions and workers on workplace health issues.

- Help in getting worker compensation and other available legal benefits.

- Social work services to help with the social, psychological, and financial problems caused by work-related health problems.

- Epidemiologic services.

Pediatric Environmental Health Specialty Unit:

We provide consultation and medical care for children with toxic environmental exposures and with diseases of suspected environmental origin. This unit serves New York, New Jersey, Puerto Rico, and the Virgin Islands.

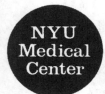

550 First Avenue (at 31st Street)
New York, NY 10016
Physician Referral: (888) 7-NYU-MED
(888-769-8633) www.nyumedicalcenter.org

SCHOOL OF
MEDICINE

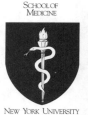

NEW YORK UNIVERSITY

INTERNAL MEDICINE

NYU Medical Center's Internal Medicine program is dedicated to treating the whole patient. Its internists meet the highest standards of the medical profession and take a comprehensive approach to each patient, addressing both the physical and mental aspects of nearly every health problem, from allergies to viruses. They combine a strong academic background with advanced medical technology to meet the diverse needs of patients in their community.

NYU's internal medicine specialists recognize that the successful care of patients requires knowledge not only of molecular medicine and pathophysiology, but also of the sciences that guide clinical decision-making, such as clinical epidemiology and behavioral medicine.

Furthermore, its numerous clinical programs, run by some of the nation's foremost physicians offer patients treatment specific to their needs – by recognizing the science behind the diagnosis.

NYU Medical Center offers cutting-edge technology, mixed with the latest in research and technique, in a multidisciplinary environment that is second to none. Below are just a few of the myriad services offered by the team.

- All primary health care needs, including physical exams.

- Comprehensive women's health care, from obstetric and gynecologic needs to osteoporosis prevention and treatment.

- Geriatric care, such as memory-loss screening for Alzheimer's disease and treatment for bone and joint problems.

- A wide range of laboratory tests, from basic blood and urine tests to screening for HIV and hepatitis, performed on-site.

- Guidance and medical treatment for substance abuse, eating disorders, obesity, and high cholesterol.

- Psychiatric care for anxiety and depression.

NYU MEDICAL CENTER

The physicians of the Division of Internal Medicine at NYU Hospitals Center treat most conditions, from addiction to rheumatoid arthritis, in an environment that is steeped in NYU's tradition of excellence and a dedication to state-of-the-art patient care and research.

This application of world-class science to bedside medicine is enhanced by interdisciplinary collaboration between departments and physicians, demonstrative of NYU Hospital Center's professionalism and dedication to teamwork and collegiality.

Physician Referral
(888) 7-NYU-MED
(888-769-8633)
www.nyumedicalcenter.org

PHYSICIAN LISTINGS

Internal Medicine

New England

Barry, Michele MD (IM) - *Spec Exp:* Travel Medicine; **Hospital:** Yale - New Haven Hosp; **Address:** 333 Cedar St, PO BOX 208025, New Haven, CT 06520-8025; **Phone:** (203) 688-2476; **Board Cert:** Internal Medicine 1980; **Med School:** Albert Einstein Coll Med 1977; **Resid:** Internal Medicine, Yale-New Haven Hosp, New Haven, CT 1978-1981; **Fellow:** Rheumatology, Yale-New Haven Hosp, New Haven, CT 1980-1981; Tropical Medicine, Walter Reed AMC, Washington, DC 1981; **Fac Appt:** Prof Medicine, Yale Univ

Beaser, Richard Seth MD (IM) - *Spec Exp:* Diabetes; **Hospital:** Beth Israel Deaconess Med Ctr - Boston; **Address:** Joslin Diabetes Med Ctr, 1 Joslin Pl, Boston, MA 02215; **Phone:** (617) 732-2675; **Board Cert:** Internal Medicine 1980; **Med School:** Boston Univ 1977; **Resid:** Internal Medicine, Mass Med Ctr, Boston, MA 1978-1980; **Fellow:** Endocrinology, Diabetes & Metabolism, Joslin Clinic, Boston, MA 1980-1981; **Fac Appt:** Asst Clin Prof Medicine, Harvard Med Sch

Horwitz, Ralph MD (IM) - *Spec Exp:* Internal Medicine - General; **Hospital:** Yale - New Haven Hosp; **Address:** 333 Cedar St, rm 1072-LMP, Box 208056, New Haven, CT 06520-8056; **Phone:** (203) 785-4119; **Board Cert:** Internal Medicine 1976; **Med School:** Penn State Univ-Hershey Med Ctr 1973; **Resid:** Internal Medicine, Royal Victoria Hosp-McGill, Montreal, Canada 1974-1975; Internal Medicine, Mass Genl Hosp, Boston, MA 1977-1978; **Fellow:** Epidemiology, Yale-New Haven Hosp, New Haven, CT 1975-1977; **Fac Appt:** Prof Medicine, Yale Univ

Koff, Raymond MD (IM) - *Spec Exp:* Hepatitis C; Liver Disease; **Hospital:** U Mass Meml Hlth Care - Worcester; **Address:** U Mass Meml Hlth Care, Shaw Bldg, Div Gastroenterology, 55 Lake Ave N, rm HA-303, Worcester, MA 01655; **Phone:** (508) 334-2806; **Board Cert:** Internal Medicine 1969; **Med School:** Albert Einstein Coll Med 1962; **Resid:** Internal Medicine, Barnes Hosp, St Louis, MO 1962-1964; **Fellow:** Research, Mass Genl Hosp, Boston, MA 1966-1969; **Fac Appt:** Prof Medicine, Univ Mass Sch Med

Loder, Elizabeth W MD (IM) - *Spec Exp:* Headache; Headache-Migraine; **Hospital:** Spauding Rehab Hosp; **Address:** 125 Nashua St, Boston, MA 02114; **Phone:** (617) 573-2493; **Board Cert:** Internal Medicine 1990; **Med School:** Univ ND Sch Med 1985; **Resid:** Internal Medicine, Faulkner Hosp, Boston, MA 1989-1990; **Fac Appt:** Medicine, Harvard Med Sch

Robinson, Dwight R. MD (IM) - *Spec Exp:* Arthritis; **Hospital:** MA Genl Hosp; **Address:** Mass Genl Hospital, WACC 730, Boston, MA 02114; **Phone:** (617) 726-7938; **Board Cert:** Internal Medicine 1968; **Med School:** Columbia P&S 1957; **Resid:** Surgery, Mass Genl Hosp, Boston, MA 1958-1959; Internal Medicine, Mass Genl Hosp, Boston, MA 1960-1961; **Fellow:** Research, Mass Genl Hosp, Boston, MA 1959-1960; Biochemistry, Brandeis Univ, Waltham, MA 1964; **Fac Appt:** Prof Medicine, Harvard Med Sch

Wood, Lawrence Crane MD (IM) - *Spec Exp:* Thyroid Disorders; **Hospital:** MA Genl Hosp; **Address:** 15 Parkman St, WACC 645, Boston, MA 02114; **Phone:** (617) 724-2700; **Board Cert:** Internal Medicine 1970; **Med School:** Univ Penn 1961; **Resid:** Internal Medicine, Univ Va Hosp, Charlottesville, VA 1962-1964; **Fellow:** Endocrinology, Univ Va Hosp, Charlottesville, VA 1964-1965; Endocrinology, Boston City Hosp, Charlottesville, MA 1968-1970

Mid Atlantic

Braunstein, Seth N MD/PhD (IM) - *Spec Exp:* Diabetes; **Hospital:** Hosp Univ Penn (page 78); **Address:** Hosp of Univ Penn, Diabetes Ctr, 3400 Spuce St, Ste I, Philadelphia, PA 19104-4219; **Phone:** (215) 662-7280; **Board Cert:** Internal Medicine 1975; **Med School:** NYU Sch Med 1972; **Resid:** Internal Medicine, Univ Penn Hosp, Philadelphia, PA 1972-1975; **Fac Appt:** Assoc Prof Medicine, Univ Penn

Cirigliano, Michael MD (IM) - *Spec Exp:* Alternative Medicine; **Hospital:** Hosp Univ Penn (page 78); **Address:** Univ Pa Clinical Practices, 3400 Sruce St, 9 Penn Tower, Philadelphia, PA 19104; **Phone:** (215) 662-3400; **Board Cert:** Internal Medicine 1994; **Med School:** Univ Penn 1990; **Resid:** Internal Medicine, Hosp Univ Penn, Philadelphia, PA 1990-1993; **Fac Appt:** Asst Prof Medicine, Univ Penn

Fisher, Laura MD (IM) - *Spec Exp:* Lyme Disease; Travel Medicine; **Hospital:** NY Presby Hosp - NY Weill Cornell Med Ctr (page 70); **Address:** 1385 York Ave, New York, NY 10021; **Phone:** (212) 717-5920; **Board Cert:** Infectious Disease 1990, Internal Medicine 1987; **Med School:** Brown Univ 1984; **Resid:** Internal Medicine, NY Hosp-Cornell Med Ctr, New York, NY 1984-1987; **Fellow:** Infectious Disease, Mass Genl Hosp, Boston, MA 1987-1989; **Fac Appt:** Asst Clin Prof Medicine, Cornell Univ-Weill Med Coll

Gitlow, Stanley MD (IM) - *Spec Exp:* Addiction Medicine; Hypertension; **Hospital:** Mount Sinai Hosp (page 68); **Address:** 50 E 89th St, New York, NY 10128-1225; **Phone:** (212) 722-5731; **Board Cert:** Internal Medicine 1977; **Med School:** SUNY Hlth Sci Ctr 1948; **Resid:** Internal Medicine, Bronx VA Hosp, Bronx, NY 1949-1950; Internal Medicine, Mount Sinai Hosp, New York, NY 1951-1952; **Fac Appt:** Clin Prof Medicine, Mount Sinai Sch Med

Rader, Daniel J MD (IM) - *Spec Exp:* Cholesterol/Lipid Disorders; **Hospital:** Hosp Univ Penn (page 78); **Address:** Cardiovascular Risk Intervention Prog, Phila Heart Inst, 39th & Market Sts, Ste 2A, Philadelphia, PA 19104; **Phone:** (215) 662-9993; **Board Cert:** Internal Medicine 1987; **Med School:** Med Coll PA Hahnemann 1984; **Resid:** Internal Medicine, Yale-New Haven Hosp, New Haven, CT 1984-1987; **Fellow:** Natl Inst Hlth, Bethesda, MD; **Fac Appt:** Assoc Prof Medicine, Univ Penn

Rivlin, Richard MD (IM) - *Spec Exp:* Cancer Prevention; Nutrition; **Hospital:** Westchester Med Ctr (page 82); **Address:** 300 E 42nd St Fl 5th, New York, NY 10017; **Phone:** (212) 551-2516; **Board Cert:** Internal Medicine 1969; **Med School:** Harvard Med Sch 1959; **Resid:** Internal Medicine, Bellevue Hosp, New York, NY 1959-1960; Internal Medicine, Johns Hopkins Hosp, Baltimore, MD 1960-1961; **Fellow:** Endocrinology, Diabetes & Metabolism, Natl Inst Hosp, Bethesda, MD 1961-1964; Internal Medicine, Johns Hopkins Hosp, Baltimore, MD 1964-1966; **Fac Appt:** Prof Medicine, Cornell Univ-Weill Med Coll

Selwyn, Peter MD (IM) - *Spec Exp:* AIDS/HIV; Addiction; Palliative Care; **Hospital:** Montefiore Med Ctr (page 67); **Address:** 3544 Jerome Ave, Fl 2, Bronx, NY 10467; **Phone:** (718) 920-4678; **Board Cert:** Family Practice 1998; **Med School:** Harvard Med Sch 1981; **Resid:** Family Practice, Montefiore Hosp, Bronx, NY 1981-1984; **Fac Appt:** Assoc Prof Medicine, Yale Univ

Seremetis, Stephanie MD (IM) - *Spec Exp:* Hemophilia/Bleeding Disorders; Women's Health; **Hospital:** Mount Sinai Hosp (page 68); **Address:** 5 E 98th St, Box 1521, New York, NY 10029; **Phone:** (212) 241-8818; **Board Cert:** Internal Medicine 1982, Hematology 1988; **Med School:** SUNY Hlth Sci Ctr 1978; **Resid:** Internal Medicine, Mount Sinai Med Ctr, New York, NY 1979-1981; **Fellow:** Hematology, Mount Sinai Med Ctr, New York, NY 1981-1983; **Fac Appt:** Assoc Prof Medicine, Mount Sinai Sch Med

Yaffe, Bruce MD (IM) - *Spec Exp:* Gastroscopy; Colonoscopy; **Hospital:** Lenox Hill Hosp (page 64); **Address:** 201 E 65th St, New York, NY 10021-6701; **Phone:** (212) 879-4700; **Board Cert:** Internal Medicine 1979, Gastroenterology 1981; **Med School:** Geo Wash Univ 1976; **Resid:** Internal Medicine, Mount Sinai Hosp, New York, NY 1977-1979; Hepatology, Mount Sinai Hosp, New York, NY 1979-1980; **Fellow:** Gastroenterology, Lenox Hill Hosp, New York, NY 1980-1982

Southeast

Carey, Timothy Stephen MD (IM) - *Spec Exp:* *Internal Medicine - General;* **Hospital:** Univ of NC Hosp (page 77); **Address:** Cecil G Sheps Ctr for Hlth Services, 725 Airport Rd, Box CB-7590, Chapel Hill, NC 27599-7590; **Phone:** (919) 966-7100; **Board Cert:** Internal Medicine 1979; **Med School:** Univ VT Coll Med 1976; **Resid:** Internal Medicine, Pacific Med Ctr, San Francisco, CA 1976-1979; **Fellow:** Internal Medicine, Univ NC Hosp, Chapel Hill, NC 1983-1985; **Fac Appt:** Prof Medicine, Univ NC Sch Med

Corbett Jr, Eugene Charles MD (IM) - *Spec Exp:* *Nutrition; Diabetes;* **Hospital:** Univ of VA Hlth Sys (page 79); **Address:** PO Box 800744, Charlottesville, VA 22908; **Phone:** (804) 924-1685; **Board Cert:** Internal Medicine 1987; **Med School:** Univ Chicago-Pritzker Sch Med 1970; **Resid:** Internal Medicine, Baltimore City Hosp, Baltimore, MD 1973-1975; **Fellow:** Research, Johns Hopkins, Baltimore, MD 1973-1975; **Fac Appt:** Asst Prof Medicine, Univ VA Sch Med

Eustace, John C MD (IM) - *Spec Exp:* *Addiction;* **Hospital:** Univ of Miami - Jackson Meml Hosp; **Address:** 9000 SW 87th Ct, Ste 112, Miami, FL 33176; **Phone:** (305) 273-7772; **Board Cert:** Internal Medicine 1978; **Med School:** Univ Miami Sch Med 1974; **Resid:** Internal Medicine, Univ Miami-Jackson Meml Hosp, Miami, FL 1975-1978

Schaberg, Dennis Ray MD (IM) - *Spec Exp:* *Staphylococcal Infections;* **Hospital:** Univ of Tenn Bowld Hosp; **Address:** Univ Tenn, Dept Internal Medicine, 956 Court Ave, rm D334, Memphis, TN 38163; **Phone:** (901) 448-5752; **Board Cert:** Internal Medicine 1978; **Med School:** Univ MO-Columbia Sch Med 1972; **Resid:** Internal Medicine, Harborview Med Ctr, Seattle, WA 1973-1974; Preventive Medicine, Ctrs For Disease Control, Atlanta, GA 1975-1977; **Fellow:** Infectious Disease, Univ Wash, Seattle, WA 1978-1979; **Fac Appt:** Prof Medicine, Univ Tenn Coll Med, Memphis

Vance, Mary Lee MD (IM) - *Spec Exp:* *Pituitary Disorders; Adrenal Tumors;* **Hospital:** Univ of VA Hlth Sys (page 79); **Address:** UVA Health System, 5840 Hospital Drive, Box 800601, Charlottesville, VA 22908-0601; **Phone:** (434) 924-2284; **Board Cert:** Internal Medicine 1980; **Med School:** Louisiana State Univ 1977; **Resid:** Internal Medicine, Baylor Univ Med Ctr, Dallas, TX 1978-1980; **Fellow:** Endocrinology, Diabetes & Metabolism, Univ Virginia Med Ctr, Charlottesville, VA 1980-1983; **Fac Appt:** Prof Medicine, Univ VA Sch Med

Midwest

Esch, Peter MD (IM) - *Spec Exp:* *Geriatric Medicine;* **Hospital:** Cleveland Clin Fdn (page 57); **Address:** 5700 Cooper Foster Park Rd, Lorain, OH 44053; **Phone:** (440) 366-8822; **Board Cert:** Internal Medicine 1977, Geriatric Medicine 1994; **Med School:** Case West Res Univ 1974; **Resid:** Internal Medicine, Hennepin Co Med Ctr, Minneapolis, MN 1974-1977

Pierach, Claus MD (IM) - *Spec Exp:* *Porphyria;* **Hospital:** Abbott - Northwestern Hosp; **Address:** Twin Cities Cancer IRB, 800 E 28th St, MC-11135, Minneapolis, MN 55407; **Phone:** (612) 863-4342; **Med School:** Germany 1959; **Fac Appt:** Prof Emeritus Medicine, Univ Minn

Sarosi, George MD (IM) - *Spec Exp:* *Infection-Respiratory; Fungal Lung Disease; Diagnostic Problems;* **Hospital:** VA Med Ctr; **Address:** 1481 W 10th St, MC 111, Indianapolis, IN 46202; **Phone:** (317) 554-0181; **Board Cert:** Internal Medicine 1970; **Med School:** Harvard Med Sch 1964; **Resid:** Internal Medicine, Univ. of Minn, Minneapolis, MN 1965-1968; **Fac Appt:** Prof Medicine, Indiana Univ

INTERNAL MEDICINE

Schwartz, Gary Lee MD (IM) - *Spec Exp:* Hypertension; Hypotension; **Hospital:** Mayo Med Ctr & Clin - Rochester, MN; **Address:** Mayo Clinic, 200 1st St SW, Rochester, MN 55905; **Phone:** (507) 284-2511; **Board Cert:** Internal Medicine 1980, Nephrology 1982; **Med School:** Univ Wisc 1977; **Resid:** Internal Medicine, Mayo Clinic, Rochester, MN 1977-1980; Nephrology, Mayo Clinic, Rochester, MN 1980-1982; **Fac Appt:** Asst Clin Prof Medicine, Mayo Med Sch

Shore, Bernard L MD (IM) - *Spec Exp:* Pulmonary Disease; **Hospital:** Barnes-Jewish Hosp (page 55); **Address:** 4652 Maryland Ave, St Louis, MO 63108-1913; **Phone:** (314) 367-3113; **Board Cert:** Internal Medicine 1980, Pulmonary Disease 1982; **Med School:** Washington Univ, St Louis 1977; **Resid:** Internal Medicine, Barnes Hosp, St Louis, MO 1978-1980; **Fellow:** Pulmonary Disease, Wash Univ Med Ctr, St Louis, MO 1980-1982; **Fac Appt:** Assoc Clin Prof Medicine, Washington Univ, St Louis

Weder, Alan B MD (IM) - *Spec Exp:* Hypertension; Vascular Medicine; **Hospital:** Univ of MI Hlth Ctr; **Address:** 325 Briarwood Cir Bldg 5, Ann Arbor, MI 48108; **Phone:** (734) 647-9000; **Board Cert:** Internal Medicine 1978; **Med School:** Hahnemann Univ 1975; **Resid:** Internal Medicine, Univ of Chicago Hosp, Chicago, IL 1976-1978; **Fac Appt:** Prof Medicine, Univ Mich Med Sch

Great Plains and Mountains

Schooley, Robert T MD (IM) - *Spec Exp:* AIDS/HIV; **Hospital:** Univ Colo HSC - Denver; **Address:** U Colo Hlth Scis Ctr, 4200 E Ninth Ave, Box B 163, Denver, CO 80262; **Phone:** (303) 315-1540; **Board Cert:** Internal Medicine 1977; **Med School:** Johns Hopkins Univ 1974; **Resid:** Internal Medicine, Johns Hopkins Univ Hospital, Baltimore, MD 1975-1976; **Fellow:** Infectious Disease, NIH/Mass. General Hospital, Boston, MA 1976-1981; **Fac Appt:** Prof Medicine, Univ Colo

Southwest

De Fronzo, Ralph Anthony MD (IM) - *Spec Exp:* Diabetes; **Hospital:** Univ of Texas Hlth & Sci Ctr; **Address:** U Tex Hlth Sci Ctr, Diabetes Div, 7703 Floyd Curl Dr, San Antonio, TX 78229-3900; **Phone:** (210) 567-6691; **Board Cert:** Internal Medicine 1975, Nephrology 1976; **Med School:** Harvard Med Sch 1969; **Resid:** Internal Medicine, Johns Hopkins Hosp, Baltimore, MD 1970-1971; **Fellow:** Endocrinology, Diabetes & Metabolism, Baltimore City Hosp-NIH, Baltimore, MD 1971-1973; Renal Disease, Hosp Univ Penn, Philadelphia, PA 1973-1975; **Fac Appt:** Prof Medicine, Univ Tex, San Antonio

Graybill, John Richard MD (IM) - *Spec Exp:* Fungal Infections; Infectious Disease; **Hospital:** Univ of Texas Hlth & Sci Ctr; **Address:** VA Hosp, 7400 Merton Mintor Blvd, rm E-703, San Antonio, TX 78284; **Phone:** (210) 617-5111; **Board Cert:** Internal Medicine 1972; **Med School:** Cornell Univ-Weill Med Coll 1966; **Resid:** Internal Medicine, Vanderbilt Univ Hosp, Nashville, TN 1967-1969; **Fellow:** Infectious Disease, Johns Hopkins Hosp, Baltimore, MD 1969-1970; **Fac Appt:** Prof Medicine, Univ Tex, San Antonio

West Coast and Pacific

Bissell Jr, Dwight Montgomery MD (IM) - *Spec Exp:* Porphyria; **Hospital:** UCSF Med Ctr; **Address:** UCSF Med Ctr-Dept Gastroenterology, 513 Parnassus Ave, rm S357, San Fransisco, CA 94143-0538; **Phone:** (415) 353-2318; **Board Cert:** Internal Medicine 1974; **Med School:** Harvard Med Sch 1967; **Resid:** Internal Medicine, Boston City Hosp-Harvard, Boston, MA 1968-1970; **Fellow:** Gastroenterology, UCSF Med Ctr, San Francisco, CA 1970-1973; **Fac Appt:** Prof Medicine, UCSF

Daar, Eric S MD (IM) - *Spec Exp:* *AIDS/HIV;* **Hospital:** LAC - Harbor - UCLA Med Ctr; **Address:** 1000 W Carson St, Box 449, Torrance, CA 90509; **Phone:** (310) 222-2467; **Board Cert:** Internal Medicine 1988; **Med School:** Georgetown Univ 1985; **Resid:** Internal Medicine, Cedars-Sinai Med Ctr, Los Angeles, CA 1985-1988

Illingworth, D Roger MD (IM) - *Spec Exp:* *Cholesterol/Lipid Disorders; Nutrition;* **Hospital:** OR Hlth Sci Univ Hosp and Clinics; **Address:** 3181 SW Sam Jackson Park Rd, MC PPV 330, Portland, OR 97201; **Phone:** (503) 494-1794; **Board Cert:** Internal Medicine 1980; **Med School:** Univ Miami Sch Med 1976; **Resid:** Internal Medicine, Oregon Hlth Sci Ctr, Portland, OR 1977-1980; **Fac Appt:** Prof Medicine, Oregon Hlth Scis Univ

Roth, Bennett E MD (IM) - *Spec Exp:* *Gastroesophageal Reflux; Inflammatory Bowel Disease/Crohn's; Irritable Bowel Syndrome;* **Hospital:** UCLA Med Ctr; **Address:** 200 UCLA Med Plaza, Ste 365A, Westwood Blvd, Los Angeles, CA 90095; **Phone:** (310) 825-1597; **Board Cert:** Internal Medicine 1972, Gastroenterology 1975; **Med School:** Hahnemann Univ 1968; **Resid:** Internal Medicine, Univ Penn, Philadelphia, PA 1969-1971; **Fellow:** Gastroenterology, UCLA Med Ctr, Los Angeles, CA 1973-1974; **Fac Appt:** Assoc Prof Medicine, UCLA

Maternal & Fetal Medicine

An obstetrician/gynecologist possesses special knowledge, skills and professional capability in the medical and surgical care of the female reproductive system and associated disorders. This physician serves as a consultant to other physicians and as a primary physician for women.

OBSTETRICS & GYNECOLOGY

An obstetrician/gynecologist who cares for, or provides consultation on, patients with complications of pregnancy. This specialist has advanced knowledge of the obstetrical, medical and surgical complications of pregnancy and their effect on both the mother and the fetus. He/she also possesses expertise in the most current diagnostic and treatment modalities used in the care of patients with complicated pregnancies.

Training required: Four years plus two years in clinical practice before certification in obstetrics and gynecology is complete *plus* additional training and examination in maternal-fetal medicine

STELLA AND JOSEPH PAYSON BIRTHING CENTER
MAIMONIDES MEDICAL CENTER

4802 Tenth Avenue • Brooklyn, NY 11219
Phone (718) 283-7048
www.maimonidesmed.org

With more than 5,000 births a year, Maimonides Medical Center's Stella and Joseph Payson Birthing Center is always bustling. The center allows patients to give birth in a warm, homelike setting equipped with advanced medical and technological support. The 11,000-square-foot facility, opened in 1997, features special delivery rooms for high-risk births and a suite of nine labor/delivery/recovery rooms for low-risk births. The facility is staffed with 40 physicians (including obstetric anesthesiologists), 27 midwives and a lactation specialist. Several physicians specialize in high-risk pregnancy, including Chairman of Obstetrics and Gynecology Howard Minkoff, MD.

Women who give birth at Maimonides also have a variety of other services available to them, including:

- A **doula** (Greek for "woman's caregiver"), who serves as a supportive companion before, during and just after childbirth. Maimonides is the only hospital in New York City that provides doulas at no cost. All doulas are trained volunteers who work under the auspices of N'shei CARES (a division of Agudah Women of America) in conjunction with the hospital's Department of Volunteer Services.
- An outstanding **Division of Neonatology and Neonatal Intensive Care Unit**, both overseen by James Pelegano, MD. Physicians are experts at handling premature births and treating all types of complications and conditions. A neonatologist is always available during high-risk deliveries and works closely with the obstetrician. Neonatal services include nutrition, physical and occupational therapy, ophthalmology and audiology.
- A **Perinatal Testing Center**, directed by Shoshana Haberman, MD, offering amniocentesis, 3-D ultrasound, fetal echocardiograms and other diagnostic exams

The center offers four monthly tours for expectant parents: one for women only (in conjunction with N'shei CARES), one for Chinese-speaking parents and two that are open to all prospective patients.

STELLA AND JOSEPH PAYSON BIRTHING CENTER

Expectant mothers come to Maimonides Medical Center because of the wide variety of specialized services designed to meet their needs. From high-risk pregnancy specialists to a state-of-the-art birthing center to a staff of certified midwives, the hospital has everything a mother-to-be could want. In addition to the services offered in the hospital, Maimonides has several outpatient sites that offer obstetric care.

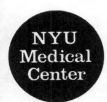

550 First Avenue (at 31st Street)
New York, NY 10016
Physician Referral: (888) 7-NYU-MED
(888-769-8633)   www.nyubaby.org

SCHOOL OF
MEDICINE

NEW YORK UNIVERSITY

MATERNAL-FETAL MEDICINE

The NYU Medical Center Program for Maternal Fetal Medicine offers prenatal care for high-risk pregnancies as well as detailed consultations before, during, and after pregnancy. Special attention is given to multifetal pregnancies and to women who have other medical conditions that complicate their pregnancy, like diabetes, heart problems, high blood pressure, and lupus, among others.

The Program's primary concern is making sure each patient delivers a healthy baby. Many of the patients referred to the specialists at NYU are able to conceive but have difficulty carrying babies to term. In response to their particular needs, NYU Medical has conducted extensive research into the causes of recurrent miscarriage and pre-term delivery, with impressive results.

Of course, the ideal time to correct fetal problems is when infants are still in the womb. Using minimally invasive tecniques, doctors at NYU Medical Center are able to repair a number of life-threatening conditions in a child before it is even born. These techniques reduce the risks of pre-term labor and the need for cesarean births.

The program's high success rates are testimony to the immediate impact research has on treatment at NYU Medical Center. This program has generated numerous new treatment modalities for high-risk obstetrics around the nation and around the world.

The Program for Maternal Fetal Medicine enjoys a close, synergistic relationship with the Prenatal Diagnostic Unit. Several of the pernatologists from the Maternal Fetal Medicine Practice provide coverage at the ultrasound unit, and refer patients for sonography and other procedures. From this partnership, residents and fellows learn state-of-the-art techniques for in-utero diagnosis and treatment, and our experienced physicians gain immediate access to the latest findings.

NYU MEDICAL CENTER

Maternal-Fetal Medicine at NYU Medical Center

- Specialized care to women with high-risk pregnancies by highly-trained Perinatologists

- Genetic counseling to provide education and genetic tests to evaluate family history

- Tests to help predict patients at risk for preterm labor and delivery, and medications for the mother

- Screening for complications, including preeclampsia, pregnancy-induced hypertension

- Nutritional counseling and education for gestational diabetes, diabetes discovered during pregnancy

Physician Referral
(888) 7-NYU-MED
(888-769-8633)
www.nyubaby.org

PHYSICIAN LISTINGS

New England

Acker, David B. MD (MF) - *Spec Exp:* Multiple Gestation; Pregnancy-High Risk; **Hospital:** Brigham & Women's Hosp; **Address:** Dept Ob/Gyn, 75 Francis St, Boston, MA 02115; **Phone:** (617) 732-5445; **Board Cert:** Obstetrics & Gynecology 1999, Maternal & Fetal Medicine 1999; **Med School:** NYU Sch Med 1968; **Resid:** Vanderbilt U Affil Hosp., Nashville, TN 1973-1974; Einstein Affil Hosp., Bronx, NY 1969-1971; **Fellow:** Maternal & Fetal Medicine, Boston Lying-In Hosp., Boston, MA 1977-1979; **Fac Appt:** Asst Prof Obstetrics & Gynecology, Harvard Med Sch

Copel, Joshua MD (MF) - *Spec Exp:* Maternal & Fetal Medicine - General; **Hospital:** Yale - New Haven Hosp; **Address:** PO Box 208063, New Haven, CT 06520-8063; **Phone:** (203) 785-2671; **Board Cert:** Maternal & Fetal Medicine 1988, Obstetrics & Gynecology 1986; **Med School:** Tufts Univ 1979; **Resid:** Obstetrics & Gynecology, Penn Hosp, Philadelphia, PA 1980-1983; **Fellow:** Maternal & Fetal Medicine, Yale-New Haven Hosp, New Haven, CT 1983-1985; **Fac Appt:** Prof Obstetrics & Gynecology, Yale Univ

Frigoletto Jr., Fredric D. MD (MF) - *Spec Exp:* Maternal & Fetal Medicine - General; **Hospital:** MA Genl Hosp; **Address:** 32 Fruit St, Bldg FND416, Boston, MA 02114; **Phone:** (617) 724-3775; **Board Cert:** Maternal & Fetal Medicine 1975, Obstetrics & Gynecology 1969; **Med School:** Boston Univ 1962; **Resid:** Obstetrics & Gynecology, Boston Womens Hosp., Boston, MA 1964-1967; Surgery, Boston City Hosp., Boston, MA 1963-1964; **Fac Appt:** Prof Obstetrics & Gynecology, Harvard Med Sch

Greene, Michael F. MD (MF) - *Spec Exp:* Pregnancy-High Risk; Multiple Gestation; Seizure Disorders-Pregnancy; **Hospital:** MA Genl Hosp; **Address:** 32 Fruit St, Blake Bldg- Fl 10, Boston, MA 02114; **Phone:** (617) 724-2229; **Board Cert:** Obstetrics & Gynecology 1997, Maternal & Fetal Medicine 1997; **Med School:** SUNY Downstate 1976; **Resid:** Obstetrics & Gynecology, Boston Womens Hosp, Boston, MA 1977-1980; **Fellow:** Maternal & Fetal Medicine, Brigham Womens Hosp, Boston, MA 1980-1982; **Fac Appt:** Assoc Prof Obstetrics & Gynecology, Harvard Med Sch

Heffner, Linda MD/PhD (MF) - *Spec Exp:* Pregnancy-High Risk; **Hospital:** Brigham & Women's Hosp; **Address:** Dept OB/GYN-Maternal & Fetal Medicine, 75 Francis St., Boston, MA 02115; **Phone:** (617) 732-4840; **Board Cert:** Maternal & Fetal Medicine 1998, Obstetrics & Gynecology 1998; **Med School:** Johns Hopkins Univ 1977; **Resid:** Obstetrics & Gynecology, Hosp Univ Penn, Philadelphia, PA 1980-1983; **Fellow:** Maternal & Fetal Medicine, Brigham-Womens Hosp., Boston, MA 1985; **Fac Appt:** Assoc Prof Obstetrics & Gynecology, Harvard Med Sch

Mid Atlantic

Bardeguez-Brown, Arlene D MD (MF) - *Spec Exp:* AIDS/HIV in Pregnancy; **Hospital:** UMDNJ-Univ Hosp-Newark; **Address:** 90 Bergen St, Ste 5100, Newark, NJ 07103; **Phone:** (973) 972-2700; **Board Cert:** Obstetrics & Gynecology 1998, Maternal & Fetal Medicine 1998; **Med School:** Univ Puerto Rico 1981; **Resid:** Obstetrics & Gynecology, Cath Med Ctr, Jamaica, NY 1981-1985; **Fellow:** Maternal & Fetal Medicine, Nassau Co Med Ctr, East Meadow, NY 1985-1987; **Fac Appt:** Assoc Prof Obstetrics & Gynecology, UMDNJ-NJ Med Sch, Newark

Chervenak, Francis Anthony MD (MF) - *Spec Exp:* Ultrasound; Pregnancy-High Risk; **Hospital:** NY Presby Hosp - NY Weill Cornell Med Ctr (page 70); **Address:** 525 E 68th St, Ste J-130, New York, NY 10021-4870; **Phone:** (212) 746-3184; **Board Cert:** Obstetrics & Gynecology 1984, Maternal & Fetal Medicine 1985; **Med School:** Jefferson Med Coll 1976; **Resid:** Obstetrics & Gynecology, NY Med Coll-Flower Fifth Ave Hosp, New York, NY 1977-1979; Obstetrics & Gynecology, St Lukes Hosp, New York, NY 1979-1981; **Fellow:** Maternal & Fetal Medicine, Yale-New Haven Hosp, New Haven, CT 1981-1983; **Fac Appt:** Prof Obstetrics & Gynecology, Cornell Univ-Weill Med Coll

Collea, Joseph Vincent MD (MF) - *Spec Exp:* Breech Birth; Multiple Gestation; **Hospital:** Georgetown Univ Hosp; **Address:** GUMC - Pasquerilla Healthcare Center, 3rd Floor, 3800 Reservoir Rd NW, Washington, DC 20007-2194; **Phone:** (202) 687-8531; **Board Cert:** Obstetrics & Gynecology 1974, Maternal & Fetal Medicine 1981; **Med School:** SUNY Syracuse 1966; **Resid:** Obstetrics & Gynecology, Johns Hopkins Hosp, Baltimore, MD 1967-1972; **Fellow:** LA CO USC Medical Center 1974-1976; **Fac Appt:** Prof Obstetrics & Gynecology, Georgetown Univ

D'Alton, Mary Elizabeth MD (MF) - *Spec Exp:* Pregnancy-High Risk; Multiple Gestation; **Hospital:** NY Presby Hosp - Columbia Presby Med Ctr (page 70); **Address:** 622 W 168 St, Ste 16-62, New York, NY 10032; **Phone:** (212) 305-6293; **Board Cert:** Obstetrics & Gynecology 1997, Maternal & Fetal Medicine 1997; **Med School:** Ireland 1976; **Resid:** Obstetrics & Gynecology, Univ Ottawa, Ontario, Canada 1977-1982; **Fellow:** Obstetrics & Gynecology, Tufts-New England Med Ctr, Boston, MA 1982-1984; **Fac Appt:** Clin Prof Obstetrics & Gynecology

Fox, Harold E MD/PhD (MF) - *Spec Exp:* Pregnancy-High Risk; **Hospital:** Johns Hopkins Hosp - Baltimore; **Address:** 600 N Wolfe St Bldg Phips - rm 264, 600 N Wolfe St, Baltimore, MD 21287; **Phone:** (410) 614-0178; **Board Cert:** Obstetrics & Gynecology 1994, Maternal & Fetal Medicine 1981; **Med School:** Univ Rochester 1972; **Resid:** Obstetrics & Gynecology, Strong Meml Hosp, Rochester, NY 1973-1975; **Fellow:** Maternal & Fetal Medicine, Univ Rochester Hosps, Rochester, NY 1975-1977; **Fac Appt:** Prof Obstetrics & Gynecology, Johns Hopkins Univ

Landers, Daniel V. MD (MF) - *Spec Exp:* Infectious Disease; **Hospital:** Magee Women's Hosp; **Address:** Magee Women's Hosp, Dept OB/GYN, 300 Halket Street, rm 2336, Pittsburgh, PA 15213; **Phone:** (412) 641-6253; **Board Cert:** Obstetrics & Gynecology 1989, Maternal & Fetal Medicine 1991; **Med School:** UCSF 1980; **Resid:** Obstetrics & Gynecology, UCSF Med Ctr, San Francisco, CA 1980-1984; **Fellow:** Maternal & Fetal Medicine, UCSF Med Ctr, San Francisco, CA 1984-1986; Infectious Disease, San Francisco General Hospital, San Francisco, CA 1986-1988; **Fac Appt:** Prof Obstetrics & Gynecology, Univ Pittsburgh

Landy, Helain Jody MD (MF) - *Spec Exp:* Genetic Disorders; Miscarriage-Recurrent; **Hospital:** Georgetown Univ Hosp; **Address:** GUMC-Pasquerilla Healthcare Ctr Dept OB/GYN, 3800 Reservoir Rd NW, Ste 3, Washington, DC 20007; **Phone:** (202) 687-8531; **Board Cert:** Obstetrics & Gynecology 1998, Maternal & Fetal Medicine 1998; **Med School:** Northwestern Univ 1982; **Resid:** Obstetrics & Gynecology, Penn Hosp, Philadelphia, PA 1982-1986; **Fellow:** Maternal & Fetal Medicine, George Washington Univ Med Ctr, Washington, DC 1986-1988; **Fac Appt:** Assoc Prof Obstetrics & Gynecology, Georgetown Univ

Lockwood, Charles MD (MF) - *Spec Exp:* Prematurity Prevention; Miscarriage-Recurrent; Multiple Gestation; **Hospital:** NYU Med Ctr (page 71); **Address:** 550 1st Ave, Ste 7N, New York, NY 10016-6402; **Phone:** (212) 263-8033; **Board Cert:** Obstetrics & Gynecology 1997, Maternal & Fetal Medicine 1997; **Med School:** Univ Penn 1981; **Resid:** Obstetrics & Gynecology, Pennsylvania Hosp, Philadelphia, PA 1981-1985; **Fellow:** Maternal & Fetal Medicine, Yale-New Haven Hosp, New Haven, CT 1985-1987; **Fac Appt:** Prof Obstetrics & Gynecology, NYU Sch Med

Mennuti, Michael MD (MF) - *Spec Exp:* Congenital Abnormalities; Pregnancy-High Risk; **Hospital:** Hosp Univ Penn (page 78); **Address:** Univ Penn Hosp, Dept OB/GYN, 3400 Spruce St, Philadelphia, PA 19104-4204; **Phone:** (215) 662-3234; **Board Cert:** Maternal & Fetal Medicine 1975, Clinical Genetics 1982; **Med School:** Georgetown Univ 1968; **Resid:** Obstetrics & Gynecology, Hosp Univ Penn, Philadelphia, PA 1969-1973; **Fellow:** Maternal & Fetal Medicine, Hosp Univ Penn, Philadelphia, PA 1975-1978; Clinical Genetics, Hosp Univ Penn, Philadelphia, PA; **Fac Appt:** Prof Obstetrics & Gynecology, Univ Penn

Nagey, David Augustus MD (MF) - *Spec Exp:* *Maternal & Fetal Medicine - General;* **Hospital:** Johns Hopkins Hosp - Baltimore; **Address:** Johns Hopkins Hosp, Women's Health Ctr, 601 Caroline St Fl 8, Baltimore, MD 21287; **Phone:** (410) 955-6700; **Board Cert:** Obstetrics & Gynecology 1991, Maternal & Fetal Medicine 1984; **Med School:** Duke Univ 1975; **Resid:** Obstetrics & Gynecology, Duke Univ Med Ctr, Durham, NC 1975-1979; **Fellow:** Maternal & Fetal Medicine, Duke Univ Med Ctr, Durham, NC 1979-1981; **Fac Appt:** Assoc Prof Obstetrics & Gynecology, Johns Hopkins Univ

Wapner, Ronald MD (MF) - *Spec Exp:* *Perinatal Medicine; Genetics;* **Hospital:** Thomas Jefferson Univ Hosp; **Address:** MCP Hahnemann University, 245 N 15th St, MS 495, Philadelphia, PA 19102; **Phone:** (215) 762-4000; **Board Cert:** Obstetrics & Gynecology 1978, Maternal & Fetal Medicine 1981; **Med School:** Jefferson Med Coll 1972; **Resid:** Obstetrics & Gynecology, Jefferson Med Coll, Philadelphia, PA 1972-1976; **Fellow:** Maternal & Fetal Medicine, Jefferson Med Coll, Philadelphia, PA 1976-1978; **Fac Appt:** Prof Obstetrics & Gynecology, Jefferson Med Coll

Southeast

Boehm, Frank Henry MD (MF) - *Spec Exp:* *Pregnancy-High Risk;* **Hospital:** Vanderbilt Univ Med Ctr (page 80); **Address:** Vanderbilt Univ Med Ctr, Dept ObGyn, B1100, Med Ctr North, Nashville, TN 37232-2519; **Phone:** (615) 322-2071; **Board Cert:** Obstetrics & Gynecology 1973, Maternal & Fetal Medicine 1976; **Med School:** Vanderbilt Univ 1965; **Resid:** Obstetrics & Gynecology, Yale-New Haven Hosp, New Haven, CT 1966-1970; **Fac Appt:** Prof Obstetrics & Gynecology, Vanderbilt Univ

Bruner, Joseph P MD (MF) - *Spec Exp:* *Fetal Surgery; Spina Bifida;* **Hospital:** Vanderbilt Univ Med Ctr (page 80); **Address:** Vanderbilt Univ Med Ctr N, Dept OB/GYN, 1161 41st Ave S, Ste B1100, Nashville, TN 37232-0001; **Phone:** (615) 322-6173; **Board Cert:** Obstetrics & Gynecology 1999, Interventional Cardiology 1999; **Med School:** Univ Nebr Coll Med 1979; **Resid:** Obstetrics & Gynecology, Letterman AMC, San Francisco, CA 1980-1983; **Fellow:** Mammography, Univ Penn Hosp, Philadelphia, PA 1986-1988; **Fac Appt:** Assoc Prof Obstetrics & Gynecology, Vanderbilt Univ

Chescheir, Nancy Custer MD (MF) - *Spec Exp:* *Ultrasound; Fetal Surgery;* **Hospital:** Univ of NC Hosp (page 77); **Address:** 214 MacNider Bldg, CB-7570, Chapel Hill, NC 27599-7516; **Phone:** (919) 966-1601; **Board Cert:** Obstetrics & Gynecology 1989, Maternal & Fetal Medicine 1990; **Med School:** Univ NC Sch Med 1982; **Resid:** Obstetrics & Gynecology, UNC Hosp, Chapel Hill, NC 1982-1986; **Fellow:** Maternal & Fetal Medicine, NC Mem Hsp-UNC, Chapel Hill, NC 1986-1988; **Fac Appt:** Assoc Prof Obstetrics & Gynecology, Univ NC Sch Med

Ferguson II, James E MD (MF) - *Spec Exp:* *Pregnancy-High Risk;* **Hospital:** Univ of VA Hlth Sys (page 79); **Address:** PO Box 800712, Charlottesville, VA 22908; **Phone:** (804) 924-2500; **Board Cert:** Obstetrics & Gynecology 1995, Maternal & Fetal Medicine 1987; **Med School:** Wake Forest Univ Sch Med 1977; **Resid:** Obstetrics & Gynecology, Bowman Gray Sch Med., Winston-Salem, NC 1980-1981; Obstetrics & Gynecology, Stanford U Med Ctr., Stanford, CA 1978-1980; **Fellow:** Maternal & Fetal Medicine, Stanford U Med Ctr., Standord, CA 1982-1984; **Fac Appt:** Asst Prof Maternal & Fetal Medicine, Univ VA Sch Med

Gabbe, Steven G MD (MF) - *Spec Exp:* *Pregnancy-High Risk; Diabetes-Gestational;* **Hospital:** Vanderbilt Univ Med Ctr (page 80); **Address:** D 3300 Medical Ctr N, Nashville, TN 37232-2104; **Phone:** (615) 322-5191; **Board Cert:** Obstetrics & Gynecology 1976, Maternal & Fetal Medicine 1977; **Med School:** Cornell Univ-Weill Med Coll 1969; **Resid:** Obstetrics & Gynecology, Boston Hosp Women, Boston, MA 1972-1974; **Fellow:** Reproductive Medicine, Boston Lying-In Hosp, Boston, MA 1972-1974; **Fac Appt:** Prof Obstetrics & Gynecology, Vanderbilt Univ

McLaren, Rodney A MD (MF) - *Spec Exp:* Prenatal Diagnosis; Amniocentesis; Pregnancy-High Risk; **Hospital:** Arlington Hosp; **Address:** Dept Maternal & Fetal Medicine, 1701 N George Mason Drive, Arlington, VA 22205; **Phone:** (703) 558-6077; **Board Cert:** Obstetrics & Gynecology 1991; **Med School:** Tufts Univ 1983; **Resid:** Obstetrics & Gynecology, LI Coll Hosp, New York, NY 1983-1987; **Fellow:** Maternal & Fetal Medicine, Georgetown Univ, Washington, DC 1989

O'Sullivan, Mary Jo MD (MF) - *Spec Exp:* Pregnancy-High Risk; **Hospital:** Univ of Miami - Jackson Meml Hosp; **Address:** 1611 NW 12th Ave, Bldg Holtz Center - rm 4070, Miami, FL 33136-1028; **Phone:** (305) 585-5610; **Board Cert:** Obstetrics & Gynecology 1970, Maternal & Fetal Medicine 1976; **Med School:** Med Coll PA Hahnemann 1963; **Resid:** Obstetrics & Gynecology, Womens Med Hosp, Philadelphia, PA 1964-1968

Thorp Jr, John Mercer MD (MF) - *Spec Exp:* Multiple Gestation; Premature Labor; Cervical Incompetence; **Hospital:** Univ of NC Hosp (page 77); **Address:** 214 MacNider Bldg, Box 7516, Dept ObGyn, Chapel Hill, NC 27599-0001; **Phone:** (919) 966-2496; **Board Cert:** Obstetrics & Gynecology 1999, Maternal & Fetal Medicine 1999; **Med School:** E Carolina Univ 1983; **Resid:** Obstetrics & Gynecology, Univ NC Hosp, Chapel Hill, NC 1983-1987; **Fellow:** Maternal & Fetal Medicine, Univ NC Hosp, Chapel Hill, NC 1987-1989; **Fac Appt:** Prof Obstetrics & Gynecology, Univ NC Sch Med

Midwest

Bartelsmeyer, James MD (MF) - *Spec Exp:* Pregnancy-High Risk; Multiple Gestation; **Hospital:** St John's Mercy Med Ctr - St Louis; **Address:** 621 S New Ballas Rd, Ste 2009-B, St. Louis, MO 63141; **Phone:** (314) 569-6882; **Board Cert:** Maternal & Fetal Medicine 1995, Obstetrics & Gynecology 1992; **Med School:** Univ IL Coll Med 1985; **Resid:** Obstetrics & Gynecology, U Ill Coll Med. Hosps., Chicago, IL 1985-1989; **Fellow:** Maternal & Fetal Medicine, Barnes Hosp.-U Wash., St. Louis, MO 1989-1991; **Fac Appt:** Assoc Prof Obstetrics & Gynecology, Washington Univ, St Louis

Dooley, Sharon L MD (MF) - *Spec Exp:* Fetal Anomaly; Pregnancy-High Risk; Multiple Gestation; **Hospital:** Northwestern Meml Hosp; **Address:** 333 E Superior St, rm 410, Chicago, IL 60611-3095; **Phone:** (312) 926-7519; **Board Cert:** Obstetrics & Gynecology 1989, Maternal & Fetal Medicine 1981; **Med School:** Univ VA Sch Med 1973; **Resid:** Obstetrics & Gynecology, Northwestern Meml Hosp, Chicago, IL 1974-1977; **Fac Appt:** Prof Obstetrics & Gynecology, Northwestern Univ

Gianopoulos, John MD (MF) - *Spec Exp:* Perinatal Medicine; Premature Labor; **Hospital:** Loyola Univ Med Ctr; **Address:** Loyola Univ Med Ctr, 2160 S 1st Ave, Bldg 103 - Ste 1019, Maywood, IL 60153; **Phone:** (708) 216-5423; **Board Cert:** Obstetrics & Gynecology 1993, Maternal & Fetal Medicine 1985; **Med School:** Loyola Univ-Stritch Sch Med 1977; **Resid:** Obstetrics & Gynecology, Loyola Univ Med Ctr, Maywood, IL 1977-1981; **Fellow:** Maternal & Fetal Medicine, Loyola Univ Med Ctr, Maywood, IL 1981-1983; **Fac Appt:** Prof Obstetrics & Gynecology, Loyola Univ-Stritch Sch Med

Hayashi, Robert H. MD (MF) - *Spec Exp:* Premature Labor; Labor-Abnormal; Pregnancy-High Risk; **Hospital:** Univ of MI Hlth Ctr; **Address:** 1500 E Medical Ctr. Dr., rm F4882, Box 0264, C.S. Mott Children's Hospital, Ann Arbor, MI 48109-0264; **Phone:** (734) 763-6295; **Board Cert:** Obstetrics & Gynecology 1989, Maternal & Fetal Medicine 1976; **Med School:** Temple Univ 1963; **Resid:** Obstetrics & Gynecology, U Mich Hosp., Ann Arbor, MI 1966-1970; **Fellow:** U Pitt Hosp., Pittsburgh, PA 1970-1972; **Fac Appt:** Prof Obstetrics & Gynecology, Univ Mich Med Sch

Hibbard, Judith MD (MF) - *Spec Exp:* *Pregnancy-High Risk; Cardiovascular Disease-Pregnancy; Ultrasound;* **Hospital:** Univ of Chicago Hosps (page 76); **Address:** Univ Chicago Hosps, Dept OB-GYN, 5841 N Maryland Ave, MC-2050, Chicago, IL 60637; **Phone:** (773) 702-5200; **Board Cert:** Obstetrics & Gynecology 1999, Maternal & Fetal Medicine 1999; **Med School:** Loyola Univ-Stritch Sch Med 1982; **Resid:** Obstetrics & Gynecology, Univ Chicago Hosp, Chicago, IL 1982-1986; **Fellow:** Maternal & Fetal Medicine, Univ Chicago Hosp, Chicago, IL 1986-1988; **Fac Appt:** Prof Obstetrics & Gynecology, Univ Chicago-Pritzker Sch Med

Hussey, Michael J MD (MF) - *Spec Exp:* *Perinatal Medicine; Tubal Ligation;* **Hospital:** Rush-Presby - St Luke's Med Ctr (page 72); **Address:** 1725 W Harrison St, Ste 408, Chicago, IL 60612; **Phone:** (312) 942-6611; **Board Cert:** Obstetrics & Gynecology 1994, Maternal & Fetal Medicine 1998; **Med School:** Univ IL Coll Med 1986; **Resid:** Obstetrics & Gynecology, Loyola Univ Med Ctr, Maywood, IL 1991-1993; **Fellow:** Maternal & Fetal Medicine, Rush Presby, Chicago, IL 1993; **Fac Appt:** Asst Prof Obstetrics & Gynecology, Rush Med Coll

Ismail, Mahmoud MD (MF) - *Spec Exp:* *Pregnancy-High Risk; Perinatal Medicine; Infections;* **Hospital:** Univ of Chicago Hosps (page 76); **Address:** 5841 S Maryland Ave, MC 2050, Chicago, IL 60637; **Phone:** (773) 702-5200; **Board Cert:** Obstetrics & Gynecology 1997, Maternal & Fetal Medicine 1997; **Med School:** Egypt 1970; **Resid:** Obstetrics & Gynecology, Wayne St Univ Affil Hosps, Detroit, MI 1973-1977; **Fellow:** Maternal & Fetal Medicine, Univ Chicago Hosps, Chicago, IL 1980-1982; **Fac Appt:** Prof Obstetrics & Gynecology, Univ Chicago-Pritzker Sch Med

Philipson, Elliot MD (MF) - *Spec Exp:* *Pregnancy-High Risk; Amniocentesis;* **Hospital:** Cleveland Clin Fdn (page 57); **Address:** 9500 Euclid Ave, Ste M66, Cleveland, OH 44195; **Phone:** (216) 445-3402; **Board Cert:** Obstetrics & Gynecology 1984, Maternal & Fetal Medicine 1990; **Med School:** Italy 1975; **Resid:** Obstetrics & Gynecology, Albany Med Ctr, Albany, NY 1977-1980; **Fellow:** Maternal & Fetal Medicine, Metro Genl Hosp, Cleveland, OH 1980-1982

Pielet, Bruce MD (MF) - *Spec Exp:* *Ultrasound; Multiple Gestation; Pregnancy-High Risk;* **Hospital:** Advocate Lutheran Gen Hosp; **Address:** 1875 Dempster St, Ste 325, Park Ridge, IL 60068; **Phone:** (847) 723-8610; **Board Cert:** Obstetrics & Gynecology 1999, Maternal & Fetal Medicine 1999; **Med School:** Loyola Univ-Stritch Sch Med 1981; **Resid:** Obstetrics & Gynecology, Univ Chicago Hosps, Chicago, IL 1981-1985; **Fellow:** Maternal & Fetal Medicine, Northwestern Univ, Chicago, IL 1985-1987

Strassner, Howard T MD (MF) - *Spec Exp:* *Fetal Transfusion; Amniocentesis;* **Hospital:** Rush-Presby - St Luke's Med Ctr (page 72); **Address:** 1725 W Harrison St, Ste 408-West, Chicago, IL 60612; **Phone:** (312) 666-0285; **Board Cert:** Obstetrics & Gynecology 1982; **Med School:** Univ Chicago-Pritzker Sch Med 1974; **Resid:** Obstetrics & Gynecology, Columbia Presby Med Ctr, New York, NY 1974-1978; **Fellow:** Maternal & Fetal Medicine, LA Co-USC Med Ctr, Los Angeles, CA 1978-1980; **Fac Appt:** Assoc Prof Obstetrics & Gynecology, Rush Med Coll

Tomich, Paul MD (MF) - *Spec Exp:* *Pregnancy-High Risk;* **Hospital:** Loyola Univ Med Ctr; **Address:** 2160 S 1st Ave Bldg 103 - rm 1013, Maywood, IL 60153; **Phone:** (708) 216-8563; **Board Cert:** Obstetrics & Gynecology 1999, Maternal & Fetal Medicine 1998; **Med School:** Loyola Univ-Stritch Sch Med 1973; **Resid:** Obstetrics & Gynecology, Mayo Clinic, Rochester, MN 1974-1978; **Fellow:** Maternal & Fetal Medicine, Barnes Hosp-Wash Univ, St Louis, MO 1978-1980; **Fac Appt:** Asst Prof Obstetrics & Gynecology, Loyola Univ-Stritch Sch Med

Treadwell, Marjorie Clarke MD (MF) - *Spec Exp:* Obstetrical Ultrasound; Pregnancy-High Risk; Fetal Therapy; **Hospital:** Hutzel Hosp - Detroit (page 59); **Address:** 4707 St Antoine, Ste 304, Detroit, MI 48201; **Phone:** (313) 745-0723; **Board Cert:** Obstetrics & Gynecology 2000, Maternal & Fetal Medicine 2000; **Med School:** Univ Mich Med Sch 1984; **Resid:** Obstetrics & Gynecology, Wayne State Univ, Detroit, MI 1984-1988; **Fellow:** Obstetrics & Gynecology, Wayne State Univ, Detroit, MI 1989-1990; **Fac Appt:** Assoc Prof Obstetrics & Gynecology, Wayne State Univ

Winn, Hung MD (MF) - *Spec Exp:* Multiple Gestation; Pregnancy-High Risk; **Hospital:** SSM St Mary's Hlth Ctr - St Louis; **Address:** 6420 Clayton Rd, Ste 559, St Louis, MO 63117; **Phone:** (314) 768-8873; **Board Cert:** Obstetrics & Gynecology 1991, Maternal & Fetal Medicine 1992; **Med School:** Univ IL Coll Med 1982; **Resid:** Obstetrics & Gynecology, Univ Illinois Hosp, Peoria, IL 1982-1986; **Fellow:** Maternal & Fetal Medicine, Yale-New Haven Hosp, New Haven, CT 1986-1988; **Fac Appt:** Prof Obstetrics & Gynecology, St Louis Univ

Great Plains and Mountains

Gibbs, Ronald Steven MD (MF) - *Spec Exp:* Maternal & Fetal Medicine - General; **Hospital:** Univ Colo HSC - Denver; **Address:** 4200 E 9th Ave, rm 4015, Denver, CO 80220; **Phone:** (303) 372-6691; **Board Cert:** Obstetrics & Gynecology 1989, Maternal & Fetal Medicine 1981; **Med School:** Univ Penn 1969; **Resid:** Obstetrics & Gynecology, Hosp Univ Penn, Philadelphia, PA 1970-1974; **Fellow:** Maternal & Fetal Medicine, Univ Tex Hlth Sci Ctr, San Antonio, TX 1976-1978; **Fac Appt:** Prof Obstetrics & Gynecology, Univ Colo

Southwest

Wilkins, Isabelle MD (MF) - *Spec Exp:* Multiple Gestation; Congenital Abnormalities; Prenatal Ultrasound; **Hospital:** St Luke's Episcopal Hosp - Houston; **Address:** Baylor College of Medicine, 6550 Fannin, Ste 901, Houston, TX 77030-2720; **Phone:** (713) 798-7593; **Board Cert:** Obstetrics & Gynecology 1996, Maternal & Fetal Medicine 1996; **Med School:** Duke Univ 1980; **Resid:** Obstetrics & Gynecology, Mount Sinai Med Ctr, New York, NY 1980-1984; **Fellow:** Maternal & Fetal Medicine, Mount Sinai Med Ctr, New York, NY 1984-1986; **Fac Appt:** Assoc Prof Obstetrics & Gynecology, Baylor Coll Med

West Coast and Pacific

Benedetti, Thomas J MD (MF) - *Spec Exp:* Prematurity Prevention; Fetal Macrosomia; **Hospital:** Univ WA Med Ctr; **Address:** 1959 NE Pacific St, Box 356460, Seattle, WA 98195; **Phone:** (206) 543-3729; **Board Cert:** Maternal & Fetal Medicine 1981, Obstetrics & Gynecology 1980; **Med School:** Univ Wash 1973; **Resid:** Obstetrics & Gynecology, LAC-USC Med Ctr, Los Angeles, CA 1974-1977; **Fellow:** Maternal & Fetal Medicine, LAC-USC Med Ctr, Los Angeles, CA 1977-1979; **Fac Appt:** Prof Obstetrics & Gynecology, Univ Wash

Druzin, Maurice L MD (MF) - *Spec Exp:* Lupus in Pregnancy; Fetal Electronic Monitors; Recurrent Miscarriage; **Hospital:** Stanford Med Ctr; **Address:** Dept OB/GYN, 300 Pasteur Dr, rm HH333, Stanford, CA 94305; **Phone:** (650) 725-8617; **Board Cert:** Maternal & Fetal Medicine 1981, Obstetrics & Gynecology 1980; **Med School:** South Africa 1970; **Resid:** Obstetrics & Gynecology, Rose Med Ctr-Univ Colo, Denver, CO 1974-1977; **Fellow:** Maternal & Fetal Medicine, USC Med Ctr, Los Angeles, CA 1977-1979; **Fac Appt:** Prof Obstetrics & Gynecology, Stanford Univ

Goldberg, James David MD (MF) - *Spec Exp:* *Prenatal Diagnosis; Fetal Therapy;* **Hospital:** CA Pacific Med Ctr - Pacific Campus; **Address:** California Pacific Med Ctr, 3700 California St, Ste G330, San Francisco, CA 94118; **Phone:** (415) 750-6400; **Board Cert:** Maternal & Fetal Medicine 1997, Clinical Genetics 1987; **Med School:** Univ Minn 1979; **Resid:** Obstetrics & Gynecology, UCSF Med Ctr, San Francisco, CA 1979-1983; **Fellow:** Maternal & Fetal Medicine, Mount Sinai Hosp, New York, NY 1983-1985; Clinical Genetics, Mount Sinai Hosp, New York, NY 1983-1985

Gravett, Michael Glen MD (MF) - *Spec Exp:* *Maternal & Fetal Medicine - General;* **Hospital:** OR Hlth Sci Univ Hosp and Clinics; **Address:** 3181 SW Sam Jackson Park Rd, rm L-458, Portland, OR 97201; **Phone:** (503) 494-2101; **Board Cert:** Maternal & Fetal Medicine 1987, Obstetrics & Gynecology 1985; **Med School:** UCLA 1977; **Resid:** Obstetrics & Gynecology, Univ Wash, Seattle, WA 1978-1981; **Fellow:** Maternal & Fetal Medicine, Univ Wash, Seattle, WA 1981-1983

Hobel, Calvin John MD (MF) - *Spec Exp:* *Prematurity Prevention; Fetal Stress;* **Hospital:** Cedars-Sinai Med Ctr; **Address:** 8700 Beverly Blvd, Ste 160, Los Angeles, CA 90048; **Phone:** (310) 423-3365; **Board Cert:** Obstetrics & Gynecology 1971, Maternal & Fetal Medicine 1975; **Med School:** Univ Nebr Coll Med 1963; **Resid:** Obstetrics & Gynecology, Harbor Genl Hosp, Torrance, CA 1964-1968; **Fellow:** Maternal & Fetal Medicine, Natl Womens Hosp, Auckland, New Zealand 1966-1967; **Fac Appt:** Prof Obstetrics & Gynecology, UCLA

Koos, Brian John MD (MF) - *Spec Exp:* *Pregnancy-High Risk; Fetal Diagnosis;* **Hospital:** UCLA Med Ctr; **Address:** 10833 Le Conte Ave, Los Angeles, CA 90095-3075; **Phone:** (310) 206-6404; **Board Cert:** Obstetrics & Gynecology 1999, Maternal & Fetal Medicine 1999; **Med School:** Loma Linda Univ 1974; **Resid:** Obstetrics & Gynecology, Brigham & Women's Hosp, Boston, MA 1976-1979; **Fellow:** Maternal & Fetal Medicine, Women's Hosp, Los Angeles, CA 1982-1983; **Fac Appt:** Prof Obstetrics & Gynecology, UCLA

NEONATAL-PERINATAL MEDICINE

(a subspecialty of OBSTETRICS AND GYNECOLOGY)

A subspecialist in neonatal-perinatal medicine is a pediatrician who is the principal care provider for sick newborn infants. Clinical expertise is used for direct patient care and for consulting with obstetrical colleagues to plan for the care of mothers who have high-risk pregnancies.

PEDIATRICS

A pediatrician is concerned with the physical, emotional and social health of children from birth to young adulthood. Care encompasses a broad spectrum of health services ranging from preventive healthcare to the diagnosis and treatment of acute and chronic diseases. The pediatrician deals with biological, social and environmental influences on the developing child and with the impact of disease and dysfunction on development.

Training required: Three years in pediatrics *plus* additional training and examination

NYU Medical Center

550 First Avenue (at 31st Street)
New York, NY 10016
Physician Referral: (888) 7-NYU-MED
(888-769-8633)   www.nyubaby.org

SCHOOL OF MEDICINE

NEW YORK UNIVERSITY

NEONATAL-PERINATAL MEDICINE

The typical NICU is full of bright lights, loud noises and round-the-clock activity. So much sensory input at such an early age can give newborn babies a lot of stress, which may have a negative impact on their development.

Recently, NYU Medical Center redesigned its NICU surroundings to provide positive early experiences – and simultaneously enhance the quality of medical care. Visitors to the NICU at Tisch Hospital will see covered incubators, drawn shades, and parents holding pre-term infants skin-to-skin in a quiet, relaxed setting. NYU School of Medicine's studies have shown dramatic decreases in length of hospitalization and in the number and severity of complications. This approach has also decreased the need for ventilator support and the risk of chronic lung disease. It has also been shown to enhance weight gain and improve overall neurological development.

Because many premature babies may be at increased risk for problems in growth and development, our Continuing Care Program is designed to follow these infants from birth through pre-school, providing evaluation and assessment of any problems as soon as they arise.

Of course, the ideal time to correct fetal problems is when infants are still in the womb. Using minimally invasive tecniques, doctors at NYU Medical Center are able to repair a number of life-threatening conditions in a child before it is even born. These techniques reduce the risks of pre-term labor and the need for cesarean births.

NYU MEDICAL CENTER

At NYU Medical Center, the new expanded Neonatal Intensive Care Unit features a more serene, family-friendly atmosphere that improves the quality of care for our smallest patients.

NYU Medical Center's statistics for survival and fewest complications are among the best in the country. Nationwide, 56% of infants born at 24 weeks' gestation survive, while at NYU Medical Center, parenting and developmentally appropriate strategies for these infants have increased the survival rate to 71%.

Physician Referral
(888) 7-NYU-MED
(888-769-8633)
www.nyubaby.org

PHYSICIAN LISTINGS

Neonatal-Perinatal Medicine

New England

Cloherty, John MD (NP) - *Spec Exp:* Neonatology; **Hospital:** Children's Hospital - Boston; **Address:** 319 Longwood Ave, Fl 4, Boston, MA 02115; **Phone:** (617) 355-7318; **Board Cert:** Pediatrics 1986, Neonatal-Perinatal Medicine 1975; **Med School:** Boston Univ 1962; **Resid:** Pediatrics, Mass Genl Hosp, Boston, MA 1967-1969; **Fellow:** Neonatal-Perinatal Medicine, Chldns Hosp, Boston, MA 1969; **Fac Appt:** Assoc Prof Pediatrics, Harvard Med Sch

Ehrenkranz, Richard MD (NP) - *Spec Exp:* Neonatology; Critical Care; **Hospital:** Yale - New Haven Hosp; **Address:** Yale Univ-Dept Ped, 333 Cedar St, Box 208064, New Haven, CT 06520-8064; **Phone:** (203) 688-2320; **Board Cert:** Neonatal-Perinatal Medicine 1979, Pediatrics 1977; **Med School:** SUNY Downstate 1972; **Resid:** Pediatrics, Yale-New Haven Hosp, New Haven, CT 1973-1974; **Fellow:** Neonatal-Perinatal Medicine, Yale Univ, New Haven, CT 1976-1978; **Fac Appt:** Prof Pediatrics, Yale Univ

Gross, Ian MD (NP) - *Spec Exp:* Breathing Disorders; **Hospital:** Yale - New Haven Hosp; **Address:** Yale Sch Med, Dept Pediatrics, 333 Cedar St, New Haven, CT 06520-3206; **Phone:** (203) 688-2320; **Board Cert:** Pediatrics 1974, Neonatal-Perinatal Medicine 1977; **Med School:** South Africa 1967; **Resid:** Pediatrics, Univ Witwatersrand Affil Hosps, Johannesburg, South Africa 1970-1971; Pediatrics, Chldns Hosp Med Ctr, Boston, MA 1971-1972; **Fellow:** Pediatrics, Harvard Med Sch, Boston, MA 1972-1973; Neonatal-Perinatal Medicine, Yale Univ Sch Med, New Haven, CT 1973-1974; **Fac Appt:** Prof Pediatrics, Yale Univ

Horbar, Jeffrey David MD (NP) - *Spec Exp:* Neonatal-Perinatal Medicine - General; **Hospital:** Fletcher Allen Hlth Care Med Ctr - Campus; **Address:** Fletcher Allen Healthcare, 111 Colchester Ave Bldg McClure, Burlington, VT 05401; **Phone:** (802) 847-0026; **Board Cert:** Pediatrics 1982, Neonatal-Perinatal Medicine 1983; **Med School:** SUNY Downstate 1977; **Resid:** Pediatrics, Med Ctr Hosp Vermont, Burlington, VT 1977-1979; **Fellow:** Obstetrics & Gynecology, Med Ctr Hosp Vermont, Burlington, VT 1979-1981

Mid Atlantic

Driscoll, John MD (NP) - *Spec Exp:* Neonatal-Perinatal Medicine - General; **Hospital:** NY Presby Hosp - Columbia Presby Med Ctr (page 70); **Address:** 3959 Broadway, Ste 114S, New York, NY 10032; **Phone:** (212) 305-2934; **Board Cert:** Pediatrics 1970, Neonatal-Perinatal Medicine 1975; **Med School:** Wake Forest Univ Sch Med 1962; **Resid:** Pediatrics, Children's Hosp, Pittsburgh, PA 1962-1963; Pediatrics, Columbia-Presbyterian Hosp, New York, NY 1967-1969; **Fellow:** Neonatal-Perinatal Medicine, Columbia-Presbyterian Hosp, New York, NY 1969-1971; **Fac Appt:** Prof Pediatrics, Columbia P&S

Hurt, Hallam MD (NP) - *Spec Exp:* Neonatology; **Hospital:** Albert Einstein Med Ctr; **Address:** Albert Einstein Med Ctr, Lifter Bldg, 5501 Old York Rd, Fl 2nd - rm 2601, Philadelphia, PA 19140; **Phone:** (215) 456-6696; **Board Cert:** Pediatrics 1976, Neonatal-Perinatal Medicine 1977; **Med School:** Univ VA Sch Med 1971; **Resid:** Pediatrics, Univ Virginia Med Ctr, Charlottesville, VA 1972-1974; **Fellow:** Neonatal-Perinatal Medicine, Univ Virginia Med Ctr, Charlottesville, VA 1974-1976; **Fac Appt:** Prof Pediatrics, Temple Univ

Lawson, Edward Earle MD (NP) - *Spec Exp:* Pregnancy-High Risk; Breathing Disorders; **Hospital:** Johns Hopkins Hosp - Baltimore; **Address:** Johns Hopkins Hospital, 600 N Wolfe St, Bldg CMSC - rm 210, Baltimore, MD 21287-3200; **Phone:** (410) 955-5259; **Board Cert:** Neonatal-Perinatal Medicine 1997, Pediatrics 1997; **Med School:** Northwestern Univ 1972; **Resid:** Pediatrics, Chldns Hosp Med Ctr, Boston, MA 1973-1975; **Fellow:** Neonatal-Perinatal Medicine, Harvard Med Sch, Boston, MA 1975-1977; **Fac Appt:** Prof Pediatrics, Univ NC Sch Med

Polin, Richard MD (NP) - *Spec Exp:* Neonatal Sepsis; **Hospital:** NY Presby Hosp - Columbia Presby Med Ctr (page 70); **Address:** 3959 Broadway BHS 115, New York, NY 10032; **Phone:** (212) 305-5827; **Board Cert:** Pediatrics 1975, Neonatal-Perinatal Medicine 1977; **Med School:** Temple Univ 1970; **Resid:** Pediatrics, Chldns Meml Hosp, Chicago, IL 1971-1972; Pediatrics, Babies Hosp-Columbia Presby, New York, NY 1972-1975; **Fellow:** Neonatal-Perinatal Medicine, Babies Hosp-Columbia Presby, New York, NY 1973-1974; **Fac Appt:** Prof Pediatrics, Columbia P&S

Southeast

Bancalari, Eduardo MD (NP) - *Spec Exp:* Neonatology; **Hospital:** Univ of Miami - Jackson Meml Hosp; **Address:** Dept Pediatrics (R-131), PO Box 016960, Miami, FL 33101; **Phone:** (305) 585-2328; **Board Cert:** Neonatal-Perinatal Medicine 1993, Pediatrics 1993; **Med School:** Chile 1966; **Resid:** Pediatrics, Hosp Luis Calvo Mackenna, Santiago, Chile 1967-1969; **Fellow:** Pediatric Cardiology, Univ Miami Med Ctr, Miami, FL 1971; **Fac Appt:** Prof Pediatrics, Univ Miami Sch Med

Boyle, Robert John MD (NP) - *Spec Exp:* Neonatology; **Hospital:** Univ of VA Hlth Sys (page 79); **Address:** UVA Hlth Sci Ctr, Dept Pediatrics, PO Box 800386, Charlottesville, VA 22908; **Phone:** (434) 924-5429; **Board Cert:** Neonatal-Perinatal Medicine 1979, Pediatrics 1978; **Med School:** Johns Hopkins Univ 1973; **Resid:** Pediatrics, Rainbow Babies Chldns Hosp 1973-1976; **Fellow:** Neonatal-Perinatal Medicine, Women's Infants Hosp 1976-1978; **Fac Appt:** Assoc Prof Pediatrics, Univ VA Sch Med

Bucciarelli, Richard L MD (NP) - *Spec Exp:* Neonatal Cardiology; **Hospital:** Shands Hlthcre at Univ of FL (page 73); **Address:** 1600 SW Archer Rd, Ste M-100, 1600 SW Archer Rd, Ste M-100, Gainesville, FL 32610; **Phone:** (352) 392-9315; **Board Cert:** Pediatric Cardiology 1977, Neonatal-Perinatal Medicine 1977; **Med School:** Univ Mich Med Sch 1972; **Resid:** Pediatrics, Shands Hosp-Univ Fla, Gainesville, FL 1974-1975; **Fellow:** Neonatal-Perinatal Medicine, Shands Hosp-Univ Fla, Gainesville, FL 1975-1977; **Fac Appt:** Prof Pediatrics, Univ Fla Coll Med

Neu, Josef MD (NP) - *Spec Exp:* Neonatal Nutrition; **Hospital:** Shands Hlthcre at Univ of FL (page 73); **Address:** Shands Healthcare-Univ Fla, 1600 SW Archer Rd, Gainesville, FL 32610; **Phone:** (352) 392-3020; **Board Cert:** Neonatal-Perinatal Medicine 1981, Pediatric Critical Care Medicine 1987; **Med School:** Univ Wisc 1975; **Resid:** Pediatrics, Johns Hopkins Hosp, Baltimore, MD 1975-1978; **Fellow:** Neonatal-Perinatal Medicine, Stanford Univ, Stanford, CA 1978-1980; **Fac Appt:** Prof Pediatrics, Univ Fla Coll Med

Sola, Augusto MD (NP) - *Spec Exp:* Neonatal-Perinatal Medicine - General; **Hospital:** Emory Univ Hosp; **Address:** Emory University, Div Neonatology, 2040 Ridgewood Drive NE, Ste 101, Atlanta, GA 30322; **Phone:** (404) 727-5765; **Board Cert:** Neonatal-Perinatal Medicine 1979, Pediatrics 1979; **Med School:** Argentina 1973; **Resid:** Pediatrics, St Vincent's Hosp, Worchester, MA 1975-1976; Pediatrics, Univ Mass Meml Med Ctr, Worchester, MA 1976-1977; **Fellow:** Neonatal-Perinatal Medicine, Univ Mass Meml Med Ctr, Worchester, MA 1977-1978; **Fac Appt:** Prof Pediatrics, Emory Univ

Stiles, Alan MD (NP) - *Spec Exp:* Neonatology; **Hospital:** Univ of NC Hosp (page 77); **Address:** 509 Burnett-Womack Bldg, Box CB7220, Chapel Hill, NC 27599; **Phone:** (919) 966-4427; **Board Cert:** Pediatrics 1984, Neonatal-Perinatal Medicine 1985; **Med School:** Univ NC Sch Med 1977; **Resid:** Pediatrics, North Carolina Meml Hosp, Chapel Hill, NC 1978-1982; **Fellow:** Neonatal-Perinatal Medicine, Chldns Hosp/Brigham Hosp, Boston, MA 1982-1985; **Fac Appt:** Prof Pediatrics, Univ NC Sch Med

Midwest

Jobe, Alan Hall MD/PhD (NP) - *Spec Exp:* Surfactant Biology; Respiritory Distress Syndrome (ARDS); Bronchopulmonary Dysplasia; **Hospital:** Cincinnati Chldns Hosp Med Ctr; **Address:** Children's Hosp Med Ctr, 3333 Burnett, Cincinnati, OH 45229-3039; **Phone:** (513) 636-8563; **Board Cert:** Pediatrics 1978, Neonatal-Perinatal Medicine 2000; **Med School:** UCSD 1973; **Resid:** Pediatrics, UCSD, San Diego, CA 1974-1975; **Fellow:** Neonatal-Perinatal Medicine, UCSD, San Diego, CA 1975-1977; **Fac Appt:** Prof Neonatal-Perinatal Medicine, Univ Cincinnati

Lemons, James A MD (NP) - *Spec Exp:* Neonatology; Perinatal Medicine; **Hospital:** Riley Chldrn's Hosp (page 588); **Address:** 699 West Drive, Bldg RR - Ste 208, Indianapolis, IN 46202-5119; **Phone:** (317) 274-4716; **Board Cert:** Pediatrics 1993, Neonatal-Perinatal Medicine 1993; **Med School:** Northwestern Univ 1969; **Resid:** Neonatal-Perinatal Medicine, U Mich Med Sch, Ann Arbor, MI 1970-1972; **Fellow:** Neonatal-Perinatal Medicine, U Colo Med Ctr 1973-1975; **Fac Appt:** Prof Pediatrics, Indiana Univ

Martin, Richard MD (NP) - *Spec Exp:* Neonatology; Neonatal Respiratory Disease; **Hospital:** Rainbow Babies & Chldns Hosp; **Address:** 11100 Euclid Ave, Cleveland, OH 44106; **Phone:** (216) 844-3387; **Board Cert:** Neonatal-Perinatal Medicine 1977, Pediatrics 1976; **Med School:** Australia 1970; **Resid:** Pediatrics, Univ Missouri, Columbia, MO 1972-1973; **Fellow:** Neonatal-Perinatal Medicine, Case West Res Univ, Cleveland, OH 1974-1975; **Fac Appt:** Prof Pediatrics, Case West Res Univ

Steinhorn, Robin MD (NP) - *Spec Exp:* Pulmonary Hypertension; Nitric Oxide Therapy; **Hospital:** Children's Mem Hosp; **Address:** 2300 Children's Plaza, Box 45, Chicago, IL 60614; **Phone:** (773) 880-4142; **Board Cert:** Neonatal-Perinatal Medicine 1997, Pediatrics 1989; **Med School:** Washington Univ, St Louis 1980; **Resid:** Obstetrics & Gynecology, Barnes Hosp, St Louis, MO 1980-1983; Pediatrics, Univ Minn, Minneapolis, MN 1983-1986; **Fellow:** Neonatal-Perinatal Medicine, Univ Minn, Minneapolis, MN 1986-1988; **Fac Appt:** Assoc Prof Neonatal-Perinatal Medicine, Northwestern Univ

Southwest

Adams, James M MD (NP) - *Spec Exp:* Lung Disease-Newborn; **Hospital:** TX Chldns Hosp - Houston; **Address:** 6621 Fannin St, Ste A340, Houston, TX 77030; **Phone:** (832) 824-1380; **Board Cert:** Pediatrics 1975, Neonatal-Perinatal Medicine 1975; **Med School:** Baylor Coll Med 1969; **Resid:** Pediatrics, Baylor Affil Hosps, Houston, TX 1971-1973; **Fellow:** Neonatal-Perinatal Medicine, Baylor Univ, Houston, TX 1973-1975; **Fac Appt:** Prof Pediatrics, Baylor Coll Med

Denson, Susan Ellen MD (NP) - *Spec Exp:* Neonatology; **Hospital:** Meml Hermann Hosp; **Address:** Univ Tex Med Sch - Peds, 6431 Fannin St, Ste 3-256, Houston, TX 77030; **Phone:** (713) 500-5726; **Board Cert:** Pediatrics 1978, Neonatal-Perinatal Medicine 1979; **Med School:** Univ Tex SW, Dallas 1972; **Resid:** Pediatrics, Univ Ariz, Tucson, AZ 1973-1974; **Fellow:** Neonatal-Perinatal Medicine, Univ Ariz, Tucson, AZ 1974-1975; Neonatal-Perinatal Medicine, Univ Tex Med Sch, Houston, TX 1975-1976; **Fac Appt:** Prof Pediatrics, Univ Tex, Houston

Escobedo, Marilyn Barnard MD (NP) - *Spec Exp:* Neonatology; **Hospital:** Chldn's Hosp at OU Med Ctr; **Address:** 940 NW 13th St, rm 2B2311, Oklahoma City, OK 73104; **Phone:** (405) 271-5215; **Board Cert:** Pediatrics 1986, Neonatal-Perinatal Medicine 1986; **Med School:** Washington Univ, St Louis 1970; **Resid:** Pediatrics, Chldns Hosp, St Louis, MO 1971-1972; Pediatrics, Chldns Hosp, St Louis, MO 1972-1973; **Fellow:** Neonatal-Perinatal Medicine, Vanderbilt Univ, Nashville, TN 1974-1976; **Fac Appt:** Prof Pediatrics, Univ Okla Coll Med

NEONATAL-PERINATAL MEDICINE

Garcia-Prats, Joseph MD (NP) - *Spec Exp:* Lung Disease-Newborn; **Hospital:** TX Chldns Hosp - Houston; **Address:** Ben Taub Genl Hosp, Dept Neonatalogy, 1504 Taub Loop, Houston, TX 77030; **Phone:** (713) 873-3515; **Board Cert:** Pediatrics 1977, Neonatal-Perinatal Medicine 1977; **Med School:** Tulane Univ 1972; **Resid:** Pediatrics, Baylor Affil Hosp, Houston, TX 1972-1975; **Fellow:** Neonatal-Perinatal Medicine, Baylor Affil Hosp, Houston, TX 1975-1977; **Fac Appt:** Assoc Prof Pediatrics, Baylor Coll Med

Odom, Michael W MD (NP) - *Spec Exp:* Neonatology; **Hospital:** Univ of Texas Hlth & Sci Ctr; **Address:** 7703 Floyd Curl Drive, Dept Ped, MC 7812, San Antonio, TX 78229; **Phone:** (210) 567-5225; **Board Cert:** Pediatrics 1987, Neonatal-Perinatal Medicine 1997; **Med School:** Univ Tex SW, Dallas 1983; **Resid:** Pediatrics, Vanderbilt Univ Affil Hosps, Nashville, TN 1983-1986; **Fellow:** Neonatal-Perinatal Medicine, Mt Zion Med Ctr Rsch Inst, San Francisco, CA 1986-1989; **Fac Appt:** Assoc Prof Pediatrics, Univ Tex, San Antonio

Perlman, Jeffrey MD (NP) - *Spec Exp:* Critically Ill Infants; Prematurity/Low Birth Weight Infants; **Hospital:** Parkland Mem Hosp; **Address:** Univ Texas SW Med Ctr at Dallas, Dept Pediatrics, 5323 Harry Hines Blvd, Dallas, TX 75390-9063; **Phone:** (214) 648-3903; **Board Cert:** Pediatrics 1983, Neonatal-Perinatal Medicine 1983; **Med School:** South Africa 1974; **Resid:** Pediatrics, Johannesburg Chlds Hosp, South Africa 1977-1979; Pediatrics, St Louis Chldns Hosp, St Louis, MO 1979-1981; **Fellow:** Neonatal-Perinatal Medicine, St Louis Chldns Hosp, St Louis, MO 1981-1983; **Fac Appt:** Assoc Prof Pediatrics, Univ Tex SW, Dallas

Seidner, Steven Richard MD (NP) - *Spec Exp:* Neonatal-Perinatal Medicine - General; **Hospital:** Univ of Texas Hlth & Sci Ctr; **Address:** Univ Texas Hlth Sci Ctr, Dept Peds, 7703 Floyd Curl Drive, MC 7812, San Antonio, TX 78229-3900; **Phone:** (210) 567-5229; **Board Cert:** Pediatrics 1987, Neonatal-Perinatal Medicine 1987; **Med School:** Univ Ariz Coll Med 1982; **Resid:** Pediatrics, Harbor-UCLA Med Ctr., Torrance, CA 1983-1985; **Fellow:** Neonatal-Perinatal Medicine, Harbor-UCLA Med Ctr., Torrance, CA 1985-1988; **Fac Appt:** Assoc Prof Pediatrics, Univ Tex, San Antonio

Tyson, Jon Edward MD (NP) - *Spec Exp:* Neonatology; Epidemiology; **Hospital:** Univ of Texas Hlth & Sci Ctr; **Address:** Univ Tex, Center Clin Research, 6431 Fannin St, MSB 2.106, Houston, TX 77030; **Phone:** (713) 500-5651; **Board Cert:** Pediatrics 1973, Neonatal-Perinatal Medicine 1975; **Med School:** Tulane Univ 1968; **Resid:** Pediatrics, Univ Tenn/Memphis Hosp, Memphis, TN 1968-1971; **Fellow:** Neonatology, McMaster Univ, Hamilton, Ont, Canada 1973-1975; **Fac Appt:** Prof Pediatrics, Univ Tex, Houston

West Coast and Pacific

Kitterman, Joseph A MD (NP) - *Spec Exp:* Neonatology; **Hospital:** UCSF Med Ctr; **Address:** UCSF Sch Med, Dept Ped, Room U-503, Box 0734, San Francisco, CA 94143-0734; **Phone:** (415) 476-7242; **Board Cert:** Pediatrics 1969, Neonatal-Perinatal Medicine 1975; **Med School:** McGill Univ 1962; **Resid:** Pediatrics, UCSF, San Francisco, CA 1965-1967; **Fellow:** Neonatal-Perinatal Medicine, UCSF, San Francisco, CA 1967-1970; **Fac Appt:** Prof Pediatrics, UCSF

Stevenson, David K MD (NP) - *Spec Exp:* Neonatology; **Hospital:** Stanford Med Ctr; **Address:** 750 Welch Rd, Ste 315, Palo Alto, CA 94304; **Phone:** (650) 723-5711; **Board Cert:** Pediatrics 1979, Neonatal-Perinatal Medicine 1997; **Med School:** Univ Wash 1975; **Resid:** Pediatrics, Univ Washington, Seattle, WA 1976-1977; **Fellow:** Neonatal-Perinatal Medicine, Stanford Univ, Stanford, CA 1977-1979; **Fac Appt:** Prof Pediatrics, Stanford Univ

NEPHROLOGY

(a subspecialty of INTERNAL MEDICINE)

An internist who treats disorders of the kidney, high blood pressure, fluid and mineral balance and dialysis of body wastes when the kidneys do not function. This specialist consults with surgeons about kidney transplantation.

INTERNAL MEDICINE

An internist is a personal physician who provides long-term, comprehensive care in the office and the hospital, managing both common and complex illness of adolescents, adults and the elderly. Internists are trained in the diagnosis and treatment of cancer, infections and diseases affecting the heart, blood, kidneys, joints and digestive, respiratory and vascular systems. They are also trained in the essentials of primary care internal medicine which incorporates an understanding of disease prevention, wellness, substance abuse, mental health and effective treatment of common problems of the eyes, ears, skin, nervous system and reproductive organs.

Training required: Three years in internal medicine *plus* additional training and examination for certification in nephrology

PHYSICIAN LISTINGS

New England

Aronson, Peter Samuel MD (Nep) - *Spec Exp:* Acid-Base Disorders; **Hospital:** Yale - New Haven Hosp; **Address:** Yale Sch Med, Sect Neph—2073-LMP, 333 Cedar St, Box 208029, New Haven, CT 06520-8029; **Phone:** (203) 785-4186; **Board Cert:** Nephrology 1976, Internal Medicine 1973; **Med School:** NYU Sch Med 1970; **Resid:** Internal Medicine, NC Meml Hosp-UNC, Chapel Hill, NC 1971-1972; **Fellow:** Nephrology, Yale Univ Sch Med, New Haven, CT 1974-1977; **Fac Appt:** Prof Medicine, Yale Univ

Brenner, Barry M MD (Nep) - *Spec Exp:* Hypertension; Diabetic Kidney Disease; Kidney Failure-Acute; **Hospital:** Brigham & Women's Hosp; **Address:** Div Renal Medicine, 75 Francis St, Boston, MA 02115; **Phone:** (617) 732-5850; **Med School:** Univ Pittsburgh 1962; **Resid:** Internal Medicine, Albert Einstein Coll Med, New York, NY 1966-1967; **Fellow:** Nephrology, Nat Inst Health, Bethesda, MD 1967; **Fac Appt:** Prof Medicine, Harvard Med Sch

Carpenter, Charles B MD (Nep) - *Spec Exp:* Transplant Medicine-Kidney; Immunogenetics; **Hospital:** Brigham & Women's Hosp; **Address:** Brigham & Women's Hosp, Dept Nephr, 75 Francis St, Boston, MA 02115; **Phone:** (617) 732-5244; **Board Cert:** Internal Medicine 1966; **Med School:** Harvard Med Sch 1958; **Resid:** Internal Medicine, Meml Hosp, New York, NY 1959-1960; Internal Medicine, Bellevue Hosp, New York, NY 1959-1960; **Fellow:** Nephrology, Peter Bent Brigham Hosp, Boston, MA 1962-1966; Pathology, Peter Bent Brigham Hosp, Boston, MA 1962-1966; **Fac Appt:** Prof Medicine, Harvard Med Sch

Coggins, Cecil MD (Nep) - *Spec Exp:* Kidney Disease; Hypertension; **Hospital:** MA Genl Hosp; **Address:** Beacon Hill, 100 Charles River Plaza, Fl 5th, Boston, MA 02114; **Phone:** (617) 726-4900; **Board Cert:** Nephrology 1975, Internal Medicine 1968; **Med School:** Harvard Med Sch 1958; **Resid:** Internal Medicine, Mass Genl Hosp, Boston, MA 1958-1959; Internal Medicine, Stanford Med Ctr, Stanford, CA 1961-1965; **Fellow:** Nephrology, Stanford Med Ctr, Stanford, CA 1962-1963; Nephrology, Mass Genl Hosp, Boston, MA 1965-1967; **Fac Appt:** Assoc Prof Medicine, Harvard Med Sch

Fang, Leslie MD (Nep) - *Spec Exp:* Kidney Failure-Chronic; **Hospital:** MA Genl Hosp; **Address:** 100 Charles River Plaza, Ste 701, Boston, MA 02114-2724; **Phone:** (617) 742-2054; **Board Cert:** Internal Medicine 1977, Nephrology 1980; **Med School:** Harvard Med Sch 1974; **Resid:** Internal Medicine, Mass Genl Hosp, Boston, MA 1975-1976; Internal Medicine, Mass Genl Hosp, Boston, MA 1979-1980; **Fellow:** Nephrology, Mass Genl Hosp, Boston, MA 1976-1978

Kliger, Alan MD (Nep) - *Spec Exp:* Kidney Disease; Kidney Disease-Metabolic; **Hospital:** Hosp of St Raphael's; **Address:** 136 Sherman Ave, New Haven, CT 06511-5238; **Phone:** (203) 787-0117; **Board Cert:** Internal Medicine 1973, Nephrology 1976; **Med School:** SUNY Syracuse 1970; **Resid:** Internal Medicine, SUNY Upstate Med Ctr, Syracuse, NY 1971-1973; **Fellow:** Nephrology, Georgetown Univ Hosp, Washington, DC 1973-1975; **Fac Appt:** Clin Prof Medicine, Yale Univ

Perrone, Ronald MD (Nep) - *Spec Exp:* Hypertension; **Hospital:** New England Med Ctr - Boston; **Address:** New England Med Ctr, 750 Washington St, Box 391, Boston, MA 02111; **Phone:** (617) 636-5866; **Board Cert:** Internal Medicine 1979, Nephrology 1982; **Med School:** Hahnemann Univ 1975; **Resid:** Internal Medicine, Grady Meml Hosp, Atlanta, GA 1976-1978; **Fellow:** Nephrology, Boston Med Ctr, Boston, MA 1979-1982; **Fac Appt:** Assoc Prof Medicine, Tufts Univ

Salant, David MD (Nep) - *Spec Exp:* Kidney Disease-Glomerular; Kidney Disease-Immunologic; **Hospital:** Boston Med Ctr; **Address:** 720 Harrison Ave, Boston, MA 02118; **Phone:** (617) 638-7480; **Board Cert:** Internal Medicine 1978, Nephrology 1980; **Med School:** South Africa 1969; **Resid:** Johannesburg Genl Hosp, South Africa 1971-1973; **Fellow:** Nephrology, Boston Univ Med Ctr., Boston, MA 1977-1978

Seifter, Julian L MD (Nep) - *Spec Exp:* Diabetic Kidney Disease; Kidney Failure-Chronic; Kidney Stones; **Hospital:** Brigham & Women's Hosp; **Address:** Brigham & Women's Hosp, Div Renal, 45 Francis St, Boston, MA 02115; **Phone:** (617) 732-7482; **Board Cert:** Nephrology 1980; **Med School:** Albert Einstein Coll Med 1975; **Resid:** Internal Medicine, Bronx Muni Hosp Ctr, Bronx, NY 1978; **Fellow:** Nephrology, Yale-New Haven Hosp, New Haven, CT 1982; **Fac Appt:** Assoc Prof Medicine, Harvard Med Sch

Tolkoff-Rubin, Nina MD (Nep) - *Spec Exp:* Transplant Medicine-Kidney; Hypertension; Kidney Failure-Acute; **Hospital:** MA Genl Hosp; **Address:** 55 Fruit St, Bldg GRB - Ste 1003J, Boston, MA 02114; **Phone:** (617) 726-3706; **Board Cert:** Nephrology 1974, Internal Medicine 1972; **Med School:** Harvard Med Sch 1968; **Resid:** Internal Medicine, Mass Genl Hosp, Boston, MA 1969-1970; Internal Medicine, Mass Genl Hosp, Boston, MA 1971-1972; **Fellow:** Nephrology, Mass Genl Hosp, Boston, MA 1970-1971; **Fac Appt:** Assoc Prof Medicine, Harvard Med Sch

Mid Atlantic

Appel, Gerald MD (Nep) - *Spec Exp:* Kidney Disease-Glomerular; Lupus Nephritis; Kidney Disease; **Hospital:** NY Presby Hosp - Columbia Presby Med Ctr (page 70); **Address:** 622 W 168th St, Ste 4124, New York, NY 10032-3720; **Phone:** (212) 305-3273; **Board Cert:** Internal Medicine 1975, Nephrology 1978; **Med School:** Albert Einstein Coll Med 1972; **Resid:** Internal Medicine, Columbia Presby, New York, NY 1972-1975; **Fellow:** Nephrology, Columbia Presby, New York, NY 1975-1976; Nephrology, Yale, New Haven, CT 1976-1978; **Fac Appt:** Clin Prof Medicine, Columbia P&S

Cohen, David Jonathan MD (Nep) - *Spec Exp:* Transplant Medicine-Kidney; Glomerulonephritis; **Hospital:** NY Presby Hosp - Columbia Presby Med Ctr (page 70); **Address:** 622 W 168th St, rm PH 4-124, New York, NY 10032-3720; **Phone:** (212) 305-3273; **Board Cert:** Internal Medicine 1980, Nephrology 1984; **Med School:** Albert Einstein Coll Med 1977; **Resid:** Internal Medicine, Mount Sinai Med Ctr, New York, NY 1977-1978; Internal Medicine, Mount Sinai Med Ctr, New York, NY 1978-1980; **Fellow:** Nephrology, Columbia Presby Med Ctr, New York, NY 1980-1981; Transplant/Immunology, Brigham & Women's Hosp, Boston, MA 1981-1983; **Fac Appt:** Assoc Prof Medicine, Columbia P&S

Dosa, Stefan MD (Nep) - *Spec Exp:* Transplant Medicine-Kidney; **Hospital:** Washington Hosp Ctr; **Address:** 730 24th St NW, Ste 17, Washington, DC 20037; **Phone:** (202) 337-7660; **Board Cert:** Internal Medicine 1980, Nephrology 1982; **Med School:** Czech Republic 1967; **Resid:** Manchester Royal Infirmary, England, UK 1972-1977; **Fellow:** Univ Cincinnati, Cincinnati, OH 1977-1979; **Fac Appt:** Assoc Clin Prof Medicine, Geo Wash Univ

Friedman, Eli A MD (Nep) - *Spec Exp:* Diabetic Kidney Disease; Transplant Medicine-Kidney; **Hospital:** Univ Hosp - Brklyn; **Address:** SUNY Hlth Sci Ctr, 450 Clarkson Ave, Box 52, Brooklyn, NY 11203; **Phone:** (718) 270-1584; **Board Cert:** Internal Medicine 1967, Nephrology 1974; **Med School:** SUNY Downstate 1957; **Resid:** Internal Medicine, Peter Bent Brigham Hosp, Boston, MA 1958-1960; **Fellow:** Nephrology, Peter Bent Brigham Hosp, Boston, MA 1960-1961; **Fac Appt:** Prof Medicine, SUNY Downstate

Johnston, James MD (Nep) - *Spec Exp:* Kidney Disease-Diabetic; Hypertension; **Hospital:** UPMC - Presbyterian Univ Hosp; **Address:** Univ of Pittsburgh Physicians, Div Renal, 3550 Terrace St, Scaife Hall, rm A915, Pittsburgh, PA 15213; **Phone:** (412) 647-7157; **Board Cert:** Internal Medicine 1982, Nephrology 1984; **Med School:** Univ Pittsburgh 1979; **Resid:** Internal Medicine, Montefiore Hosp, Pittsburgh, PA 1980-1982; **Fellow:** Nephrology, Brigham & Women's Hosp, Boston, MA 1983-1986; Nephrology, Univ Pittsburgh Med Ctr, Pittsburgh, PA 1982-1983; **Fac Appt:** Assoc Prof Nephrology, Univ Pittsburgh

Madaio, Michael P MD (Nep) - *Spec Exp:* *Lupus Nephritis; Kidney Disease-Glomerular;* **Hospital:** Hosp Univ Penn (page 78); **Address:** Renal Electrolyte/Hypertension Div, 3400 Spruce St, Philadelphia, PA 19104; **Phone:** (215) 662-2638; **Board Cert:** Internal Medicine 1977, Nephrology 1980; **Med School:** Albany Med Coll 1974; **Resid:** Internal Medicine, Med Coll Va, Richmond, VA 1975-1978; **Fellow:** Nephrology, Boston Univ, Boston, MA 1978-1981; Tufts Univ, Boston, MA 1981-1982; **Fac Appt:** Prof Medicine, Univ Penn

Piraino, Beth Marie MD (Nep) - *Spec Exp:* *Kidney Failure; Hypertension;* **Hospital:** UPMC - Presbyterian Univ Hosp; **Address:** UPMC Montefiore-Univ Pittsburgh Phys, Div Renal, 3459 Fifth Ave, Pittsburgh, PA 15213; **Phone:** (412) 383-4899; **Board Cert:** Internal Medicine 1980, Nephrology 1982; **Med School:** Med Coll PA Hahnemann 1977; **Resid:** Internal Medicine, Presby Univ Hosp, Pittsburgh, PA 1978-1980; **Fellow:** Nephrology, Presby Univ Hosp, Pittsburgh, PA 1980-1982; **Fac Appt:** Prof Medicine, Univ Pittsburgh

Rakowski, Thomas A MD (Nep) - *Spec Exp:* *Polycystic Kidney Disease; Kidney Disease-Glomerular;* **Hospital:** Georgetown Univ Hosp; **Address:** 3800 Reservoir Rd NW, PHC Bldg- Fl 6, Washington, DC 20007; **Phone:** (202) 687-9183; **Board Cert:** Nephrology 1974, Internal Medicine 1972; **Med School:** Hahnemann Univ 1969; **Resid:** Internal Medicine, Georgetown Univ, Washington, DC 1970-1971; **Fellow:** Nephrology, Georgetown Univ, Washington, DC 1971-1972

Scheel Jr, Paul Joseph MD (Nep) - *Spec Exp:* *Kidney Failure;* **Hospital:** Johns Hopkins Hosp - Baltimore; **Address:** 1830 E Monument St, Ste 412, Baltimore, MD 21205; **Phone:** (410) 955-7658; **Board Cert:** Internal Medicine 1990, Nephrology 1997; **Med School:** Georgetown Univ 1987; **Resid:** Internal Medicine, Johns Hopkins Hosp, Baltimore, MD 1987-1990; **Fellow:** Nephrology, Johns Hopkins Hosp, Baltimore, MD 1990-1992; **Fac Appt:** Assoc Prof Medicine, Johns Hopkins Univ

Scheinman, Steven J MD (Nep) - *Spec Exp:* *Kidney Stones; Bartter's Syndrome; Gitelman's Sydrome;* **Hospital:** Univ. Hosp. SUNY Upstate Med. Univ.; **Address:** Div Nephrology, 750 S Adams St, Syracuse, NY 13210; **Phone:** (315) 464-5290; **Board Cert:** Infectious Disease 1980, Nephrology 1984; **Med School:** Yale Univ 1977; **Resid:** Internal Medicine, Yale New Haven Hosp, New Haven, CT 1978-1990; Internal Medicine, Upstate Med Ctr, Syracuse, NY 1980-1981; **Fellow:** Nephrology, Upstate Med Ctr, Syracuse, NY 1981-1983; Nephrology, Yale New Haven Hosp, New Haven, CT 1983-1984; **Fac Appt:** Prof Medicine, SUNY Syracuse

Townsend, Raymond R MD (Nep) - *Spec Exp:* *Hypertension; Renal Artery Stenosis;* **Hospital:** Hosp Univ Penn (page 78); **Address:** Renal Electrolyte/Hypertension Div, 3400 Spruce St, Philadelphia, PA 19104; **Phone:** (215) 662-2638; **Board Cert:** Internal Medicine 1982, Nephrology 1984; **Med School:** Hahnemann Univ 1979; **Resid:** Internal Medicine, Allegheny Genl Hosp, Pittsburgh, PA 1980-1982; **Fellow:** Nephrology, Temple Univ Hosp, Philadelphia, PA 1982-1984; **Fac Appt:** Assoc Prof Medicine, Univ Penn

Umans, Jason MD/PhD (Nep) - *Spec Exp:* *Hypertension; Kidney Disease;* **Hospital:** Georgetown Univ Hosp; **Address:** 3800 Reservoir Rd NW, PHC Bldg- Fl 6, Washington, DC 20007; **Phone:** (202) 687-9183; **Board Cert:** Internal Medicine 1988, Nephrology 1990; **Med School:** Cornell Univ-Weill Med Coll 1984; **Resid:** Internal Medicine, Univ Chicago Hosps, Chicago, IL 1984-1987; **Fellow:** Nephrology, Univ Chicago Hosps, Chicago, IL 1987-1988; **Fac Appt:** Assoc Prof Nephrology, Georgetown Univ

Wilcox, Christopher S MD (Nep) - *Spec Exp:* Hypertension-Renovascular/Adrenal; Hypertension-Drug Resistent; **Hospital:** Georgetown Univ Hosp; **Address:** Georgetown Univ Med Ctr - Pasquerilla Healthcare Ctr, 3800 Reservoir Rd NW, Bldg PHC - Fl 6th, Washington, DC 20007-2113; **Phone:** (202) 687-8539; **Board Cert:** Internal Medicine 1983, Nephrology 1986; **Med School:** England 1968; **Resid:** Internal Medicine, Middlesex Hosp, London, England 1970-1971; Nephrology, Middlesex Hosp, London, England 1971-1972; **Fellow:** Nephrology, Middlesex Hosp, London, England 1972-1975; **Fac Appt:** Prof Nephrology, Georgetown Univ

Williams, Gail S MD (Nep) - *Spec Exp:* Kidney Failure-Chronic; Transplant Medicine-Kidney; **Hospital:** NY Presby Hosp - Columbia Presby Med Ctr (page 70); **Address:** 161 Ft. Washington Ave, Ste 351, Atchley Pavilion, New York, NY 10032; **Phone:** (212) 305-5376; **Board Cert:** Internal Medicine 1972, Nephrology 1974; **Med School:** Columbia P&S 1968; **Resid:** Internal Medicine, Columbia Presby Hosp, New York, NY 1970-1972; **Fellow:** Nephrology, Columbia Presby Hosp, New York, NY 1972-1973; **Fac Appt:** Assoc Clin Prof Medicine, Columbia P&S

Southeast

Bolton, Warren Kline MD (Nep) - *Spec Exp:* Kidney Disease-Glomerular; Kidney Disease; **Hospital:** Univ of VA Hlth Sys (page 79); **Address:** Univ of VA Hlth Scis Ctr, Box 800 133, Charlottesville, VA 22908; **Phone:** (804) 924-5125; **Board Cert:** Internal Medicine 1972, Nephrology 1974; **Med School:** Univ VA Sch Med 1969; **Resid:** Internal Medicine, Boston City Hosp, Chicago, IL 1970-1971; **Fellow:** Nephrology, Univ Chicago, Boston, MA 1971-1973; **Fac Appt:** Prof Medicine, Univ VA Sch Med

Bourgoignie, Jacques MD (Nep) - *Spec Exp:* Hypertension; Kidney Failure-Chronic; **Hospital:** Univ of Miami - Jackson Meml Hosp; **Address:** Div Nephrology & Hypertension, 1600 NW 10th Ave Bldg RMSB - rm 7168, MC R-126, Miami, FL 33136; **Phone:** (305) 243-6251; **Med School:** Belgium 1958; **Resid:** Internal Medicine, Catholic Univ- Louvain Hosp, Belgium 1958-1961; **Fellow:** VA Med Ctr, St Louis, MO 1963-1965; Nephrology, Wash Univ, St Louis, MO 1965-1968; **Fac Appt:** Prof Medicine, Univ Miami Sch Med

Buckalew Jr., Vardaman Moore MD (Nep) - *Spec Exp:* Hypertension; Kidney Disease; **Hospital:** Wake Forest Univ Baptist Med Ctr (page 81); **Address:** Wake Forest Univ Baptist Med Ctr, Medical Center Blvd, Winston Salem, NC 27157; **Phone:** (336) 716-2062; **Board Cert:** Internal Medicine 1966; **Med School:** Univ Penn **Resid:** Internal Medicine, Hosp Univ Penn, Philadelphia, PA 1958-1962; **Fellow:** Nephrology, Hosp Univ Penn, Philadelphia, PA 1964-1967; **Fac Appt:** Prof Nephrology, Wake Forest Univ Sch Med

Coffman, Thomas Myron MD (Nep) - *Spec Exp:* Transplant Medicine-Kidney; Hypertension; **Hospital:** Duke Univ Med Ctr (page 60); **Address:** Duke Univ Med Center, Box 3014, Durham, NC 27710; **Phone:** (919) 286-6947; **Board Cert:** Nephrology 1988, Internal Medicine 1983; **Med School:** Ohio State Univ 1980; **Resid:** Internal Medicine, Duke Univ Med Ctr, Durham, NC 1980-1983; **Fellow:** Nephrology, Duke Univ Med Ctr, Durham, NC 1983-1985; **Fac Appt:** Prof Medicine, Duke Univ

Falk, Ronald J MD (Nep) - *Spec Exp:* Kidney Disease-Glomerular; Lupus Nephritis; Vasculitis; **Hospital:** Univ of NC Hosp (page 77); **Address:** 349 MacNider Bldg, CB7155, Chapel Hill, NC 27599-7155; **Phone:** (919) 966-2561; **Board Cert:** Internal Medicine 1980, Nephrology 1982; **Med School:** Univ NC Sch Med 1977; **Resid:** Internal Medicine, Univ NC Sch Med, Chapel Hill, NC 1978-1980; Nephrology, Univ NC Sch Med, Chapel Hill, NC 1980-1981; **Fellow:** Research, Univ Minn, Minneapolis, MN 1981-1983; **Fac Appt:** Prof Medicine, Univ NC Sch Med

Gluck, Stephen MD (Nep) - *Spec Exp:* Kidney Disease-Glomerular; Diabetic Kidney Disease; Hypertensive Kidney Disease; **Hospital:** Shands Hlthcre at Univ of FL (page 73); **Address:** Univ Florida, Div Nephrology & Transplantation, 1600 SW Archer Rd, Box 100224, Gainesville, FL 32610-0224; **Phone:** (352) 392-4008; **Board Cert:** Internal Medicine 1980, Nephrology 1984; **Med School:** UCLA 1977; **Resid:** Internal Medicine, Columbia Presby Med Ctr, New York, NY 1977-1980; **Fellow:** Nephrology, Columbia Presby Med Ctr, New York, NY 1980-1983; **Fac Appt:** Prof Nephrology, Univ Fla Coll Med

Harris, Raymond C MD (Nep) - *Spec Exp:* Kidney Disease; Hypertension; **Hospital:** Vanderbilt Univ Med Ctr (page 80); **Address:** Vanderbilt Univ Med Ctr, C3121 Medical Center North, Nashville, TN 37232; **Phone:** (615) 322-2150; **Board Cert:** Internal Medicine 1981, Nephrology 1986; **Med School:** Emory Univ 1978; **Resid:** Internal Medicine, UCSF Med Ctr, San Francisco, CA 1979-1981; **Fellow:** Nephrology, Brigham & Womens Hosp, Boston, MA 1982-1986; **Fac Appt:** Prof Medicine, Vanderbilt Univ

Hoffman, David MD (Nep) - *Spec Exp:* Kidney Disease; Dialysis Care; **Hospital:** Baptist Hosp - Miami; **Address:** Miami Kidney Group, 7900 SW 57th Ave, Ste 21, South Miami, FL 33143-5546; **Phone:** (305) 662-3984; **Board Cert:** Internal Medicine 1976, Nephrology 1978; **Med School:** Univ Tenn Coll Med, Memphis 1971; **Resid:** Internal Medicine, Univ Miami Project to Cure Paralysis, Miami, FL 1972-1973; **Fellow:** Nephrology, Univ Miami Project to Cure Paralysis, Miami, FL 1975-1977

Okusa, Mark D MD (Nep) - *Spec Exp:* Kidney Failure-Chronic; Nephrotic Syndrome; **Hospital:** Univ of VA Hlth Sys (page 79); **Address:** Univ of VA Hlth Sci Ctr, Div Nephrology, Lee St, Box 800-133, Charlottesville, VA 22908-0133; **Phone:** (804) 924-5125; **Board Cert:** Internal Medicine 1985, Nephrology 1988; **Med School:** Med Coll VA 1982; **Resid:** Internal Medicine, Med Coll Virginia, Richmond, VA 1983-1985; **Fellow:** Nephrology, Yale Univ Sch Med, New Haven, CT 1985-1988; **Fac Appt:** Assoc Prof Medicine, Univ VA Sch Med

Roth, David MD (Nep) - *Spec Exp:* Transplant Medicine-Kidney; Kidney Failure-Chronic; **Hospital:** Univ of Miami - Jackson Meml Hosp; **Address:** Nephrology and Hypertension, 1600 NW 10th Ave, Bldg RMSB - rm 7168, Miami, FL 33101; **Phone:** (305) 243-6251; **Board Cert:** Internal Medicine 1980, Nephrology 1982; **Med School:** SUNY Downstate 1977; **Resid:** Internal Medicine, Univ Miami-Jackson Meml Hosp, Miami, FL 1977-1980; **Fellow:** Nephrology, Univ Miami-Jackson Meml Hosp, Miami, FL 1980-1982; **Fac Appt:** Prof Medicine, Univ Miami Sch Med

Schwab, Steve Joseph MD (Nep) - *Spec Exp:* Polycystic Kidney Disease; Kidney Failure; **Hospital:** Duke Univ Med Ctr (page 60); **Address:** Duke Univ Med Ctr, Box 3014, Durham, NC 27710; **Phone:** (919) 684-3355; **Board Cert:** Internal Medicine 1982, Nephrology 1986; **Med School:** Univ MO-Columbia Sch Med 1979; **Resid:** Internal Medicine, Univ Kans Med Ctr, Kansas City, KS 1980-1982; **Fellow:** Nephrology, Wash Univ-Barnes Hosp, St Louis, MO 1982-1984; **Fac Appt:** Prof Medicine, Duke Univ

Weiner, Irving David MD (Nep) - *Spec Exp:* Kidney Disease; Acid-Base Disorders; Kidney Stones; **Hospital:** Shands Hlthcre at Univ of FL (page 73); **Address:** Shands at Univ Florida, Dept Neph, PO Box 100224, Gainesville, FL 32610-0224; **Phone:** (352) 392-4008; **Board Cert:** Internal Medicine 1987, Nephrology 1990; **Med School:** Vanderbilt Univ 1984; **Resid:** Internal Medicine, Univ Texas Hlth Sci Ctr, San Antonio, TX 1984-1987; **Fac Appt:** Assoc Prof Medicine, Univ Fla Coll Med

Midwest

Black, Henry R MD (Nep) - *Spec Exp:* *Hypertension; Nephrotic Syndrome; Cholesterol/Lipid Disorder;* **Hospital:** Rush-Presby - St Luke's Med Ctr (page 72); **Address:** 1700 W Van Buren, Ste 470, Chicago, IL 60612; **Phone:** (312) 942-5910; **Board Cert:** Internal Medicine 1972, Nephrology 1974; **Med School:** NYU Sch Med 1967; **Resid:** Internal Medicine, Johns Hopkins Hosp, Baltimore, MD 1967-1968; Internal Medicine, Yale-New Haven Hosp, New Haven, CT 1971-1972; **Fellow:** Nephrology, Yale-New Haven Hosp, New Haven, CT 1972-1974

Brazy, Peter C MD (Nep) - *Spec Exp:* *Kidney Disease; Kidney Disease-Metabolic; Phosphate Homeostasis;* **Hospital:** Univ WI Hosp & Clins; **Address:** J5/223 UW Hosp, 600 Highland Ave, Madison, WI 53792; **Phone:** (608) 263-6808; **Board Cert:** Nephrology 1984, Internal Medicine 1978; **Med School:** Washington Univ, St Louis 1972; **Resid:** Internal Medicine, Barnes Hosp, St Louis, MO 1973-1974; **Fellow:** Nephrology, Duke Univ Med Ctr, Durham, NC 1976-1978; **Fac Appt:** Asst Prof Medicine, Univ Wisc

Coe, Fredric MD (Nep) - *Spec Exp:* *Medical Prevention of Kidney Stones; Fluid and Electrolyte Disorders; Kidney Stones;* **Hospital:** Univ of Chicago Hosps (page 76); **Address:** 5841 S Maryland Ave, MS 5100, Chicago, IL 60637; **Phone:** (773) 702-1475; **Board Cert:** Internal Medicine 1968; **Med School:** Univ Chicago-Pritzker Sch Med 1961; **Resid:** Internal Medicine, Michael Reese Hosp, Chicago, IL 1961-1965; **Fellow:** Nephrology, Univ Texas SW, Dallas, TX 1967-1969; **Fac Appt:** Prof Medicine, Univ Chicago-Pritzker Sch Med

Delmez, James Albert MD (Nep) - *Spec Exp:* *Kidney Disease;* **Hospital:** Barnes-Jewish Hosp (page 55); **Address:** 4921 Pakview Pl Fl 5 - Ste C, St Louis, MO 63110; **Phone:** (314) 362-7603; **Board Cert:** Internal Medicine 1976, Nephrology 1982; **Med School:** Univ Rochester 1973; **Resid:** Internal Medicine, Barnes Hosp, St Louis, MO 1974-1976; **Fellow:** Nephrology, Barnes Hosp, St Louis, MO 1976-1978; **Fac Appt:** Prof Medicine, Washington Univ, St Louis

Hruska, Keith Anthony MD (Nep) - *Spec Exp:* *Kidney Disease-Pediatric;* **Hospital:** St Louis Children's Hospital; **Address:** St Louis Chldn's Hospital, Dept Pediatrics, 660 S Euclid Ave, Box 8208, St Louis, MO 63110; **Phone:** (314) 286-2772; **Board Cert:** Internal Medicine 1972, Nephrology 1976; **Med School:** Creighton Univ 1969; **Resid:** Internal Medicine, NY Hosp-Cornell, New York, NY 1970-1971; Internal Medicine, Barnes Hosp-Wash U, St Louis, MO 1971-1972; **Fellow:** Nephrology, Barnes Hosp-Wash Univ, St Louis, MO 1972-1974

Josephson, Michelle Ann MD (Nep) - *Spec Exp:* *Transplant Medicine-Kidney;* **Hospital:** Univ of Chicago Hosps (page 76); **Address:** 5841 S Maryland Ave, MC-5100, Chicago, IL 60637; **Phone:** (773) 702-6134; **Board Cert:** Internal Medicine 1986, Nephrology 1990; **Med School:** Univ Penn 1983; **Resid:** Internal Medicine, Univ Chicago Hosps, Chicago, IL 1984-1986; **Fellow:** Nephrology, Univ Chicago, Chicago, IL 1987-1991; **Fac Appt:** Asst Prof Medicine, Univ Chicago-Pritzker Sch Med

Kasiske, Bertram MD (Nep) - *Spec Exp:* *Transplant Medicine-Kidney; Kidney Disease-Geriatric;* **Hospital:** Hennepin Cnty Med Ctr; **Address:** Dept Nephrology, 701 Park Ave S, Minneapolis, MN 55415-1623; **Phone:** (612) 347-6088; **Board Cert:** Internal Medicine 1980, Nephrology 1982; **Med School:** Univ Iowa Coll Med 1976; **Resid:** Internal Medicine, Hennepin Co Med Ctr, Minneapolis, MN 1976-1980; **Fellow:** Nephrology, Hennepin Co Med Ctr, Minneapolis, MN 1980-1983; **Fac Appt:** Prof Medicine, Univ Minn

Lewis, Edmund J MD (Nep) - *Spec Exp:* *Lupus Nephritis; Diabetic Kidney Disease;* **Hospital:** Rush-Presby - St Luke's Med Ctr (page 72); **Address:** 1426 W Washington Blvd, Chicago, IL 60607; **Phone:** (312) 850-8434; **Board Cert:** Internal Medicine 1969; **Med School:** Univ British Columbia Fac Med 1962; **Resid:** Internal Medicine, Johns Hopkins Hosp, Baltimore, MD 1962-1965; **Fellow:** Nephrology, Peter Bent Brigham Hosp, Boston, MA 1965-1966; Research, Peter Bent Brigham Hosp, Boston, MA 1968-1969; **Fac Appt:** Prof Medicine, Rush Med Coll

Owen, William F. MD (Nep) - *Spec Exp:* *Kidney Failure;* **Hospital:** Brigham & Women's Hosp; **Address:** 1620 Waukegan Rd, McGaw Park, IL 60085; **Phone:** (847) 473-6307; **Board Cert:** Internal Medicine 1984, Nephrology 1986; **Med School:** Tufts Univ 1980; **Resid:** Internal Medicine, Brigham Womens Hosp, Boston, MA 1981-1983; **Fellow:** Nephrology, Brigham Womens Hosp, Boston, MA 1983-1984; **Fac Appt:** Asst Prof Nephrology, Harvard Med Sch

Paganini, Emil MD (Nep) - *Spec Exp:* *Kidney Failure-Chronic; Kidney Failure-Acute;* **Hospital:** Cleveland Clin Fdn (page 57); **Address:** Cleveland Clinic Foundation, 9500 Euclid Ave, Cleveland, OH 44195; **Phone:** (216) 444-5792; **Board Cert:** Internal Medicine 1977; **Med School:** Italy 1973; **Resid:** Internal Medicine, Winthrop Univ Hosp, Mineola, NY 1975-1977; **Fellow:** Nephrology, Cleveland Clin Fdn, Cleveland, OH 1977-1979

Pohl, Marc MD (Nep) - *Spec Exp:* *Hypertension; Kidney Disease; Diabetes;* **Hospital:** Cleveland Clin Fdn (page 57); **Address:** 9500 Euclid Ave, Cleveland, OH 44195; **Phone:** (216) 444-6776; **Board Cert:** Internal Medicine 1972, Nephrology 1978; **Med School:** Case West Res Univ 1966; **Resid:** Internal Medicine, Univ Hosps Cleveland 1967-1968; Internal Medicine, Mass Genl Hosp, Boston, MA 1970-1971

Roguska-Kyts, Jadwiga MD (Nep) - *Spec Exp:* *Kidney Disease;* **Hospital:** Northwestern Meml Hosp; **Address:** 201 E Huron Street, Ste 11-205, Chicago, IL 60611; **Phone:** (312) 926-3626; **Board Cert:** Internal Medicine 1987, Nephrology 1976; **Med School:** Poland 1958; **Resid:** Internal Medicine, Northwestern Meml Hosp, Chicago, IL 1960-1962; **Fellow:** Nephrology, Northwestern Meml Hosp, Chicago, IL 1963-1965; **Fac Appt:** Assoc Prof Medicine, Northwestern Univ

Somerville, James MD (Nep) - *Spec Exp:* *Nephrology - General;* **Hospital:** Fairview-Univ Med Ctr - Univ Campus; **Address:** InterMed Consultants, 6363 France Ave S, Ste 400, Edina, MN 55435; **Phone:** (952) 920-2070; **Board Cert:** Nephrology 1982, Critical Care Medicine 1987; **Med School:** Univ MD Sch Med 1975; **Resid:** Internal Medicine, Hennepin Co Med Ctr, Minneapolis, MN 1975-1978; **Fellow:** Nephrology, Hennepin Co Med Ctr, Minneapolis, MN 1979-1980

Swartz, Richard D MD (Nep) - *Spec Exp:* *Kidney Failure; Dialysis Care;* **Hospital:** Univ of MI Hlth Ctr; **Address:** 3914 Taubman Ctr, Box 0364, 1500 E Med Ctr Drive, Ann Arbor, MI 48109-0364; **Phone:** (734) 936-4890; **Board Cert:** Internal Medicine 1975, Nephrology 1977; **Med School:** Univ Mich Med Sch 1970; **Resid:** Internal Medicine, Boston City Hosp, Boston, MA 1971-1975; Nephrology, Beth Israel Hosp, Boston, MA 1975-1977; **Fac Appt:** Prof Nephrology, Univ Mich Med Sch

Textor, Stephen C MD (Nep) - *Spec Exp:* *Transplant Medicine-Kidney; Hypertension; Renal Artery Stenosis;* **Hospital:** Mayo Med Ctr & Clin - Rochester, MN; **Address:** 200 1st St SW, Rochester, MN 55905; **Phone:** (507) 284-4841; **Board Cert:** Internal Medicine 1977, Nephrology 1980; **Med School:** UCLA 1973; **Resid:** Internal Medicine, Boston City Hosp, Boston, MA 1974-1977; **Fellow:** Nephrology, Boston Univ, Boston, MA 1977-1978; Internal Medicine, Fogarty Inst, Lausanne, Switzerland 1979; **Fac Appt:** Prof Medicine, Mayo Med Sch

NEPHROLOGY

Torres, Vincente Esbarranch MD (Nep) - *Spec Exp:* Polycystic Kidney Disease; **Hospital:** Mayo Med Ctr & Clin - Rochester, MN; **Address:** Mayo Clinic, Eisenberg Bldg, 200 1st St SW, rm S24, Rochester, MN 55905; **Phone:** (507) 266-7093; **Board Cert:** Internal Medicine 1977, Nephrology 1980; **Med School:** Spain 1969; **Resid:** Internal Medicine, Mayo Grad Sch Med, Rochester, MN 1975-1977; **Fellow:** Nephrology, Mayo Grad Sch Med, Rochester, MN 1977-1979; **Fac Appt:** Prof Medicine, Mayo Med Sch

Venkat, K K MD (Nep) - *Spec Exp:* Transplant Medicine-Kidney; Kidney Disease; **Hospital:** Henry Ford Hosp; **Address:** Henry Ford Hospital, 2799 W Grand Blvd, rm CFP5, Detroit, MI 48202-2689; **Phone:** (313) 916-2702; **Board Cert:** Internal Medicine 1977, Nephrology 1978; **Med School:** India 1970; **Resid:** Internal Medicine, Henry Ford Hosp, Detroit, MI 1975-1976; **Fellow:** Nephrology, Henry Ford Hosp, Detroit, MI 1976-1978

Zimmerman, Stephen W MD (Nep) - *Spec Exp:* Transplant Medicine-Kidney; Kidney Failure-Chronic; **Hospital:** Univ WI Hosp & Clins; **Address:** VA Hospital, 2500 Overlook Terrace, Rm B3060, Madison, WI 53705; **Phone:** (608) 263-6808; **Board Cert:** Nephrology 1972, Internal Medicine 1972; **Med School:** Univ Wisc 1966; **Resid:** Internal Medicine, Univ Wisconsin, Madison, WI 1967-1969; **Fellow:** Nephrology, Univ Wisconsin, Madison, WI 1969-1970; Research, Univ Wisconsin, Madison, WI 1972-1974; **Fac Appt:** Prof Nephrology, Univ Wisc

Great Plains and Mountains

Berl, Tomas MD (Nep) - *Spec Exp:* Fluid/Electrolyte Balance; **Hospital:** Univ Colo HSC - Denver; **Address:** Univ Colo Med Ctr, Dept Med Renal Div, 4200 E 9th Ave, rm C281, Denver, CO 80220-3706; **Phone:** (303) 372-8156; **Board Cert:** Internal Medicine 1972, Nephrology 1976; **Med School:** NYU Sch Med 1968; **Resid:** Internal Medicine, Bronx Muni Hosp, Bronx, NY 1969-1970; **Fellow:** Renal Disease, Moffit Hosp-UCSF, San Francisco, CA 1970-1971

Schrier, Robert William MD (Nep) - *Spec Exp:* Nephrology - General; **Hospital:** Univ Colo HSC - Denver; **Address:** U Colo Med Ctr-Dept Medicine, 4200 E 9th Ave, Ste B 178, Denver, CO 80220; **Phone:** (303) 315-7765; **Board Cert:** Nephrology, Internal Medicine; **Med School:** Indiana Univ 1962; **Resid:** Internal Medicine, Univ WA Med Ctr 1963-1965; Internal Medicine, Brigham & Women's Hospital 1965-1966; **Fac Appt:** Prof Medicine, Univ Colo

Southwest

Alpern, Robert MD (Nep) - *Spec Exp:* Nephrology - General; **Hospital:** Parkland Mem Hosp; **Address:** Dept of Nephrology, 5323 Harry Hines Blvd, Dallas, TX 75390-9003; **Phone:** (214) 648-2509; **Board Cert:** Internal Medicine 1979, Nephrology 1982; **Med School:** Univ Chicago-Pritzker Sch Med 1976; **Resid:** Internal Medicine, Columbia-Presby Hosp, New York, NY 1976-1977; **Fellow:** Nephrology, Univ California San Fran Med Ctr, San Francisco, CA 1979-1982; **Fac Appt:** Prof Medicine, Univ Tex SW, Dallas

Barcenas, Camilo Gustavo MD (Nep) - *Spec Exp:* Transplant Medicine-Kidney; **Hospital:** St Luke's Episcopal Hosp - Houston; **Address:** 6624 Fannin, Ste 2510, Houston, TX 77030; **Phone:** (713) 791-2648; **Board Cert:** Internal Medicine 1973, Nephrology 1974; **Med School:** Nicaragua 1968; **Resid:** Internal Medicine, Baylor Med Coll, Houston, TX 1970-1972; **Fellow:** Nephrology, UTSW Hosps, Dallas, TX 1972-1974; **Fac Appt:** Clin Prof Medicine, Baylor Coll Med

Brennan, Thomas Stephen MD (Nep) - *Spec Exp:* Transplant Medicine-Kidney & Pancreas; Kidney Stones; Kidney Failure-Chronic; **Hospital:** Methodist Hosp - Houston; **Address:** 2256 Holcombe Blvd, Houston, TX 77030; **Phone:** (713) 790-9080; **Board Cert:** Internal Medicine 1983, Nephrology 1988; **Med School:** Loyola Univ-Stritch Sch Med 1979; **Resid:** Internal Medicine, Loyola Univ Med Ctr, Maywood, IL 1980-1983; **Fellow:** Nephrology, Univ Wash-Barnes Hosp, St. Louis, MO 1983-1986; **Fac Appt:** Assoc Clin Prof Medicine, Baylor Coll Med

Kasinath, Balakuntalam S MD (Nep) - *Spec Exp:* Nephrology - General; **Hospital:** Univ of Texas Hlth & Sci Ctr; **Address:** Univ Texas Hlth & Sci Ctr, Dept Med/Div Nephrology, 7703 Floyd Curl Drive, MC 7882, San Antonio, TX 78229-3900; **Phone:** (210) 567-4700; **Board Cert:** Internal Medicine 1980, Nephrology 1982; **Med School:** India 1975; **Resid:** Internal Medicine, Ill Masonic Med Ctr, Chicago, IL 1977-1980; **Fellow:** Nephrology, Univ Chicago Hosp, Chicago, IL 1980-1983; **Fac Appt:** Prof Medicine, Univ Tex, San Antonio

Olivero, Juan Jose MD (Nep) - *Spec Exp:* Kidney Failure; Fluid/Electrolyte Balance; Hypertension; **Hospital:** Methodist Hosp - Houston; **Address:** 6560 Fannin, Bldg Scurlock - Ste 2206, Houston, TX 77030; **Phone:** (713) 790-4615; **Board Cert:** Internal Medicine 1974, Nephrology 1976; **Med School:** Guatemala 1970; **Resid:** Internal Medicine, Baylor Affil Hosps, Houston, TX 1971-1973; Internal Medicine, Ben Taub Genl Hosp, Houston, TX 1973-1974; **Fellow:** Nephrology, Baylor Affil Hosps, Houston, TX 1974-1975; **Fac Appt:** Clin Prof Medicine, Baylor Coll Med

Suki, Wadi MD (Nep) - *Spec Exp:* Transplant Medicine-Kidney; Kidney Stones; Lupus Kidney Disease; **Hospital:** Methodist Hosp - Houston; **Address:** 2256 Holcombe Blvd, Houston, TX 77030; **Phone:** (713) 790-9080; **Board Cert:** Internal Medicine 1967, Nephrology 1972; **Med School:** Sudan 1959; **Resid:** Internal Medicine, Parkland Meml Hosp, Dallas, TX 1961-1963; **Fellow:** Hypertension, Univ Texas SW, Dallas, TX 1959-1961; Nephrology, Univ Texas SW, Dallas, TX 1963-1965; **Fac Appt:** Clin Prof Medicine, Baylor Coll Med

Wesson, Donald MD (Nep) - *Spec Exp:* Nephrology - General; **Hospital:** Univ Med Ctr - Lubbock; **Address:** Texas Tech Univ Hlth Sci Ctr, Dept Med, Div Nephrology, 3601 4th St, Lubbock, TX 79430; **Phone:** (806) 743-2521; **Board Cert:** Internal Medicine 1981, Nephrology 1986; **Med School:** Baylor Coll Med 1978; **Resid:** Internal Medicine, Baylor Coll Med Hosp, Houston, TX 1979-1981; **Fellow:** Nephrology, Univ Illinois Med Ctr, Chicago, IL 1981-1983; **Fac Appt:** Prof Medicine, Texas Tech Univ

West Coast and Pacific

Ahmad, Suhail MD (Nep) - *Spec Exp:* Hypertension; Kidney Failure-Chronic; Kidney Stones; **Hospital:** Univ WA Med Ctr; **Address:** 2150 N 107th St, Ste 160, Seattle, WA 98133; **Phone:** (206) 363-5090; **Med School:** India 1968; **Resid:** Internal Medicine, Univ Allahabad, Allahabad, India 1968-1971; **Fellow:** Nephrology, Univ Washington, Seattle, WA 1976-1978; **Fac Appt:** Assoc Prof Medicine, Univ Wash

Amend Jr, William JC MD (Nep) - *Spec Exp:* Transplant Medicine-Kidney; **Hospital:** UCSF Med Ctr; **Address:** UCSF, Div Nephrology, 513 Parnassus Ave, Box 0532, San Francisco, CA 94143; **Phone:** (415) 476-2172; **Board Cert:** Internal Medicine 1972, Nephrology 1974; **Med School:** Cornell Univ-Weill Med Coll 1967; **Resid:** Internal Medicine, UCSF Hosp, San Francisco, CA 1968-1969; Internal Medicine, Mass Genl Hosp, Boston, MA 1971-1972; **Fellow:** Nephrology, Peter Bent Brigham Hosp, Boston, MA 1972-1973; **Fac Appt:** Prof Nephrology, UCSF

Bennett, William M MD (Nep) - *Spec Exp:* Polycystic Kidney Disease; Transplant Medicine-Kidney; Drug Toxicity-Kidneys; **Hospital:** Legacy Good Samaritan Hosp and Med Ctr; **Address:** Legacy Good Samaritan Hosp, Transplant Svcs NSC430, 1040 NW 22nd, Portland, OR 97210; **Phone:** (503) 413-7349; **Board Cert:** Internal Medicine 1988, Nephrology 1972; **Med School:** Northwestern Univ 1963; **Resid:** Internal Medicine, Northwestern Univ, Chicago, IL 1963-1965; Internal Medicine, Ore Hlth Sci Univ, Portland, OR 1965-1966; **Fellow:** Nephrology, Mass Genl Hosp, Boston, MA 1968-1970; **Fac Appt:** Prof Medicine, Oregon Hlth Scis Univ

Couser, William MD (Nep) - *Spec Exp:* Kidney Disease-Glomerular; Nephrotic Syndrome; **Hospital:** Univ WA Med Ctr; **Address:** UWMC, Div of Nephrology, 1959 NE Pacific St Bldg HSB - rm BB-1265, Seattle, WA 98195; **Phone:** (206) 543-3792; **Board Cert:** Nephrology 1973, Internal Medicine 1971; **Med School:** Harvard Med Sch 1965; **Resid:** Internal Medicine, Univ of CA Med Cter, San Francisco, CA 1965-1967; Internal Medicine, Boston City Hosp, Boston, MA 1969-1970; **Fellow:** Nephrology, Boston City Hosp, Boston, MA 1970-1971; Nephrology, Univ of Chicago, Chicago, IL 1971-1973; **Fac Appt:** Prof Medicine, Univ Wash

Ellison, David H MD (Nep) - *Spec Exp:* Bartter's Syndrome; Gitelman's Syndrome; Hypertension; **Hospital:** OR Hlth Sci Univ Hosp and Clinics; **Address:** Div Nephrology/Hypertension, 3314 SW US Veterans Hospital Rd, PP262, Portland, OR 97201; **Phone:** (503) 494-8490; **Board Cert:** Internal Medicine 1981, Nephrology 1986; **Med School:** Rush Med Coll 1978; **Resid:** Internal Medicine, Oregon Hlth Scis Univ, Portland, OR 1978-1981; **Fellow:** Research, Oregon Hlth Scis Univ, Portland, OR 1981-1982; Nephrology, Yale Univ Sch Med, New Haven, CT 1982-1985; **Fac Appt:** Prof Medicine, Oregon Hlth Scis Univ

Kaysen, George Alan MD/PhD (Nep) - *Spec Exp:* Kidney Disease-Metabolic; Kidney Failure-Chronic; **Hospital:** Univ CA - Davis Med Ctr; **Address:** UC Davis Med Ctr, Div Nephr, TB 136, Davis, CA 95616; **Phone:** (530) 752-4010; **Board Cert:** Internal Medicine 1975, Nephrology 1980; **Med School:** Albert Einstein Coll Med 1972; **Resid:** Internal Medicine, Bronx Muni Hosp, Bronx, NY 1973-1975; **Fellow:** Renal Disease, Bronx Muni Hosp, Bronx, NY 1975-1977; **Fac Appt:** Prof Medicine, UC Davis

Kopple, Joel David MD (Nep) - *Spec Exp:* Kidney Disease-Nutrition; Nutrition in Kidney Diseas; **Hospital:** LAC - Harbor - UCLA Med Ctr; **Address:** UCLA Med Ctr, 1000 W Carson St, Box 406, Torrance, CA 90509; **Phone:** (310) 222-3891; **Board Cert:** Internal Medicine 1969, Nephrology 1974; **Med School:** Univ IL Coll Med 1962; **Resid:** Internal Medicine, Wadsworth VA Hosp, Los Angeles, CA 1963-1966; **Fellow:** Nephrology, Wadsworth VA Hosp Ctr, Los Angeles, CA 1966-1967; **Fac Appt:** Prof Medicine, UCLA

Massry, Shaul Gourgi MD (Nep) - *Spec Exp:* Hypertension; Parathyroid Disease; Kidney Disease-Metabolic; **Hospital:** LAC & USC Med Ctr; **Address:** 1355 San Pablo St, Ste 100, Los Angeles, CA 90033; **Phone:** (323) 442-5100; **Board Cert:** Internal Medicine 1973, Nephrology 1974; **Med School:** Israel 1954; **Resid:** Internal Medicine, Beilinson Med Ctr., Israel 1962-1965; **Fellow:** Renal Disease, Cedars-Sinai Med Ctr., Los Angeles, CA 1966-1968; **Fac Appt:** Prof Medicine, Univ SC Sch Med

Myers, Bryan David MD (Nep) - *Spec Exp:* Kidney Disease; Hypertension; **Hospital:** Stanford Med Ctr; **Address:** 900 Wilbur, rm W-2002, Palo Alto, CA 94305; **Phone:** (650) 723-6961; **Med School:** South Africa 1959; **Fac Appt:** Prof Medicine, Stanford Univ

Omachi, Rodney S MD (Nep) - *Spec Exp:* Dialysis Care; **Hospital:** UCSF Med Ctr; **Address:** 400 Parnassus Ave, Ste A429, San Francisco, CA 94143; **Phone:** (415) 353-2318; **Board Cert:** Internal Medicine 1973, Nephrology 1974; **Med School:** Harvard Med Sch 1968; **Resid:** Internal Medicine, Mass Genl Hosp, Boston, MA 1969-1970; **Fellow:** Nephrology, Natl Inst Hlth, Bethesda, MD 1970-1973; Nephrology, UCSF, San Franciscio, CA 1973-1974; **Fac Appt:** Clin Prof Nephrology, UCSF

Riordan, John William MD (Nep) - *Spec Exp:* Internal Medicine; **Hospital:** CA Pacific Med Ctr - Pacific Campus; **Address:** 2100 Webster St, Ste 412, San Francisco, CA 94115; **Phone:** (415) 923-3815; **Board Cert:** Internal Medicine 1990, Nephrology 1994; **Med School:** Univ Tex Med Br, Galveston 1987; **Resid:** Internal Medicine, Univ TX Hlth Sci Ctr, San Antonio, TX 1988-1990; **Fellow:** Nephrology, UCSF, San Francisco, CA 1991-1995

Saleh, Saleh MD (Nep) - *Spec Exp:* Kidney Stones; **Hospital:** UCLA Med Ctr; **Address:** 100 UCLA Med Plaza, Ste 690, Los Angeles, CA 90095; **Phone:** (310) 824-0088; **Board Cert:** Internal Medicine 1983, Nephrology 1984; **Med School:** McGill Univ 1977; **Resid:** Internal Medicine, Royal Victoria Hosp, Montreal, Canada 1978-1979; **Fellow:** Nephrology, UCLA Ctr Hlth Scis, Los Angeles, CA 1981-1984; **Fac Appt:** Assoc Clin Prof Medicine, UCLA

Scandling Jr, John David MD (Nep) - *Spec Exp:* Transplant Medicine-Kidney; **Hospital:** Stanford Med Ctr; **Address:** 750 Welch Rd, Ste 200, Palo Alto, CA 94304; **Phone:** (650) 725-9891; **Board Cert:** Internal Medicine 1981, Nephrology 1984; **Med School:** Med Coll VA 1978; **Resid:** Internal Medicine, W Va Univ Hosp, Morgantown, VA 1979-1981; **Fellow:** Nephrology, Univ Rochester, Rochester, NY 1981-1983; **Fac Appt:** Prof Medicine, Stanford Univ

NEUROLOGICAL SURGERY

A neurological surgeon provides the operative and non-operative management (i.e., prevention, diagnosis, evaluation, treatment, critical care and rehabilitation) of disorders of the central, peripheral and autonomic nervous systems, including their supporting structures and vascular supply; the evaluation and treatment of pathological processes which modify function or activity of the nervous system; and the operative and non-operative management of pain. A neurological surgeon treats patients with disorders of the nervous system; disorders of the brain, meninges, skull and their blood supply, including the extracranial carotid and vertebral arteries; disorders of the pituitary gland; disorders of the spinal cord, meninges and vertebral column, including those which may require treatment by spinal fusion or instrumentation; and disorders of the cranial and spinal nerves throughout their distribution.

Training required: Seven years (including general surgery)

NYU Medical Center

550 First Avenue (at 31st Street)
New York, NY 10016
Physician Referral: (888) 7-NYU-MED
(888-769-8633)   www.nyumedicalcenter.org

SCHOOL OF
MEDICINE

NEW YORK UNIVERSITY

NEUROSURGERY

The Department of Neurosurgery at NYU Medical Center offers the most advanced surgical procedures available anywhere in the world, along with compassionate care and supportive services for patients and their families. In an environment of leading-edge research and medical education, the department's interdisciplinary team of physicians, nurses, and allied health professionals are world-renowned for their highly specialized training and their down-to-earth approach to clinical care. The department also is home to some of the most sophisticated equipment in the region.

Because neurosurgery encompasses the surgical treatment of disorders of the entire nervous system and its coverings – the brain, spinal cord, skull, scalp, and vertebral column – many physicians subspecialize in a particular aspect of the field. At NYU Medical Center, neurosurgeons treat a broad range of conditions, including tumors, vascular disorders, Parkinson's disease, and epilepsy, among others.

THE CENTER FOR THE STUDY AND TREATMENT OF MOVEMENT DISORDERS

The Center for Study and Treatment of Movement Disorders provides surgical care for patients with Parkinson's disease and other movement disorders. Its highly focused surgeons perform pallidotomy surgery when a patient suffers from severe stiffness, rigidity, and movement difficulties; and thalamotomy for those with disabling tremor. One of the center's most innovative treatments is deep brain stimulation, used to relieve the disabling symptoms of Parkinson's disease. NYU's neurosurgeons perform these procedures using the latest computer technology in conjunction with electrophysiologic monitoring.

THE GAMMA KNIFE

In the recent past, patients with brain abnormalities considered too deep or too delicate to reach with a scalpel had little reason for hope. But with the Gamma Knife, neurosurgeons at NYU Medical Center can now remove deep-seated tumors, vascular malformations, and other sites of dysfunction with outstanding results. The Leksell Gamma Knife® – a revolutionary tool developed in Sweden for performing stereotactic radiosurgery – is the latest such technology in the New York and New England regions. Aided by three-dimensional MRI technology that pinpoints the problem area, the neurosurgeon uses the Gamma Knife to bombard its target with precise doses of radiation.

NYU MEDICAL CENTER

The Tumor Surgery Program at NYU Medical Center treats patients referred from all over the world. The program is committed to the development and application of minimally invasive methods for the complete removal of brain tumors. With an emphasis on noninvasive brain mapping via magnetoencephalotomography (MEG) and functional MRI, NYU's neurosurgeons are able to plan a surgical approach that minimizes risk and ensures the best possible outcome. Stereotactic volumetric resection, a method developed by Patrick J. Kelly, MD – Professor and Chairman of Neurosurgery – assures exceptionally thorough surgical removal of the tumor.

Physician Referral
(888) 7-NYU-MED
(888-769-8633)
www.nyumedicalcenter.org

PHYSICIAN LISTINGS

Neurological Surgery

New England

Black, Peter MD/PhD (NS) - *Spec Exp:* Seizure Surgery; Brain & Spinal Cord Tumors; Intra Operative MRI Surgery; **Hospital:** Brigham & Women's Hosp; **Address:** Brigham & Women's Hosp, Dept Neurosurg, 75 Francis St, Boston, MA 02115; **Phone:** (617) 355-7795; **Board Cert:** Neurological Surgery 1984; **Med School:** McGill Univ 1970; **Resid:** Surgery, Mass Genl Hosp, Boston, MA 1971-1972; Neurological Surgery, Mass Genl Hosp, Boston, MA 1975-1978; **Fellow:** Neurological Oncology, Mass Genl Hosp, Boston, MA 1975-1976; **Fac Appt:** Prof Neurological Surgery, Harvard Med Sch

Borges, Lawrence F. MD (NS) - *Spec Exp:* Spinal Surgery; **Hospital:** MA Genl Hosp; **Address:** Divison of Neurosurgery, 32 Fruit St, Boston, MA 02114-2620; **Phone:** (617) 726-6156; **Board Cert:** Neurological Surgery 1986; **Med School:** Johns Hopkins Univ 1977; **Resid:** Neurological Surgery, Mass Genl Hosp, Boston, MA 1978-1983; **Fac Appt:** Assoc Prof Surgery, Harvard Med Sch

Chapman, Paul H. MD (NS) - *Spec Exp:* Neurosurgery-Pediatric; Stereotactic Radiosurgery; **Hospital:** MA Genl Hosp; **Address:** 55 Fruit St, rm GRB-502, Boston, MA 02114; **Phone:** (617) 726-3887; **Board Cert:** Neurological Surgery 1976; **Med School:** Harvard Med Sch 1964; **Resid:** Surgery, Mass Genl Hosp, Boston, MA 1965-1966; Neurological Surgery, Mass Genl Hosp, Boston, MA 1968-1972; **Fellow:** Neurological Surgery, Hosp Sick Chldn, Tornto, Canada 1972; **Fac Appt:** Assoc Prof Surgery, Harvard Med Sch

Cosgrove, G. Rees MD (NS) - *Spec Exp:* Epilepsy/Seizure Disorders; Brain Tumors; **Hospital:** MA Genl Hosp; **Address:** 15 Parkman St, Ste 331, Boston, MA 02114; **Phone:** (617) 724-0357; **Board Cert:** Neurological Surgery 1989; **Med School:** Queens Univ 1980; **Resid:** Neurological Surgery, Montreal Neur Inst, Canada 1981-1986; **Fac Appt:** Assoc Prof Surgery, Harvard Med Sch

Nazzaro, Jules M. MD (NS) - *Spec Exp:* Parkinson's Disease; Movement Disorders; Stereotactic Radiosurgery; **Hospital:** Boston Med Ctr; **Address:** 720 Harrison Ave, Ste 710, Boston, MA 02118; **Phone:** (617) 638-8993; **Board Cert:** Neurological Surgery 1996; **Med School:** Albert Einstein Coll Med 1984; **Resid:** Neurology, NYU Med Ctr, New York, NY 1985-1991; **Fellow:** Nephrology, Meml Sloan-Kettering Cancer Ctr, New York, NY 1991-1992; **Fac Appt:** Asst Prof Neurological Surgery, Boston Univ

Ojemann, Robert G. MD (NS) - *Spec Exp:* Brain Tumors; Spinal Cord Tumors; Acoustic Nerve Tumors; **Hospital:** MA Genl Hosp; **Address:** Mass Genl Dept of Neurosurgery, 55 Fruit Street, Boston, MA 02114-2621; **Phone:** (617) 726-2936; **Board Cert:** Neurological Surgery 1964; **Med School:** Univ Iowa Coll Med 1955; **Resid:** Sports Medicine, Baylor University, Houston, TX 1956-1957; Neurological Surgery, Mass Genl Hosp, Boston, MA 1957-1966; **Fac Appt:** Prof Surgery, Harvard Med Sch

Piepmeier, Joseph MD (NS) - *Spec Exp:* Neuro-Oncology; Brain & Spinal Cord Tumors; **Hospital:** Yale - New Haven Hosp; **Address:** Dept Neurological Surgery, 333 Cedar St, TMP-410, New Haven, CT 06520; **Phone:** (203) 785-2791; **Board Cert:** Neurological Surgery 1984; **Med School:** Univ Tenn Coll Med, Memphis 1975; **Resid:** Neurological Surgery, Yale-New Haven Hosp, New Haven, CT 1977-1982; **Fac Appt:** Prof Neurological Surgery, Yale Univ

Scott, R. Michael MD (NS) - *Spec Exp:* Moya Moya; Brain Tumors; Cerebrovascular Disease; **Hospital:** Children's Hospital - Boston; **Address:** Children's Hosp, Dept Neurosurgery, 300 Longwood Ave, Bldg Bader - Ste 319, Boston, MA 02115-5724; **Phone:** (617) 355-6011; **Board Cert:** Neurological Surgery 1976; **Med School:** Temple Univ 1966; **Resid:** Neurological Surgery, Massachusetts General Hospital, Boston, MA 1969-1973; **Fac Appt:** Prof Surgery, Harvard Med Sch

Shucart, William A MD (NS) - *Spec Exp:* Pituitary Surgery; **Hospital:** New England Med Ctr - Boston; **Address:** 750 Washington St, Box 178, Boston, MA 02111; **Phone:** (617) 636-5858; **Board Cert:** Neurological Surgery 1973; **Med School:** Univ MO-Columbia Sch Med 1961; **Resid:** Neurological Surgery, Colum-Presby Hosp, New York, NY 1967-1970; Neurological Surgery, Hosp Sick Chldn, Toronto Canada 1970-1971

Spencer, Dennis D MD (NS) - *Spec Exp:* Epilepsy/Seizure Disorders; **Hospital:** Yale - New Haven Hosp; **Address:** Dept Neurosurgery, 333 Cedar St Bldg TMP-4, New Haven, CT 06520; **Phone:** (203) 785-2811; **Board Cert:** Neurological Surgery 1980; **Med School:** Washington Univ, St Louis 1971; **Resid:** Surgery, Barnes Hosp, St Louis, MO 1971-1972; Neurological Surgery, Yale-New Haven Hosp, New Haven, CT 1972-1976; **Fac Appt:** Prof Neurological Surgery, Yale Univ

Woodard, Eric J MD (NS) - *Spec Exp:* Spinal Surgery; **Hospital:** Brigham & Women's Hosp; **Address:** Brigham & Women's Hosp, Div Neurosurgery, 75 Francis St, Boston, MA 02115; **Phone:** (617) 732-6003; **Board Cert:** Neurological Surgery 1997; **Med School:** Penn State Univ-Hershey Med Ctr 1985; **Resid:** Neurological Surgery, Emory Univ Affil Hosps, Atlanta, GA 1986-1991; **Fellow:** Spine Surgery, Med Coll Wisc, Milwaukee, WI 1986-1991; **Fac Appt:** Asst Clin Prof Neurological Surgery, Harvard Med Sch

Mid Atlantic

Albright, Leland MD (NS) - *Spec Exp:* Neurosurgery-Pediatric; Spasticity & Movement Disorders; Brain Tumors; **Hospital:** Chldn's Hosp of Pittsbrgh; **Address:** Children's Hosp- Pittsburgh, Dept Neurosurgery, 3705 5th Ave, Ste 3705, Pittsburgh, PA 15213-2524; **Phone:** (412) 692-8142; **Board Cert:** Neurological Surgery 1981; **Med School:** Louisiana State Univ 1969; **Resid:** Surgery, Barnes Hosp, St Louis, MO 1970-1971; **Fellow:** Neurological Surgery, National Inst of Hlth, Bethesda, MD 1971-1974; Neurological Surgery, Univ Pittsburgh, Pittsburgh, PA 1974-1978; **Fac Appt:** Neurological Surgery, Univ Pittsburgh

Baltuch, Gordon MD/PhD (NS) - *Spec Exp:* Movement Disorders; Parkinson's Disease; Epilepsy/Seizure Disorders; **Hospital:** Pennsylvania Hosp (page 78); **Address:** Penn Neurological Institute/Silverstein 5, 3400 Spruce St, Philadelphia, PA 19104; **Phone:** (215) 662-7788; **Board Cert:** Neurological Surgery 1998; **Med School:** McGill Univ 1986; **Resid:** Neurological Surgery, Montreal Neuro Inst, Montreal, Canada; **Fac Appt:** Asst Prof Neurological Surgery, Univ Penn

Benjamin, Vallo MD (NS) - *Spec Exp:* Spinal Surgery; Skull Base Surgery; Acoustic Neuroma; **Hospital:** NYU Med Ctr (page 71); **Address:** 530 First Ave, Ste 7W, New York, NY 10016; **Phone:** (212) 263-5013; **Board Cert:** Neurological Surgery 1967; **Med School:** Iran 1958; **Resid:** Neurological Surgery, Bellevue Hosp, New York, NY 1960-1964; **Fellow:** Neurological Surgery, NYU Med Ctr, New York, NY 1965-1966; **Fac Appt:** Prof Neurological Surgery, NYU Sch Med

Brem, Henry MD (NS) - *Spec Exp:* Brain Tumors/ Skull Base Tumors; Spinal Cord Tumors; Pituitary Tumors; **Hospital:** Johns Hopkins Hosp - Baltimore; **Address:** Johns Hopkins Med Ctr-Dept NeuroSurg, 600 N Wolfe St Bldg Meyer 7-109, Baltimore, MD 21287; **Phone:** (410) 955-2248; **Board Cert:** Neurological Surgery 1986; **Med School:** Harvard Med Sch 1978; **Resid:** Neurological Surgery, Columbia-Presby Ctr, New York, NY 1979-1984; **Fellow:** Neurological Surgery, Johns Hopkins Hosp, Baltimore, MD 1979-1980; **Fac Appt:** Prof Neurological Surgery, Johns Hopkins Univ

Camins, Martin B MD (NS) - *Spec Exp:* Spinal Surgery; Brain Tumors; **Hospital:** Mount Sinai Hosp (page 68); **Address:** 205 E 68th St, Ste T1C, New York, NY 10021-5735; **Phone:** (212) 570-0100; **Board Cert:** Neurological Surgery 1980; **Med School:** Univ Hlth Sci/Chicago Med Sch 1969; **Resid:** Neurology, Columbia-Presby, New York, NY 1970-1971; Neurological Surgery, Columbia-Presby, New York, NY 1971-1975; **Fellow:** Neurological Surgery, Nat Hosp, London, England 1973; Neurological Surgery, New York Univ Med Ctr, New York, NY 1976-1977; **Fac Appt:** Assoc Prof Neurological Surgery, Mount Sinai Sch Med

Caputy, Anthony J. MD (NS) - *Spec Exp:* Epilepsy/Seizure Disorders; Spinal Surgery; **Hospital:** Inova Fairfax Hosp; **Address:** Geo Wash Univ, Dept Neuro Surg, 2150 Pennsylvania Ave NW, Fl 7-420, Washington, DC 20037; **Phone:** (202) 994-9226; **Board Cert:** Neurological Surgery 1989; **Med School:** Univ VA Sch Med 1980; **Resid:** Neurological Surgery, Georgetown Univ, Washington, DC 1981-1986; **Fac Appt:** Assoc Clin Prof Neurological Surgery, Univ MD Sch Med

Carmel, Peter MD (NS) - *Spec Exp:* Brain Tumors-Pediatric; Skull Base Surgery; **Hospital:** UMDNJ-Univ Hosp-Newark; **Address:** 90 Bergen St, Ste 1700, Newark, NJ 07103-2499; **Phone:** (973) 972-2323; **Board Cert:** Neurological Surgery 1969; **Med School:** NYU Sch Med 1960; **Resid:** Neurological Surgery, Columbia Presby Med Ctr, New York, NY 1963-1967; Neurological Surgery, Neuro-Inst-Columbia Presbyterian, New York, NY 1963-1967; **Fac Appt:** Prof Neurological Surgery, UMDNJ-NJ Med Sch, Newark

Carson, Benjamin S MD (NS) - *Spec Exp:* Brain Injury; Brain & Spinal Cord Tumors; **Hospital:** Johns Hopkins Hosp - Baltimore; **Address:** 600 N Wolfe St, Harvey 811, Baltimore, MD 21287-8811; **Phone:** (410) 955-7888; **Board Cert:** Neurological Surgery 1988; **Med School:** Univ Mich Med Sch 1977; **Resid:** Neurological Surgery, Johns Hopkins Hosp, Baltimore, MD 1978-1983; **Fellow:** Pediatric Neurological Surgery, Queen Elizabeth II Med Ctr, Western Australia 1983-1984; **Fac Appt:** Assoc Prof Neurological Surgery, Johns Hopkins Univ

Dennis, Gary Creed MD (NS) - *Spec Exp:* Brain & Spinal Surgery; Pain Management; *Subarachnoid Hemorrhage;* **Hospital:** Howard Univ Hosp; **Address:** Howard U Hosp, 2041 Georgia Ave NW, Ste 5B-47, Washington, DC 20060; **Phone:** (202) 865-6681; **Board Cert:** Neurological Surgery 1983; **Med School:** Howard Univ 1976; **Resid:** Neurological Surgery, Baylor Affil Hosps, Houston, TX 1977-1981; **Fac Appt:** Assoc Prof Surgery, Howard Univ

Eisenberg, Howard M MD (NS) - *Spec Exp:* Acoustic Nerve Tumors; Head & Spinal Cord Injury; Epilepsy/Seizure Disorders; **Hospital:** University of MD Med Sys; **Address:** Univ MD Sch Med, Dept Neuro, 22 S Greene St, Ste 512D, Baltimore, MD 21201-1544; **Phone:** (410) 328-3514; **Board Cert:** Neurological Surgery 1973; **Med School:** SUNY Downstate 1964; **Resid:** Surgery, New York Hosp, New York, NY 1965-1966; Neurological Surgery, Peter Bent Brigham Hosp, Boston, MA 1966-1970; **Fellow:** Harvard Univ, Boston, MA 1969-1970; **Fac Appt:** Prof Neurological Surgery, Univ MD Sch Med

Epstein, Fred Jacob MD (NS) - *Spec Exp:* Spinal Cord Tumors-Pediatric; Brain Stem Tumors-Pediatric; **Hospital:** Beth Israel Med Ctr - Singer Div (page 58); **Address:** 170 East End Ave, rm 521, New York, NY 10128; **Phone:** (212) 870-9600; **Board Cert:** Neurological Surgery 1972; **Med School:** NY Med Coll 1963; **Resid:** Surgery, Montefiore Hosp, New York, NY 1964-1965; Neurological Surgery, NYU Med Ctr, New York, NY 1965-1970; **Fac Appt:** Prof Neurological Surgery, Albert Einstein Coll Med

Flamm, Eugene MD (NS) - *Spec Exp:* *Aneurysm-Cerebral; Spinal Cord Lesions; Vascular Brain/Spine Problems;* **Hospital:** Beth Israel Med Ctr - Singer Div (page 58); **Address:** Inst for Neurl & Neurosurg, 170 E End Ave, New York, NY 10128; **Phone:** (212) 870-7960; **Board Cert:** Neurological Surgery 1973; **Med School:** SUNY Buffalo 1962; **Resid:** Surgery, NY Hosp, New York, NY 1963-1964; Neurological Surgery, NYU Med Ctr, New York, NY 1966-1970; **Fellow:** Neurological Surgery, Univ Zurich, Zurich, Switzerland 1970-1971; **Fac Appt:** Prof Neurological Surgery, Albert Einstein Coll Med

Germano, Isabelle M MD (NS) - *Spec Exp:* *Brain Tumors; Movement Disorders; Epilepsy;* **Hospital:** Mount Sinai Hosp (page 68); **Address:** 5 E 98th St, Box 1136, New York, NY 10029-6504; **Phone:** (212) 241-9638; **Board Cert:** Neurological Surgery 1995; **Med School:** Italy 1984; **Resid:** Neurological Surgery, UCSF Med Ctr, San Francisco, CA 1988-1990; Neurological Surgery, Albert Einstein Coll Med, New York, NY 1990-1993; **Fac Appt:** Assoc Prof Neurological Surgery, Mount Sinai Sch Med

Grady, M Sean MD (NS) - *Spec Exp:* *Cerebrovascular Disease; Stroke;* **Hospital:** Hosp Univ Penn (page 78); **Address:** Hosp Univ Penn, Dept Neurosurgery, 3400 Spruce St Bldg Silverstein Fl 5, Philadelphia, PA 19104; **Phone:** (215) 662-3487; **Board Cert:** Neurological Surgery 1990; **Med School:** Georgetown Univ 1981; **Resid:** Neurological Surgery, Univ Virginia, Charlottesville, VA 1981-1987; **Fac Appt:** Assoc Prof Neurological Surgery, Univ Penn

Hodge Jr., Charles J. MD (NS) - *Spec Exp:* *Vascular Neurosurgery;* **Hospital:** Upstate Univ Med Hosp; **Address:** 750 E Adams St, Neurosurgery Dept, Jacobson Hall, 6th Fl, Syracuse, NY 13210; **Phone:** (315) 464-4470; **Board Cert:** Neurological Surgery 1977; **Med School:** Columbia P&S 1967; **Resid:** Surgery, Yale-New Haven Hosp, New Haven, CT 1968-1969; Neurological Surgery, SUNY Upstate Med Ctr, Syracuse, NY 1969-1974; **Fac Appt:** Prof Neurological Surgery, SUNY Syracuse

Hopkins, Leo Nelson MD (NS) - *Spec Exp:* *Cerebrovascular Disease; Endovascular Surgery;* **Hospital:** Millard Fillmore Hosp; **Address:** Millard Fillmore Hosp, Neurosurgery Dept, 3 Gates Cir, Buffalo, NY 14209; **Phone:** (716) 887-5210; **Board Cert:** Neurological Surgery 1977; **Med School:** Albany Med Coll 1969; **Resid:** Neurological Surgery, SUNY Buffalo, Buffalo, NY 1971-1975; **Fac Appt:** Prof Neurological Surgery, SUNY Buffalo

Jacobson, Jeff MD (NS) - *Spec Exp:* *Acoustic Nerve Tumors;* **Hospital:** Washington Hosp Ctr; **Address:** 3 Washington Cir NW, Ste 306, Washington, DC 20037; **Phone:** (202) 223-1060; **Board Cert:** Neurological Surgery 1988; **Med School:** Geo Wash Univ 1977; **Resid:** Surgery, Geo Wash U, Washington, DC 1977-1978; Neurological Surgery, Geo Wash U, Washington, DC 1978-1983; **Fac Appt:** Neurological Surgery, Geo Wash Univ

Jho, Hae-Dong MD/PhD (NS) - *Spec Exp:* *Minimally Invasive Neurosurgery;* **Hospital:** Allegheny General Hosp; **Address:** Institute for Minimally Invasive Neurosurgery, 420 E North Ave, Ste 312, Pittsburgh, PA 15212-4746; **Phone:** (412) 359-6110; **Board Cert:** Neurological Surgery 1991; **Med School:** Korea 1971; **Resid:** Neurological Surgery, Hanyang Univ Hosp, Seoul, South Korea 1975-1979; Neurological Surgery, Univ Pittsburgh, Pittsburgh, PA 1985-1989; **Fellow:** Microneurosurgery, Univ Pittsburgh, Pittsburgh, PA 1983-1984; Surgery, Univ Pittsburgh, Pittsburgh, PA 1984-1985; **Fac Appt:** Prof Neurological Surgery, Med Coll PA Hahnemann

Kelly, Patrick J MD (NS) - *Spec Exp:* *Brain Tumors; Stereotactic Radiosurgery; Movement Disorders;* **Hospital:** NYU Med Ctr (page 71); **Address:** NYU Dept Neurological Surgery, 530 1st Ave, Ste 8R, New York, NY 10016; **Phone:** (212) 263-8002; **Board Cert:** Neurological Surgery 1978; **Med School:** SUNY Buffalo 1966; **Resid:** Neurological Surgery, Northwestern, Chicago, IL 1970-1972; Neurological Surgery, Univ TX Med Hosp, Galveston, TX 1972-1974; **Fellow:** Neurological Surgery, St Anne Hosp, Paris, France 1977; **Fac Appt:** Prof Neurological Surgery, NYU Sch Med

Khan, Agha S MD (NS) - *Spec Exp:* Skull Base Surgery; Spinal Surgery; **Hospital:** Maryland Genl Hosp; **Address:** 2411 W Belvedere Ave, Ste 402, Baltimore, MD 21215; **Phone:** (410) 601-8314; **Board Cert:** Neurological Surgery 1995; **Med School:** Pakistan 1979; **Resid:** Surgery, Washington Hosp Ctr, Washington, DC 1982-1983; Neurological Surgery, Univ Wisconsin Hosp & Clinic, Madison, WI 1983-1990

Kobrine, Arthur MD/PhD (NS) - *Spec Exp:* Spinal Cord Surgery; Brain & Spinal Cord Tumors; **Hospital:** Georgetown Univ Hosp; **Address:** 2440 M St NW, Ste 315, Washington, DC 20037-1404; **Phone:** (202) 293-7136; **Board Cert:** Neurological Surgery 1976; **Med School:** Northwestern Univ **Resid:** Neurological Surgery, Northwestern, Chicago, IL 1969-1970; Neurological Surgery, Walter Reed Genl Hosp, Washington, DC 1970-1973; **Fellow:** Physiology, Geo Wash Univ, Washington, DC 1979; **Fac Appt:** Clin Prof Neurological Surgery, Georgetown Univ

Lavyne, Michael H MD (NS) - *Spec Exp:* Spinal Surgery; Skull Base Surgery; Acoustic Neuroma; **Hospital:** NY Presby Hosp - NY Weill Cornell Med Ctr (page 70); **Address:** 523 E 72nd St, New York, NY 10021; **Phone:** (212) 717-0200; **Board Cert:** Neurological Surgery 1982; **Med School:** Cornell Univ-Weill Med Coll 1972; **Resid:** Neurological Surgery, Mass Genl Hosp, Boston, MA 1974-1979; **Fellow:** Neurology, Beth Israel, Boston, MA 1973-1974; **Fac Appt:** Asst Clin Prof Surgery, Cornell Univ-Weill Med Coll

Long, Donlin M MD/PhD (NS) - *Spec Exp:* Skull Base Tumors; Acoustic Nerve Tumors; Spinal Diseases; **Hospital:** Johns Hopkins Hosp - Baltimore; **Address:** Johns Hopkins Hospital, 600 N Wolfe St Bldg Carnegie - rm 466, Baltimore, MD 21287-7709; **Phone:** (410) 955-2251; **Board Cert:** Neurological Surgery 1968; **Med School:** Univ MO-Columbia Sch Med 1959; **Resid:** Neurological Surgery, Univ Minnesota Hosp, Minneapolis, MN 1960-1964; Peter Bent Brigham Hosp, Boston, MA 1965; **Fac Appt:** Prof Neurological Surgery, Johns Hopkins Univ

Lunsford, L Dade MD (NS) - *Spec Exp:* Stereotactic Radiosurgery; Movement Disorders; **Hospital:** UPMC - Presbyterian Univ Hosp; **Address:** UPMC Presbyterian, 200 Lothrop St, Ste B400, Pittsburgh, PA 15213; **Phone:** (412) 647-3685; **Board Cert:** Neurological Surgery 1983; **Med School:** Columbia P&S 1974; **Resid:** Neurological Surgery, Univ Pittsburgh, Pittsburgh, PA 1975-1980; **Fellow:** Stereo Neurological Surgery, Karolinska Hospital, Stockholm, Sweden 1980-1981; **Fac Appt:** Prof Neurological Surgery, Univ Pittsburgh

Mangiardi, John MD (NS) - *Spec Exp:* Brain Tumors; Spinal Surgery; Aneurysm-Cerebral; **Hospital:** Lenox Hill Hosp (page 64); **Address:** 50 E 72 St, New York, NY 10021-4246; **Phone:** (212) 879-1919; **Board Cert:** Neurological Surgery 1987; **Med School:** Wayne State Univ 1976; **Resid:** Neurological Surgery, NYU Med Ctr, New York, NY 1978-1983; **Fac Appt:** Prof Neurological Surgery, NYU Sch Med

Marion, Donald W MD (NS) - *Spec Exp:* Trauma-Brain Injury; Spinal Surgery; Brain Tumors; **Hospital:** UPMC - Presbyterian Univ Hosp; **Address:** 200 Lothrop St, Ste B400, Pittsburgh, PA 15213-2582; **Phone:** (412) 647-0956; **Board Cert:** Neurological Surgery 1993; **Med School:** UCSF 1982; **Resid:** Surgery, Univ Pittsburgh Med Ctr, Pittsburgh, PA 1982-1983; Neurological Surgery, Univ Pittsburgh Med Ctr, Pittsburgh, PA 1983-1989; **Fellow:** Neurological Trauma, Med Coll Virginia, Charlottesville, VA 1989-1990; **Fac Appt:** Prof Neurological Surgery, Univ Pittsburgh

Maroon, Joseph C MD (NS) - *Spec Exp:* Minimally Invasive Surgery; Microdiscectomy; Concussion/Sports-Related; **Hospital:** UPMC - Presbyterian Univ Hosp; **Address:** UPMC Presbyterian, Dept Neurological Surgery, 200 Lothrop St, Ste 5-C, Pittsburgh, PA 15213; **Phone:** (412) 647-3604; **Board Cert:** Neurological Surgery 1973; **Med School:** Indiana Univ 1965; **Resid:** Surgery, Georgetown Univ Hosp, Washington, DC 1966-1967; Neurological Surgery, Indiana Univ Med Ctr, Indianapolis, IN 1967-1971; **Fellow:** Neurological Surgery, Radcliffe Infirm/Oxford Univ, Oxford, England 1968-1969; Microneurosurgery, Univ Vermont, Burlington, VT 1971-1972; **Fac Appt:** Clin Prof Neurological Surgery, Univ Pittsburgh

McCormick, Paul MD (NS) - *Spec Exp:* Spinal Surgery; **Hospital:** NY Presby Hosp - Columbia Presby Med Ctr (page 70); **Address:** 710 W 168th St, Ste 406, New York, NY 10032-2603; **Phone:** (212) 305-7976; **Board Cert:** Neurological Surgery 1993; **Med School:** Columbia P&S 1982; **Resid:** Neurological Surgery, Columbia Presby Med Ctr, New York, NY 1984-1989; **Fellow:** Neurological Surgery, Natl Inst Hlth, Bethesda, MD 1982-1983; Spine Surgery, Med Coll Wisc, Milwaukee, WI 1989-1990; **Fac Appt:** Prof Neurological Surgery, Columbia P&S

Milhorat, Thomas H MD (NS) - *Spec Exp:* Syringomyelia; Chiari's Deformity; Hydrocephalus; **Hospital:** N Shore Univ Hosp at Manhasset; **Address:** North Shore Univ Hosp-Manhasset Dept Neurosurgery, 300 Community Drive, Manhasset, NY 11030; **Phone:** (516) 562-3020; **Board Cert:** Neurological Surgery 1972; **Med School:** Cornell Univ-Weill Med Coll 1961; **Resid:** Surgery, NY Hosp-Cornel Med Ctr, New York, NY 1961-1963; Neurological Surgery, NY Hosp-Cornel Med Ctr, New York, NY 1965-1969; **Fellow:** Neurological Surgery, Nat Inst Hlth, Bethesda, MD 1963-1965; **Fac Appt:** Prof Neurological Surgery, SUNY Downstate

Murali, Raj MD (NS) - *Spec Exp:* Trigeminal Neuralgia; Skull Base Surgery; Spinal Surgery-Neck; **Hospital:** St Vincent Cath Med Ctrs - Manhattan (page 75); **Address:** 153 W 11th St, Ste NR 8, New York, NY 10011-8305; **Phone:** (212) 604-7767; **Board Cert:** Neurological Surgery 1982; **Med School:** India 1968; **Resid:** Neurological Surgery, Royal Infirm-U Edinburgh, United Kingdom 1968-1974; Neurological Surgery, NYU Med Ctr, NY, NY 1974-1979; **Fac Appt:** Prof Neurological Surgery, NY Med Coll

Pollack, Ian MD (NS) - *Spec Exp:* Neurosurgery-Pediatric; Brain Tumors; Craniofacial Surgery; **Hospital:** Chldn's Hosp of Pittsbrgh; **Address:** Children's Hosp of Pittsburgh, Dept of Neurosurgery, 3705 Fifth Ave, Ste 3670A, Pittsburgh, PA 15213; **Phone:** (412) 692-5881; **Board Cert:** Neurological Surgery 1996; **Med School:** Johns Hopkins Univ 1984; **Resid:** Univ Pittsburgh Sch Med 1985-1991; **Fellow:** Hosp Sick Chldn, Toronto, Canada 1991-1991; **Fac Appt:** Prof Neurological Surgery, Univ Pittsburgh

Post, Kalmon MD (NS) - *Spec Exp:* Pituitary Surgery; Acoustic Nerve Tumors; **Hospital:** Mount Sinai Hosp (page 68); **Address:** 5 E 98th St, Fl 7, New York, NY 10029-6501; **Phone:** (212) 241-0933; **Board Cert:** Neurological Surgery 1978; **Med School:** NYU Sch Med 1967; **Resid:** Surgery, Bellevue Hosp, New York, NY 1968-1969; Neurological Surgery, Bellevue Hosp, New York, NY 1971-1975; **Fac Appt:** Prof Neurological Surgery, Mount Sinai Sch Med

Sen, Chandra Nath MD (NS) - *Spec Exp:* Brain Tumors; Skull Base Surgery; **Hospital:** St Luke's - Roosevelt Hosp Ctr - Roosevelt Div (page 58); **Address:** 1000 10th Ave Fl 5 - Ste G41, New York, NY 10019; **Phone:** (212) 523-6720; **Board Cert:** Neurological Surgery 1989; **Med School:** India 1976; **Resid:** Surgery, Univ. of Wisconsin, Madison 1978-1980; Neurological Surgery, Univ. of Wisconsin, Madison 1980-1985; **Fellow:** Microsurgery, Univ. of Pittsburg 1985-1986; **Fac Appt:** Prof Neurological Surgery

Solomon, Robert A MD (NS) - *Spec Exp:* Aneurysm-Cerebral; Arteriovenous Malformation; **Hospital:** NY Presby Hosp - Columbia Presby Med Ctr (page 70); **Address:** 710 W 168th St, Ste 439, New York, NY 10032; **Phone:** (212) 305-4118; **Board Cert:** Neurological Surgery 1988; **Med School:** Johns Hopkins Univ 1980; **Resid:** Neurological Surgery, Neuro Inst-Columbia Univ, New York, NY 1981-1986; **Fac Appt:** Prof Neurological Surgery, Columbia P&S

Stieg, Philip E MD/PhD (NS) - *Spec Exp:* Aneurysm-Cerebral; Acoustic Nerve Tumors; Skull Base Surgery; **Hospital:** NY Presby Hosp - NY Weill Cornell Med Ctr (page 70); **Address:** 520 E 70th St, STARR 651, New York, NY 10021-9800; **Phone:** (212) 746-4684; **Board Cert:** Neurological Surgery 1992; **Med School:** Med Coll Wisc 1983; **Resid:** Neurological Surgery, Dallas Chldns Hosp/Parkland Meml Hosp, Dallas, TX 1984-1988; **Fellow:** Neurological Biology, Karolinska Inst, Stockholm, Sweden 1987-1988; **Fac Appt:** Prof Neurological Surgery, Cornell Univ-Weill Med Coll

Southeast

Branch Jr, Charles L MD (NS) - *Spec Exp:* Spinal Surgery; Disc Disease; Stereotactic Radiosurgery; **Hospital:** Wake Forest Univ Baptist Med Ctr (page 81); **Address:** Wake Forest Univ Baptist Med Ctr, Medical Center Blvd, Winston Salem, NC 27157-1029; **Phone:** (336) 716-4038; **Board Cert:** Neurological Surgery 1991; **Med School:** Univ Tex SW, Dallas 1981; **Resid:** Neurological Surgery, NC Bapt Hosp, Winston Salem, NC 1982-1987; **Fac Appt:** Assoc Prof Neurological Surgery, Wake Forest Univ Sch Med

Cahill, David W MD (NS) - *Spec Exp:* Spinal Surgery; **Hospital:** Tampa Genl Hosp; **Address:** 4 Columbia Drive, Ste 730, Tampa, FL 33606-3568; **Phone:** (813) 259-0965; **Board Cert:** Neurological Surgery 1985, Neurology 1983; **Med School:** Univ VA Sch Med 1976; **Resid:** Neurological Surgery, Univ Maryland Hosp, Baltimore, MD 1978-1983; Neurology, Univ Maryland Hosp, Baltimore, MD 1977-1979; **Fac Appt:** Prof Neurological Surgery, Univ S FL Coll Med

Day, Arthur L MD (NS) - *Spec Exp:* Cerebrovascular Disease; Cranial/Orbital Tumors; Carotid Artery Disease; **Hospital:** Shands Hlthcre at Univ of FL (page 73); **Address:** Shands Univ Florida, Dept Neuro Surg, 1600 SW Archer Rd, Box 100265, Gainesville, FL 32610-0265; **Phone:** (352) 392-4331; **Board Cert:** Neurological Surgery 1980; **Med School:** Louisiana State Univ 1972; **Resid:** Neurological Surgery, Shands-Univ Florida Hosp, Gainesville, FL 1973-1977; **Fellow:** Neurological Pathology, Shands-Univ Florida Hosp, Gainesville, FL 1977-1978; **Fac Appt:** Prof Neurological Surgery, Univ Fla Coll Med

Faillace, Walter MD (NS) - *Spec Exp:* Hydrocephalus; Spinal Disorders; Trauma; **Hospital:** Shands Jacksonville; **Address:** 653 W 8th St, Ste 1, Jacksonville, FL 32209-6511; **Phone:** (904) 244-3950; **Board Cert:** Neurological Surgery 1991; **Med School:** Italy 1980; **Resid:** Surgery, Jewish Hosp Med Ctr, Brooklyn, NY 1980-1982; Neurological Surgery, Univ Rochester Sch Med, Rochester, NY 1982-1987; **Fellow:** Pediatrics, Chldns Hosp Mich-Wayne State, Detroit, MI 1987-1988; **Fac Appt:** Assoc Prof Neurological Surgery, Univ Fla Coll Med

Ferraz, Francisco M MD (NS) - *Spec Exp:* Brain Tumors; Spinal Surgery; Cervical Spine Surgery; **Hospital:** Arlington Hosp; **Address:** 611 S Carlin Springs Rd, Ste 105, Arlington, VA 22204; **Phone:** (703) 845-1552; **Board Cert:** Neurological Surgery 1987; **Med School:** Brazil 1975; **Resid:** Neurological Surgery, Georgetown Univ Affil Hosp, Washington, DC 1977-1982

Freeman, Thomas B MD (NS) - *Spec Exp:* Parkinson's Disease; Neural Transplantation; Spinal Surgery; **Hospital:** Tampa Genl Hosp; **Address:** 4 Columbia Dr, Ste 730, Tampa, FL 33606; **Phone:** (813) 259-0889; **Board Cert:** Neurological Surgery 1993; **Med School:** Johns Hopkins Univ 1981; **Resid:** Neurological Surgery, NYU Med Ctr, New York, NY 1982-1988; **Fac Appt:** Prof Neurological Surgery, Univ S Fla Coll Med

Friedman, William A MD (NS) - *Spec Exp:* Stereotactic Radiosurgery; Brain Tumors; Parkinson's Disease; **Hospital:** Shands Hlthcre at Univ of FL (page 73); **Address:** Dept Surgery, 1600 SW Archer Rd, Box 100265, Gainesville, FL 32610-0265; **Phone:** (352) 392-4331; **Board Cert:** Neurological Surgery 1984; **Med School:** Ohio State Univ 1976; **Resid:** Neurological Surgery, Shands-Univ Florida Hosp, Gainesville, FL 1977-1982; **Fac Appt:** Prof Neurological Surgery, Univ Fla Coll Med

Green, Barth MD (NS) - *Spec Exp:* Spinal Surgery; **Hospital:** Univ of Miami - Jackson Meml Hosp; **Address:** Univ Miami, Dept Neuro Surg, 1095 NW 14th Terr, Miami, FL 33136; **Phone:** (305) 243-3254; **Board Cert:** Neurological Surgery 1978; **Med School:** Indiana Univ 1969; **Resid:** Neurological Surgery, Northwestern Univ Sch Med, Chicago, IL 1970-1975; **Fac Appt:** Prof Neurological Surgery, Univ Miami Sch Med

Hadley, Mark N MD (NS) - *Spec Exp:* Spinal Surgery; Spinal Surgery-Degenerative; **Hospital:** Univ of Ala Hosp at Birmingham; **Address:** Univ Alabama-Birmingham Sch Med, Div Neurosurgery, 1813 6th Ave S, Birmingham, AL 35294; **Phone:** (205) 934-1439; **Board Cert:** Neurological Surgery 1992; **Med School:** Albany Med Coll 1982; **Resid:** Neurological Surgery, St Josephs Hosp Med Ctr, Phoenix, AZ 1983-1988; **Fac Appt:** Prof Neurological Surgery, Univ Ala

Heros, Roberto MD (NS) - *Spec Exp:* Cerebrovascular Disease; **Hospital:** Jackson Meml Hosp; **Address:** 1095 NW Fourteen Terr, MC D-46, Miami, FL 33136; **Phone:** (305) 243-6672; **Board Cert:** Neurological Surgery 1978; **Med School:** Univ Tenn Coll Med, Memphis 1968; **Resid:** Surgery, Mass Genl Hosp, Boston, MA 1969-1970; Neurological Surgery, Mass Genl Hosp, Boston, MA 1972-1976; **Fac Appt:** Prof Neurological Surgery, Univ Miami Sch Med

Kelly Jr, David L MD (NS) - *Spec Exp:* Disc Disease; Spine Surgery-Degenerative; **Hospital:** Wake Forest Univ Baptist Med Ctr (page 81); **Address:** Wake Forest Univ Baptist Med Ctr, Med Ctr Blvd, Winston Salem, NC 27157-1029; **Phone:** (336) 716-4049; **Board Cert:** Neurological Surgery 1967; **Med School:** Univ NC Sch Med 1959; **Resid:** Neurological Surgery, Chldns Hospital, Boston, MA 1962-1963; Neurological Surgery, NC Bapt Hosp, Winston Salem, NC 1960-1962; **Fellow:** Neurological Physiology, Wash Univ, St Louis, MO 1963-1964; **Fac Appt:** Prof Neurological Surgery, Wake Forest Univ Sch Med

Laws Jr., Edward R MD (NS) - *Spec Exp:* Pituitary Surgery; Epilepsy/Seizure Disorders; Brain Tumors; **Hospital:** Univ of VA Hlth Sys (page 79); **Address:** Univ VA Hlth Scis Ctr, Dept Neurosurg, Box 800212, Charlottesville, VA 22908-0212; **Phone:** (434) 924-2650; **Board Cert:** Neurological Surgery 1974; **Med School:** Johns Hopkins Univ 1963; **Resid:** Neurological Surgery, Johns Hopkins Hosp, Baltimore, MD 1966-1971; **Fac Appt:** Prof Neurological Surgery, Univ VA Sch Med

Morrison, Glenn MD (NS) - *Spec Exp:* Neurosurgery-Pediatric; Craniofacial Surgery; Hydrocephalus; **Hospital:** Miami Children's Hosp; **Address:** Medical Arts Bldg, 3200 SW 60th Ct, Ste 301, Miami, FL 33155-4071; **Phone:** (305) 662-8386; **Board Cert:** Neurological Surgery 1976; **Med School:** Case West Res Univ 1967; **Resid:** Neurological Surgery, Case Western Univ Hosp, Cleveland, OH 1970-1974; **Fac Appt:** Prof Neurological Surgery, Univ Miami Sch Med

O'Brien, Mark S MD (NS) - *Spec Exp:* Hydrocephalus-Pediatric; Brain & Spinal Cord Tumors-Pediatric; **Hospital:** Chldn's Hlthcre of Atlanta - Scottish Rite; **Address:** 1900 Century Blvd NE, Ste 4, Atlanta, GA 30345; **Phone:** (404) 321-9234; **Board Cert:** Neurological Surgery 1971; **Med School:** St Louis Univ 1959; **Resid:** Neurology, Charity Hosp, New Orleans, LA 1962-1963; Neurological Surgery, St Vincents Hosp Med Ctr, New York, NY 1963-1965; **Fellow:** Neuroradiology, Albert Einstein Sch Med, Bronx, NY 1968-1969; **Fac Appt:** Prof Surgery, Emory Univ

Oakes, W Jerry MD (NS) - *Spec Exp:* *Neurosurgery-Pediatric; Chiari's Deformity;* **Hospital:** Children's Hospital - Birmingham; **Address:** Children's Hospital of Alabama, 1600 7th Ave S Bldg ACC - rm 400, Birmingham, AL 35233; **Phone:** (205) 939-9653; **Board Cert:** Neurological Surgery 1981; **Med School:** Duke Univ 1972; **Resid:** Neurological Surgery, Duke Hosp, Durham, NC 1972-1978; **Fellow:** Neurological Surgery, Hosp for Sick Chldn, Toronto, Canada 1975; Neurological Surgery, Great Ormond St Hosp, London, England 1978-1979; **Fac Appt:** Prof Neurological Surgery, Univ Ala

Rhoton Jr, Albert L MD (NS) - *Spec Exp:* *Pituitary Surgery; Acoustic Nerve Tumors; Trigeminal Neuralgia;* **Hospital:** Shands Hlthcre at Univ of FL (page 73); **Address:** Shands-Univ Florida Hosp, Dept Neurological Surgery, 1600 SW Archer Blvd, Box 100265, Gainesville, FL 32610-0265; **Phone:** (352) 392-4331; **Board Cert:** Neurological Surgery 1968; **Med School:** Univ Wash 1959; **Resid:** Surgery, Columbia Presby Med Ctr, New York, NY 1960-1961; Neurological Surgery, Barnes Hosp, St Louis, MO 1962-1965; **Fellow:** Neurological Anatomy, Natl Inst Neuro Disorder-NIH, Bethesda, MD 1965; **Fac Appt:** Prof Neurological Surgery, Univ Fla Coll Med

Rodts Jr, Gerald E MD (NS) - *Spec Exp:* *Spinal Surgery;* **Hospital:** Emory Univ Hosp; **Address:** Neoro Spine Inst, Emory Univ, 478 Peachtree St, Ste 607A, Atlanta, GA 30308; **Phone:** (404) 686-8101; **Board Cert:** Neurological Surgery 1998; **Med School:** Columbia P&S 1987; **Resid:** Neurological Surgery, UCLA Med Ctr, Los Angeles, CA 1988-1994; **Fellow:** Spine Surgery, Emory Univ Hosp, Atlanta, GA 1994-1995; **Fac Appt:** Assoc Prof Neurological Surgery, Emory Univ

Rosomoff, Hubert L MD (NS) - *Spec Exp:* *Pain Management;* **Hospital:** South Shore Hosp - Miami Bch; **Address:** Univ Miami Comprehensive Pain & Rehab Ctr, 600 Alton Rd, Ste 932, Miami Beach, FL 33139; **Phone:** (305) 532-7246; **Board Cert:** Neurological Surgery 1961; **Med School:** Hahnemann Univ 1952; **Resid:** Neurological Surgery, Neurology Inst-Columbia Presbyterian, New York, NY 1953-1959; **Fac Appt:** Prof Neurological Surgery, Univ Miami Sch Med

Sekhar, Laligam N MD (NS) - *Spec Exp:* *Aneurysm-Cerebral; Brain Tumors/Skull Base Tumors; Arteriovenous Malformations;* **Hospital:** Inova Fairfax Hosp; **Address:** 3301 Woodburn Rd, Ste 202, Annandale, VA 22003-7301; **Phone:** (703) 641-5911; **Board Cert:** Neurological Surgery 1986; **Med School:** India 1973; **Resid:** Neurology, Univ Cincinnati Med Ctr, Cincinnati, OH 1976-1977; Neurology, Univ Pittsburgh Med Ctr, Pittsburgh, PA 1977-1982; **Fellow:** Cerebrovascular Neurosurgery, Norstadt Krankenhaus, Hannover, W Germany 1982-1983; Neurological Surgery, Univ Zurich Hospital, Zurich, Switzerland 1983; **Fac Appt:** Clin Prof Neurological Surgery, Geo Wash Univ

Swaid, Swaid MD (NS) - *Spec Exp:* *Neurological Surgery - General;* **Hospital:** Healthsouth Med Ctr - Birmingham; **Address:** 1201 11th Ave S, Ste 500, Birmingham, AL 35205; **Phone:** (205) 930-8400; **Board Cert:** Neurological Surgery 1983; **Med School:** Univ Ala 1976; **Resid:** Neurological Surgery, Univ Alabama Sch Med., Birmingham, AL 1977-1981

Tulipan, Noel B MD (NS) - *Spec Exp:* *Pediatric Neurosurgery; Fetal Neurosurgery; Spina Bifida;* **Hospital:** Vanderbilt Univ Med Ctr (page 80); **Address:** Vanderbilt Univ Med Ctr N, Dept Nerosurgery, Med Ctr North, Ste T4224, Nashville, TN 37232; **Phone:** (615) 322-6875; **Board Cert:** Neurological Surgery 1989; **Med School:** Johns Hopkins Univ 1977; **Fac Appt:** Assoc Prof Neurological Surgery, Vanderbilt Univ

Midwest

Atkinson, John MD (NS) - *Spec Exp:* Pituitary Surgery; Brain Hemorrhage; Cerebrovascular Disease; **Hospital:** Mayo Med Ctr & Clin - Rochester, MN; **Address:** Dept Neurosurgery, 200 1st St SW, Rochester, MN 55905; **Phone:** (507) 284-2376; **Board Cert:** Neurological Surgery 1992; **Med School:** Univ Ala 1984; **Resid:** Neurological Surgery, Mayo Clinic, Rochester, MN 1985-1990; **Fac Appt:** Assoc Prof Neurological Surgery, Mayo Med Sch

Barnett, Gene H MD (NS) - *Spec Exp:* Brain Tumors; Stereotactic Radiosurgery; **Hospital:** Cleveland Clin Fdn (page 57); **Address:** Cleveland Clinic, Dept Surgery, 9500 Euclid Ave, rm S80, Cleveland, OH 44195-0001; **Phone:** (216) 444-5381; **Board Cert:** Neurological Surgery 1990; **Med School:** Case West Res Univ 1980; **Resid:** Neurological Surgery, Cleveland Clinic, Cleveland, OH 1981-1986; **Fellow:** Neurology, Cleveland Clinic, Cleveland, OH 1981-1982; Research, Mass Genl Hosp-Harvard, Boston, MA 1986-1987

Batjer, H Hunt MD (NS) - *Spec Exp:* Aneurysm-Cerebral; Arteriovenous Malformations; Stroke; **Hospital:** Northwestern Meml Hosp; **Address:** 675 N St. Clair, Ste 20-100, Chicago, IL 60611; **Phone:** (312) 695-8143; **Board Cert:** Neurological Surgery 1986; **Med School:** Univ Tex SW, Dallas 1977; **Resid:** Neurological Surgery, Parkland Meml, Dallas, TX 1978-1981; **Fellow:** Neurological Surgery, Univ West Ont, Ontario, Canada 1981-1982; **Fac Appt:** Prof Neurological Surgery, Northwestern Univ

Bauer, Jerry MD (NS) - *Spec Exp:* Pain-Back & Neck; Brain Tumors; Sciatica; **Hospital:** Advocate Lutheran Gen Hosp; **Address:** Ctr Brain & Spine Surg-Parkside Ctr, 1875 Dempster St, Ste 605, Park Ridge, IL 60068; **Phone:** (847) 698-1088; **Board Cert:** Neurological Surgery 1981; **Med School:** Univ IL Coll Med 1974; **Resid:** Neurological Surgery, Northwestern, Chicago, IL 1974-1975; Neurological Surgery, Univ Illinois Hosp, Chicago, IL 1975-1979; **Fac Appt:** Asst Clin Prof Neurological Surgery, Univ IL Coll Med

Benzel, Edward C MD (NS) - *Spec Exp:* Spinal Surgery; **Hospital:** Cleveland Clin Fdn (page 57); **Address:** Cleveland Clinic, Dept Neurosurgery, 9500 Euclid Ave, MC S80, Cleveland, OH 44195; **Phone:** (216) 445-5514; **Board Cert:** Neurological Surgery 1986; **Med School:** Univ Wisc 1974; **Resid:** Neurological Surgery, Univ Wisconsin Med Ctr, Madison, WI 1976-1980; **Fellow:** Spinal Cord Injury Medicine, Wood VA Med Ctr, Milwaukee, WI 1980-1981; **Fac Appt:** Prof Neurological Surgery, Case West Res Univ

Brown, Frederick MD (NS) - *Spec Exp:* Spinal Surgery; Pain-Chronic; Spasticity Surgery; **Hospital:** Univ of Chicago Hosps (page 76); **Address:** 5841 S Maryland Ave, MS 3026, Chicago, IL 60637; **Phone:** (773) 702-2123; **Board Cert:** Neurological Surgery 1982; **Med School:** Ohio State Univ 1972; **Resid:** Neurological Surgery, Univ Chicago Hosps, Chicago, IL 1973-1978; **Fac Appt:** Assoc Prof Neurological Surgery, Univ Chicago-Pritzker Sch Med

Chandler, William F MD (NS) - *Spec Exp:* Pituitary Surgery; Brain Tumors; **Hospital:** Univ of MI Hlth Ctr; **Address:** 1500 E Med Center Drive, Ste 2124D, Ann Arbor, MI 48109; **Phone:** (734) 936-5020; **Board Cert:** Neurological Surgery 1980; **Med School:** Univ Mich Med Sch 1971; **Resid:** Neurological Surgery, Michigan Hosp, Detroit, MI 1972-1977; **Fac Appt:** Prof Neurological Surgery, Univ Mich Med Sch

Dacey Jr., Ralph Gerald MD (NS) - *Spec Exp:* Vascular Neurosurgery; Aneurysm-Cerebral; **Hospital:** Barnes-Jewish Hosp (page 55); **Address:** Barnes-Jewish Hospital, 660 S Euclid Ave, Box Campus - 8057, St. Louis, MO 63110; **Phone:** (314) 362-5039; **Board Cert:** Neurological Surgery 1985, Internal Medicine 1978; **Med School:** Univ VA Sch Med 1974; **Resid:** Neurological Surgery, Univ VA, Charolettesville, VA 1977-1983; Internal Medicine, Strong Meml Hosp, Rochester 1975-1977; **Fac Appt:** Prof Neurological Surgery, Washington Univ, St Louis

Dempsey, Robert J. MD (NS) - *Spec Exp:* Vascular Neurosurgery; Aneurysm-Cerebral; Stroke; **Hospital:** Univ WI Hosp & Clins; **Address:** Univ Wisconsin Hosp, Dept Neurosurgery, 600 Highland Ave Bldg CSC - rm K4822, Madison, WI 53792; **Phone:** (608) 263-9585; **Board Cert:** Neurological Surgery 1985; **Med School:** Univ Chicago-Pritzker Sch Med 1977; **Resid:** Neurological Surgery, Univ Wisconsin Hosp, Madison, WI 1978-1983; **Fac Appt:** Prof Neurological Surgery, Univ Wisc

Diaz, Fernando G MD (NS) - *Spec Exp:* Neck & Carotid Reconstruction; Carotid Artery Disease; **Hospital:** Harper Hosp (page 59); **Address:** Harper Professional Bldg, 4160 John R, Ste 930, Detroit, MI 48201; **Phone:** (248) 784-3667; **Board Cert:** Neurological Surgery 1980; **Med School:** Mexico 1968; **Resid:** Surgery, Univ Kansas Med Ctr, Kansas City, MO 1971-1973; Neurological Surgery, Univ Minn Med Ctr, Minneapolis, MN 1973-1978; **Fellow:** Cerebrovascular Disease, Univ Minn, Minneapolis, MN 1978-1979; **Fac Appt:** Prof Neurological Surgery, Wayne State Univ

Grubb Jr, Robert L MD (NS) - *Spec Exp:* Cerebrovascular Disease; Skull Base Tumors; Trigeminal Neuralgia; **Hospital:** Barnes-Jewish Hosp (page 55); **Address:** Washington Univ School of Med, One Barnes-Jewish Hospital Plaza, St. Louis, MO 63110; **Phone:** (314) 362-3577; **Board Cert:** Neurological Surgery 1976; **Med School:** Univ NC Sch Med 1965; **Resid:** Surgery, Barnes Hosp, St Louis, MO 1966-1967; Neurological Surgery, Barnes Hosp, St Louis, MO 1969-1973; **Fellow:** Neurological Surgery, Natl Inst Hlth, Bethesda, MD 1968-1969; **Fac Appt:** Prof Neurological Surgery, Univ Wash

Gutierrez, Francisco A MD (NS) - *Spec Exp:* Brain Tumors; Cerebrovascular Disease; **Hospital:** Northwestern Meml Hosp; **Address:** 201 E Huron St, Ste 9-160, Chicago, IL 60611; **Phone:** (312) 926-3490; **Board Cert:** Neurological Surgery 1976; **Med School:** Colombia 1965; **Resid:** Neurological Surgery, San Juan de Dios Hosp, Bogota, Columbia 1967; Neurological Surgery, Northwestern Meml Hosp, Chicago, IL 1969-1973; **Fac Appt:** Asst Prof Neurological Surgery, Northwestern Univ

Hekmatpanah, Javad MD (NS) - *Spec Exp:* Brain Tumors; Spinal Stenosis; Chiari's Deformity; **Hospital:** Univ of Chicago Hosps (page 76); **Address:** 5841 S Maryland Ave, MC 3026, Chicago, IL 60637; **Phone:** (773) 702-6157; **Board Cert:** Neurological Surgery 1966, Neurology 1967; **Med School:** Iran 1956; **Resid:** Neurology, Wisconsin Genl Hosp-Univ Wisconsin, Milwaukee, WI 1958-1961; Neurological Surgery, Univ Chicago Hosp, Chicago, IL 1961-1964; **Fac Appt:** Prof Neurological Surgery, Univ Chicago-Pritzker Sch Med

Hoff, Julian T MD (NS) - *Spec Exp:* Brain & Spinal Surgery; Disc Disease-Lumbar; Neurofibromatosis; **Hospital:** Univ of MI Hlth Ctr; **Address:** Univ Mich Med Ctr, Dept NS, 1500 N Med Ctr Drive, Ste 2128, Ann Arbor, MI 48109-0338; **Phone:** (734) 936-5015; **Board Cert:** Neurological Surgery 1973; **Med School:** Cornell Univ-Weill Med Coll 1962; **Resid:** Neurological Surgery, NY Hosp, New York, NY 1966-1970; Surgery, NY Hosp, New York, NY 1963-1964; **Fellow:** Anesthesiology, Cardio Vascular Inst UCSF, San Francisco, CA 1970; Neurological Science, Univ of Glasgow, Glasgow, Scotland 1972-1974; **Fac Appt:** Prof Neurological Surgery, Univ Mich Med Sch

Kranzler, Leonard I MD (NS) - *Spec Exp:* Brain Tumors; **Hospital:** Advocate IL Masonic Med Ctr; **Address:** 3000 N Halstead St, Ste 701, Chicago, IL 60657; **Phone:** (773) 296-6666; **Board Cert:** Neurological Surgery 1974; **Med School:** Northwestern Univ 1963; **Resid:** Neurological Surgery, Northwestern Univ, Chicago, IL 1964-1969; Neurological Surgery, Chldns Meml Hosp, Chicago, IL 1966-1967; **Fellow:** Neurological Surgery, Zurich, Switzerland 1971; **Fac Appt:** Assoc Clin Prof Neurological Surgery, Univ Chicago-Pritzker Sch Med

Levy, Robert M MD (NS) - *Spec Exp:* Stereotactic Radiosurgery; Brain Tumors; Pain-Chronic; **Hospital:** Northwestern Meml Hosp; **Address:** 233 E Erie St, Ste 614, Chicago, IL 60611-5935; **Phone:** (312) 695-8143; **Board Cert:** Neurological Surgery 1991; **Med School:** Stanford Univ 1981; **Resid:** Neurological Surgery, UCSF, San Francisco, CA 1982-1987; **Fellow:** Neurological Surgery, UCSF, San Francisco, CA 1983-1986; **Fac Appt:** Prof Neurological Surgery, Northwestern Univ

Luerssen, Thomas G. MD (NS) - *Spec Exp:* Neurosurgery-Pediatric; **Hospital:** Riley Chldrn's Hosp (page 588); **Address:** 702 Barnhill Drive, Ste 1730, Indianapolis, IN 46202; **Phone:** (317) 274-5000; **Board Cert:** Neurological Surgery 1985; **Med School:** Indiana Univ 1976; **Resid:** Neurological Surgery, Ind Univ Hosp, Indianapolis, IN 1977-1981; **Fellow:** Pediatric Neurological Surgery, Childrens Hospital, Philadelphia, PA 1983-1984; **Fac Appt:** Prof Neurological Surgery, Indiana Univ

Luken, Martin MD (NS) - *Spec Exp:* Cervical Spine Surgery; Chiari's Deformity; **Hospital:** Rush-Presby - St Luke's Med Ctr (page 72); **Address:** 71 W 156th St, Ste 208, Harvey, IL 60426; **Phone:** (708) 331-6669; **Board Cert:** Neurological Surgery 1983; **Med School:** Columbia P&S 1973; **Resid:** Surgery, Univ IL Med Ctr, Chicago, NY 1975-1976; Neurological Surgery, Neurology Inst-Columbia Presbyterian, Chicago, IL 1976-1980

Malik, Ghaus MD (NS) - *Spec Exp:* Trigeminal Neuralgia; Vascular Neurosurgery; Tumors-Complex Brain & Spinal Cord; **Hospital:** Henry Ford Hosp; **Address:** 2799 W Grand Blvd, Detroit, MI 48202; **Phone:** (313) 916-2241; **Board Cert:** Neurological Surgery 1978; **Med School:** Pakistan 1968; **Resid:** Neurological Surgery, Henry Ford Hosp, Detroit, MI 1971-1975; Surgery, Henry Ford Hosp, Detroit, MI 1970-1971

Mayberg, Marc MD (NS) - *Spec Exp:* Pituitary Surgery; Stroke/Cerebrovascular Disease; Skull Base Tumors; **Hospital:** Cleveland Clin Fdn (page 57); **Address:** Cleveland Clinic Foundation, 9500 Euclid Ave, rm S80, Cleveland, OH 44195-0002; **Phone:** (216) 445-4430; **Board Cert:** Neurological Surgery 1988; **Med School:** Mayo Med Sch 1978; **Resid:** Neurological Surgery, Mass Genl Hosp, Boston, MA 1979-1984; **Fellow:** Neurological Surgery, Natl Hosp for Nervous Dis, London 1985; **Fac Appt:** Prof Surgery, Ohio State Univ

Menezes, Arnold MD (NS) - *Spec Exp:* Neurosurgery-Pediatric; Craniocervical Abnormalities; **Hospital:** Univ of IA Hosp and Clinics; **Address:** Dept Neurosurgery, 200 Hawkins Drive Bldg JPP - rm 1841, Iowa City, IA 52242; **Phone:** (319) 356-2768; **Board Cert:** Neurological Surgery 1976; **Med School:** India 1967; **Resid:** Surgery, Univ of Iowa Hosp, Iowa City, IA 1969-1970; Neurological Surgery, Univ of Iowa Hosp, Iowa City, IA 1970-1974; **Fellow:** Child Neurology, Univ of Iowa Hosp, Iowa City, IA 1973; **Fac Appt:** Prof Neurological Surgery, Univ Iowa Coll Med

Nagib, Mahmoud MD (NS) - *Spec Exp:* Neurological Surgery - General; **Hospital:** Chldns Hosp and Clinics - Minneapolis; **Address:** 305 Piper Bldg, 800 E 28th Street, Minneapolis, MN 55407-3723; **Phone:** (612) 871-7278; **Board Cert:** Neurological Surgery 1985; **Resid:** Neurological Surgery, Univ Minnesota Hosps, Minneapolis, MN 1977-1982; **Fellow:** Neurological Physiology, Univ Oslo, Oslo, Norway 1975-1976; **Fac Appt:** Asst Clin Prof Neurological Surgery, Univ Minn

Ondra, Stephen MD (NS) - *Spec Exp:* Spinal Surgery; **Hospital:** Northwestern Meml Hosp; **Address:** 675 N St Claire St, Ste 20-100, Chicago, IL 60611; **Phone:** (312) 695-8143; **Board Cert:** Neurological Surgery 1994; **Med School:** Rush Med Coll 1984; **Resid:** Neurological Surgery, Walter Reed Army Med Ctr, Washington, DC 1985-1990; **Fac Appt:** Assoc Prof Neurological Surgery, Northwestern Univ

Piepgras, David MD (NS) - *Spec Exp:* Vascular Neurosurgery; **Hospital:** Mayo Med Ctr & Clin - Rochester, MN; **Address:** Dept Neurologic Surgery, 200 W First St SW, Rochester, MN 55905; **Phone:** (507) 284-3331; **Board Cert:** Neurological Surgery 1977; **Med School:** Univ Minn 1965; **Resid:** Surgery, Hennipin Co Genl Hosp, Minneapolis, MN 1969-1970; Neurological Surgery, Mayo Clinic, Rochester, MN 1970-1974; **Fac Appt:** Prof Neurological Surgery, Mayo Med Sch

Rezai, Ali R MD (NS) - *Spec Exp:* Parkinson's Disease; Pain-Chronic; **Hospital:** Cleveland Clin Fdn (page 57); **Address:** Cleveland Clinic, Dept Neurosurgery-Desk S80, 9500 Euclid Ave, Cleveland, OH 44195-0001; **Phone:** (216) 444-4720; **Board Cert:** Neurological Surgery 1992; **Med School:** Univ SC Sch Med 1989; **Resid:** Neurological Surgery, NYU Med Ctr, New York, NY 1991-1997; **Fellow:** Neurological Surgery, Univ Toronto Med Ctr, Canada 1997-1998

Rosenblum, Mark MD (NS) - *Spec Exp:* Brain Tumors; Spinal Surgery; Infections of Nervous System; **Hospital:** Henry Ford Hosp; **Address:** Henry Ford Hospital, K11, 2799 W Grand Blvd, Detroit, MI 48202; **Phone:** (313) 916-1340; **Board Cert:** Neurological Surgery 1982; **Med School:** NY Med Coll 1969; **Resid:** Surgery, UCLA, Los Angeles, CA 1972-1973; Neurological Surgery, UC San Francisco Med Ctr, San Francisco, CA 1973-1979; **Fac Appt:** Prof Neurological Surgery, Case West Res Univ

Ruge, John MD (NS) - *Spec Exp:* Neurosurgery-Pediatric; Brain Tumors; Pain-Facial; **Hospital:** Advocate Lutheran Gen Hosp; **Address:** 1875 Dempster St, Ste 605, Park Ridge, IL 60608; **Phone:** (847) 698-1088; **Board Cert:** Neurological Surgery 1993; **Med School:** Northwestern Univ 1983; **Resid:** Neurological Surgery, Northwestern Meml Hosp, Chicago, IL 1983-1989; **Fellow:** Pediatric Neurological Surgery, Children's Hosp, Chicago, IL 1989-1990; **Fac Appt:** Asst Prof Surgery, Univ IL Coll Med

Selman, Warren R MD (NS) - *Spec Exp:* Stroke-Microsurgery; Pituitary Surgery; **Hospital:** Univ Hosp of Cleveland; **Address:** 11100 Euclid Ave, Dept Neurosurgery, Cleveland, OH 44106; **Phone:** (216) 844-5745; **Board Cert:** Neurological Surgery 1986; **Med School:** Case West Res Univ 1977; **Resid:** Neurological Surgery, Univ Hosp Cleveland, Cleveland, OH 1978-1984; **Fellow:** Research, Univ Hosp Cleveland, Cleveland, OH 1978-1980; Neurological Surgery, Mayo Clin, Rochester, MN 1984; **Fac Appt:** Prof Neurological Surgery, Case West Res Univ

Traynelis, Vincent C MD (NS) - *Spec Exp:* Spinal Surgery; **Hospital:** Univ of IA Hosp and Clinics; **Address:** Univ Iowa Hosp & Clinic, Dept Neurosurgery, 200 Hawkins Drive, Iowa City, IA 52242; **Phone:** (319) 356-2774; **Board Cert:** Neurological Surgery 1992; **Med School:** Univ Iowa Coll Med 1983; **Resid:** Neurological Surgery, West Virginia Med Ctr, Morgantown, WV 1984-1989; **Fac Appt:** Prof Neurological Surgery, Univ Iowa Coll Med

Great Plains and Mountains

Apfelbaum, Ronald I MD (NS) - *Spec Exp:* Spinal Surgery; **Hospital:** Univ Utah Hosp and Clin; **Address:** University of Utah Hosp, Dept Neurosurgery, 50 N Medical Drive, rm 3B409, Salt Lake City, UT 84132-1001; **Phone:** (801) 581-6908; **Board Cert:** Neurological Surgery 1976; **Med School:** Hahnemann Univ 1965; **Resid:** Surgery, Montefiore Med Ctr, Bronx, NY 1968-1969; Neurological Surgery, Montefiore Med Ctr, Bronx, NY 1969-1974; **Fac Appt:** Prof Neurological Surgery, Univ Utah

Awad, Issam A MD (NS) - *Spec Exp:* Neurovascular Surgery; Stroke; Cerebrovascular Disease; **Hospital:** Univ Colo HSC - Denver; **Address:** 4200 E Ninth Ave, Campus Box C-307, Denver, CO 80262; **Phone:** (303) 315-1310; **Board Cert:** Neurological Surgery 1988; **Med School:** Loma Linda Univ 1980; **Resid:** Neurological Surgery, Cleveland Clin, Cleveland, OH 1981-1985; **Fellow:** Neurological Vascular Surgery, Barrow Neur Inst, Pheonix, AZ 1985-1986; **Fac Appt:** Prof Neurological Surgery, Yale Univ

Walker, Marion L. MD (NS) - *Spec Exp:* Neurosurgery-Pediatric; Hydrocephalus; Brain Tumors; **Hospital:** Primary Children's Med Ctr; **Address:** Primary Chldns Med Ctr, Div Ped Neurosurg, 100 N Medical Dr, Salt Lake City, UT 84113-1103; **Phone:** (801) 588-3400; **Board Cert:** Surgery 1979; **Med School:** Univ Tenn Coll Med, Memphis 1969; **Resid:** Neurological Surgery, St Joseph's Hosp, Phoenix, AZ 1971-1976; **Fellow:** Pediatric Neurological Surgery, Hosp for Sick Chldn, Toronto, Ontario 1972-1973; **Fac Appt:** Prof Neurological Surgery, Univ Utah

Winston, Ken R. MD (NS) - *Spec Exp:* Neurosurgery-Pediatric; Craniosynostosis; Epilepsy/Seizure Disorders; **Hospital:** Chldn's Hosp - Denver; **Address:** 1056 E 19th Ave, Box B330, Denver, CO 80218; **Phone:** (303) 861-6100; **Board Cert:** Neurological Surgery 1973; **Med School:** Univ Tenn Coll Med, Memphis 1963; **Resid:** Surgery, Colorado General Hosp, Denver, CO 1966-1967; Neurological Surgery, Colorado General Hospital, Denver, CO 1967-1971; **Fac Appt:** Prof Neurological Surgery, Univ Colo

Southwest

Al-Mefty, Ossama MD (NS) - *Spec Exp:* Skull Base Surgery; Neuro-Oncology; Cerebrovascular Disease; **Hospital:** UAMS; **Address:** University Hospital of Arkansas for Medical Sciences, 4301 W Markham Slot 507, Little Rock, AR 72205; **Phone:** (501) 686-8757; **Board Cert:** Neurological Surgery 1980; **Med School:** Syria 1972; **Resid:** Surgery, Med Coll Ohio, Toledo, OH 1973-1974; Neurological Surgery, West Va Med Ctr, WV 1974-1978; **Fac Appt:** Prof Neurological Surgery, Univ Ark

Clifton, Guy MD (NS) - *Spec Exp:* Head Injury; Spinal Cord Surgery; **Hospital:** Meml Hermann Hosp; **Address:** Univ Texas Med Sch-Houston, Dept Neuro Surg, 6431 Fannin St , Ste 7.148, Houston, TX 77030; **Phone:** (713) 500-6135; **Board Cert:** Neurological Surgery 1983; **Med School:** Univ Tex Med Br, Galveston 1975; **Resid:** Neurological Surgery, Univ Texas Med Branch, Galveston, TX 1976-1980; **Fac Appt:** Prof Neurological Surgery, Univ Tex, Houston

Hankinson, Hal L. MD (NS) - *Spec Exp:* Brain Tumors; **Hospital:** Presbyterian Hospital - Albuquerque; **Address:** New Mexico Neurosurgery, 522 Lomas Blvd NE, Albuquerque, NM 87102-2454; **Phone:** (505) 247-4253; **Board Cert:** Neurological Surgery 1977; **Med School:** Tulane Univ 1967; **Resid:** Neurological Surgery, UC San Francisco, San Francisco, CA 1970-1975; **Fac Appt:** Clin Prof Neurological Surgery, Univ New Mexico

Harper, Richard L MD (NS) - *Spec Exp:* Spinal Surgery; Brain Tumors & Hemifacial Spasms; **Hospital:** Methodist Hosp - Houston; **Address:** 6560 Fannin St, Ste 1200, Houston, TX 77030; **Phone:** (713) 790-1211; **Board Cert:** Neurological Surgery 1983; **Med School:** Baylor Coll Med 1971; **Resid:** Baylor Hosps, Houston, TX 1974-1978

Hassenbusch, Samuel J MD/PhD (NS) - *Spec Exp:* Pain Management; Stereotactic Radiosurgery; Intratumoral Chemotherapy; **Hospital:** Univ of TX MD Anderson Cancer Ctr, The; **Address:** 1515 Holcombe Blvd, Box 442, Houston, TX 77030; **Phone:** (713) 792-2400; **Board Cert:** Neurological Surgery 1992; **Med School:** Johns Hopkins Univ 1978; **Resid:** Surgery, Johns Hopkins Univ, Baltimore, MD 1979-1980; Neurological Surgery, Johns Hopkins Univ, Baltimore, MD 1980-1988; **Fellow:** Research, Keck Foundation-UCSF, San Francisco, CA 1985-1986; **Fac Appt:** Assoc Prof Neurological Surgery, Univ Tex, Houston

Loftus, Christopher M. MD (NS) - *Spec Exp:* Cerebrovascular Disease; Carotid Artery,Gamma Knife Surgery; Brain Aneurysm/AVM Surgery; **Hospital:** Univ OK Hlth Sci Ctr; **Address:** Univ OK Hlth Sci Ctr, Dept Neurosurgery, 711 Stanton L Young Blvd, Ste 206, Oklahoma City, OK 73104; **Phone:** (405) 271-4912; **Board Cert:** Neurological Surgery 1987; **Med School:** SUNY Downstate 1979; **Resid:** Neurological Surgery, Columbia Presby Med Ctr, New York, NY 1980-1985; **Fac Appt:** Prof Neurological Surgery, Univ Okla Coll Med

Papadopoulos, Stephen M. MD (NS) - *Spec Exp:* Spinal Surgery; Stealth Guided Surgery; Stereotactic Radiosurgery; **Hospital:** St Joseph's Hosp & Med Ctr - Phoenix; **Address:** 2910 N 3rd Ave, Phoenix, AZ 85013; **Phone:** (602) 406-3159; **Board Cert:** Neurological Surgery 1991; **Med School:** UCSD 1978; **Resid:** Neurological Surgery, U Mich., Ann Arbor, MI 1983-1988; **Fellow:** Neurological Surgery, Barrow Neur. Inst., Phoenix, AZ 1989; **Fac Appt:** Assoc Prof Neurological Surgery, Univ Mich Med Sch

Samson, Duke MD (NS) - *Spec Exp:* Vascular Neurosurgery; Cerebrovascular Disease; **Hospital:** Zale Lipshy Univ Hosp; **Address:** U Tex SW Med Ctr @ Dallas, Dept Neuro Surg, 5303 Harry Hines Blvd, MC-8855, Dallas, TX 75390-8855; **Phone:** (214) 648-3529; **Board Cert:** Neurological Surgery 1978; **Med School:** Washington Univ, St Louis 1969; **Resid:** Neurological Surgery, Ctr Medico-Chirurgical Fech, Paris, France 1972-1973; **Fellow:** Neurological Surgery, U Tex SW, Dallas, TX 1970-1975; **Fac Appt:** Prof Neurological Surgery, Univ Tex SW, Dallas

Sonntag, Volker MD (NS) - *Spec Exp:* Spinal Surgery; **Hospital:** St Joseph's Hosp & Med Ctr - Phoenix; **Address:** Barrow Neurosurgical Assocs, Ltd, 2910 N Third Ave, Phoenix, AZ 85013; **Phone:** (602) 406-3458; **Board Cert:** Neurological Surgery 1980; **Med School:** Univ Ariz Coll Med 1971; **Resid:** Neurological Surgery, Tufts-New Eng Med Ctr, Boston, MA 1972-1977; **Fac Appt:** Clin Prof Neurological Surgery, Univ Ariz Coll Med

Spetzler, Robert MD (NS) - *Spec Exp:* Cerebrovascular Neurosurgery; **Hospital:** St Joseph's Hosp & Med Ctr - Phoenix; **Address:** Barrow Neurosurgical Assocs, 2910 N Third Ave, Phoenix, AZ 85013; **Phone:** (602) 406-3489; **Board Cert:** Neurological Surgery 1979; **Med School:** Northwestern Univ 1971; **Resid:** Neurological Surgery, UCSF Med Ctr, San Francisco, CA 1972-1976; **Fac Appt:** Prof Surgery, Univ Ariz Coll Med

West Coast and Pacific

Adler Jr, John R MD (NS) - *Spec Exp:* Stereotactic Radiosurgery; **Hospital:** Stanford Med Ctr; **Address:** Stanford Univ Med Ctr, 300 Pastuer Dr, Ste R155, Palo Alto, CA 94304-2203; **Phone:** (650) 723-5573; **Board Cert:** Neurological Surgery 1990; **Med School:** Harvard Med Sch 1980; **Resid:** Neurological Surgery, Chldns Hosp, Boston, MA 1981-1987; Neurological Surgery, Mass Genl Hosp, Boston, MA 1984-1985; **Fellow:** Cerebrovascular Disease, Karolinska Inst, Stockholm, Sweden 1985-1986; **Fac Appt:** Prof Neurological Surgery, Stanford Univ

Apuzzo, Michael L J MD (NS) - *Spec Exp:* Brain Tumors; Epilepsy/Seizure Disorders; Stereotactic Neurosurgery; **Hospital:** LAC & USC Med Ctr; **Address:** 1200 N State St, rm 5046, Los Angeles, CA 90033-1029; **Phone:** (323) 226-7421; **Board Cert:** Neurological Surgery 1975; **Med School:** Boston Univ 1965; **Resid:** Neurological Surgery, Hartford Hosp, Hartford, CT 1966; Neurological Surgery, Hartford Hosp, Hartford, CT 1970-1973; **Fellow:** Neurological Physiology, Yale Univ Hosp, New Haven, CT 1971; **Fac Appt:** Prof Neurological Surgery, USC Sch Med

Batzdorf, Ulrich MD (NS) - *Spec Exp:* Chiari's Deformity; Syringomyelia; Spinal Cord Tumors; **Hospital:** UCLA Med Ctr; **Address:** UCLA Med Ctr, Box 956901, Los Angeles, CA 90095-6901; **Phone:** (310) 825-5079; **Board Cert:** Neurological Surgery 1968; **Med School:** NY Med Coll 1955; **Resid:** Surgery, Univ Maryland Hosp, Baltimore, MD 1958-1960; Neurological Surgery, UCLA Ctr Hlth Sci, Los Angeles, CA 1963-1965; **Fellow:** Pathology, UCSF-Moffit Hosp, San Francisco, CA 1961-1962; **Fac Appt:** Prof Neurological Surgery, UCLA

Berger, Mitchel Stuart MD (NS) - *Spec Exp:* Brain Tumors-Adult & Pedatric; **Hospital:** UCSF Med Ctr; **Address:** UCSF, Dept of Neurological Surgery, 505 Parnassus Avenue, M-786, San Francisco, CA 94143-0112; **Phone:** (415) 502-7673; **Board Cert:** Neurological Surgery 1991; **Med School:** Univ Miami Sch Med 1979; **Resid:** Neurological Surgery, Univ CA SF Sch Med, San Francisco, CA 1979-1985; **Fellow:** Surgery, Univ CA SF Sch Med, San Francisco, CA 1985

Black, Keith Lanier MD (NS) - *Spec Exp:* Brain Tumors; **Hospital:** Cedars-Sinai Med Ctr; **Address:** 8631 W Third St, Ste 800, Los Angeles, CA 90048; **Phone:** (310) 423-7900; **Board Cert:** Neurological Surgery 1990; **Med School:** Univ Mich Med Sch 1981; **Resid:** Neurological Surgery, U Mich Med Ctr, Ann Arbor, MI 1982-1987; **Fac Appt:** Prof Neurological Surgery, UC Irvine

Burchiel, Kim James MD (NS) - *Spec Exp:* Pain Management; Stereotactic Radiosurgery; Epilepsy/Seizure Disorders; **Hospital:** OR Hlth Sci Univ Hosp and Clinics; **Address:** Dept Neuro Surgery-L472, 3181 SW Sam Jackson Park Rd, Portland, OR 97201; **Phone:** (503) 494-4314; **Board Cert:** Neurological Surgery 1984; **Med School:** UCSD 1976; **Resid:** Neurological Surgery, Univ Washington, Seattle, WA 1977-1982; **Fac Appt:** Assoc Prof Neurological Surgery, Oregon Hlth Scis Univ

Dogali, Michael MD (NS) - *Spec Exp:* Parkinson's Disease; Pain/Seizures; Seizures; **Hospital:** USC Univ Hosp - R K Eamer Med Plz; **Address:** USC Unv Hosp- USC Health Care Consultation Ctr, 1510 San Pablo St, Ste 268, Los Angeles, CA 90033; **Phone:** (323) 442-1799; **Board Cert:** Neurological Surgery 1980; **Med School:** McGill Univ 1970; **Resid:** Surgery, Duke University, Durham, NC 1970-1971; Neurological Surgery, Montreal Neuro Inst, Monteal, Quebec 1971-1976; **Fac Appt:** Prof Neurological Surgery, USC Sch Med

Ellenbogen, Richard MD (NS) - *Spec Exp:* Neurosurgery-Pediatric; Chiari's Deformity; **Hospital:** Chldns Hosp and Regl Med Ctr - Seattle; **Address:** 4800 Sand Point Way NE, MS CH-50, Seattle, WA 98105; **Phone:** (206) 526-2544; **Board Cert:** Neurological Surgery 1992; **Med School:** Brown Univ 1983; **Resid:** Neurological Surgery, Brigham&Womens Hosp, Boston, MA 1984-1989; **Fac Appt:** Asst Prof Neurological Surgery, Univ MD Sch Med

Giannotta, Steven L MD (NS) - *Spec Exp:* Aneurysm-Cerebral; Skull Base Tumors; Acoustic Neuroma; **Hospital:** USC Univ Hosp - R K Eamer Med Plz; **Address:** 1510 San Pablo St, Ste 268, Los Angeles, CA 90033; **Phone:** (323) 442-5757; **Board Cert:** Neurological Surgery 1980; **Med School:** Univ Mich Med Sch 1972; **Resid:** Neurological Surgery, Univ Michigan, Ann Arbor, MI 1973-1978; **Fac Appt:** Prof Neurological Surgery, USC Sch Med

Greene Jr, Clarence S MD (NS) - *Spec Exp:* Neurosurgery-Pediatric; **Hospital:** Long Beach Meml Med Ctr; **Address:** 2865 Atlantic Ave, Ste 202, Long Beach, CA 90806; **Phone:** (562) 426-4121; **Board Cert:** Neurological Surgery 1984; **Med School:** Howard Univ 1974; **Resid:** Neurological Surgery, Childrens Hosp, Boston, MA 1977-1981; Neurological Surgery, Peter Bent Brigham Hosp, Boston, MA 1977-1981; **Fellow:** Child Neurology, Childrens Hosp, Boston, MA 1984

Heilbrun, M Peter MD (NS) - *Spec Exp:* Stereotactic Radiosurgery; **Hospital:** Stanford Med Ctr; **Address:** Stanford Univ, Dept Neurosurgery, 300 Pasteur Drive, rm R200, Stanford, CA 94305; **Phone:** (650) 723-5574; **Board Cert:** Neurological Surgery 1973; **Med School:** SUNY Buffalo 1962; **Resid:** Surgery, Barnes Hosp, St Louis, MO 1963-1964; **Fellow:** Neurological Surgery, Univ Washington, St Louis, MO 1966-1967

Loeser, John D MD (NS) - *Spec Exp:* Pain Management; **Hospital:** Univ WA Med Ctr; **Address:** 1959 NE Pacific St, Box 356470, Seattle, WA 98195; **Phone:** (206) 543-3570; **Board Cert:** Neurological Surgery 1970; **Med School:** NYU Sch Med 1961; **Resid:** Neurological Surgery, Univ Wash, Seattle, WA 1962-1967; **Fac Appt:** Prof Anesthesiology, Univ Wash

McComb, J Gordon MD (NS) - *Spec Exp:* Neurosurgery-Pediatric; **Hospital:** Chldns Hosp - Los Angeles; **Address:** Children's Hosp, Queen of Angels Bldg, 1300 N Vermont Ave, Ste 906, Los Angeles, CA 90027-6005; **Phone:** (323) 663-8128; **Board Cert:** Neurological Surgery 1976; **Med School:** Univ Miami Sch Med 1965; **Resid:** Neurological Surgery, Chldns Hosp/Brigham Hosp, Boston, MA 1969-1973; Pediatrics, Chldns Hosp, Los Angeles, CA 1966-1967; **Fellow:** Physiology, Univ Coll London, London, UK 1973-1974; **Fac Appt:** Prof Neurological Surgery, USC Sch Med

Pitts, Lawrence H MD (NS) - *Spec Exp: Acoustic Nerve Tumors; Skull Base Surgery; Spinal Surgery;* **Hospital:** UCSF Med Ctr; **Address:** 400 Parnassus Ave, Ste A808, San Francisco, CA 94143-0350; **Phone:** (415) 353-2071; **Board Cert:** Neurological Surgery 1978; **Med School:** Case West Res Univ 1969; **Resid:** Neurological Surgery, UCSF, SanFrancisco, CA 1969-1975; **Fac Appt:** Prof Neurological Surgery, UCSF

Shaffrey, Christopher I MD (NS) - *Spec Exp: Spinal Surgery; Spinal Surgery-Pediatric;* **Hospital:** Univ WA Med Ctr; **Address:** 1959 NE Pacific St, Dept Neurological Surgery, Box 356470, Seattle, WA 98195; **Phone:** (206) 543-3570; **Board Cert:** Neurological Surgery 1997, Orthopaedic Surgery 1997; **Med School:** Univ VA Sch Med 1986; **Resid:** Neurological Surgery, Univ Virginia Med Ctr, Charlottesville, VA 1987-1992; Orthopaedic Surgery, Univ Virginia Med Ctr, Charlottesville, VA 1992-1995; **Fellow:** Spine Surgery, Univ Virginia Med Ctr, Charlottesville, VA 1995-1996; **Fac Appt:** Assoc Prof Neurological Surgery, Univ Wash

Steinberg, Gary K MD/PhD (NS) - *Spec Exp: Aneurysm-Cerebral; Moyamoya Syndrome-Adult; Arteriovenous Malformations;* **Hospital:** Stanford Med Ctr; **Address:** Stanford Univ Hosp, Dept Neurosurg, 300 Pasteur Drive, rm R281, Stanford, CA 94305-5327; **Phone:** (650) 723-5575; **Board Cert:** Neurological Surgery 1989; **Med School:** Stanford Univ 1980; **Resid:** Neuropathology, Stanford Univ, Palto Alto, CA 1981-1982; Neurological Surgery, Stanford Univ, Palto Alto, CA 1982-1987; **Fellow:** Cerebrovascular Neurosurgery, Univ West Ontario, Ontario, Canada 1984-1985; **Fac Appt:** Assoc Prof Neurological Surgery, Stanford Univ

Weiss, Martin Harvey MD (NS) - *Spec Exp: Brain Tumors; Spinal Cord Tumors;* **Hospital:** USC Univ Hosp - R K Eamer Med Plz; **Address:** LAC-USC Med Ctr, 1200 N State St, Ste 5046, Los Angeles, CA 90033-1029; **Phone:** (323) 226-7421; **Board Cert:** Neurological Surgery 1972; **Med School:** Cornell Univ-Weill Med Coll 1963; **Resid:** Surgery, US Army Hosp, West Point, NY 1964-1966; Neurological Surgery, Univ Hosp, Cleveland, OH 1966-1970; **Fellow:** Neurological Surgery, NIH-Univ Hosp, Cleveland, OH 1969-1970; **Fac Appt:** Prof Neurological Surgery, USC Sch Med

Winn, H Richard MD (NS) - *Spec Exp: Cerebrovascular Disease; Arteriovenous Malformations;* **Hospital:** Univ WA Med Ctr; **Address:** 700 Ninth Ave, Ste 311, Seattle, WA 98104; **Phone:** (206) 521-1833; **Board Cert:** Neurological Surgery 1979; **Med School:** Univ Penn 1968; **Resid:** Surgery, Univ Hosp, Cleveland, OH 1969-1970; Neurological Surgery, Univ VA, Charlottesville, VA 1970-1974; **Fac Appt:** Prof Neurological Surgery, Univ Wash

NEUROLOGY

A neurologist specializes in the diagnosis and treatment of all types of disease or impaired function of the brain, spinal cord, peripheral nerves, muscles and autonomic nervous system, as well as the blood vessels that relate to these structures. A child neurologist has special skills in the diagnosis and management of neurologic disorders of the neonatal period, infancy, early childhood and adolescence.

Training required: Four years

Certification in the following subspecialty requires additional training and examination.

Spinal Cord Injury Medicine: A physician who addresses the prevention, diagnosis, treatment and management of traumatic spinal cord injury and non-traumatic etiologies of spinal cord dysfunction by working in an interdisciplinary manner. Care is provided to patients of all ages on a lifelong basis and covers related medical, physical, psychological and vocational disabilities and complications.

CONTINUUM HEALTH PARTNERS, INC.
NEUROSCIENCES EXPERTISE

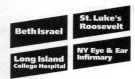

Phone (800) 420-4004

The partner hospitals of Continuum Health Partners have extensive clinical expertise in the challenging fields of neurology and neurosurgery. Our physicians are recognized authorities who establish care protocols, chart new venues in therapy and develop the technologies that set the standards in the field.

At Beth Israel Medical Center, The Hyman-Newman Institute for Neurology and Neurosurgery (The INN) is dedicated to care for children and adults with disorders of the brain, spinal cord, peripheral nerves and muscles. The founding clinicians of the INN had a vision of humanistic care that marries emotional and spiritual well being together with expert clinical care provided by world-recognized experts.

The Stanley S. Lamm Institute for Child Neurology and Developmental Medicine at Long Island College Hospital provides comprehensive care for children with neurodevelopmental disabilities. Care begins at diagnosis and continues with ongoing treatment and therapeutic intervention throughout a child's life—it includes neurologic care, physical and occupational therapy and speech and language pathology.

The Center for Cranial Base Therapy and the Minimally Invasive Spine Center offer advanced surgical treatments for tumors of the skull base, spine and spinal cord at Roosevelt Hospital. These neurosurgeons are also experts in surgery for acoustic neuromas and treatment of trigeminal neuralgia and hemifacial spasm.

Stroke prevention programs are located throughout Continuum's Manhattan and Brooklyn locations, offering 24-hour diagnosis and treatment, including use of clot busting thrombolitic medications.

PHYSICIAN REFERRAL SERVICE

For a referral to an expert physician in neurology or neurosurgery, call us at 1-800-420-4004 or visit us on the web at www.WeHealNewYork.org.

THE MOUNT SINAI HOSPITAL
NEUROLOGY AND NEUROSURGERY

One Gustave L. Levy Place (Fifth Avenue and 98th Street)
New York, NY 10029-6574   Phone: (212) 241-6500
Physician Referral: 1-800-MD-SINAI (637-4624)
www.mountsinai.org

A selection of our programs and services include:

The Neurosciences and Restorative Care Center
We provide adult inpatient care in neurology, neurosurgery, and orthopedics as well as plastic surgery and joint replacement. Specific programs and services are offered for the diagnosis and treatment of stroke, movement disorders, such as Parkinson's Disease, multiple sclerosis and myasthenia gravis, brain tumors, neuroAIDS, epilepsy, and degenerative disc disease. Ambulatory services are also available.

Autonomic Disorders Research and Treatment Program
Since 1985, we have been offering a comprehensive program committed to research, education, and care for patients with confirmed or suspected autonomic disorders every year.

The Clinical Program for Cerebrovascular Disorders
We provide expertise in the evaluation, treatment, and rehabilitation of patients with cerebrovascular diseases. Complementing the highly experienced team of medical experts are state-of-the-art facilities for surgical and endovascular treatment of cerebrovascular pathologies, a specialized Neurointensive Care Unit, and a brand new inpatient stroke unit. Video-telemedicine is utilized for the early diagnosis and treatment of stroke.

Division of Neuromuscular Diseases
It is our mission to provide unparalleled diagnosis, treatment, and compassionate care of patients with disorders in neuromuscular transmission, diseases of the muscles, or peripheral nerve problems.

The MDA/ALS Program
This clinic, dedicated to Muscular Dystrophy and Amyotrophic Lateral Sclerosis, provides comprehensive, multidimensional, and seamless patient- and family-centered care for those afflicted with these disorders.

The Robert and John M. Bendheim Parkinson's Disease Center
One of the world's first major centers for the study of Parkinson's Disease, we are a nucleus for multi-disciplinary translational research studies and a forum for collaboration. The center offers state-of-the-art research programs, fostering the development of new medical and surgical therapies for the disease.

THE MOUNT SINAI HOSPITAL

The Department of Neurology at The Mount Sinai hospital is the oldest neurology department in the country. From the beginning, it has been an intensively productive center for research and patient care, and over the past century, it has seen its reputation for excellence grow.

The Department of Neurosurgery at The Mount Sinai Hospital was established in 1910 and stands as an internationally renowned, independent department.

The residency program began in 1946 and is a nationally recognized center of excellence.

Areas of expertise exist in skull-base, cerebrovascular, pituitary, acoustic, spinal reconstruction, epilepsy, radiosurgery, stereotactic, primary brain tumor surgery, and neuroendoscopy.

Neurosurgery Research
- Clinical Programs & Case Presentations
- Cerebrovascular Laboratory
- Skull Base Dissection Laboratory
- Spinal Cord Injury Laboratory
- Epilepsy Laboratory
- Pituitary Endocrine Laboratory

NewYork-Presbyterian
The University Hospitals of Columbia and Cornell
Columbia Weill Cornell Neuroscience Centers

The Neurological Institute of New York at
Columbia Presbyterian Medical Center
710 West 168th Street
New York, NY 10032

NewYork Weill Cornell Neuroscience Institute at
NewYork Weill Cornell Medical Center
525 East 68th Street
New York, NY 10021

OVERVIEW:

The Columbia Weill Cornell Neuroscience Centers are consistently ranked among the top providers of neurological services in the United States, according to *U.S. News & World Report*. The Centers provide the most innovative, up-to-date treatments to combat the full range of neurological disorders, including:

- Stroke and Cerebrovascular Services – Diagnoses and treatments of Stroke (brain attack), Aneurysms, and Arteriovenous Malformations (AVMs) by leading neurologists, neurosurgeons and interventional neuroradiologists.

- Epilepsy – Comprehensive Epilepsy Centers provide round-the-clock surveillance of adults and children in monitoring unit and functional brain mapping to identify source of a seizure and the most effective treatment.

- Pediatric Neurology – Expertise and state-of-the-art care tailored to special needs of children.

- Spinal Disorders – The Spine Center integrates physicians specializing in neurology, neurosurgery, neuroradiology, orthopedics, physiatry (rehabilitative medicine) and anesthesiology/pain management, as well as physical and occupational therapy.

- Neuro-Oncology – Neuro-oncologists of the Herbert Irving Comprehensive Cancer Center, one of a select group of National Cancer Institute - designated cancer centers, utilize the latest techniques for improving patient survival and qualify of life.

- Neuro-Immunology – One of the country's largest Multiple Sclerosis treatment and research programs.

- Neuro-Infectious Diseases – Rapid diagnosis and a wide range of experts.

- Neuromuscular Diseases –Diagnosis and appropriate therapies for improving pain management and quality of life.

- Movement Disorders – Largest regional program offering latest protocols and Deep Brain Stimulation Surgery to reduce/eliminate tremors.

- Memory Disorders – A premier center offering standard and investigational treatments to help slow or reverse progression of symptoms.

Physician Referral: For physician referral or to learn more about Columbia Weill Cornell Neuroscience Centers call toll free **1-877-NYP-WELL** (1-877-697-9355) or visit our website at **www.nypneuro.com**.

HIGHLIGHTS INCLUDE:

- Leading interventional neuroradiology service providing minimally invasive endovascular surgery, including Vertebroplasty, GDC Coils, embolization, balloon angioplasty and stenting and endovascular thrombolysis.

- Participating in FDA CREST-approved trial evaluating carotid stenting as opposed to carotid endarterectomy surgery and clot extraction.

- Country's largest program for Parkinson's Disease and other movement disorders; provides deep brain stimulation surgery for controlling Parkinson's.

- One of few centers offering Gamma Knife, a non-invasive radiosurgical technique for tumors, tremors, and AVMs – some once considered untreatable.

- Only multidisciplinary academic neurointensive care units in the greater New York area.

- One of 28 specialized Alzheimer's Disease Research Centers sponsored by the National Institute on Aging.

NYU Medical Center

550 First Avenue (at 31st Street)
New York, NY 10016
Physician Referral: (888) 7-NYU-MED
(888-769-8633) www.nyumedicalcenter.org

SCHOOL OF
MEDICINE

NEW YORK UNIVERSITY

NEUROLOGY

Dedicated to exceptional patient care, advanced scientific research, and high-quality graduate education, the Department of Neurology at NYU Medical Center evaluates and treats children and adults with a broad spectrum of neurological diseases. Specialty groups within the department deliver integrated care to patients with behavioral disorders and dementia, brain tumor, genetic and degenerative diseases, headache and pain syndromes, movement disorders including Parkinson's disease, multiple sclerosis, neuromuscular diseases, and diseases of children. NYU Medical Center is home to the largest multiple sclerosis program in New York.

The clinical mission especially benefits from a 30-bed neurorehabilitation unit, a state-of-the-art neurophysiology laboratory, and neurogenetics testing facility, each conducted under departmental auspices.

NYU COMPREHENSIVE EPILEPSY CENTER

Among the department's core programs is the NYU Comprehensive Epilepsy Center – the largest epilepsy program in the Eastern United States. The center offers testing, evaluation, treatment, drug trials, alternative therapies, and surgical intervention for patients with all forms of epilepsy. Beyond control of seizures, the center aims to improve quality of life by addressing problems of social isolation and helping patients achieve gratification at school, at work, at home, and in their communities.

At present, medications adequately control about 75 percent of those who suffer from recurrent epileptic seizures. But when medications fail to bring these debilitating seizures under control, a patient may be a candidate for surgery.

In the past two decades, enormous strides in understanding, technology, and surgical techniques have made surgery a safe and effective option for patients with intractable seizure disorders. Key to surgical success is functional mapping, which involves testing the brain to make sure it is safe to remove the tissues that are responsible for the seizures. Using a variety of imaging technologies, including MRI, PET, and SPECT, NYU's epileptologists are able to visualize abnormal anatomy and physiology and define a surgical target. Video-EEG recording is the most important test of all for characterizing and localizing seizures.

The most common surgical procedure for epilepsy is temporal lobe resection, often involving the removal of the deepest temporal structures. A low incidence of permanent complications makes this surgery a safe and attractive option when appropriate. At NYU, temporal lobe resection is performed without removing the patient's hair, using computer-assisted navigation and microscopic techniques. Patients are normally able to leave the hospital in 4 to 5 days. Vagus nerve stimulation (VNS), a reversible technique that was approved by the FDA in 1997, is just one of several additional surgical options for patients with particular types of seizures.

NYU MEDICAL CENTER

Brain diseases can cause intellectual impairments of profound complexity. The diagnosis and management of the cognitive disabilities accompanying traumatic brain injury or such diseases as stroke, Alzheimer's disease, epilepsy, and systemic illness often require an integrated approach. The Cognitive Neurology Program is an outpatient specialty clinic that serves adults with brain-based memory, perceptual, cognitive, or emotional impairments. Its specialists work closely with other branches of the Department of Neurology, and have close ties with Rusk Institute for Rehabilitation Medicine, where patients receive cognitive rehabilitation and speech therapy.

Physician Referral
(888) 7-NYU-MED

(888-769-8633)

www.nyumedicalcenter.org

SHANDS NEUROLOGICAL CENTER AT THE UNIVERSITY OF FLORIDA

SHANDS AT THE UNIVERSITY OF FLORIDA

1600 SW Archer Road, Gainesville, FL 32610
Patient referral: 800.749.7424
Physician-to-physician referral: 800.633.2122 Website: www.shands.org

SPECIALIZED SERVICES

The Shands Neurological Center at UF is one of the most advanced centers in the nation for the diagnosis and treatment of brain and spinal cord disorders. The center also is the Southeast's leading referral center for diagnosis and treatment of pituitary tumors and pediatric brain tumors.

The Comprehensive Epilepsy Program at Shands Neurological Center at UF offers a multidisciplinary approach to the diagnosis and treatment of patients with intractable epilepsy. The program is staffed by a team of UF physicians, psychologists and research scientists, as well as Shands at UF neuroscience nurses, EEG technologists and social workers.

UF physicians provide expert treatment and services including:
- Pallidotomy procedure using stereotactic neurosurgery for Parkinson's disease
- Stereotactic Radiosurgery: the LINAC Scalpel for arteriovenous malformations, brain tumors and intracranial disorders
- Medical evaluation and a full range of diagnostic services and treatment options, including resective surgery and vagus nerve stimulation offered in the center's comprehensive Adult and Pediatric Epilepsy Program
- Inpatient and outpatient surgical and medical treatments for cranial nerve disorders, including trigeminal neuralgia and hemifacial spasm
- Treatment for stroke, neuromuscular disorders, movement disorders, and memory disorders
- Evaluation and treatment for adult and pediatric sleep disorders
- Skull base surgery including acoustic neuromas, meningiomas and other cranial base lesions
- Pediatric neurosurgery including spinal tumors, brain tumors, congenital diseases (spina bifida, craniofacial abnormalities and neurofibromatosis), vascular disease, peripheral nerve injuries, spasticity and trauma
- Comprehensive evaluation and a full range of diagnostic services and treatment options, including neuropsychological testing, neurorehabilitation and physical therapy, at the center's Mild Traumatic Brain Injury Clinic

PHYSICIAN REFERRAL

The Shands Consultation Center is your link to UF physicians at the Shands Neurological Center at UF. For more information or to schedule an appointment, please call 800.749.7424 or visit our Web site at shands.org.

WORLD-CLASS NEUROLOGICAL AND NEUROSURGICAL CARE

The University of Florida faculty who practice at the Shands Neurological Center at UF offer some of the world's most advanced neurological and neurosurgical care for the diagnosis and treatment of a wide range of medical problems. The team includes nationally and internationally recognized neurosurgeons, neurologists and specialists in every discipline, from basic scientists to pathologists, radiologists, anesthesiologists and psychologists, to nurses and pharmacists. The Shands Neurological Center at UF historically ranks among the nation's best by *U.S. News & World Report.*

PENN NEUROLOGICAL INSTITUTE
UNIVERSITY OF PENNSYLVANIA
HEALTH SYSTEM

1-800-789-PENN
Philadelphia, PA
www.pennhealth.com

OVERVIEW

The Neurological Institute of the University of Pennsylvania Health System provides comprehensive medical and surgical care for people with disorders of the brain, spinal cord, and peripheral nervous system. We coordinate the clinical activities of the Departments of Neurology and Neurosurgery to ensure smooth delivery of care for complex neurological disorders, including cerebrovascular disease, epilepsy, cancer of the brain and nervous system, neuromuscular diseases and disorders of the spine. Our specialists are backed up by the most extensive neuro-diagnostic and imaging facilities in the region as well as one of the nation's foremost research programs in clinical and basic neuroscience.

The University of Pennsylvania has a history of excellence in the treatment of neurological diseases dating back to the establishment of the Department of Neurology in 1874. *The Best Doctors in America* lists more neurologists and neurosurgeons from the University of Pennsylvania Medical Center than from any other Delaware Valley hospital or medical center. In addition, the Hospital of the University of Pennsylvania was ranked highest in the region and in the top 10 nationally for medical and surgical treatment of neurological disorders by *U.S. News & World Report*.

EXCELLENCE AND EXPERTISE

The Parkinson's Disease and Movement Disorders Center is committed to providing exceptional patient care, education, social support services and ongoing research into the causes of Parkinson's disease.

Five internationally recognized neurologists treat more than 2,000 patients annually. The team also consists of a neurosurgeon, neuropsychologists, nurses, a social worker, physical and occupational therapists and speech pathologists who provide a multidimensional approach to patient care.

Research is an important and ongoing mission of the Parkinson's Disease and Movement Disorders Center, which actively pursues the investigation of the disease as well as exploration of new medications.

The Multiple Sclerosis Center specializes in quality, state-of-the-art care with a personal approach. The comprehensive multidisciplinary team caring for you includes neurologists, nurse-practitioners and specialists from other disciplines who are available for consultation in the management of genitourinary complications, spasticity and pain. Our program has existed for more than two decades, and basic research to investigate the origin and development of multiple sclerosis has taken place at Penn since 1963.

For direct connection to one of our Penn physicians, call PennLine **1-800-635-7780**.

PROGRAMS

- ALS
- The Center for Cranial Base Surgery
- The Cognitive Neurology Program
- The Head Injury Center
- The Interventional Neuro-Center
- The Memory Disorders Clinic
- Multiple Sclerosis Center
- Neuro Intensive Care
- The Neurogenetics Center
- Neuromuscular Disorders Program
- The Neuro-Ophthalmology Service
- The Neuropsychology Service
- The Parkinson's Disease and Movement Disorders Center
- The Penn Epilepsy Center
- Penn Center for Sleep Disorders
- The Spine Center
- The Stroke Center

LOCATIONS

Penn Neurological Institute at University of Pennsylvania Medical Center
34th and Spruce Streets
Philadelphia, PA 19104

Penn Neurological Institute at Pennsylvania Hospital
8th and Spruce Streets
Philadelphia, PA 19107

UNIVERSITY OF VIRGINIA HEALTH SYSTEM
NEUROSCIENCES SERVICE CENTER
Charlottesville, Va   www.med.virginia.edu/neurosciences

PROVIDING THE FINEST PATIENT CARE

We are Virginia's foremost research and treatment center for disorders affecting the nervous system. Our neurosurgery and neurology departments are among the nation's top 20 centers ranked by *U.S. News & World Report*. We offer superb diagnosis and treatment for strokes, headaches, dementias, movement disorders, brain and spine tumors, and all neurological disorders, diseases and injuries.

PROGRAMS & CENTERS

The **Comprehensive Epilepsy Program** provides complete neurological care and neurosurgery through its coordinated team approach and its ability to apply every available diagnostic and treatment option to achieve remission of seizures.

The **Movement Disorders Program** delivers expert neurological and neurosurgical care to patients with Parkinson's disease and related disorders, Huntington's disease, ataxia and many other diseases and syndromes.

The **Neuromuscular Disease Program** is devoted to treating and studying peripheral neuropathies, neuromuscular junction disorders, myopathies and motor neuron diseases in our dedicated neuromuscular clinics. The program provides inpatient consultation services, electrodiagnostic and electromyographic evaluations and clinical treatment trials.

The **Comprehensive Stroke Center** is establishing a new standard of care for stroke patients through its intensive program of clinical research and specialized treatment protocols. The Center is able to treat patients suffering from all cerebrovascular diseases in a comprehensive and coordinated manner and offers the latest vascular neurosurgical techniques. Patients recover on the Stroke Unit—dedicated rooms with specially trained staff.

The **Spine Center** offers the full range of care for patients requiring elective or emergency spine surgery. The Spine Center provides focused care through a multidisciplinary staff of physicians, nurses, therapists and social workers.

The **Neuro-Oncology Program** for brain and spinal tumors has assembled a remarkable staff of neuro-oncologists, neurosurgeons, radiation oncologists, neuro-psychologists and neuro-pathologists.

Likewise, the **Neuro-Endocrine Center** is internationally known and offers technologies such as Gamma Knife™ surgery for successful, noninvasive treatment of pituitary tumors.

RESEARCH

The UVa Neurosciences Service Center is pioneering new surgical therapies, treatment methods and medical therapies. Current clinical trials, which give patients access to promising new treatments, are being conducted for epilepsy, movement disorders, memory disorders, multiple sclerosis and stroke.

REFERRAL

Our physicians maintain close relationships with referring physicians. We apprise referring and primary care physicians of Neurosciences clinic and inpatient visits over the course of the patient's admission, treatments, operations and discharge process.

To schedule a Neurology appointment at UVa Health System, call 434-924-5304. For Neurosurgery, call 800-362-2203. UVa Neurosciences: www.med.virginia.edu/neurosciences

WESTCHESTER MEDICAL CENTER
WORLD-CLASS MEDICINE THAT'S NOT A WORLD AWAY.®

Valhalla Campus • Valhalla, NY 10595 • (914) 493-7211

Website: www.worldclassmedicine.com

OVERVIEW

Today doctors at Westchester Medical Center's Neuroscience Center are saving the lives of patients for whom there was no hope only a short time ago. World-class neurosurgeons work in concert with neurologists to provide innovative and outstanding care for medical problems that can carry a frightening stigma, such as brain tumors, epilepsy, stroke and motion disorders like Parkinson's disease. The Neuroscience Center has dedicated nursing, intensive care and operating facilities. The staff works closely with specialists from related departments, offering hope for longer and better lives to hundreds of adults and children from throughout the tri-state area. The Neuroscience Center offers several specialized programs, including adult and pediatric Brain Tumor Treatment programs, Pediatric Neurosurgery, a Birth Defects Center, motion disorder treatment including the subthalamic implantation device, Epilepsy Monitoring and Surgery and a dedicated unit for stroke research, treatment and management, one of only a few such centers in the state.

The latest technological advances are used by doctors at the Neuroscience Center to deal with disorders that require the most delicate and precise treatment. At the forefront of medical technology, Westchester Medical Center recently became the fifth hospital in the nation to offer Novalis® Shaped Beam Surgery—the least invasive and most precise treatment option available to patients diagnosed with cancer, brain tumors, and neurologic and vascular disorders. This revolutionary system, comprised of four state-of-the-art radiosurgery and radiotherapy applications, custom shapes the treatment beam to better target affected tissue while protecting healthy tissue.

The Neuroscience Center also includes the expertise of psychiatrists from our own Behavioral Health Center and the talents of a team of in-house rehabilitation specialists, including physicians from the Kessler Institute.

NEUROSCIENCE CENTER

At the forefront of medical technology, Westchester Medical Center recently became the fifth hospital in the nation to offer Novalis® Shaped Beam Surgery — the least invasive and most precise treatment option available to patients diagnosed with cancer, brain tumors, and neurologic and vascular disorders. This revolutionary system, comprised of four state-of-the-art radiosurgery and radiotherapy applications, custom shapes the treatment beam to better target affected tissue while protecting healthy tissue.

For more information on Novalis® Shaped Beam Surgery:
Call 1-866-BEAM CENTER

Neuroscience Center
Westchester Medical Center

Physician Listings

New England

Caplan, Louis Robert MD (N) - *Spec Exp: Stroke;* **Hospital:** Beth Israel Deaconess Med Ctr - Boston; **Address:** Dept Neurology, 330 Brookline Ave, Boston, MA 02111; **Phone:** (617) 667-0571; **Board Cert:** Neurology 1972; **Med School:** Univ MD Sch Med 1962; **Resid:** Neurology, Boston City Hosp., Boston, MA 1966-1967; Neurology, Boston City Hosp., Boston, MA 1967-1969; **Fellow:** Neurology, Harvard, Boston, MA 1966-1970; **Fac Appt:** Prof Neurology, Tufts Univ

Cole, Andrew J. MD (N) - *Spec Exp: Epilepsy/Seizure Disorders;* **Hospital:** MA Genl Hosp; **Address:** 55 Fruit St, Bldg VBK - Ste 830, Boston, MA 02114; **Phone:** (617) 726-3311; **Board Cert:** Neurology 1987, Clinical Neurophysiology 1992; **Med School:** Dartmouth Med Sch 1982; **Resid:** Neurology, Neoro Inst-McGill, Montreal, Canada 1983-1986; **Fellow:** Electroencephalography, Neuro Inst-McGill, Montreal, Canada 1986-1987; Neurological Surgery, Johns Hopkins Hospital, Baltimore, MD 1987-1988; **Fac Appt:** Asst Prof Neurology, Harvard Med Sch

Easton, J Donald MD (N) - *Spec Exp: Stroke;* **Hospital:** Rhode Island Hosp; **Address:** 110 Lockwood St, Ste 324, Providence, RI 02903; **Phone:** (401) 444-8795; **Board Cert:** Neurology 1971; **Med School:** Univ Wash 1964; **Resid:** Neurology, NY Hosp-Cornell Med Ctr, New York, NY 1965-1968; **Fac Appt:** Prof Neurology, Brown Univ

Feldman, Robert G MD (N) - *Spec Exp: Movement Disorders; Parkinson's Disease;* **Hospital:** Boston Med Ctr; **Address:** 720 Harrison Ave, Ste 707, Boston, MA 02118; **Phone:** (617) 638-8456; **Board Cert:** Neurology 1965; **Med School:** Univ Cincinnati 1958; **Resid:** Neurology, Yale New Haven Med Ctr, New Haven, CT 1959-1962; **Fellow:** Neurology, Yale Univ, New Haven, CT 1962-1963; **Fac Appt:** Prof Neurology, Boston Univ

Feldmann, Edward MD (N) - *Spec Exp: Cerebrovascular Disease; Stroke;* **Hospital:** Rhode Island Hosp; **Address:** 110 Lockwood St, Ste 322, Providence, RI 02903-4801; **Phone:** (401) 444-8806; **Board Cert:** Neurology 1988; **Med School:** Harvard Med Sch 1983; **Resid:** Neurology, NY Hosp, Cornell Med Ctr, New York, NY 1984-1987; **Fellow:** Neurology, Tufts New Eng Med Ctr, Boston, MA 1987-1988; **Fac Appt:** Assoc Prof Neurology, Brown Univ

Fink, J. Stephen MD (N) - *Spec Exp: Parkinson's Disease; Movement Disorders;* **Hospital:** Boston Med Ctr; **Address:** 720 Harrison Ave, Ste 707, Boston, MA 02118; **Phone:** (617) 638-8456; **Board Cert:** Neurology 1985; **Med School:** Cornell Univ-Weill Med Coll 1980; **Resid:** Neurology, Mass Genl Hosp, Boston, MA 1981-1984; **Fac Appt:** Prof Neurology, Harvard Med Sch

Hafler, David A. MD (N) - *Spec Exp: Multiple Sclerosis;* **Hospital:** Brigham & Women's Hosp; **Address:** 77 Louis Pasteur Ave Bldg HIM - Ste 786, , Boston, MA 02115; **Phone:** (617) 525-5330; **Board Cert:** Neurology 1987; **Med School:** Univ Miami Sch Med 1978; **Resid:** Neurology, NY Hosp-Cornell Med Ctr, New York, NY 1979-1982; **Fellow:** Neurological Immunology, Harvard Med Sch, Boston, MA 1982-1984; **Fac Appt:** Assoc Prof Neurology, Harvard Med Sch

Hochberg, Fred MD (N) - *Spec Exp: Brain Tumors; Occupational Movement Disorders;* **Hospital:** MA Genl Hosp; **Address:** One Hawthorne Pl, Ste 105, Boston, MA 02114-2698; **Phone:** (617) 726-8657; **Board Cert:** Neurology 1976; **Med School:** Case West Res Univ 1967; **Resid:** Neurology, Cleveland Metro Genl Hosp, Cleveland, OH 1968-1970; Neuropathology, Mass Genl Hosp, Boston, MA 1972-1974; **Fac Appt:** Assoc Prof Neurology, Harvard Med Sch

Kase, Carlos S. MD (N) - *Spec Exp: Stroke; Seizure Disorders;* **Hospital:** Boston Med Ctr; **Address:** 720 Harrison Ave, Ste 707, Roxbury, MA 02018; **Phone:** (617) 638-8456; **Board Cert:** Neurology 1980; **Med School:** Chile 1967; **Resid:** Neurology, Mass Genl Hospital, Boston, MA 1972-1973; Neurology, Mass Genl Hospital, Boston, MA 1977-1978; **Fac Appt:** Prof Neurology, Boston Univ

Kistler, John Philip MD (N) - *Spec Exp:* Stroke; **Hospital:** MA Genl Hosp; **Address:** Mass Genl Hosp, Stroke Service, 55 Fruit St, Bldg VBK - rm 802, Boston, MA 02114-2696; **Phone:** (617) 726-8459; **Board Cert:** Internal Medicine 1970, Neurology 1976; **Med School:** Columbia P&S 1964; **Resid:** Internal Medicine, Columbia Presby Hosp, New York, NY 1966-1968; Neurology, Mass Genl Hosp-Harvard Med Sch, New York, NY 1972-1975; **Fellow:** Neurology, Mass Genl Hos, Boston, MA 1971-1972; **Fac Appt:** Prof Neurology, Harvard Med Sch

Koroshetz, Walter J. MD (N) - *Spec Exp:* Stroke; Huntington's Disease; Movement Disorders; **Hospital:** MA Genl Hosp; **Address:** Dept of Neurology & Neurointensive Care, 55 Fruit Street, VBK 915, Boston, MA 02114-2696; **Phone:** (617) 726-8459; **Board Cert:** Internal Medicine 1982, Neurology 1986; **Med School:** Univ Chicago-Pritzker Sch Med 1979; **Resid:** Internal Medicine, Univ Chicago Med Ctr, Chicago, IL 1980-1981; Internal Medicine, Mass Genl Hosp, Boston, MA 1981-1982; **Fellow:** Neurology, Mass Genl Hosp, Boston, MA 1985-1987; Research, Mass Genl Hosp, Boston, MA 1989; **Fac Appt:** Asst Prof Medicine, Harvard Med Sch

Ropper, Allan MD (N) - *Spec Exp:* Trauma Neurology; Guillain-Barre Syndrome; Neurology-Intensive Care; **Hospital:** St Elizabeth's Med Ctr; **Address:** St. Elizabeth Hosp, Dept of Neurology, 736 Cambridge St, Boston, MA 02135; **Phone:** (617) 789-3300; **Board Cert:** Neurology 1980, Critical Care Medicine 1987, Internal Medicine 1977; **Med School:** Cornell Univ-Weill Med Coll 1974; **Resid:** Neurology, Mass Genl Hosp, Boston, MA 1976-1979; Internal Medicine, Univ California- San Francisco, San Francisco, CA 1975-1976; **Fac Appt:** Prof Neurology, Tufts Univ

Samuels, Martin Allen MD (N) - *Spec Exp:* Neurological Aspects of Systemic Disease; **Hospital:** Brigham & Women's Hosp; **Address:** BWH, Dept Neurology, 75 Francis St, Bldg Armory 2, Boston, MA 02115; **Phone:** (617) 732-5355; **Board Cert:** Neurology 1978, Internal Medicine 1974; **Med School:** Univ Cincinnati 1971; **Resid:** Internal Medicine, Boston City Hosp, Boston, MA 1972-1975; Neurology, Mass Genl Hosp, Boston, MA 1973-1977; **Fellow:** Neurological Pathology, Mass Genl Hosp, Boston, MA 1975-1976; **Fac Appt:** Prof Neurology, Harvard Med Sch

Selkoe, Dennis MD (N) - *Spec Exp:* Alzheimer's Disease; Neurobiology; **Hospital:** Brigham & Women's Hosp; **Address:** Brigham & Women's Hosp, Ctr for Neurol Dis, 77 Louis Pasteur Ave, Ste HIM 730, Boston, MA 02115-5716; **Phone:** (617) 525-5200; **Board Cert:** Neurology 1977; **Med School:** Univ VA Sch Med 1969; **Resid:** Neurology, Peter Bent Brigham, Boston, MA 1972-1975; **Fellow:** Neurological Biology, Chldns Hosp Med Ctr, Boston, MA 1975-1978; **Fac Appt:** Prof Neurology, Harvard Med Sch

Spencer, Susan S MD (N) - *Spec Exp:* Epilepsy/Seizure Disorders; **Hospital:** Yale - New Haven Hosp; **Address:** Yale Univ Sch Med, Dept Neurology, 333 Cedar St, New Haven, CT 06510-3206; **Phone:** (203) 785-3865; **Board Cert:** Neurology 1980; **Med School:** Univ Rochester 1974; **Resid:** Neurology, Yale-New Haven Hosp, New Haven, CT 1975-1978; **Fellow:** Epilepsy, Yale Univ-Yale New Haven Hosp, New Haven, CT 1978-1980; **Fac Appt:** Prof Neurology, Yale Univ

Vollmer, Timothy Lee MD (N) - *Spec Exp:* Multiple Sclerosis; **Hospital:** Yale - New Haven Hosp; **Address:** 40 Temple St, Ste 7-I, New Haven, CT 06510; **Phone:** (203) 785-4085; **Board Cert:** Neurology 1991; **Med School:** Stanford Univ 1983; **Resid:** Neurology, Stanford Univ Hosp, Stanford, CA 1984-1987; **Fellow:** Neurological Immunology, Stanford Univ Sch Med, Stanford, CA 1985-1986; **Fac Appt:** Assoc Prof Neurology, Yale Univ

Weiner, Howard MD (N) - *Spec Exp:* Multiple Sclerosis; Autoimmune Disease; **Hospital:** Brigham & Women's Hosp; **Address:** 75 Francis St, Boston, MA 02115; **Phone:** (617) 732-7432; **Board Cert:** Neurology 1978; **Med School:** Univ Colo 1969; **Resid:** Internal Medicine, Beth Israel, Boston, MA 1970-1971; Neurology, Longwood Prog, Boston, MA 1971-1974; **Fellow:** Immunology, Univ Colo, Denver, CO 1974-1976; **Fac Appt:** Prof Neurology, Harvard Med Sch

Young, Anne MD (N) - *Spec Exp:* Huntington's Disease; Parkinson's Disease; Movement Disorders; **Hospital:** MA Genl Hosp; **Address:** Mass Genl Hosp, Dept of Neurology, 32 Fruit Street, VBK 915, Boston, MA 02114; **Phone:** (617) 726-5532; **Board Cert:** Neurology 1981; **Med School:** Johns Hopkins Univ 1973; **Resid:** Neurology, UCSF, San Francisco, CA 1975-1978; **Fac Appt:** Prof Neurology, Harvard Med Sch

Mid Atlantic

Apatoff, Brian R MD/PhD (N) - *Spec Exp:* Multiple Sclerosis; Neuro-Immunology; Lyme Disease; **Hospital:** NY Presby Hosp - NY Weill Cornell Med Ctr (page 70); **Address:** 520 E 70th St, New York, NY 10021; **Phone:** (212) 746-4504; **Board Cert:** Neurology 1991; **Med School:** Univ Chicago-Pritzker Sch Med 1984; **Resid:** Neurology, Columbia Presby Med Ctr, New York, NY 1987-1990; **Fellow:** Multiple Sclerosis, Neuro Inst-Columbia Univ, New York, NY 1990-1992; **Fac Appt:** Assoc Prof Neurology, Cornell Univ-Weill Med Coll

Asbury, Arthur K MD (N) - *Spec Exp:* Peripheral Neuropathy; Guillain-Barre Syndrome; **Hospital:** Hosp Univ Penn (page 78); **Address:** Univ Penn Hosp, Dept Neurology, 3400 Spruce St, Philadelphia, PA 19104; **Phone:** (215) 662-2629; **Board Cert:** Neurology 1967; **Med School:** Univ Cincinnati 1958; **Resid:** Neurology, Mass Genl Hosp, Boston, MA 1960-1963; Internal Medicine, Mass Genl Hosp, Boston, MA 1959-1960; **Fellow:** Neurology, Mass Genl Hosp, Boston, MA 1963-1965; **Fac Appt:** Prof Emeritus Neurology, Univ Penn

Beal, Myron Flint MD (N) - *Spec Exp:* Huntington's Disease; Alzheimer's Disease; Neurodegenerative Disease; **Hospital:** NY Presby Hosp - NY Weill Cornell Med Ctr (page 70); **Address:** 520 E 70th St, New York, NY 10021-9800; **Phone:** (212) 746-6575; **Board Cert:** Internal Medicine 1979, Neurology 1982; **Med School:** Univ VA Sch Med 1976; **Resid:** Internal Medicine, New York Hosp-Cornell Med Ctr, New York, NY 1977-1978; Neurology, Mass Genl Hosp, Boston, MA 1978-1981; **Fac Appt:** Prof Neurology, Cornell Univ-Weill Med Coll

Bernad, Peter MD (N) - *Spec Exp:* Stroke; Headache-Migraine; Head Injury; **Hospital:** Inova Fairfax Hosp; **Address:** 2112 F St NW, Ste 303, Washington, DC 20037; **Phone:** (202) 728-0099; **Board Cert:** Internal Medicine 1979, Neurology 1981; **Med School:** McGill Univ 1974; **Resid:** Internal Medicine, Univ Southern California, Los Angeles, CA 1975-1976; Neurology, Mass Genl Hosp-Harvard, Boston, MA 1976-1979; **Fellow:** Neurological Muscular Disease, Natl Inst Hlth, Bethesda, MD 1979-1981; **Fac Appt:** Assoc Clin Prof Neurology, Geo Wash Univ

Braun, Carl MD (N) - *Spec Exp:* Cerebrovascular Disease; Neuromuscular Disorders; Headache; **Hospital:** St Luke's - Roosevelt Hosp Ctr - Roosevelt Div (page 58); **Address:** 1090 Amsterdam Ave, Ste 5F, New York, NY 10025-1737; **Phone:** (212) 523-3650; **Board Cert:** Neurology 1972; **Med School:** Univ Penn 1962; **Resid:** Internal Medicine, St Luke's Roosevelt Hosp Ctr, New York, NY 1962-1963; Neurology, Columbia-Presby Med Ctr, New York, NY 1964-1967; **Fac Appt:** Clin Prof Neurology, Columbia P&S

Brust, John C MD (N) - *Spec Exp:* Stroke; Substance Abuse; **Hospital:** Harlem Hosp Ctr; **Address:** 506 Lenox Ave, rm 16-101, New York, NY 10037-1802; **Phone:** (212) 939-4244; **Board Cert:** Neurology 1971; **Med School:** Columbia P&S 1962; **Resid:** Internal Medicine, Columbia Presby, New York, NY 1965-1966; Neurology, Columbia Presby, New York, NY 1966-1969; **Fac Appt:** Clin Prof Neurology, Columbia P&S

Caronna, John J MD (N) - *Spec Exp:* Stroke; Cerebrovascular Disease; **Hospital:** NY Presby Hosp - NY Weill Cornell Med Ctr (page 70); **Address:** Cornell Univ, Dept Neurology, 520 E 70th St, Ste 607, New York, NY 10021; **Phone:** (212) 746-2304; **Board Cert:** Neurology 1974; **Med School:** Cornell Univ-Weill Med Coll 1965; **Resid:** Internal Medicine, NY Hosp, New York, NY 1965-1967; Neurology, NY Hosp, New York, NY 1969-1971; **Fellow:** Neurology, NY Hosp, New York, NY 1972-1973; **Fac Appt:** Prof Neurology, Cornell Univ-Weill Med Coll

Charney, Jonathan MD (N) - *Spec Exp:* Headache; Stroke; **Hospital:** Mount Sinai Hosp (page 68); **Address:** 1111 Park Ave, Ste 1A, New York, NY 10128-1234; **Phone:** (212) 831-2886; **Board Cert:** Neurology 1977; **Med School:** NY Med Coll 1969; **Resid:** Neurology, Meth Hosp-Baylor, Dallas, TX 1970-1971; Neurology, Columbia-Presby Med Ctr, New York, NY 1971-1973; **Fac Appt:** Asst Prof Neurology, Mount Sinai Sch Med

Cook, Stuart MD (N) - *Spec Exp:* Infectious & Demyelinating Diseases; **Hospital:** UMDNJ-Univ Hosp-Newark; **Address:** 65 Bergen St, Ste 1535, Newark, NJ 07107; **Phone:** (973) 972-4400; **Board Cert:** Neurology 1970; **Med School:** Univ VT Coll Med 1962; **Resid:** Neurology, Albert Einstein Coll Meded Ctr, Bronx, NY 1965-1968; **Fac Appt:** Prof Neurology, UMDNJ-NJ Med Sch, Newark

Cornblath, David R. MD (N) - *Spec Exp:* Peripheral Neuropathy; **Hospital:** Johns Hopkins Hosp - Baltimore; **Address:** 600 N Wolfe St, Baltimore, MD 21287-6965; **Phone:** (410) 955-2229; **Board Cert:** Neurology 1982, Clinical Neurophysiology 1994; **Med School:** Case West Res Univ 1977; **Resid:** Neurology, Hosp Univ Penn, Philadelphia, PA 1978-1981; **Fellow:** Neurology, Hosp Univ Penn, Philadelphia, PA 1981-1982; **Fac Appt:** Prof Neurology, Johns Hopkins Univ

Coyle, Patricia K MD (N) - *Spec Exp:* Multiple Sclerosis; Neuro-Immunology; Lyme Disease; **Hospital:** Stony Brook Univ Hosp; **Address:** SUNY Stony Brook, Dept Neurology, HSC T12-020, Stony Brook, NY 11794-8121; **Phone:** (631) 444-2599; **Board Cert:** Neurology 1978; **Med School:** Johns Hopkins Univ 1974; **Resid:** Neurology, Johns Hopkins Hosp, Baltimore, MD 1975-1978; **Fellow:** Neurological Immunology, Johns Hopkins Hosp, Blatimore, MD 1978-1980; **Fac Appt:** Prof Neurology, SUNY Stony Brook

De Angelis, Lisa MD (N) - *Spec Exp:* Neuro-Oncology; **Hospital:** Mem Sloan Kettering Cancer Ctr; **Address:** 1275 York Ave, New York, NY 10021-6007; **Phone:** (212) 639-7123; **Board Cert:** Neurology 1986; **Med School:** Columbia P&S 1980; **Resid:** Neurology, Columbia Presby, New York, NY 1981-1984; **Fellow:** Neurological Oncology, Neuro Inst Presby Hosp, New York, NY 1984-1985; Neurological Oncology, Meml Sloan-Kettering Cancer Ctr, New York, Ny 1985-1986; **Fac Appt:** Prof Neurology, Cornell Univ-Weill Med Coll

DeKosky, Steven T. MD (N) - *Spec Exp:* Alzheimer's Disease; **Hospital:** UPMC - Presbyterian Univ Hosp; **Address:** Univ Pittsburgh Physicians, 3471 Fifth Ave, Ste 811, Pittsburgh, PA 15213-2593; **Phone:** (412) 692-4622; **Board Cert:** Neurology 1979; **Med School:** Univ Fla Coll Med 1974; **Resid:** Internal Medicine, Johns Hopkins Univ Med Ctr, Gainesville, FL 1974-1975; Neurology, Univ Florida Hlth Sci Ctr, Gainesville, FL 1975-1978; **Fellow:** Neurological Chemistry, Univ Virginia Hlth Sci Ctr, Charlottesville, VA 1978-1979; **Fac Appt:** Prof Neurology, Univ Pittsburgh

Devinsky, Orrin MD (N) - *Spec Exp:* Epilepsy; **Hospital:** NYU Med Ctr (page 71); **Address:** 403 E 34th St, FL 4, New York, NY 10016-4972; **Phone:** (212) 263-8871; **Board Cert:** Neurology 1987; **Med School:** Harvard Med Sch 1983; **Resid:** Neurology, NY-Cornell Med Ctr, New York, NY 1983-1986; **Fellow:** Epilepsy, Natl Inst Health, Bethesda, MD 1986-1988; **Fac Appt:** Prof Neurology, NYU Sch Med

Dewberry, Robert Gerard MD (N) - *Spec Exp:* Neurology - General; **Hospital:** Maryland Genl Hosp; **Address:** 827 Linden Ave, Baltimore, MD 21201; **Phone:** (410) 225-8290; **Board Cert:** Neurology 1982; **Med School:** Univ MD Sch Med 1987; **Resid:** Neurology, Barnes Hospital, St. Louis, MO 1988-1991; **Fellow:** Neurological Muscular Disease, Univ VA Hosp, Charlottesville, VA 1991-1993

Dichter, Marc A MD (N) - *Spec Exp:* Epilepsy/Seizure Disorders; **Hospital:** Hosp Univ Penn (page 78); **Address:** 3400 Spruce St, Dept Neurology, 2 Ravdin, Philadelphia, PA 19104; **Phone:** (215) 349-5166; **Board Cert:** Neurology 1978; **Med School:** NYU Sch Med 1969; **Resid:** Neurology, Beth Israel Hosp, Boston, MA 1972-1975; Neurology, Chlsn Hosp/PB Brgham Hosp-Harvard, Boston, MA 1972-1975; **Fac Appt:** Prof Neurology, Univ Penn

Drachman, Daniel Bruce MD (N) - *Spec Exp:* Muscular Dystrophy; Neuromuscular Disorders; **Hospital:** Johns Hopkins Hosp - Baltimore; **Address:** Johns Hopkins Med Ctr, 600 N Wolfe St, Bldg Meyer - Fl 5119, Baltimore, MD 21287; **Phone:** (410) 955-5406; **Board Cert:** Neurology 1963; **Med School:** NYU Sch Med 1956; **Resid:** Neuropathology, Mallory Inst Path/Boston City Hosp., Boston, MA 1959-1960; **Fellow:** Neurology, Harvard Med Sch., Boston, MA 1957-1960; **Fac Appt:** Prof Neurology, Johns Hopkins Univ

Fahn, Stanley MD (N) - *Spec Exp:* Movement Disorders; Parkinson's Disease; **Hospital:** NY Presby Hosp - Columbia Presby Med Ctr (page 70); **Address:** 710 W 168th St, Fl 3rd - rm 350, New York, NY 10032; **Phone:** (212) 305-5277; **Board Cert:** Neurology 1958; **Med School:** UCSF 1958; **Resid:** Neurology, Columbia Presby Hosp, New York, NY 1959-1962; **Fac Appt:** Prof Neurology, Columbia P&S

French, Jacqueline MD (N) - *Spec Exp:* Epilepsy/Seizure Disorders; **Hospital:** Hosp Univ Penn (page 78); **Address:** Hosp Univ Penn, Dept Neurology, 3400 Spruce St, Philadelphia, PA 19104; **Phone:** (215) 349-5565; **Board Cert:** Neurology 1987; **Med School:** Brown Univ 1982; **Resid:** Neurological Surgery, Mount Sinai Hosp, New York, NY 1982-1986; **Fellow:** Epilepsy, Mount Sinai Hosp, New York, NY 1986-1988; Epilepsy, Yale Univ, New Haven, CT 1988-1989; **Fac Appt:** Assoc Prof Neurology, Univ Penn

Galetta, Steven MD (N) - *Spec Exp:* Neuro-Ophthalmology; Optic Nerve Diseases; Multiple Sclerosis; **Hospital:** Hosp Univ Penn (page 78); **Address:** Hosp Univ Penn, Dept Neurology, 3400 Spruce St, Philadelphia, PA 19104; **Phone:** (215) 662-3606; **Board Cert:** Neurology 1988; **Med School:** Cornell Univ-Weill Med Coll 1983; **Resid:** Neurology, Univ Penn Med Ctr, Philadelphia, PA 1984-1987; **Fellow:** Neurological Ophthalmology, Bascom Palmer Eye Inst, Miami, FL 1987-1988; **Fac Appt:** Prof Neurology, Univ Penn

Gendelman, Seymour MD (N) - *Spec Exp:* Parkinson's Disease; Dementia; **Hospital:** Mount Sinai Hosp (page 68); **Address:** 5 E 98th St, Fl 7, New York, NY 10029-6501; **Phone:** (212) 241-8172; **Board Cert:** Neurology 1971; **Med School:** Geo Wash Univ 1964; **Resid:** Neurology, Mount Sinai, New York, NY 1965-1968; **Fac Appt:** Clin Prof Neurology, Mount Sinai Sch Med

Gizzi, Martin MD/PhD (N) - *Spec Exp:* Neuro-Ophthalmology; Balance Disorders; Progressive Supranuclear Palsy (PSP); **Hospital:** JFK Med Ctr - Edison; **Address:** 65 James St, Edison, NJ 08820-3947; **Phone:** (732) 321-7010; **Board Cert:** Neurology 1990; **Med School:** Univ Miami Sch Med 1985; **Resid:** Neurology, Mount Sinai, New York, NY 1986-1989; **Fellow:** Neurological Ophthalmology, Mount Sinai, New York, NY 1989-1991; **Fac Appt:** Prof Neurology, Seton Hall Coll Med

Golbe, Lawrence MD (N) - *Spec Exp:* Parkinson's Disease; Progressive Supranuclear Palsy (PSP); Movement Disorders; **Hospital:** Robert Wood Johnson Univ Hosp @ New Brunswick; **Address:** 97 Paterson St, rm 208, New Brunswick, NJ 08901-2160; **Phone:** (732) 235-7729; **Board Cert:** Neurology 1984; **Med School:** NYU Sch Med 1978; **Resid:** Neurology, Bellevue Hosp, New York, NY 1980-1983; Internal Medicine, Hahnemann, Philadelphia, PA 1978-1980; **Fac Appt:** Prof Neurology, UMDNJ-RW Johnson Med Sch

Goodgold, Albert MD (N) - *Spec Exp:* Parkinson's Disease & Movement Disorders; Spinal Root & Cord Disorders; **Hospital:** NYU Med Ctr (page 71); **Address:** NYU Medical Center, 530 First Ave, Ste 5A, New York, NY 10016; **Phone:** (212) 263-7205; **Med School:** Switzerland 1955; **Resid:** Neurology, Bellevue Hosp, New York, NY 1957-1960; **Fac Appt:** Prof Neuroradiology, NYU Sch Med

Griffin, John Wesley MD (N) - *Spec Exp:* Neuropathy; **Hospital:** Johns Hopkins Hosp - Baltimore; **Address:** 600 N Wolfe St Bldg Meyer - rm 6-113, Baltimore, MD 21287-7613; **Phone:** (410) 955-2227; **Board Cert:** Neurology 1976, Internal Medicine 1974; **Med School:** Stanford Univ 1968; **Resid:** Neurology, Johns Hopkins Hosp, Baltimore, MD 1970-1973; Internal Medicine, Johns Hopkins Hosp, Baltimore, MD 1969-1970; **Fac Appt:** Prof Neurology, Johns Hopkins Univ

Hiesiger, Emile MD (N) - *Spec Exp:* Pain Management; Neuro-Oncology; **Hospital:** NYU Med Ctr (page 71); **Address:** 530 1st Ave, Ste 5A, New York, NY 10016; **Phone:** (212) 263-6123; **Board Cert:** Neurology 1983; **Med School:** NY Med Coll 1978; **Resid:** Neurology, New York Univ, New York, NY 1979-1982; **Fellow:** Neurology, Mem Sloan-Kettering Cancer Ctr, New York, NY 1982-1984; **Fac Appt:** Assoc Clin Prof Neurology, NYU Sch Med

Hurtig, Howard MD (N) - *Spec Exp:* Parkinson's Disease; Movement Disorders; **Hospital:** Pennsylvania Hosp (page 78); **Address:** Penn Neurological Inst, 330 S 9th St Fl 2, Philadelphia, PA 19107; **Phone:** (215) 829-6500; **Board Cert:** Neurology 1976; **Med School:** Tulane Univ 1966; **Resid:** Internal Medicine, New York Hosp- Cornell Med Ctr., New York, NY 1966-1968; Neurology, Hosp Univ Penn, Philadelphia, PA 1970-1973; **Fac Appt:** Prof Neurology, Univ Penn

Johnson, Kenneth P MD (N) - *Spec Exp:* Multiple Sclerosis; **Hospital:** University of MD Med Sys; **Address:** Maryland Ctr for Multiple Sclerosis, 11 S Paca St Fl 4, Baltimore, MD 21201; **Phone:** (410) 328-6484; **Board Cert:** Neurology 1968; **Med School:** Jefferson Med Coll 1959; **Resid:** Neurology, Buffalo Genl Hosp, Buffalo, NY 1960-1961; Neurology, Univ Hosp, Cleveland, OH 1963-1965; **Fellow:** Neurology, Univ Case West Res, Cleveland, OH 1965-1968; **Fac Appt:** Prof Neurology, Univ MD Sch Med

Jordan, Barry D MD (N) - *Spec Exp:* Traumatic Brain Injury; Sports Neurology; Sports Medicine; **Hospital:** Burke Rehab Hosp; **Address:** Burke Rehabilitation Hosp, 785 Mamaroneck Ave, White Plains, NY 10605; **Phone:** (914) 597-2831; **Board Cert:** Neurology 1989; **Med School:** Harvard Med Sch 1981; **Resid:** Neurology, New York Hosp, New York, NY 1982-1985; New York Hosp, New York, NY 1985-1989; **Fellow:** Hosp Spec, New York, NY 1986-1987; UCLA Med Ctr, Los Angeles, CA 1997-1998

Kolodny, Edwin H MD (N) - *Spec Exp:* Neurology - General; **Hospital:** NYU Med Ctr (page 71); **Address:** 403 E 34 St Fl 2, New York, NY 10016-6402; **Phone:** (212) 263-7755; **Board Cert:** Clinical Genetics 1987, Neurology 1971; **Med School:** NYU Sch Med 1962; **Resid:** Internal Medicine, Bellevue Hosp, New York, NY 1962-1964; Neurology, Mass Genl Hosp, Boston, MA 1964-1967; **Fellow:** Nat Inst Neurol Dis & Stroke, Bethesda, MD 1967-1970; **Fac Appt:** Prof Neurology, NYU Sch Med

Krumholz, Allan MD (N) - *Spec Exp:* *Epilepsy/Seizure Disorders;* **Hospital:** University of MD Med Sys; **Address:** 22 S Greene St., Baltimore, MD 21201-1544; **Phone:** (410) 328-6266; **Board Cert:** Neurology 1977, Clinical Neurophysiology 1996; **Med School:** Univ Hlth Sci/Chicago Med Sch 1970; **Resid:** Neurology, Johns Hopkins Hosp, Baltimore, MD 1972-1975; Internal Medicine, Baltimore City Hospital, Baltimore, MD 1971-1972; **Fellow:** Electroencephalography, Johns Hopkins Hosp, Baltimore, MD 1980; **Fac Appt:** Prof Neurology, Univ MD Sch Med

Levine, David MD (N) - *Spec Exp:* *Dementia; Stroke;* **Hospital:** NYU Med Ctr (page 71); **Address:** 400 E 34th St, Ste RIRM- 311, New York, NY 10016-4901; **Phone:** (212) 263-7744; **Board Cert:** Neurology 1976; **Med School:** Harvard Med Sch 1968; **Resid:** Neurology, Mass Genl Hosp, Boston, MA 1971-1974; **Fellow:** Neurology, Mass Genl Hosp, Boston, MA 1974-1976; **Fac Appt:** Prof Neurology, NYU Sch Med

Levine, Steven R MD (N) - *Spec Exp:* *Stroke; Cerebrovascular Disease;* **Hospital:** Mount Sinai Hosp (page 68); **Address:** Mount Sinai Sch Med, Dept Neurology, Stroke Program, 1 Gustave Levy Pl, Box 1137, New York, NY 10029-6574; **Phone:** (212) 241-9443; **Board Cert:** Neurology 1986; **Med School:** Med Coll Wisc 1981; **Resid:** Neurology, Univ Mich Hosp, Ann Arbor, MI 1982-1985; **Fellow:** Cerebrovascular Disease, Henry Ford Hosp, Detroit, MI 1985-1987; **Fac Appt:** Prof Neurology, Mount Sinai Sch Med

Logigian, Eric L MD (N) - *Spec Exp:* *Neuromuscular Disease; Electromyography; Lyme Disease;* **Hospital:** Strong Memorial Hosp - URMC; **Address:** Univ Rochester, Dept of Neurology, 601 Elmwood Ave, Box 673, Rochester, NY 14642; **Phone:** (716) 275-4568; **Board Cert:** Neurology 1985, Clinical Neurophysiology 1999; **Med School:** Boston Univ 1978; **Resid:** Internal Medicine, Beth Israel Hosp, Boston, MA 1979-1981; Neurology, Mass Genl Hosp, Boston, MA 1981-1984; **Fellow:** Clinical Neurophysiology, Mass General Hosp, Boston, MA 1984-1985; **Fac Appt:** Prof Neurology, Univ Rochester

Lublin, Fred MD (N) - *Spec Exp:* *Multiple Sclerosis;* **Hospital:** Mount Sinai Hosp (page 68); **Address:** Corrine Goldsmith Dickenson Ctr for Multiple Sclerosis, 5 E 98th St, New York, NY 10029-6574; **Phone:** (212) 241-6854; **Board Cert:** Neurology 1977; **Med School:** Jefferson Med Coll 1972; **Resid:** Neurology, New York Hosp/Cornell, New York, NY 1973-1976; **Fac Appt:** Prof Neurology, Mount Sinai Sch Med

Max, Mitchell Bruce MD (N) - *Spec Exp:* *Pain Management;* **Hospital:** Natl Inst of Hlth - Clin Ctr; **Address:** Natl Inst of Hlth, 3C405 Bldg 10, Bethesda, MD 20892; **Phone:** (301) 496-5483; **Board Cert:** Neurology 1982, Internal Medicine 1978; **Med School:** Harvard Med Sch 1974; **Resid:** Internal Medicine, Univ Chicago Hosp, Chicago, IL 1974-1976; Neurology, NY Presby- Cornell Med Ctr, New York, NY 1979-1982; **Fellow:** Neurology, Meml Sloan Kettering Cancer Ctr, New York, NY

Mohr, Jay Preston MD (N) - *Spec Exp:* *Aphasia; Stroke;* **Hospital:** NY Presby Hosp - Columbia Presby Med Ctr (page 70); **Address:** Columbia Presbyterian, Dept Neur-Neuro Inst, 710 W 168 St, rm 514, New York, NY 10032-2603; **Phone:** (212) 305-8033; **Board Cert:** Neurology 1971; **Med School:** Univ VA Sch Med 1963; **Resid:** Neurology, Columbia Presby Med Ctr, New York, NY 1965-1966; Neurology, Mass Genl Hosp, Boston, MA 1966-1968; **Fellow:** Neurology, Mass Genl Hosp, Boston, MA 1967-1969; **Fac Appt:** Clin Prof Neurology, Columbia P&S

Morrell, Martha J MD (N) - *Spec Exp:* *Epilepsy; Epilepsy-Women's Issues; Epilepsy-Surgery;* **Hospital:** NY Presby Hosp - Columbia Presby Med Ctr (page 70); **Address:** 710 W 168th St, Fl 7, New York, NY 10032; **Phone:** (212) 305-1742; **Board Cert:** Neurology 1989, Clinical Neurophysiology 1992; **Med School:** Stanford Univ 1984; **Resid:** Neurology, Univ Penn Hosp, Philadelphia, PA 1985-1988; **Fellow:** Epilepsy, Univ Penn Hosp, Philadelphia, PA 1988-1990; **Fac Appt:** Prof Neurology, Columbia P&S

Olanow, C Warren MD (N) - *Spec Exp:* Parkinson's Disease; Movement Disorders; **Hospital:** Mount Sinai Hosp (page 68); **Address:** 5 E 98th St Fl 6, New York, NY 10029; **Phone:** (212) 241-4623; **Board Cert:** Neurology 1970; **Med School:** Univ Toronto 1965; **Resid:** Neurology, Toronto Genl Hosp, Toronto, Canada 1967-1968; Neurology, Columbia Presby, New York, NY 1968-1970; **Fellow:** Neurological Anatomy, Columbia Presby, New York, NY 1970-1971; **Fac Appt:** Neurology, Mount Sinai Sch Med

Pedley, Timothy A MD (N) - *Spec Exp:* Epilepsy/Seizure Disorders; **Hospital:** NY Presby Hosp - Columbia Presby Med Ctr (page 70); **Address:** 710 W 168th St Fl 14 - rm 1401, New York, NY 10032; **Phone:** (212) 305-6489; **Board Cert:** Neurology 1975, Clinical Neurophysiology 1993; **Med School:** Yale Univ 1969; **Resid:** Neurology, Stanford Hosp & Cln, Stanford, CA 1970-1973; **Fellow:** Clinical Neurophysiology, Stanford Hosp & Cln, Stanford, CA 1973-1975; **Fac Appt:** Prof Neurology, Columbia P&S

Petito, Frank MD (N) - *Spec Exp:* Multiple Sclerosis; Headache; Lyme Disease; **Hospital:** NY Presby Hosp - NY Weill Cornell Med Ctr (page 70); **Address:** 525 E 68th St, Ste 615, New York, NY 10021; **Phone:** (212) 746-2309; **Board Cert:** Neurology 1972; **Med School:** Columbia P&S 1967; **Resid:** Neurology, NY Hosp-Cornell Univ, New York, NY 1967-1971; **Fac Appt:** Prof Neurology, Cornell Univ-Weill Med Coll

Plum, Fred MD (N) - *Spec Exp:* Coma; Stroke; **Hospital:** NY Presby Hosp - NY Weill Cornell Med Ctr (page 70); **Address:** 525 E 70th St, Ste 607, New York, NY 10021; **Phone:** (212) 746-6141; **Board Cert:** Neurology 1956; **Med School:** Cornell Univ-Weill Med Coll 1947; **Resid:** Internal Medicine, NY Hosp-Cornell Univ, New York, NY 1948-1949; Neurology, NY Hosp-Cornell Univ, New York, NY 1949-1950; **Fellow:** Neurology, Bellevue Psyc Inst, New York, NY 1950-1951; **Fac Appt:** Prof Neurology, Cornell Univ-Weill Med Coll

Posner, Jerome MD (N) - *Spec Exp:* Neuro-Oncology; Brain Tumors; **Hospital:** Mem Sloan Kettering Cancer Ctr; **Address:** 1275 York Ave, New York, NY 10021-6007; **Phone:** (212) 639-7047; **Board Cert:** Neurology 1962; **Med School:** Univ Wash 1955; **Resid:** Neurology, Univ WA Affil Hosp, Seattle, WA 1955-1959; **Fellow:** Neurology, Univ WA Affil Hosp, Seattle, WA 1961-1963; **Fac Appt:** Prof Neurology, Cornell Univ-Weill Med Coll

Pula, Thaddeus MD (N) - *Spec Exp:* Neurophysiology; Electromyography & Nerve Conduction; **Hospital:** Maryland Genl Hosp; **Address:** Maryland Genl Hosp Div Neur, 827 Linden Ave, Baltimore, MD 21201-4606; **Phone:** (410) 225-8290; **Board Cert:** Clinical Neurophysiology 1994, Neurology 1981; **Med School:** Univ MD Sch Med 1976; **Resid:** Internal Medicine, Mercy Hosp Med Ctr

Relkin, Norman MD/PhD (N) - *Spec Exp:* Alzheimer's Disease; Dementia; Memory Disorders; **Hospital:** NY Presby Hosp - NY Weill Cornell Med Ctr (page 70); **Address:** New York Weill Cornell Med Ctr, 525 E 68th St, rm LC807, New York, NY 10021; **Phone:** (212) 746-2441; **Board Cert:** Neurology 1992; **Med School:** Albert Einstein Coll Med 1987; **Resid:** Neurology, NY Hosp-Cornell Med Ctr., New York, NY 1988-1991; **Fellow:** Behavioral Neurology, NY Hosp-Cornell Med Ctr, New York, NY 1991-1992; **Fac Appt:** Asst Prof Neurology, Cornell Univ-Weill Med Coll

Richert, John R MD (N) - *Spec Exp:* Multiple Sclerosis; Neuro-Immunology; **Hospital:** Georgetown Univ Hosp; **Address:** 3800 Reservoir Rd NW, Washington, DC 20007-2196; **Phone:** (202) 687-8525; **Board Cert:** Neurology 1978; **Med School:** Univ Rochester 1970; **Resid:** Internal Medicine, Rochester-Strong Meml Hosp, Rochester, NY 1971-1972; Neurology, Mayo Clinic, Rochester, MN 1974-1977; **Fellow:** Multiple Sclerosis, Natl Inst Hlth, Bethesda, MD 1977-1980; **Fac Appt:** Prof Neurology, Georgetown Univ

Sage, Jacob MD (N) - *Spec Exp:* Neurology - General; **Hospital:** Robert Wood Johnson Univ Hosp @ New Brunswick; **Address:** UMDNJ, Dept Neurology, 125 Paterson St, New Brunswick, NJ 08903-1962; **Phone:** (732) 235-7731; **Board Cert:** Neurology 1979; **Med School:** Univ Pittsburgh 1972; **Resid:** Neurology, Pittsburgh Hosp, Pittsburgh, PA 1978; **Fellow:** Neurological Chemistry, New York Hosp-Cornell Univ, New York, NY 1978-1980; **Fac Appt:** Prof Neurology, UMDNJ-RW Johnson Med Sch

Schold Jr., S. Clifford MD (N) - *Spec Exp:* Brain Tumors; **Hospital:** UPMC - Presbyterian Univ Hosp; **Address:** Univ Pitts Cancer Inst, 3471 5th Ave, Ste 802, Pittsburgh, PA 15213; **Phone:** (412) 692-2600; **Board Cert:** Neurology 1980; **Med School:** Univ Ariz Coll Med 1973; **Resid:** Neurology, Colo Med Ctr, Denver, CO 1974-1977; **Fellow:** Neurological Oncology, Sloan-Kettering Cancer Ctr, New York, NY 1977-1978

Shoulson, Ira MD (N) - *Spec Exp:* Parkinson's Disease; Movement Disorders; Huntington's Disease; **Hospital:** Strong Memorial Hosp - URMC; **Address:** 919 Westfall Rd, Bldg C - Ste 220, Rochester, NY 14618; **Phone:** (716) 275-2585; **Board Cert:** Internal Medicine 1974, Neurology 1980; **Med School:** Univ Rochester 1971; **Resid:** Internal Medicine, Strong Meml Hospital, Rochester, MN 1972-1973; Neurology, Strong Meml Hosp, Rochester, MN 1975-1977; **Fellow:** Neurology, Natl Inst Hlth, Bethesda, MD 1973-1975; **Fac Appt:** Prof Neurology, Univ Rochester

Sirdofsky, Michael D MD (N) - *Spec Exp:* Neuromuscular Disorders; Electrodiagnosis-EEG, EMG; **Hospital:** Georgetown Univ Hosp; **Address:** 3800 Reservoir Rd NW, Washington, DC 20007; **Phone:** (202) 687-8525; **Board Cert:** Neurology 1981; **Med School:** Georgetown Univ 1976; **Resid:** Neurology, Georgetown Univ Hosp, Washington, DC 1977-1980; **Fac Appt:** Assoc Prof Neurology, Georgetown Univ

Stern, Matthew MD (N) - *Spec Exp:* Parkinson's Disease; Movement Disorders; Botox Therapy; **Hospital:** Pennsylvania Hosp (page 78); **Address:** Dept Neurology, 330 S 9th St Fl 2, Philadelphia, PA 19107; **Phone:** (215) 829-6500; **Board Cert:** Neurology 1983; **Med School:** Duke Univ 1970; **Resid:** Neurology, Hosp Univ Penn, Philadelphia, PA 1979-1982

Swerdlow, Michael MD (N) - *Spec Exp:* Myasthenia Gravis; **Hospital:** Montefiore Med Ctr (page 67); **Address:** 3400 Bainbridge Ave, Ste 5A, Bronx, NY 10467-2401; **Phone:** (718) 920-4178; **Board Cert:** Neurology 1975; **Med School:** Univ Penn 1967; **Resid:** Internal Medicine, Mount Sinai Hosp, New York, NY 1967-1969; Neurology, Albert Einstein Coll, Bronx, NY 1969-1972; **Fac Appt:** Prof Neurology, Albert Einstein Coll Med

Vas, George A MD (N) - *Spec Exp:* Stroke; **Hospital:** Univ Hosp - Brklyn; **Address:** 450 Clarkson Ave, Ste A, Brooklyn, NY 11203-2056; **Phone:** (718) 270-1950; **Board Cert:** Internal Medicine 1973, Neurology 1977; **Med School:** Univ Pittsburgh 1970; **Resid:** Internal Medicine, New York Hosp-Cornell Univ, New York, NY 1971-1972; Neurology, New York Hosp-Cornell Univ, New York, NY 1972-1975; **Fac Appt:** Prof SUNY Downstate

Wechsler, Lawrence Richard MD (N) - *Spec Exp:* Neurophysiology; Stroke; Transcranial Doppler; **Hospital:** UPMC - Presbyterian Univ Hosp; **Address:** Lillian Kaufman Bldg, 3471 5th Ave, Ste 810, Pittsburgh, PA 15213; **Phone:** (412) 692-4920; **Board Cert:** Neurology 1984, Clinical Neurophysiology 1994; **Med School:** Univ Penn 1978; **Resid:** Internal Medicine, Presby-Univ Hosp, Pittsburgh, PA 1979-1980; Neurology, Mass Genl Hosp, Boston, MA 1980-1983; **Fellow:** Neurological Physiology, Mass Genl Hosp, Boston, MA 1983-1984; Cerebrovascular Disease, Mass Genl Hosp, Boston, MA 1984-1985; **Fac Appt:** Prof Neurology, Univ Pittsburgh

Weinberg, Harold MD (N) - ***Spec Exp:*** *Headache; Spinal Disorders; Neuromuscular Disorders;* **Hospital:** NYU Med Ctr (page 71); **Address:** 650 1st Ave, Fl 4, New York, NY 10016-3240; **Phone:** (212) 213-9339; **Board Cert:** Neurology 1983; **Med School:** Albert Einstein Coll Med 1978; **Resid:** Neurology, Columbia-Presby Med Ctr, New York, NY 1979-1982; **Fellow:** Neurological Muscular Disease, Columbia-Presby Med Ctr, New York, NY 1982; **Fac Appt:** Assoc Prof Neurology, NYU Sch Med

Weiner, William J. MD (N) - ***Spec Exp:*** *Movement Disorders; Parkinson's Disease; Huntington's Disease;* **Hospital:** University of MD Med Sys; **Address:** Univ Maryland Med System, Dept Neurology, 22 S Greene St, rm N4W46, Baltimore, MD 21201; **Phone:** (410) 328-6484; **Board Cert:** Neurology 1975; **Med School:** Univ IL Coll Med 1969; **Resid:** Neurology, Univ Minn, Minneapolis, MN 1970-1971; Neurology, Rush-Presby Med Ctr, Chicago, IL 1971-1973; **Fac Appt:** Prof Neurology, Univ Miami Sch Med

Zimmerman, Earl Abram MD (N) - ***Spec Exp:*** *Movement Disorders; Alzheimer's Disease;* **Hospital:** Albany Medical Center; **Address:** Albany Med Ctr-Neurology, 47 New Scotland Ave, MC-342, Albany, NY 12208; **Phone:** (518) 262-5226; **Board Cert:** Neurology 1970, Internal Medicine 1970; **Med School:** Univ Penn 1963; **Resid:** Internal Medicine, Columbia Presby Hosp, New York, NY 1964-1965; Neurology, Presby Hosp., New York, NY 1965-1968; **Fellow:** Endocrinology, Diabetes & Metabolism, Columbia Presby Hosp, New York, NY 1970-1972

Southeast

Adams, Robert Joseph MD (N) - ***Spec Exp:*** *Stroke;* **Hospital:** Med Coll of GA Hosp and Clin; **Address:** Med Coll of Georgia, Dept Neuro, 1429 Harper St, rm HF1154, Augusta, GA 30912; **Phone:** (706) 721-4670; **Board Cert:** Neurology 1987; **Med School:** Univ Ark 1980; **Resid:** Neurology, Med Coll GA, Augusta, GA 1982-1985; **Fac Appt:** Assoc Prof Neurology, Med Coll GA

Berger, Joseph MD (N) - ***Spec Exp:*** *Multiple Sclerosis; AIDS/HIV; Infectious & Demyelinating Diseases;* **Hospital:** Univ Kentucky Med Ctr; **Address:** Dept Neurology, Kentucky Clinic, Rm L-445, Lexington, KY 40536; **Phone:** (859) 323-5661; **Board Cert:** Neurology 1983, Internal Medicine 1977; **Med School:** Jefferson Med Coll 1974; **Resid:** Internal Medicine, Georgetown Univ Hosp, Washington, DC 1975-1977; Neurology, Jackson Meml Hosp, Miami, FL 1978-1981; **Fac Appt:** Prof Emeritus Neurology, Univ KY Coll Med

Corbett, James MD (N) - ***Spec Exp:*** *Neuro-Ophthalmology; Pseudotumor Cerebri; Multiple Sclerosis;* **Hospital:** Univ Hosps & Clins - Mississippi; **Address:** Univ Mississippi Med Ctr Neuro Grp, 2500 N State St, Jackson, MS 39216; **Phone:** (601) 984-5501; **Board Cert:** Neurology 1974; **Med School:** Univ Hlth Sci/Chicago Med Sch 1966; **Resid:** Internal Medicine, Rhode Island Hosp, Providence, RI 1967-1968; Neurology, Univ Hosp-CWRU, Cleveland, OH 1968-1971; **Fac Appt:** Prof Neurology, Univ Miss

De Long, Mahlon R. MD (N) - ***Spec Exp:*** *Parkinson's Disease; Movement Disorders;* **Hospital:** Emory Univ Hosp; **Address:** 1639 Pierce St, Ste 6000, Dept Neurology, Atlanta, GA 30322; **Phone:** (404) 727-3818; **Board Cert:** Neurology 1980; **Med School:** Harvard Med Sch 1966; **Resid:** Neurology, Johns Hopkins Hosp, Baltimore, MD 1973-1976; Internal Medicine, Boston City Hosp, Boston, MA 1967-1968; **Fellow:** Neurology, NIMH, Bethesda, MD 1968-1973; **Fac Appt:** Prof Neurology

Dokson, Joel MD (N) - ***Spec Exp:*** *Parkinson's Disease; Stroke;* **Hospital:** Mount Sinai Med Ctr; **Address:** 4302 Alton Rd, Ste 680, Miami Beach, FL 33140-2877; **Phone:** (305) 538-1877; **Board Cert:** Neurology 1973; **Med School:** Univ Miami Sch Med 1967; **Resid:** Neurology, Mount Sinai Hosp, New York, NY 1968-1971

Finkel, Michael MD (N) - *Spec Exp:* Lower Extremity Movement Disorders; ADHD; Headaches in Women; **Hospital:** Cleveland Clin FL; **Address:** Cleveland Clinic-Florida Naples, 6101 Pine Ridge Rd, Naples, FL 34119; **Phone:** (941) 348-4000; **Board Cert:** Neurology 1979; **Med School:** Washington Univ, St Louis 1973; **Resid:** Neurology, Strong Meml Hosp, Rochester, NY 1974-1977

Glass, Jonathan MD (N) - *Spec Exp:* Neuropathology; Neoromuscular Disorders; Peripheral Neuropathy; **Hospital:** Emory Univ Hosp; **Address:** Emory Univ Sch Med, Dept Neurology, 1639 Pierce Dr, WMRB Bldg, Ste 6000, Atlanta, GA 30322; **Phone:** (404) 727-3507; **Board Cert:** Neurology 1990, Clinical Neurophysiology 1996, Neuropathology 1997; **Med School:** Univ VT Coll Med 1985; **Resid:** Neurology, Johns Hopkins Univ, Baltimore, MD 1986-1989; **Fellow:** Neuropathology, Johns Hopkins Univ, Baltimore, MD 1989-1991; **Fac Appt:** Assoc Prof Neurology, Emory Univ

Goldstein, Larry Bruce MD (N) - *Spec Exp:* Stroke; Carotid Artery Disease; **Hospital:** Duke Univ Med Ctr (page 60); **Address:** Duke University Medical Center, Box 3651, Durham, NC 27710; **Phone:** (919) 684-3801; **Board Cert:** Neurology 1987; **Med School:** Mount Sinai Sch Med 1981; **Resid:** Neurology, Mt Sinai Hosp, New York, NY 1982-1985; **Fellow:** Cerebrovascular Disease, Duke U Med Ctr, Durham, NC 1985-1986; **Fac Appt:** Assoc Prof Neurology, Duke Univ

Haley Jr, Elliott Clarke MD (N) - *Spec Exp:* Stroke; **Hospital:** Univ of VA Hlth Sys (page 79); **Address:** PO Box 800394, Charlottesville, VA 22908; **Phone:** (804) 924-8041; **Board Cert:** Neurology 1985, Internal Medicine 1978; **Med School:** Tulane Univ 1974; **Resid:** Internal Medicine, Univ Virginia Hosp, Charlottesville, VA 1976-1978; Neurology, Univ Virginia Hosp, Charlottesville, VA 1979-1982; **Fellow:** Cerebrovascular Disease, Mass Genl Hosp, Boston, MA 1983-1984

Heilman, Kenneth MD (N) - *Spec Exp:* Behavioral Neurology; Memory Disorders; **Hospital:** Shands Hlthcre at Univ of FL (page 73); **Address:** Hlth Ctr Univ Fla Coll Med, Dept Neur, Box 100236, Gainesville, FL 32610-0236; **Phone:** (352) 392-3491; **Board Cert:** Neurology 1973; **Med School:** Univ VA Sch Med 1963; **Resid:** Bellevue Hosp Ctr, New York, NY 1964-1965; Neurology, Boston City Hosp, Boston, MA 1967-1970; **Fac Appt:** Prof Neurology, Univ Fla Coll Med

Hess, David Charles MD (N) - *Spec Exp:* Stroke; **Hospital:** Med Coll of GA Hosp and Clin; **Address:** Dept Neurology, 1120 15th St, rm BI-3080, Augusta, GA 30912; **Phone:** (706) 721-1691; **Board Cert:** Neurology 1990, Internal Medicine 1986; **Med School:** Univ MD Sch Med 1983; **Resid:** Internal Medicine, Allegheny Genl Hosp, Pittsburgh, PA 1984-1985; Neurology, Med Coll Georgia, Augusta, GA 1986-1989; **Fellow:** Cerebrovascular Disease, Med Coll Georgia, Augusta, GA 1989-1990; **Fac Appt:** Assoc Prof Neurology, Med Coll GA

Hurwitz, Barrie MD (N) - *Spec Exp:* Multiple Sclerosis; Parkinson's Disease; Stroke/Cerebrovascular Disease; **Hospital:** Duke Univ Med Ctr (page 60); **Address:** 122 Baker House, Box 3184, Durham, NC 27710; **Phone:** (919) 684-4126; **Board Cert:** Neurology 1979, Internal Medicine 1974; **Med School:** Africa 1968; **Resid:** Internal Medicine, Johannesburg Genl, Johannesburg 1971-1973; Neurology, Sloan Kettering hosp, New York, NY 1974-1977; **Fellow:** Neurology, Cornell, New York, NY 1974-1976; **Fac Appt:** Assoc Prof Medicine, Duke Univ

Kirshner, Howard S MD (N) - *Spec Exp:* Stroke; Aphasia; Rehabilitation; **Hospital:** Vanderbilt Univ Med Ctr (page 80); **Address:** Med Ctr South, 2100 Pierce Ave, Fl 362, Nashville, TN 37212-3162; **Phone:** (615) 936-1354; **Board Cert:** Neurology 1980; **Med School:** Harvard Med Sch 1972; **Resid:** Internal Medicine, Mass Genl Hosp, Boston, MA 1972-1973; Neurology, Mass Genl Hosp, Boston, MA 1975-1978; **Fellow:** Neurological Science, Natl Inst Hlth, Bethesda, MD 1973-1975; **Fac Appt:** Prof Neurology, Vanderbilt Univ

Koller, William C MD (N) - *Spec Exp:* Movement Disorders; Parkinson's Disease; **Hospital:** Univ of Miami - Jackson Meml Hosp; **Address:** Dept Neurology, 2nd Fl, 1501 NW Ninth Ave, Ste 1001, Miami, FL 33136; **Phone:** (305) 243-2235; **Board Cert:** Neurology 1982; **Med School:** Northwestern Univ 1976; **Resid:** Neurology, Rush-Presby-St Lukes Med Ctr, Chicago, IL 1977-1980; **Fac Appt:** Prof Neurology, Univ Miami Sch Med

Kurtzke, Robert MD (N) - *Spec Exp:* Electromyography; Nerve/Muscle Disorders; **Hospital:** Inova Fairfax Hosp; **Address:** Neur Ctr Fairfax Ltd, 3020 Hamaker Ct Ste 400, Fairfax, VA 22031-2220; **Phone:** (703) 876-0800; **Board Cert:** Clinical Neurophysiology 1994, Neurology 1990; **Med School:** Georgetown Univ 1985; **Resid:** Neurology, Neurology Inst-Columbia Presbyterian, New York, NY 1988-1989; Neurology, Neur Inst, New York, NY 1986-1989; **Fellow:** Neurological Muscular Disease, Duke Med Ctr, Durham, NC 1989-1990; **Fac Appt:** Neurology, Georgetown Univ

Lopez, Raul MD (N) - *Spec Exp:* Headache; **Hospital:** Mercy Hosp - Miami, FL; **Address:** 3661 S Miami Ave, Ste 209, Miami, FL 33133-4206; **Phone:** (305) 856-8942; **Board Cert:** Neurology 1970; **Med School:** Univ Fla Coll Med 1963; **Resid:** Internal Medicine, Univ Florida Med Ctr, Gainesville, FL 1963-1965; Neurology, Univ Florida Med Ctr, Gainesville, FL 1967-1968; **Fellow:** Neurology, Univ Florida Med Ctr, Gainesville, FL 1965-1967

Morgenlander, Joel Charles MD (N) - *Spec Exp:* Neurology - General; **Hospital:** Duke Univ Med Ctr (page 60); **Address:** Duke Univ Med Ctr, Box 3394, Durham, NC 27710-0001; **Phone:** (919) 684-6887; **Board Cert:** Neurology 1992; **Med School:** Univ Pittsburgh 1986; **Resid:** Neurology, Duke Univ, Durham, NC 1987-1990; **Fellow:** Neurological Muscular Disease, Duke Univ, Durham, NC 1990-1991; **Fac Appt:** Assoc Prof Neurology, Univ Pittsburgh

Nadeau, Stephen E MD (N) - *Spec Exp:* Dementia; Cerebrovascular Disease; Collagen Vascular Disease; **Hospital:** Shands Hlthcre at Univ of FL (page 73); **Address:** The Brain Inst, 100 S Newell Dr, rm L3-100, Gainesville, FL 32610; **Phone:** (352) 392-3491; **Board Cert:** Neurology 1984; **Med School:** Univ Fla Coll Med 1977; **Resid:** Neurology, Shands Teaching Hosp, Gainesville, FL 1978-1981; **Fellow:** Behavioral Neurology, Shands Teaching Hosp, Gainesville, FL 1981-1982; **Fac Appt:** Prof Neurology, Univ Fla Coll Med

Newman, Nancy Jean MD (N) - *Spec Exp:* Neuro-Ophthalmology; **Hospital:** Emory Univ Hosp; **Address:** Emory Eye Center, 1365-B Clifton RD NE, Atlanta, GA 30322; **Phone:** (404) 778-5360; **Board Cert:** Neurology 1989; **Med School:** Harvard Med Sch 1984; **Resid:** Neurology, Mass Genl Hosp, Boston, MA 1985-1988; **Fellow:** Neurological Ophthalmology, Mass EE Infirm, Boston, MA 1988-1989; **Fac Appt:** Prof Neurology, Emory Univ

Nolan, Bruce A MD (N) - *Spec Exp:* Sleep Disorders/Apnea; **Hospital:** Univ of Miami - Jackson Meml Hosp; **Address:** Univ Miami Sleep Disorder Ctr, 1201 NW 16th St, rm A212, Miami, FL 33101-6960; **Phone:** (305) 324-3371; **Board Cert:** Neurology 1974; **Med School:** Wayne State Univ 1966; **Resid:** Neurology, Univ Miami Med Ctr, Miami, FL 1967-1970; **Fac Appt:** Assoc Prof Neurology, Univ Miami Sch Med

Rothrock, John MD (N) - *Spec Exp:* Aneurysm; Headache; **Hospital:** Univ of S Ala Med Ctr; **Address:** Univ S Alabama Med Ctr, 3401 Medical Park Dr, Bldg 3 - Ste 205, Mobile, AL 36693; **Phone:** (251) 660-5108; **Board Cert:** Neurology 1984; **Med School:** Univ VA Sch Med 1977; **Resid:** Neurology, Univ Ariz Med Ctr, Tucson, AZ 1978-1981; **Fac Appt:** Prof Neurology, Univ S Ala Coll Med

Sadowsky, Carl Howard MD (N) - *Spec Exp:* Memory Disorders; **Hospital:** St Mary's Med Ctr - W Palm Bch; **Address:** 5205 Greenwood Ave, Ste 200, West Palm Beach, FL 33407-2493; **Phone:** (561) 845-0500; **Board Cert:** Neurology 1977; **Med School:** Cornell Univ-Weill Med Coll 1971; **Resid:** Internal Medicine, Dartmouth-Hitchcock Med Ctr, Hanover, NH 1972-1973; Neurology, Dartmouth-Hitchcock Med Ctr, Hanover, NH 1973-1976; **Fac Appt:** Asst Clin Prof Neurology, Nova SE Univ, Coll Osteo Med

Schatz, Norman Joseph MD (N) - *Spec Exp:* Neuro-Ophthalmology; **Hospital:** Mount Sinai Med Ctr; **Address:** 325 Alhambra Cir, Coral Gable, FL 33134; **Phone:** (305) 442-3355; **Board Cert:** Neurology 1969; **Med School:** Hahnemann Univ 1961; **Resid:** Neurology, Jefferson Hosp, Philadelphia, PA 1962-1965; **Fellow:** Neurological Ophthalmology, Univ Miami Project to Cure Paralysis, Miami, FL 1965-1966; **Fac Appt:** Clin Prof Neurology, Univ Penn

Sethi, Kapil MD (N) - *Spec Exp:* Parkinson's Disease; Movement Disorders; Botox Therapy; **Hospital:** Med Coll of GA Hosp and Clin; **Address:** Neurology Dept, 1120 15th St Bldg HB 2060, Augusta, GA 30912; **Phone:** (706) 721-2798; **Board Cert:** Neurology 1987; **Med School:** India 1976; **Resid:** Neurology, Pgimer, Chandigarh, India 1979-1981; Neurology, Med Coll Georgia, Augusta, GA 1983-1985; **Fac Appt:** Prof Neurology, Med Coll GA

Troost, Bradley Todd MD (N) - *Spec Exp:* Headache; Neuro-Ophthalmology; Dizziness; **Hospital:** Wake Forest Univ Baptist Med Ctr (page 81); **Address:** Wake Forest Baptist Med Ctr, Med Center Blvd, Winston Salem, NC 27157-1078; **Phone:** (336) 716-3429; **Board Cert:** Neurology 1972; **Med School:** Harvard Med Sch 1963; **Resid:** Neurology, Univ Colo Med Ctr, Denver, CO 1966-1969; **Fellow:** Ophthalmology, UCSF Med Ctr, San Francisco, CA 1969-1970; **Fac Appt:** Prof Neurology, Wake Forest Univ Sch Med

Valenstein, Edward MD (N) - *Spec Exp:* Neuromuscular Disorders; Amyotrophic Lateral Sclerosis(ALS); **Hospital:** Shands Hlthcre at Univ of FL (page 73); **Address:** 1600 SW Archer Rd, Box 100236, Gainesville, FL 32610-0236; **Phone:** (352) 392-3491; **Board Cert:** Neurology 1974, Clinical Neurophysiology 1996; **Med School:** Albert Einstein Coll Med 1967; **Resid:** Neurology, Boston City Hosp, Boston, MA 1968-1971; **Fac Appt:** Prof Neurology, Univ Fla Coll Med

Vitek, Jerrold Lee MD (N) - *Spec Exp:* Movement Disorders; **Hospital:** Emory Univ Hosp; **Address:** Dept Neurology, Clinic A, 1365 Clifton Drive NE Fl 3, Atlanta, GA 30322; **Phone:** (404) 778-4278; **Board Cert:** Neurology 1992; **Med School:** Univ Minn 1984; **Resid:** Neurology, Johns Hopkins Univ, Baltimore, MD 1985-1988; **Fac Appt:** Assoc Prof Neurology, Emory Univ

Watts, Ray Lannon MD (N) - *Spec Exp:* Parkinson's Disease; Movement Disorders; **Hospital:** Emory Univ Hosp; **Address:** Emory Univ Sch Med, Dept Neur, 1639 Pierce Drive, Ste 6000, Atlanta, GA 30322; **Phone:** (404) 727-5002; **Board Cert:** Neurology 1985; **Med School:** Washington Univ, St Louis 1980; **Resid:** Neurology, Mass Genl Hosp, Boston, MA 1981-1984; **Fellow:** Electromyography, Mass Genl Hosp, Boston, MA 1982-1983; **Fac Appt:** Neurology, Emory Univ

Wooten, George Frederick MD (N) - *Spec Exp:* Movement Disorders; Parkinson's Disease; Tremor; **Hospital:** Univ of VA Hlth Sys (page 79); **Address:** Box 800394, UVA Med Ctr, Dept Neurology The McKim Hall, Charlottesville, VA 22908; **Phone:** (804) 924-8369; **Board Cert:** Neurology 1977; **Med School:** Cornell Univ-Weill Med Coll 1970; **Resid:** Neurology, NY Hosp-Cornell Med, New York, NY 1974-1977; **Fellow:** Pharmacology, Natl Inst Mental Hlth-NIHMH, Bethesda, MD 1971-1974; **Fac Appt:** Prof Neurology, Univ VA Sch Med

Midwest

Adams Jr., Harlold Pomeroy MD (N) - *Spec Exp:* Stroke; **Hospital:** Univ of IA Hosp and Clinics; **Address:** Dept Neurology, 200 Hawkins Drive, rm 2148-RCP, Iowa City, IA 52242; **Phone:** (319) 356-4110; **Board Cert:** Neurology 1977; **Med School:** Northwestern Univ 1970; **Resid:** Neurology, Univ Iowa Hosp, Iowa City, IA 1971-1974; **Fac Appt:** Prof Neurology, Univ Iowa Coll Med

Ahlskog, J. Eric MD (N) - *Spec Exp:* Parkinson's Disease; Movement Disorders; **Hospital:** Mayo Med Ctr & Clin - Rochester, MN; **Address:** Mayo Clinic, Dept Neur, 200 First St SW, Rochester, MN 55905; **Phone:** (507) 538-1038; **Board Cert:** Neurology 1984; **Med School:** Dartmouth Med Sch 1976; **Resid:** Internal Medicine, Univ Chicago Hosps Clins, Chicago, IL 1977-1978; Neurology, Mayo Grad Sch Med, Rochester, MN 1978-1981; **Fac Appt:** Prof Neurology, Mayo Med Sch

Arnason, Barry G W MD (N) - *Spec Exp:* Multiple Sclerosis; Guillain-Barre Syndrome; Myasthenia Gravis; **Hospital:** Univ of Chicago Hosps (page 76); **Address:** 5758 S Maryland Ave, MC-2030, Chicago, IL 60637; **Phone:** (773) 702-6386; **Board Cert:** Neurology 1971; **Med School:** Univ Manitoba 1957; **Resid:** Neurology, Mass Genl Hosp, Boston, MA 1958-1959; Neurology, Mass Genl Hosp, Boston, MA 1961-1962; **Fac Appt:** Prof Neurology, Univ Chicago-Pritzker Sch Med

Brooks, Benjamin MD (N) - *Spec Exp:* Neuromuscular Disorders; Multiple Sclerosis; **Hospital:** Univ WI Hosp & Clins; **Address:** Univ Wisc Hosp, Dept Neurology, 600 Highland Ave, rm H6-558, Madison, WI 53792; **Phone:** (608) 263-5421; **Board Cert:** Neurology 1978, Internal Medicine 1974; **Med School:** Harvard Med Sch 1970; **Resid:** Neurology, Mass Genl Hosp, Bethesda, MD 1972-1974; Neurology, Natl Inst Neuro Disorders & Stroke-NIH, Boston, MA 1974-1976; **Fellow:** Neurological Virus, Johns Hopkins, Baltimore, MD 1976-1978; **Fac Appt:** Prof Neurology, Univ Wisc

Brunstrom, Janice E MD (N) - *Spec Exp:* Cerebral Palsy; Pediatric Neurology; **Hospital:** St Louis Children's Hospital; **Address:** St Louis Children's Hosp, Dept Child Neurology, One Children's Place, St Louis, MO 63110; **Phone:** (314) 454-6120; **Board Cert:** Pediatrics 1992, Child Neurology 1994; **Med School:** Med Coll VA 1987; **Resid:** Neurology, St Louis Chldn's Hosp, St Louis, MO 1988-1989; Neurology, Barnes Jewish Hosp, St Louis, MO 1989-1990; **Fellow:** Child Neurology, St Louis Chldn's Hosp, St Louis, MO 1990-1995

Burke, Allan M MD (N) - *Spec Exp:* Cerebrovascular Disease; Neural Imaging; **Hospital:** Northwestern Meml Hosp; **Address:** 150 E Huron St, Ste 803, Chicago, IL 60611-2912; **Phone:** (312) 944-0063; **Board Cert:** Neurology 1982; **Med School:** Columbia P&S 1976; **Resid:** Internal Medicine, NY Hosp, New York, NY 1976-1978; Neurology, Columbia-Presby Med Ctr, New York, NY 1978-1981; **Fellow:** Cerebrovascular Disease, Univ Penn Med Ctr, Philadelphia, PA 1981-1983; **Fac Appt:** Assoc Clin Prof Neurology, Northwestern Univ

Burns, R Stanley MD (N) - *Spec Exp:* Movement Disorders; Ataxia; Neurodegenerative Disease; **Hospital:** St John's Hosp - Springfield; **Address:** 751 N Rutledge, Ste 2300, Springfield, IL 62702; **Phone:** (217) 545-8249; **Board Cert:** Neurology 1985; **Med School:** Univ Minn 1969; **Resid:** Internal Medicine, Huntington Meml Hosp, Pasadena, CA 1970-1971; Neurology, UC Irvine Med Ctr, Irvine, CA 1975-1978; **Fellow:** Clinical Pharmacology, Natl Inst Genl Med Sci, Bethesda, MD 1978-1980; **Fac Appt:** Prof Neurology, Southern IL Univ

Cohen, Jeffrey Alan MD (N) - *Spec Exp:* Multiple Sclerosis; Neuro-Immunology; **Hospital:** Cleveland Clin Fdn (page 57); **Address:** The Cleveland Clin, Mellen Ctr, U10, 9500 Euclid Ave, Cleveland, OH 44195; **Phone:** (216) 445-8110; **Board Cert:** Neurology 1985; **Med School:** Univ Chicago-Pritzker Sch Med 1980; **Resid:** Neurology, Hosp Univ Penn, Philadelphia, PA 1981-1984; **Fellow:** Neurological Immunology, Hosp Univ Penn, Philadelphia, PA 1984-1987

Cutrer, F Michael MD (N) - *Spec Exp:* Headache; **Hospital:** Mayo Med Ctr & Clin - Rochester, MN; **Address:** Mayo Clinic, Dept Neurology, 200 First St NW, Rochester, MN 55905; **Phone:** (507) 284-4409; **Board Cert:** Neurology 1993; **Med School:** Univ Minn 1988; **Resid:** Neurology, UCLA Med Ctr, Los Angeles, CA 1989-1992; **Fellow:** Headache Medicine, Mass Genl Hosp, Boston, MA 1992-1994; **Fac Appt:** Asst Prof Neurology, Mayo Med Sch

Elias, Stanton B MD (N) - *Spec Exp:* Multiple Sclerosis; Myasthenia Gravis; **Hospital:** Henry Ford Hosp; **Address:** Henry Ford Hosp, Dept Neur, 2799 W Grand Blvd, Fl K-11, Detroit, MI 48202-2689; **Phone:** (313) 916-7207; **Board Cert:** Neurology 1979; **Med School:** Univ Pittsburgh 1972; **Resid:** Neurology, Duke Univ, Durham, NC 1973-1976; **Fellow:** Neurology, Duke Univ, Durham, NC 1976-1977

Farlow, Martin MD (N) - *Spec Exp:* Alzheimer's Disease; Neurodegenerative Disorders; Multiple Sclerosis; **Hospital:** IN Univ Hosp (page 63); **Address:** IN Univ Hosp & Med Ctr - Indianapolis, 550 N University Blvd, Indianapolis, IN 46202; **Phone:** (317) 274-2291; **Board Cert:** Neurology 1988; **Med School:** Indiana Univ 1979; **Resid:** Neurology, Indiana Univ, Indianapolis, IN 1980-1983; **Fac Appt:** Prof Neurology, Indiana Univ

Feldman, Eva L. MD/PhD (N) - *Spec Exp:* Neuromuscular Disorders; Amyotrophic Lateral Sclerosis(ALS); Neuropathy; **Hospital:** Univ of MI Hlth Ctr; **Address:** 1500 E Med Center Drive, Ste 1324, Box 0322, Ann Arbor, MI 48109-0322; **Phone:** (734) 936-9020; **Board Cert:** Neurology 1988; **Med School:** Univ Mich Med Sch 1983; **Resid:** Neurology, Johns Hopkins Hosp, Baltimore, MD 1984-1987; **Fellow:** Neurology, Univ Mich, Ann Arbor, MI 1987-1988; **Fac Appt:** Prof Neurology, Univ Mich Med Sch

Fox, Jacob H MD (N) - *Spec Exp:* Alzheimer's Disease; Dementia; **Hospital:** Rush-Presby - St Luke's Med Ctr (page 72); **Address:** Rush Presby-St Lukes Med Ctr, Dept Neurology, 710 S Paulina St, Chicago, IL 60612; **Phone:** (312) 942-8729; **Board Cert:** Neurology 1974; **Med School:** Univ IL Coll Med 1967; **Resid:** Neurology, Barnes Hosp, St Louis, MO 1968-1971; **Fac Appt:** Prof Neurology, Rush Med Coll

Furlan, Anthony J MD (N) - *Spec Exp:* Stroke; Thrombolytic Therapy-Stroke; **Hospital:** Cleveland Clin Fdn (page 57); **Address:** 9500 Euclid Ave, Ste S91, Cleveland, OH 44195-0001; **Phone:** (216) 444-5535; **Board Cert:** Neurology 1979; **Med School:** Loyola Univ-Stritch Sch Med 1973; **Resid:** Neurology, Cleveland Clinic, Cleveland, OH 1974-1977; **Fellow:** Cerebrovascular Disease, Mayo Clinic, Rochester, MN 1977-1978; **Fac Appt:** Assoc Prof Neurology, Ohio State Univ

Gilman, Sid MD (N) - *Spec Exp:* Movement & Cognitive Disorders; Alzheimer's Disease; Ataxia; **Hospital:** Univ of MI Hlth Ctr; **Address:** Univ Michigan Med Ctr, Dept Neur, 1500 E Med Ctr Dr, 1914 Taubman Ctr, Ann Arbor, MI 48109-0316; **Phone:** (734) 936-9070; **Board Cert:** Neurology 1966; **Med School:** UCLA 1957; **Resid:** Neurology, Boston City Hosp-Harvard, Boston, MA 1960-1963; **Fellow:** Neurological Physiology, Boston City Hosp-Harvard, Boston, MA 1963-1965; **Fac Appt:** Prof Neurology, Univ Mich Med Sch

Goetz, Christopher MD (N) - *Spec Exp:* Movement Disorders; Parkinson's Disease; Dyskinesias; **Hospital:** Rush-Presby - St Luke's Med Ctr (page 72); **Address:** 1725 W Harrison St, Ste 755, Chicago, IL 60612-3835; **Phone:** (312) 563-2030; **Board Cert:** Neurology 1982; **Med School:** Rush Med Coll 1975; **Resid:** Neurology, Rush Presby-St Luke's Med Ctr, Chicago, IL 1975-1976; Neurology, Michael Reese Med Ctr, Chicago, IL 1976-1977; **Fellow:** Neurology, Rush-Presby-St Luke's Med Ctr, Chicago, IL 1976-1979; **Fac Appt:** Prof Neurology, Rush Med Coll

Greenberg, Harry S. MD (N) - *Spec Exp:* Neuro-Oncology; Brain Tumors; **Hospital:** Univ of MI Hlth Ctr; **Address:** Taubman Ctr 1914-0316, 1500 E Med Ctr Dr, Ann Arbor, MI 48109-0316; **Phone:** (734) 936-9055; **Board Cert:** Neurology 1980; **Med School:** SUNY Syracuse 1973; **Resid:** Neurology, Stanford Hosp, Stanford, CA 1974-1977; **Fellow:** Medical Oncology, Sloan Kettering Cancer Ctr, New York, NY 1979; **Fac Appt:** Prof Neurology, Univ Mich Med Sch

Hubble, Jean Pintar MD (N) - *Spec Exp:* Movement Disorders; Parkinson's Disease; Neuro-Pharmacology; **Hospital:** Ohio St Univ Med Ctr; **Address:** 1581 Dodd, Ste 371, Columbus, OH 43210-1257; **Phone:** (614) 688-4048; **Board Cert:** Neurology 1988; **Med School:** Univ Kans 1983; **Resid:** Neurology, Ohio State Univ Med Ctr, Columbus, OH 1984-1988; **Fellow:** Neuropharmacology, Ohio State Univ Med Ctr, Columbus, OH 1987-1989; **Fac Appt:** Assoc Clin Prof Neurology, Ohio State Univ

Kincaid, John C MD (N) - *Spec Exp:* Pain-Facial; Neuromuscular Disease; Electromyography; **Hospital:** IN Univ Hosp (page 63); **Address:** Indiana U Hosp, 550 N University Blvd, Indianapolis, IN 46202; **Phone:** (317) 274-0311; **Board Cert:** Neurology 1982, Clinical Neurophysiology 1997; **Med School:** Indiana Univ 1975; **Resid:** Neurology, Indiana U, Indianapolis, IN 1976-1979; **Fellow:** Electromyography, Mayo Clin, Rochester, MN 1980; **Fac Appt:** Prof Neurology, Indiana Univ

Kotagal, Suresh MD (N) - *Spec Exp:* Sleep Disorders-Children; Epilepsy/Seizure Disorders; Neurodegenerative Disorders; **Hospital:** Mayo Med Ctr & Clin - Rochester, MN; **Address:** Mayo Clinic, 200 First St SW, Rochester, MN 55905; **Phone:** (507) 284-2901; **Board Cert:** Pediatrics 1979, Neurology-Child Neurology 1982; **Med School:** India 1974; **Resid:** Child Neurology, St Louis U, St Louis, MO 1976-1979; Pediatrics, Chldns Hosp Mich, Detroit, MI 1975-1976; **Fellow:** Sleep Medicine, Stanford U, Stanford, CA 1982; **Fac Appt:** Prof Neurology, Mayo Med Sch

Lisak, Robert Philip MD (N) - *Spec Exp:* Multiple Sclerosis; Myasthenia Gravis; Vasclitis of the Nervous System; **Hospital:** Harper Hosp (page 59); **Address:** Wayne State Univ Sch Med, 4201 St Antoine, Hlth Ctr 8D, Detroit, MI 48201; **Phone:** (313) 745-4275; **Board Cert:** Neurology 1975; **Med School:** Columbia P&S 1965; **Resid:** Internal Medicine, Bronx Muni Hosp-Einstein, Bronx, NY 1968-1969; Neurology, Hosp Univ Penn, Philadelphia, PA 1969-1972; **Fac Appt:** Prof Neurology, Wayne State Univ

Mahowald, Mark W MD (N) - *Spec Exp:* Sleep Apnea; Sleep Disorders; **Hospital:** Hennepin Cnty Med Ctr; **Address:** Minnesota Regl Sleep Disordr Ctr, 701 Park Ave S, Minneapolis, MN 55415; **Phone:** (612) 347-6288; **Board Cert:** Neurology 1976; **Med School:** Univ Minn 1968; **Resid:** Neurology, Fairview Univ Med Ctr, Minneapolis, MN 1971-1974; **Fac Appt:** Prof Neurology, Univ Minn

Mendell, Jerry R MD (N) - *Spec Exp:* Neuromuscular Disorders; **Hospital:** Ohio St Univ Med Ctr; **Address:** 1654 Upham Drive Bldg Means - rm 445, Columbus, OH 43210; **Phone:** (614) 293-4962; **Board Cert:** Neurology 1972; **Med School:** Univ Tex SW, Dallas 1966; **Resid:** Neurology, NY Neur Inst, New York, NY 1967-1969; Neurology, Natl Inst Hlth, Bethesda, MD 1969-1970; **Fellow:** Neurological Muscular Disease, Natl Inst Hlth, Bethesda, MD 1970-1972; **Fac Appt:** Prof Neurology, Ohio State Univ

Mesulam, Marek Marsel MD (N) - *Spec Exp:* Alzheimer's Disease; Tourette's Syndrome; Dementia; **Hospital:** Northwestern Meml Hosp; **Address:** 675 N St Claire St, Ste 20-100, Chicago,, IL 60611; **Phone:** (312) 695-9627; **Board Cert:** Neurology 1977; **Med School:** Harvard Med Sch 1972; **Resid:** Neurology, Boston City Hosp, Boston, MA 1973-1976

Montgomery Jr, Erwin B MD (N) - *Spec Exp:* Parkinson's Disease; **Hospital:** Cleveland Clin Fdn (page 57); **Address:** Cleveland Clinic, Dept Neurology - Desk S90, 9500 Euclid Ave, Cleveland, OH 44195; **Phone:** (216) 445-1108; **Board Cert:** Neurology 1982; **Med School:** SUNY Buffalo 1976; **Resid:** Neurology, Wahington Univ Med Ctr, St Louis, MO 1977-1980; **Fellow:** Neurological Physiology, Washington Univ Med Ctr, St Louis, MO 1980-1981

Morris, John MD (N) - *Spec Exp:* Alzheimer's Disease; **Hospital:** Barnes-Jewish Hosp (page 55); **Address:** Memory Diagnostic Ctr., 4488 Forest Park, Ste 160, St Louis, MO 63108; **Phone:** (314) 286-1967; **Board Cert:** Internal Medicine 1979, Neurology 1985; **Med School:** Univ Rochester 1974; **Resid:** Internal Medicine, Akron Genl Med Ctr, Akron, OH 1977-1979; Neurology, Cleveland Metro Genl Hosp, Cleveland, OH 1979-1982; **Fellow:** Neuropharmacology, Washington Univ, St Louis, MO 1982-1985; **Fac Appt:** Prof Neurology, Washington Univ, St Louis

Pascuzzi, Robert MD (N) - *Spec Exp:* Neuromuscular Disease; Amyotrophic Lateral Sclerosis(ALS); **Hospital:** IN Univ Hosp (page 63); **Address:** Indiana U Med Ctr Dept Neur, 1050 Walnut St, Indianapolis, IN 46202; **Phone:** (317) 630-6146; **Board Cert:** Neurology 1984; **Med School:** Indiana Univ 1979; **Resid:** Neurology, Univ Va Med Ctr, Charlottesville, VA 1980-1983; **Fellow:** Neurological Muscular Disease, Univ Va Med Ctr, Charlottesville, VA 1983-1985; **Fac Appt:** Prof Neurology, Indiana Univ

Perlmutter, Joel S MD (N) - *Spec Exp:* Parkinson's Disease; Movement Disorders; **Hospital:** Barnes-Jewish Hosp (page 55); **Address:** 660 S Euclid Ave, Box CB8111, St Louis, MO 63110; **Phone:** (314) 362-6908; **Board Cert:** Neurology 1985; **Med School:** Univ MO-Columbia Sch Med 1979; **Resid:** Neurology, Banres Hosp-Wash Univ, St Louis, MO 1980-1983; **Fellow:** Neurology, Barnes Hosp-Wash Univ, St Louis, MO 1983-1984; **Fac Appt:** Assoc Prof Neurology, Washington Univ, St Louis

Porth, Karen MD (N) - *Spec Exp:* Muscular Dystrophy; Electromyography; **Hospital:** Fairview Southdale Hosp; **Address:** Minneapolis Clin of Neuro-Southdale, 6363 France Ave S, Ste 200, Edina, MN 55435-2145; **Phone:** (952) 920-7200; **Board Cert:** Neurology 1988; **Med School:** Univ Cincinnati 1983; **Resid:** Psychiatry, Univ Pittsburgh, Pittsburgh, PA 1984-1987

Reder, Anthony T MD (N) - *Spec Exp:* Multiple Sclerosis; Dementia; Myasthenia Gravis; **Hospital:** Univ of Chicago Hosps (page 76); **Address:** Center for Advanced Medicine, 5758 S Maryland Ave, Chicago, IL 60637-1426; **Phone:** (773) 702-6204; **Board Cert:** Neurology 1984; **Med School:** Univ Mich Med Sch 1978; **Resid:** Neurology, Univ Minn Hosps, Minneapolis, MN 1979-1982; **Fellow:** Neurological Immunology, Univ Chicago, Chicago, IL 1982-1984; **Fac Appt:** Assoc Prof Neurology, Univ Chicago-Pritzker Sch Med

Reed, Robert L MD (N) - *Spec Exp:* Multiple Sclerosis; Stroke; **Hospital:** Good Samaritan Hosp - Cincinnati; **Address:** 111 Wellington Pl, Cincinnati, OH 45219; **Phone:** (513) 241-2370; **Board Cert:** Neurology 1975; **Med School:** Univ Cincinnati 1966; **Resid:** Internal Medicine, Mayo Grad Sch Med, Rochester, MN 1969-1970; Neurology, Mayo Grad Sch Med, Rochester, MN 1970-1973

Rogers, Lisa R DO (N) - *Spec Exp:* Neuro-Oncology; **Hospital:** Henry Ford Hosp; **Address:** Henry Fd Hosp Dept Neur, 2799 W Grand Blvd Fl K-11, Detroit, MI 48202; **Phone:** (313) 916-8662; **Board Cert:** Neurology 1982; **Med School:** Kirksville Coll Osteo Med 1976; **Resid:** Neurology, Cleveland Clinic Fdn, Cleveland, OH 1977-1980; **Fellow:** Neurological Oncology, Meml-Sloan Kettering Cancer Ctr, New York, NY 1980-1982

Roos, Karen MD (N) - *Spec Exp:* Neurofibromatosis; Infectious Diseases-CNS; **Hospital:** IN Univ Hosp (page 63); **Address:** Indiana U Med Ctr, 550 N University Blvd, rm 4411, Indianapolis, IN 46202; **Phone:** (317) 278-6785; **Board Cert:** Neurology 1986; **Med School:** Hahnemann Univ 1981; **Resid:** Neurology, Univ VA, Charlottesville, VA 1982-1985; **Fac Appt:** Prof Neurology, Indiana Univ

Roos, Raymond MD (N) - *Spec Exp:* Amyotrophic Lateral Sclerosis(ALS); Multiple Sclerosis; **Hospital:** Univ of Chicago Hosps (page 76); **Address:** Dept Neurology, 5841 S Maryland Ave, MC-2030, Chicago, IL 60637; **Phone:** (773) 702-6390; **Board Cert:** Neurology 1976; **Med School:** SUNY Downstate 1968; **Resid:** Neurology, Johns Hopkins Hosp, Baltimore, MD 1971-1974; **Fellow:** Neurology, Natl Inst of Neur Dis and Stroke, Bethesda, MD 1969-1971; Neurology, Johns Hospkins Hosp, Baltimore, MD 1974-1976; **Fac Appt:** Prof Neurology, Univ Chicago-Pritzker Sch Med

Rubin, Susan MD (N) - *Spec Exp:* Multiple Sclerosis in Women; Epilepsy in Pregnancy; Headache-Migraine in Women; **Hospital:** Glenbrook Hosp; **Address:** Glenbrook Hospital, Dept of Neurology, 2100 Pfingsten Road, Glenview, IL 60025-1393; **Phone:** (847) 657-5875; **Board Cert:** Neurology 1996; **Med School:** Univ IL Coll Med 1988; **Resid:** Neurology, Northwestern Meml Hosp, Chicago, IL 1990-1993; **Fellow:** Neurology, Northwestern Meml Hosp, Chicago, IL 1993-1994; **Fac Appt:** Neurology, Northwestern Univ

Sagar, Stephen M MD (N) - *Spec Exp:* Neuro-Oncology; **Hospital:** Univ Hosp of Cleveland; **Address:** Univ Hosp Cleveland, Hanna House, 11100 Euclid Ave Fl 5, Cleveland, OH 44106; **Phone:** (216) 844-7510; **Board Cert:** Internal Medicine 1976, Neurology 1979; **Med School:** Harvard Med Sch 1972; **Resid:** Internal Medicine, Peter Bent Brigham Hosp, Boston, MA 1973-1974; Neurology, Mass Genl Hosp, Boston, MA 1974-1977; **Fellow:** Neurology, Chldns Hosp Med Ctr, Boston, MA 1978-1979; **Fac Appt:** Prof Neurology, Case West Res Univ

Saper, Joel R MD (N) - *Spec Exp:* Headache; Pain-Chronic after Head Injury; **Hospital:** St Joseph Mercy Hosp - Ann Arbor; **Address:** Michigan Head Pain & Neurological Inst, 3120 Professional Drive, Ann Arbor, MI 48104-5131; **Phone:** (734) 677-6000; **Board Cert:** Neurology 1975; **Med School:** Univ IL Coll Med 1969; **Resid:** Neurology, Mich Hosp & Med Ctr, Ann Arbor, MI 1970-1973; **Fac Appt:** Clin Prof Neurology, Mich State Univ

Schapiro, Randall MD (N) - *Spec Exp:* Multiple Sclerosis; **Hospital:** Fairview-Univ Med Ctr - Univ Campus; **Address:** 701 25th Ave S, Ste 200, Minneapolis, MN 55454; **Phone:** (612) 672-6100; **Board Cert:** Neurology 1976; **Med School:** Univ Minn 1970; **Resid:** Internal Medicine, Wadsworth VA Hosp, Los Angeles, CA 1971-1972; Neurology, Univ Minnesota Hosp, Minneapolis, MN 1972-1975; **Fac Appt:** Clin Prof Neurology, Univ Minn

Siddique, Teepu MD (N) - *Spec Exp:* Amyotrophic Lateral Sclerosis(ALS); Muscular Dystrophy; **Hospital:** Northwestern Meml Hosp; **Address:** Northwestern Med Fac Fdn, 675 N St Clair Galter 20-100, Chicago, IL 60611-5935; **Phone:** (312) 695-5886; **Board Cert:** Neurology 1980; **Med School:** Pakistan 1973; **Resid:** Neurology, UMDNJ-RW Johnson Med Sch, Plainfield, NJ 1976-1979; **Fellow:** Electromyography, Hosp Special Surg-Cornell Med Ctr, New York, NY 1979-1980; Neurological Muscular Disease, Natl Inst Hlth, Bethesda, MD 1980-1981; **Fac Appt:** Prof Neurology, Northwestern Univ

Swanson, Jerry W MD (N) - *Spec Exp:* Headache; **Hospital:** Mayo Med Ctr & Clin - Rochester, MN; **Address:** Mayo Clinic, Dept Neurology, 200 First St NW, Rochester, MN 55905; **Phone:** (507) 284-4409; **Board Cert:** Neurology 1984; **Med School:** Northwestern Univ 1977; **Resid:** Neurology, Mayo Clinic, Rochester, MN 1978-1982; **Fellow:** Electroencephalography, Mayo Clinic, Rochester, MN 1983; **Fac Appt:** Assoc Prof Neurology, Mayo Med Sch

Taylor, Frederick R MD (N) - *Spec Exp:* Headache; **Hospital:** Methodist Hosp - Minnesota; **Address:** Park Nicollet Headache Clinic, E-500 Meadowbrook Bldg, 6490 Excelsior Blvd, Minneapolis, MN 55426; **Phone:** (952) 993-3639; **Board Cert:** Pediatrics 1982, Neurology 1985; **Med School:** Univ New Mexico 1977; **Resid:** Pediatrics, Univ Wisc Hlth Sci Ctr, Madison, WI 1978-1980; Neurology, Univ Wisc Hlth Sci Ctr, Madison, WI 1980-1983; **Fac Appt:** Assoc Prof Neurology, Univ Minn

Taylor, Fredrick R MD (N) - *Spec Exp:* Headache; Electromyography; **Hospital:** Methodist Hosp - Minnesota; **Address:** Park Nicollet Clinic, 6490 Excelsior Blvd, Ste E500, Minneapolis, MN 55426-4700; **Phone:** (952) 993-3494; **Board Cert:** Pediatrics 1982, Neurology-Child Neurology 1985, Clinical Neurophysiology 1996; **Med School:** Univ New Mexico 1977; **Resid:** Pediatrics, Univ Wisc Affil Hosps, WI 1978-1980; Neurology, Univ Wisc Affil Hosps, WI 1980-1983; **Fellow:** Clinical Neurophysiology, Univ Wisc Affil Hosps, WI 1983-1984

Wiebers, David O MD (N) - *Spec Exp:* Stroke; Aneurysm-Cerebral; **Hospital:** Mayo Med Ctr & Clin - Rochester, MN; **Address:** Mayo Clinic, Dept Neur, 200 First St SW, Rochester, MN 55905; **Phone:** (507) 284-9735; **Board Cert:** Neurology 1984; **Med School:** Univ Nebr Coll Med 1975; **Resid:** Neurology, Mayo Clin, Rochester, MN 1976-1980; **Fac Appt:** Prof Neurology, Mayo Med Sch

Windebank, Anthony J. MD (N) - *Spec Exp:* Peripheral Neuropathy; Amyotrophic Lateral Sclerosis(ALS); Multiple Sclerosis; **Hospital:** Mayo Med Ctr & Clin - Rochester, MN; **Address:** Mayo Clinic, Dept of Neurology, 200 1st St SW, Rochester, MN 55905; **Phone:** (507) 284-2233; **Board Cert:** Neurology 1982; **Med School:** England 1974; **Resid:** Neurology, Mayo Grad Sch Med, Rochester, MN 1977-1981; Internal Medicine, Radcliffe Infirm, Oxford, England 1976-1977; **Fac Appt:** Prof Nephrology, Mayo Med Sch

Wright, Robert B MD (N) - *Spec Exp:* Myasthenia Gravis; Migraine; **Hospital:** Rush-Presby - St Luke's Med Ctr (page 72); **Address:** 1725 W Harrison St, Fl 11th - Ste 1118, Chicago, IL 60612; **Phone:** (312) 942-5936; **Board Cert:** Neurology 1988; **Med School:** Univ IL Coll Med 1982; **Resid:** Internal Medicine, Rush Presby-St Luke's Med Ctr, Chicago, IL 1983-1986; **Fellow:** Neurology, Rush Presby-St Luke's Med Ctr, Chicago, IL 1986-1987

Great Plains and Mountains

Cilo, Mark P MD (N) - *Spec Exp:* Brain Injury; **Hospital:** Craig Hospital; **Address:** 3425 S Clarkson St, Englewood, CO 80110-2811; **Phone:** (303) 789-8220; **Board Cert:** Neurology 1979; **Med School:** Mount Sinai Sch Med 1972; **Resid:** Neurology, Mount Sinai Hosp, New York, NY 1973-1976; **Fellow:** Spinal Cord & Brain Injury Rehab, Craig Hosp, Englewood, NJ 1977-1978; **Fac Appt:** Asst Clin Prof Medicine, Univ Colo

Kelts, K Alan MD/PhD (N) - *Spec Exp:* Child Neurology; Sleep Disorders; Neuromuscular Disorders; **Hospital:** Rapid City Reg Hosp; **Address:** Black Hills Neurology, 2929 5th St, Ste 240, Rapid City, SD 57701; **Phone:** (605) 341-3770; **Board Cert:** Pediatrics 1977, Child Neurology 1978; **Med School:** Univ Rochester 1971; **Resid:** Pediatrics, Chldns Oregon & Univ Hosps, Seattle, WA 1971-1973; Child Neurology, Colorado Med Ctr, Denver, CO 1973-1976; **Fellow:** Neurological Muscular Disease, Muscular Dystrophy Assn of America 1974-1975; **Fac Appt:** Clin Prof Neurology, Univ SD Sch Med

Ringel, Steven MD (N) - *Spec Exp:* Neuromuscular Disorders; **Hospital:** Univ Colo HSC - Denver; **Address:** Univ CO Hlth Sci Ctr Dept Neur, 4200 E Ninth Ave, Box B 185, Denver, CO 80262; **Phone:** (303) 315-7221; **Board Cert:** Neurology 1974; **Med School:** Univ Mich Med Sch 1968; **Resid:** Neurology, Rush-Presby-St Lukes Med Hosp, Denver, CO 1968-1972; **Fellow:** Neurology, Natl Inst Neuro Dis-NIH, Bethesda, MD 1974-1976; **Fac Appt:** Prof Neurology, Univ Colo

Southwest

Carter, John E MD (N) - *Spec Exp:* *Neuro-Ophthalmology;* **Hospital:** Univ of Texas Hlth & Sci Ctr; **Address:** Univ Texas Hlth &Sci Ctr, Dept Med, 7703 Floyd Curl, MC 7883, San Antonio, TX 78229-3900; **Phone:** (210) 567-4615; **Board Cert:** Neurology 1978; **Med School:** Univ Ark 1969; **Resid:** Neurology, Boston Univ, Boston, MA 1974-1978; Neurological Ophthalmology, Tufts Univ, Boston, MA 1978-1979; **Fac Appt:** Assoc Prof Neurology, Univ Tex, San Antonio

Couch Jr, James R MD/PhD (N) - *Spec Exp:* *Headache; Stroke;* **Hospital:** Presby Hosp - Oklahoma City; **Address:** 711 S L Young Blvd, Ste 215, Oklahoma City, OK 73104; **Phone:** (405) 271-4113; **Board Cert:** Neurology 1974, Clinical Neurophysiology 1992; **Med School:** Baylor Coll Med 1965; **Resid:** Neurology, Washington Univ Med Ctr, St Louis, MO 1969-1972; **Fellow:** Neuropharmacology, Natl Inst Hlth, Bethesda, MD 1967-1969; **Fac Appt:** Prof Neurology, Univ Okla Coll Med

Coull, Bruce MD (N) - *Spec Exp:* *Stroke; Cerebrovascular Disease;* **Hospital:** Univ Med Ctr; **Address:** 707 N Alvernon, Ste 201, Tuscon, AZ 85711; **Phone:** (520) 694-1450; **Board Cert:** Neurology 1979; **Med School:** Univ Pittsburgh 1972; **Resid:** Neurology, Stanford Univ, Stanford, CA 1973-1976

Ferrendelli, James A MD (N) - *Spec Exp:* *Epilepsy/Seizure Disorders; Neuropharmacology; Geriatric Neurology;* **Hospital:** Meml Hermann Hosp; **Address:** Univ Tex-Houston, Dept Neur, 6431 Fannin St, Ste 7044, Houston, TX 77030-1501; **Phone:** (713) 500-7100; **Board Cert:** Neurology 1973; **Med School:** Univ Colo 1962; **Resid:** Neurology, Cleveland Metro Genl Hosp, Cleveland, OH 1965-1968; **Fellow:** Neuropharmacology, Washington Univ Med Sch, St Louis, MO 1968-1971; **Fac Appt:** Prof Neurology, Univ Tex, Houston

Fox, Peter Thornton MD (N) - *Spec Exp:* *PET Scans;* **Hospital:** Univ of Texas Hlth & Sci Ctr; **Address:** Univ Texas Hlth Sci Ctr, Research Imaging Ctr, 7703 Floyd Curl Drive, MS 6240, San Antonio, TX 78229-3900; **Phone:** (210) 567-8150; **Board Cert:** Neurology 1985; **Med School:** Georgetown Univ 1979; **Resid:** Neurology, Washington Univ, St Louis, MO 1980-1983; **Fellow:** Radiotracer Imaging, Washington Univ, St Louis, MO 1983-1984; **Fac Appt:** Prof Neurology, Univ Tex, San Antonio

Garcia, Carlos MD (N) - *Spec Exp:* *Muscular Dystrophy; Myasthenia Gravis;* **Hospital:** Tulane Univ Med Ctr Hosp & Clinic; **Address:** Tulane Univ Med Ctr, 1430 Tulane Ave, New Orleans, LA 70112-2699; **Phone:** (504) 588-5231; **Board Cert:** Neuropathology 1974, Neurology 1976; **Med School:** Colombia 1961; **Resid:** Pathology, Univ Hosp - Cali, Cali, Colombia 1960-1962; Neurology, Louisiana Med Ctr, New Orleans, LA 1965-1967; **Fellow:** Neuropathology, Louisiana Med Ctr, New Orleans, LA 1962-1965; **Fac Appt:** Prof Neurology, Tulane Univ

Grotta, James MD (N) - *Spec Exp:* *Stroke;* **Hospital:** Meml Hermann Hosp; **Address:** Meml Hermann Hlthcare Sys, 6410 Fannin St, Houston, TX 77030; **Phone:** (713) 704-0780; **Board Cert:** Neurology 1978; **Med School:** Univ VA Sch Med 1971; **Resid:** Neurology, Univ Colorado Hlth Sci Ctr, Denver, CO 1974-1977; **Fellow:** Diagnostic Radiology, Mass Genl Hosp, Boston, MA 1978-1979; **Fac Appt:** Prof Neurology, Univ Tex, Houston

Hart, Robert G. MD (N) - *Spec Exp:* *Stroke;* **Hospital:** Univ Hosp-San Antonio; **Address:** Univ Texas Hlth & Sci Ctr, Dept Neurology, 7703 Floyd Curl Dr, San Antonio, TX 78229-3900; **Phone:** (210) 617-5161; **Board Cert:** Neurology 1985; **Med School:** Univ MO-Columbia Sch Med 1977; **Resid:** Neurology, Univ Hosp & Clinic, Columbia, MO 1978-1981; **Fellow:** Stroke, Oregon Hlth Sci Ctr, Portland, OR 1981-1982; **Fac Appt:** Prof Neurology, Univ Tex, San Antonio

Infante, Ernesto MD (N) - *Spec Exp:* Amyotrophic Lateral Sclerosis(ALS); Cervical Disc Disease; **Hospital:** Methodist Hosp - Houston; **Address:** Diagnostic Clinic of Houston, 6448 Fannin St Fl 12, Houston, TX 77030; **Phone:** (713) 797-9191; **Board Cert:** Neurology 1973; **Med School:** Spain 1964; **Resid:** Neurology, Univ Minn Hosps, Minneapolis, MN 1966-1969; **Fellow:** Electromyography, Mayo Clinic, Rochester, MN 1969-1970; **Fac Appt:** Assoc Clin Prof Neurology, Univ Tex, Houston

Jackson, John Kevin MD (N) - *Spec Exp:* Neuro-Psychiatry; Neuro-Behavioral Disorder; **Hospital:** Tulane Univ Med Ctr Hosp & Clinic; **Address:** Tulane Medical Center, 1415 Tulane Ave, New Orleans, LA 70112; **Phone:** (504) 588-5231; **Med School:** Tulane Univ 1990; **Resid:** Neurology, Tulane Univ Sch of Med, New Orleans, LA 1991-1994

Jankovic, Joseph MD (N) - *Spec Exp:* Movement Disorders; Parkinson's Disease; Tourette's Syndrome; **Hospital:** Methodist Hosp - Houston; **Address:** Baylor Coll Med, Dept Neur, Smith Twr #1801, 6550 Fannin St, Houston, TX 77030-2717; **Phone:** (713) 798-5998; **Board Cert:** Neurology 1979; **Med School:** Univ Ariz Coll Med 1973; **Resid:** Neurology, Columbia-Presby Med Ctr, New York, NY 1974-1977; **Fac Appt:** Prof Neurology, Baylor Coll Med

Knoefel, Janice E MD (N) - *Spec Exp:* Neurology-Geriatric; **Hospital:** Univ NM Hosp; **Address:** New Mexico VA Hlth Care Sys, 1501 San Pedro SE, MC 111K, Albuquerque, NM 87108-5128; **Phone:** (505) 256-2795; **Board Cert:** Neurology 1983; **Med School:** Ohio State Univ 1977; **Resid:** Internal Medicine, Univ Cincinnati Med Ctr, Cincinnati, OH 1978-1979; Neurology, Boston Univ Med Ctr, Boston, MA 1979-1982; **Fellow:** Geriatric Medicine, Boston Univ Med Ctr, Boston, MA 1982-1983; **Fac Appt:** Assoc Prof Neurology, Univ New Mexico

Levin, Victor Alan MD (N) - *Spec Exp:* Brain Tumors; **Hospital:** Univ of TX MD Anderson Cancer Ctr, The; **Address:** 1515 Holcombe Blvd, #431, Houston, TX 77030-4009; **Phone:** (713) 792-8297; **Board Cert:** Neurology 1976; **Med School:** Univ Wisc 1966; **Resid:** Neurology, Mass Genl Hosp, Boston, MA 1969-1972; **Fac Appt:** Prof Neurology, Univ Tex, Houston

Shapiro, William R. MD (N) - *Spec Exp:* Neuro-Oncology; **Hospital:** St Joseph's Hosp & Med Ctr - Phoenix; **Address:** Barrow Neurology Clinics, 500 W Thomas Rd, Ste 300, Phoenix, AZ 85013; **Phone:** (602) 406-6262; **Board Cert:** Neurology 1969; **Med School:** UCSF 1961; **Resid:** Internal Medicine, Univ Wash osp, Seattle, WA 1962-1963; Neurology, Ny Hosp-Cornell Med Ctr, New York, NY 1963-1966; **Fellow:** Neurological Oncology, National Inst Hlth, Bethesda, MD 1966-1969; **Fac Appt:** Prof Neurology, Univ Ariz Coll Med

Sherman, David MD (N) - *Spec Exp:* Cerebrovascular Disease; Stroke; **Hospital:** Univ of Texas Hlth & Sci Ctr; **Address:** Univ TX Hlth Scis Ctr, Dept Med, 7703 Floyd Curl Dr, San Antonio, TX 78229-3900; **Phone:** (210) 617-5161; **Board Cert:** Neurology 1976; **Med School:** Univ Okla Coll Med 1967; **Resid:** Internal Medicine, Baylor Affil Hosp, Houston, TX 1968-1969; Neurology, UCSD Med Ctr, San Diego, CA 1971-1974; **Fac Appt:** Prof Neurology, Univ Tex, San Antonio

Weisberg, Leon MD (N) - *Spec Exp:* Stroke; **Hospital:** Tulane Univ Med Ctr Hosp & Clinic; **Address:** Tulane Medical Center, 1415 Tulane Ave, New Orleans, LA 70112-2605; **Phone:** (504) 588-5231; **Board Cert:** Neurology 1975; **Med School:** Columbia P&S 1968; **Resid:** Neurology, New York Hosp, New York, NY 1969-1972

Wolinsky, Jerry MD (N) - *Spec Exp:* Multiple Sclerosis; **Hospital:** Meml Hermann Hosp; **Address:** Univ Texas Med Sch, 6431 Fannin St, Ste 7044, Houston, TX 77030; **Phone:** (713) 500-7135; **Board Cert:** Neurology 1975; **Med School:** Univ IL Coll Med 1969; **Resid:** Neurology, UCSF MED cTR, San Francisco, CA 1970-1973; **Fellow:** Neuropathology, VA Hosp, San Francisco, CA 1973-1975; **Fac Appt:** Prof Neurology, Univ Tex, Houston

453

West Coast and Pacific

Adornato, Bruce T. MD (N) - *Spec Exp:* Sleep Disorders/Apnea; Neuropathy; Stroke; **Hospital:** Stanford Med Ctr; **Address:** 1101 Welch Rd, Ste C5, Palo Alto, CA 94304; **Phone:** (650) 324-4300; **Board Cert:** Internal Medicine 1975, Neurology 1978; **Med School:** UCSD 1972; **Resid:** Internal Medicine, UCSF-Moffitt Hosp, San Francisco, CA 1973-1974; Neurology, UCSF-Moffitt Hosp, San Francisco, CA 1974-1976; **Fellow:** Neurology, Natl Inst Hlth, Bethesda, MD 1976-1978; **Fac Appt:** Clin Prof Neurology, Stanford Univ

Albers, Gregory William MD (N) - *Spec Exp:* Cerebrovascular Disease; Stroke; **Hospital:** Stanford Med Ctr; **Address:** Stanford Stroke Ctr, 701 Welch Rd, Ste 325, Palo Alto, CA 94304-1702; **Phone:** (650) 723-4448; **Board Cert:** Neurology 1990; **Med School:** UCSD 1984; **Resid:** Neurology, Standford Univ Med Ctr, Stanford, CA 1984-1988; **Fellow:** Stroke, Standford Univ Med Ctr, Stanford, CA 1988-1989; **Fac Appt:** Assoc Prof Neurology, Stanford Univ

Aminoff, Michael J MD (N) - *Spec Exp:* Movement Disorders; Parkinson's Disease; Clinical Neurophysiology; **Hospital:** UCSF Med Ctr; **Address:** 505 Parnassus Ave, Fl 3 - rm M348, San Francisco, CA 94143; **Phone:** (415) 353-1986; **Board Cert:** Neurology 1982, Clinical Neurophysiology 1992; **Med School:** England 1965; **Resid:** Neurology, Middlesex Hosp, London, England 1970-1971; Neurology, Natl Hosp Queen Sq, London, England 1971-1972; **Fac Appt:** Prof Neurology, UCSF

Armon, Carmel MD (N) - *Spec Exp:* Epilepsy/Seizure Disorders; Amyotrophic Lateral Sclerosis(ALS); **Hospital:** Loma Linda Univ Behav Med Ctr - Redlands; **Address:** 11370 Anderson St, Ste 2400, Loma Linda, CA 92354; **Phone:** (909) 558-2037; **Board Cert:** Neurology 1990, Clinical Neurophysiology 1992; **Med School:** Israel 1980; **Resid:** Neurology, Mayo Clinic, Rochester, MN 1984-1988; **Fellow:** Neurology, Mayo Clinic, Rochester, MN 1988-1989; Clinical Neurophysiology, Duke Univ Med Ctr, Durham, NC 1989-1991; **Fac Appt:** Assoc Prof Neurology, Loma Linda Univ

Bourdette, Dennis MD (N) - *Spec Exp:* Multiple Sclerosis; **Hospital:** OR Hlth Sci Univ Hosp and Clinics; **Address:** Oregon Health Science U Hosp, 3181 Sam Javkson Park Rd, Portland, OR 97201; **Phone:** (503) 494-5759; **Board Cert:** Neurology 1985; **Med School:** UC Davis 1978; **Resid:** Neurology, Oregon Hlth Sci U, Portland, OR 1979-1982; **Fellow:** Neurological Immunology, VA Med Ctr, Portland, OR 1982-1985; **Fac Appt:** Assoc Prof Neurology, Oregon Hlth Scis Univ

Bowen, James MD (N) - *Spec Exp:* Multiple Sclerosis; **Hospital:** Univ WA Med Ctr; **Address:** UWMC - Neurology Clinic, 1959 NE Pacific St, Seattle, WA 98195-0001; **Phone:** (206) 598-3344; **Board Cert:** Neurology 1990; **Med School:** Johns Hopkins Univ 1982; **Resid:** Internal Medicine, Univ Washington Med Ctr, Seattle, WA 1983-1984; Neurology, Univ Washington Med Ctr, Seattle, WA 1984-1987; **Fac Appt:** Asst Prof Neurology, Univ Wash

Chui, Helena Chang MD (N) - *Spec Exp:* Stroke; Dementia/Alzheimer's; **Hospital:** Rancho Los Amigos Natl Rehab Ctr; **Address:** Rancho Los Amigos Med Ctr-JPI Building, 7601 E Imperial Hwy, Ste 3 - rm 3135, Downey, CA 90242; **Phone:** (562) 401-7713; **Board Cert:** Neurology 1984; **Med School:** Johns Hopkins Univ 1977; **Resid:** Neurology, Univ Iowa Med Ctr, Iowa City, IA 1979-1981; **Fellow:** Behavioral Neurology, Univ Iowa Med Ctr, Iowa City, IA 1978-1979; **Fac Appt:** Prof Neurology, USC Sch Med

Cloughesy, Timothy Francis MD (N) - *Spec Exp:* Neuro-Oncology; Seizure Disorders; **Hospital:** UCLA Med Ctr; **Address:** UCLA Neurological Services, 300 UCLA Medical Plaza, Ste B200, Los Angeles, CA 90095; **Phone:** (310) 825-5321; **Board Cert:** Neurology 1993; **Med School:** Tulane Univ 1987; **Resid:** Neurology, UCLA Med Ctr, Los Angeles, CA 1986-1991; **Fellow:** Neurological Oncology, Meml Sloan-Kettering Canc Ctr, New York, NY 1992; **Fac Appt:** Asst Clin Prof Neurology, UCLA

454

Cummings, Jeffrey Lee MD (N) - *Spec Exp:* Neuro-Psychiatry; Parkinson's Disease; **Hospital:** UCLA Med Ctr; **Address:** 710 Westwood Plaza, rm 2-232, Los Angeles, CA 90095; **Phone:** (310) 206-5238; **Board Cert:** Neurology 1979; **Med School:** Univ Wash 1974; **Resid:** Neurology, Boston, MA 1975-1978; **Fellow:** Behavioral Neurology and Psychiatry, Boston, MA 1978-1979; **Fac Appt:** Assoc Prof Neurology, UCLA

De Giorgio, Christopher M MD (N) - *Spec Exp:* Neurology - General; **Hospital:** LAC - Olive View - UCLA Med Ctr; **Address:** Olive View Med Ctr, 14445 Olive View Drive, Sylmar, CA 91342; **Phone:** (818) 364-3104; **Board Cert:** Neurology 1987; **Med School:** Loyola Univ-Stritch Sch Med 1981

Dobkin, Bruce H MD (N) - *Spec Exp:* Stroke; Spinal Cord Injury; Neurologic Rehabilitation; **Hospital:** UCLA Med Ctr; **Address:** UCLA-RNRC, Dept Neuro, 710 Westwood Plaza, Ste 1129, Los Angeles, CA 90095-1769; **Phone:** (310) 206-6500; **Board Cert:** Neurology 1979; **Med School:** Temple Univ 1973; **Resid:** Neurology, UCLA Med Ctr, Los Angeles, CA 1973-1977; **Fac Appt:** Prof Neurology, UCLA

Engel, William King MD (N) - *Spec Exp:* Neurology - General; **Hospital:** Good Samaritan Hosp - Los Angeles; **Address:** 637 S Lucas Ave, Los Angeles, CA 90017; **Phone:** (213) 743-1612; **Board Cert:** Neurology 1962; **Med School:** McGill Univ 1955; **Resid:** Neurology, Natl Inst Hlth, Bethesda, MD 1956-1959; Neurology, Natl Hosp, London, England 1959-1960; **Fellow:** Neurology, Natl Inst Hlth, Bethesda, MD 1960-1961; **Fac Appt:** Prof Neuropathology, USC Sch Med

Engstrom, John Walter MD (N) - *Spec Exp:* Spinal Deformities; **Hospital:** UCSF Med Ctr; **Address:** UCSF, Dept of Neurology, 400 Parnassus Ave, Bldg ACC - Fl 8 - rm A887, Box 0348, MC-0348, San Francisco, CA 94143-0348; **Phone:** (415) 353-2273; **Board Cert:** Neurology 1991, Clinical Neurophysiology 1992; **Med School:** Stanford Univ 1981; **Resid:** Internal Medicine, Johns Hopkins, Baltimore, MD 1981-1984; Neurology, UCSF, San Francisco, CA 1984-1988; **Fellow:** Neurology, UCSF, San Francisco, CA 1988-1989; **Fac Appt:** Assoc Prof Neurology, UCSF

Fisher, Mark MD (N) - *Spec Exp:* Stroke; Cerebrovascular Disease; **Hospital:** UCI Med Ctr; **Address:** UC Irvine Med Ctr, Dept Neur, 101 The City Drive S Bldg S5 - rm 121, Orange, CA 92868; **Phone:** (714) 456-6808; **Board Cert:** Neurology 1981; **Med School:** Univ Cincinnati 1975; **Resid:** Neurology, UCLA-Wadsworth VA Hosp, Los Angeles, CA 1976-1979; **Fellow:** Neurology, UCLA-Wadsworth VA Hosp, Los Angeles, CA 1979-1980; **Fac Appt:** Prof Neurology, UC Irvine

Fisher, Robert MD (N) - *Spec Exp:* Epilepsy/Seizure Disorders; **Hospital:** Stanford Med Ctr; **Address:** 300 Pasteur Drive, rm A-343, Stanford, CA 94305-5235; **Phone:** (650) 498-3056; **Board Cert:** Clinical Neurophysiology 1992, Neurology 1983; **Med School:** Stanford Univ 1977; **Resid:** Internal Medicine, Stanford Univ, Stanford, CA 1977-1979; Neurology, Johns Hopkins, Baltimore, MD 1979-1982

Goodin, Douglas MD (N) - *Spec Exp:* Multiple Sclerosis; **Hospital:** UCSF Med Ctr; **Address:** 350 Parnassus Ave, Ste 908, San Francisco, CA 94117; **Phone:** (415) 514-1684; **Board Cert:** Clinical Neurophysiology 1992, Neurology 1985; **Med School:** UC Irvine 1978; **Resid:** Neurology, U Calif Hosps, San Francisco, CA 1979-1981; **Fac Appt:** Assoc Prof Neurology, UCSF

Graves, Michael Clark MD (N) - *Spec Exp:* Amyotrophic Lateral Sclerosis(ALS); **Hospital:** UCLA Med Ctr; **Address:** 300 Medical Plaza, Ste B200, Los Angeles, CA 90095; **Phone:** (310) 825-7266; **Board Cert:** Neurology 1977; **Med School:** Stanford Univ 1970; **Resid:** Internal Medicine, UC San Diego, San Diego, CA 1971-1972; Neurology, Johns Hopkins Hosp, Baltimore, MD 1972-1975; **Fellow:** Rockefeller Univ Hosp, New York, NY; **Fac Appt:** Assoc Prof Neurology, UCLA

Gress, Daryl Ray MD (N) - Spec Exp: *Critical Care; Stroke; Pain-Back;* **Hospital:** UCSF Med Ctr; **Address:** 505 Parnassus Ave, Ste M830, Box 0114, San Francisco, CA 94143-0348; **Phone:** (415) 353-1489; **Board Cert:** Neurology 1989; **Med School:** Washington Univ, St Louis 1982; **Resid:** Internal Medicine, Johns Hopkins Hosp, Baltimore, MD 1983-1984; Neurology, Mass Genl Hosp, Boston, MA 1984-1987; **Fellow:** Neurological Surgery, Mass Genl Hosp, Boston, MA 1987-1988; **Fac Appt:** Assoc Prof Neurology, UCSF

Hauser, Stephen Lawrence MD (N) - Spec Exp: *Multiple Sclerosis;* **Hospital:** UCSF - Mount Zion Med Ctr; **Address:** 350 Parnassus Ave, Ste 908, San Francisco, CA 94117; **Phone:** (415) 514-1684; **Board Cert:** Neurology 1981; **Med School:** Harvard Med Sch 1975; **Resid:** Neurology, Mass Genl Hosp, Boston, MA 1977-1980; Internal Medicine, NY Presby - Cornell, New York, NY 1976-1977; **Fellow:** Neurology, Harvard, Boston, MA 1977-1980; **Fac Appt:** Prof Neurology, UCSF

Langston, J William MD (N) - Spec Exp: *Parkinson's Disease; Movement Disorders; Tremor;* **Hospital:** Parkinson's Inst/Movement Disorders Treatmt Ctr; **Address:** The Parkinsons Institute, 1170 Morse Ave, Sunnyvale, CA 94089; **Phone:** (408) 734-2800; **Board Cert:** Neurology 1986; **Med School:** Univ MO-Kansas City 1967; **Resid:** Neurology, Stanford Univ, Stanford, CA 1971-1974; **Fellow:** Neurological Muscular Disease, Stanford Univ, Stanford, CA 1974

Nutt Jr, John G. MD (N) - Spec Exp: *Movement Disorders; Parkinson's Disease;* **Hospital:** OR Hlth Sci Univ Hosp and Clinics; **Address:** MC OP-32, 3181 SW Sam Jackson Park Rd, Portland, OR 97201; **Phone:** (503) 494-7772; **Board Cert:** Neurology 1978; **Med School:** Baylor Coll Med 1970; **Resid:** Neurology, Univ Wash, Seattle, WA 1973-1976; **Fellow:** Pharmacology, Nuero Inst Neuro Disorders Stroke, Bethesda, MD 1976-1978; **Fac Appt:** Prof Neurology, Oregon Hlth Scis Univ

Olney, Richard Koch MD (N) - Spec Exp: *Amyotrophic Lateral Sclerosis(ALS); Peripheral Neuropathy;* **Hospital:** UCSF Med Ctr; **Address:** UCSF Medical Ctr, Dept Neurology, 350 Parnassus Ave, Ste 500, San Francisco, CA 94117; **Phone:** (415) 476-7581; **Board Cert:** Neurology 1980, Clinical Neurophysiology 1994; **Med School:** Baylor Coll Med 1973; **Resid:** Psychiatry, UCLA, Los Angeles, CA 1974-1976; Neurology, Oregon Hlth Scis Univ, Portland, OR 1976-1979; **Fac Appt:** Prof Neurology, UCSF

Seybold, Marjorie MD (N) - Spec Exp: *Myasthenia Gravis; Neuromuscular Disorders; Neuro-Ophthalmology;* **Hospital:** VA San Diego Hlthcre Sys; **Address:** 3350 La Jolla Village Dr., Ste 127 Neurology, San Diego, CA 92161-0002; **Phone:** (858) 552-8585; **Board Cert:** Neurology 1971; **Med School:** Temple Univ 1965; **Resid:** Neurology, Mayo Grad School, Rochester, MN 1966-1969; **Fellow:** Neurological Ophthalmology, Johns Hopkins Hosp, Baltimore, MD 1970-1971

Shults, Clifford Walter MD (N) - Spec Exp: *Parkinson's Disease; Movement Disorders;* **Hospital:** UCSD Healthcare; **Address:** VA Med Ctr, MC 127, 3350 La Jolla Vlg Drive, San Diego, CA 92161; **Phone:** (858) 552-8585; **Board Cert:** Neurology 1985; **Med School:** Univ Tenn Coll Med, Memphis 1977; **Resid:** Internal Medicine, Univ Calif Med Ctr, San Francisco, CA 1977-1979; Neurology, Albert Einstein Coll Med, Bronx, NY 1979-1982; **Fellow:** Movement Disorders, Natl Inst Hlth, Bethesda, MD 1982-1985; **Fac Appt:** Prof Neurology, UCSD

Smith, Wade S MD/PhD (N) - Spec Exp: *Stroke; Pain-Back & Shoulder;* **Hospital:** UCSF Med Ctr; **Address:** UCSF, Dept Neurology, 505 Parnassus Ave, Box 0114, San Francisco, CA 94143; **Phone:** (415) 353-1489; **Board Cert:** Neurology 1996; **Med School:** Univ Wash 1989; **Resid:** Neurology, UCSF-Moffitt Hosp, San Francisco, CA 1990-1993; **Fellow:** Critical Care Medicine, UCSF-Moffitt Hosp, San Francisco, CA 1993-1994; **Fac Appt:** Asst Clin Prof Neurology, UCSF

Spence, Alexander Morton MD (N) - *Spec Exp:* Neuro-Oncology; **Hospital:** Univ WA Med Ctr; **Address:** Univ Wash, Dept Neur, 1959 NE Pacific St, MS 356465, Seattle, WA 98195-0001; **Phone:** (206) 543-2342; **Board Cert:** Neurology 1971; **Med School:** Univ Chicago-Pritzker Sch Med 1965; **Resid:** Neurology, Chldns Hosp, Boston, MA 1966-1969; Neuropathology, Stanford Univ Med Ctr, Standford, CA 1971-1974; **Fac Appt:** Prof Neurology, Univ Wash

Tanner, Caroline M MD/PhD (N) - *Spec Exp:* Parkinson's Disease; Movement Disorders; Dystonia; **Hospital:** Parkinson's Inst/Movement Disorders Treatmt Ctr; **Address:** The Parkinsons Institute, 1170 Morse Ave, Sunnyvale, CA 94089; **Phone:** (408) 734-2800; **Board Cert:** Neurology 1982; **Med School:** Loyola Univ-Stritch Sch Med 1976; **Resid:** Neurology, Rush-Presby-St Luke's Med Ctr, Chicago, IL 1977-1980; **Fellow:** Neurological Pharmacology, Rush-Presby-St Luke's Med Ctr, Chicago, IL 1980-1982

Tetrud, James W MD (N) - *Spec Exp:* Movement Disorders; Parkinson's Disease; Tremor; **Hospital:** Parkinson's Inst/Movement Disorders Treatmt Ctr; **Address:** 1170 Morse Ave, Sunnyvale, CA 94089; **Phone:** (408) 734-2800; **Board Cert:** Neurology 1981; **Med School:** NYU Sch Med 1973; **Resid:** Internal Medicine, Vet Affairs Med Ctr-West Los Angeles, Los Angeles, CA 1973-1974; Neurology, Vet Affairs Med Ctr-West Los Angeles, Los Angeles, CA 1974-1978

Vijayan, Nazhivath MD (N) - *Spec Exp:* Headache; **Hospital:** Univ CA - Davis Med Ctr; **Address:** UC Davis Med Ctr, Neurosciences Clinic-ACC, 4860 Y St, Ste 0100, Sacramento, CA 95817; **Phone:** (916) 734-3588; **Board Cert:** Neurology 1974; **Med School:** India 1964; **Resid:** Internal Medicine, Trivandrum Med Coll, India 1965-1967; Neurology, UC Davis Med Ctr, Sacramento, CA 1968-1971; **Fac Appt:** Prof Neurology, UC Davis

Weiner, Leslie P MD (N) - *Spec Exp:* Multiple Sclerosis; Amyotrophic Lateral Sclerosis(ALS); **Hospital:** USC Univ Hosp - R K Eamer Med Plz; **Address:** USC Hlthcare Consultation Ctr Dept Neur, 1975 Zonal Ave Bldg KAM - rm 410, Los Angeles, CA 90033; **Phone:** (323) 442-3020; **Board Cert:** Neurology 1969; **Med School:** Univ Cincinnati 1961; **Resid:** Neurology, Baltimore City Hosp, Baltimore, MD 1962-1963; Neurology, Johns Hopkins Hosp, Baltimore, MD 1963-1965; **Fellow:** Neurology, Johns Hopkins Univ, Baltimore, MD 1967-1969; **Fac Appt:** Prof Neurology, Univ SC Sch Med

NUCLEAR MEDICINE

A nuclear medicine specialist employs the properties of radioactive atoms and molecules in the diagnosis and treatment of disease, and in research. Radiation detection and imaging instrument systems are used to detect disease as it changes the function and metabolism of normal cells, tissues and organs. A wide variety of diseases can be found in this way, usually before the structure of the organ involved by the disease can be seen to be abnormal by any other techniques. Early detection of coronary artery disease (including acute heart attack); early cancer detection and evaluation of the effect of tumor treatment; diagnosis of infection and inflammation anywhere in the body; and early detection of blood clot in the lungs, are all possible with these techniques. Unique forms of radioactive molecules can attack and kill cancer cells (e.g., lymphoma, thyroid cancer) or can relieve the severe pain of cancer that has spread to bone.

The nuclear medicine specialist has special knowledge in the biologic effects of radiation exposure, the fundamentals of the physical sciences and the principles and operation of radiation detection and imaging instrumentation systems.

Training required: Three years

NYU Medical Center

550 First Avenue (at 31st Street)
New York, NY 10016
Physician Referral: (888) 7-NYU-MED
(888-769-8633) www.nyumedicalcenter.org

SCHOOL OF MEDICINE

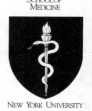

NEW YORK UNIVERSITY

NUCLEAR MEDICINE

Nuclear Medicine is an integral part of patient care, offering safe, painless, and cost-effective techniques to image the body and provides diagnosis, management, treatment, and prevention of disease.

The Division of Nuclear Medicine in the Department of Radiology at NYU Medical Center is an integral component of its world-renowned multidisciplinary care. Offering the latest in technological expertise to medical specialties from pediatrics to cardiology to oncology to psychiatry, nuclear medicine truly cuts across all fields to deliver life-saving diagnoses. There are nearly one hundred different nuclear medicine imaging procedures available, and not a major organ system which is not imaged by Positron Emission Tomography (PET) scans.

PET scans are simple imaging studies that allow physicians to view the metabolic function of various organs and tissues in the body. Patients receive a simple injection in the arm of radiolabeled sugar. One hour later patients lie on the imaging table of the scanner while images are taken.

NYU Medical Center houses some of the most advanced radiology equipment in the world, including remote-controlled digital fluoroscopy and advanced digital subtraction angiography with three-dimensional capabilities. There are six high-field, large bore Magnetic Resonance Imaging (MRI) units, an open MRI unit, 10 Computed Tomography (CT) units (seven of which are the latest spiral units) and one of the largest concentration of Single-Photon Emission Computed Tomography (SPECT) gamma cameras in the United States. Over 90% of the reports at Tisch Hospital are dictated directly into the radiology information system using computerized voice recognition technology.

NYU MEDICAL CENTER

The NYU Department of Radiology has a large and distinguished faculty. In a recent year, department members wrote 146 peer-reviewed scientific papers as well as 11 complete texts and 55 chapters for other academic texts. Among the faculty are officers of national and regional scientific and professional societies, members of selective societies, and frequent peer reviewers and editors of professional journals.

Physician Referral
(888) 7-NYU-MED
(888-769-8633)
www.nyumedicalcenter.org

Physician Listings

Nuclear Medicine

Mid Atlantic

Alavi, Abass MD (NuM) - *Spec Exp:* Brain Cancer; Pulmonary Imaging; **Hospital:** Hosp Univ Penn (page 78); **Address:** Univ of PA Med Ctr, Div of Nuclear Med, Donner Bldg, 3400 Spruce St, rm 110, Philadelphia, PA 19104; **Phone:** (215) 662-3014; **Board Cert:** Nuclear Medicine 1973, Internal Medicine 1972; **Med School:** Iran 1964; **Resid:** Internal Medicine, Albert Einstein Med Ctr, Philadelphia, PA 1967-1968; Hematology, Univ of PA Hlth Syst, Philadelphia, PA 1969-1970; **Fellow:** Nuclear Medicine, Hosp of Univ of PA, Philadelphia, PA 1971-1973; **Fac Appt:** Prof Radiology, Univ Penn

Carrasquillo, Jorge Amilcar MD (NuM) - *Spec Exp:* Nuclear Medicine - General; **Hospital:** Natl Inst of Hlth - Clin Ctr; **Address:** 9000 Rockville Pike #10, Bethesda, MD 20892-0001; **Phone:** (301) 496-5675; **Board Cert:** Nuclear Medicine 1982, Internal Medicine 1977; **Med School:** Univ Puerto Rico 1974; **Resid:** Internal Medicine, Univ Dist Hosp, San Juan, Puerto Rico 1976-1977; Nuclear Medicine, Univ Wash Hosp, Seattle, WA 1980-1982

Goldsmith, Stanley J MD (NuM) - *Spec Exp:* Thyroid Cancer; Neuroendocrine Disorders; PET Imaging; **Hospital:** NY Presby Hosp - NY Weill Cornell Med Ctr (page 70); **Address:** 520 E 70th St Bldg Starr - rm 221, New York, NY 10021-9800; **Phone:** (212) 746-4588; **Board Cert:** Endocrinology 1972, Nuclear Medicine 1972, Internal Medicine 1969; **Med School:** SUNY Downstate 1962; **Resid:** Internal Medicine, Kings Co Hosp, Brooklyn, NY 1965-1967; **Fellow:** Endocrinology, Diabetes & Metabolism, Mt Sinai Hosp, New York, NY 1967-1968; Nuclear Medicine, Bronx VA Hosp, Bronx, NY 1968-1969; **Fac Appt:** Prof Radiology, Cornell Univ-Weill Med Coll

Larson, Steven MD (NuM) - *Spec Exp:* Thyroid Cancer; PET Imaging; **Hospital:** Mem Sloan Kettering Cancer Ctr; **Address:** 1275 York Ave, Box 77, New York, NY 10021; **Phone:** (212) 639-7373; **Board Cert:** Nuclear Medicine 1972, Internal Medicine 1973; **Med School:** Univ Wash 1965; **Resid:** Internal Medicine, Virginia Mason Hosp, Seattle, WA 1968-1970; Nuclear Medicine, Natl Inst Hlth, Bethesda, MD 1970-1972; **Fac Appt:** Prof Nuclear Medicine, Cornell Univ-Weill Med Coll

Majd, Massoud MD (NuM) - *Spec Exp:* Nuclear Medicine-Pediatric; **Hospital:** Chldns Natl Med Ctr - DC; **Address:** 111 Michigan Ave NW, Washington, DC 20010-2916; **Phone:** (202) 884-5088; **Board Cert:** Radiology 1972, Nuclear Medicine 1973; **Med School:** Iran 1960; **Resid:** Radiology, Georgetown Hosp, Washington, DC 1962-1965; **Fac Appt:** Prof Radiology, Geo Wash Univ

Neumann, Ronald D MD (NuM) - *Spec Exp:* Nuclear Medicine - General; **Hospital:** Natl Inst of Hlth - Clin Ctr; **Address:** NIH/Clinical Ctr Fl 10, Box 1C-401, 10 Center Dr, MSC 1180, Bethesda, MD 20892-1180; **Phone:** (301) 496-6455; **Board Cert:** Nuclear Medicine 1979; **Med School:** Yale Univ 1974; **Resid:** Pathology, Yale-New Haven Hosp, New Haven, CT 1974-1977; Nuclear Medicine, Yale-New Haven Hosp, New Haven, CT 1977-1979

Strashun, Arnold M MD (NuM) - *Spec Exp:* Neurologic Imaging; Nuclear Cardiology; **Hospital:** Univ Hosp - Brklyn; **Address:** 450 Clarkson Ave Fl 2, Box 1210, Brooklyn, NY 11203; **Phone:** (718) 245-3692; **Board Cert:** Internal Medicine 1977, Nuclear Medicine 1979; **Med School:** Baylor Coll Med 1974; **Resid:** Internal Medicine, Baylor Med Ctr, Dallas, TX 1974-1975; Internal Medicine, Texas Med, Houston, TX 1975-1977; **Fellow:** Nuclear Medicine, VA Med Ctr, Bronx, NY; Nuclear Medicine, Mount Sinai Hosp, New York, NY; **Fac Appt:** Prof Radiology, SUNY Downstate

Van Heertum, Ronald Lanny MD (NuM) - *Spec Exp:* PET Imaging; SPECT Imaging; **Hospital:** NY Presby Hosp - Columbia Presby Med Ctr (page 70); **Address:** Dept of Radiology, 177 Fort Washington Ave, rm MHB2131, New York, NY 10032; **Phone:** (212) 305-7132; **Board Cert:** Radiology 1971, Nuclear Medicine 1973; **Med School:** UMDNJ-NJ Med Sch, Newark 1966; **Resid:** Radiology, St Vincents Hosp Med Ctr, New York, NY 1967-1970; **Fellow:** Neuroradiology, St Vincents Hosp Med Ctr, New York, NY 1970-1971; Nuclear Medicine, SUNY-Upstate Med Ctr, Syracuse, NY 1974-1975; **Fac Appt:** Prof Radiology, Columbia P&S

Wahl, Richard L MD (NuM) - *Spec Exp:* Radioimmunotherapy of Cancer; PET Imaging; **Hospital:** Johns Hopkins Hosp - Baltimore; **Address:** Johns Hopkins OPD Dept, Div Nuclear Medicine, 601 N Caroline St, rm 3223, Baltimore, MD 21287-0817; **Phone:** (410) 614-3764; **Board Cert:** Diagnostic Radiology 1982, Nuclear Radiology 1983, Nuclear Medicine 1985; **Med School:** Washington Univ, St Louis 1978; **Resid:** Diagnostic Radiology, Mallinckrodt Inst, St. Louis, MO 1979-1982; **Fellow:** Nuclear Radiology, Mallinckrodt Inst, St. Louis, MO 1982-1983; **Fac Appt:** Prof Radiology, Johns Hopkins Univ

Southeast

Alazraki, Naomi Parver MD (NuM) - *Spec Exp:* Nuclear Oncology; **Hospital:** VA Med Ctr - Atlanta; **Address:** VAMC Atlanta, 1670 Clairmont Rd, rm 115, Decatur, GA 30033; **Phone:** (404) 728-7629; **Board Cert:** Nuclear Medicine 1972, Diagnostic Radiology 1972; **Med School:** Albert Einstein Coll Med 1966; **Resid:** Radiology, Univ Hospital, San Diego, CA 1968-1971; **Fac Appt:** Prof Radiology, Emory Univ

Coleman, Ralph Edward MD (NuM) - *Spec Exp:* PET Imaging; Tumors; **Hospital:** Duke Univ Med Ctr (page 60); **Address:** Duke Univ Med Ctr, Erwin Rd, Box 3949, Durham, NC 27710; **Phone:** (919) 684-7244; **Board Cert:** Nuclear Medicine 1974, Internal Medicine 1973; **Med School:** Washington Univ, St Louis 1968; **Resid:** Internal Medicine, Royal Victoria, Montreal, Canada 1969-1970; **Fellow:** Nuclear Medicine, Mallinckrodt Institute of Radiology, St Louis, MO 1972-1974; **Fac Appt:** Prof Radiology, Duke Univ

Dubovsky, Eva V MD/PhD (NuM) - *Spec Exp:* Renal Nuclear Medicine; Thyroid Disease; **Hospital:** Univ of Ala Hosp at Birmingham; **Address:** Univ Ala Hosp, Div NuM, 619 19th St S, Birmingham, AL 35249; **Phone:** (205) 934-2140; **Board Cert:** Nuclear Medicine 1973; **Med School:** Czech Republic 1957; **Resid:** Internal Medicine, Univ Hosp-Charles Univ, Prague, Czech Republic 1957-1963; Nuclear Medicine, VA Med Ctr, Birmingham, AL 1970-1972; **Fellow:** Endocrinology, Diabetes & Metabolism, Univ Hosp-Charles Univ, Prague, Czech Republic 1963-1965; Endocrinology, Diabetes & Metabolism, Univ Hosp-Univ Ala Sch Med, Birmingham, AL 1968-1970; **Fac Appt:** Prof Radiology, Univ Ala

Partain, Clarence Leon MD (NuM) - *Spec Exp:* MRI; Nuclear Radiology; **Hospital:** Vanderbilt Univ Med Ctr (page 80); **Address:** Vanderbilt University Med Ctr, Dept Rad, Rm RR1223, MCN, Nashville, TN 37232-2675; **Phone:** (615) 343-3588; **Board Cert:** Nuclear Medicine 1979, Diagnostic Radiology 1980, Nuclear Radiology 1981; **Med School:** Washington Univ, St Louis 1975; **Resid:** Diagnostic Radiology, Univ North Carolina, Chapel Hill, NC 1975-1979; Nuclear Medicine, Univ North Carolina, Chapel Hill, NC 1975-1979; **Fac Appt:** Prof Radiology, Vanderbilt Univ

Sandler, Martin P MD (NuM) - *Spec Exp:* Nuclear Endocrinology; Cardiac Imaging; **Hospital:** Vanderbilt Univ Med Ctr (page 80); **Address:** Vanderbilt Univ Med Ctr, Dept Radiology, MCN, Nashville, TN 37232; **Phone:** (615) 343-3585; **Board Cert:** Nuclear Medicine 1983; **Med School:** South Africa 1972; **Resid:** Groote Schur Hosp, Cape Town, Johannesburg; **Fellow:** Endocrinology, Diabetes & Metabolism, Vanderbilt Univ, Nashville, TN; Nuclear Medicine, Vanderbilt Univ, Nashville, TN; **Fac Appt:** Prof Radiology, Vanderbilt Univ

Midwest

Siegel, Barry MD (NuM) - *Spec Exp:* Cancer Detection & Staging; PET Imaging; **Hospital:** Barnes-Jewish Hosp (page 55); **Address:** 510 S Kingshighway Blvd, West Pavilion, St Louis, MO 63110-1076; **Phone:** (314) 362-2809; **Board Cert:** Diagnostic Radiology 1977, Nuclear Medicine 1973; **Med School:** Washington Univ, St Louis 1969; **Resid:** Diagnostic Radiology, Mallinckrodt Inst of Rad, St Louis, MO 1970-1973; **Fellow:** Nuclear Medicine, Mallinckrodt Inst of Rad, St Louis, MO 1973; **Fac Appt:** Prof Radiology, Washington Univ, St Louis

Silberstein, Edward B. MD (NuM) - *Spec Exp:* Prostate Cancer Pain; Lymphoma; Thyroid Cancer; **Hospital:** Univ Hosp - Cincinnati; **Address:** Univ Hosp-Cincinnati, Mont Reid Pavilion, 234 Goodman Ave, rm G26, Cincinnati, OH 45219; **Phone:** (513) 584-9032; **Board Cert:** Internal Medicine 1980, Nuclear Medicine 1972, Hematology 1972, Medical Oncology 1981; **Med School:** Harvard Med Sch 1962; **Resid:** Internal Medicine, Univ Cincinnati Hospital, Cleveland, OH 1963-1967; **Fellow:** Hematology, New England Med Ctr, Boston, MA 1967-1968; **Fac Appt:** Prof Medicine, Univ Cincinnati

Southwest

Podoloff, Donald MD (NuM) - *Spec Exp:* Prostate Cancer; Breast Cancer; **Hospital:** Univ of TX MD Anderson Cancer Ctr, The; **Address:** UT MD Anderson Cancer Ctr, 1515 Holcombe Blvd, Box 83, Houston, TX 77030; **Phone:** (713) 745-1160; **Board Cert:** Internal Medicine 1969, Diagnostic Radiology 1973, Nuclear Medicine 1975, Nuclear Radiology 1975; **Med School:** SUNY Downstate 1964; **Resid:** Internal Medicine, Beth Israel Med Ctr, New York, NY 1965-1968; Radiology, Wilford Hall USAF Med Ctr, Lackland AFB, TX 1970-1973; **Fac Appt:** Prof Nuclear Radiology, Univ Tex, Houston

West Coast and Pacific

Scheff, Alice M MD (NuM) - *Spec Exp:* Breast Imaging; Thyroid Imaging; Neurologic Imaging; **Hospital:** Santa Clara Valley Med Ctr; **Address:** 751 S Bascom Ave, San Jose, CA 95128; **Phone:** (408) 885-6970; **Board Cert:** Nuclear Medicine 1982, Nuclear Radiology 1983; **Med School:** Penn State Univ-Hershey Med Ctr 1978; **Resid:** Diagnostic Radiology, Penn State-Hershey Med Ctr, Hershey, PA 1978-1982; Nuclear Medicine, Penn State-Hershey Med Ctr, Hershey, PA 1978-1982; **Fellow:** Magnetic Resonance Imaging, Long Beach Meml Med Ctr, Long Beach, CA 1993

Schelbert, Heinrich R MD/PhD (NuM) - *Spec Exp:* Cardiology; Clinical Medicine; **Hospital:** UCLA Med Ctr; **Address:** 23-148 CHS, Ste B2-085J, Box 956948, Los Angeles, CA 90095-1735; **Phone:** (310) 825-3076; **Board Cert:** Nuclear Medicine 1976; **Med School:** Germany 1964; **Resid:** Internal Medicine, Mercy Med Ctr, Philadelphia, PA 1967-1968; Cardiology (Cardiovascular Disease), Univ of Duesseldorf Sch of Med, Germany 1971-1972; **Fellow:** Nuclear Medicine, UC San Diego Sch of Med, San Diego, CA 1972-1973; Cardiology (Cardiovascular Disease), UC San Diego Sch of Med, San Diego, CA 1968-1969; **Fac Appt:** Prof Radiology, UCLA

Strauss, H William MD (NuM) - *Spec Exp:* Nuclear Medicine - General; **Hospital:** Stanford Med Ctr; **Address:** Stanford Univ Sch Med, Div Nuc Med, 300 Pasteur Drive, rm H-010, MS 5281, Stanford, CA 94305; **Phone:** (650) 725-7441; **Board Cert:** Nuclear Medicine 1972; **Med School:** SUNY Downstate 1965; **Resid:** Internal Medicine, Downstate Med Ctr, Brooklyn, NY 1966-1967; Internal Medicine, Bellevue Hosp, New York, NY 1967-1968; **Fellow:** Nuclear Medicine, Johns Hopkins Hosp, Baltimore, MD 1968-1970; **Fac Appt:** Prof Radiology, Stanford Univ

Waxman, Alan D MD (NuM) - *Spec Exp: PET Imaging-Brain; Thyroid Cancer; Cancer Detection & Staging;* **Hospital:** Cedars-Sinai Med Ctr; **Address:** Cedars-Sinai Med Ctr, 8700 Beverly Blvd, rm A041, Los Angeles, CA 90048-1804; **Phone:** (310) 423-4216; **Board Cert:** Nuclear Medicine 1972; **Med School:** USC Sch Med 1963; **Resid:** Nuclear Medicine, Wadsworth VA Hosp, Los Angeles, CA 1964-1965; **Fellow:** Internal Medicine, Natl Inst Hlth, Bethesda, MD 1965-1967; **Fac Appt:** Clin Prof Radiology, USC Sch Med

OBSTETRICS & GYNECOLOGY

An obstetrician/gynecologist possesses special knowledge, skills and professional capability in the medical and surgical care of the female reproductive system and associated disorders. This physician serves as a consultant to other physicians and as a primary physician for women.

Training required: Four years *plus* two years in clinical practice before certification is complete

NYU Medical Center

550 First Avenue (at 31st Street)
New York, NY 10016
Physician Referral: (888) 7-NYU-MED
(888-769-8633) www.nyumedicalcenter.org

SCHOOL OF
MEDICINE

NEW YORK UNIVERSITY

WOMEN'S HEALTH

NYU Medical Center supports a comprehensive group of programs and services designed specifically for women's medical needs. Services range from primary care to the most specialized clinical care programs available in the nation. Supported by the most sophisticated research and advanced training at NYU School of Medicine, the Department of Obstetrics and Gynecology at NYU Medical Center offers a unique, abundant blend of high quality therapies and regimens, as well as leading-edge research technologies and methods.

Along with routine gynecological care, many other services are offered including: pelvic ultrasound; aspiration of breast cysts; evaluation of infertility, including the special needs of same-sex couples; colposcopy (a diagnostic evaluation of abnormal pap smears); LEEP (a loop electrosurgical procedure used to diagnose and treat cervical cancer); cryotherapy for vaginal warts; and bone density testing for osteoporosis prevention and treatment.

The Obstetrics program also offers a broad range of services. Among these are prenatal care that gives equal emphasis to the well-being of the mother and of the fetus; fetal monitoring through ultrasound and other techniques; childbirth preparedness and breastfeeding classes; and consultation for high-risk pregnancies, including treatment for women who experience recurrent pregnancy loss.

At NYU Medical Center, the backbone of patient care is the continued research into gynecologic diseases. With world-class faculty leading clinical investigations into disorders that can occur at any stage of a woman's life, doctors at NYU Medical Center are equipped with the latest findings to treat women throughout their lives.

NYU MEDICAL CENTER

Women's Health at NYU Medical Center

- Obstetrics
- Gynecology
- Maternal-Fetal Medicine
- Gynecologic Oncology
- Reproductive Endocrinology and Infertility
- Reconstructive Pelvic Surgery and Urogynecology
- Endoscopic Pelvic Surgery and Family Planning
- Ultrasound Imaging
- Gynecological Pathology

Physician Referral
(888) 7-NYU-MED
(888-769-8633)
www.nyumedicalcenter.org

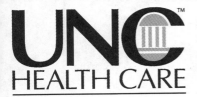

Department of Obstetrics and Gynecology
The University of North Carolina Health Care System
101 Manning Drive Chapel Hill, NC 27514

www.unchealthcare.org

CARING FOR WOMEN ... FOR LIFE

Under the leadership of Valerie Parisi, MD, MPH, the Department of Obstetrics and Gynecology at the University of North Carolina at Chapel Hill School of Medicine and UNC Hospitals is committed to providing comprehensive care to the women of North Carolina and beyond.

WOMEN'S WELLNESS

The department's clinical program, known as UNC Women's Wellness and Specialty Services, offers a continuous, coordinated and personalized approach to preventive and specialty care in both clinical practice and in health education.

WOMEN'S PRIMARY HEALTH CARE

Helping women achieve and maintain wellness is an important emphasis of the Women's Primary Health Care Division, which provides full screening and preventive care counseling. The availability of its nurse midwifery program underscores the department's commitment to a wellness perspective to women's health care.

WOMEN'S SPECIALTY SERVICES

Beyond these services, the department offers exemplary women's specialty services. These include comprehensive cancer care, diagnostic and treatment programs for infertility, evaluation and treatment of pelvic floor dysfunction/urinary incontinence and of chronic pelvic pain. The department's maternal-fetal specialists provide diagnosis and treatment of complicated pregnancies. In all of its activities, clinical care, cutting edge research and advocacy, the department embraces its motto, "Caring for Women . . . for Life."

To request an appointment, call (919) 966-7890.

MATERNAL & INFANT HEALTH

A particularly innovative program is the Center for Maternal and Infant Health. The center, a collaborative effort with the UNC Department of Pediatrics, is designed to help families whose pregnancies are complicated by birth defects. The center works to develop integrated, patient-centered plans for the diagnosis and treatment of birth defects; it features a care coordinator model to help parents understand their child's conditions and the various prenatal and infant care options. Visit the center's Web site at www.mombaby.org.

Physician Listings

Obstetrics & Gynecology

New England

Baker, Emily MD (ObG) - **Spec Exp:** *Maternal-Fetal Medicine; Obstetric Ultrasound;* **Hospital:** Dartmouth - Hitchcock Med Ctr; **Address:** One Medical Center Drive, Lebanaon, NH 03756; **Phone:** (603) 650-8370; **Board Cert:** Obstetrics & Gynecology 1993, Maternal & Fetal Medicine 1997; **Med School:** Stanford Univ **Resid:** Obstetrics & Gynecology, Univ of Chicago Hospitals, Chicago, IL 1986-1990; Maternal & Fetal Medicine, UUniv of Washington Med Ctr, Seattle, WA 1990-1991; **Fellow:** Maternal & Fetal Medicine, St. Margaret's Hosp - Tufts Univ, Boston, MA 1991-1992

Hunt, Robert Bridger MD (ObG) - **Spec Exp:** *Pelvic Reconstruction;* **Hospital:** New England Baptist; **Address:** 319 Longwood Ave, Boston, MA 02115-5728; **Phone:** (617) 731-6111; **Board Cert:** Obstetrics & Gynecology 1975; **Med School:** Med Univ SC 1964; **Resid:** Obstetrics & Gynecology, Brigham & Womens Hosp, Boston, MA 1969-1971; Surgery, Mary Imogene Bassett Hosp, Cooperstown, NY 1967-1968; **Fac Appt:** Asst Clin Prof Obstetrics & Gynecology, Harvard Med Sch

Jackson, Neil MD (ObG) - **Spec Exp:** *Uro-Gynecology;* **Hospital:** Women & Infants Hosp - Rhode Island; **Address:** Center for Womens Surg.-Dir. Uro-Gyn, 695 Eddy St, Providence, RI 02903; **Phone:** (401) 453-7560; **Board Cert:** Obstetrics & Gynecology 1972; **Med School:** Boston Univ 1962; **Resid:** Natl Naval Med Ctr, Bethesda, MD 1966-1969; **Fac Appt:** Clin Prof Obstetrics & Gynecology, Brown Univ

Naftolin, Frederick MD (ObG) - **Spec Exp:** *Neuro-Endocrinology; Reproductive Endocrinology; Menopause Problems;* **Hospital:** Yale - New Haven Hosp; **Address:** 20 York St, rm 335FMB, New Haven, CT 06504-8900; **Phone:** (203) 785-4003; **Board Cert:** Obstetrics & Gynecology 1972; **Med School:** UCSF 1961; **Resid:** Obstetrics & Gynecology, UCLA Med Ctr, Los Angeles, CA 1962-1966; **Fellow:** Reproductive Endocrinology, Univ Wash, Seattle, WA 1966-1968; Obstetrics & Gynecology, UCLA Med Ctr, Los Angeles, CA 1968-1970; **Fac Appt:** Prof Obstetrics & Gynecology, Yale Univ

Reilly, Raymond J MD (ObG) - **Spec Exp:** *Gynecologic Surgery;* **Hospital:** Brigham & Women's Hosp; **Address:** 1 Brookline Pkwy, Ste 522, Brookline, MA 02445; **Phone:** (617) 731-3400; **Board Cert:** Obstetrics & Gynecology 1969; **Med School:** Ireland 1958; **Resid:** Obstetrics & Gynecology, Johns Hopkins Hosp., Baltimore, MD 1962-1964; **Fac Appt:** Assoc Prof Obstetrics & Gynecology, Harvard Med Sch

Mid Atlantic

Amstey, Marvin S. MD (ObG) - **Spec Exp:** *Infectious Disease; Vulva Disease/Neoplasia;* **Hospital:** Via Hlth Sys-Genesee Hosp; **Address:** 220 Alexander St, Ste 604, Rochester, NY 14607; **Phone:** (716) 232-1069; **Board Cert:** Obstetrics & Gynecology 1989; **Med School:** Duke Univ 1964; **Resid:** Obstetrics & Gynecology, Strong Meml Hosp, Rochester, NY 1967-1971; **Fellow:** Virology, Natl Inst Hlth, Bethesda, MD 1965-1967; **Fac Appt:** Prof Obstetrics & Gynecology, Univ Rochester

Baxi, Laxmi V MD (ObG) - **Spec Exp:** *Pregnancy-High Risk; Miscarriage-Recurrent; Multiple Gestation;* **Hospital:** NY Presby Hosp - Columbia Presby Med Ctr (page 70); **Address:** Columbia Presby Med Ctr, Dept OB/GYN, 161 Ft Washington Ave, Fl 3 - Ste 336, New York, NY 10032-3713; **Phone:** (212) 305-5899; **Board Cert:** Obstetrics & Gynecology 1995, Maternal & Fetal Medicine 1997; **Med School:** India 1962; **Resid:** Obstetrics & Gynecology, King Edward M. Hosp, Bombay, India 1963-1969; Obstetrics & Gynecology, St Peter's Med Ctr-Rutgers Univ NJ, New Brunswick, NJ 1976-1977; **Fellow:** Maternal & Fetal Medicine, Columbia-Presbyterian Med Ctr, New York, NY 1977-1979; **Fac Appt:** Prof Obstetrics & Gynecology, Columbia P&S

Berkowitz, Richard MD (ObG) - *Spec Exp:* Obstetrics & Gynecology - General; **Hospital:** Mount Sinai Hosp (page 68); **Address:** 5 E 98th St, Fl 2, New York, NY 10029; **Phone:** (212) 241-5681; **Board Cert:** Obstetrics & Gynecology 1974, Maternal & Fetal Medicine 1979; **Med School:** NYU Sch Med 1965; **Resid:** Obstetrics & Gynecology, NY Hosp-Cornell Univ, New York, NY 1968-1972; **Fac Appt:** Prof Obstetrics & Gynecology, Mount Sinai Sch Med

Bieber, Eric J MD (ObG) - *Spec Exp:* Fibroids; Endoscopy; Infertility; **Hospital:** Geisinger Hlth Sys; **Address:** 100 N Academy Ave, Danville, PA 17822-2920; **Phone:** (570) 271-5620; **Board Cert:** Obstetrics & Gynecology 1994, Reproductive Endocrinology 1998; **Med School:** Loyola Univ-Stritch Sch Med 1986; **Resid:** Obstetrics & Gynecology, Rush Presby-St Lukes Med Ctr, Chicago, IL 1987-1990; **Fellow:** Reproductive Endocrinology, Univ Chicago, Chicago, IL 1990-1993

Boyce, John G MD (ObG) - *Spec Exp:* Gynecologic Cancer; **Hospital:** Univ Hosp - Brklyn; **Address:** 450 Clarkson Ave, Box 24, Brooklyn, NY 11203; **Phone:** (718) 270-2081; **Board Cert:** Obstetrics & Gynecology 1991, Gynecologic Oncology 1974; **Med School:** Univ British Columbia Fac Med 1962; **Resid:** Obstetrics & Gynecology, Kings Co Hosp, Brooklyn, NY 1963-1967; **Fellow:** Gynecologic Oncology, Kings Co Hosp, Brooklyn, NY 1967-1969; **Fac Appt:** Prof Obstetrics & Gynecology, SUNY Hlth Sci Ctr

Cundiff, Geoffrey Williams MD (ObG) - *Spec Exp:* Pelvic Reconstruction; Urogynecology; Endoscopy; **Hospital:** Johns Hopkins Hosp - Baltimore; **Address:** 600 N Wolfe, Bldg Harvey - rm 319, Baltimore, MD 21287; **Phone:** (410) 614-2870; **Board Cert:** Obstetrics & Gynecology 1996; **Med School:** Univ Tex SW, Dallas 1989; **Resid:** Obstetrics & Gynecology, Parkland Memorial Hospital/ Univ Tex SW Med Ctr, Dallas, TX 1990-1993; **Fellow:** Urogynecology, Greater Baltimore Med Ctr, Baltimore, MD 1993-1994; Reconstructive Pelvic Surgery, Duke Univ Med Ctr, Durham, NC 1994-1995; **Fac Appt:** Asst Prof Obstetrics & Gynecology, Johns Hopkins Univ

Divon, Michael Y MD (ObG) - *Spec Exp:* Maternal & Fetal Medicine; Pregnancy-High Risk; **Hospital:** Lenox Hill Hosp (page 64); **Address:** 130 E 77th St Fl 2 Black Hall, New York, NY 10021; **Phone:** (212) 434-2160; **Board Cert:** Obstetrics & Gynecology 1993; **Med School:** Israel 1982; **Resid:** Obstetrics & Gynecology, Rambam Med Ctr, Israel 1979-1983; **Fellow:** Perinatal Medicine, USC, Los Angeles, CA 1983-1985; Perinatal Medicine, Albert Einstein, Bronx, NY 1987-1989; **Fac Appt:** Clin Prof Maternal & Fetal Medicine, Albert Einstein Coll Med

Evans, Mark Ira MD (ObG) - *Spec Exp:* Reproductive Genetics; **Hospital:** Hahnemann Univ Hosp; **Address:** 245 N 15th St, MS 495, Philadelphia, PA 19102-1192; **Phone:** (215) 762-1720; **Board Cert:** Obstetrics & Gynecology 1999, Clinical Genetics 1984; **Med School:** SUNY Downstate 1978; **Resid:** Obstetrics & Gynecology, Lying-In Hosp/U Chicago, Chicago, IL 1979-1982; **Fellow:** Clinical Genetics, Natl Inst Hlth Bethesda, Bethesada, MD 1982-1984

Goldstein, Martin MD (ObG) - *Spec Exp:* Incontinence; Laparoscopic Hysterectomy; Laser Myomectomy; **Hospital:** Mount Sinai Hosp (page 68); **Address:** 40 E 84th St, New York, NY 10128-1314; **Phone:** (212) 472-6500; **Board Cert:** Obstetrics & Gynecology 1973; **Med School:** SUNY Hlth Sci Ctr 1966; **Resid:** Obstetrics & Gynecology, Mount Sinai, New York, NY 1967-1971; **Fac Appt:** Assoc Clin Prof Obstetrics & Gynecology, Mount Sinai Sch Med

Ledger, William MD (ObG) - *Spec Exp:* AIDS/HIV in Pregnancy; Infectious Disease; **Hospital:** NY Presby Hosp - NY Weill Cornell Med Ctr (page 70); **Address:** New York Weill Cornell Med Ctr, 525 E 68th St, Ste J130, New York, NY 10021; **Phone:** (212) 746-3009; **Board Cert:** Obstetrics & Gynecology 1967; **Med School:** Univ Penn 1958; **Resid:** Obstetrics & Gynecology, Temple Univ Hosp, Philadelphia, PA 1961-1964; **Fac Appt:** Prof Obstetrics & Gynecology, Cornell Univ-Weill Med Coll

Minkoff, Howard L MD (ObG) - *Spec Exp:* AIDS/HIV in Pregnancy; **Hospital:** Maimonides Med Ctr (page 65); **Address:** Maimonides Med Ctr, Dept Ob-Gyn, 4802 Tenth Ave, Brooklyn, NY 11219; **Phone:** (718) 283-7048; **Board Cert:** Obstetrics & Gynecology 1995, Maternal & Fetal Medicine 1983; **Med School:** Penn State Univ-Hershey Med Ctr 1975; **Resid:** Obstetrics & Gynecology, Kings Co Hosp Ctr, Brooklyn, NY 1976-1979; Obstetrics & Gynecology, SUNY Hlth Sci Ctr, Brooklyn, NY 1979-1981; **Fellow:** Maternal & Fetal Medicine, Kings Co Hosp Ctr, Brooklyn, NY 1979-1981; **Fac Appt:** Prof Obstetrics & Gynecology, SUNY Hlth Sci Ctr

Porges, Robert MD (ObG) - *Spec Exp:* Gynecologic Repair After Childbirth; Pelvic Organ Prolapse Repair; Laparoscopic Assist Vaginal Hysterectomy; **Hospital:** NYU Med Ctr (page 71); **Address:** 530 1st Ave, Ste 5H, New York, NY 10016-6402; **Phone:** (212) 263-6362; **Board Cert:** Obstetrics & Gynecology 1963; **Med School:** SUNY Downstate 1955; **Resid:** Obstetrics & Gynecology, Mount Sinai, New York, NY 1956-1957; Obstetrics & Gynecology, Bronx Muncipal Hosp, Bronx, NY 1957-1960; **Fac Appt:** Prof Obstetrics & Gynecology, NYU Sch Med

Sanz, Luis E MD (ObG) - *Spec Exp:* Uro-Gynecology; Hysteroscopic Surgery; Laparoscopic Surgery; **Hospital:** Georgetown Univ Hosp; **Address:** 5530 Wisconsin Ave, Ste 645, Chevy Chase, MD 20815; **Phone:** (301) 652-7679; **Board Cert:** Obstetrics & Gynecology 1982; **Med School:** Georgetown Univ 1976; **Resid:** Obstetrics & Gynecology, Georgetown Univ, Washington, DC 1977-1980; **Fellow:** Advanced Pelvic Surgery, Georgetown Univ, Washington, DC 1980-1982; **Fac Appt:** Prof Obstetrics & Gynecology, Georgetown Univ

Scialli, Anthony R MD (ObG) - *Spec Exp:* Reproductive Toxicology; Menopause Problems; Bone Densitometry; **Hospital:** Georgetown Univ Hosp; **Address:** 3800 Reservoir Rd NW, PHC Bldg-Fl 3, Washington, DC 20007; **Phone:** (202) 687-8531; **Board Cert:** Obstetrics & Gynecology 1981; **Med School:** Albany Med Coll 1975; **Resid:** Obstetrics & Gynecology, Geo Wash Univ Hosp, Washington, DC 1975-1979; **Fellow:** Reproductive Medicine, Repro Toxic Ctr, Washington, DC 1982-1984; **Fac Appt:** Prof Obstetrics & Gynecology, Georgetown Univ

Sweet, Richard Lance MD (ObG) - *Spec Exp:* Sexually Transmitted Diseases; **Hospital:** Magee Women's Hosp; **Address:** 300 Halket St Fl 2, Pittsburgh, PA 15213; **Phone:** (412) 641-4200; **Board Cert:** Obstetrics & Gynecology 1975; **Med School:** Univ Mich Med Sch 1966; **Resid:** Obstetrics & Gynecology, Univ Mich, Ann Arbor 1969-1973

Witter, Frank Robert MD (ObG) - *Spec Exp:* Pregnancy-High Risk; Multiple Gestation; **Hospital:** Johns Hopkins Hosp - Baltimore; **Address:** 601 N Caroline St Fl 8, Baltimore, MD 21287; **Phone:** (410) 955-6700; **Board Cert:** Maternal & Fetal Medicine 1987, Obstetrics & Gynecology 1985; **Med School:** Univ Chicago-Pritzker Sch Med 1976; **Resid:** Obstetrics & Gynecology, Johns Hopkins Hosp, Baltimore, MD 1977-1980; **Fellow:** Clinical Pharmacology, Johns Hopkins Hosp, Baltimore, MD 1982-1984; Maternal & Fetal Medicine, Johns Hopkins Hosp, Baltimore, MD 1980-1982; **Fac Appt:** Assoc Prof Obstetrics & Gynecology, Johns Hopkins Univ

Wylen, Michele MD (ObG) - *Spec Exp:* Gynecology-Adolescent; Menopause Problems; **Hospital:** Georgetown Univ Hosp; **Address:** 3800 Reservoir Rd NW, Washington, DC 20007; **Phone:** (202) 687-8531; **Board Cert:** Obstetrics & Gynecology 1999; **Med School:** Georgetown Univ 1988; **Resid:** Obstetrics & Gynecology, Georgetown Univ, Washington, DC 1990-1992

Young, Bruce MD (ObG) - *Spec Exp:* Fetal Minimally Invasive Surgery; Infertility; Miscarriage; **Hospital:** NYU Med Ctr (page 71); **Address:** 530 1st Ave, Ste 5G, New York, NY 10016; **Phone:** (212) 263-6359; **Board Cert:** Obstetrics & Gynecology 1970, Maternal & Fetal Medicine 1975; **Med School:** NYU Sch Med 1963; **Resid:** Obstetrics & Gynecology, New York Univ Med Ctr, New York, NY 1964-1968; **Fellow:** Reproductive Endocrinology, New York Univ Med Ctr, New York, NY 1968; **Fac Appt:** Prof Obstetrics & Gynecology, NYU Sch Med

Southeast

Duff, W Patrick MD (ObG) - *Spec Exp: Pregnancy-High Risk; Infectious Disease;* **Hospital:** Shands Hlthcre at Univ of FL (page 73); **Address:** 807 NW 57th St, Gainesville, FL 32605; **Phone:** (352) 392-6200; **Board Cert:** Obstetrics & Gynecology 1999, Maternal & Fetal Medicine 1999; **Med School:** Georgetown Univ 1974; **Resid:** Obstetrics & Gynecology, Walter Reed Med Ctr, Washington, DC 1974-1978; **Fellow:** Maternal & Fetal Medicine, UT - San Antonio, San Antonio, TX 1981-1983; **Fac Appt:** Prof Obstetrics & Gynecology, Univ S Fla Coll Med

Filip, Stanley John MD (ObG) - *Spec Exp: Obstetrics & Gynecology - General;* **Hospital:** Duke Univ Med Ctr (page 60); **Address:** Duke Univ Med Ctr, Dept Ob/Gyn, Box 3840, Durham, NC 27710; **Phone:** (919) 684-9696; **Board Cert:** Obstetrics & Gynecology 1985; **Med School:** Mount Sinai Sch Med 1979; **Resid:** Obstetrics & Gynecology, Univ Colo Hlth Scis Ctr, Denver, CO 1980-1983

Gluck, Paul MD (ObG) - *Spec Exp: Gynecology; Menopause Problems;* **Hospital:** Baptist Hosp - Miami; **Address:** 8950 N Kendall Dr, Ste 507, Miami, FL 33176-2132; **Phone:** (305) 279-3773; **Board Cert:** Obstetrics & Gynecology 1978; **Med School:** NYU Sch Med 1972; **Resid:** Obstetrics & Gynecology, Univ of Miami Jackson Meml Hosp, Miami, FL 1972-1976; **Fac Appt:** Assoc Clin Prof Obstetrics & Gynecology, Univ Miami Sch Med

Hager, William David MD (ObG) - *Spec Exp: Yeast Infection-Chronic; Salpingitis; Infectious Disease;* **Hospital:** Univ Kentucky Med Ctr; **Address:** Physicians for Women, 2620 Wilhite Drive, Lexington, KY 40503; **Phone:** (606) 278-0363; **Board Cert:** Obstetrics & Gynecology 1993; **Med School:** Univ KY Coll Med 1972; **Resid:** Obstetrics & Gynecology, Univ Kentucky Med Ctr, Lexington, KY 1976; **Fac Appt:** Prof Obstetrics & Gynecology, Univ KY Coll Med

McLeod, Allan G W MD (ObG) - *Spec Exp: Pelvic Reconstruction; Pelvic Prolapse Repair;* **Hospital:** Univ of Miami - Jackson Meml Hosp; **Address:** 1611 NW 12th Ave, Bldg Holtz - rm 7007, Miami, FL 33136; **Phone:** (305) 585-5160; **Board Cert:** Obstetrics & Gynecology 1981; **Med School:** Scotland 1952; **Resid:** Obstetrics & Gynecology, Western Hosp, Doncaster, England 1956-1957; Obstetrics & Gynecology, Southern Genl Hosp, Glasgow, Scotland 1957-1959; **Fac Appt:** Prof Obstetrics & Gynecology, Univ Miami Sch Med

Morgan, Linda S MD (ObG) - *Spec Exp: Gynecologic Cancer;* **Hospital:** Shands Hlthcre at Univ of FL (page 73); **Address:** 2000 SW Archer Rd, Women's Health Clinic PO Box 100294, Gainesville, FL 32610; **Phone:** (352) 392-2893; **Board Cert:** Obstetrics & Gynecology 1982, Gynecologic Oncology 1983; **Med School:** Med Coll PA Hahnemann 1975; **Resid:** Obstetrics & Gynecology, Shands Hosp, Gainesville, FL 1975-1979; **Fellow:** Gynecologic Oncology, Mass Genl Hosp, Boston, MA 1979-1981; **Fac Appt:** Prof Obstetrics & Gynecology, Univ Fla Coll Med

Nahmias, Jaime Pablo MD (ObG) - *Spec Exp: Reproductive Endocrinology; Infertility-Female;* **Hospital:** Univ of Miami & Clinics/Sylvestor Comp Cancer Ctr; **Address:** Univ of Miami Med Group, Dept of OB/GYN, 1611 NW 12th Ave Bldg Holtz - rm 7007, Maimi, FL 33136; **Phone:** (305) 585-5160; **Board Cert:** Obstetrics & Gynecology 1996; **Med School:** Chile 1978; **Resid:** Obstetrics & Gynecology, Jackson Meml Hosp Univ Miami, Miami, Fl 1986-1988; **Fellow:** Reproductive Endocrinology, Jackson Meml Hosp Univ Miami, Miami, Fl 1991-1994; **Fac Appt:** Asst Prof Obstetrics & Gynecology, Univ Miami Sch Med

Steege, John Francis MD (ObG) - *Spec Exp:* Laparoscopic Surgery (Advanced); Gynecologic Surgery-Benign; **Hospital:** Univ of NC Hosp (page 77); **Address:** Univ NC-Dept OB, Box MacNider 7570, Chapel Hill, NC 27599-7570; **Phone:** (919) 966-7764; **Board Cert:** Obstetrics & Gynecology 1978; **Med School:** Yale Univ 1972; **Resid:** Obstetrics & Gynecology, Yale - New Haven Hosp, New Haven, CT 1973-1976; **Fac Appt:** Prof Obstetrics & Gynecology, Univ NC Sch Med

Underwood, Paul MD (ObG) - *Spec Exp:* Pelvic Reconstructive Surg; Menopause; **Hospital:** Med Univ Hosp Authority; **Address:** 96 Jonathan Lucas St, Charleston, SC 29425; **Phone:** (843) 792-5300; **Board Cert:** Obstetrics & Gynecology 1967, Medical Oncology 1974; **Med School:** Med Univ SC 1959; **Resid:** Obstetrics & Gynecology, Medcial University of South Carolina, Charleston, SC; **Fellow:** Gynecologic Oncology, MD Anderson Tumor Institute, Houston, TX; **Fac Appt:** Prof Obstetrics & Gynecology, Med Univ SC

Midwest

Beer, Alan Earl MD (ObG) - *Spec Exp:* Infertility-Female; Reproductive Immunology; **Hospital:** Highland Park Hosp; **Address:** Chicago Medical School, 3333 Green Bay Rd, North Chicago, IL 60064; **Phone:** (847) 578-3233; **Board Cert:** Obstetrics & Gynecology 1971; **Med School:** Indiana Univ 1962; **Resid:** Obstetrics & Gynecology, U Penn Med Ctr, Philadelphia, PA 1965-1969; **Fellow:** Reproductive Immunology, U Penn Med Ctr, Philadelphia, PA 1968-1970; **Fac Appt:** Prof Obstetrics & Gynecology, Univ Chicago-Pritzker Sch Med

Elias, Sherman MD (ObG) - *Spec Exp:* Prenatal Diagnosis; **Hospital:** Univ of IL at Chicago Med Ctr; **Address:** 820 S Wood St, MC 808, Chicago, IL 60612; **Phone:** (312) 413-2040; **Board Cert:** Clinical Genetics 1982, Obstetrics & Gynecology 1996; **Med School:** Univ KY Coll Med 1976; **Resid:** Obstetrics & Gynecology, Michael Reese Hosp, Chicago, IL 1972-1973; Obstetrics & Gynecology, Univ Louisville, Louisville, KY 1973-1976; **Fellow:** Clinical Genetics, Yale, New Haven, CT 1974-1975; Clinical Genetics, Northwestern Univ, Chicigo, IL 1976-1978; **Fac Appt:** Prof Obstetrics & Gynecology, Univ IL Coll Med

Galask, Rudolph P. MD (ObG) - *Spec Exp:* Vulva Disease/Neoplasia; Infectious Disease; **Hospital:** Univ of IA Hosp and Clinics; **Address:** Dept Ob/Gyn, 200 Hawkins Drive Fl 2nd - rm BT-2004-E, Iowa City, IA 52242; **Phone:** (319) 353-6323; **Board Cert:** Obstetrics & Gynecology 1972; **Med School:** Univ Iowa Coll Med 1964; **Resid:** Obstetrics & Gynecology, Univ Iowa, Iowa City, IA 1967-1970

Gonik, Bernard MD (ObG) - *Spec Exp:* Maternal & Fetal Medicine; **Hospital:** Sinai-Grace Hosp - Detroit (page 59); **Address:** 6071 W Outer Drive, Detroit, MI 48235; **Phone:** (313) 966-1880; **Board Cert:** Obstetrics & Gynecology 1995, Maternal & Fetal Medicine 1987; **Med School:** Mich State Univ 1978; **Resid:** Obstetrics & Gynecology, Univ Texas Med Sch, Houston, TX 1978-1982; **Fellow:** Maternal & Fetal Medicine, Univ Texas Med Sch, Houston, TX 1982-1985; **Fac Appt:** Asst Prof Medicine, Univ Tex, Houston

Gonzalez-Loya, Juan MD (ObG) - *Spec Exp:* Obstetrics & Gynecology - General; **Hospital:** Loyola Univ Med Ctr; **Address:** 2511 S Pulaski Rd, Chicago, IL 60623-3732; **Phone:** (773) 522-3056; **Board Cert:** Obstetrics & Gynecology 1999; **Med School:** Mexico 1959; **Resid:** Internal Medicine, Metropolitan Hosp Ctr, New York, NY

Johnson, Timothy R.B. MD (ObG) - *Spec Exp: Fetal Assessment; Prenatal Diagnosis;* **Hospital:** Univ of MI Hlth Ctr; **Address:** Dept of Obstetrics & Gynecology, 1500 E Med Ctr Dr, rm L4000, Box 0276, Ann Arbor, MI 48109-0999; **Phone:** (734) 764-8123; **Board Cert:** Obstetrics & Gynecology 2001, Maternal & Fetal Medicine 2001; **Med School:** Univ VA Sch Med 1975; **Resid:** Obstetrics & Gynecology, Univ Michigan Med Ctr, Ann Arbor, MI 1976-1979; **Fellow:** Maternal & Fetal Medicine, Johns Hopkins Hosp, Baltimore, MD 1979-1981; **Fac Appt:** Prof Obstetrics & Gynecology, Univ Mich Med Sch

Levine, Elliot Mark MD (ObG) - *Spec Exp: Sexual Transmitted Disease; Sexual Dysfunction; Vulvar Problems;* **Hospital:** Advocate IL Masonic Med Ctr; **Address:** 3000 N Halsted St, Ste 209B, Chicago, IL 60657; **Phone:** (773) 296-3300; **Board Cert:** Obstetrics & Gynecology 1984; **Med School:** Univ Hlth Sci/Chicago Med Sch 1978; **Resid:** Obstetrics & Gynecology, Illinois Masonic Med Ctr, Chicago, IL 1978-1982; **Fac Appt:** Asst Prof Obstetrics & Gynecology, Rush Med Coll

Linn, Edward S MD (ObG) - *Spec Exp: Menopause Problems; Infectious Disease-Gynecologic; Contraception;* **Hospital:** Advocate Lutheran Gen Hosp; **Address:** Advocate Med Grp-Parkside Ctr, 1875 Dempster St, Ste 665, Park Ridge, IL 60068; **Phone:** (847) 825-1590; **Board Cert:** Obstetrics & Gynecology 1994; **Med School:** Univ Chicago-Pritzker Sch Med 1974; **Resid:** Obstetrics & Gynecology, Michael Reese Hosp, Chicago, IL 1974-1978

Merritt, Diane MD (ObG) - *Spec Exp: Gynecology-Adolescent; Gynecology-Pediatric; Endometriosis;* **Hospital:** Barnes-Jewish Hosp (page 55); **Address:** 2 Maternity, 4911 Barnes Jewish Plaza, Fl 2, St. Louis, MO 63110; **Phone:** (314) 747-1454; **Board Cert:** Obstetrics & Gynecology 1984; **Med School:** NYU Sch Med 1975; **Resid:** Obstetrics & Gynecology, Barnes Hospital University Washington, St. Louis, MO 1977-1980; Surgery, Barnes Hospital University Washington, St. Louis, MO 1976-1977; **Fac Appt:** Prof Obstetrics & Gynecology, Washington Univ, St Louis

Moawad, Atef H MD (ObG) - *Spec Exp: Pregnancy-High Risk; Premature Labor;* **Hospital:** Univ of Chicago Hosps (page 76); **Address:** 5841 S Maryland Ave, MC 2050, Chicago, IL 60637; **Phone:** (773) 702-5200; **Board Cert:** Obstetrics & Gynecology 2000; **Med School:** Egypt 1957; **Resid:** Obstetrics & Gynecology, Thomas Jefferson Univ Hosp, Philadelphia, PA 1961-1964; **Fellow:** Maternal & Fetal Medicine, Case Western Reserve, Cleveland, OH 1965-1966; Obstetrics & Gynecology, Univ Lund Hosps, Lund, Sweden 1966-1967; **Fac Appt:** Prof Obstetrics & Gynecology, Univ Chicago-Pritzker Sch Med

Muraskas, Erik MD (ObG) - *Spec Exp: Obstetrics & Gynecology - General;* **Hospital:** Loyola Univ Med Ctr; **Address:** 2160 S 1st Ave, Maywood, IL 60153; **Phone:** (708) 216-3816; **Board Cert:** Obstetrics & Gynecology 1990; **Med School:** Loyola Univ-Stritch Sch Med 1981; **Resid:** Obstetrics & Gynecology, Loyola U-Stritch Sch Med, Maywood, IL 1981-1985; **Fac Appt:** Asst Prof Obstetrics & Gynecology, Loyola Univ-Stritch Sch Med

Olive, David MD (ObG) - *Spec Exp: Infertility-IVF; Endometriosis;* **Hospital:** Univ WI Hosp & Clins; **Address:** Ob/Gyn Dept, H4-630-CSC Bldg, 600 Highland Ave, Madison, WI 53792-6188; **Phone:** (608) 263-1218; **Board Cert:** Obstetrics & Gynecology 1995, Reproductive Endocrinology 1995; **Med School:** Baylor Coll Med 1979; **Resid:** Obstetrics & Gynecology, Northwestern Univ Hosps, Chicago, IL 1980-1983; **Fellow:** Reproductive Endocrinology, Duke Univ Med Ctr, Durham, NC 1983-1985; **Fac Appt:** Prof Obstetrics & Gynecology, Univ Wisc

Sciarra, John J MD (ObG) - *Spec Exp: Gynecologic Surgery;* **Hospital:** Northwestern Meml Hosp; **Address:** Dept Ob/Gyn, 333 E Superior St, Chicago, IL 60611; **Phone:** (312) 926-7504; **Board Cert:** Obstetrics & Gynecology 1979; **Med School:** Columbia P&S 1957; **Resid:** Obstetrics & Gynecology, Columbia-Presby Hosp, New York, NY 1958-1964; **Fac Appt:** Prof Obstetrics & Gynecology, Northwestern Univ

Socol, Michael MD (ObG) - *Spec Exp:* Diabetes in Pregnancy; Multiple Gestation; Premature Labor; **Hospital:** Northwestern Meml Hosp; **Address:** Northwestern Univ Hosp, 333 E Superior St, Ste 410, Chicago, IL 60611-3056; **Phone:** (312) 695-7542; **Board Cert:** Obstetrics & Gynecology 1979, Maternal & Fetal Medicine 1981; **Med School:** Univ IL Coll Med 1974; **Resid:** Obstetrics & Gynecology, Univ Illinois Med Ctr, Chicago, IL 1974-1977; **Fellow:** Maternal & Fetal Medicine, USC Med Ctr, Los Angeles, CA 1977-1979; **Fac Appt:** Prof Obstetrics & Gynecology, Northwestern Univ

Tan, Merita R.C. MD (ObG) - *Spec Exp:* Menstrual Disorders; Laser Surgery; **Hospital:** Northwestern Meml Hosp; **Address:** 680 N Lake Shore Dr, Ste 1424, Chicago, IL 60611; **Phone:** (312) 482-8484; **Board Cert:** Obstetrics & Gynecology 1995; **Med School:** Univ Hlth Sci/Chicago Med Sch 1989; **Resid:** Obstetrics & Gynecology, Cook Co Hosp, Chicago, IL 1989-203

Toig, Randall MD (ObG) - *Spec Exp:* Pregnancy-Advanced Maternal Age; Osteoporosis; **Hospital:** Northwestern Meml Hosp; **Address:** Dept Ob/Gyn, 680 N Lake Shore Dr, Ste 830, Chicago, IL 60611; **Phone:** (312) 440-1600; **Board Cert:** Obstetrics & Gynecology 1985; **Med School:** Univ Pittsburgh 1977; **Resid:** Obstetrics & Gynecology, Northwestern Meml Hosp, Chicago, IL 1978-1982

Walters, Mark MD (ObG) - *Spec Exp:* Uro-Gynecology; Vaginal Reconstructive surgery; **Hospital:** Cleveland Clin Fdn (page 57); **Address:** 9500 Euclid Ave, rm A81, Cleveland, OH 44195; **Phone:** (216) 445-6586; **Board Cert:** Obstetrics & Gynecology 1996; **Med School:** Ohio State Univ 1980; **Resid:** Obstetrics & Gynecology, New England Med Ctr, Boston, MA 1980-1984

Great Plains and Mountains

Bury, Robert MD (ObG) - *Spec Exp:* Infertility; Laser Surgery; Microsurgery; **Hospital:** St. Alexius Med Ctr - Bismarck; **Address:** 401 N Ninth St, Bismarck, ND 58501; **Phone:** (701) 530-6000; **Board Cert:** Obstetrics & Gynecology 1981; **Med School:** Baylor Coll Med **Resid:** Obstetrics & Gynecology, Baylor Affil Hosp, Houston, TX 1975-1979; **Fac Appt:** Clin Prof Obstetrics & Gynecology, Univ ND Sch Med

Southwest

Carr, Bruce MD (ObG) - *Spec Exp:* Infertility-Female; **Hospital:** Zale Lipshy Univ Hosp; **Address:** 5323 Harry Hines Blvd, rm J6-114, Dallas, TX 75390-9032; **Phone:** (214) 648-2784; **Board Cert:** Obstetrics & Gynecology 1999, Reproductive Endocrinology 1999; **Med School:** Univ Mich Med Sch 1971; **Resid:** Obstetrics & Gynecology, Parkland Meml Hosp, Dallas, TX 1972-1975; **Fellow:** Reproductive Endocrinology, Univ Texas SW Med Ctr, Dallas, TX 1978-1980; **Fac Appt:** Prof Obstetrics & Gynecology, Univ Tex SW, Dallas

Faro, Sebastian MD/PhD (ObG) - *Spec Exp:* Infections in Pregnancy; Gynecologic Infections; Sexually Transmitted Diseases; **Hospital:** Woman's Hosp TX; **Address:** 7400 Fannin, Ste 1160, Houston, TX 77054; **Phone:** (713) 799-8994; **Board Cert:** Obstetrics & Gynecology 1991; **Med School:** Creighton Univ 1975; **Resid:** Obstetrics & Gynecology, Creighton Univ, Omaha, NE 1975-1978; **Fac Appt:** Clin Prof Obstetrics & Gynecology, Univ Tex, Houston

Simpson, Joe Leigh MD (ObG) - *Spec Exp:* Prenatal Diagnosis; Ovarian Failure-Recurrent; Spontaneous Abortion; **Hospital:** Methodist Hosp - Houston; **Address:** Baylor Coll Med, 6550 Fannin St, Ste 901, Houston, TX 77030-2717; **Phone:** (713) 798-8360; **Board Cert:** Obstetrics & Gynecology 1989, Clinical Genetics 1982; **Med School:** Duke Univ 1968; **Resid:** Obstetrics & Gynecology, New York Hosp, New York, NY 1969-1973; **Fac Appt:** Prof Obstetrics & Gynecology, Baylor Coll Med

Smith, Harriet Olivia MD (ObG) - *Spec Exp:* *Gynecologic Oncology;* **Hospital:** Univ NM Hosp; **Address:** 2211 Lomas NE, Albuquerque, NM 87106; **Phone:** (505) 272-4051; **Board Cert:** Obstetrics & Gynecology 1987, Gynecologic Oncology 1996; **Med School:** Med Coll GA 1980; **Resid:** Obstetrics & Gynecology, Medical College of Georgia, Augusta, GA 1982-1985; Gynecologic Oncology, MD Anderson Hospital, Houston, TX 1986; **Fellow:** Gynecologic Oncology, Albert Einstein College of Medicine, Bronx, NY 1993; Reconstructive Pelvic Surgery, Emory University Hospital, Atlanta, GA 1986; **Fac Appt:** Assoc Prof Obstetrics & Gynecology, Univ New Mexico

West Coast and Pacific

DeCherney, Alan Hersh MD (ObG) - *Spec Exp:* *Infertility-Female; Reproductive Endocrinology;* **Hospital:** UCLA Med Ctr; **Address:** 10833 Le Conte Ave, rm 27-117 CHS, Los Angeles, CA 90095; **Phone:** (310) 794-1884; **Board Cert:** Obstetrics & Gynecology 1989, Reproductive Endocrinology 1979; **Med School:** Temple Univ 1967; **Resid:** Obstetrics & Gynecology, Hosp Univ Penn, Philadelphia, PA 1968-1972

Eschenbach, David Arthur MD (ObG) - *Spec Exp:* *Gynecologic Surgery; Infectious Disease; Vaginal Disorders;* **Hospital:** Univ WA Med Ctr; **Address:** WHCC, 4245 Roosevelt Way NE, Seattle, WA 98105; **Phone:** (206) 543-2444; **Board Cert:** Obstetrics & Gynecology 1975; **Med School:** Univ Wisc 1968; **Resid:** Obstetrics & Gynecology, Univ Wash Hosp, Seattle, WA 1969-1973; **Fellow:** Infectious Disease, Univ Wash Hosp, Seattle, WA 1972-1974; **Fac Appt:** Prof Obstetrics & Gynecology, Univ Wash

Novy, Miles MD (ObG) - *Spec Exp:* *Transabdominal Cervical Cerclage (TCIC); Reproductive Endocrinology;* **Hospital:** OR Hlth Sci Univ Hosp and Clinics; **Address:** 1750 SW Harbor Way, Portland, OR 97201; **Phone:** (503) 418-3700; **Board Cert:** Maternal & Fetal Medicine 1975, Obstetrics & Gynecology 1972; **Med School:** Harvard Med Sch 1963; **Resid:** Obstetrics & Gynecology, Boston Hosp Women, Boston, MA 1964-1965; **Fellow:** Maternal & Fetal Medicine, Univ Oregon, Portland, OR 1965-1967; **Fac Appt:** Prof Obstetrics & Gynecology, Oregon Hlth Scis Univ

Platt, Lawrence David MD (ObG) - *Spec Exp:* *Maternal & Fetal Medicine; Ultrasound;* **Hospital:** Cedars-Sinai Med Ctr; **Address:** 8635 W 3rd St, Ste 160, Los Angeles, CA 90048; **Phone:** (310) 423-7433; **Board Cert:** Obstetrics & Gynecology 1979, Maternal & Fetal Medicine 1981; **Med School:** Wayne State Univ 1972; **Resid:** Obstetrics & Gynecology, Sinai Hosp, Detroit, MI 1973-1975; Obstetrics & Gynecology, Sinai Hosp, Detroit, MI 1975-1976; **Fellow:** Maternal & Fetal Medicine, USC Med Ctr, Los Angeles, CA 1976-1978

Ophthalmology

An ophthalmologist has the knowledge and professional skills needed to provide comprehensive eye and vision care. Ophthalmologists are medically trained to diagnose, monitor and medically or surgically treat all ocular and visual disorders. This includes problems affecting the eye and its component structures, the eyelids, the orbit and the visual pathways. In so doing, an ophthalmologist prescribes vision services, including glasses and contact lenses.

Training required: Four years

DEPARTMENT OF OPHTHALMOLOGY
THE NEW YORK EYE & EAR INFIRMARY

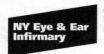

NY Eye & Ear Infirmary

Affiliated Teaching
Hospital of New York
Medical College

310 East 14th Street (corner Second Avenue)
New York, NY 10003
212-979-4000 • FAX: 212-228-0664
Physician Referral: 1-800-449-HOPE (4673)
website: www.nyee.edu

Continuum Health Partners, Inc.

PROVIDING EXCEPTIONAL EYE CARE

The Department of Ophthalmology is the region's most comprehensive center for the delivery of primary through tertiary eye care. It is also by far the largest provider of eye care in the metropolitan area – with some 82,000 outpatient visits and 14,000 surgical cases performed each year. More than 250 board certified ophthalmologists located throughout New York City and its tri-state area comprise the attending Medical Staff.

IN A HIGHLY SPECIALIZED SETTING

As a specialty hospital, the Infirmary is uniquely qualified to handle the most complicated cases. It serves as a nationwide referral center with a commitment to teaching, research, and high-technology based patient care. Computerized ocular imaging equipment including optical coherence tomography, corneal topography/modeling, and retinal tomography assist in the earliest and most accurate diagnosis of diseases such as glaucoma and macular degeneration. Highly experienced staff using state-of-the-art instrumentation have made the Infirmary's 17 operating rooms a national benchmark in efficiency in eye surgery cases.

FOR PATIENTS OF ALL AGES

Staff at the Infirmary are sensitive to the specific needs of patients of all ages, especially senior citizens – who comprise the vast majority of the Infirmary's 7,500 yearly cataract patients as well as individuals receiving treatment for age-related macular degeneration – and young children, now 25 percent of all patients treated here. For those rare cases of children who have a disease ordinarily associated with age, the Infirmary runs New York's only Pediatric Glaucoma Service. Active adults of all ages utilize the New York Eye Trauma Center and the Vision Correction Center.

While most of the 4,500 procedures performed each year in the Vision Center are LASIK, others include PRK, Intacs, and scleral expansion for presbyopia reversal. New wavefront measurement technology provides customized treatment and potential rehabilitation for patients with vision irregularities.

CLINICAL SERVICES

Ambulatory Care Services

Comprehensive Eye Care

Cornea & Refractive Surgery

Eye Trauma

Glaucoma

Low Vision

Neuro-Ophthalmology

Oculoplastic & Orbital Surgery

Ocular Tumor

Pediatric Ophthalmology & Strabismus

Retinal-Vitreal

Uveitis

FACILITIES

Ambulatory Surgery Center

Eye Trauma Center

Vision Correction Center

ABOUT THE NEW YORK EYE AND EAR INFIRMARY

Founded in 1820, it is the nation's oldest, continuously operating specialty hospital. More than 10 million people have sought treatment here since its inception.

Physician Listings

Ophthalmology

New England

Aiello, Lloyd MD (Oph) - *Spec Exp:* Diabetic Eye Disease/Retinopathy; **Hospital:** Beth Israel Deaconess Med Ctr - Boston; **Address:** Beetham Eye Inst-Joslin Diabetes Ctr, 1 Joslin Pl, Boston, MA 02215-5397; **Phone:** (617) 732-2520; **Board Cert:** Ophthalmology 1966; **Med School:** Boston Univ 1960; **Resid:** Ophthalmology, Mass Eye & Ear Inf, Boston, MA 1962-1964; **Fac Appt:** Assoc Clin Prof Ophthalmology, Harvard Med Sch

Foster, Charles Stephen MD (Oph) - *Spec Exp:* Uveitis; Corneal Disease; Cataract Surgery; **Hospital:** Mass Eye & Ear Infirmary; **Address:** 243 Charles St, Boston, MA 02114-3002; **Phone:** (617) 573-3591; **Board Cert:** Ophthalmology 1976; **Med School:** Duke Univ 1969; **Resid:** Ophthalmology, Wash Univ - Barnes Hosp, St Louis, MO 1972-1975; **Fellow:** Cornea, Mass EE Infirm - Harvard, Boston, MA 1975-1976; Ocular Immunology, Mass EE Infirm - Harvard, Boston, MA 1976-1977; **Fac Appt:** Prof Ophthalmology, Harvard Med Sch

Jakobiec, Frederick A. MD (Oph) - *Spec Exp:* Eye & Orbital Tumors/Cancer; Eyelid & Conjunctival Tumors; **Hospital:** Mass Eye & Ear Infirmary; **Address:** Mass EE Infirm-Chairman Oph., 243 Charles St, Boston, MA 02114-3002; **Phone:** (617) 573-3526; **Board Cert:** Ophthalmology 1975, Anatomic Pathology 1978; **Med School:** Harvard Med Sch 1971; **Resid:** Ophthalmology, Harkness Eye Inst, New York, NY 1969-1973; Pathology, Columbia P&S, New York, NY 1969-1973; **Fellow:** Columbia P&S, New York, NY 1969-1970

Mitchell, Paul Ralph MD (Oph) - *Spec Exp:* Ophthalmology-Pediatric; **Hospital:** Hartford Hosp; **Address:** 366 Colt Hwy, Farmington, CT 06032-2547; **Phone:** (860) 409-0449; **Board Cert:** Ophthalmology 1977; **Med School:** Geo Wash Univ 1970; **Resid:** Ophthalmology, Wills Eye Hosp, Philadelphia, PA 1973-1976; **Fellow:** Ophthalmology, Chldns Hosp MC/Geo Wash, Washington, DC 1976-1977; **Fac Appt:** Asst Clin Prof Ophthalmology, Univ Conn

Petersen, Robert Allen MD (Oph) - *Spec Exp:* Ophthalmology-Pediatric; **Hospital:** Children's Hospital - Boston; **Address:** Children's Hosp, Dept of Oph, Fegan-4, 300 Longwood Ave, Boston, MA 02115; **Phone:** (617) 355-6415; **Board Cert:** Ophthalmology 1967; **Med School:** Columbia P&S 1959; **Resid:** Internal Medicine, Presby Hosp, New York, NY 1960-1961; Ophthalmology, Mass EE Infirm, Boston, MA 1962-1966; **Fellow:** Ophthalmology, Columbia Presby Hosp, New York, NY 1961-1962; Research, MAss EE Infirm, Boston, MA 1962-1963; **Fac Appt:** Asst Prof Ophthalmology, Harvard Med Sch

Robb, Richard M MD (Oph) - *Spec Exp:* Strabismus; Cataract-Congenital; Lacrimal Gland Disorders; **Hospital:** Children's Hospital - Boston; **Address:** Chldns Hosp, Dept Oph, 300 Longwood Ave, Boston, MA 02115; **Phone:** (617) 355-6412; **Board Cert:** Ophthalmology 1967; **Med School:** Univ Penn 1960; **Resid:** Ophthalmology, Mass EE Infirm, Boston, MA 1961-1965; **Fac Appt:** Prof Emeritus Ophthalmology, Harvard Med Sch

Steinert, Roger F MD (Oph) - *Spec Exp:* Refractive, Cataract Surgery; Cornea Transplant; **Hospital:** Mass Eye & Ear Infirmary; **Address:** 50 Staniford St, Ste 600, Boston, MA 02114-2517; **Phone:** (617) 367-4800; **Board Cert:** Ophthalmology 1982; **Med School:** Harvard Med Sch 1977; **Resid:** Ophthalmology, Mass EE Infirm., Boston, MA 1978-1981; **Fac Appt:** Asst Clin Prof Ophthalmology, Harvard Med Sch

Walton, David S MD (Oph) - *Spec Exp:* Glaucoma-Pediatric; Cataract-Pediatric; Neuro-Ophthalmology; **Hospital:** Mass Eye & Ear Infirmary; **Address:** 2 Longfellow Pl, Ste 201, Boston, MA 02114; **Phone:** (617) 227-3011; **Board Cert:** Ophthalmology 1969, Pediatrics 1983; **Med School:** Duke Univ 1961; **Resid:** Ophthalmology, MA EE Infirm, Boston, MA 1964-1967; **Fac Appt:** Asst Prof Ophthalmology, Harvard Med Sch

Mid Atlantic

Abramson, David Harold MD (Oph) - *Spec Exp:* Eye Tumors/Cancer; **Hospital:** New York Eye & Ear Infirm (page 69); **Address:** 70 E 66th St, New York, NY 10021; **Phone:** (212) 744-1700; **Board Cert:** Ophthalmology 1975; **Med School:** Albert Einstein Coll Med 1969; **Resid:** Ophthalmology, Edward S Harkness Eye Inst, New York, NY 1970-1974; **Fellow:** Ocular Oncology, Columbia Presby Med Ctr, New York, NY 1974-1975; **Fac Appt:** Clin Prof Ophthalmology, Cornell Univ-Weill Med Coll

Aronian, Dianne D MD (Oph) - *Spec Exp:* Ophthalmology-Pediatric; Retinopathy of Prematurity; **Hospital:** NY Presby Hosp - NY Weill Cornell Med Ctr (page 70); **Address:** 155 E 72nd St, New York, NY 10021; **Phone:** (212) 534-4404; **Board Cert:** Ophthalmology 1977; **Med School:** Cornell Univ-Weill Med Coll 1972; **Resid:** Ophthalmology, New York Hosp, New York 1973-1976; **Fac Appt:** Assoc Prof Ophthalmology, Cornell Univ-Weill Med Coll

Behrens, Myles MD (Oph) - *Spec Exp:* Neuro-Ophthalmology; **Hospital:** NY Presby Hosp - Columbia Presby Med Ctr (page 70); **Address:** 635 W 165th St, New York, NY 10032-3701; **Phone:** (212) 305-5415; **Board Cert:** Ophthalmology 1971; **Med School:** Columbia P&S 1962; **Resid:** Internal Medicine, Columbia Presby Hosp, New York, NY 1963-1964; Ophthalmology, Columbia Presby Hosp, New York, NY 1967-1970; **Fellow:** Neurological Ophthalmology, Univ of California San Fran Hosp, San Francisco, CA 1970-1971; **Fac Appt:** Prof Ophthalmology, Columbia P&S

Biglan, Albert William MD (Oph) - *Spec Exp:* Ophthalmology-Pediatric; **Hospital:** Chldn's Hosp of Pittsbrgh; **Address:** 22 Landmark North, Ste 300, 20397 Route 19 North, Cranberry Township, PA 16066; **Phone:** (724) 772-3388; **Board Cert:** Ophthalmology 1977; **Med School:** SUNY Buffalo 1968; **Resid:** Ophthalmology, EE Hosp - Univ Pitt, Pittsburgh, PA 1973-1976; **Fellow:** Pediatric Ophthalmology, Indiana Univ Med Ctr, Indianapolis, IN 1977; **Fac Appt:** Assoc Prof Ophthalmology, Univ Pittsburgh

Burde, Ronald MD (Oph) - *Spec Exp:* Ischemic/Optic/Neuropathy; Glaucoma; Pseudotumor Cerebri; **Hospital:** Montefiore Med Ctr (page 67); **Address:** 111 E 210th St, Bronx, NY 10467-2401; **Phone:** (718) 920-6665; **Board Cert:** Ophthalmology 1970; **Med School:** Jefferson Med Coll 1964; **Resid:** Ophthalmology, Washington Univ Hosp, St Louis, MO 1965-1968; **Fellow:** Neurological Ophthalmology, Washington Hosp, St Louis, MO 1968-1970; **Fac Appt:** Prof Ophthalmology, Albert Einstein Coll Med

Caputo, Anthony R MD (Oph) - *Spec Exp:* Ophthalmology-Pediatric; Strabismus; **Hospital:** Columbus Hosp; **Address:** 556 Eagle Rock Ave, Ste 203, Roseland, NJ 07068-1500; **Phone:** (973) 228-3111; **Board Cert:** Ophthalmology 1976; **Med School:** Italy 1969; **Resid:** Ophthalmology, UMDNJ-Univ Hosp, Newark, NJ 1971-1974; **Fellow:** Ophthalmology, Wills Eye Hosp, Philadelphia, PA 1974-1975; **Fac Appt:** Prof Ophthalmology, UMDNJ-NJ Med Sch, Newark

Chang, Stanley MD (Oph) - *Spec Exp:* Retina/Vitreous Surgery; **Hospital:** NY Presby Hosp - Columbia Presby Med Ctr (page 70); **Address:** 635 W 165th St, New York, NY 10032; **Phone:** (212) 305-9535; **Board Cert:** Ophthalmology 1979; **Med School:** Columbia P&S 1974; **Resid:** Ophthalmology, Mass Eye & Ear Infirmary, Boston, MA 1976-1978; **Fellow:** Vitreoretinal Surgery, Bascom Palmer Eye Institute, Miami, FL 1978-1979; **Fac Appt:** Prof Ophthalmology, Columbia P&S

Del Priore, Lucian MD/PhD (Oph) - *Spec Exp:* Retina/Vitreous Surgery; Macular Degeneration; Retinal Transplant; **Hospital:** NY Presby Hosp - Columbia Presby Med Ctr (page 70); **Address:** Harkness Eye Inst, 635 W 165th St, New York, NY 10032; **Phone:** (212) 305-2923; **Board Cert:** Ophthalmology 1989; **Med School:** Univ Rochester 1982; **Resid:** Ophthalmology, Wilmer Eye Inst/Johns HopkinsHosp, Baltimore, MD 1984-1987; **Fellow:** Glaucoma, Wilmer Eye Inst/Johns Hopkins Hosp, Baltimore, MD 1987-1988; Vitreoretinal Surgery, Wilmer Eye Inst/Johns Hopkins Hosp, Baltimore, MD 1988-1989; **Fac Appt:** Assoc Prof Ophthalmology, Columbia P&S

Della Rocca, Robert MD (Oph) - *Spec Exp:* Eyelid Reconstruction; Oculoplastic Surgery; Thyroid Eye Disease; **Hospital:** New York Eye & Ear Infirm (page 69); **Address:** 310 E 14th St, Bldg South - rm 319, New York, NY 10003; **Phone:** (212) 979-4575; **Board Cert:** Ophthalmology 1975; **Med School:** Creighton Univ 1967; **Resid:** Ophthalmology, NY Eye & Ear Infirm, New York, NY 1970-1973; **Fellow:** Oculoplastic Surgery, Albany Med Ctr, New York, NY 1973

Diamond, Gary Richard MD (Oph) - *Spec Exp:* Eye Diseases-Pediatric; Strabismus; Amblyopia; **Hospital:** St Christopher's Hosp for Children; **Address:** St. Christopher's Hosp for Chldn, Div Oph, Front Street at Erie Ave, Philadelphia, PA 19134-1095; **Phone:** (215) 427-8120; **Board Cert:** Ophthalmology 1979; **Med School:** Johns Hopkins Univ 1974; **Resid:** Ophthalmology, Wilmer Inst-Johns Hopkins, Baltimore, MD 1975-1979; Ophthalmology, Chldns Hosp Med Ctr, Washington, DC 1978-1979; **Fellow:** Pediatric Ophthalmology, Harkness Eye Inst, Baltimore, MD 1978-1979; **Fac Appt:** Prof Ophthalmology, Hahnemann Univ

Dodick, Jack M MD (Oph) - *Spec Exp:* Cataract Surgery; Laser Vision Surgery; **Hospital:** Manhattan Eye, Ear & Throat Hosp; **Address:** 535 Park Ave, New York, NY 10021-8167; **Phone:** (212) 288-7638; **Board Cert:** Ophthalmology 1969; **Med School:** Univ Toronto 1963; **Resid:** Ophthalmology, Manhattan Eye & Ear Infirmary, New York, NY 1964-1967; **Fellow:** Cataract & Implant, NY Med Coll, New York, NY 1967-1968; **Fac Appt:** Clin Prof Ophthalmology, Columbia P&S

Eagle, Ralph C MD (Oph) - *Spec Exp:* Ophthalmic Pathology; **Hospital:** Wills Eye Hosp; **Address:** Wills Eye Hosp, Ophthalmic Pathology Lab, 900 Walnut St Fl 4, Philadelphia, PA 19107; **Phone:** (215) 928-3280; **Board Cert:** Ophthalmology 1976; **Med School:** Univ Penn 1970; **Resid:** Ophthalmology, Scheie Eye Inst, Philadelphia, PA 1972-1975; **Fellow:** Ophthalmic Pathology, AFIP, Washington, DC 1976-1978; **Fac Appt:** Prof Ophthalmology, Jefferson Med Coll

Eggers, Howard M MD (Oph) - *Spec Exp:* Ophthalmology-Pediatric; Strabismus; **Hospital:** NY Presby Hosp - Columbia Presby Med Ctr (page 70); **Address:** 635 W 165th St, New York, NY 10032; **Phone:** (212) 305-5409; **Board Cert:** Ophthalmology 1978; **Med School:** Columbia P&S 1971; **Resid:** Ophthalmology, Harkness Inst - Presby Hosp, New York, NY 1972-1975; **Fac Appt:** Prof Ophthalmology, Columbia P&S

Feldon, Steven E MD (Oph) - *Spec Exp:* Neuro-Ophthalmology; Orbital Surgery; Strabismus; **Hospital:** Rochester Gen Hosp; **Address:** 601 Elmwood Ave, Box 659, Rochester, NY 14642; **Phone:** (323) 342-6488; **Board Cert:** Ophthalmology 1979; **Med School:** Albert Einstein Coll Med 1973; **Resid:** Ophthalmology, Mass Eye & Ear, Boston, MA 1975-1978; **Fellow:** Ophthalmology, UCSF Med Ctr, San Francisco, CA 1978-1979

Flynn, John T MD (Oph) - *Spec Exp:* Pediatric Ophthalmology; Strabismus; Retinopathy of Prematurity; **Hospital:** NY Presby Hosp - Columbia Presby Med Ctr (page 70); **Address:** Harkness Eye Inst, 635 W 165th St, New York, NY 10032; **Phone:** (212) 305-3908; **Board Cert:** Ophthalmology 1967; **Med School:** Northwestern Univ 1956; **Resid:** Ophthalmology, NY Cornell Med Ctr, New York, NY 1961-1964; **Fellow:** Strabismus, Natl Inst Hlth, Bethesda, MD 1964-1965; **Fac Appt:** Prof Ophthalmology, Columbia P&S

Fuchs, Wayne MD (Oph) - *Spec Exp:* Diabetic Eye Disease/Retinopathy; Macular Disease/Degeneration; **Hospital:** Mount Sinai Hosp (page 68); **Address:** 121 E 60th St, Fl 5, New York, NY 10022; **Phone:** (212) 319-8205; **Board Cert:** Ophthalmology 1985; **Med School:** Mount Sinai Sch Med 1979; **Resid:** Ophthalmology, Mount Sinai Hosp, New York, NY 1980-1983; **Fellow:** Ophthalmology, NY Cornell Med Ctr, New York, NY 1983-1984; **Fac Appt:** Assoc Clin Prof Ophthalmology, Mount Sinai Sch Med

Gentile, Ronald MD (Oph) - *Spec Exp:* Retina/Vitreous Surgery; Diabetic Eye Disease; Macular Degeneration; **Hospital:** New York Eye & Ear Infirm (page 69); **Address:** 2nd Ave at 14th St, Bldg South - Ste 319, New York, NY 10003-4201; **Phone:** (212) 979-4120; **Board Cert:** Ophthalmology 1997; **Med School:** SUNY Downstate 1991; **Resid:** Ophthalmology, NY Eye & Ear Infirmary, New York, NY 1992-1995; **Fellow:** Vitreoretinal Surgery & Disease, Kresge Eye Inst, Detroit, MI 1996-1998; **Fac Appt:** Asst Prof Ophthalmology, NY Med Coll

Goldberg, Morton MD (Oph) - *Spec Exp:* Macular Disease/Degeneration; Diabetic Eye Disease/Retinopathy; **Hospital:** Johns Hopkins Hosp - Baltimore; **Address:** Johns Hopkins Hosp, Maumenee Bldg 727, 600 N Wolfe St, Baltimore, MD 21287-9278; **Phone:** (410) 955-6846; **Board Cert:** Ophthalmology 1968; **Med School:** Harvard Med Sch 1962; **Resid:** Ophthalmology, Wilmer Oph Inst, Baltimore, MD 1963-1966; **Fellow:** Ophthalmology, Wilmer Oph Inst, Baltimore, MD 1966-1967; Research, Johns Jopkins Hosp, Baltimore, MD 1966-1967; **Fac Appt:** Prof Ophthalmology, Johns Hopkins Univ

Green, William Richard MD (Oph) - *Spec Exp:* Ophthalmic Pathology; Retinal Disorders; **Hospital:** Johns Hopkins Hosp - Baltimore; **Address:** Johns Hopkins Hosp, Eye Path Lab-Maumenee Bldg, 600 N Wolfe St, rm 427, Baltimore, MD 21287-9248; **Phone:** (410) 955-3455; **Board Cert:** Ophthalmology 1965, Anatomic Pathology 1970; **Med School:** Univ Louisville Sch Med 1959; **Resid:** Ophthalmology, Wills Eye Hosp, Philadelphia, PA 1961-1963; Anatomic Pathology, Temple Univ, Philadelphia, PA 1967-1968; **Fellow:** Ophthalmology, Natl Inst Neuro Dis-Blindness 1963-1965; **Fac Appt:** Prof Ophthalmology, Johns Hopkins Univ

Guyer, David MD (Oph) - *Spec Exp:* Macular Disease/Degeneration; Diabetic Eye Disease/Retinopathy; **Hospital:** NYU Med Ctr (page 71); **Address:** 519 E 72nd St, rm 203, New York, NY 10021-4028; **Phone:** (212) 861-9797; **Board Cert:** Ophthalmology 1991; **Med School:** Johns Hopkins Univ 1986; **Resid:** Ophthalmology, Wilmer Eye Inst/ Johns Hopkins, Baltimore, MS 1987-1990; **Fellow:** Vitreoretinal Surgery, Mass EE Infirm/Harvard Med Sch, Boston, MA 1990-1992; **Fac Appt:** Prof Ophthalmology, NYU Sch Med

Guyton, David Lee MD (Oph) - *Spec Exp:* Optics; Strabismus; **Hospital:** Johns Hopkins Hosp - Baltimore; **Address:** Wilmer Eye Inst, rm 233, 600 N Wolfe St, Baltimore City, MD 21287-9028; **Phone:** (410) 955-8314; **Board Cert:** Ophthalmology 1977; **Med School:** Harvard Med Sch 1969; **Resid:** Ophthalmology, Johns Hopkins Hospital, Baltimore, MD 1973-1976; **Fellow:** Pediatric Ophthalmology, Baylor College of Medicine, Houston, TX 1976-1977; **Fac Appt:** Prof Ophthalmology, Johns Hopkins Univ

Hall, Lisabeth MD (Oph) - *Spec Exp:* Ophthalmology-Pediatric; Strabismus; Diplopia; **Hospital:** New York Eye & Ear Infirm (page 69); **Address:** 310 E 14th St, Bldg South - Fl 2, New York, NY 10003-4201; **Phone:** (212) 979-4375; **Board Cert:** Ophthalmology 1998; **Med School:** SUNY Stony Brook 1992; **Resid:** Ophthalmology, Manhattan Eye & Ear Infirm, New York, NY 1993-1996; **Fellow:** Ophthalmology, Jules Stein Eye Inst/UCLA, Los Angeles, LA 1996-1997; **Fac Appt:** Asst Clin Prof Ophthalmology, NY Med Coll

Hersh, Peter MD (Oph) - *Spec Exp: Corneal Disease; LASIK-Refractive Surgery; Cataract Surgery;* **Hospital:** Hackensack Univ Med Ctr; **Address:** 300 Frank W Burr Blvd, Teaneck, NJ 07666; **Phone:** (201) 883-0505; **Board Cert:** Ophthalmology 1987; **Med School:** Johns Hopkins Univ 1982; **Resid:** Ophthalmology, Lenox Hill Hosp, New York, NY 1982-1983; Ophthalmology, Mass Eye & Ear Infirm, Boston, MA 1983-1986; **Fellow:** Cornea External Disease, Mass Eye & Ear Infirm, Boston, MA 1986-1987; **Fac Appt:** Prof Ophthalmology, UMDNJ-NJ Med Sch, Newark

Hornblass, Albert MD (Oph) - *Spec Exp: Eyelid Surgery; Lacrimal Gland Disorders; Orbital Tumors;* **Hospital:** Manhattan Eye, Ear & Throat Hosp; **Address:** Oculoplastic Surgery, 130 E 67th St, New York, NY 10021; **Phone:** (212) 879-6824; **Board Cert:** Ophthalmology 1970, Plastic Surgery 1972; **Med School:** Univ Cincinnati 1964; **Resid:** Ophthalmology, SUNY Hlth Sci Ctr, Brooklyn, NY 1965-1969; **Fellow:** Plastic Surgery, Manhattan Eye, Ear, & Throat Hosp, New York, NY 1971-1972; **Fac Appt:** Clin Prof Ophthalmology, NYU Sch Med

Jaafar, Mohamad S MD (Oph) - *Spec Exp: Pediatric Ophthalmology; Strabismus-Adults & Children; Glaucoma-Pediatric;* **Hospital:** Chldns Natl Med Ctr - DC; **Address:** Dept of Ophthalmology, 111 Michigan Ave NW, Washington, DC 20010-2970; **Phone:** (202) 884-3017; **Board Cert:** Ophthalmology 1997; **Med School:** Lebanon 1978; **Resid:** Ophthalmology, Am U Beirut Med Ctr, Beirut, Lebanon 1978-1981; Ophthalmology, Washington Hosp Ctr, Washington, DC 1989-1994; **Fellow:** Pediatric Ophthalmology, Chldns Hosp, Boston, MA 1981-1982; Pediatric Ophthalmology, Baylor Coll Med, Houston, TX 1982-1983; **Fac Appt:** Prof Ophthalmology, Geo Wash Univ

Katowitz, James A MD (Oph) - *Spec Exp: Oculoplastic & Orbital Surgery; Ophthalmology-Pediatric; Cornea Plastic Surgery;* **Hospital:** Chldn's Hosp of Philadelphia; **Address:** Chldn's Hosp, Div Oph Wood Bldg 1st FL, 34th St & Civic Center Blvd, Philadelphia, PA 19104; **Phone:** (215) 590-2791; **Board Cert:** Ophthalmology 1969; **Med School:** Univ Penn 1963; **Resid:** Ophthalmology, Hosp Penn, Philadelphia, PA 1964-1967; **Fellow:** Oculoplastic Surgery, Queen Victoria Hosp, London, England 1967-1968; Oculoplastic Surgery, Moorfield Eye Hosp, London, England 1967-1968; **Fac Appt:** Prof Ophthalmology, Univ Penn

Kupersmith, Mark MD (Oph) - *Spec Exp: Neuro-Ophthalmology;* **Hospital:** New York Eye & Ear Infirm (page 69); **Address:** 170 East End Ave, rm 535, New York, NY 10128; **Phone:** (212) 870-9418; **Board Cert:** Ophthalmology 1981, Neurology 1981; **Med School:** Northwestern Univ 1974; **Resid:** Neurology, NYU Med Ctr, New York, NY 1974-1978; Ophthalmology, NYU Med Ctr, New York, NY 1976-1980

Laibson, Peter R MD (Oph) - *Spec Exp: Corneal Disease;* **Hospital:** Wills Eye Hosp; **Address:** Wills Eye Hospital, 900 Walnut St, Fl 3rd, Philadelphia, PA 19107; **Phone:** (215) 928-3180; **Board Cert:** Ophthalmology 1965; **Med School:** SUNY Downstate 1959; **Resid:** Ophthalmology, Wills Eye Hosp, Philadelphia, PA 1961-1964; **Fellow:** Mass EE Infirm, Boston, MA 1964-1965; **Fac Appt:** Prof Emeritus Ophthalmology, Jefferson Med Coll

Liebmann, Jeffrey MD (Oph) - *Spec Exp: Glaucoma;* **Hospital:** New York Eye & Ear Infirm (page 69); **Address:** 310 E 14th St, Ste 3, New York, NY 10003-4201; **Phone:** (212) 477-7540; **Board Cert:** Ophthalmology 1989; **Med School:** Boston Univ 1983; **Resid:** Ophthalmology, SUNY Downstate, Brooklyn, NY 1984-1987; **Fellow:** Glaucoma, NY EE Infirm, New York, NY 1988; **Fac Appt:** Assoc Clin Prof Ophthalmology, NY Med Coll

Lisman, Richard MD (Oph) - *Spec Exp:* Ophthalmic Plastic Surgery; Cosmetic Eyelid Surgery; Eyelid Reconstruction; **Hospital:** NYU Med Ctr (page 71); **Address:** 635 Park Ave, New York, NY 10021; **Phone:** (212) 585-1405; **Board Cert:** Ophthalmology 1981; **Med School:** NYU Sch Med 1976; **Resid:** Ophthalmology, Manhattan EE Hosp, New York, NY 1977-1980; **Fellow:** Ophthalmic Plastic Surgery, NY Eye & Ear Infirm, New York, NY 1980-1981; Plastic Surgery, Manhattan EE&T Hosp, New York, NY 1981-1982; **Fac Appt:** Clin Prof Ophthalmology, NYU Sch Med

Mackool, Richard MD (Oph) - *Spec Exp:* LASIK-Refractive Surgery; Cataract Surgery; **Hospital:** New York Eye & Ear Infirm (page 69); **Address:** Mackool Eye Inst & Laser Ctr, 31-27 41st St, Astoria, NY 11103; **Phone:** (718) 728-3400; **Board Cert:** Ophthalmology 1975; **Med School:** Boston Univ 1968; **Resid:** Ophthalmology, New York EE Infirm, New York, NY 1970-1973; **Fac Appt:** Asst Clin Prof Ophthalmology, NY Med Coll

Magramm, Irene MD (Oph) - *Spec Exp:* Ophthalmology-Pediatric; Strabismus; Cataract Surgery; **Hospital:** Manhattan Eye, Ear & Throat Hosp; **Address:** 225 E 64th St, New York, NY 10021; **Phone:** (212) 644-5100; **Board Cert:** Ophthalmology 1987; **Med School:** Cornell Univ-Weill Med Coll 1981; **Resid:** Ophthalmology, North Shore Univ Hosp, Manhasset, NY 1982-1985; **Fellow:** Pediatric Ophthalmology, Manhattan Ear, Eye & Throat Hosp, New York, NY 1985-1986; **Fac Appt:** Ophthalmology, Cornell Univ-Weill Med Coll

Mandel, Eric MD (Oph) - *Spec Exp:* LASIK-Refractive Surgery; Corneal Disease & Transplant; **Hospital:** New York Eye & Ear Infirm (page 69); **Address:** 211 E 70th St, New York, NY 10021-5106; **Phone:** (212) 734-0111; **Board Cert:** Ophthalmology 1988; **Med School:** SUNY Stony Brook 1982; **Resid:** Ophthalmology, Lenox Hill Hosp, New York, NY 1983-1986; **Fellow:** Cornea External Disease, Mass EE Infirm, Boston, MA 1986-1987

Medow, Norman MD (Oph) - *Spec Exp:* Cataract-Pediatric; Glaucoma-Pediatric; Corneal Disease-Pediatric; **Hospital:** Manhattan Eye, Ear & Throat Hosp; **Address:** 225 E 64th St, Ste 6, New York, NY 10021-6690; **Phone:** (212) 644-5100; **Board Cert:** Ophthalmology 1975; **Med School:** SUNY Hlth Sci Ctr 1966; **Resid:** Ophthalmology, Manhattan Eye, Ear & Throat Hosp, New York, NY 1969-1972; **Fac Appt:** Assoc Clin Prof Ophthalmology, Cornell Univ-Weill Med Coll

Metz, Henry MD (Oph) - *Spec Exp:* Ophthalmology-Pediatric; **Hospital:** Rochester Gen Hosp; **Address:** 1425 Portland Ave, Rochester, NY 14621-3001; **Phone:** (585) 922-4787; **Board Cert:** Ophthalmology 1967; **Med School:** SUNY Downstate 1961; **Resid:** Ophthalmology, Strong Meml Hosp, Rochester, NY 1962-1966; **Fellow:** Strabismus, Smith-Kettlewell Inst Vis, San Franscico, CA 1968-1969

Miller, Neil MD (Oph) - *Spec Exp:* Neuro-Ophthalmology; **Hospital:** Johns Hopkins Hosp - Baltimore; **Address:** Johns Hopkins - Wilmer Eye Inst, 600 N Wolfe Bldg Maumenee - rm B109, Baltimore, MD 21287-0001; **Phone:** (410) 955-8679; **Board Cert:** Ophthalmology 1976; **Med School:** Johns Hopkins Univ 1971; **Resid:** Ophthalmology, Johns Hopkins Hosp, Baltimore, MD 1972-1975; **Fellow:** Neurological Ophthalmology, UC San Francisco, San Francisco, CA 1975; **Fac Appt:** Prof Ophthalmology, Johns Hopkins Univ

Mills, Monte D MD (Oph) - *Spec Exp:* Ophthalmology-Pediatric; Eye Muscle Disorders; Strabismus; **Hospital:** Chldn's Hosp of Philadelphia; **Address:** Children's Hosp of Philadelphia, Richard D Wood Bldg, 34th and Civic Center Blvd Fl 1, Philadelphia, PA 19104; **Phone:** (215) 590-5761; **Board Cert:** Ophthalmology 1993; **Med School:** Baylor Coll Med 1988; **Resid:** Ophthalmology, Mass E&E Infirm, Boston, MA 1989-1992; **Fellow:** Pediatric Ophthalmology, Chldn's Hosp, Boston, MA 1992-1993; **Fac Appt:** Prof Ophthalmology, Univ Penn

Muldoon, Thomas O MD (Oph) - *Spec Exp:* Retina/Vitreous Surgery; Macular Disease/Degeneration; Diabetic Eye Disease/Retinopathy; **Hospital:** New York Eye & Ear Infirm (page 69); **Address:** 310 E 14th St, New York, NY 10003-4201; **Phone:** (212) 979-4595; **Board Cert:** Ophthalmology 1971; **Med School:** Univ Rochester 1962; **Resid:** Surgery, St Lukes Hosp, New York, NY 1965-1966; Ophthalmology, New York EE Infirm, New York, NY 1966-1969; **Fellow:** Strabismus, New York EE Infirm, New York, NY 1969-1970; **Fac Appt:** Assoc Clin Prof Ophthalmology, NY Med Coll

Olitsky, Scott Eric MD (Oph) - *Spec Exp:* Ophthalmology-Pediatric; Strabismus; **Hospital:** Chldn's Hosp of Buffalo; **Address:** Chldns Hosp, Dept Oph, 219 Bryant, Ste 2C, Buffalo, NY 14222; **Phone:** (716) 878-7567; **Board Cert:** Ophthalmology 1993; **Med School:** Jefferson Med Coll 1988; **Resid:** Ophthalmology, SUNY Buffalo, Buffalo, NY 1989-1992; **Fellow:** Pediatric Ophthalmology, Wills Eye Hosp, Philadelphia, PA 1992-1993; **Fac Appt:** Assoc Prof Ophthalmology, SUNY Buffalo

Podos, Steven M MD (Oph) - *Spec Exp:* Glaucoma; **Hospital:** Mount Sinai Hosp (page 68); **Address:** 1 Gustave Levy Pl, Box 1183, New York, NY 10029; **Phone:** (212) 241-6752; **Board Cert:** Ophthalmology 1968; **Med School:** Harvard Med Sch 1962; **Resid:** Ophthalmology, Washington Univ-Barnes Hosp, St Louis, MO 1963-1967; **Fac Appt:** Prof Ophthalmology, Mount Sinai Sch Med

Quigley, Harry Alan MD (Oph) - *Spec Exp:* Glaucoma; **Hospital:** Johns Hopkins Hosp - Baltimore; **Address:** 600 N Wolfe St, Maumenee B-110, 601 N Broadway St, Baltimore, MD 21287; **Phone:** (410) 955-6052; **Board Cert:** Ophthalmology 1976; **Med School:** Johns Hopkins Univ 1971; **Resid:** Ophthalmology, Wilmer Inst-Johns Hopkins, Baltimore, MD 1972-1975; **Fellow:** Ophthalmology, Bascom Palmer Eye Inst., Miami, FL 1975-1977; **Fac Appt:** Prof Ophthalmology, Johns Hopkins Univ

Quinn, Graham Earl MD (Oph) - *Spec Exp:* Ophthalmology-Pediatric; Eye Growth/Development; **Hospital:** Chldn's Hosp of Philadelphia; **Address:** Children's Hospital of Philadelphia - Division of Ophthalmology, 34th st & Civic Center Blvd Fl 9, Philadelphia, PA 19104; **Phone:** (215) 590-4594; **Board Cert:** Ophthalmology 1979; **Med School:** Duke Univ 1973; **Resid:** Pathology, Cleveland Metro Genl Hosp 1974-1975; Ophthalmology, Univ Penn 1975-1978; **Fellow:** Chldns Hosp Philadelphia, PA 1978-1979; **Fac Appt:** Prof Ophthalmology, Univ Penn

Raab, Edward MD (Oph) - *Spec Exp:* Ophthalmology-Pediatric; Strabismus; Glaucoma; **Hospital:** Mount Sinai Hosp (page 68); **Address:** 5 E 98th St, Fl 7, New York, NY 10029-6501; **Phone:** (212) 369-0988; **Board Cert:** Ophthalmology 1966; **Med School:** NYU Sch Med 1958; **Resid:** Mount Sinai, New York, NY 1961-1964; **Fellow:** Pediatric Ophthalmology, Children's Hosp, Washington, DC 1966-1967; **Fac Appt:** Prof Ophthalmology, Mount Sinai Sch Med

Reynolds, James D. MD (Oph) - *Spec Exp:* Ophthalmology-Pediatric; Strabismus; **Hospital:** Chldn's Hosp of Buffalo; **Address:** Children's Hospital - Department of Ophthalmology, 219 Bryant St, Buffalo, NY 14222; **Phone:** (716) 878-7567; **Board Cert:** Ophthalmology; **Med School:** SUNY Buffalo 1978; **Resid:** Erie CO Medical Center, Buffalo, NY 1978-1981; **Fellow:** Ophthalmology, Pittsburgh EE Hospital 1981-1982; **Fac Appt:** Prof Ophthalmology, SUNY Buffalo

Ritch, Robert MD (Oph) - *Spec Exp:* Glaucoma; **Hospital:** New York Eye & Ear Infirm (page 69); **Address:** 310 E 14th St, rm 304S, New York, NY 10003-4201; **Phone:** (212) 477-7540; **Board Cert:** Ophthalmology 1977; **Med School:** Albert Einstein Coll Med 1972; **Resid:** Ophthalmology, Mount Sinai Hosp, New York, NY 1973-1976; **Fellow:** Glaucoma, Mount Sinai Hosp, New York, NY 1976-1978; **Fac Appt:** Clin Prof Ophthalmology, NY Med Coll

Rosen, Richard MD (Oph) - *Spec Exp:* Diabetic Eye Disease/Retinopathy; Macular Disease/Degeneration; **Hospital:** New York Eye & Ear Infirm (page 69); **Address:** 310 E 14th St, Ste 319, New York, NY 10003-4201; **Phone:** (212) 979-4288; **Board Cert:** Ophthalmology 1991; **Med School:** Univ Miami Sch Med 1985; **Resid:** Ophthalmology, New York EE Infirm, New York, NY 1986-1989; **Fellow:** Ophthalmology, New York EE Infirm, New York, NY 1989-1991

Savino, Peter MD (Oph) - *Spec Exp:* Neuro-Ophthalmology; **Hospital:** Wills Eye Hosp; **Address:** Wills Eye Hosp, Neuro Dept, 900 Walnut St, Fl 2nd, Philadelphia, PA 19107; **Phone:** (215) 928-3130; **Board Cert:** Ophthalmology 1975; **Med School:** Italy 1968; **Resid:** Ophthalmology, Georgetown Med Ctr, Washington, DC 1970-1973; **Fellow:** Neurological Ophthalmology, Bascom Palmer Eye Inst, Miami, FL 1973-1974

Sergott, Robert C MD (Oph) - *Spec Exp:* Neuro-Ophthalmology; **Hospital:** Wills Eye Hosp; **Address:** Dept Neuro-Opthalmology, 900 Walnut St Fl 2, Philadelphia, PA 19107; **Phone:** (215) 928-3130; **Board Cert:** Ophthalmology 1982; **Med School:** Johns Hopkins Univ 1975; **Resid:** Internal Medicine, Mary Imogene Bassett Hospital, Cooperstown, NY 1975-1976; Ophthalmology, Jackson Memorial Hospital, Miami, FL 1979-1980; **Fellow:** Ophthalmology, Jackson Memorial Hospital, Miami, FL 1979-1980

Shabto, Uri MD (Oph) - *Spec Exp:* Retinopathy of Prematurity; Macular Degeneration; Diabetic Eye Disease/Retinopathy; **Hospital:** New York Eye & Ear Infirm (page 69); **Address:** 310 E 14th St Bldg South Fl 419, New York, NY 10003-4201; **Phone:** (212) 677-2000; **Board Cert:** Ophthalmology 1991; **Med School:** Harvard Med Sch 1986; **Resid:** Ophthalmology, New York Eye & Ear Infirmary, New York, NY 1988-1990; **Fellow:** Vitreoretinal Surgery, Montefiore Hosp Med Ctr, Bronx, NY 1990-1991; **Fac Appt:** Asst Prof Ophthalmology, NYU Sch Med

Shields, Jerry MD (Oph) - *Spec Exp:* Eye Tumors/Cancer; Ophthalmology-Pediatric; **Hospital:** Wills Eye Hosp; **Address:** 9th & Walnut Sts, 2nd Fl, Philadelphia, PA 19107; **Phone:** (215) 928-3105; **Board Cert:** Ophthalmology 1972; **Med School:** Univ Mich Med Sch 1964; **Resid:** Ophthalmology, Wills Eye Hosp, Philadelphia, PA 1967-1970; **Fellow:** Ophthalmology, Wills Eye Hosp, Philadelphia, PA 1970-1972

Simon, John W MD (Oph) - *Spec Exp:* Ophthalmology-Pediatric; Strabismus; **Hospital:** Albany Medical Center; **Address:** Albany Med Ctr, Dept Ped Opth, 35 Hackett Blvd, Albany, NY 12208; **Phone:** (518) 262-2500; **Board Cert:** Ophthalmology 1981; **Med School:** Mount Sinai Sch Med 1976; **Resid:** Ophthalmology, Mt Sinai Hosp, New York, NY 1977-1980; **Fellow:** Pediatric Ophthalmology, Wills Eye Hosp, Philadelphia, PA 1980-1981; **Fac Appt:** Prof Ophthalmology, Albany Med Coll

Stark, Walter J MD (Oph) - *Spec Exp:* Corneal Disease & Transplant; Cataract Surgery; Refractive Surgery; **Hospital:** Johns Hopkins Hosp - Baltimore; **Address:** Johns Hopkins Sch Med-Wilmer Opth Inst, 600 N Wolfe St, Maumenee 327, Baltimore, MD 21287-0005; **Phone:** (410) 955-5490; **Board Cert:** Ophthalmology 1973; **Med School:** Univ Okla Coll Med 1967; **Resid:** Ophthalmology, Wilmer Inst-Johns Hopkins, Baltimore, MD 1968-1971; **Fac Appt:** Prof Ophthalmology, Johns Hopkins Univ

Stern, Kathleen MD (Oph) - *Spec Exp:* Strabismus; Ophthalmology-Pediatric; **Hospital:** NY Presby Hosp - NY Weill Cornell Med Ctr (page 70); **Address:** 485 Park Ave, New York, NY 10022-1228; **Phone:** (212) 753-6464; **Board Cert:** Ophthalmology 1983; **Med School:** Harvard Med Sch 1978; **Resid:** Ophthalmology, Manhattan Eye, Ear & Throat Hosp, New York, NY 1979-1982; **Fellow:** Neuropathology, NY Hosp, New York, NY 1982-1983; **Fac Appt:** Asst Clin Prof Ophthalmology, Cornell Univ-Weill Med Coll

Walsh, Joseph MD (Oph) - *Spec Exp:* Diabetic Eye Disease; Macular Degeneration; Retinal Disorders; **Hospital:** New York Eye & Ear Infirm (page 69); **Address:** 310 E 14th St Bldg S Fl 3, New York, NY 10003-4201; **Phone:** (212) 979-4447; **Board Cert:** Ophthalmology 1976; **Med School:** Georgetown Univ 1966; **Resid:** Ophthalmology, New York Eye & Ear Infirm, New York, NY 1970-1973; **Fellow:** Retina, Montefiore Hosp Med Ctr, Bronx, NY 1973-1974; **Fac Appt:** Prof Ophthalmology, NY Med Coll

Wang, Frederick MD (Oph) - *Spec Exp:* Pediatric Ophthalmology; Strabismus; Eye Alignment Disorders; **Hospital:** New York Eye & Ear Infirm (page 69); **Address:** 30 E 40th St, Ste 405, New York, NY 10016-1201; **Phone:** (212) 684-3980; **Board Cert:** Ophthalmology 1980, Pediatrics 1978; **Med School:** Albert Einstein Coll Med 1972; **Resid:** Pediatrics, Jacobi Med Ctr, Bronx, NY 1973-1974; Ophthalmology, Albert Einstein, Bronx, NY 1976-1979; **Fellow:** Pediatric Ophthalmology, Children's Hosp, Washington, DC 1980; **Fac Appt:** Clin Prof Ophthalmology, Albert Einstein Coll Med

Yannuzzi, Lawrence MD (Oph) - *Spec Exp:* Retina/Vitreous Surgery; Macular Disease/Degeneration; Diabetic Eye Disease/Retinopathy; **Hospital:** Manhattan Eye, Ear & Throat Hosp; **Address:** 519 E 72nd St, Ste 203, New York, NY 10021-4028; **Phone:** (212) 861-9797; **Board Cert:** Ophthalmology 1970; **Med School:** Boston Univ 1964; **Resid:** Ophthalmology, Manhattan Eye, Ear & Throat Hosp, New York, NY 1965-1968; **Fac Appt:** Prof Ophthalmology, Columbia P&S

Zaidman, Gerald MD (Oph) - *Spec Exp:* Laser Vision Surgery; Cornea Transplant; Cataract Surgery; **Hospital:** Westchester Med Ctr (page 82); **Address:** Macy Pavilion, Dept Opth, Rm 1100, Westchester Medical Center, Valhalla, NY 10595; **Phone:** (914) 493-1599; **Board Cert:** Ophthalmology 1981; **Med School:** Albert Einstein Coll Med 1975; **Resid:** Ophthalmology, Beth Abraham Hosp, Westchester, NY 1976-1977; Ophthalmology, Lenox Hill Hosp, New York, NY 1977-1980; **Fellow:** Cornea External Disease, Univ Pitts, Pittsburgh, PA 1980-1982; **Fac Appt:** Assoc Prof Ophthalmology, NY Med Coll

Southeast

Aaberg Sr, Thomas Marshall MD (Oph) - *Spec Exp:* Retina/Vitreous Surgery; **Hospital:** Emory Univ Hosp; **Address:** Emory Eye Clinic, Dept Opth, 1365B Clifton Rd NE, Atlanta, GA 30322; **Phone:** (404) 778-4456; **Board Cert:** Ophthalmology 1967; **Med School:** Harvard Med Sch 1961; **Resid:** Ophthalmology, Mass EE Infirm, Boston, MA 1962-1966; **Fellow:** Bascom-Palmer Eye Inst, Miami, FL 1968-1969; **Fac Appt:** Prof Ophthalmology, Emory Univ

Alfonso, Eduardo MD (Oph) - *Spec Exp:* Corneal & External Eye Disease; **Hospital:** Anne B Leach Eye Hosp; **Address:** Bascom Palmer Eye Inst, 900 NW 17th St, Miami, FL 33136-1119; **Phone:** (305) 326-6366; **Board Cert:** Ophthalmology 1985; **Med School:** Yale Univ 1980; **Resid:** Ophthalmology, Bascom Palmer Eye Inst-U Miami, Miami, FL 1981-1984; **Fellow:** Ophthalmology, Mass Eye & Ear Hosp, Boston, MA 1984-1986; **Fac Appt:** Prof Ophthalmology, Univ Miami Sch Med

Anderson, Douglas R MD (Oph) - *Spec Exp:* Glaucoma; **Hospital:** Anne B Leach Eye Hosp; **Address:** Bascom Palmer Eye Inst, 900 NW 17th St, Miami, FL 33136-1119; **Phone:** (305) 326-6146; **Board Cert:** Ophthalmology 1970; **Med School:** Washington Univ, St Louis 1962; **Resid:** Ophthalmology, UCSF Hosp, San Francisco, CA 1965-1968; **Fellow:** Ophthalmology, Mass Eye & Ear Infirm-Howe Lab, Boston, MA 1968-1969; **Fac Appt:** Prof Ophthalmology, Univ Miami Sch Med

Buckley, Edward G MD (Oph) - *Spec Exp:* *Eye Diseases-Pediatric; Strabismus; Cataracts-Pediatric;* **Hospital:** Duke Univ Med Ctr (page 60); **Address:** Duke Univ Med Ctr - Eye Ctr, PO Box 3802 DUEC, Durham, NC 27710; **Phone:** (919) 684-6084; **Board Cert:** Ophthalmology 1982; **Med School:** Duke Univ 1977; **Resid:** Ophthalmology, Duke Univ Eye Ctr, Durham, NC 1978-1981; **Fellow:** Ophthalmology, Bascom Palmer Eye Inst, Miami, FL 1981-1983; **Fac Appt:** Prof Ophthalmology, Duke Univ

Capo, Hilda MD (Oph) - *Spec Exp:* *Ophthalmology-Pediatric; Strabismus; Neuro-Ophthalmology;* **Hospital:** Anne B Leach Eye Hosp; **Address:** Bascom Plamer Eye Inst, 900 NW 17th St, Miami, FL 33136; **Phone:** (305) 326-6555; **Board Cert:** Ophthalmology 1989; **Med School:** Puerto Rico 1982; **Resid:** Ophthalmology, Univ PR Med Sch, San Juan, Puerto Rico 1984-1987; **Fellow:** Neurological Ophthalmology, NYU Med Ctr, New York, NY 1988-1989; Pediatric Ophthalmology, Johns Hopkins Hosp, Baltimore, MD 1987-1988; **Fac Appt:** Asst Clin Prof Ophthalmology, Univ Miami Sch Med

Culbertson, William MD (Oph) - *Spec Exp:* *LASIK-Refractive Surgery; Corneal Disease & Surgery; Cataract Surgery;* **Hospital:** Anne B Leach Eye Hosp; **Address:** Bascom Palmer Eye Inst, 900 NW 17th St, Miami, FL 33136-1119; **Phone:** (305) 326-6364; **Board Cert:** Ophthalmology 1976; **Med School:** Emory Univ 1970; **Resid:** Ophthalmology, Vanderbilt Univ Hosp, Nashville, TN 1971-1974; **Fellow:** Ophthalmology, Bascom Palmer Eye Inst, Miami, FL 1978-1979; **Fac Appt:** Prof Ophthalmology, Univ Miami Sch Med

Driebe Jr, William T MD (Oph) - *Spec Exp:* *Cornea Transplant; Lens Implant Complications;* **Hospital:** Shands Hlthcre at Univ of FL (page 73); **Address:** Shands Hlthcare Univ FL, 1600 SW Archer Rd, Box 100284, Gainesville, FL 32610-0284; **Phone:** (352) 392-3451; **Board Cert:** Ophthalmology 1984; **Med School:** Univ VA Sch Med 1979; **Resid:** Ophthalmology, Shands Hlthcare Univ FL, Gainesville, FL 1980-1983; **Fellow:** Bascom Palmer Eye Inst, Miami, FL 1983-1984; **Fac Appt:** Prof Ophthalmology, Univ Fla Coll Med

Fagien, Steven MD (Oph) - *Spec Exp:* *Oculoplastic Surgery;* **Hospital:** Boca Raton Comm Hosp; **Address:** 1000 NW 9th Ct, Ste 104, Boca Raton, FL 33486-2268; **Phone:** (561) 393-9898; **Board Cert:** Ophthalmology 1988; **Med School:** Univ Fla Coll Med 1983; **Resid:** Ophthalmology, Univ IL Michael Reese Hosp, Chicago, IL 1987-1988; **Fellow:** Ophthalmology, Shands Hosp - Univ FL, Gainesville, FL 1984-1987; **Fac Appt:** Assoc Clin Prof Ophthalmology, Univ Fla Coll Med

Flynn, Harry W MD (Oph) - *Spec Exp:* *Retina/Vitreous Surgery; Diabetic Eye Disease/Retinopathy;* **Hospital:** Anne B Leach Eye Hosp; **Address:** 900 NW 17th St, Miami, FL 33136; **Phone:** (305) 326-6118; **Board Cert:** Ophthalmology 1976; **Med School:** Univ VA Sch Med 1971; **Resid:** Ophthalmology, Univ VA Hosp, Charlottesville, VA 1972-1975; **Fellow:** Retina, Pacific Med Ctr, San Francisco, CA 1975-1976; **Fac Appt:** Prof Ophthalmology, Univ Miami Sch Med

Forster, Richard K MD (Oph) - *Spec Exp:* *Cornea Transplant; Cataract Surgery;* **Hospital:** Anne B Leach Eye Hosp; **Address:** 900 NW 17th St, Miami, FL 33125; **Phone:** (305) 326-6373; **Board Cert:** Ophthalmology 1971; **Med School:** Boston Univ 1963; **Resid:** Ophthalmology, Bascom Palmer Eye Inst, Miami, FL 1966-1969; **Fac Appt:** Prof Ophthalmology, Univ Miami Sch Med

Freedman, Sharon MD (Oph) - *Spec Exp:* *Ophthalmology-Pediatric; Glaucoma-Congenital/Pediatric;* **Hospital:** Duke Univ Med Ctr (page 60); **Address:** Duke Eye Center, DUMC 3082, Durham, NC 27710; **Phone:** (919) 684-4584; **Board Cert:** Ophthalmology 1991; **Med School:** Harvard Med Sch 1985; **Resid:** Ophthalmology, Chldns Hosp., Boston, MA 1986-1989; **Fellow:** Glaucoma, Duke Eye Ctr., Durham, NC 1990-1992; Pediatric Ophthalmology, Chldns Hosp., Boston, MA 1989-1990; **Fac Appt:** Asst Prof Ophthalmology, Duke Univ

Gass, John Donald MD (Oph) - *Spec Exp:* Retinal Disorders; **Hospital:** Vanderbilt Univ Med Ctr (page 80); **Address:** Vanderbilt Univ, Dept Oph, Med Ctr East, 2115 21st Ave S, Nashville, TN 37232-8808; **Phone:** (615) 936-2100; **Board Cert:** Ophthalmology 1963; **Med School:** Vanderbilt Univ 1957; **Resid:** Ophthalmology, Wilmer Inst-Johns Hopkins, Baltimore, MD 1958-1963; **Fellow:** Ophthalmic Pathology, Armed Forces Institute, Washington, DC 1961-1962; **Fac Appt:** Prof Ophthalmology, Vanderbilt Univ

Gills Jr, James P MD (Oph) - *Spec Exp:* Cataract Surgery- Lens Implant; Refractive Surgery; Glaucoma; **Hospital:** Helen Ellis Memorial Hosp; **Address:** St Luke's Cataract and Laser Inst, 43309 US Highway 19 N, Tarpon Springs, FL 34689-6221; **Phone:** (727) 938-2020; **Board Cert:** Ophthalmology 1967; **Med School:** Duke Univ 1959; **Resid:** Ophthalmology, Johns Hopkins Hosp, Baltimore, MD 1962-1965; Ophthalmology, DuKe Univ Med Ctr, Durham, NC 1965-1968; **Fac Appt:** Clin Prof Ophthalmology, Univ S Fla Coll Med

Glaser, Joel MD (Oph) - *Spec Exp:* Neuro-Ophthalmology; Orbital Diseases; **Hospital:** Mercy Hosp - Miami, FL; **Address:** 801 Arthur Godfrey Rd, Ste 402, Miami Beach, FL 33140; **Phone:** (305) 442-3355; **Board Cert:** Ophthalmology 1968; **Med School:** Duke Univ 1963; **Resid:** Ophthalmology, Univ Miami Med Coll, Miami, FL 1964-1965; **Fellow:** Neurological Ophthalmology, Univ California San Fran Med Ctr, San Francisco, CA 1969-1970

Grossniklaus, Hans E MD (Oph) - *Spec Exp:* Ophthalmic Pathology; Eye Melanoma; Macular Degeneration; **Hospital:** Emory Univ Hosp; **Address:** Emory Eye Center, BT428, 1365 Clifton Rd, Atlanta, GA 30322; **Phone:** (404) 778-4611; **Board Cert:** Ophthalmology 1985, Anatomic Pathology 1987; **Med School:** Ohio State Univ 1980; **Resid:** Ophthalmology, Case West Res Univ Hosp, Cleveland, OH 1981-1984; Pathology, Case West Res Univ Hosp, Cleveland, OH 1985-1987; **Fellow:** Ophthalmological Pathology, Johns Hopkins Hosp, Baltimore MD, MD 1984-1985; **Fac Appt:** Prof Ophthalmology

Haik, Barrett MD (Oph) - *Spec Exp:* Eye Tumors/Cancer; **Hospital:** St Jude Children's Research Hosp; **Address:** 920 Madison Ave, Ste 915, Memphis, TN 38103; **Phone:** (901) 448-6650; **Board Cert:** Ophthalmology 1981; **Med School:** Louisiana State Univ 1976; **Resid:** Ophthalmology, Columbia-Presby/Harkness Eye Inst, New York, NY 1977-1980; **Fac Appt:** Prof Ophthalmology, Univ Tenn Coll Med, Memphis

Hess, J Bruce MD (Oph) - *Spec Exp:* Ophthalmology-Pediatric; Strabismus; **Hospital:** All Children's Hosp; **Address:** 880 6th St S, Ste 350, St Petersburg, FL 33701; **Phone:** (727) 892-4393; **Board Cert:** Ophthalmology 1978; **Med School:** Baylor Coll Med 1971; **Resid:** Ophthalmology, Geisinger Med Ctr, Danville, PA 1974-1977; **Fellow:** Ophthalmology, Wills Eye Hosp, Philadelphia, PA 1977-1978; **Fac Appt:** Assoc Prof Ophthalmology, Univ S FL Coll Med

Holliday, James N MD/PhD (Oph) - *Spec Exp:* Corneal Disease; **Hospital:** Meth Healthcare Central - Memphis Hosp; **Address:** 1795 N Germantown Pkwy, Cordova, TN 38016; **Phone:** (901) 759-9757; **Board Cert:** Ophthalmology 1994; **Med School:** Duke Univ 1987; **Resid:** Ophthalmology, UC Irvine Med Ctr, Orange, CA 1989-1992; **Fellow:** Anterior Segment - External Disease, Mayo Clinic, Rochester, MN 1992-1993

Lambert, Scott MD (Oph) - *Spec Exp:* Ophthalmology-Pediatric; Strabismus; Cataract-Pediatric; **Hospital:** Chldn's Hlthcre of Atlanta - Scottish Rite; **Address:** Emory Eye Ctr, Dept Ped Opth, 1365B Clifton Rd Ste 4500, Atlanta, GA 30322; **Phone:** (404) 778-3431; **Board Cert:** Ophthalmology 1989; **Med School:** Yale Univ 1983; **Resid:** Ophthalmology, UCSF, San Francisco, CA 1984-1987; **Fellow:** Pediatric Ophthalmology, Hosp Sick Chldn, London, England 1987-1988; **Fac Appt:** Prof Ophthalmology, Emory Univ

Lee, Paul P MD (Oph) - *Spec Exp:* *Glaucoma;* **Hospital:** Duke Univ Med Ctr (page 60); **Address:** Duke Univ Eye Ctr, Erwin Rd, Wadsworth Bldg, Box 3802, Durham, NC 27710; **Phone:** (919) 681-2793; **Board Cert:** Ophthalmology 1991; **Med School:** Univ Mich Med Sch 1986; **Resid:** Ophthalmology, Wilmer Eye Inst/Johns Hopkins, Baltimore, MD 1987-1990; **Fellow:** Glaucoma, Mass EE Infirm, Boston, MA 1990-1991; **Fac Appt:** Prof Ophthalmology, Duke Univ

McCord, Clinton MD (Oph) - *Spec Exp:* *Eyelid Surgery; Oculoplastic Surgery;* **Hospital:** Promina Piedmont Hosp; **Address:** 3200 Downwood Cir, Ste 640, Atlanta, GA 30327; **Phone:** (404) 351-0051; **Board Cert:** Ophthalmology 1968; **Med School:** Emory Univ 1961; **Fellow:** Oculoplastic Surgery, Man Eye&Ear Inst, New York, NY 1966-1967

McKeown, Craig A MD (Oph) - *Spec Exp:* *Ophthalmology - General;* **Address:** Bascolm Palmer Eye Institute, 900 NW 17th St, Miami, FL 33136; **Phone:** (800) 329-7000; **Board Cert:** Ophthalmology 1982; **Med School:** Northwestern Univ 1971; **Resid:** Ophthalmology, Walter Reed Med Ctr, Washington, DC 1977-1980; **Fellow:** Pediatric Ophthalmology, Chldns Hosp Natl Med Ctr, Washington, DC 1983-1984; Pediatric Ophthalmology, Wilmer Inst-Johns Hospkins, Baltimore, MD 1984-1985

Meredith, Travis MD (Oph) - *Spec Exp:* *Retina/Vitreous Surgery;* **Hospital:** Univ of NC Hosp (page 77); **Address:** 617 Burnett-Womack Bldg, Box CB#7040, Chapel Hill, NC 27599-7040; **Phone:** (919) 966-5296; **Board Cert:** Ophthalmology 1976; **Med School:** Johns Hopkins Univ 1969; **Resid:** Wilmer Inst-Johns Hopkins, Baltimore, MD 1970-1971; Wilmer Inst-Johns Hopkins, Baltimore, MD 1973-1975; **Fellow:** Vitreoretinal Surgery, Med Coll Wisc, Milwaukee, WI 1975-1976; **Fac Appt:** Clin Prof Ophthalmology, Univ Wash

Nussbaum, Julian MD (Oph) - *Spec Exp:* *Diabetic Eye Disease/Retinopathy; Macular Degeneration;* **Hospital:** Med Coll of GA Hosp and Clin; **Address:** 1120 15th St Bldg BA 2701, Augusta, GA 30912; **Phone:** (706) 721-1148; **Board Cert:** Ophthalmology 1981; **Med School:** Univ Miami Sch Med 1976; **Resid:** Internal Medicine, Jackson Memorial, Miami, FL 1976-1977; Ophthalmology, Medical College Of Georgia, Augusta, GA 1977-1980; **Fellow:** Ophthalmology, Retina Foundation, Boston, MA 1980-1982; Ophthalmology, Mass Eye & Ear, Boston, MA 1980-1982; **Fac Appt:** Prof Ophthalmology, Med Coll GA

Palmberg, Paul MD/PhD (Oph) - *Spec Exp:* *Glaucoma;* **Hospital:** Anne B Leach Eye Hosp; **Address:** 900 NW 17th St, Miami, FL 33136; **Phone:** (305) 326-6386; **Board Cert:** Ophthalmology 1976; **Med School:** Northwestern Univ 1970; **Resid:** Ophthalmology, Washington Univ, St Louis, MO 1971-1974; Ophthalmology, Barnes Hosp, St Louis, MO 1976-1977; **Fellow:** Glaucoma, Univ Washington, St Louis, MO 1974-1976; **Fac Appt:** Prof Ophthalmology, Univ Miami Sch Med

Parrish, Richard K MD (Oph) - *Spec Exp:* *Glaucoma; Cataract Surgery; Anterior Segment Surgery;* **Hospital:** Anne B Leach Eye Hosp; **Address:** 900 NW 17th St, Fl 4th, Miami, FL 33136; **Phone:** (305) 326-6389; **Board Cert:** Ophthalmology 1981; **Med School:** Indiana Univ 1976; **Resid:** Ophthalmology, Wills Eye Hosp, Philadelphia, PA 1977-1980; **Fellow:** Ophthalmology, Bascom Palmer Eye Inst, Miami, FL 1980-1982; **Fac Appt:** Prof Ophthalmology, Univ Miami Sch Med

Pollard, Zane F MD (Oph) - *Spec Exp:* *Ophthalmology-Pediatric; Strabismus;* **Hospital:** Chldns Hlthcare of Atlanta - Eggleston; **Address:** 5455 Meridian Mark Rd, Ste 220, Atlanta, GA 30342; **Phone:** (404) 255-2419; **Board Cert:** Ophthalmology 1975; **Med School:** Tufts Univ 1966; **Resid:** Surgery, UC San Francisco, San Francisco, CA 1967-1968; Ophthalmology, USC, Los Angeles, CA 1970-1973; **Fellow:** Pediatric Ophthalmology, Wills Eye Hosp, Philadelphia, PA 1974-1975

Pollock, Stephen MD (Oph) - *Spec Exp:* *Neuro-Ophthalmology; Optic Nerve Disorders;* **Hospital:** Duke Univ Med Ctr (page 60); **Address:** 3802 Erwing Rd, Durham, NC 27710-3802; **Phone:** (919) 684-4417; **Board Cert:** Ophthalmology 1986; **Med School:** Univ IL Coll Med 1981; **Resid:** Ophthalmology, U Ill EE Infirm., Chicago, IL 1982-1987; **Fellow:** Ophthalmology, Wilmer Inst./Johns Hopkins, Baltimore, MD 1985-1986; **Fac Appt:** Assoc Prof Ophthalmology, Duke Univ

Sternberg Jr, Paul MD (Oph) - *Spec Exp:* *Retina/Vitreous Surgery; Macular Disease/Degeneration;* **Hospital:** Emory Univ Hosp; **Address:** 1365-B Clifton Rd, Atlanta, GA 30322; **Phone:** (404) 778-3690; **Board Cert:** Ophthalmology 1985; **Med School:** Univ Chicago-Pritzker Sch Med 1979; **Resid:** Ophthalmology, Johns Hopkins Hosp, Baltimore, MD 1980-1983; **Fellow:** Vitreoretinal Surgery, Duke Univ, Durham, NC 1983-1984; **Fac Appt:** Prof Ophthalmology, Emory Univ

Stulting, R. Doyle MD (Oph) - *Spec Exp:* *Corneal Disease & Transplant; Laser Vision Surgery; Cataract Surgery;* **Hospital:** Emory Univ Hosp; **Address:** Dept Ophthalmology, 1365B Clifton Rd NE, Atlanta, GA 30322; **Phone:** (404) 778-5818; **Board Cert:** Ophthalmology 1982; **Med School:** Duke Univ 1976; **Resid:** Internal Medicine, Barnes Hosp, St Louis, MO 1976-1978; Ophthalmology, Bascom Palmer Eye Inst, Miami, FL 1978-1981; **Fellow:** Cornea, Emory Univ Clinic, Atlanta, GA 1981-1982; **Fac Appt:** Prof Ophthalmology, Emory Univ

Tse, David MD (Oph) - *Spec Exp:* *Oculoplastic & Orbital Surgery; Eyelid Repair; Lacrimal Gland Disorders;* **Hospital:** Anne B Leach Eye Hosp; **Address:** Bascom Palmer Eye Inst, 900 NW 17th St, Miami, FL 33136-1119; **Phone:** (305) 326-6086; **Board Cert:** Ophthalmology 1983; **Med School:** Univ Miami Sch Med 1976; **Resid:** Ophthalmology, LAC/USC Med Ctr, Los Angeles, CA 1979-1981; **Fellow:** Oculoplastic Surgery, Univ Iowa, Iowa City, IA 1981-1982

Waring III, George Oral MD (Oph) - *Spec Exp:* *Cataract Surgery; Cornea Transplant; LASIK-Refractive Surgery;* **Hospital:** Emory Univ Hosp; **Address:** Emory Clinic, Dept Oph, 1365-B Clifton Rd NE, Atlanta, GA 30322-1013; **Phone:** (404) 778-4190; **Board Cert:** Ophthalmology 1975; **Med School:** Baylor Coll Med 1967; **Resid:** Ophthalmology, Wills Eye Hosp, Philadelphia, PA 1970-1973; **Fellow:** Cornea External Disease, Wills Eye Hosp, Philadelphia, PA 1972-1974; **Fac Appt:** Prof Ophthalmology, Emory Univ

Midwest

Abrams, Gary W MD (Oph) - *Spec Exp:* *Retina/Vitreous Surgery;* **Hospital:** Hutzel Hosp - Detroit (page 59); **Address:** Kresge Eye Institute, 4717 St Antoine St, Detroit, MI 48201; **Phone:** (313) 577-8900; **Board Cert:** Ophthalmology 1977; **Med School:** Univ Okla Coll Med 1968; **Resid:** Ophthalmology, Med Coll Wisc Affil Hosps, Milwaukee, WI 1973-1976; **Fellow:** Vitreoretinal Surgery, Bascom Palmer Eye Inst, Miami, FL 1976-1978; **Fac Appt:** Prof Ophthalmology, Wayne State Univ

Albert, Daniel M. MD (Oph) - *Spec Exp:* *Eye Tumors/Cancer; Ophthalmic Pathology;* **Hospital:** Univ WI Hosp & Clins; **Address:** U Wisc Med Sch-Dept. Ophthalmology and Visual Sciences, 600 Highland Ave, Bldg CSC - Ste F4 - rm 336, Madison, WI 53792; **Phone:** (608) 636-6070; **Board Cert:** Ophthalmology 1969; **Med School:** Penn State Univ-Hershey Med Ctr 1962; **Resid:** Ophthalmology, University of Penn, Philadelphia, PA 1963-1966; Neurological Ophthalmology, Natl Inst Hlth, Bethesda, MD 1966-1968; **Fellow:** Pathology, Natl Inst Hlth, Bethesda, MD 1968-1969; **Fac Appt:** Prof Ophthalmology, Univ Wisc

OPHTHALMOLOGY

Alward, Wallace MD (Oph) - *Spec Exp:* Glaucoma; **Hospital:** Univ of IA Hosp and Clinics; **Address:** 200 Hawkins Drive, Iowa City, IA 52242; **Phone:** (319) 356-3938; **Board Cert:** Ophthalmology 1987; **Med School:** Ohio State Univ 1976; **Resid:** Ophthalmology, Univ Louisville, Louisville, KY 1983-1986; **Fellow:** Ophthalmology, Univ Miami-Bascom Palmer Eye, Miami, FL 1986-1987; **Fac Appt:** Prof Ophthalmology, Univ Iowa Coll Med

Archer, Steven M MD (Oph) - *Spec Exp:* Ophthalmology-Pediatric; **Hospital:** Univ of MI Hlth Ctr; **Address:** 1000 Wall St, Ann Arbor, MI 48105-1912; **Phone:** (734) 764-7558; **Board Cert:** Ophthalmology 1986; **Med School:** Univ Chicago-Pritzker Sch Med 1978; **Resid:** Ophthalmology, Univ Chicago, Chicago, IL 1981-1984; **Fellow:** Pediatric Ophthalmology, Indiana Univ, Indianapolis, IN 1984-1986; **Fac Appt:** Asst Prof Ophthalmology, Univ Mich Med Sch

Baker, John D MD (Oph) - *Spec Exp:* Ophthalmology-Pediatric; **Hospital:** Chldns Hosp of Michigan (page 59); **Address:** 2355 Monroe Blvd, Dearborn, MI 48124; **Phone:** (313) 561-1777; **Board Cert:** Ophthalmology 1974; **Med School:** Wayne State Univ 1967; **Resid:** Internal Medicine, Detroit General Hospital, Detroit, MI 1968-1971; **Fellow:** Pediatric Ophthalmology, Childrens Hospital DC, Washington, DC 1972; **Fac Appt:** Clin Prof Ophthalmology, Wayne State Univ

Burke, Miles Joseph MD (Oph) - *Spec Exp:* Ophthalmology-Pediatric; Strabismus-Adult & Child; Amblyopia; **Hospital:** Cincinnati Chldns Hosp Med Ctr; **Address:** 10475 Montgomery Rd, Ste 4F, Cincinnati, OH 45242-5200; **Phone:** (513) 984-4949; **Board Cert:** Ophthalmology 1979; **Med School:** Univ Ariz Coll Med 1974; **Resid:** Ophthalmology, U Michigan, Ann Arbor, MI 1975-1978; **Fellow:** Wills Eye Hosp, Philadelphia, PA 1978-1979; **Fac Appt:** Assoc Prof Ophthalmology, Univ Cincinnati

Cibis, Gerhard W MD (Oph) - *Spec Exp:* Ophthalmology-Pediatric; Strabismus; **Hospital:** Chldns Mercy Hosps & Clinics; **Address:** 4620 J C Nichols Pkwy, Ste 421, Kansas City, MO 64112; **Phone:** (816) 561-0306; **Board Cert:** Ophthalmology 1976; **Med School:** Washington Univ, St Louis 1968; **Resid:** Ophthalmology, Univ Iowa, Iowa City, IA 1972-1975; Ophthalmology, Univ Iowa, Iowa City, IA 1969-1970; **Fellow:** Pediatric Ophthalmology, Univ Miami Project to Cure Paralysis 1976-1977; **Fac Appt:** Clin Prof Ophthalmology, Univ Kans

Del Monte, Monte A MD (Oph) - *Spec Exp:* Ophthalmology-Pediatric; **Hospital:** Univ of MI Hlth Ctr; **Address:** 1000 Wall St, Ann Arbor, MI 48105-1912; **Phone:** (734) 764-3111; **Board Cert:** Ophthalmology 1982; **Med School:** Johns Hopkins Univ 1974; **Resid:** Pediatrics, Chldns Hosp Med Ctr, Boston, MA 1975-1977; Ophthalmology, Wilmer Eye Inst, Baltimore, MD 1978-1981; **Fellow:** Ophthalmology, Wilmer Eye Inst, Baltimore, MD 1977-1978; Pediatric Ophthalmology, Chldns Hosp, Washington, DC 1981

Feder, Robert S MD (Oph) - *Spec Exp:* Corneal Disease; LASIK-Refractive Surgery; **Hospital:** Northwestern Meml Hosp; **Address:** 675 N St Clair St, Fl 15, Chicago, IL 60611; **Phone:** (312) 695-8150; **Board Cert:** Ophthalmology 1983; **Med School:** Northwestern Univ 1978; **Resid:** Ophthalmology, Barnes Hosp-Wash Univ, St Louis, MO 1979-1982; **Fellow:** Cornea External Disease, Univ Iowa, Iowa City, IA 1982-1983; **Fac Appt:** Assoc Prof Ophthalmology, Northwestern Univ

France, Thomas D MD (Oph) - *Spec Exp:* Ophthalmology-Pediatric; Strabismus; Vision Development; **Hospital:** Univ WI Hosp & Clins; **Address:** Univ Station Clinics, Dept Oph, 2880 University Ave, Madison, WI 53705; **Phone:** (608) 263-6414; **Board Cert:** Ophthalmology 1971; **Med School:** Northwestern Univ 1962; **Resid:** Ophthalmology, UCSF, San Francisco, CA 1966-1969; **Fellow:** Pediatric Ophthalmology, DC Chldns Hosp, Washington, DC 1969-1970; Pediatric Ophthalmology, Hosp for Sick Chldn, London, England 1970; **Fac Appt:** Prof Ophthalmology, Univ Wisc

Holland, Edward J. MD (Oph) - *Spec Exp:* Corneal Disease; Refractive Surgery; Cataract Surgery; **Hospital:** Univ Hosp - Cincinnati; **Address:** 10494 Montgomery Rd, Cincinnati, OH 45242; **Phone:** (800) 544-5133; **Board Cert:** Ophthalmology 1986; **Med School:** Loyola Univ-Stritch Sch Med 1981; **Resid:** Ophthalmology, Univ Minn Med Ctr, Minneapolis, MN 1982-1985; Ophthalmology, Univ Iowa, Iowa City, IA 1985-1986; **Fellow:** Ocular Immunology, Natl Eye Inst, Bethesda, MD 1986-1987; **Fac Appt:** Clin Prof Ophthalmology, Univ Cincinnati

Kass, Michael A MD (Oph) - *Spec Exp:* Glaucoma; **Hospital:** Barnes-Jewish Hosp (page 55); **Address:** 660 S Euclid Ave, Box 8096, St Louis, MO 63110-1010; **Phone:** (314) 362-3937; **Board Cert:** Ophthalmology 1974; **Med School:** Northwestern Univ 1966; **Resid:** Ophthalmology, Washington Univ Med Ctr, St Louis, MO 1969-1972; **Fellow:** Glaucoma, Washington Univ Med Ctr, St Louis, MO 1972-1973; **Fac Appt:** Prof Ophthalmology, Washington Univ, St Louis

Krachmer, Jay H. MD (Oph) - *Spec Exp:* Corneal Disease; **Hospital:** Fairview-Univ Med Ctr - Univ Campus; **Address:** Univ Minn Med Sch, Dept Oph, 420 Delaware St SE, MMC 493, Minneapolis, MN 55455; **Phone:** (612) 625-4400; **Board Cert:** Ophthalmology 1972; **Med School:** Tulane Univ 1966; **Resid:** Ophthalmology, Univ Hosp, Iowa City, IA 1967-1970; **Fac Appt:** Prof Ophthalmology, Univ Minn

Krueger, Ronald MD (Oph) - *Spec Exp:* Corneal Disease; Refractive Surgery; **Hospital:** Cleveland Clin Fdn (page 57); **Address:** Cole Eye Institute,Cleveland Clinic Foundation, 9500 Euclid Ave, Ste i-32, Cleveland, OH 44195; **Phone:** (216) 444-8158; **Board Cert:** Ophthalmology 1992; **Med School:** UMDNJ-NJ Med Sch, Newark 1987; **Resid:** Internal Medicine, Colombia Presby Med Ctr, New York, NY 1988-1991; **Fellow:** Ophthalmology, U So. Calif Dohery Eye Inst, Los Angeles, CA 1992-1993; U Okla Hlth Sci Ctr Dean A. McGee Eye Ins., Oklahoma City, OK 1991; **Fac Appt:** Asst Prof Ophthalmology, St Louis Univ

Kushner, Burton J MD (Oph) - *Spec Exp:* Ophthalmology-Pediatric; Strabismus (Adult & Pediatric); **Hospital:** Univ WI Hosp & Clins; **Address:** Univ Wisc, Dept Ped Oph, 2870 University Ave, Ste 206, Madison, WI 53705-3611; **Phone:** (608) 263-6414; **Board Cert:** Ophthalmology 1975; **Med School:** Northwestern Univ 1969; **Resid:** Ophthalmology, Univ Wisc Hosp, Madison, WI 1970-1973; **Fellow:** Ophthalmology, Bascom Palmer Eye Inst, Miami, FL 1973-1974; **Fac Appt:** Prof Ophthalmology, Univ Wisc

Lewis, Hilel MD (Oph) - *Spec Exp:* Retina/Vitreous Surgery; Macular Degeneration; **Hospital:** Cleveland Clin Fdn (page 57); **Address:** Cleveland Clinic, Dept Ophthalmology-Desk i30, 9500 Euclid Ave, Cleveland, OH 44195-0001; **Phone:** (216) 444-0430; **Board Cert:** Ophthalmology 1990; **Med School:** Mexico 1980; **Resid:** Ophthalmology, Jules Stein Eye Inst-UCLA, Los Angeles, CA 1983-1986; **Fellow:** Ocular Pathology, Jules Stein Eye Inst-UCLA, Los Angeles, CA 1982-1983; Vitreoretinal Surgery, Med Coll Wisc, Milwaukee, WI 1986-1987; **Fac Appt:** Assoc Prof Ophthalmology, UCLA

Lichter, Paul R. MD (Oph) - *Spec Exp:* Cataract Surgery; Glaucoma; **Hospital:** Univ of MI Hlth Ctr; **Address:** 1000 Wall St, rm 740, Box 0714, Ann Arbor, MI 48105-1912; **Phone:** (734) 763-5874; **Board Cert:** Ophthalmology 1970; **Med School:** Univ Mich Med Sch 1964; **Resid:** Ophthalmology, U Mich. Med Ctr., Ann Arbor, MI 1965-1968; **Fellow:** Ophthalmology, UC San Francisco, San Francisco, CA 1968-1969; **Fac Appt:** Prof Ophthalmology, Univ Mich Med Sch

Lindstrom, Richard Lyndon MD (Oph) - *Spec Exp:* Corneal Disease; Cataract Surgery; Refractive Surgery; **Hospital:** Phillips Eye Inst; **Address:** 710 E 24th St, Ste 106, Minneapolis, MN 55404; **Phone:** (800) 526-7632; **Board Cert:** Ophthalmology 1978; **Med School:** Univ Minn 1972; **Resid:** Internal Medicine, Abbott-Northwestern Med Ctr, Minneapolis, MN 1973; Ophthalmology, Fairview Univ Med Ctr, Minneapolis, MN 1974-1978; **Fac Appt:** Prof Ophthalmology, Univ Minn

Mets, Marilyn MD (Oph) - *Spec Exp: Ophthalmology-Pediatric; Ophthalmology-Genetics;* **Hospital:** Children's Mem Hosp; **Address:** 2300 N Children's Plaza, Chicago, IL 60614; **Phone:** (773) 880-4000; **Board Cert:** Ophthalmology 1981; **Med School:** Geo Wash Univ 1976; **Resid:** Ophthalmology, Cleveland Clinic Fdn, Cleveland, OH 1977-1980; **Fellow:** Ophthalmology, Natl Chldns Hosp, Washington, DC 1980-1981; **Fac Appt:** Assoc Prof Ophthalmology, Northwestern Univ

Miller, Marilyn T MD (Oph) - *Spec Exp: Eye Diseases-Hereditary; Ophthalmology-Pediatric;* **Hospital:** Univ of IL at Chicago Eye and Ear Infi; **Address:** 1855 W Taylor St, Ste 205, Chicago, IL 60612-7242; **Phone:** (312) 996-7445; **Board Cert:** Ophthalmology 1966; **Med School:** Univ IL Coll Med 1959; **Resid:** Ophthalmology, U IL Hosps, Chicago, IL 1961-1964; IL Eye & Ear Infirmary, Chicago, IL 1964; **Fellow:** Ophthalmology, IL Eye & Ear Infirmary, Chicago, IL 1965-1967; **Fac Appt:** Prof Ophthalmology, Univ IL Coll Med

Pepose, Jay MD (Oph) - *Spec Exp: LASIK-Refractive Surgery; Glaucoma; Corneal & External Eye Disease;* **Hospital:** Barnes-Jewish Hosp (page 55); **Address:** 16216 Baxter Rd, Ste 205, Chesterfield, MO 63017; **Phone:** (636) 728-0111; **Board Cert:** Ophthalmology 1989; **Med School:** UCLA 1982; **Resid:** Ophthalmology, Johns Hopkins Hospital, Baltimore, MD 1984-1987; **Fellow:** Georgetown U Med Ctr, Washington, DC 1987-1988; **Fac Appt:** Prof Ophthalmology, Washington Univ, St Louis

Price, Ronald MD (Oph) - *Spec Exp: Ophthalmology-Pediatric; Strabismus (Eye Muscle Disorders);* **Hospital:** Univ Hosp of Cleveland; **Address:** Univ Ophth Assocs, 1611 S Green Rd, Ste 306-C, Cleveland, OH 44121; **Phone:** (216) 382-8022; **Board Cert:** Ophthalmology 1971; **Med School:** Columbia P&S 1965; **Resid:** Ophthalmology, Univ Louisville Hosps, Louisville, KY 1966-1970; **Fellow:** Pediatric Ophthalmology, DC Chldns Hosp, Washington, DC 1970-1971; **Fac Appt:** Asst Clin Prof Ophthalmology, Case West Res Univ

Putterman, Allen M MD (Oph) - *Spec Exp: Oculoplastic Surgery; Oculoplastic Surgery; Eyelid Surgery;* **Hospital:** Michael Reese Hosp & Med Ctr; **Address:** 111 N Wabash Ave, Ste 1722, Chicago, IL 60602-2002; **Phone:** (312) 372-2256; **Board Cert:** Ophthalmology 1971; **Med School:** Univ Wisc 1963; **Resid:** Ophthalmology, Michael Reese Hosp, Chicago, IL 1966-1969; **Fellow:** Oculoplastic Surgery, Manhattan Eye/Ear Infirm, New York, NY 1969-1970; **Fac Appt:** Prof Ophthalmology, Univ IL Coll Med

Rogers, Gary L MD (Oph) - *Spec Exp: Strabismus (Adult & Pediatric);* **Hospital:** Chldn's Hosp - Columbus, OH; **Address:** 555 S 18th St, Ste 4C, Columbus, OH 43205-2654; **Phone:** (614) 224-6222; **Board Cert:** Ophthalmology 1974; **Med School:** Ohio State Univ 1968; **Resid:** Ophthalmology, Mt Sinai Hosp, Cleveland, OH 1969-1972; **Fellow:** Pediatric Ophthalmology, Chldns Natl Med Ctr, Washington, DC 1973-1974; **Fac Appt:** Clin Prof Ophthalmology, Ohio State Univ

Rosenberg, Michael A MD (Oph) - *Spec Exp: Refractive Surgery; Cataract Surgery; Eye Muscle Surgery;* **Hospital:** Northwestern Meml Hosp; **Address:** Northwestern Med Faculty Foundation, 675 N St Clair, Ste 15-150, Chicago, IL 60611; **Phone:** (312) 695-8150; **Board Cert:** Ophthalmology 1975; **Med School:** Northwestern Univ 1967; **Resid:** Ophthalmology, Bascom Palmer Eye Inst, Miami, FL 1970-1973; **Fellow:** Neurological Ophthalmology, Univ Calif, San Franicsco, CA 1973-1974; Refractive Surgery, Univ Monterrey 1998; **Fac Appt:** Assoc Clin Prof Ophthalmology, Northwestern Univ

Samuelson, Thomas MD (Oph) - *Spec Exp: Glaucoma;* **Hospital:** Phillips Eye Inst; **Address:** 710 E 24th St, Ste 106, Minneapolis, MN 55404; **Phone:** (612) 874-9982; **Board Cert:** Ophthalmology 1991; **Med School:** Univ Minn 1985; **Resid:** Ophthalmology, Univ South Fla, Tampa, FL 1987-1990; **Fellow:** Glaucoma, Wills Eye Hosp, Philadelphia, PA 1990-1991; **Fac Appt:** Assoc Clin Prof Ophthalmology, Univ Minn

Scott, William MD (Oph) - *Spec Exp:* *Ophthalmology-Pediatric;* **Hospital:** Univ of IA Hosp and Clinics; **Address:** Dept Ophthalmology, 200 Hawkins Drive Bldg PFP - Ste 11290-H, Iowa City, IA 52242; **Phone:** (319) 356-0382; **Board Cert:** Ophthalmology 1972; **Med School:** Univ Iowa Coll Med 1964; **Resid:** Ophthalmology, Univ Iowa Hosps, Iowa City, IA 1967-1970; **Fellow:** Smith-Kettlewell Inst Vision, San Francisco, CA 1971

Stone, Edwin MD (Oph) - *Spec Exp:* *Retinal Disorders; Eye Diseases-Hereditary;* **Hospital:** Univ of IA Hosp and Clinics; **Address:** Dept Ophthalmology, 200 Hawkins Drive Bldg PFP Fl 1, Iowa City, IA 52242; **Phone:** (319) 356-2864; **Board Cert:** Ophthalmology 1990; **Med School:** Baylor Coll Med 1985; **Resid:** Ophthalmology, Univ Iowa Hosps & Clins, Iowa City, IA 1986-1989; **Fellow:** Retina, Univ Iowa Hosps & Clins, Iowa City, IA 1990-1992; **Fac Appt:** Assoc Prof Ophthalmology, Univ Iowa Coll Med

Traboulsi, Elias Iskan MD (Oph) - *Spec Exp:* *Ophthalmology-Pediatric; Eye Diseases; Glaucoma-Pediatric;* **Hospital:** Cleveland Clin Fdn (page 57); **Address:** 9500 Euclid Ave, Ste 132, Cleveland, OH 44195; **Phone:** (216) 444-4363; **Board Cert:** Clinical Genetics 1987, Ophthalmology 1991; **Med School:** American Univ of Beirut 1982; **Resid:** Ophthalmology, American Univ Beirut Hosp, Beirut, Lebanon 1982-1985; Ophthalmology, Georgetown Hosp, Washington, DC 1986-1989; **Fellow:** Ophthalmology, Johns Hopkins Hosp, Baltimore, MD 1985-1986; Pediatric Ophthalmology, Chldns Hosp, Washington, DC 1989-1990

Trese, Michael T MD (Oph) - *Spec Exp:* *Retina/Vitreous Surgery;* **Hospital:** William Beaumont Hosp; **Address:** 3535 W 13 Mile Rd, Ste 632, Royal Oak, MI 48073-6704; **Phone:** (248) 288-2280; **Board Cert:** Ophthalmology 1981; **Med School:** Geo Wash Univ 1976; **Resid:** Ophthalmology, Jules Stein Eye Inst-UCLA, Los Angeles, CA 1977-1980; **Fellow:** Retina, Duke Univ Med Ctr, Durham, NC 1980-1981; **Fac Appt:** Assoc Clin Prof Ophthalmology, Wayne State Univ

Tychsen, Lawrence MD (Oph) - *Spec Exp:* *Ophthalmology-Pediatric;* **Hospital:** St Louis Children's Hospital; **Address:** 1 Children's Pl, Ste 2S89, St. Louis, MO 63110; **Phone:** (314) 454-6026; **Board Cert:** Ophthalmology 1984; **Med School:** Georgetown Univ 1979; **Resid:** Ophthalmology, Univ Iowa Hosp, Iowa City, IA 1980-1983; **Fellow:** Pediatric Ophthalmology, Univ Calif Med Ctr, San Francisco, CA 1984-1985

Younge, Brian R MD (Oph) - *Spec Exp:* *Neuro-Ophthalmology; Temporal Arteritis; Ocular Palsies;* **Hospital:** Mayo Med Ctr & Clin - Rochester, MN; **Address:** Mayo Clinic, 200 First St SW, Rochester, MN 55905-0001; **Phone:** (507) 284-4567; **Board Cert:** Ophthalmology 1974; **Med School:** Univ Alberta 1965; **Resid:** Ophthalmology, Montreal Genl Hosp, Montreal, Canada 1969-1972; **Fellow:** Neurological Ophthalmology, Mayo Clinic, Rochester, MN 1973-1974; **Fac Appt:** Assoc Prof Ophthalmology, Mayo Med Sch

Great Plains and Mountains

Bateman, Jane Bronwyn MD (Oph) - *Spec Exp:* *Ophthalmology-Pediatric; Medical Genetics;* **Hospital:** Chldn's Hosp - Denver; **Address:** 1056 E 19th Ave, Box B-430, Denver, CO 80218; **Phone:** (303) 861-6062; **Board Cert:** Ophthalmology 1979, Clinical Genetics 1982; **Med School:** Coll Physicians & Surgeons 1974; **Fellow:** Ophthalmology, UCLA Med Ctr, Los Angeles, CA 1978; Pediatric Ophthalmology, Chldn's Natl Med Ctr, Washington, DC 1979

Crandall, Alan S MD (Oph) - *Spec Exp:* *Glaucoma; Cataract Surgery;* **Hospital:** Univ Utah Hosp and Clin; **Address:** Univ Utah Hosp, Moran Eye Ctr, 50 N Medical Dr, Salt Lake City, UT 84132; **Phone:** (801) 581-2769; **Board Cert:** Ophthalmology 1977; **Med School:** Univ Utah 1973; **Resid:** Ophthalmology, Univ Penn, Philadelphia, PA 1973-1976; **Fellow:** Glaucoma, Scheie Eye Inst, Philadelphia, PA 1981; **Fac Appt:** Prof Ophthalmology, Univ Utah

OPHTHALMOLOGY

Durrie, Daniel MD (Oph) - *Spec Exp:* *LASIK-Refractive Surgery; Corneal Disease;* **Hospital:** St Luke's Hosp; **Address:** 5520 College Blvd Fl 2 - Ste 201, Overland Park, KS 66211; **Phone:** (913) 491-3737; **Board Cert:** Ophthalmology 1979; **Med School:** Univ Nebr Coll Med 1975; **Resid:** Ophthalmology, Univ Nebr Med Coll, Omaha, NE 1976-1979; **Fac Appt:** Asst Clin Prof Ophthalmology, Univ Nebr Coll Med

Southwest

Boniuk, Milton MD (Oph) - *Spec Exp:* *Oculoplastic Surgery; Eye Tumors/Cancer;* **Hospital:** Methodist Hosp - Houston; **Address:** 6560 Fannin St, Ste 902, Houston, TX 77030; **Phone:** (713) 798-5955; **Board Cert:** Ophthalmology 1960; **Med School:** Dalhousie Univ 1956; **Resid:** Ophthalmology, Wills Eye Hosp, Philadelphia, PA 1957-1959; **Fellow:** Pathology, AFIP, Washington, DC 1959-1961; **Fac Appt:** Prof Ophthalmology, Baylor Coll Med

Ellis Jr, George S MD (Oph) - *Spec Exp:* *Ophthalmology-Pediatric; Eye & Muscle Motility;* **Hospital:** Children's Hospital - New Orleans; **Address:** Chldns Hosp, 200 Henry Clay Ave, Ste 305A, New Orleans, LA 70118; **Phone:** (504) 896-9426; **Board Cert:** Ophthalmology 1982; **Med School:** Tulane Univ 1977; **Resid:** Ophthalmology, Duke Univ-Eye Ctr, Durham, NC 1979-1982; Pediatric Ophthalmology, Hall Eye Clinic, Atlanta, NC 1982; **Fellow:** Pediatric Ophthalmology, Chldns Hosp, Washington, DC 1982-1983; **Fac Appt:** Clin Prof Ophthalmology, Tulane Univ

Eustis, Horatio Sprague MD (Oph) - *Spec Exp:* *Ophthalmology-Pediatric;* **Hospital:** Ochsner Found Hosp; **Address:** Ochsner Clinic, Dept Ophthamology, 1514 Jefferson Hwy, Fl 10, New Orleans, LA 70121; **Phone:** (504) 842-3995; **Board Cert:** Ophthalmology 1985; **Med School:** Louisiana State Univ 1980; **Resid:** Ophthalmology, La State Univ Eye Ctr, New Orleans, LA 1981-1984; **Fellow:** Pediatric Ophthalmology, Hosp Sick Chldn, Toronto, Canada 1984-1985; Pediatric Ophthalmology, Chldns Hosp, Washington, DC 1985; **Fac Appt:** Clin Prof Ophthalmology, Louisiana State Univ

Holladay, Jack T. MD (Oph) - *Spec Exp:* *LASIK-Refractive Surgery; Cataract Surgery; Eye Surgery-Lens;* **Hospital:** Meml Hermann Hosp; **Address:** 5420 Dashwood, Ste 207, Houston, TX 77081; **Phone:** (713) 668-7337; **Board Cert:** Ophthalmology 1979; **Med School:** Univ Tex, Houston 1974; **Resid:** Ophthalmology, Univ Tex Hlth Sci Ctr, Houston, TX 1974-1975; **Fac Appt:** Assoc Prof Ophthalmology, Univ Tex, Houston

Koch, Douglas D MD (Oph) - *Spec Exp:* *Cataract Surgery; Refractive Surgery; Corneal Disease;* **Hospital:** Methodist Hosp - Houston; **Address:** 6565 Fannin, MC-NC205, Houston, TX 77030; **Phone:** (713) 798-6443; **Board Cert:** Ophthalmology 1982; **Med School:** Harvard Med Sch 1977; **Resid:** Baylor Coll Med, Houston, TX 1978-1981; **Fellow:** Moorfields Eye Hosp., London, UK 1981-1982; Baylor Coll of Med 1982; **Fac Appt:** Prof Ophthalmology, Baylor Coll Med

Lambert, H. Michael MD (Oph) - *Spec Exp:* *Retina/Vitreous Surgery; Macular Disease/Degeneration; Diabetic Eye Disease/Retinopathy;* **Hospital:** Methodist Hosp - Houston; **Address:** Retina and Vitreous of Texas, 6500 Fannin, Ste 1100, Houston, TX 77030; **Phone:** (713) 799-9975; **Board Cert:** Ophthalmology 1983; **Med School:** Baylor Coll Med 1977; **Resid:** Ophthalmology, Wilford Hall USAF Med Ctr, San Antonio, TX 1979-1982; **Fellow:** Vitreoretinal Surgery, Duke Univ Eye Ctr, Durham, NC 1982-1983; **Fac Appt:** Assoc Clin Prof Ophthalmology, Baylor Coll Med

Mazow, Malcolm L. MD (Oph) - *Spec Exp:* *Strabismus-Adult; Ophthalmology-Pediatric;* **Hospital:** Meml Hermann Hosp; **Address:** 2855 Gramercy St, Houston, TX 77025; **Phone:** (713) 668-6828; **Board Cert:** Ophthalmology 1967; **Med School:** Univ Tex Med Br, Galveston 1961; **Resid:** Ophthalmology, Univ Iowa Hosp, Iowa City, IA 1962-1965; **Fellow:** Strabismus, Univ Iowa Hospital, Iowa City, IA 1965-1966; **Fac Appt:** Clin Prof Ophthalmology, Univ Tex, Houston

McCulley, James P MD (Oph) - *Spec Exp:* Corneal & External Eye Disease; Laser Vision Surgery; Cataract Surgery; **Hospital:** Zale Lipshy Univ Hosp; **Address:** Univ Texas SW Med School, 5323 Harry Hines Blvd, Dallas, TX 75390-9057; **Phone:** (214) 648-2020; **Board Cert:** Ophthalmology 1974; **Med School:** Washington Univ, St Louis 1968; **Resid:** Ophthalmology, Mass EE Infirmary, Boston, MA 1969-1973; **Fellow:** Cornea, Cornea Rsch-Retina Fdtn, Boston, MA 1973-1974; Cornea, Mass EE Infirmary, Boston, MA 1973-1974; **Fac Appt:** Prof Ophthalmology, Univ Tex SW, Dallas

McDonald, Marguerite B. MD (Oph) - *Spec Exp:* Refractive Surgery; **Hospital:** Meml Med Ctr - Baptist Campus; **Address:** Southern Vision Ins, 2820 Napleon Ave, Ste 750, New Orleans, LA 70115; **Phone:** (504) 896-1240; **Board Cert:** Ophthalmology 1981; **Med School:** Columbia P&S 1976; **Resid:** Ophthalmology, Manhattan EET Hosp., New York, NY 1977-1980; **Fellow:** Cornea, LSU Eye Ctr, New Orleans, LA 1980-1981; **Fac Appt:** Clin Prof Ophthalmology, Tulane Univ

Mims III, James Luther MD (Oph) - *Spec Exp:* Ophthalmology-Pediatric; Strabismus-Pediatric; **Hospital:** Baptist Med Ctr - San Antonio; **Address:** 311 Camden St, Ste 511, San Antonio, TX 78215; **Phone:** (210) 225-0084; **Board Cert:** Ophthalmology 1977; **Med School:** Tulane Univ 1968; **Resid:** Ophthalmology, Wills Eye Hosp, Philadelphia, PA 1973-1976; **Fellow:** Pediatric Ophthalmology, Wills Eye Hosp, Philadelphia, PA 1976-1977; **Fac Appt:** Clin Prof Ophthalmology, Univ Tex, San Antonio

Parks, Marshall M MD (Oph) - *Spec Exp:* Ophthalmology - General; **Hospital:** Chldns Med Ctr of Dallas; **Address:** 8201 Preston Rd, Ste 140A, Dallas, TX 75225; **Phone:** (214) 369-6434; **Board Cert:** Ophthalmology 1951; **Med School:** St Louis Univ 1943; **Resid:** Ophthalmology, Naval Med Ctr, San Diego, CA; **Fac Appt:** Clin Prof Ophthalmology, Geo Wash Univ

Piest, Kenneth L MD (Oph) - *Spec Exp:* Ophthalmic Plastic Surgery; **Hospital:** N Central Baptist Hosp; **Address:** 540 Madison Oak, Ste 450, San Antonio, TX 78258; **Phone:** (210) 494-8859; **Board Cert:** Ophthalmology 1991; **Med School:** Univ IL Coll Med 1984; **Resid:** Ophthalmology, Univ Tex Hlth Scis Ctr, San Antonio, TX 1985-1986; **Fellow:** Ophthalmological Pathology, Univ Utah, Salt Lake City, UT 1985-1986; Ophthalmic Plastic Surgery, Chldns Hosp/Sheie Eye Inst/Univ Penn, Philadelphia, PA 1989-1991; **Fac Appt:** Assoc Clin Prof Ophthalmology, Univ Tex, San Antonio

Richard, James Marshall MD (Oph) - *Spec Exp:* Ophthalmology-Pediatric; **Hospital:** Chldn's Hosp at OU Med Ctr; **Address:** 11013 Hefner Pointe Drive, Oklahoma City, OK 73120-5050; **Phone:** (405) 751-2020; **Board Cert:** Ophthalmology 1979; **Med School:** Univ Okla Coll Med 1974; **Resid:** Obstetrics & Gynecology, Baylor Coll Med, Houston, TX 1975-1978; **Fellow:** Pediatric Ophthalmology, Childns Hosp, Washington, DC 1978-1979; Ophthalmology, Johns Hopkins Hosp, Baltimore, MD 1970-1980; **Fac Appt:** Clin Prof Ophthalmology, Univ Okla Coll Med

Wilhelmus, Kirk R MD (Oph) - *Spec Exp:* Ophthalmology - General; **Hospital:** Methodist Hosp - Houston; **Address:** Cullen Eye Inst, 6500 Fannin St, Ste 1501, Houston, TX 77030; **Phone:** (713) 798-6100; **Board Cert:** Ophthalmology 1981; **Med School:** Vanderbilt Univ 1975; **Resid:** Ophthalmology, Baylor Coll Med, Houston, TX 1976-1979; **Fellow:** Cornea External Disease, Moorfields Eye Hosp, London, England 1979-1981; **Fac Appt:** Prof Ophthalmology, Baylor Coll Med

West Coast and Pacific

Arnold, Anthony C MD (Oph) - *Spec Exp:* Neuro-Ophthalmology; **Hospital:** UCLA Med Ctr; **Address:** 100 Stein Plaza, Los Angeles, CA 90095-7065; **Phone:** (310) 825-4344; **Board Cert:** Ophthalmology 1980; **Med School:** UCLA 1975; **Resid:** Ophthalmology, Jules Stein Eye Inst. UCLA, Los Angeles, CA 1976-1979; **Fellow:** Ophthalmology, Jules Stein Eye Inst UCLA, Los Angeles, CA 1982-1983; **Fac Appt:** Clin Prof Ophthalmology, UCLA

Baylis, Henry I MD (Oph) - *Spec Exp:* Oculoplastic Surgery; Cosmetic Surgery-Complications; **Hospital:** UCLA Med Ctr; **Address:** 1551 Ocean Ave, Ste 200, Santa Monica, CA 90401; **Phone:** (310) 207-0300; **Board Cert:** Ophthalmology 1969; **Med School:** Univ Mich Med Sch 1960; **Resid:** Ophthalmology, UCLA Med Ctr, Los Angeles, CA 1963-1966; **Fellow:** Oculoplastic Surgery, Manhattan EET Hosp, New York, NY 1966-1967; **Fac Appt:** Clin Prof Ophthalmology, UCLA

Binder, Perry Scott MD (Oph) - *Spec Exp:* Refractive Surgery; **Hospital:** Sharp Mem Hosp; **Address:** 8910 Univ Center Lane, Ste 800, San Diego, CA 92122; **Phone:** (858) 455-6800; **Board Cert:** Ophthalmology 1975; **Med School:** Northwestern Univ 1969; **Resid:** Ophthalmology, USC Med Ctr, Los Angeles, CA 1970-1973; **Fellow:** U Fla Hosp, Gainesville, FL 1973-1974; **Fac Appt:** Assoc Clin Prof Ophthalmology, UCSD

Borchert, Mark S MD (Oph) - *Spec Exp:* Ophthalmology-Pediatric; Vision-Unexplained Loss; Optic Nerve Disorders; **Hospital:** Chldns Hosp - Los Angeles; **Address:** Childrens Hospital - Division of Ophthalmology, 4650 Sunset Blvd, MC-88, Los Angeles, CA 90027-6062; **Phone:** (323) 669-2344; **Board Cert:** Ophthalmology 1989; **Med School:** Baylor Coll Med 1983; **Resid:** Ophthalmology, USC, Los Angeles, CA 1984-1987; **Fellow:** Ophthalmology, Harvard, Boston, MA 1987-1988; **Fac Appt:** Assoc Prof Ophthalmology, USC Sch Med

Boxrud, Cynthia Ann MD (Oph) - *Spec Exp:* Oculoplastic Surgery; Ophthalmic Tumors; Orbital Diseases; **Hospital:** UCLA Med Ctr; **Address:** 2021 Santa Monica Blvd, Ste 700E, Santa Monica, CA 90404; **Phone:** (310) 829-9060; **Board Cert:** Ophthalmology 1997; **Med School:** Case West Res Univ 1986; **Resid:** Ophthalmology, NYU-Bellevue Hosp Ctr, New York, NY 1987-1990; **Fellow:** Opthalmologic Oncololgy, NY Hosp Cornell Med Ctr, New York, NY 1990-1992; Ophthalmic Plastic Surgery, UCLA - Jules Stein Eye Inst, Los Angeles, CA 1992-1993

Caprioli, Joseph MD (Oph) - *Spec Exp:* Glaucoma; **Hospital:** UCLA-Sepulveda VA Grtr LA Hlth Care Sys; **Address:** UCLA- Jules Stein, 100 Stein Plaza, rm 2-273, Los Angeles, CA 90095-7006; **Phone:** (310) 794-9442; **Board Cert:** Ophthalmology 1985; **Med School:** SUNY Buffalo 1979; **Resid:** Ophthalmology, Yale-New Haven Hosp., New Haven, CT 1980-1983; **Fellow:** Ophthalmology, Wills Eye Hosp., Philadelphia, PA 1983-1984; **Fac Appt:** Prof Ophthalmology, UCLA

Char, Devron H MD (Oph) - *Spec Exp:* Eye Tumors/Cancer; Thyroid Eye Disease; **Hospital:** CA Pacific Med Ctr - Pacific Campus; **Address:** 45 Castro St, Ste 309, San Francisco, CA 94114; **Phone:** (415) 522-0700; **Board Cert:** Ophthalmology 1978; **Med School:** Univ Minn 1970; **Resid:** Internal Medicine, Mass Genl Hosp, Boston, MA 1970-1972; Medical Oncology, Natl Cancer Inst, Bethesda, MD 1972-1974; **Fellow:** Ophthalmology, UCSF, San Francisco, CA 1974-1977; Ophthalmology, UCSF, San Francisco, CA 1977-1978; **Fac Appt:** Prof Ophthalmology, Stanford Univ

Choy, Andrew Eng MD (Oph) - *Spec Exp:* Eye Motility-Pediatric; Oculoplastic & Orbital Surgery; **Hospital:** Long Beach Meml Med Ctr; **Address:** 4100 Long Beach Blvd, Ste 108, Long Beach, CA 90807-2619; **Phone:** (562) 426-3925; **Board Cert:** Ophthalmology 1976; **Med School:** USC Sch Med 1969; **Resid:** Neurology, Los Angeles Co-USC Med Ctr, Los Angeles, CA 1970-1971; Ophthalmology, Bellevue Hosp Ctr-NYU, New York, NY 1971-1974; **Fellow:** Columbia-Presby Med Ctr, New York, NY 1974-1975; **Fac Appt:** Assoc Clin Prof Ophthalmology, UCLA

Day, Susan H MD (Oph) - *Spec Exp:* Ophthalmology-Pediatric; Strabismus; **Hospital:** CA Pacific Med Ctr - Pacific Campus; **Address:** 2340 Clay St, Ste 100, San Francisco, CA 94115; **Phone:** (415) 202-1500; **Board Cert:** Ophthalmology 1980; **Med School:** Louisiana State Univ 1975; **Resid:** Internal Medicine, Letterman Army Med Ctr, San Francisco, CA 1975-1976; Ophthalmology, California Pacific Med Ctr, San Francisco, CA 1976-1979; **Fellow:** Sick Chldns Hosp, London, England 1979-1980

De Juan Jr, Eugene MD (Oph) - *Spec Exp:* Retina/Vitreous Surgery; **Hospital:** USC Univ Hosp - R K Eamer Med Plz; **Address:** 1450 Saint Pablo St, Ste 3600, Los Angeles, CA 90033; **Phone:** (323) 442-6335; **Board Cert:** Ophthalmology 1985; **Med School:** Univ S Ala Coll Med 1979; **Resid:** Ophthalmology, Johns Hopkins Hosp, Baltimore, DC 1980-1983; **Fellow:** Vitreoretinal Surgery, Duke Univ Eye Ctr, Durham, NC 1983-1984; **Fac Appt:** Prof Ophthalmology, Johns Hopkins Univ

Demer, Joseph L MD/PhD (Oph) - *Spec Exp:* Ophthalmology-Pediatric; Strabismus; Nystagmus; **Hospital:** UCLA Med Ctr; **Address:** Jules Stein Eye Institute, 100 Stein Plaza, MC 700219, Los Angeles, CA 90095-7002; **Phone:** (310) 825-5931; **Board Cert:** Ophthalmology 1988; **Med School:** Johns Hopkins Univ 1983; **Resid:** Ophthalmology, Baylor Coll Med, Houston, TX 1984-1987; **Fellow:** Pediatric Ophthalmology, Texas Chldns Hosp, Houston, TX 1987-1988; **Fac Appt:** Prof Ophthalmology, UCLA

Fein, William MD (Oph) - *Spec Exp:* Oculoplastic Surgery; Lacrimal Gland Disorders; Orbital Surgery; **Hospital:** Cedars-Sinai Med Ctr; **Address:** 415 N Crescent Drive, Ste 200, Beverly Hills, CA 90210-4860; **Phone:** (310) 859-0760; **Board Cert:** Ophthalmology 1969; **Med School:** UC Irvine 1960; **Resid:** Ophthalmology, Los Angeles Co General Hospital, Los Angeles, CA 1963-1966; **Fellow:** Ophthalmology, Manhattan EE&T Infirm, New York, NY 1966-1967; **Fac Appt:** Assoc Clin Prof Ophthalmology, USC Sch Med

Granet, David Bruce MD (Oph) - *Spec Exp:* Ophthalmology-Pediatric; Sports Vision; **Hospital:** UCSD Healthcare; **Address:** UCSD-Ratner Chldns Eye Ctr, 9415 Campus Point Dr, La Jolla, CA 92093-0946; **Phone:** (858) 534-7440; **Board Cert:** Ophthalmology 1994; **Med School:** Yale Univ 1987; **Resid:** Ophthalmology, Bellevue Hosp-NYU, New York, NY 1988-1991; **Fellow:** Pediatric Ophthalmology, Chldns Hosp, Philadelphia, PA 1991-1993; **Fac Appt:** Asst Prof Ophthalmology, UCSD

Hoyt, Creig S MD (Oph) - *Spec Exp:* Amblyopia; Strabismus; **Hospital:** UCSF Med Ctr; **Address:** 400 Parnassus Ave, Ste 702A, Box 0344, San Francisco, CA 94143; **Phone:** (415) 353-2289; **Board Cert:** Ophthalmology 1978; **Med School:** Cornell Univ-Weill Med Coll 1968; **Resid:** Neurology, UCSF, San Francisco, CA 1969-1970; Ophthalmology, UCSF, San Francisco, CA 1970; **Fellow:** Pediatric Ophthalmology, Chldns Hosp, Melbourne, Australia 1977-1977; **Fac Appt:** Prof Ophthalmology, UCSF

Hoyt, William Fletcher MD (Oph) - *Spec Exp:* Neuro-Ophthalmology; Retinal Disease; **Hospital:** UCSF Med Ctr; **Address:** 533 Parnassus Ave, Ste U521, San Fransisco, CA 94143-0001; **Phone:** (415) 476-1130; **Board Cert:** Ophthalmology 1958; **Med School:** UCSF 1950; **Resid:** Ophthalmology, UCSF Hosp, San Francisco, CA 1953-1956; **Fellow:** Neurological Ophthalmology, Johns Hopkins Hosp, Baltimore, MD 1958-1958; **Fac Appt:** Prof Ophthalmology, UCSF

Irvine, John Alexander MD (Oph) - *Spec Exp:* Corneal & External Eye Disease; **Hospital:** USC Univ Hosp - R K Eamer Med Plz; **Address:** 1450 San Pablo St, Los Angeles, CA 90033; **Phone:** (323) 442-6335; **Board Cert:** Ophthalmology 1989; **Med School:** USC Sch Med 1982; **Resid:** Ophthalmology, Mass EE Infirm/Harvard, Boston, MA 1983-1986; **Fellow:** Cornea External Disease, Mass EE Infirm, Boston, MA 1986-1987; **Fac Appt:** Prof Ophthalmology, USC Sch Med

Isenberg, Sherwin Jay MD (Oph) - *Spec Exp:* Strabismus; Ophthalmology-Pediatric; **Hospital:** LAC - Harbor - UCLA Med Ctr; **Address:** 100 Stein Plaza, Los Angeles, CA 90095-7000; **Phone:** (310) 825-8840; **Board Cert:** Ophthalmology 1978; **Med School:** UCLA 1973; **Resid:** Ophthalmology, Illinois Ear & Eye Infirmary, Chicago, IL 1974-1977; **Fellow:** Pediatric Ophthalmology, Chldns Hosp Natl Med Ctr, Washington, DC 1977-1978; **Fac Appt:** Prof Ophthalmology, UCLA

OPHTHALMOLOGY

Kramer, Steven G MD (Oph) - *Spec Exp:* Corneal Disease; Cataracts; **Hospital:** UCSF Med Ctr; **Address:** University of California San Francisco, 10 Kirkham St, rm K301, San Francisco, CA 94143-0730; **Phone:** (415) 476-1921; **Board Cert:** Ophthalmology 1971; **Med School:** Case West Res Univ 1965; **Resid:** Ophthalmology, U Chicago Hosps, Chicago, IL 1966-1969; **Fellow:** USPHS, Chicago, IL 1970-1971; **Fac Appt:** Prof Ophthalmology, UCSF

Mahon, Kathleen MK MD (Oph) - *Spec Exp:* Ophthalmology-Pediatric; **Hospital:** Sunrise Hosp & Med Ctr/Sunrise Chldn's Hosp; **Address:** 3201 S Maryland Pkwy, Ste 400, Las Vegas, NV 89109; **Phone:** (702) 731-3333; **Board Cert:** Ophthalmology 1980; **Med School:** Univ New Mexico 1975; **Resid:** Ophthalmology, Univ FL Med Ctr, Gainsville, FL 1976-1979; **Fellow:** Pediatric Ophthalmology, Univ Tex Hlth Sci Ctr, Houston, TX 1979-1980; **Fac Appt:** Clin Prof Ophthalmology, Univ Nevada

Maloney, Robert Keller MD (Oph) - *Spec Exp:* Refractive Surgery; LASIK-Refractive Surgery; **Hospital:** UCLA Med Ctr; **Address:** Maloney Vision Institute, 10921 Wilshire Blvd, Ste 900, Los Angeles, CA 90024-4002; **Phone:** (310) 208-3937; **Board Cert:** Ophthalmology 1991; **Med School:** UCSF 1985; **Resid:** Ophthalmology, Johns Hopkins Hosp, Baltimore, MD 1986-1989; **Fellow:** Refractive Surgery, Emory Univ Hosp, Atlanta, GA 1989-1991; **Fac Appt:** Assoc Clin Prof Ophthalmology, UCLA

Manche, Edward Emanuel MD (Oph) - *Spec Exp:* LASIK-Refractive Surgery; Corneal Disease & Transplant; **Hospital:** Stanford Med Ctr; **Address:** 900 Blake Wilbur Dr, rm W3002, Stanford, CA 94305; **Phone:** (650) 498-7020; **Board Cert:** Ophthalmology 1996; **Med School:** Albert Einstein Coll Med 1990; **Resid:** Ophthalmology, UMDNJ-NJ Med Sch, Newark, NJ 1991-1994; **Fellow:** Cornea External Disease, Jules Stein Eye Inst-UCLA, Los Angeles, CA 1994-1996; **Fac Appt:** Assoc Prof Ophthalmology, Stanford Univ

Marmor, Michael F MD (Oph) - *Spec Exp:* Eye Diseases-Neurophysiologic; **Hospital:** Stanford Med Ctr; **Address:** Stanford Med Ctr, Dept Oph, 300 Pasteur Rd, rm A157, Stanford, CA 94305-5308; **Phone:** (650) 723-5517; **Board Cert:** Ophthalmology 1974; **Med School:** Harvard Med Sch 1966; **Resid:** Ophthalmology, Mass EE Infirm, Boston, MA 1970-1973; **Fellow:** Neurological Physiology, Natl Inst Mental Hlth, Bethesda, MD 1967-1970; **Fac Appt:** Assoc Prof Ophthalmology, Stanford Univ

Masket, Samuel MD (Oph) - *Spec Exp:* Cataract Surgery; **Hospital:** West Hills Med Ctr; **Address:** 2080 Century Park E, Ste 911, Los Angeles, CA 90067; **Phone:** (310) 229-1220; **Board Cert:** Ophthalmology 1974; **Med School:** NY Med Coll 1968; **Resid:** Ophthalmology, Metro Hosp Ctr, New York, NY 1969-1973; **Fellow:** Ophthalmology, Columbia Presby Med Ctr, NewYork, NY; **Fac Appt:** Asst Clin Prof Ophthalmology, UCLA

Minckler, Donald Saier MD (Oph) - *Spec Exp:* Glaucoma; **Hospital:** LAC & USC Med Ctr; **Address:** Doheny Eye Inst, 1450 San Pablo St, Fl 4, Los Angeles, CA 90033-4507; **Phone:** (323) 442-6415; **Board Cert:** Ophthalmology 1975, Pathology 1978; **Med School:** Oregon Hlth Scis Univ 1964; **Resid:** Anatomic Pathology, Univ Wash Med Ctr, Seattle, WA 1968-1970; Ophthalmology, Univ Wash Med Ctr, Seattle, Wa 1970-1973; **Fellow:** Pathology, Armed Forces Inst Path, Washington, DC 1973-1975; Glaucoma, Shaffer Assocs-UCSF, San Francisco, CA 1981-1982; **Fac Appt:** Prof Ophthalmology, Univ SC Sch Med

Mondino, Bartly John MD (Oph) - *Spec Exp:* Corneal & External Eye Disease; **Hospital:** UCLA Med Ctr; **Address:** 100 Stein Plaza, MC-70019, Los Angeles, CA 90095; **Phone:** (310) 825-5053; **Board Cert:** Ophthalmology 1976; **Med School:** Stanford Univ 1971; **Resid:** Ophthalmology, NY Hosp/Cornell Univ, New York, NY 1972-1975; **Fellow:** Univ Pittsburgh Eye & Ear Hosp, Pittsburgh, PA 1975-1976; **Fac Appt:** Prof Ophthalmology, UCLA

Murphree, A. Linn MD (Oph) - *Spec Exp: Ophthalmology-Pediatric; Eye Diseases-Hereditary;* **Hospital:** Chldns Hosp - Los Angeles; **Address:** Chldns Hosp - Div Oph, 4650 W Sunset Blvd, MS 88, Los Angeles, CA 90027-6016; **Phone:** (323) 669-2299; **Board Cert:** Ophthalmology 1978; **Med School:** Baylor Coll Med 1972; **Resid:** Clinical Genetics, Baylor Heed, Houston, TX 1972-1973; Ophthalmology, Baylor College Medicine, Houston, TX 1973-1976; **Fellow:** Ophthalmology, Wilmer Inst/Johns Hopkins, Baltimore, MD 1976-1977; **Fac Appt:** Prof Ophthalmology, USC Sch Med

Nesburn, Anthony B MD (Oph) - *Spec Exp: Corneal Disease; Laser Vision Surgery; Herpes;* **Hospital:** Cedars-Sinai Med Ctr; **Address:** Cedars-Sinai Med Ctr, Dept Opthalmology, 8635 W 3rd St, Ste 390W, Los Angeles, CA 90048-6101; **Phone:** (310) 652-1133; **Board Cert:** Ophthalmology 1969; **Med School:** Harvard Med Sch 1960; **Resid:** Ophthalmology, Mass Eye & Ear Infirm, Boston, MA 1966-1968; **Fellow:** Virology, Harvard, Boston, MA 1964-1965; **Fac Appt:** Clin Prof Ophthalmology, UCLA

Palmer, Earl A. MD (Oph) - *Spec Exp: Ophthalmology-Pediatric; Retinopathy of Prematurity; Strabismus;* **Hospital:** OR Hlth Sci Univ Hosp and Clinics; **Address:** 3375 SW Terwilliger Blvd, Portland, OR 97201; **Phone:** (503) 494-7675; **Board Cert:** Ophthalmology 1976, Pediatrics 1975; **Med School:** Duke Univ 1966; **Resid:** Pediatrics, Univ Colo Med Ctr, Denver, CO 1967-1968; Ophthalmology, Oreg Hlth Scis Univ, Portland, OR 1971-1974; **Fellow:** Pediatric Ophthalmology, Univ Colo Med Ctr, Denver, CO 1966-1967; **Fac Appt:** Prof Ophthalmology, Oregon Hlth Scis Univ

Paul, Theodore Otis MD (Oph) - *Spec Exp: Ophthalmology-Pediatric; Strabismus;* **Hospital:** CA Pacific Med Ctr - Pacific Campus; **Address:** 909 Hyde St, Ste 518, San Francisco, CA 94109; **Phone:** (415) 563-1515; **Board Cert:** Ophthalmology 1974; **Med School:** UCLA 1967; **Resid:** Ophthalmology, Naval Hospital, San Diego, CA 1969-1972; **Fellow:** Ophthalmology, California Pacific Medical Center, San Francisco, CA 1973-1974

Rao, Narsing Adupa MD (Oph) - *Spec Exp: Uveitis/AIDS; Eye Pathology;* **Hospital:** USC Univ Hosp - R K Eamer Med Plz; **Address:** 1450 San Pablo St, Bldg DVRC-211, Los Angeles, CA 90033-4581; **Phone:** (323) 342-6645; **Board Cert:** Ophthalmology 1977, Pathology 1974; **Med School:** India 1967; **Resid:** Ophthalmology, Georgetown Hosp, Washington, DC 1972-1975; Pathology, Georgetown Hosp, Washington, DC 1969-1972; **Fac Appt:** Prof Ophthalmology, USC Sch Med

Salz, James Joseph MD (Oph) - *Spec Exp: Eye Laser Surgery (LASIK); Cataract Surgery;* **Hospital:** Cedars-Sinai Med Ctr; **Address:** 444 S San Vicente Blvd, Ste 704, Los Angeles, CA 90048-5901; **Phone:** (323) 653-3800; **Board Cert:** Ophthalmology 1971; **Med School:** Duke Univ 1965; **Resid:** Ophthalmology, Los Angeles Co-USC Med Ctr., Los Angeles, CA 1966-1969; **Fac Appt:** Clin Prof Ophthalmology, USC Sch Med

Serafano, Donald N MD (Oph) - *Spec Exp: LASIK-Refractive Surgery; Cataract Surgery; Lens Implants;* **Hospital:** Los Alamitos Med Ctr; **Address:** 10861 Cherry St, Ste 204, Box 250, Los Alamitos, CA 90720-5403; **Phone:** (562) 598-3160; **Board Cert:** Ophthalmology 1978; **Med School:** Wayne State Univ 1971; **Resid:** Ophthalmology, Mayo Clinic, Rochester, MN 1975-1978; **Fac Appt:** Assoc Clin Prof Ophthalmology, USC Sch Med

Shorr, Norman MD (Oph) - *Spec Exp: Oculoplastic Surgery; Reoperative Surgery-Blepharoplasty; Cosmetic Surgery-Eyelid & Forehead;* **Hospital:** UCLA Med Ctr; **Address:** 435 N Roxbury Dr, Ste 104, Beverly Hills, CA 90210-5003; **Phone:** (310) 278-1839; **Board Cert:** Ophthalmology 1976; **Med School:** Univ Miami Sch Med 1969; **Resid:** Ophthalmology, Jules Stein Eye Inst-UCLA, Los Angeles, CA 1972-1975; **Fellow:** Ophthalmic Plastic Surgery, UCLA Med Ctr, Los Angeles, CA 1975-1976; **Fac Appt:** Clin Prof Ophthalmology, UCLA

Smith, Ronald E MD (Oph) - *Spec Exp:* *Corneal Disease; External Disease;* **Hospital:** USC Univ Hosp - R K Eamer Med Plz; **Address:** Doheny Eye Medical Group, 1450 San Pablo, Ste DEI-5706, Los Angeles, CA 90033; **Phone:** (323) 442-6424; **Board Cert:** Ophthalmology 1974; **Med School:** Johns Hopkins Univ 1967; **Resid:** Wilmer Oph. Inst./Johns Hopkins, Baltimore, MD; **Fellow:** Francis I Proctor Fdn/UCSF, San Francisco, CA

Stout, J Timothy MD/PhD (Oph) - *Spec Exp:* *Retinal Disorders-Pediatric; Retina/Vitreous Surgery; Retinopathy of Prematurity;* **Hospital:** OR Hlth Sci Univ Hosp and Clinics; **Address:** 3375 SW Terwilliger Blvd, Portland, OR 97201; **Phone:** (503) 494-2435; **Board Cert:** Ophthalmology 1999; **Med School:** Baylor Coll Med 1989; **Resid:** Ophthalmology, Doheny Eye Inst, Los Angeles, CA 1990-1993; **Fellow:** Moorfields Eye Hosp, London, England 1993-1994; Doheny Eye Inst, Los Angeles, CA 1994-1995; **Fac Appt:** Assoc Clin Prof Ophthalmology, Oregon Hlth Scis Univ

Teplick, Stanley MD (Oph) - *Spec Exp:* *Refractive Surgery; Cataract Surgery;* **Address:** 9989 SW Nimbus Ave, Beaverton, OR 97008; **Phone:** (503) 520-0800; **Board Cert:** Ophthalmology 1983; **Med School:** Hahnemann Univ 1977; **Resid:** Ophthalmology, Mayo Clinic, Rochester, MN 1979-1981

Turner, Stephen Gordon MD (Oph) - *Spec Exp:* *Refractive Surgery; Glaucoma; Cornea & Cataract Surgery;* **Hospital:** Eden Med Ctr; **Address:** Turner Eye Inst Med Grp, 420 Estudillo Ave, San Leandro, CA 94577-4908; **Phone:** (510) 614-1515; **Board Cert:** Ophthalmology 1977; **Med School:** Baylor Coll Med 1968; **Resid:** Ophthalmology, UCSF Med Ctr, San Francisco, CA 1971-1975; **Fellow:** Ophthalmology, St John Ophthalmic Hosp, Jerusalem, Israel 1974-1975; **Fac Appt:** Asst Clin Prof Ophthalmology, UCSF

Weiss, Avery MD (Oph) - *Spec Exp:* *Ophthalmology-Pediatric; Strabismus and Amblyopia;* **Hospital:** Chldns Hosp and Regl Med Ctr - Seattle; **Address:** 4800 Sand Point Way NE, MS CH-61, Seattle, WA 98105; **Phone:** (206) 526-2100; **Board Cert:** Ophthalmology 1981; **Med School:** Univ Miami Sch Med 1974; **Resid:** Internal Medicine, Barnes Hosp, St Louis, MO 1974-1976; Ophthalmology, Barnes Hosp, St Louis, MO 1977-1980; **Fellow:** Research, Barnes Hosp, St Louis, MO 1976-1977; Pediatric Ophthalmology, Chldns Hosp Natl Med Ctr, Washington, DC 1980-1981; **Fac Appt:** Assoc Prof Ophthalmology, Univ Wash

Wright, Kenneth W MD (Oph) - *Spec Exp:* *Ophthalmology-Pediatric;* **Hospital:** Cedars-Sinai Med Ctr; **Address:** 8631 W 3rd St, Ste 304-E, Los Angeles, CA 90048; **Phone:** (310) 652-6420; **Board Cert:** Ophthalmology 1983; **Med School:** Boston Univ **Resid:** Ophthalmology, USC Med Ctr, Los Angeles, CA 1978-1981; **Fellow:** Pediatric Ophthalmology, Johns Hopkins, Baltimore, MD 1981; **Fac Appt:** Asst Prof Ophthalmology, UC Irvine

Yoshizumi, Marc Osamu MD (Oph) - *Spec Exp:* *Retinal Disorders; Eye Trauma;* **Hospital:** UCLA Med Ctr; **Address:** 200 Stein Plaza, rm 3519, Los Angeles, CA 90095; **Phone:** (310) 825-4749; **Board Cert:** Ophthalmology 1978; **Med School:** Yale Univ 1970; **Resid:** Ophthalmology, Mass EE Infirm/Harvard, Boston, MA 1974-1977; Neuropathology, Oxford Univ, Oxford, England 1970-1971; **Fellow:** Retina, Harvard Med Sch, Boston, MA 1977-1978; **Fac Appt:** Prof Ophthalmology, UCLA

ORTHOPAEDIC SURGERY

An orthopaedic surgeon is trained in the preservation, investigation and restoration of the form and function of the extremities, spine and associated structures by medical, surgical and physical means.

An orthopaedic surgeon is involved with the care of patients whose musculoskeletal problems include congenital deformities, trauma, infections, tumors, metabolic disturbances of the musculoskeletal system, deformities, injuries and degenerative diseases of the spine, hands, feet, knee, hip, shoulder and elbow in children and adults. An orthopaedic surgeon is also concerned with primary and secondary muscular problems and the effects of central or peripheral nervous system lesions of the musculoskeletal system.

Training required: Five years (including general surgery training) plus two years in clinical practice before final certification is achieved

Barnes-Jewish Hospital

BJC HealthCare℠

the primary adult hospital for
Washington University School of Medicine

216 S. Kingshighway
St. Louis, MO 63110
314-TOP-DOCS
(314-867-3627)
or toll free 1-866-867-3627
www.barnesjewish.org

ORTHOPAEDIC MEDICINE

offering specialized physicians, complete care

Because of their commitment to excellence in research, education and patient care, the Washington University specialists at Barnes-Jewish Hospital are able to provide the highest level of orthopaedic care. Our specialists are known for:

- *Adult Reconstruction and Joint Replacement* – Providing comprehensive care for all degenerative disorders of the hip and knee with a major focus on total joint replacement (arthroplasty)

- *Foot and Ankle* – Treating all types of foot and ankle disorders and deformities

- *Hand and Wrist* – Providing outpatient procedures that include treatment for carpal tunnel syndrome, trigger finger, Dupytrens contracture and ganglion cyst as well as tendon repair. Inpatient procedures include fracture care, care of the rheumatoid hand, and microsurgery and reconstructive surgery of the hand and wrist

- *Musculoskeletal Oncology* – Providing diagnosis and treatment of patients with benign, malignant and metastatic diseases of the musculoskeletal system

- *Physiatry* – Providing comprehensive, nonoperative care of musculoskeletal injuries and conditions with particular interest in conditions and injuries of the foot and ankle, neck, back and spine

- *Shoulder and Elbow* – Developing many arthroscopic procedures including a technique to treat frozen shoulder syndrome and a rare procedure to treat early arthritis in the elbow

- *Spine* – Pioneering surgeries that straighten the spines of patients who have previously undergone unsuccessful spinal surgeries and performing advanced degree spinal cord monitoring

- *Sports Medicine* – Specializing in comprehensive pediatric, adolescent and adult sports medicine for athletes of all levels, from professional to amateur level

- *Trauma* – Handling any orthopaedic trauma in our Level I Trauma Center.

Advancing Medicine. Touching Lives.

"Our goal is to establish a model for exceptional orthopaedic clinical care, research and education."

— Richard H. Gelberman, MD
Chief, Orthopaedics

If you need an orthopaedic specialist, go straight to the top. Call **314-TOP-DOCS** (314-867-3627) or toll free 1-866-867-3627. **www.barnesjewish.org**

DUKE ORTHOPAEDIC SERVICES

Durham, North Carolina • 1-888-ASK-DUKE • <u>dukehealth.org</u>

 DUKE UNIVERSITY HEALTH SYSTEM

Ranked sixth in the nation by *U.S.News & World Report*, Duke Orthopaedic Services offers comprehensive, individualized care for all injuries and diseases of the musculoskeletal system.

The program's 20 surgeons include recognized experts in nearly all orthopaedic subspecialties, who perform a collective 5,000 surgeries annually. The team also includes rheumatologists, specialized anesthesiologists, therapists, and other caregivers who work together to ensure that patients receive the best treatment, pain relief, and rehabilitation available.

PROGRAM HIGHLIGHTS

The **Orthopaedic Oncology Program**—part of the world-renowned Duke Comprehensive Cancer Center—uses sophisticated techniques to diagnose and treat musculoskeletal tumors. Surgical specialties include minimally invasive diagnostic biopsies that limit subsequent complications, limb-sparing surgery for bone and soft-tissue tumors, and limb salvage and reconstruction of skeletal defects.

The Back and Spine Clinic brings together leading orthopaedists, neurosurgeons, physical therapists, and psychologists to diagnose bone and muscle conditions and coordinate personalized treatment plans for people with debilitating back pain and disorders of the spine.

The Total Joint Center performs some 700 hip and knee replacements annually, and also includes specialists highly experienced in treating the shoulder, elbow, ankle, and other joints. Novel techniques—many pioneered at Duke—are used to delay the need for an artificial joint, including vascularized bone grafting, arthroscopy of the hip and knee, and osteotomy. Physician-scientists are also examining new technologies to improve the longevity of total joint implants.

Duke's **Pediatric Orthopaedic Services** include spine and hip surgery, treatment for club feet, trauma treatment, the Ilizarov method for limb lengthening, deformity correction, and specialty clinics for scoliosis, myelodysplasia, cerebral palsy, and pediatric amputees.

Duke orthopaedists also include recognized experts in areas such as **Reconstructive Microsurgery, Hand and Foot Surgery,** and **Trauma Surgery**. The Hand and Microsurgery group have done pioneering clinical and research work in replantation of amputated extremities and elective microsurgical reconstruction of extremities, while the Foot Service is known for outpatient surgical procedures designed to speed the return to athletic activities.

SPORTS MEDICINE AT DUKE

The Duke Sports Medicine Center takes a multidisciplinary approach to treating athletes and other active individuals whose physical abilities have been limited due to injury, disease, or the normal process of aging. It features the South's only sports medicine clinic dedicated exclusively to meeting the needs of active women.

Staffed by a core of nationally recognized orthopaedic surgeons, the Sports Medicine team also includes primary care and pediatric sports medicine physicians, rheumatologists, a sports psychologist, and physical therapists. Together, they provide comprehensive evaluation and treatment of the complex factors that affect performance, with the goal of helping each individual heal, rebuild strength, and enhance performance.

The Center also includes the Michael W. Krzyzewski Human Performance Lab, where researchers are discovering new ways to prevent sports injuries.

Visit the Center online at **dukesportsmedicine.com**

DEPARTMENT OF ORTHOPAEDIC SURGERY AND MUSCULOSKELETAL SERVICES

MAIMONIDES MEDICAL CENTER

4802 Tenth Avenue • Brooklyn, NY 11219
Phone (718) 283-7400   Fax (718) 283-6199
www.maimonidesmed.org

PHYSICAL REHABILITATION

Operating from state-of-the-art outpatient facilities, Maimonides' rehabilitation team offers physiatry; physical, occupational and speech therapy; therapeutic massage; hand therapy; weight loss programs; wellness and health enhancement; pool therapy; pulmonary rehabilitation; and post-mastectomy rehabilitation.

PEDIATRIC ORTHOPAEDICS

Maimonides provides care for children with orthopaedic problems—from simple fractures to complex congenital afflictions. Areas of expertise include the treatment of Blount's disease, club foot, long bone fractures, growth plate injuries and neuromuscular disorders such as cerebral palsy and muscular dystrophy.

BROOKLYN SPINE CENTER

Led by the internationally renowned spine surgeon Jean Pierre Farcy, MD, this division is dedicated to all aspects of spine care, including surgery, research and teaching. Backed by leading-edge technology and a highly respected staff of surgeons, Maimonides offers patients comprehensive management and treatment of all back- and neck-related problems.

THE KNEE CENTER

The center is led by Ronald P. Grelsamer, MD, a pioneer in the areas of hip reconstruction and sports medicine. Physicians work with patients to design a treatment plan tailored to their specific needs—from skilled physical therapy to complex surgery.

THE HAND AND UPPER EXTREMITY CENTER

Under the direction of Jack Choueka, MD, the hand center cares for all upper extremity disorders, including carpal tunnel syndrome, arthritis, fractures, rotator cuff tears and sports injuries. Techniques include minimally invasive arthroscopic and endoscopic surgery. The center provides on-site physical and occupational therapy.

ORTHOPAEDIC SURGERY AND MUSCULOSKELETAL SERVICES

Maimonides Medical Center operates one of the most comprehensive orthopaedics departments in the New York region. The department, led by Allan Strongwater, MD, includes Rehabilitation Medicine and Podiatry to provide patients with highly integrated and coordinated care. Our clinicians are dedicated to helping patients improve mobility and function while minimizing the pain and discomfort of bone, joint, muscle and ligament problems.

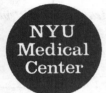

NYU Medical Center
550 First Avenue (at 31st St.), New York, NY 10016
Physician Referral: (888) 7-NYU-MED (888-769-8633)
www.nyumedicalcenter.org

Hospital for Joint Diseases
301 East 17th Street (at 2nd Ave.), New York, NY 10003
Physician Referral: (888) HJD-DOCS (888-453-3627)
www.jointdiseases.com

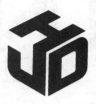

NYU-HOSPITAL FOR JOINT DISEASES ORTHOPAEDIC SERVICES

Leaders in the treatment of adult and children's bone and joint disorders.

The NYU-Hospital for Joint Diseases Department of Orthopaedic Surgery Offers the Following Services and Treatments:

- General Orthopaedics
- Hip and Knee Replacement Center
- Arthroscopic Surgery
- Bone Tumor Service
- Foot and Ankle Surgery
- Hand Surgery
- Limb Lengthening and Bone Growth
- Occupational and Industrial Orthopaedic Care
- Sports Medicine
- Pediatric Orthopaedics
- Shoulder Institute
- Center for Neuromuscular and Developmental Disorders
- The Geriatric Hip Fracture Program
- The Scoliosis Program
- The Spine Center
- The Harkness Center for Dance Injuries
- 24-Hour Immediate Orthopaedic Care

NYU-Hospital for Joint Diseases Orthopaedics provides care at NYU Tisch Hospital, Hospital for Joint Diseases, Manhattan VA, Jamaica Hospital, and Bellevue Hospital Center, where more than 12,000 surgical procedures are performed each year. The orthopaedic faculty maintains offices in all five boroughs as well as in Rockland County and New Jersey.

NYU MEDICAL CENTER

The NYU-Hospital for Joint Diseases Department of Orthopaedic Surgery is the largest and most accomplished in the region for the diagnosis and treatment of musculoskeletal disorders as well as in research and education. The clinical expertise of the faculty represents all subspecialty areas of orthopaedic surgery, including spine, total joint replacement, sports medicine and arthroscopy, pediatric orthopaedics, shoulder, hand, and foot-and-ankle.

Physician Referral
(888) 7-NYU-MED
(888-769-8633)
www.nyumedicalcenter.org

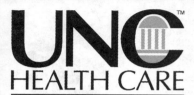

Department of Orthopaedics
The University of North Carolina Health Care System
101 Manning Drive Chapel Hill, NC 27514

www.unchealthcare.org

THE MUSCULOSKELETAL SERVICE AT UNC

The Musculoskeletal Service at UNC consists of 28 physicians who provide state-of-the-art patient care in a dozen clinical subspecialties. These include pediatric orthopaedics; sports medicine; joint replacements; musculoskeletal oncology; surgery of the hand, foot, upper extremity and spine; pain management; trauma; rheumatology; and physical medicine and rehabilitation. The Adult Reconstructive Service is staffed by faculty members with special expertise in joint replacement, surgery of the spine, and surgery of the hand and foot. The faculty in Pediatric Orthopaedics have particular interests in birth defects and congenital deformities, scoliosis, neuromuscular diseases, oncology, and hemophilia. Trauma includes sports medicine and post-traumatic reconstruction, as well as acute trauma.

PATIENT CARE AND RESEARCH

Research conducted by Musculoskeletal Service faculty plays a very important role in the quality of care given to patients. Ongoing studies are focused on areas such as arthritis, osteoporosis, joint replacements, mechanism of sports injuries and the assessment of human physical performance.

A GROWING SERVICE

Each year, approximately 30,000 patients are seen in the Orthopaedic Clinics at UNC, and more than 6,800 operative procedures are performed at UNC Hospitals. The number of patient visits to the Musculoskeletal Service is growing by more than 10 percent a year. In the 2001 fiscal year, on-site clinic visits increased by 14 percent, and operations performed on-site increased by 13 percent.

To request an appointment, call (919) 966-7890.

SPORTS MEDICINE

UNC is a leader in sports medicine. In addition to caring for the UNC Tar Heel teams, we also provide the highest quality care to professional and recreational athletes. Our orthopaedists have served as the team physicians for USA teams at the Olympic and Pan American Games as well as for the world championships in basketball, soccer and swimming. We have a dedicated team of specialists who have special interests and expertise in treating sports-related problems of the shoulder, knee, hand, foot and ankle. At UNC the patient always comes first.

PHYSICIAN LISTINGS

Orthopaedic Surgery

New England

Bierbaum, Benjamin MD (OrS) - *Spec Exp:* Hip Replacement; Knee Surgery; **Hospital:** New England Baptist; **Address:** 830 Boylston St, Ste 106, Chestnut Hill, MA 02467; **Phone:** (617) 277-1205; **Board Cert:** Orthopaedic Surgery 1993; **Med School:** Univ Iowa Coll Med 1960; **Resid:** Orthopaedic Surgery, Harvard Med Ctr, Boston, MA 1964-1967; Orthopaedic Surgery, Mass Genl Hosp, Boston, MA 1966; **Fellow:** Hip Surgery, Mass Genl Hosp, Boston, MA 1967-1968; **Fac Appt:** Clin Prof Orthopaedic Surgery, Tufts Univ

Boland Jr., Arthur L MD (OrS) - *Spec Exp:* Knee Surgery; Sports Medicine; **Hospital:** MA Genl Hosp; **Address:** 10 Hawthorne Pl, Ste 114, Boston, MA 02114; **Phone:** (617) 726-6917; **Board Cert:** Orthopaedic Surgery 1971; **Med School:** Cornell Univ-Weill Med Coll 1961; **Resid:** Surgery, NY Hosp-Cornell Med Ctr, New York, NY 1962-1963; Orthopaedic Surgery, Chldns Hosp Med Ctr, Boston, MA 1965-1969

Brick, Gregory MD (OrS) - *Spec Exp:* Hip & Knee Replacement; Spinal Surgery; Hip & Knee Replacement; **Hospital:** Brigham & Women's Hosp; **Address:** Brigham and Womens, Dept Orthopaedics, 75 Francis St, Boston, MA 02115; **Phone:** (617) 732-5386; **Board Cert:** Orthopaedic Surgery 1984; **Med School:** New Zealand 1976; **Fellow:** Brigham & Women's Hospital, Boston, MA 1985-1986; Orthopaedic Surgery, Vanderbuilt University Medical Center, Nashville, TN 1986-1987; **Fac Appt:** Assoc Clin Prof Orthopaedic Surgery, Harvard Med Sch

Browner, Bruce D MD (OrS) - *Spec Exp:* Fractures-Complex; Osteomyelitis; **Hospital:** Univ of Conn Hlth Ctr, John Dempsey Hosp; **Address:** 10 Talcott Notch Rd, Ste 100, Farmington, CT 06034-4037; **Phone:** (860) 679-6655; **Board Cert:** Orthopaedic Surgery 1997; **Med School:** SUNY Downstate 1973; **Resid:** Orthopaedic Surgery, Albany Med Ctr, Albany, NY 1973-1978; **Fellow:** Trauma, Albany Med Ctr, Albany, NY 1974-1975

Friedlaender, Gary MD (OrS) - *Spec Exp:* Bone Tumors; Limb Surgery; Fractures-Non Union; **Hospital:** Yale - New Haven Hosp; **Address:** Yale Univ Sch Med, Dept Ortho Surg, Box 208071, New Haven, CT 06520-8071; **Phone:** (203) 737-5656; **Board Cert:** Orthopaedic Surgery 1975; **Med School:** Univ Mich Med Sch 1969; **Resid:** Orthopaedic Surgery, Michigan Med Ctr, Ann Arbor, MI 1970-1971; Orthopaedic Surgery, Yale Med Ctr, New Haven, CT 1971-1974; **Fellow:** Muscular Skel Onc, Mass Genl Hosp, Boston, MA 1983; **Fac Appt:** Prof Orthopaedic Surgery, Yale Univ

Gebhardt, Mark MD (OrS) - *Spec Exp:* Musculoskeletal Tumors; Bone Tumors; **Hospital:** MA Genl Hosp; **Address:** 55 Fruit St, Gray Bldg-rm 606, Boston, MA 02114-2696; **Phone:** (617) 724-3700; **Board Cert:** Orthopaedic Surgery 1992; **Med School:** Univ Cincinnati 1975; **Resid:** Surgery, Univ Pittsburg Hlth Ctr, Pittsburgh, PA 1976-1977; Orthopaedic Surgery, Harvard Med Sch, Boston, MA 1978-1982; **Fellow:** Pediatric Orthopedic Surgery, Mass Genl Hosp-Boston Chldns Hosp, Boston, MA 1982-1983; **Fac Appt:** Assoc Prof Orthopaedic Surgery, Harvard Med Sch

Goldberg, Michael Jay MD (OrS) - *Spec Exp:* Orthopaedic Surgery-Pediatric; Congenital Malformations & Syndromes; Cerebral Palsy; **Hospital:** New England Med Ctr - Boston; **Address:** 750 Washington St, Box 202, Boston, MA 02111-1533; **Phone:** (617) 636-7922; **Board Cert:** Orthopaedic Surgery 1992; **Med School:** SUNY Downstate 1964; **Resid:** Surgery, Presby Hosp, New York, NY 1965-1966; Orthopaedic Surgery, Boston Hosps, Boston, MA 1967-1970; **Fac Appt:** Prof Orthopaedic Surgery, Tufts Univ

Jokl, Peter MD (OrS) - *Spec Exp:* Knee Surgery; Sports Medicine; **Hospital:** Yale - New Haven Hosp; **Address:** Yale Sports Medicine, Dept Orthopaedics, 800 Howard Ave, New Haven, CT 06519; **Phone:** (203) 785-2579; **Board Cert:** Orthopaedic Surgery 1974; **Med School:** Yale Univ 1968; **Resid:** Orthopaedic Surgery, Yale-New Haven Hosp, New Haven, CT 1969-1972; **Fac Appt:** Prof Orthopaedic Surgery, Yale Univ

Jupiter, Jesse B MD (OrS) - *Spec Exp:* Upper Extremity Trauma; Hand Surgery; **Hospital:** MA Genl Hosp; **Address:** 15 Parkman St Bldg WACC - rm 527, Boston, MA 02114-2698; **Phone:** (617) 726-8530; **Board Cert:** Orthopaedic Surgery 1982; **Med School:** Yale Univ 1972; **Resid:** Surgery, Mass Genl Hosp, Boston, MA 1975-1976; Orthopaedic Surgery, Mass Genl Hosp, Boston, MA 1976-1979; **Fellow:** Hand Surgery, Univ Louisville, Louisville, KY 1981; **Fac Appt:** Assoc Prof Orthopaedic Surgery, Harvard Med Sch

Kasser, James MD (OrS) - *Spec Exp:* Orthopaedic Surgery-Pediatric; **Hospital:** Children's Hospital - Boston; **Address:** Children's Hosp, Dept Orthopaedic Surgery, 300 Longwood Ave, Ste Hunnewell-2, Boston, MA 02115; **Phone:** (617) 355-6021; **Board Cert:** Orthopaedic Surgery 1984; **Med School:** Tufts Univ 1976; **Resid:** Orthopaedic Surgery, Tufts, Boston, MA 1978-1981; **Fellow:** Pediatric Orthopedic Surgery, Dupont Institute, Wilmington, DE; **Fac Appt:** Prof Orthopaedic Surgery, Harvard Med Sch

Lipson, Stephen Jay MD (OrS) - *Spec Exp:* Spinal Surgery; **Hospital:** Beth Israel Deaconess Med Ctr - Boston; **Address:** 133 Brookline Ave, Boston, MA 02215; **Phone:** (617) 421-5966; **Board Cert:** Orthopaedic Surgery 1980; **Med School:** Harvard Med Sch 1972; **Resid:** Surgery, Mass General Hosp, Boston, MA 1973-1974; Orthopaedic Surgery, Harvard Med Sch, Boston, MA 1974-1977; **Fac Appt:** Assoc Prof Orthopaedic Surgery, Harvard Med Sch

Micheli, Lyle J MD (OrS) - *Spec Exp:* Sports Medicine; Dance/Ballet Injuries; **Hospital:** Beth Israel Deaconess Med Ctr - Boston; **Address:** Children's Hospital, Div Sports Medicine, 300 Longwell Bldg Honnewell - Ste 202, Boston, MA 02115-5737; **Phone:** (617) 355-6028; **Board Cert:** Orthopaedic Surgery 1973; **Med School:** Harvard Med Sch 1966; **Resid:** Surgery, U Hospitals, Cleveland, OH 1967; Orthopaedic Surgery, Mass Genl Hospital, Boston, MA 1968-1972; **Fac Appt:** Assoc Clin Prof Orthopaedic Surgery, Harvard Med Sch

Reilly, Donald T. MD (OrS) - *Spec Exp:* Hip & Knee Replacement; **Hospital:** New England Baptist; **Address:** 125 Parker Hill Ave, Boston, MA 02120; **Phone:** (617) 232-6025; **Board Cert:** Orthopaedic Surgery 1984; **Med School:** Case West Res Univ 1975; **Resid:** Orthopaedic Surgery, Harvard 1977-1981

Scheller, Arnold MD (OrS) - *Spec Exp:* Sports Medicine; **Hospital:** New England Baptist; **Address:** 840 Winter St, Waltham, MA 02451; **Phone:** (781) 487-9444; **Board Cert:** Orthopaedic Surgery 1980; **Med School:** Rush Med Coll 1980; **Resid:** Orthopaedic Surgery, New England Hosp, Boston, MA 1981-1983; **Fac Appt:** Asst Clin Prof Orthopaedic Surgery, Tufts Univ

Scott, Richard David MD (OrS) - *Spec Exp:* Hip Replacement; Knee Replacement; **Hospital:** Brigham & Women's Hosp; **Address:** 125 Parker Hill Ave, Boston, MA 02120-2847; **Phone:** (617) 738-9151; **Board Cert:** Orthopaedic Surgery 1975; **Med School:** Temple Univ 1968; **Resid:** Orthopaedic Surgery, Mass General Hosp, Boston, MA 1971-1974; **Fellow:** Orthopaedic Surgery, Mass General Hosp, Boston, MA 1974; **Fac Appt:** Prof Orthopaedic Surgery, Harvard Med Sch

Thornhill, Thomas S MD (OrS) - *Spec Exp:* Hip & Knee Replacement; Arthritis; **Hospital:** Brigham & Women's Hosp; **Address:** 75 Francis St, Boston, MA 02115; **Phone:** (617) 732-5383; **Board Cert:** Internal Medicine 1973, Orthopaedic Surgery 1978; **Med School:** Cornell Univ-Weill Med Coll 1970; **Resid:** Internal Medicine, Peter Brent Brigham Hosp, Boston, MA 1970-1972; Orthopaedic Surgery, Harvard Combined Prog, Boston, MA 1975-1978; **Fac Appt:** Prof Orthopaedic Surgery, Harvard Med Sch

Zarins, Bertram MD (OrS) - *Spec Exp:* Knee Injuries; Arthroscopic Surgery; Sports Medicine; **Hospital:** MA Genl Hosp; **Address:** 15 Parkman St, Ste 514, Boston, MA 02114; **Phone:** (617) 726-3421; **Board Cert:** Orthopaedic Surgery 1994; **Med School:** SUNY Syracuse 1967; **Resid:** Surgery, Johns Hopkins Hosp, Baltimore, MD 1968-1969; Orthopaedic Surgery, Boston Hosp, Boston, MA 1970-1973; **Fellow:** Sports Medicine, Mass Genl Hosp, Boston, MA 1976; **Fac Appt:** Assoc Clin Prof Orthopaedic Surgery, Harvard Med Sch

Mid Atlantic

Balderston, Richard MD (OrS) - *Spec Exp:* Scoliosis; **Hospital:** Pennsylvania Hosp (page 78); **Address:** 800 Spruce St, Fl 1, Philadelphia, PA 19107; **Phone:** (215) 829-2222; **Board Cert:** Orthopaedic Surgery 1985; **Med School:** Univ Penn 1977; **Resid:** Orthopaedic Surgery, Hosp Univ Penn, Philadelphia, PA 1978-1982; **Fellow:** Spine Surgery, Univ Minn Affil Hosp, Minneapolis, MN 1982-1983; **Fac Appt:** Assoc Prof Orthopaedic Surgery, Univ Penn

Baratz, Mark E MD (OrS) - *Spec Exp:* Hand Surgery; Upper Extremity Surgery; **Hospital:** Allegheny General Hosp; **Address:** Allegheny Profl Bldg, 490 E North Ave, Ste 500, Pittsburgh, PA 15212; **Phone:** (412) 359-5196; **Board Cert:** Orthopaedic Surgery 1993, Hand Surgery 1994; **Med School:** Univ Pittsburgh 1984; **Resid:** Orthopaedic Surgery, Univ Hlth Ctr PA, Pittsburgh, PA 1987-1990; **Fellow:** Orthopaedic Surgery, Univ Hlth Ctr PA, Pittsburgh, PA 1985-1987; Hand Surgery, Med Coll of PA, Pittsburgh, PA 1990-1991; **Fac Appt:** Assoc Prof Orthopaedic Surgery, Med Coll PA Hahnemann

Bartolozzi, Arthur R. MD (OrS) - *Spec Exp:* Sports Medicine; **Hospital:** Pennsylvania Hosp (page 78); **Address:** 800 Spruce St, Fl 1, Philadelphia, PA 19107; **Phone:** (215) 829-2222; **Board Cert:** Orthopaedic Surgery 2000; **Med School:** UCSD 1981; **Resid:** Orthopaedic Surgery, Hosp Univ Penn, Philadelphia, PA 1982-1986; **Fellow:** Sports Medicine, UCLA Med Ctr, Los Angeles, CA 1986-1987; **Fac Appt:** Assoc Prof Orthopaedic Surgery, Univ Penn

Bauman, Phillip MD (OrS) - *Spec Exp:* Dance/Sports Medicine; Foot & Ankle Surgery; Knee Arthroscopy; **Hospital:** St Luke's - Roosevelt Hosp Ctr - Roosevelt Div (page 58); **Address:** 343 W 58th St, rm 1, Orthopaedic Associates of New York, New York, NY 10019; **Phone:** (212) 765-2260; **Board Cert:** Orthopaedic Surgery 1990; **Med School:** Columbia P&S 1981; **Resid:** St Luke's-Roosevelt Hosp Ctr, New York, NY 1981-1983; Orthopaedic Surgery, Columbia-Presby, New York, NY 1984-1987; **Fac Appt:** Asst Prof Orthopaedic Surgery, Columbia P&S

Benevenia, Joseph MD (OrS) - *Spec Exp:* Musculoskeletal Tumors; **Hospital:** UMDNJ-Univ Hosp-Newark; **Address:** 90 Bergen St, Ste 1200, Newark, NJ 07103; **Phone:** (973) 972-2150; **Board Cert:** Orthopaedic Surgery 1992; **Med School:** UMDNJ-NJ Med Sch, Newark 1984; **Resid:** Orthopaedic Surgery, UMDNJ-NJ Med Sch., Newark, NJ 1985-1988; **Fellow:** Orthopedic Oncology, Case Western Reserve Univ, Cleveland, OH 1990-1991; **Fac Appt:** Asst Prof Orthopaedic Surgery, UMDNJ-NJ Med Sch, Newark

Bigliani, Louis MD (OrS) - *Spec Exp:* Shoulder Surgery; Sports Medicine; **Hospital:** NY Presby Hosp - Columbia Presby Med Ctr (page 70); **Address:** 622 W 168th St, New York, NY 10032; **Phone:** (212) 305-5564; **Board Cert:** Orthopaedic Surgery 1979; **Med School:** Loyola Univ-Stritch Sch Med 1973; **Resid:** Surgery, St Lukes Hosp, New York, NY 1972-1974; Orthopaedic Surgery, Columbia Presby Med Ctr, New York, NY 1974-1977; **Fac Appt:** Prof Orthopaedic Surgery, Columbia P&S

Blaha, J David MD (OrS) - *Spec Exp:* Hip & Knee Replacement; **Hospital:** WV Univ Hosp - Ruby Memorial; **Address:** West Virginia Univ Hosp, PO Box 782, Morgantown, WV 26506-9196; **Phone:** (304) 598-4830; **Board Cert:** Orthopaedic Surgery 1979; **Med School:** Univ Mich Med Sch 1973; **Resid:** Surgery, Univ Mich, Ann Arbor, MI 1974-1975; Orthopaedic Surgery, Univ Mich, Ann Arbor, MI 1975-1978; **Fellow:** Joint Replacement Surgery, Univ London, London, England 1979-1980; **Fac Appt:** Prof Orthopaedic Surgery, W VA Univ

Boachie, Oheneba MD (OrS) - *Spec Exp:* Spinal Surgery; Scoliosis; **Hospital:** Hosp For Special Surgery (page 62); **Address:** Dept Orth Surgery, 535 E 70th St, New York, NY 10021; **Phone:** (212) 606-1948; **Board Cert:** Orthopaedic Surgery 2000; **Med School:** Columbia P&S 1980; **Resid:** Surgery, St Vincents Hosp, New York, NY 1981-1982; Orthopaedic Surgery, Hosp Spec Surg, New York, NY 1983-1986; **Fellow:** Orthopaedic Pathology, Hosp Spec Surg, New York, NY 1982-1983; Spine Surgery, Twin Cities Scol Ctr, Minneapolis, MN 1986-1987; **Fac Appt:** Assoc Clin Prof Surgery, Cornell Univ-Weill Med Coll

Booth, Robert MD (OrS) - *Spec Exp:* Knee Replacement; **Hospital:** Pennsylvania Hosp (page 78); **Address:** 800 Spruce St, Fl 1, Philadelphia, PA 19107; **Phone:** (215) 829-2214; **Board Cert:** Orthopaedic Surgery 1978; **Med School:** Univ Penn 1971; **Resid:** Surgery, Penn Hosp, Philadelphia, PA 1972-1973; Orthopaedic Surgery, Penn Hosp, Philadelphia, PA 1973-1977; **Fac Appt:** Clin Prof Orthopaedic Surgery, Jefferson Med Coll

Bradley, James P. MD (OrS) - *Spec Exp:* Sports Medicine; **Hospital:** UPMC - Presbyterian Univ Hosp; **Address:** Med Arts Bldg, 200 Delafield Ave, Ste 4010, Pittsburgh, PA 15215; **Phone:** (412) 661-5500; **Board Cert:** Orthopaedic Surgery 1990; **Med School:** Georgetown Univ 1982; **Resid:** Orthopaedic Surgery, Univ Hlth Ctr of Pitts, Pittsburgh, PA 1984-1987; Surgery, Univ TN, Chattanooga, TN 1982-1984; **Fellow:** Sports Medicine, Kerlan-Jobe Orth Clinic, Inglewood, CA 1987-1988; **Fac Appt:** Asst Clin Prof Orthopaedic Surgery, Univ Pittsburgh

Brushart, Thomas M MD (OrS) - *Spec Exp:* Hand Surgery; **Hospital:** Johns Hopkins Hosp - Baltimore; **Address:** 601 N Caroline St, Baltimore, MD 21287-0882; **Phone:** (410) 955-9663; **Board Cert:** Orthopaedic Surgery 1985, Hand Surgery 1989; **Med School:** Harvard Med Sch 1978; **Resid:** Orthopaedic Surgery, Harvard Univ, Boston, MA 1978-1981; **Fellow:** Hand Surgery, Curtis Hand Ctr, Baltimore, MD 1982-1983; **Fac Appt:** Prof Orthopaedic Surgery, Johns Hopkins Univ

Buly, Robert L MD (OrS) - *Spec Exp:* Hip Replacement/Reconstruction; Minimally Invasive Hip Surgery; Arthritis Surgery; **Hospital:** Hosp For Special Surgery (page 62); **Address:** Hospital for Special Surgery, 535 E 70th St, New York, NY 10021; **Phone:** (212) 606-1971; **Board Cert:** Orthopaedic Surgery 1993; **Med School:** Cornell Univ-Weill Med Coll 1985; **Resid:** Orthopaedic Surgery, Hosp for Special Surg, New York, NY 1986-1990; **Fellow:** Hip Surgery, Mueller Fdn, Bern Switzerland 1990-1991; Joint Reconstruction, Case Western Univ Hosp, Cleveland, OH 1991-1992; **Fac Appt:** Asst Prof Orthopaedic Surgery, Cornell Univ-Weill Med Coll

Burgess, Andrew MD (OrS) - *Spec Exp:* Trauma; **Hospital:** University of MD Med Sys; **Address:** 22 S Greene St, Ste S11B, Baltimore, MD 21201; **Phone:** (410) 328-6280; **Board Cert:** Orthopaedic Surgery 1980; **Med School:** Albany Med Coll 1975; **Resid:** Orthopaedic Surgery, Albany Med Coll, Albany, NY 1976-1979; **Fellow:** Trauma, MD Inst Emer Med, Baltimore, MD 1981-1982; **Fac Appt:** Asst Prof Surgery, Univ MD Sch Med

Cammisa Jr, Frank P MD (OrS) - *Spec Exp:* Spinal Surgery; Spinal Nucleoplasty; **Hospital:** Hosp For Special Surgery (page 62); **Address:** 523 E 72nd St, Fl 3, New York, NY 10021; **Phone:** (212) 606-1946; **Board Cert:** Orthopaedic Surgery 1990; **Med School:** Coll Physicians & Surgeons 1982; **Resid:** Surgery, Columbia-Presby Hosp, New York, NY 1982-1983; Orthopaedic Surgery, Hosp For Special Surgery, New York, NY 1983-1987; **Fellow:** Spine Surgery, Jackson Meml Hosp, Miami, FL 1987-1988; **Fac Appt:** Assoc Prof Orthopaedic Surgery, Cornell Univ-Weill Med Coll

Crossett, Lawrence MD (OrS) - *Spec Exp:* *Shoulder Surgery;* **Hospital:** UPMC - Presbyterian Univ Hosp; **Address:** Univ Orth, 3471 Fifth Ave Ste 1010, Pittsburgh, PA 15213; **Phone:** (412) 687-3900; **Board Cert:** Orthopaedic Surgery 2000; **Med School:** Temple Univ 1981; **Resid:** Orthopaedic Surgery, Shriners Hosp Crippled Chldn 1983-1984; Orthopaedic Surgery, Temple Univ, Philadelphia, PA 1984-1986; **Fac Appt:** Asst Prof Orthopaedic Surgery, Univ Pittsburgh

Delahay, John Norris MD (OrS) - *Spec Exp:* *Trauma; Orthopaedic Surgery-Pediatric;* **Hospital:** Georgetown Univ Hosp; **Address:** 3800 Reservoir Rd NW, PHC Bldg, Ground FL, Washington, DC 20007; **Phone:** (202) 687-1438; **Board Cert:** Orthopaedic Surgery 1975; **Med School:** Georgetown Univ 1969; **Resid:** Orthopaedic Surgery, Georgetown Univ Hosp, Washington, DC 1970-1974; **Fac Appt:** Prof Orthopaedic Surgery, Georgetown Univ

Deland, Jonathan T MD (OrS) - *Spec Exp:* *Foot & Ankle Surgery; Sports Medicine; Rheumatoid Arthritis-Reconstruction;* **Hospital:** Hosp For Special Surgery (page 62); **Address:** 523 E 72nd St, Ste 516, New York, NY 10021; **Phone:** (212) 606-1665; **Board Cert:** Orthopaedic Surgery 1992; **Med School:** Columbia P&S 1980; **Resid:** Orthopaedic Surgery, St Luke's-Roosevelt Hosp Ctr, Boston, MA 1980-1982; Orthopaedic Surgery, Mass Genl Hosp, Boston, MA 1982-1987; **Fac Appt:** Asst Prof Surgery, Cornell Univ-Weill Med Coll

Dines, David Michael MD (OrS) - *Spec Exp:* *Shoulder Surgery;* **Hospital:** N Shore Univ Hosp at Manhasset; **Address:** 935 Northern Blvd, Ste 303, Great Neck, NY 11021; **Phone:** (516) 482-1037; **Board Cert:** Orthopaedic Surgery 1980; **Med School:** UMDNJ-NJ Med Sch, Newark 1974; **Resid:** Surgery, NY Hosp-Cornell Med Ctr, New York, NY 1975-1976; Orthopaedic Surgery, Hosp for Special Surg, New York, NY 1976-1979; **Fac Appt:** Assoc Clin Prof Orthopaedic Surgery, Albert Einstein Coll Med

Donaldson III, William F MD (OrS) - *Spec Exp:* *Spinal Surgery;* **Hospital:** UPMC - Presbyterian Univ Hosp; **Address:** Univ Pitts Med Ctr, Dept Orth, 3471 5th Ave, Ste 1010, Pittsburgh, PA 15213; **Phone:** (412) 605-3218; **Board Cert:** Orthopaedic Surgery 1998; **Med School:** Rush Med Coll 1980; **Resid:** Surgery, Rush Presby-St Luke's Med Ctr, Chicago, IL 1980-1981; Orthopaedic Surgery, Hosp Special Surg, New York, NY 1981-1985; **Fellow:** Spine Surgery, Hosp Special Surg, New York, NY 1985-1986; **Fac Appt:** Asst Prof Orthopaedic Surgery, Univ Pittsburgh

Errico, Thomas MD (OrS) - *Spec Exp:* *Spinal Surgery; Spinal Microdiscectomy; Scoliosis;* **Hospital:** NYU Med Ctr (page 71); **Address:** 530 1st Ave, Ste 8U, NYU Medical Ctr, New York, NY 10016-6402; **Phone:** (212) 263-7182; **Board Cert:** Orthopaedic Surgery 1986; **Med School:** UMDNJ-NJ Med Sch, Newark 1978; **Resid:** Orthopaedic Surgery, New York Univ Med Ctr, New York, NY 1979-1983; **Fellow:** Univ Toronto, Toronto, Canada 1983-1984; **Fac Appt:** Assoc Clin Prof Orthopaedic Surgery, NYU Sch Med

Farcy, Jean-Pierre MD (OrS) - *Spec Exp:* *Spinal Surgery; Spinal Nucleoplasty;* **Hospital:** Maimonides Med Ctr (page 65); **Address:** 1301 57th St, Brooklyn, NY 11219; **Phone:** (718) 283-6520; **Med School:** France 1967; **Resid:** Orthopaedic Surgery, Univ Marseilles Med Ctr, France 1961-1967; **Fellow:** Orthopaedic Surgery, Columbia Presby Med Ctr, New York, NY 1981-1983; **Fac Appt:** Assoc Clin Prof Orthopaedic Surgery, NYU Sch Med

Feldman, David Steven MD (OrS) - *Spec Exp:* *Limb Deformity; Scoliosis; Cerebral Palsy;* **Hospital:** Hosp For Joint Diseases (page 61); **Address:** Hosp for Joint Diseases, 301 E 17th St, Ste 413A, New York, NY 10003; **Phone:** (212) 598-6699; **Board Cert:** Orthopaedic Surgery 1996; **Med School:** Albert Einstein Coll Med 1988; **Resid:** Orthopaedic Surgery, Hosp for Joint Diseases/NYU Med Ctr, New York, NY 1989-1993; **Fellow:** Pediatric Surgery, Hosp For Sick Chldn, Toronto, Canada 1993-1994; **Fac Appt:** Asst Prof Orthopaedic Surgery, NYU Sch Med

ORTHOPAEDIC SURGERY

Flatow, Evan MD (OrS) - *Spec Exp: Shoulder Replacement; Shoulder Injuries; Shoulder Surgery-Arthroscopic;* **Hospital:** Mount Sinai Hosp (page 68); **Address:** 5 E 98th St, FL 9, Box 1188, New York, NY 10029; **Phone:** (212) 241-1663; **Board Cert:** Orthopaedic Surgery 1989; **Med School:** Columbia P&S 1981; **Resid:** Surgery, St Luke's Roosevelt Hosp, New York, NY 1982-1983; Orthopaedic Surgery, Columbia-Presby Med Ctr, New York, NY 1983-1985; **Fellow:** Shoulder Surgery, Columbia-Presby Med Ctr, New York, NY 1986-1987; **Fac Appt:** Prof Orthopaedic Surgery, Columbia P&S

Frassica, Frank John MD (OrS) - *Spec Exp: Orthopaedic Surgery - General;* **Hospital:** Johns Hopkins Hosp - Baltimore; **Address:** 601 N Caroline St, rm 5212, Baltimore, MD 21287-0882; **Phone:** (410) 955-9300; **Board Cert:** Orthopaedic Surgery 1990; **Med School:** Univ SC Sch Med 1982; **Resid:** Orthopaedic Surgery, Mayo Clinic, Rochester, MN 1983-1987; **Fellow:** Orthopaedic Surgery, Mayo Clinic, Rochester, MN 1987-1988; **Fac Appt:** Prof Orthopaedic Surgery, Johns Hopkins Univ

Fu, Freddie MD (OrS) - *Spec Exp: Sports Medicine;* **Hospital:** UPMC - Presbyterian Univ Hosp; **Address:** Presbyterian Univ Hospital, Kaufmann Bldg, 3471 5th Ave, Ste 1011, Pittsburgh, PA 15213; **Phone:** (412) 605-3265; **Board Cert:** Orthopaedic Surgery 1984; **Med School:** Dartmouth Med Sch 1977; **Resid:** Orthopaedic Surgery, U Pittsburgh, Pittsburgh, PA 1979-1982; **Fellow:** Orthopaedic Surgery, U Pittsburgh, Pittsburgh, PA 1978-1979; **Fac Appt:** Prof Orthopaedic Surgery, Univ Pittsburgh

Grant, Richard E MD (OrS) - *Spec Exp: Hip & Knee Replacement; Spinal Surgery-Low Back;* **Hospital:** Howard Univ Hosp; **Address:** 1160 Varnum St NW Bldg DePaul - Ste 104, Washington, DC 20017; **Phone:** (202) 269-7383; **Board Cert:** Orthopaedic Surgery 1992; **Med School:** Howard Univ 1976; **Resid:** Orthopaedic Surgery, Wilford Hall Med Ctr-Lackland, San Antonio, TX 1980-1984; **Fellow:** Joint Arthroplasty, Ohio State Univ Hosp, Columbus, OH 1985; Spinal Cord Injury Medicine, St Lukes/Baylor Univ, Houston, TX 1986; **Fac Appt:** Assoc Prof Surgery, Howard Univ

Greisamer, Ronald MD (OrS) - *Spec Exp: Patella Problems; Sports Medicine; Hip & Knee Reconstruction;* **Hospital:** Maimonides Med Ctr (page 65); **Address:** 345 E 37th St, Ste 317A, New York, NY 10016-3256; **Phone:** (212) 535-4848; **Board Cert:** Orthopaedic Surgery 1987; **Med School:** Columbia P&S 1979; **Resid:** Surgery, Columbia Presby Med Ctr, New York, NY 1981-1984; **Fellow:** Orthopaedic Surgery, Columbia Presby Med Ctr, New York, NY 1984-1985

Hamilton, William MD (OrS) - *Spec Exp: Dance Medicine; Foot & Ankle Surgery; Sports Medicine;* **Hospital:** St Luke's - Roosevelt Hosp Ctr - Roosevelt Div (page 58); **Address:** 343 W 58th St, New York, NY 10019-1173; **Phone:** (212) 765-2260; **Board Cert:** Orthopaedic Surgery 1971; **Med School:** Columbia P&S 1964; **Resid:** Surgery, St Luke's-Roosevelt Hosp Ctr, New York, NY 1965-1966; Orthopaedic Surgery, Columbia-Presby Hosp, New York, NY 1966-1969; **Fellow:** Pediatric Orthopaedics, Newington Chldrn's Hosp, Newington, CT 1969-1970; **Fac Appt:** Clin Prof Orthopaedic Surgery, Columbia P&S

Hannafin, Jo MD/PhD (OrS) - *Spec Exp: Sports Medicine-Women;* **Hospital:** Hosp For Special Surgery (page 62); **Address:** 535 E 70th St, New York, NY 10021; **Phone:** (212) 606-1469; **Board Cert:** Orthopaedic Surgery 1994; **Med School:** Albert Einstein Coll Med 1985; **Resid:** Surgery, Montefiore Hosp Med Ctr, Bronx, NY 1986-1990; Orthopaedic Surgery, Montefiore Hosp Med Ctr, Bronx, NY 1990-1991; **Fellow:** Sports Medicine, Hosp Special Surg-Cornell Med Coll, New York, NY 1990-1992; **Fac Appt:** Asst Prof Surgery, Cornell Univ-Weill Med Coll

Hausman, Michael R MD (OrS) - *Spec Exp:* Hand Reconstruction; Elbow Reconstruction; Arthroscopic Surgery; **Hospital:** Mount Sinai Hosp (page 68); **Address:** 5 E 98th St, Box 1188, New York, NY 10029-6501; **Phone:** (212) 241-1658; **Board Cert:** Orthopaedic Surgery 1989, Hand Surgery 1990; **Med School:** Yale Univ 1979; **Resid:** Surgery, Yale-New Haven Hosp, New Haven, CT 1980-1981; Orthopaedic Surgery, Yale-New Haven Hosp, New Haven, CT 1982-1985; **Fellow:** Hand Surgery, Roosevelt Hosp, New York, NY 1986-1987; **Fac Appt:** Assoc Clin Prof Orthopaedic Surgery, Mount Sinai Sch Med

Healey, John MD (OrS) - *Spec Exp:* Bone Tumors; **Hospital:** Mem Sloan Kettering Cancer Ctr; **Address:** 1275 York Ave, Ste A-342, Ave, New York, NY 10021; **Phone:** (212) 639-7610; **Board Cert:** Orthopaedic Surgery 1997; **Med School:** Univ VT Coll Med 1978; **Resid:** Orthopaedic Surgery, Hosp for Spec Surg, New York, NY 1979-1983; **Fellow:** Orthopedic Oncology, Meml Sloan Kettering Cancer Ctr, New York, NY 1983-1984; Orthopaedic Surgery, Hosp For Spec Surg, New York, NY 1983-1984; **Fac Appt:** Assoc Prof Orthopaedic Surgery, Cornell Univ-Weill Med Coll

Helfet, David L MD (OrS) - *Spec Exp:* Fractures-Complex; Trauma; **Hospital:** Hosp For Special Surgery (page 62); **Address:** 535 E 70th St, New York, NY 10021; **Phone:** (212) 606-1888; **Board Cert:** Orthopaedic Surgery 1984; **Med School:** South Africa 1975; **Resid:** Surgery, Edendale Hosp, Pietermaritzburg, South Africa 1975-1977; Orthopaedic Surgery, Johns Hopkins, Baltimore, MD 1977-1981; **Fellow:** Orthopaedic Surgery, Inselspita Hosp, Bern, Switzerland 1981; Orthopaedic Surgery, UCLA Med Ctr, Los Angeles, CA 1981-1982; **Fac Appt:** Prof Orthopaedic Surgery, Cornell Univ-Weill Med Coll

Hotchkiss, Robert MD (OrS) - *Spec Exp:* Hand Surgery; Wrist Arthroscopy; **Hospital:** Hosp For Special Surgery (page 62); **Address:** 523 E 72nd St, Ste 441, New York, NY 10021; **Phone:** (212) 606-1964; **Board Cert:** Orthopaedic Surgery 2000, Hand Surgery 2000; **Med School:** Johns Hopkins Univ 1980; **Resid:** Surgery, Johns Hopkins Hosp, Baltimore, MD 1981-1982; Orthopaedic Surgery, Johns Hopkins Hosp, Baltimore, MD 1982-1985; **Fellow:** Hand Surgery, Union Meml Hosp, Baltimore, MD 1986-1987; **Fac Appt:** Assoc Prof Orthopaedic Surgery, Cornell Univ-Weill Med Coll

Johnson, Carl A MD (OrS) - *Spec Exp:* Knee Surgery; **Hospital:** Johns Hopkins Hosp - Baltimore; **Address:** Johns Hopkins Univ, Dept Orth Surg, 4940 Eastern Ave, Baltimore, MD 21287-0881; **Phone:** (410) 550-0453; **Board Cert:** Orthopaedic Surgery 1983; **Med School:** Johns Hopkins Univ 1976; **Resid:** Surgery, Johns Hopkins Hosp, Baltimore, MD 1977-1978; Orthopaedic Surgery, Johns Hopkins Hosp, Baltimore, MD 1978-1981; **Fac Appt:** Assoc Prof Orthopaedic Surgery, Johns Hopkins Univ

Lane, Joseph MD (OrS) - *Spec Exp:* Metabolic Bone Disease; Kyphoplasty for Osteoporosis; **Hospital:** Hosp For Special Surgery (page 62); **Address:** 535 E 70th St, Hospital for Special Surgery,Dept Ortho Surg, New York, NY 10021; **Phone:** (212) 606-1172; **Board Cert:** Orthopaedic Surgery 1974; **Med School:** Harvard Med Sch 1965; **Resid:** Orthopaedic Surgery, Hosp Univ Penn, Philadelphia, PA 1969-1973; Surgery, Hosp Univ Penn, Philadelphia, PA 1966-1967; **Fac Appt:** Prof Orthopaedic Surgery, Cornell Univ-Weill Med Coll

Lauerman, William MD (OrS) - *Spec Exp:* Spinal Deformities-Adult & Pediatric; Spinal Surgery; **Hospital:** Georgetown Univ Hosp; **Address:** 3800 Reservoir Rd NW, 1 Gorman - Spine Surgery Clinic, Washington, DC 20007; **Phone:** (202) 687-0655; **Board Cert:** Orthopaedic Surgery 1990; **Med School:** Georgetown Univ 1982; **Resid:** Orthopaedic Surgery, Georgetown Univ Med Ctr, Washington, DC 1982-1987; **Fellow:** Orthopaedic Surgery, Univ Minn-Twin Cities Scoliosis Ctr, Minneapolis, MN 1987-1988; **Fac Appt:** Assoc Prof Orthopaedic Surgery, Georgetown Univ

521

McAfee, Paul C MD (OrS) - *Spec Exp:* Spinal Surgery; Scoliosis; **Hospital:** St Joseph Med Ctr; **Address:** Scoliosis & Spine Ctr, 7505 Osler Drive, Ste 104, Towson, MD 21204; **Phone:** (410) 337-8888; **Board Cert:** Orthopaedic Surgery 1997; **Med School:** SUNY Syracuse 1979; **Resid:** Orthopaedic Surgery, SUNY Upstate Med Ctr, Syracuse, NY 1980-1984; **Fellow:** Spine Surgery, Case West Res Univ Hosps, OH 1984-1986; **Fac Appt:** Assoc Prof Orthopaedic Surgery, Johns Hopkins Univ

Myerson, Mark MD (OrS) - *Spec Exp:* Foot & Ankle Surgery; **Hospital:** Union Memorial Hosp - Baltimore; **Address:** 3333 N Calvert St, Ste 100, Baltimore, MD 21218; **Phone:** (410) 554-2866; **Board Cert:** Orthopaedic Surgery 1999; **Med School:** South Africa 1979; **Resid:** Orthopaedic Surgery, Johns Hopkins Hosp Univ MD, Baltimore, MD 1982-1985; Surgery, Sinai Hospital, Baltimore, MD 1980-1981; **Fellow:** Foot/Ankle Reconstruction, Hospital Joint Disease, New York, NY 1986

Nicholas, Stephen MD (OrS) - *Spec Exp:* Sports Medicine; Shoulder & Knee Surgery; Arthroscopic Surgery; **Hospital:** Lenox Hill Hosp (page 64); **Address:** 130 E 77th St, New York, NY 10021-1803; **Phone:** (212) 737-3301; **Board Cert:** Orthopaedic Surgery 1994; **Med School:** NY Med Coll 1986; **Resid:** Orthopaedic Surgery, Hosp For Special Surgery, New York, NY 1987-1991; **Fellow:** Sports Medicine, Lenox Hill Hosp, New York, NY 1991-1992

O'Leary, Patrick MD (OrS) - *Spec Exp:* Spinal Surgery; **Hospital:** Lenox Hill Hosp (page 64); **Address:** 1160 Park Ave, New York, NY 10128; **Phone:** (212) 249-8100; **Board Cert:** Orthopaedic Surgery 1976; **Med School:** Ireland 1968; **Resid:** Surgery, Roosevelt Hosp., New York, NY 1969-1972; Orthopaedic Surgery, Hosp Spec Surg-Cornell, New York, NY 1972-1975; **Fellow:** Spine Surgery, Univ Toronto Genl Hosp, Toronto, Canada 1975-1976; **Fac Appt:** Assoc Clin Prof Orthopaedic Surgery, Cornell Univ-Weill Med Coll

Osterman Jr, Arthur Lee MD (OrS) - *Spec Exp:* Hand Surgery; Wrist Arthroscopy; Neuromuscular Disorders; **Hospital:** Thomas Jefferson Univ Hosp; **Address:** Philadelphia Hand Center, 700 S Henderson Rd, Ste 200, King of Prussia, PA 19406; **Phone:** (610) 768-4467; **Board Cert:** Orthopaedic Surgery 1980, Hand Surgery 1990; **Med School:** Univ Penn 1973; **Resid:** Orthopaedic Surgery, Hosp Univ Penn, Philadelphia, PA 1974-1978; Orthopaedic Surgery, Hosp Univ Penn, Philadelphia, PA 1977-1978; **Fellow:** Hand Surgery, Hosp Univ Penn, Philadelphia, PA 1978-1979; Microvascular Surgery, Duke Univ Med Ctr, Durham, NC 1979-1980; **Fac Appt:** Prof Surgery, Jefferson Med Coll

Palmer, Andrew MD (OrS) - *Spec Exp:* Hand Surgery; **Hospital:** Univ. Hosp.- SUNY Upstate Med. Univ.; **Address:** SUNY Hlth Sci Ctr, Dept Orth, 550 Harrison Street, Ste 100, Syracuse, NY 13202-3096; **Phone:** (315) 464-4472; **Board Cert:** Orthopaedic Surgery 1978, Hand Surgery 1998; **Med School:** SUNY Syracuse 1972; **Resid:** Orthopaedic Surgery, Univ Mich, Ann Arbor, MI 1973-1976; **Fellow:** Hand Surgery, Mayo Clinic, Rochester, MN 1976; **Fac Appt:** Prof Orthopaedic Surgery, SUNY Syracuse

Ranawat, Chitranjan MD (OrS) - *Spec Exp:* Hip Surgery; Knee Surgery; Arthroscopic Surgery; **Hospital:** Lenox Hill Hosp (page 64); **Address:** 130 E 77th St, FL 11, New York, NY 10021-1851; **Phone:** (212) 434-4700; **Board Cert:** Orthopaedic Surgery 1969; **Med School:** India 1962; **Resid:** Surgery, MY Hosp, Indore, India 1959-1963; Orthopaedic Surgery, Albany Med Ctr, Albany, NY 1964-1965; **Fellow:** Orthopaedic Surgery, Hospital Special Surgery, New York, NY 1967-1969; **Fac Appt:** Prof Orthopaedic Surgery, Cornell Univ-Weill Med Coll

Rokito, Andrew MD (OrS) - *Spec Exp:* *Shoulder & Elbow Surgery; Ankle & Knee Surgery; Arthroscopic Surgery;* **Hospital:** Hosp For Joint Diseases (page 61); **Address:** 305 2nd Ave, Ste C-4, New York, NY 10003; **Phone:** (212) 598-6008; **Board Cert:** Orthopaedic Surgery 1996; **Med School:** Boston Univ 1988; **Resid:** Orthopaedic Surgery, Hosp Joint Diseases, New York, NY 1989-1993; **Fellow:** Orthopaedic Surgery, Kerlan-Jobe Clin, Inglewood, CA 1993-1994; **Fac Appt:** Asst Prof Orthopaedic Surgery, NYU Sch Med

Rosenwasser, Melvin MD (OrS) - *Spec Exp:* *Carpal Tunnel Syndrome; Hand Surgery;* **Hospital:** NY Presby Hosp - Columbia Presby Med Ctr (page 70); **Address:** 161 Fort Washington Ave, rm 251, New York, NY 10032; **Phone:** (212) 305-8036; **Board Cert:** Orthopaedic Surgery 1985, Hand Surgery 1989; **Med School:** Columbia P&S 1976; **Resid:** Surgery, St Lukes Roosevelt, New York, NY 1976-1979; Orthopaedic Surgery, Columbia Presby Med Ctr, New York, NY 1979-1982; **Fellow:** Hand Surgery, Columbia Presby Med Ctr, New York, NY 1982-1983; **Fac Appt:** Asst Prof Orthopaedic Surgery, Columbia P&S

Rosier, Randy MD/PhD (OrS) - *Spec Exp:* *Bone Disorders-Metabolic;* **Hospital:** Strong Memorial Hosp - URMC; **Address:** 601 Elmwood Ave, Box 655, Rochester, NY 14642; **Phone:** (716) 275-3100; **Board Cert:** Orthopaedic Surgery 2007; **Med School:** Univ Rochester 1978; **Resid:** Univ Iowa, Iowa City, IA 1979-1981; **Fellow:** Univ Iowa, Iowa City, IA 1982-1983

Rothman, Richard MD (OrS) - *Spec Exp:* *Hip & Knee Replacement;* **Hospital:** Thomas Jefferson Univ Hosp; **Address:** 925 Chesnut St, Fl 5, Rothman Inst, Philadelphia, PA 19107; **Phone:** (215) 955-3458; **Board Cert:** Orthopaedic Surgery 1970; **Med School:** Univ Penn 1962; **Resid:** Orthopaedic Surgery, Jefferson Hosp, Philadelphia, PA 1963-1968; **Fac Appt:** Prof Orthopaedic Surgery, Jefferson Med Coll

Roye, David MD (OrS) - *Spec Exp:* *Orthopaedic Surgery-Pediatric; Scoliosis;* **Hospital:** NY Presby Hosp - Columbia Presby Med Ctr (page 70); **Address:** Columbia Presby, Dept Ped Surg, 3959 Broadway Bldg 8 North, New York, NY 10032; **Phone:** (212) 305-5475; **Board Cert:** Orthopaedic Surgery 1981; **Med School:** Columbia P&S 1975; **Resid:** Orthopaedic Surgery, Columbia P&S, New York, NY 1976-1979; **Fellow:** Orthopaedic Surgery, Hosp For Sick Chldrn, Toronto, Canada 1979-1980; **Fac Appt:** Prof Orthopaedic Surgery, Columbia P&S

Salvati, Eduardo Augustin MD (OrS) - *Spec Exp:* *Hip Surgery; Hip & Knee Replacement;* **Hospital:** Hosp For Special Surgery (page 62); **Address:** Hosp for Spec Surg, 535 E 70th Street, New York, NY 10021-4872; **Phone:** (212) 606-1472; **Board Cert:** Orthopaedic Surgery 1972; **Med School:** Argentina 1963; **Resid:** Orthopaedic Surgery, Univ of Florence Orth Clinic, Florence, Italy 1963-1965; Orthopaedic Surgery, Hosp Buenos Aires, Buenos Aires, Argentina 1966-1969; **Fellow:** Hip Surgery, Hosp For Spec Surg, New York, NY 1969-1972; **Fac Appt:** Clin Prof Orthopaedic Surgery, Cornell Univ-Weill Med Coll

Sandhu, Harvinder S MD (OrS) - *Spec Exp:* *Spinal Fusion Disorders; Spinal Surgery;* **Hospital:** Hosp For Special Surgery (page 62); **Address:** 523 E 72nd St, New York, NY 10021; **Phone:** (212) 606-1798; **Med School:** Northwestern Univ 1987; **Resid:** Orthopaedic Surgery, UCLA Med Ctr, Los Angeles, CA 1987-1989; Orthopaedic Surgery, Univ Hosp-SUNY Hlth Sci Ctr, Brooklyn, NY 1989-1991

Scott, W Norman MD (OrS) - *Spec Exp:* *Knee Injuries; Knee Replacement; Sports Medicine;* **Hospital:** Beth Israel Med Ctr - Singer Div (page 58); **Address:** 170 East End Ave Fl 4, New York, NY 10128-7603; **Phone:** (212) 870-9740; **Board Cert:** Orthopaedic Surgery 1978; **Med School:** Cornell Univ-Weill Med Coll 1972; **Resid:** Surgery, St Luke's-Roosevelt Hosp Ctr, New York, NY 1973-1974; Orthopaedic Surgery, Hosp for Special Surgery, New York, NY 1974-1977; **Fac Appt:** Clin Prof Orthopaedic Surgery, Cornell Univ-Weill Med Coll

Sculco, Thomas Peter MD (OrS) - *Spec Exp: Hip & Knee Replacement; Arthroscopic Surgery; Minimally Invasive Hip Replacement;* **Hospital:** Hosp For Special Surgery (page 62); **Address:** 535 E 70th St, Ste 238, New York, NY 10021; **Phone:** (212) 606-1475; **Board Cert:** Orthopaedic Surgery 1976; **Med School:** Columbia P&S 1969; **Resid:** Surgery, St Luke's Rooselvelt, New York, NY 1970-1971; Orthopaedic Surgery, Hosp For Spec Surg, New York, NY 1971-1974; **Fellow:** Orthopaedic Surgery, London Hosp, London, England 1974-1975; **Fac Appt:** Prof Surgery, Cornell Univ-Weill Med Coll

Sherman, Orrin MD (OrS) - *Spec Exp: Knee Injuries/Ligament Surgery; Shoulder Surgery; Arthroscopic Surgery;* **Hospital:** NYU Med Ctr (page 71); **Address:** 530 1st Ave, Fl 8U, New York, NY 10016-6402; **Phone:** (212) 263-8961; **Board Cert:** Orthopaedic Surgery 1997; **Med School:** Geo Wash Univ 1978; **Resid:** Orthopaedic Surgery, NYU Med Ctr, New York, NY 1979-1983; **Fellow:** Sports Medicine, So Cal Med Ctr, Van Nuys, CA 1983-1984; **Fac Appt:** Asst Prof Orthopaedic Surgery, NYU Sch Med

Spivak, Jeffrey MD (OrS) - *Spec Exp: Spinal Surgery; Scoliosis;* **Hospital:** Hosp For Joint Diseases (page 61); **Address:** Hospital for Joint Diseases, Spine Center, 301 E 17th St, Ste 400, New York, NY 10003-3804; **Phone:** (212) 598-6696; **Board Cert:** Orthopaedic Surgery 1995; **Med School:** Cornell Univ-Weill Med Coll 1986; **Resid:** Orthopaedic Surgery, Hosp for Joint Diseases, New York, NY 1987-1992; **Fellow:** Spine Surgery, Thomas Jefferson Med Ctr, Philadelphia, PA 1992-1993; **Fac Appt:** Asst Prof Orthopaedic Surgery, NYU Sch Med

Sponseller, Paul D MD (OrS) - *Spec Exp: Cerebral Palsy; Scoliosis; Orthopaedic Surgery-Pediatric;* **Hospital:** Johns Hopkins Hosp - Baltimore; **Address:** 601 N Caroline St, Box 0882, Baltimore, MD 21287-0882; **Phone:** (410) 955-1795; **Board Cert:** Orthopaedic Surgery 2000; **Med School:** Univ Mich Med Sch 1980; **Resid:** Orthopaedic Surgery, Univ Wisc Hosp, Madison, WI 1980-1985; **Fellow:** Pediatric Orthopedic Surgery, Chldns Hosp, Boston, MA 1985-1986; **Fac Appt:** Prof Orthopaedic Surgery, Johns Hopkins Univ

Springfield, Dempsey MD (OrS) - *Spec Exp: Bone Tumors;* **Hospital:** Mount Sinai Hosp (page 68); **Address:** 5 E 98th St Fl 9, Box 1188, New York, NY 10029; **Phone:** (212) 241-8311; **Board Cert:** Orthopaedic Surgery 1992; **Med School:** Univ Fla Coll Med 1971; **Resid:** Orthopaedic Surgery, Univ Florida/Shands, Gainesville, FL 1972-1978; **Fellow:** Orthopaedic Surgery, Univ Florida/Shands, Gainesville, FL 1978-1979; **Fac Appt:** Prof Orthopaedic Surgery, Mount Sinai Sch Med

Strongwater, Allan MD (OrS) - *Spec Exp: Orthopaedic Surgery-Pediatric;* **Hospital:** Maimonides Med Ctr (page 65); **Address:** 927 49th St, Brooklyn, NY 11219-2923; **Phone:** (718) 283-7400; **Board Cert:** Orthopaedic Surgery 1986; **Med School:** Rush Med Coll 1978; **Resid:** Orthopaedic Surgery, Yale-New Haven Hosp, New Haven, CT 1978-1983; Orthopaedic Surgery, Hosp Joint Diseases, New York, NY 1983-1984; **Fac Appt:** Clin Prof Orthopaedic Surgery, SUNY Hlth Sci Ctr

Tischler, Henry MD (OrS) - *Spec Exp: Hip Replacement; Knee Replacement;* **Hospital:** Univ Hosp - Brklyn; **Address:** 506 6th St, Brooklyn, NY 11215; **Phone:** (718) 246-8700; **Board Cert:** Orthopaedic Surgery 1995; **Med School:** SUNY Downstate 1985; **Resid:** Orthopaedic Surgery, SUNY Downstate, Brooklyn, NY 1986-1990; **Fellow:** Orthopaedic Surgery, Tampa Gen Hosp/Fla Osteo Inst, Tampa, FL 1990-1991; **Fac Appt:** Asst Prof Orthopaedic Surgery, SUNY Hlth Sci Ctr

Waller, John F MD (OrS) - *Spec Exp: Foot Surgery; Ankle Surgery;* **Hospital:** Lenox Hill Hosp (page 64); **Address:** 133 E 58th St, Fl 14, New York, NY 10022-1258; **Phone:** (212) 583-2920; **Board Cert:** Orthopaedic Surgery 1979; **Med School:** NY Med Coll 1971; **Resid:** Orthopaedic Surgery, Lenox Hill Hosp, New York, NY 1974-1977; **Fellow:** Orthopaedic Surgery, Hosp For Special Surg, New York, NY 1978-1979

Wapner, Keith Leslie MD (OrS) - *Spec Exp:* *Foot Surgery;* **Hospital:** Hahnemann Univ Hosp; **Address:** The Farm Journal Bldg 5th FL., 230 W Washington Square, Philadelphia, PA 19106; **Phone:** (215) 829-3668; **Board Cert:** Orthopaedic Surgery 1999; **Med School:** Temple Univ 1980; **Resid:** Surgery, Hosp Univ Penn, Philadelphia, PA 1980-1981; Orthopaedic Surgery, Hosp Univ Penn, Philadelphia, PA 1981-1985; **Fellow:** Joint Reconstruction, Ohio St Univ Med Ctr, Columbus, OH 1985; Foot/Ankle Reconstruction, UCSF Med Ctr, San Francisco, CA 1986; **Fac Appt:** Prof Orthopaedic Surgery, Hahnemann Univ

Warren, Russell MD (OrS) - *Spec Exp:* *Knee Replacement; Shoulder Reconstruction & Replacement; Sports Medicine;* **Hospital:** Hosp For Special Surgery (page 62); **Address:** 535 E 70th St, New York, NY 10021-4892; **Phone:** (212) 606-1178; **Board Cert:** Orthopaedic Surgery 1974; **Med School:** SUNY Syracuse 1966; **Resid:** Surgery, St Luke's Hosp, New York, NY 1966-1968; Orthopaedic Surgery, Hosp For Special Surgery, New York, NY 1970-1973; **Fellow:** Shoulder Surgery, Columbia-Presby Med Ctr, New York, NY 1976; **Fac Appt:** Prof Orthopaedic Surgery, Cornell Univ-Weill Med Coll

Wickiewicz, Thomas MD (OrS) - *Spec Exp:* *Shoulder Surgery; Sports Medicine;* **Hospital:** Hosp For Special Surgery (page 62); **Address:** 525 E 71th St, New York, NY 10021; **Phone:** (212) 606-1450; **Board Cert:** Orthopaedic Surgery 1984; **Med School:** UMDNJ-NJ Med Sch, Newark 1976; **Resid:** Orthopaedic Surgery, Hosp for Special Surg, New York, NY 1977-1981; **Fellow:** Sports Medicine, UCLA, Los Angeles, CA 1981-1982; **Fac Appt:** Prof Orthopaedic Surgery, Cornell Univ-Weill Med Coll

Wiesel, Sam W MD (OrS) - *Spec Exp:* *Spinal Surgery;* **Hospital:** Georgetown Univ Hosp; **Address:** 3800 Reservoir Rd, Washington, DC 20007-2113; **Phone:** (202) 687-5203; **Board Cert:** Orthopaedic Surgery 1977; **Med School:** Univ Penn 1971; **Resid:** Orthopaedic Surgery, Univ Penn, Philadelphia, PA 1972-1973; **Fellow:** Orthopaedic Surgery, Univ Penn, Philadelphia, PA 1973-1976

Zuckerman, Joseph MD (OrS) - *Spec Exp:* *Shoulder Surgery; Hip & Knee Replacement; Minimally Invasive Surgery;* **Hospital:** Hosp For Joint Diseases (page 61); **Address:** Hosp for Joint Disease, Dept Orth, 301 E 17th St, Fl 14, New York, NY 10003-3804; **Phone:** (212) 598-6674; **Board Cert:** Orthopaedic Surgery 1992; **Med School:** Med Coll Wisc 1978; **Resid:** Orthopaedic Surgery, Univ WA Med Ctr, Seattle, WA 1979-1983; **Fellow:** Arthritis Surgery, Brigham & Woman's Hosp, Boston, MA 1983-1984; Shoulder Surgery, Mayo Clinic, Rochester, MN 1984; **Fac Appt:** Prof Orthopaedic Surgery, NYU Sch Med

Southeast

Beaty, James Harold MD (OrS) - *Spec Exp:* *Clubfoot; Orthopaedic Surgery-Pediatric; Cerebral Palsy;* **Hospital:** Campbell Clin; **Address:** Cambell Clinic, 910 Madison Ave, Memphis, TN 38103; **Phone:** (901) 759-3125; **Board Cert:** Orthopaedic Surgery 1995; **Med School:** Univ Tenn Coll Med, Memphis 1976; **Resid:** Surgery, Baptist Meml Hosp, Memphis, TN 1978-1979; Orthopaedic Surgery, Campbell Clin Fdn, Memphis, TN 1979-1981; **Fellow:** Pediatric Orthopedic Surgery, Alfred I Dupont Inst, Wilmington, DE 1981-1982; **Fac Appt:** Prof Orthopaedic Surgery, Univ Tenn Coll Med, Memphis

Cuckler, John MD (OrS) - *Spec Exp:* *Hip & Knee Replacement;* **Hospital:** Univ of Ala Hosp at Birmingham; **Address:** UAB Div Orthopaedics Bldg MEB - rm 508, 1813 6th Ave S, Birmingham, AL 35294; **Phone:** (205) 975-2663; **Board Cert:** Orthopaedic Surgery 1981; **Med School:** NYU Sch Med 1975; **Resid:** Orthopaedic Surgery, Hosp Univ Penn, Philadelphia, PA; **Fac Appt:** Prof Orthopaedic Surgery, Univ Ala

Curl, Walton Wright MD (OrS) - *Spec Exp: Sports Medicine;* **Hospital:** Wake Forest Univ Baptist Med Ctr (page 81); **Address:** 131 Miller St, Winston Salem, NC 27103; **Phone:** (336) 716-8091; **Board Cert:** Orthopaedic Surgery 1980; **Med School:** Duke Univ 1973; **Resid:** Orthopaedic Surgery, Letterman Army Med Ctr, San Francisco, CA 1975-1978; **Fellow:** Sports Medicine, Keller Army Hosp, West Point, NY 1978-1979; **Fac Appt:** Asst Prof Orthopaedic Surgery, Wake Forest Univ Sch Med

Eismont, Frank MD (OrS) - *Spec Exp: Spinal Surgery;* **Hospital:** Univ of Miami - Jackson Meml Hosp; **Address:** Univ Miami Sch Med, Dept Orth Surg, PO Box 016960, Miami, FL 33101; **Phone:** (305) 243-3000; **Board Cert:** Orthopaedic Surgery 1994; **Med School:** Univ Rochester 1973; **Resid:** Orthopaedic Surgery, Case Western Res Univ Hosp, Cleveland, OH 1975-1978; **Fellow:** Spine Surgery, Case Western Res Univ Hosp, Cleveland, OH 1978-1979; Spine Surgery, PA Hosp, Philadelphia, PA 1979-1980

Garrett, William MD (OrS) - *Spec Exp: Sports Medicine; Shoulder & Knee Surgery; Shoulder & Knee Reconstruction;* **Hospital:** Univ of NC Hosp (page 77); **Address:** Univ NC Sch Med, Dept Orthopaedics, Burnett Womack Bldg Rm 236 - CB 7055, Chapel Hill, NC 27599-7055; **Phone:** (919) 962-6637; **Board Cert:** Orthopaedic Surgery 1985; **Med School:** Duke Univ 1976; **Resid:** Orthopaedic Surgery, Duke Univ Med Ctr, Durham, NC 1976-1982; **Fac Appt:** Prof Orthopaedic Surgery, Univ NC Sch Med

Goldner, Richard MD (OrS) - *Spec Exp: Orthopaedic Surgery - General;* **Hospital:** Duke Univ Med Ctr (page 60); **Address:** Duke Univ Med Ctr, Dept Orth Surg, Box 3480, Durham, NC 27710; **Phone:** (919) 684-6461; **Board Cert:** Orthopaedic Surgery 1982, Hand Surgery 2000; **Med School:** Duke Univ 1974; **Resid:** Orthopaedic Surgery, Univ Virginia, Charlottesville, VA 1976-1980; Surgery, Duke Univ Med Ctr, Durham, NC 1975-1976; **Fellow:** Hand Surgery, Duke Univ Med Ctr, Durham, NC 1980-1981; **Fac Appt:** Assoc Prof Orthopaedic Surgery, Duke Univ

Green, Neil Edward MD (OrS) - *Spec Exp: Orthopaedic Surgery-Pediatric; Scoliosis & Kyphosis;* **Hospital:** Vanderbilt Univ Med Ctr (page 80); **Address:** Medical Center North, rm D4207, Nashville, TN 37232-0001; **Phone:** (615) 322-7133; **Board Cert:** Orthopaedic Surgery 1992; **Med School:** Albany Med Coll 1968; **Resid:** Surgery, Duke Univ Med Ctr, Durham, NC 1969-1970; Orthopaedic Surgery, Duke Univ Med Ctr, Durham, NC 1970-1974; **Fac Appt:** Prof Orthopaedic Surgery, Vanderbilt Univ

Grober, Ronald S MD (OrS) - *Spec Exp: Orthopaedic Surgery - General;* **Hospital:** Atlantic Med Ctr - Daytona; **Address:** 2000 Nebraska Ave, Ft Pierce, FL 34950-4833; **Phone:** (561) 464-3657; **Board Cert:** Orthopaedic Surgery 1973; **Med School:** Albert Einstein Coll Med 1962; **Resid:** Orthopaedic Surgery, Jacksonville Hosp, Jacksonville, FL 1967-1971; Orthopaedic Surgery, Naval Hosp, Philadelphia, PA 1965-1966; **Fellow:** Internal Medicine, Philadelphial Genl Hosp, Philadelphia, PA 1962-1963

Johnson, Darren Lee MD (OrS) - *Spec Exp: Knee Injuries; Sports Medicine;* **Hospital:** Univ Kentucky Med Ctr; **Address:** Dept Orthopaedic Surgery, 740 S Limestone, Ste K-401, Lexington, KY 40536-0284; **Phone:** (859) 257-4969; **Board Cert:** Orthopaedic Surgery 1995; **Med School:** UCLA 1987; **Resid:** Orthopaedic Surgery, LA Co-USC Med Ctr, Los Angeles, CA 1988-1992; **Fellow:** Sports Medicine, Univ Pittsburgh, Pittsburgh, PA 1992-1993; **Fac Appt:** Assoc Prof Orthopaedic Surgery, Univ KY Coll Med

Minkoff, Jeffrey MD (OrS) - *Spec Exp: Sports Medicine; Arthroscopy; Disorders of the Patella Femoral Joint;* **Hospital:** Cleveland Clin FL; **Address:** Cleveland Clinic, Dept Ortho Surgery, 3000 W Cypress Creek Rd, Ft Lauderdale, FL 33309; **Phone:** (954) 659-5432; **Board Cert:** Orthopaedic Surgery 1973; **Med School:** SUNY Downstate 1967; **Resid:** Orthopaedic Surgery, Bronx Muni Hosp, New York, NY 1968-1969; Orthopaedic Surgery, Lenox Hill Hosp, New York, NY 1969-1972

Perry, James MD (OrS) - *Spec Exp:* Hip Replacement; Knee Replacement; **Hospital:** St Luke's Hosp; **Address:** 4203 Belfort Rd, Ste 315, Jacksonville, FL 32216; **Phone:** (904) 296-0400; **Board Cert:** Orthopaedic Surgery 1982; **Med School:** Univ Fla Coll Med 1975; **Resid:** Orthopaedic Surgery, Dartmouth Affil Hosps, Hanover, NH 1976-1979; **Fellow:** Sports Medicine, Boston Chldns Hosp, Boston, MA; **Fac Appt:** Asst Prof Orthopaedic Surgery, Univ Fla Coll Med

Pettrone, Frank A MD (OrS) - *Spec Exp:* Sports Medicine; Shoulder & Knee Surgery; **Hospital:** Arlington Hosp; **Address:** 1635 N George Mason Drive, Ste 310, Arlington, VA 22205; **Phone:** (703) 525-6100; **Board Cert:** Orthopaedic Surgery 1975; **Med School:** Georgetown Univ 1969; **Resid:** Orthopaedic Surgery, Georgetown Hosp, Washington, DC 1970-1974

Poehling, Gary G. MD (OrS) - *Spec Exp:* Orthopaedic Surgery - General; **Hospital:** Wake Forest Univ Baptist Med Ctr (page 81); **Address:** 131 Miller St, Winston Salem, NC 27103; **Phone:** (336) 716-8091; **Board Cert:** Orthopaedic Surgery 1977, Hand Surgery 1989; **Med School:** Marquette Sch Med 1968; **Resid:** Orthopaedic Surgery, Duke Med Ctr., Durham, NC 1972-1976; Surgery, Duke Med Ctr., Durham, NC 1969-1970; **Fac Appt:** Prof Medicine, Wake Forest Univ Sch Med

Rechtine, Glenn MD (OrS) - *Spec Exp:* Spinal Surgery; **Hospital:** Shands Hlthcre at Univ of FL (page 73); **Address:** Shands Hlthcare, Univ Florida, 1600 Archer Rd, Box 100246, Gainesville, FL 32610; **Phone:** (352) 265-9400; **Board Cert:** Orthopaedic Surgery 1982; **Med School:** Univ S Fla Coll Med 1975; **Resid:** Orthopaedic Surgery, NRMC, Portsmouth, VA 1977-1980; **Fellow:** Spine Surgery, Case West Res Univ, Cleveland, OH 1980-1981; **Fac Appt:** Prof Orthopaedic Surgery, Univ Fla Coll Med

Scarborough, Mark MD (OrS) - *Spec Exp:* Bone Tumors; Sarcoma; **Hospital:** Shands Hlthcre at Univ of FL (page 73); **Address:** Shands Hlthcare Univ FL, 1600 SW Archer Rd, Box 100246, Gainesville, FL 32610-0246; **Phone:** (352) 392-4251; **Board Cert:** Orthopaedic Surgery 1993; **Med School:** Univ Fla Coll Med 1985; **Resid:** Orthopaedic Surgery, UT Med Ctr, Galveston, TX 1985-1990; **Fellow:** Orthopaedic Surgery, Mass Genl Hosp, Boston, MA 1990-1991; **Fac Appt:** Assoc Prof Orthopaedic Surgery, Univ Fla Coll Med

Spengler, Dan M MD (OrS) - *Spec Exp:* Spinal Surgery; **Hospital:** Vanderbilt Univ Med Ctr (page 80); **Address:** Vanderbilt Univ Med Ctr North, 1161 21st Ave S, rm D4221, Nashville, TN 37232-2550; **Phone:** (615) 343-6364; **Board Cert:** Orthopaedic Surgery 1974; **Med School:** Univ Mich Med Sch 1966; **Resid:** Orthopaedic Surgery, Univ Mich Med Ctr, Ann Arbor, MI 1967-1973; **Fellow:** Orthopaedic Surgery, Case West Res Hosp, Cleveland, OH 1973-1974; **Fac Appt:** Prof Orthopaedic Surgery, Vanderbilt Univ

Spindler, Kurt Paul MD (OrS) - *Spec Exp:* Sports Medicine; Arthroscopic Surgery; **Hospital:** Vanderbilt Univ Med Ctr (page 80); **Address:** Vanderbilt Sports Med Ctr, 2601 Jess Neely Dr, McGugin Ctr, Nashville, TN 37212; **Phone:** (615) 343-1685; **Board Cert:** Orthopaedic Surgery 1993; **Med School:** Univ Penn 1985; **Resid:** Orthopaedic Surgery, Univ Penn, Philadelphia, PA 1986-1990; **Fellow:** Sports Medicine, Cleveland Clinic Fdn, Cleveland, OH 1990-1991; **Fac Appt:** Assoc Prof Orthopaedic Surgery, Vanderbilt Univ

Taft, Timothy MD (OrS) - *Spec Exp:* Sports Medicine; Ligament Injuries; Shoulder Impingement Syndrome; **Hospital:** Univ of NC Hosp (page 77); **Address:** UNC Orthopaedics, CB # 7055, Chapel Hill, NC 27599-7055; **Phone:** (919) 962-6637; **Board Cert:** Orthopaedic Surgery 1976; **Med School:** Univ MO-Columbia Sch Med 1969; **Resid:** Orthopaedic Surgery, Univ North Carolina Hosps, Chapel Hill, NC 1970-1974; Orthopaedic Surgery, North Carolina Ortho Hosp, Gastonia, NC 1972; **Fac Appt:** Prof Orthopaedic Surgery, Univ NC Sch Med

Uribe, John MD (OrS) - *Spec Exp: Shoulder & Elbow Surgery; Arthroscopic Surgery; Sports Medicine;* **Hospital:** Healthsouth Doctor's Hosp; **Address:** 1150 Campo Sano Ave, Ste 200, Coral Gables, FL 33146-6960; **Phone:** (305) 669-3320; **Board Cert:** Orthopaedic Surgery 1982; **Med School:** Univ NC Sch Med 1976; **Resid:** Orthopaedic Surgery, Jackson Meml Hosp-Univ Miami, Miami, FL 1977-1981; **Fellow:** Sports Medicine, Hughston Sports Med Hosp, Columbus, OH 1984-1985; **Fac Appt:** Assoc Prof Orthopaedic Surgery, Univ Miami Sch Med

Vail, Thomas Parker MD (OrS) - *Spec Exp: Hip & Knee Replacement; Arthritis;* **Hospital:** Duke Univ Med Ctr (page 60); **Address:** Duke Univ Med Ctr, PO Box 3332, Durham, NC 27710; **Phone:** (919) 684-6166; **Board Cert:** Orthopaedic Surgery 1994; **Med School:** Loyola Univ-Stritch Sch Med 1985; **Resid:** Thoracic Surgery, Duke Univ Med Ctr, Durham, NC 1986-1987; Orthopaedic Surgery, Duke Univ Med Ctr, Durham, NC 1987-1991; **Fellow:** Sports Medicine, North Amer/Euro Trav Prgm 1991-1992; **Fac Appt:** Assoc Prof Orthopaedic Surgery, Duke Univ

Webb, Lawrence MD (OrS) - *Spec Exp: Trauma; Foot & Ankle Surgery;* **Hospital:** Wake Forest Univ Baptist Med Ctr (page 81); **Address:** Wake Forest Baptist Med Ctr, Med Center Blvd, Winston Salem, NC 27157-1070; **Phone:** (336) 716-3606; **Board Cert:** Orthopaedic Surgery 1997; **Med School:** Temple Univ 1978; **Resid:** Orthopaedic Surgery, Bowman Gray Sch Med Ctr, Winston-Salem, NC 1979-1983; **Fellow:** Trauma, Harborview Med Ctr, Seattle, WA 1983-1984; **Fac Appt:** Assoc Prof Medicine, Wake Forest Univ Sch Med

Weiner, Richard MD (OrS) - *Spec Exp: Knee Surgery; Shoulder Surgery; Trauma;* **Hospital:** St Mary's Med Ctr - W Palm Bch; **Address:** 733 US Highway 1, North Palm Beach, FL 33403-4508; **Phone:** (561) 840-1090; **Board Cert:** Orthopaedic Surgery 1993; **Med School:** Univ Penn 1986; **Resid:** Orthopaedic Surgery, UMDNJ-Univ Hosp-Newark, Newark, NJ 1987-1991

Midwest

Aamoth, Gordon MD (OrS) - *Spec Exp: Limb Surgery;* **Hospital:** Abbott - Northwestern Hosp; **Address:** Minneapolis Ortho & Arth Inst, 825 S 8th St, Ste 550, Minneapolis, MN 55404; **Phone:** (612) 333-5000; **Board Cert:** Orthopaedic Surgery 1992; **Med School:** Northwestern Univ 1966; **Resid:** Orthopaedic Surgery, Moffitt Hosp-UCSF, San Francisco, CA 1973; **Fac Appt:** Clin Prof Surgery, Univ Minn

Bach Jr, Bernard R MD (OrS) - *Spec Exp: Sports Medicine; Knee Surgery; Ligament Injuries-ACL;* **Hospital:** Rush-Presby - St Luke's Med Ctr (page 72); **Address:** 1725 W Harrison St, Ste 1063, Chicago, IL 60612; **Phone:** (312) 243-4244; **Board Cert:** Orthopaedic Surgery 2000; **Med School:** Univ Cincinnati 1979; **Resid:** Surgery, New England Deaconess Hosp, Boston, MA 1980-1981; Orthopaedic Surgery, Mass Genl Hosp, Boston, MA 1981-1985; **Fellow:** Sports Medicine, Hosp Special Surg, New York, NY 1985-1986; **Fac Appt:** Prof Orthopaedic Surgery, Rush Med Coll

Bergfeld, John MD (OrS) - *Spec Exp: Sports Medicine;* **Hospital:** Cleveland Clin Fdn (page 57); **Address:** 9500 Euclid Ave, Ste A41, Cleveland, OH 44195-5027; **Phone:** (216) 444-2618; **Board Cert:** Orthopaedic Surgery 1972; **Med School:** Temple Univ 1964; **Resid:** Orthopaedic Surgery, Cleveland Clinic, Cleveland, OH 1966-1970; Surgery, Cleveland Clinic, Cleveland, OH 1966

Bohlman, Henry H MD (OrS) - *Spec Exp: Spinal Surgery;* **Hospital:** Univ Hosp of Cleveland; **Address:** 11100 Euclid Ave, Cleveland, OH 44106-1736; **Phone:** (216) 844-1025; **Board Cert:** Orthopaedic Surgery 1972; **Med School:** Univ MD Sch Med 1964; **Resid:** Surgery, Baltimore U Hosp, Baltimore, MD 1964-1966; Orthopaedic Surgery, Johns Hopkins Hosp, Baltimore, MD 1966-1970; **Fellow:** Spine Surgery, Johns Hopkins Hosp, Baltimore, MD 1967-1968; **Fac Appt:** Prof Orthopaedic Surgery, Case West Res Univ

Bridwell, Keith MD (OrS) - *Spec Exp:* Scoliosis; Spinal Surgery; **Hospital:** Barnes-Jewish Hosp (page 55); **Address:** Washington Univ Sch Med, Dept Orthopedic Surgery, 1 Barnes Hospital Plaza, Ste 11300, St. Louis, MO 63110; **Phone:** (314) 362-4080; **Board Cert:** Orthopaedic Surgery 1985; **Med School:** Washington Univ, St Louis 1977; **Resid:** Orthopaedic Surgery, Barnes Hosptial, St. Louis, MO 1978-1981; **Fellow:** Scoliosis, Rush Med Coll, Chicago, IL 1982; **Fac Appt:** Prof Orthopaedic Surgery, Washington Univ, St Louis

Callaghan, John J MD (OrS) - *Spec Exp:* Hip & Knee Replacement; Sports Medicine; **Hospital:** Univ of IA Hosp and Clinics; **Address:** Dept Orthopaedics, 200 Hawkins Drive, Iowa City, IA 52242; **Phone:** (319) 356-3110; **Board Cert:** Orthopaedic Surgery 1985; **Med School:** Loyola Univ-Stritch Sch Med 1978; **Resid:** Orthopaedic Surgery, Univ IA Hosp Clin, Iowa City, IA 1979-1983; **Fellow:** Orthopaedic Surgery, Hosp Special Surg, New York, NY 1983-1984; **Fac Appt:** Prof Orthopaedic Surgery, Univ Iowa Coll Med

Cofield, Robert H MD (OrS) - *Spec Exp:* Shoulder Surgery; **Hospital:** Mayo Med Ctr & Clin - Rochester, MN; **Address:** Dept of Orthopedic Surgery, 200 1st St SW, Rochester, MN 55905; **Phone:** (507) 284-2511; **Board Cert:** Orthopaedic Surgery 1976; **Med School:** Univ KY Coll Med 1969; **Resid:** Surgery, Charity Hosp - Tulane Div, New Orleans, LA 1969-1971; Orthopaedic Surgery, Mayo Clinic, Rochester, MN 1971-1975; **Fac Appt:** Prof Orthopaedic Surgery, Mayo Med Sch

Gage, James MD (OrS) - *Spec Exp:* Orthopaedic Surgery-Pediatric; **Hospital:** Gillette Chldn's Specialty Hlthcre; **Address:** Pediatric Orthopedic Associates, 200 E University Ave, St Paul, MN 55101; **Phone:** (651) 290-8707; **Board Cert:** Orthopaedic Surgery 1983; **Med School:** Northwestern Univ 1964; **Resid:** Orthopaedic Surgery, Minneapolis VA Hosp, Minneapolis, MN 1967-1971; **Fac Appt:** Prof Orthopaedic Surgery, Univ Minn

Galante, Jorge O MD (OrS) - *Spec Exp:* Knee & Hip Surgery; Hip & Knee Replacement; **Hospital:** Rush-Presby - St Luke's Med Ctr (page 72); **Address:** 1725 W Harrison St, Ste 1063, Chicago, IL 60612; **Phone:** (312) 243-4244; **Board Cert:** Orthopaedic Surgery 1968; **Med School:** Argentina 1958; **Resid:** Orthopaedic Surgery, Michael Reese Hosp, Chicago, IL 1959-1961; **Fellow:** Orthopaedic Surgery, Univ Goteborg, Sweden 1964-1967; **Fac Appt:** Prof Orthopaedic Surgery, Rush Med Coll

Goitz, Henry MD (OrS) - *Spec Exp:* Sports Medicine; Arthroscopic Surgery; **Hospital:** Med Coll of Ohio Hosps; **Address:** 3065 Arlington Ave Bldg Dowling Hall - rm 2440, Toledo, OH 43614-5807; **Phone:** (419) 383-4020; **Board Cert:** Orthopaedic Surgery 1995; **Med School:** Rutgers Univ 1985; **Resid:** Surgery, Univ Virginia, Charlottesville, VA 1986-1987; Orthopaedic Surgery, Univ Virginia, Charlottesville, VA 1987-1991; **Fellow:** Hand Surgery, Univ Virginia, Charlottesville, VA 1991; Sports Medicine, Am Sports Med Inst, Birmingham, AL 1992; **Fac Appt:** Prof Orthopaedic Surgery, Med Coll OH

Goldberg, Victor M MD (OrS) - *Spec Exp:* Hip & Knee Replacement; Arthritis; **Hospital:** Univ Hosp of Cleveland; **Address:** Case Western Res Univ, Dept Ortho Surg, 11100 Euclid Ave, Cleveland, OH 44106-2602; **Phone:** (216) 844-3044; **Board Cert:** Orthopaedic Surgery 1973; **Med School:** SUNY Downstate 1964; **Resid:** Surgery, Univ Hosp, Cleveland, OH 1965-1966; Orthopaedic Surgery, Spl Surg Hosp, New York, NY 1968-1971; **Fac Appt:** Prof Orthopaedic Surgery, Case West Res Univ

Goldstein, Wayne MD (OrS) - *Spec Exp:* Hip Replacement; Knee Replacement; **Hospital:** Advocate Lutheran Gen Hosp; **Address:** 150 N River Rd, Ste 160, Des Plaines, IL 60016; **Phone:** (847) 375-3000; **Board Cert:** Orthopaedic Surgery 1986; **Med School:** Univ IL Coll Med 1978; **Resid:** Orthopaedic Surgery, Univ IL Med Ctr, Chicago, IL 1979-1983; **Fellow:** Orthopaedic Surgery, Harvard Med Ctr, Cambridge, MA 1983-1984; **Fac Appt:** Asst Clin Prof Orthopaedic Surgery, Univ Chicago-Pritzker Sch Med

Graf, Ben K MD (OrS) - *Spec Exp:* Sports Medicine; **Hospital:** Univ WI Hosp & Clins; **Address:** 600 Highland Ave, rm K4-735, Madison, WI 53792; **Phone:** (608) 263-8850; **Board Cert:** Orthopaedic Surgery 1998; **Med School:** Univ Wisc 1979; **Resid:** Univ Wisconsin Hosps, Madison, WI 1980-1984; **Fellow:** Sports Medicine, Long Beach Meml Hosp 1984-1985; **Fac Appt:** Assoc Prof Surgery, Univ Wisc

Hensinger, Robert MD (OrS) - *Spec Exp:* Orthopaedic Surgery-Pediatric; Spinal Surgery-Pediatric; **Hospital:** Univ of MI Hlth Ctr; **Address:** Univ Michigan Med Ctr, Dept Ortho Surg, 2912 Taubman Ctr, 1500 E Medical Ctr Dr, Ann Arbor, MI 48109-0328; **Phone:** (734) 936-5780; **Board Cert:** Orthopaedic Surgery 1992; **Med School:** Univ Mich Med Sch 1964; **Resid:** Orthopaedic Surgery, Univ Michigan, Ann Arbor, MI 1965-1966; Orthopaedic Surgery, Univ Michigan, Ann Arbor, MI 1968-1971; **Fellow:** Pediatric Orthopedic Surgery, Al DuPont Inst, Wilmington, NC 1971-1972

Iannotti, Joseph MD (OrS) - *Spec Exp:* Shoulder Surgery; **Hospital:** Cleveland Clin Fdn (page 57); **Address:** 9500 Euclid Ave/Desk A41, Cleveland, OH 44195; **Phone:** (216) 445-5151; **Board Cert:** Orthopaedic Surgery 1987; **Med School:** Northwestern Univ 1979; **Resid:** Orthopaedic Surgery, Hosp U Penn, Philadelphia, PA 1980-1984; **Fellow:** Orthopaedic Surgery, Hosp U Penn, Philadelphia, PA 1984-1985

Lock, Terrence Ralph MD (OrS) - *Spec Exp:* Sports Medicine; **Hospital:** Henry Ford Hosp; **Address:** 6525 2nd Ave, Detroit, MI 48202; **Phone:** (313) 972-4065; **Board Cert:** Orthopaedic Surgery 1991; **Med School:** Wayne State Univ 1983; **Resid:** Orthopaedic Surgery, Wayne St Univ Sch Med, Detroit, MI 1984-1988; **Fellow:** Sports Medicine, Mass Genl Hosp, Boston, MA 1988-1989

Mallory, Thomas MD (OrS) - *Spec Exp:* Hip & Knee Replacement; **Hospital:** Ohio St Univ Med Ctr; **Address:** 720 E Broad St, Columbus, OH 43215; **Phone:** (614) 221-6331; **Board Cert:** Orthopaedic Surgery 1972; **Med School:** Ohio State Univ 1965; **Resid:** Orthopaedic Surgery, Ohio State Univ Hosp, Colombus, OH 1966-1970; **Fellow:** Hip Surgery, Harvard Med Sch, Boston, MA 1970-1971; **Fac Appt:** Asst Clin Prof Orthopaedic Surgery, Ohio State Univ

Manoli II, Arthur MD (OrS) - *Spec Exp:* Foot & Ankle Surgery; **Hospital:** St Joseph Mercy - Oakland; **Address:** 44555 Woodward Ave, Ste 105, Pontiac, MI 48341-5032; **Phone:** (248) 858-6773; **Board Cert:** Orthopaedic Surgery 1992; **Med School:** Univ Mich Med Sch 1970; **Resid:** Surgery, Oakwood Hosp, Dearborn, MI 1971-1972; Orthopaedic Surgery, Wayne St Univ Affil Hosps, Detroit, MI 1972-1975; **Fellow:** Ankle and Foot Surgery, Univ Wash/Vanderbilt Univ, Seattle, WA 1989-1990

Martell, John Mark MD (OrS) - *Spec Exp:* Hip & Knee Replacement; Knee Surgery; **Hospital:** Univ of Chicago Hosps (page 76); **Address:** 5841 S Maryland Ave, MC 3079, Chicago, IL 60637; **Phone:** (773) 702-7297; **Board Cert:** Orthopaedic Surgery 1991; **Med School:** Univ Chicago-Pritzker Sch Med 1983; **Resid:** Orthopaedic Surgery, U Chicago Med Ctr, Chicago, IL 1984-1988; **Fellow:** Joint Replacement Surgery, Rush Presby-St Luke's Med Ctr, Chicago, IL 1988-1989; **Fac Appt:** Asst Prof Orthopaedic Surgery, Univ Chicago-Pritzker Sch Med

Nuber, Gordon MD (OrS) - *Spec Exp:* *Shoulder Reconstruction; Cartilage Problems; Elbow Surgery;* **Hospital:** Northwestern Meml Hosp; **Address:** Northwestern Orth Inst, 680 N Lakeshore Dr, Ste 1028, Chicago, IL 60611; **Phone:** (312) 664-6848; **Board Cert:** Orthopaedic Surgery 1986; **Med School:** Wayne State Univ 1978; **Resid:** Orthopaedic Surgery, Northwestern Meml Hosp, Chicago, IL 1978-1983; **Fellow:** Sports Medicine, Natl Hlth Inst, Ingelwood, CA 1983-1984; **Fac Appt:** Clin Prof Orthopaedic Surgery, Northwestern Univ

Riew, K Daniel MD (OrS) - *Spec Exp:* *Cervical Spine Surgery; Minimally Invasive Surgery-Spine; Spinal Microsurgery;* **Hospital:** Barnes-Jewish Hosp (page 55); **Address:** 1 Barnes-Jewish Hosp Plaza, West Pavilion, Ste 11300, St. Louis, MO 63110; **Phone:** (314) 747-2500; **Board Cert:** Internal Medicine 1987, Orthopaedic Surgery 1997; **Med School:** Case West Res Univ 1984; **Resid:** Internal Medicine, NY Hosp - Cornell Med Ctr, New York, NY 1984-1987; Orthopaedic Surgery, George Wash Univ Med Ctr, Washington, DC 1990-1994; **Fellow:** Spine Surgery, Case Western, Cleveland, OH 1994-1995; **Fac Appt:** Assoc Prof Orthopaedic Surgery, Washington Univ, St Louis

Saltzman, Charles Louis MD (OrS) - *Spec Exp:* *Foot & Ankle Surgery;* **Hospital:** Univ of IA Hosp and Clinics; **Address:** Dept Orthopaedic Surgery, 200 Hawkins, MC 01017-JPP, Iowa City, IA 52242; **Phone:** (319) 356-7149; **Board Cert:** Orthopaedic Surgery 1993; **Med School:** Univ NC Sch Med 1985

Schafer, Michael F MD (OrS) - *Spec Exp:* *Sports Medicine; Spinal Surgery; Scoliosis;* **Hospital:** Northwestern Meml Hosp; **Address:** 675 N St. Clair, Ste 17-100, Chicago, IL 60611-5968; **Phone:** (312) 695-6800; **Board Cert:** Orthopaedic Surgery 1983; **Med School:** Univ Iowa Coll Med 1967; **Resid:** Orthopaedic Surgery, Northwestern Univ Hospitals, Chicago, IL 1968-1972; **Fellow:** Spine Surgery, Natl Fdn Traveling Fellowship, Sydney, Australia 1972; **Fac Appt:** Prof Orthopaedic Surgery, Northwestern Univ

Shelbourne, K Donald MD (OrS) - *Spec Exp:* *Sports Medicine; Knee Surgery;* **Hospital:** Methodist Hosp - Indianapolis (page 66); **Address:** 1815 N Capitol Ave, Ste 530, Indianapolis, IN 46202-1288; **Phone:** (317) 924-8636; **Board Cert:** Orthopaedic Surgery 1984; **Med School:** Indiana Univ 1976; **Resid:** Orthopaedic Surgery, Indiana Univ Hosp, Indianapolis, IN 1977-1981; **Fellow:** Sports Medicine, Univ of WI, Madison, WI 1981-1982; **Fac Appt:** Assoc Clin Prof Orthopaedic Surgery, Indiana Univ

Simon, Michael MD (OrS) - *Spec Exp:* *Bone Tumors; Soft Tissue Tumors; Sarcoma;* **Hospital:** Univ of Chicago Hosps (page 76); **Address:** 5841 S Maryland Ave, MC 3079, Chicago, IL 60637; **Phone:** (773) 702-6144; **Board Cert:** Orthopaedic Surgery 1975; **Med School:** Univ Mich Med Sch 1967; **Resid:** Surgery, Univ Mich Med Ctr, Ann Arbor, MI 1968-1969; Orthopaedic Surgery, Univ Mich Med Ctr, Ann Arbor, MI 1971-1974; **Fellow:** Orthopedic Oncology, Univ Fla, Gainesville, FL 1974-1975; **Fac Appt:** Prof Surgery, Univ Chicago-Pritzker Sch Med

Stulberg, Samuel David MD (OrS) - *Spec Exp:* *Shoulder Replacement; Hip & Knee Replacement; Arthritic Reconstruction;* **Hospital:** Northwestern Meml Hosp; **Address:** 680 N Lake Shore Drive, Ste 1028, Chicago, IL 60611; **Phone:** (312) 664-6848; **Board Cert:** Orthopaedic Surgery 1977; **Med School:** Univ Mich Med Sch 1969; **Resid:** Orthopaedic Surgery, Mass Genl Hosp, Boston, MA 1970-1971; Orthopaedic Surgery, Harvard Med Ctr, Boston, MA 1972-1974; **Fellow:** Research, Sick Childrens Hosp, Toronto, Canada 1975-1976; **Fac Appt:** Prof Orthopaedic Surgery, Northwestern Univ

Swiontkowski, Marc F MD (OrS) - *Spec Exp:* *Osteomyelitis; Fractures-Non Union; Trauma;* **Hospital:** Fairview-Univ Med Ctr - Univ Campus; **Address:** Univ Minn Med Sch, Mayo Meml Bldg, 420 Delaware St SE, MMC-492, Minneapolis, MN 55455; **Phone:** (612) 625-1177; **Board Cert:** Orthopaedic Surgery 1998; **Med School:** USC Sch Med 1979; **Resid:** Orthopaedic Surgery, Univ Washington Med Ctr, Seattle, WA 1980-1984; **Fac Appt:** Prof Orthopaedic Surgery, Univ Minn

Weinstein, Stuart L MD (OrS) - *Spec Exp:* Scoliosis/Spine Deformities; Developmental Hip Dysplasia; Hip Disorders-Pediatric; **Hospital:** Univ of IA Hosp and Clinics; **Address:** 200 Hawkins Drive, rm 01026, Iowa City, IA 52242; **Phone:** (319) 356-1872; **Board Cert:** Orthopaedic Surgery 1995; **Med School:** Univ Iowa Coll Med 1972; **Resid:** Orthopaedic Surgery, Univ Iowa Coll Med, Iowa City, IA 1973-1976; **Fac Appt:** Prof Orthopaedic Surgery, Univ Iowa Coll Med

Wixson, Richard L MD (OrS) - *Spec Exp:* Hip & Knee Replacement; **Hospital:** Northwestern Meml Hosp; **Address:** 676 N St Clair, Ste 450, Chicago, IL 60611; **Phone:** (312) 943-7850; **Board Cert:** Orthopaedic Surgery 1979; **Med School:** Univ Wisc 1972; **Resid:** Orthopaedic Surgery, Henry Ford Hosp, Boston, MA 1974-1977; Orthopaedic Surgery, New Eng Bapt Hosp, Boston, MA 1978-1979; **Fellow:** Orthopaedic Surgery, Mass Genl Hosp, Boston, MA 1977; **Fac Appt:** Clin Prof Orthopaedic Surgery, Northwestern Univ

Zdeblick, Thomas MD (OrS) - *Spec Exp:* Spinal Surgery; **Hospital:** Univ WI Hosp & Clins; **Address:** rm K4/739, 600 Highland Ave Bldg CSC, Madison, WI 53792; **Phone:** (608) 265-3207; **Board Cert:** Orthopaedic Surgery 1991; **Med School:** Tufts Univ 1982; **Resid:** Orthopaedic Surgery, Case West Res Univ, Cleveland, OH 1984-1988; **Fellow:** Spine Surgery, Johns Hopkins Univ, Baltimore, MD 1988-1989; **Fac Appt:** Assoc Prof Orthopaedic Surgery, Univ Wisc

Great Plains and Mountains

Coughlin, Michael MD (OrS) - *Spec Exp:* Foot & Ankle Surgery; **Hospital:** St Alphonsus Reg Med Ctr; **Address:** 901 N Curtis, Ste 503, Boise, ID 83706-1343; **Phone:** (208) 377-1000; **Board Cert:** Orthopaedic Surgery 1980; **Med School:** Oregon Hlth Scis Univ 1974; **Resid:** Orthopaedic Surgery, UCSF Med Ctr, San Fransisco, CA 1975-1978; **Fellow:** Foot Surgery, Samuel Merrit Hosp 1978-1979; **Fac Appt:** Clin Prof Orthopaedic Surgery, Oregon Hlth Scis Univ

Dunn, Harold K MD (OrS) - *Spec Exp:* Hip Reconstruction-Adult; Knee Reconstruction-Knee; **Hospital:** Univ Utah Hosp and Clin; **Address:** 50 N Medical Dr, Salt Lake City, UT 84132-0001; **Phone:** (801) 581-2041; **Board Cert:** Orthopaedic Surgery 1983; **Med School:** Baylor Coll Med 1963; **Resid:** Orthopaedic Surgery, U NM Affil Hosp, Alberquerque, NM 1966-1967; Orthopaedic Surgery, Baylor Coll Med, Houston, TX 1967-1969; **Fac Appt:** Prof Orthopaedic Surgery, Univ Utah

Neff, James R MD (OrS) - *Spec Exp:* Musculoskeletal Tumors; **Hospital:** Nebraska Hlth Sys - Clarkson; **Address:** Dept Orth Surg, 981080 Nebraska Med Ctr., Omaha, NE 68198-1080; **Phone:** (402) 559-8000; **Board Cert:** Orthopaedic Surgery 1974; **Med School:** Univ Kans 1966; **Resid:** Surgery, U Mich Hosp, Ann Arbor, MI 1967-1968; Orthopaedic Surgery, U Mich Hosp, Ann Arbor, MI 1970-1973; **Fellow:** Fla Univ 1973-1974; **Fac Appt:** Prof Orthopaedic Surgery, Univ Nebr Coll Med

Paulos, Leon MD (OrS) - *Spec Exp:* Sports Medicine; Shoulder & Knee Surgery; **Hospital:** TOSH - The Ortho Spec Hosp; **Address:** 5848 S 300 E, Murray, UT 84107; **Phone:** (801) 314-4006; **Board Cert:** Orthopaedic Surgery 1980; **Med School:** Univ Utah 1973; **Resid:** Orthopaedic Surgery, Univ Utah Sch Med, Salt Lake City, UT 1974-1978; **Fellow:** Sports Medicine, Atlanta Sports Med Fdn, Atlanta, GA 1978; Sports Medicine, Univ Hosp - Cincinatti, Cincinatti, OH 1979; **Fac Appt:** Asst Clin Prof Orthopaedic Surgery, Univ Utah

Rosenberg, Thomas D MD (OrS) - *Spec Exp:* Knee Surgery; Sports Medicine; **Hospital:** TOSH - The Ortho Spec Hosp; **Address:** Rosenberg-Cooley Clinic, 1820 Sidewinder Drive, Park City, UT 84060; **Phone:** (435) 655-6600; **Board Cert:** Orthopaedic Surgery 1979; **Med School:** Univ Utah 1973; **Resid:** Orthopaedic Surgery, Univ Utah Affil Hosps, Salt Lake City, UT 1973-1978; Sports Medicine, Univ WI Hosp & Clinics, Madison, WI 1977-1978

Wiedel, Jerome D MD (OrS) - *Spec Exp:* Orthopaedic Surgery - General; **Hospital:** Univ Colo HSC - Denver; **Address:** 1665 N Ursula St, Denver, CO 80262-0001; **Phone:** (720) 848-1900; **Board Cert:** Orthopaedic Surgery 1993; **Med School:** Univ Nebr Coll Med 1964; **Resid:** Orthopaedic Surgery, Univ Colorado Med Ctr, Denver, CO 1967-1971; **Fellow:** Adult Reconstruction, Robert Jones-A Hunt Ortho Hosp, Oswestry, England 1971-1972; **Fac Appt:** Prof Orthopaedic Surgery, Univ Colo

Southwest

Aronson, James MD (OrS) - *Spec Exp:* Ilizarov Procedure; Hip Disorders; Clubfoot; **Hospital:** Arkansas Chldns Hosp; **Address:** 800 Marshall St, Slot 839, Little Rock, AR 72202; **Phone:** (501) 320-1468; **Board Cert:** Orthopaedic Surgery 1997; **Med School:** Univ Pittsburgh 1975; **Resid:** Surgery, Maine Med Ctr, Portland, ME 1976-1977; Orthopaedic Surgery, Duke U Med Ctr, Durham, NC 1978-1982; **Fellow:** Pediatric Orthopedic Surgery, Alfred I DuPont Inst, Wilmington, DE 1983; **Fac Appt:** Prof Orthopaedic Surgery, Univ Ark

Brodsky, James White MD (OrS) - *Spec Exp:* Foot Surgery; **Hospital:** Baylor Univ Medical Ctr; **Address:** 411 N Washington Ave, Ste 7000, Dallas, TX 75246-1777; **Phone:** (214) 823-7090; **Board Cert:** Orthopaedic Surgery 1998; **Med School:** Case West Res Univ 1979; **Resid:** Orthopaedic Surgery, Bellevue Hosp Ctr/NYU, New York, NY 1980-1981; Orthopaedic Surgery, Baylor Coll Med, Houston, TX 1981-1984; **Fellow:** Ankle and Foot Surgery, USC/LAC Hosp, Los Angeles, CA 1984-1985; **Fac Appt:** Assoc Clin Prof Orthopaedic Surgery, Univ Tex SW, Dallas

Bucholz, Robert MD (OrS) - *Spec Exp:* Trauma; **Hospital:** Parkland Mem Hosp; **Address:** 5353 Harry Hines Blvd, Dallas, TX 75390-8883; **Phone:** (214) 648-3870; **Board Cert:** Orthopaedic Surgery 1994; **Med School:** Yale Univ 1973; **Resid:** Orthopaedic Surgery, Yale-New Haven Hosp, New Haven, CT 1974-1977; **Fac Appt:** Prof Orthopaedic Surgery, Univ Tex SW, Dallas

Dabezies, Eugene MD (OrS) - *Spec Exp:* Hand Surgery; **Hospital:** Univ Med Ctr - Lubbock; **Address:** 3502 9th St, Ste 450, Lubbock, TX 79415; **Phone:** (806) 743-4263; **Board Cert:** Orthopaedic Surgery 1992; **Med School:** Tulane Univ 1960; **Resid:** Orthopaedic Surgery, Charity Hosp, New Orleans, LA 1961-1965; **Fac Appt:** Prof Orthopaedic Surgery, Texas Tech Univ

Mabrey, Jay D MD (OrS) - *Spec Exp:* Knee Replacement & Revision; Hip Replacement & Revision; Arthroscopy-Hip; **Hospital:** Univ of Texas Hlth & Sci Ctr; **Address:** Univ TX Hlth Sci Ctr. Dept of Orthopaedics, 7703 Floyd Curl Drive, San Antonio, TX 78229-3900; **Phone:** (210) 567-5125; **Board Cert:** Orthopaedic Surgery 2000; **Med School:** Cornell Univ-Weill Med Coll 1981; **Resid:** Orthopaedic Surgery, Duke U MC, Durham, NC 1983-1987; Surgery, Duke U MC, Durham, NC 1982-1983; **Fellow:** Hosp Special Surg., New York, NY 1990-1991; **Fac Appt:** Assoc Prof Orthopaedic Surgery, Univ Tex, San Antonio

Nelson, Carl MD (OrS) - *Spec Exp:* Hip Surgery; Hip & Knee Replacement; **Hospital:** UAMS; **Address:** Univ Arkansas Med Scis, 4301 West Markham , MS 531, Little Rock, AR 72205; **Phone:** (501) 686-5505; **Board Cert:** Orthopaedic Surgery 1969; **Med School:** Indiana Univ 1959; **Resid:** Internal Medicine, Los Angeles Co Genl Hosp, Los Angeles, CA 1960-1961; Surgery, Cleveland Clin Fdn, Cleveland, OH 1962-1963; **Fellow:** Orthopaedic Surgery, Cleveland Clin Fdn, Cleveland, OH 1963-1966; **Fac Appt:** Prof Orthopaedic Surgery, Univ Ark

Rockwood Jr, Charles A MD (OrS) - *Spec Exp:* Shoulder Surgery; **Hospital:** Univ Hosp-San Antonio; **Address:** Univ Hosp, Dept Orth Surg, 7703 Floyd Curl Dr, San Antonio, TX 78229-3900; **Phone:** (210) 567-5125; **Board Cert:** Orthopaedic Surgery 1994; **Med School:** Univ Okla Coll Med 1956; **Resid:** Orthopaedic Surgery, Univ Oklahoma Med Ctr, Oklahoma City, OK 1957-1961; **Fellow:** Shoulder Surgery, Columbia Presby Med Ctr, New York, NY; **Fac Appt:** Prof Orthopaedic Surgery, Univ Tex, San Antonio

ORTHOPAEDIC SURGERY

Trick, Lorence Wain MD (OrS) - *Spec Exp:* Hip & Knee Replacement; Joint Revision; **Hospital:** SW Texas Methodist Hosp; **Address:** 414 Navarro St, Ste 1128, San Antonio, TX 78205; **Phone:** (210) 351-6500; **Board Cert:** Orthopaedic Surgery 1973; **Med School:** Geo Wash Univ 1967; **Resid:** Orthopaedic Surgery, Wilford Hall USAF Med Ctr, San Antonio, TX 1968-1972; **Fellow:** Orthopaedic Surgery, New England Baptist Med Ctr, Boston, MA 1973; **Fac Appt:** Clin Prof Orthopaedic Surgery, Univ Tex, San Antonio

Wirth, Michael A MD (OrS) - *Spec Exp:* Shoulder Surgery; **Hospital:** Univ of Texas Hlth & Sci Ctr; **Address:** UT Hlth & Sci Ctr, Dept Orth, 7703 Floyd Curl Dr, San Antonio, TX 78229-3900; **Phone:** (210) 567-5135; **Board Cert:** Orthopaedic Surgery 1993; **Med School:** Oregon Hlth Scis Univ 1985; **Resid:** Orthopaedic Surgery, UT Hlth Sci Ctr, San Antonio, TX 1986-1990; **Fellow:** Shoulder Surgery, Charles Rockwood Jr MD, San Antonio, TX 1990-1991; **Fac Appt:** Prof Orthopaedic Surgery, Univ Tex, San Antonio

West Coast and Pacific

Anderson, Lesley J MD (OrS) - *Spec Exp:* Knee Injuries-Women; Knee Cartilage Problems; Shoulder Surgery; **Hospital:** CA Pacific Med Ctr - Pacific Campus; **Address:** 2100 Webster St, Ste 309, San Francisco, CA 94115; **Phone:** (415) 923-3029; **Board Cert:** Orthopaedic Surgery 1987; **Med School:** Penn State Univ-Hershey Med Ctr 1976; **Resid:** Orthopaedic Surgery, UCLA Med Ctr, Los Angeles, CA 1979-1983; **Fellow:** Knee Surgery, Blazina Orthopedic Clinic, Sherman Oaks, CA 1983-1984

Bradford, David S MD (OrS) - *Spec Exp:* Scoliosis/Spine Deformities; Spinal Surgery; **Hospital:** UCSF Med Ctr; **Address:** 500 Parnassus Ave Fl 3, Box 0728, San Francisco, CA 94143-0728; **Phone:** (415) 476-2280; **Board Cert:** Orthopaedic Surgery 1988; **Med School:** Univ Penn 1962; **Resid:** Orthopaedic Surgery, Columbia-Presbyterian Med Ctr, New York, NY 1966-1968; **Fellow:** Orthopaedic Surgery, Columbia-Presbyterian Med Ctr, New York, NY 1968-1969; **Fac Appt:** Prof Orthopaedic Surgery, UCSF

Brage, Michael MD (OrS) - *Spec Exp:* Foot & Ankle Surgery; **Hospital:** UCSD Healthcare; **Address:** Univ CA San Diego, Dept Ortho, 200 W Arbor Rd, MS 8894, San Diego, CA 92103-8894; **Phone:** (858) 657-8200; **Board Cert:** Orthopaedic Surgery 1994; **Med School:** Univ IL Coll Med 1986; **Resid:** University Chicago, Chicago, IL 1986-1991; **Fellow:** University Washington, Seattle, WA 1991-1992; **Fac Appt:** Asst Clin Prof Surgery, UCSD

Cannon Jr, W Dilworth MD (OrS) - *Spec Exp:* Sports Medicine; Knee Surgery; **Hospital:** UCSF Med Ctr; **Address:** 1701 Divisadero St, Ste 240, San Francisco, CA 94115-1351; **Phone:** (415) 353-7566; **Board Cert:** Orthopaedic Surgery 1972; **Med School:** Columbia P&S 1963; **Resid:** Surgery, St Vincents Hosp, New York, NY 1963-1965; Orthopaedic Surgery, NY Ortho Hosp, New York, NY 1967-1970; **Fellow:** Orthopaedic Surgery, Royal Nat Ortho Hosp, London England 1970-1971; **Fac Appt:** Clin Prof Orthopaedic Surgery, UCSF

Chambers, Richard Byron MD (OrS) - *Spec Exp:* Diabetes-Amputation; **Hospital:** Rancho Los Amigos Natl Rehab Ctr; **Address:** 7601 E Imperial Hwy, rm 145-HB, Downey, CA 90242; **Phone:** (562) 401-7225; **Board Cert:** Orthopaedic Surgery 1977; **Med School:** Columbia P&S 1971; **Resid:** Orthopaedic Surgery, Hosp for Special Surgery, New York, NY; Surgery, Harlem Hosp, New York, NY

Dillingham, Michael Francis MD (OrS) - *Spec Exp:* *Orthopaedic Surgery - General;* **Hospital:** Stanford Med Ctr; **Address:** 2884 Sand Hill Rd, Ste 110, Menlo Park, CA 94025; **Phone:** (650) 851-4900; **Board Cert:** Physical Medicine & Rehabilitation 1979, Orthopaedic Surgery 1977; **Med School:** Stanford Univ 1971; **Resid:** Internal Medicine, Santa Clara Valley Med Ctr, San Jose, CA 1975-1977; Orthopaedic Surgery, Standford, Stanford, CA 1972-1975; **Fellow:** Orthopaedic Surgery, Santa Clara Valley Med Ctr, San Jose, CA 1975-1976; **Fac Appt:** Clin Prof Orthopaedic Surgery, Stanford Univ

Dorr, Lawrence Douglas MD (OrS) - *Spec Exp:* *Hip & Knee Replacement;* **Hospital:** Centinela Hosp Med Ctr; **Address:** The Arthritis Institute, 501 E Hardy St, Ste 300, Inglewood, CA 90301; **Phone:** (310) 695-4800; **Board Cert:** Orthopaedic Surgery 1978; **Med School:** Univ Iowa Coll Med 1967; **Resid:** Orthopaedic Surgery, Los Angeles Co-USC Sch Med, Los Angeles, CA 1974-1976; **Fellow:** Joint Replacement Surgery, Hosp Spec Surg, New York, NY 1976-1977

Eckardt, Jeffrey J MD (OrS) - *Spec Exp:* *Bone Tumors; Soft Tissue Tumors; Limb Salvage Surgery;* **Hospital:** UCLA Med Ctr; **Address:** UCLA Med Ctr, Dept OrS, 10833 LeConte Ave, Los Angeles, CA 90095-6902; **Phone:** (310) 206-6503; **Board Cert:** Orthopaedic Surgery 1981; **Med School:** Cornell Univ-Weill Med Coll 1971; **Resid:** Orthopaedic Surgery, UCLA, Los Angeles, CA 1975-1979; **Fellow:** Orthopedic Oncology, Mayo Clinic, Rochester, MN 1979-1980; **Fac Appt:** Prof Orthopaedic Surgery, UCLA

Finerman, Gerald MD (OrS) - *Spec Exp:* *Sports Medicine; Hip & Knee Replacement;* **Hospital:** UCLA Med Ctr; **Address:** Dep Orthopaedic Surgery, 10833 Le Conte Ave, rm 76-131, Los Angeles, CA 90095; **Phone:** (310) 825-6019; **Board Cert:** Orthopaedic Surgery 1971; **Med School:** Johns Hopkins Univ 1962; **Resid:** Surgery, Johns Hopkins Hosp, Baltimore, MD 1963-1964; Orthopaedic Surgery, Johns Hopkins Hosp, Baltimore, MD 1966-1969; **Fac Appt:** Prof Orthopaedic Surgery, UCLA

Garfin, Steven R MD (OrS) - *Spec Exp:* *Spinal Surgery;* **Hospital:** UCSD Healthcare; **Address:** Univ California-San Diego, Dept Orthopedic Surgery, 200 W Arbor Drive, rm 8894, San Diego, CA 92103-8894; **Phone:** (619) 543-2542; **Board Cert:** Orthopaedic Surgery 1982; **Med School:** Univ Minn 1972; **Resid:** Orthopaedic Surgery, UCSD Med Ctr, San Diego, CA 1975-1979; **Fellow:** Spine Surgery, Univ Penn Hosp, Philadelphia, PA 1980-1981; **Fac Appt:** Prof Orthopaedic Surgery, UCSD

Goodman, Stuart Barry MD/PhD (OrS) - *Spec Exp:* *Arthritis; Joint Replacement;* **Hospital:** Stanford Med Ctr; **Address:** Div Orthopaedic Surgery, 300 Pasteur, rm R-I44, Stanford, CA 94305-5341; **Phone:** (650) 723-7072; **Board Cert:** Orthopaedic Surgery 1998; **Med School:** Univ Toronto 1978; **Resid:** Orthopaedic Surgery, Univ of Toronto, Toronto, Canada 1979-1984; **Fellow:** Orthopaedic Surgery, Univ of Toronto, Toronto, Canada 1984-1985; **Fac Appt:** Prof Orthopaedic Surgery, Stanford Univ

Hansen Jr., Sigvard MD (OrS) - *Spec Exp:* *Foot & Ankle Surgery;* **Hospital:** Univ WA Med Ctr; **Address:** Dept Orthopaedics, 325 9th Ave, Box 359798, Seattle, WA 98104; **Phone:** (206) 731-4487; **Board Cert:** Orthopaedic Surgery 1993; **Med School:** Univ Wash 1961; **Resid:** Orthopaedic Surgery, Univ Washington Affiliation Hosp, Seattle, WA 1965-1969; **Fellow:** Orthopaedic Surgery, Sheffield Chldrns Hosp, England 1970; **Fac Appt:** Prof Orthopaedic Surgery, Univ Wash

Lowenberg, David W MD (OrS) - *Spec Exp:* *Osteomyelitis; Ilizarov Procedure;* **Hospital:** CA Pacific Med Ctr - Pacific Campus; **Address:** 2351 Clay St, Ste 134, San Francisco, CA 94115; **Phone:** (415) 600-3835; **Board Cert:** Orthopaedic Surgery 1992; **Med School:** UCLA 1985; **Resid:** Orthopaedic Surgery, UCSF, San Francisco, CA 1986-1990; **Fac Appt:** Prof Orthopaedic Surgery, UCSF

535

Luck Jr, James Vernon MD (OrS) - *Spec Exp:* Hemophilla Related Disease; Hip & Knee Replacement; Musculoskeletal Tumors; **Hospital:** Orthopaedic Hosp; **Address:** 2300 S Flower St, Ste 200, Los Angeles, CA 90007-2660; **Phone:** (213) 749-8255; **Board Cert:** Orthopaedic Surgery 1975; **Med School:** USC Sch Med 1967; **Resid:** Orthopaedic Surgery, Orthopaedic Hosp, Los Angeles, CA 1968-1973; **Fellow:** Orthopedic Oncology, Orthopaedic Hosp, Los Angeles, CA 1973-1974; Reconstructive Surgery, Rancho Los Amigos, Downey, CA 1973-1974

Patzakis, Michael J MD (OrS) - *Spec Exp:* Rheumatological Surgery; **Hospital:** USC Univ Hosp - R K Eamer Med Plz; **Address:** 1200 N State St GNH3900, Los Angeles, CA 90033-4525; **Phone:** (323) 226-7201; **Board Cert:** Orthopaedic Surgery 1983; **Med School:** Ohio State Univ **Resid:** Orthopaedic Surgery, Los Angeles Co-USC Med Ctr, Los Angeles, CA 1964-1968; **Fellow:** Rheumatology, Univ CO Med Ctr, Denver, CO 1968-1969; **Fac Appt:** Prof Orthopaedic Surgery, USC Sch Med

Peterson, Davis C MD (OrS) - *Spec Exp:* Spinal Surgery; Scoliosis; Trauma; **Hospital:** Alaska Native Medical Ctr; **Address:** 3260 Providence Drive, Ste 200, Anchorage, AK 99508-4603; **Phone:** (907) 563-3145; **Board Cert:** Orthopaedic Surgery 1999; **Med School:** Baylor Coll Med 1980; **Resid:** Orthopaedic Surgery, Madigan Med Ctr, Tacoma, WA 1982-1986; **Fellow:** Spine Surgery, St Luke's Med Ctr, Houston, TX 1989-1990

Sangeorzan, Bruce J. MD (OrS) - *Spec Exp:* Foot & Ankle Surgery; **Hospital:** Univ WA Med Ctr; **Address:** 325 9th Ave, Box 359798, Seattle, WA 98104-2499; **Phone:** (206) 731-3466; **Board Cert:** Orthopaedic Surgery 2000; **Med School:** Wayne State Univ 1981; **Resid:** Orthopaedic Surgery, Wayne State U, Detroit, MI 1982-1986; **Fellow:** Adult Orthopedic Surgery, U Wash, Seattle, WA 1986-1987; **Fac Appt:** Prof Orthopaedic Surgery, Univ Wash

Schmalzried, Thomas P MD (OrS) - *Spec Exp:* Hip Replacement; **Hospital:** Orthopaedic Hosp; **Address:** 2400 S Flower St, Los Angeles, CA 90007-2629; **Phone:** (213) 742-1075; **Board Cert:** Orthopaedic Surgery 1993; **Med School:** UCLA 1984; **Resid:** Orthopaedic Surgery, UCLA Med Ctr, Los Angeles, CA 1985-1990; **Fellow:** Orthopaedic Surgery, UCLA Med Ctr, Los Angeles, CA 1986-1987; Hip Surgery, Mass Genl Hosp - Harvard U, Boston, MA 1990-1991; **Fac Appt:** Asst Prof Orthopaedic Surgery, UCLA

Schurman, David J MD (OrS) - *Spec Exp:* Orthopaedic Surgery - General; **Hospital:** Stanford Med Ctr; **Address:** 300 Pasteur Drive, Ste R144, Stanford, CA 94305-5341; **Phone:** (650) 723-5643; **Board Cert:** Orthopaedic Surgery 1994; **Med School:** Columbia P&S 1965; **Resid:** Surgery, Mount Sinai Hosp, New York, NY 1966-1967; Orthopaedic Surgery, UCLA Med Ctr, Los Angeles, CA 1967-1972; **Fellow:** Orthopaedic Surgery, UCLA Med Ctr, Los Angeles, CA 1972-1973; **Fac Appt:** Prof Orthopaedic Surgery, Stanford Univ

Tolo, Vernon Thorpe MD (OrS) - *Spec Exp:* Spinal Deformity-Pediatric; Skeletal Dysplasias; **Hospital:** Chldns Hosp - Los Angeles; **Address:** Chldns Hosp LA, 4650 W Sunset Blvd, MC-69, Los Angeles, CA 90027-6062; **Phone:** (323) 669-4658; **Board Cert:** Orthopaedic Surgery 1977; **Med School:** Johns Hopkins Univ 1968; **Resid:** Orthopaedic Surgery, Johns Hopkins Hosp, Baltimore, MD 1972-1975; **Fellow:** Pediatric Orthopedic Surgery, Hosp Sick Chldn, Toronto, Canada 1975-1976; **Fac Appt:** Prof Orthopaedic Surgery, USC Sch Med

Watkins, Robert Green MD (OrS) - *Spec Exp:* Spinal Surgery; **Hospital:** USC Univ Hosp - R K Eamer Med Plz; **Address:** 1510 San Pablo St, Ste 700, Los Angeles, CA 90033; **Phone:** (323) 442-5300; **Board Cert:** Orthopaedic Surgery 1982; **Med School:** Univ Tenn Coll Med, Memphis 1969; **Resid:** Orthopaedic Surgery, LAC-USC Med Ctr, Los Angeles, CA; **Fellow:** Spine Surgery, Jones-Hunt Orth Hosp, Oswestry, UK; **Fac Appt:** Assoc Prof Orthopaedic Surgery, USC Sch Med

Otolaryngology

An otolaryngologist-head and neck surgeon provides comprehensive medical and surgical care for patients with diseases and disorders that affect the ears, nose, throat, the respiratory and upper alimentary systems and related structures of the head and neck.

An otolaryngologist diagnoses and provides medical and/or surgical therapy or prevention of diseases, allergies, neoplasms, deformities, disorders and/or injuries of the ears, nose, sinuses, throat, respiratory and upper alimentary systems, face, jaws and the other head and neck systems. Head and neck oncology, facial plastic and reconstructive surgery and the treatment of disorders of hearing and voice are fundamental areas of expertise.

Certification in the following subspecialty requires additional training and examination.

Plastic Surgery within the Head and Neck: An otolaryngologist with additional training in plastic and reconstructive procedures within the head, face, neck and associated structures, including cutaneous head and neck oncology and reconstruction, management of maxillofacial trauma, soft tissue repair and neural surgery.

This field is diverse and involved a wide age range of patients, from the newborn to the aged. While both cosmetic and reconstructive surgeries are practiced, there are many additional procedures which interface with them.

Training required: Five years

THE MOUNT SINAI HOSPITAL
EAR, NOSE, AND THROAT – OTOLARYNGOLOGY

5 East 98th Street, 8th Floor
New York, NY 10029-6574   Phone: (212) 241-9410
Physician Referral: 1-800-MD-SINAI (637-4624)
www.mountsinai.org

We offer a comprehensive variety of programs:

Audiology Program – All aspects of audiology are covered, including the performance and interpretation of audiograms, brainstem evoked potentials, otoacoustic emission testing, neonatal hearing screening, and evaluations for assisted listening devices.

Cranial Base Surgery – Interdisciplinary teams provide expertise in the diagnosis and treatment of tumors, vascular lesions, and trauma at the base of the brain.

Facial Plastic and Cosmetic Surgery – Our reconstructive facial surgeons and specialists in facial cosmetic surgery use state-of-the-art endoscopic techniques.

Head and Neck Oncologic Surgery – With one of the world's leading programs, Mount Sinai is on the cutting edge of head and neck cancer therapy, reconstruction, and rehabilitation.

Head and Neck Reconstructive Surgery – The Department has some of the most experienced reconstructive surgeons in the world, specializing in microvascular free tissue transfer.

Hearing, Facial Nerve, and Balance Disorders – Multidisciplinary teams provide treatment for a broad range of adult and pediatric otologic and neuro-otologic disorders.

Maxillofacial Prosthodontics – Complete services to restore speech and chewing abilities and minimize cosmetic defects.

Nasal and Sinus Surgery – Renowned rhinologists treat all inflammatory and infectious diseases of the nose and sinuses.

Oral and Maxillofacial Surgery – All treatment options are provided for patients with congenital, acquired, or traumatic problems of the oral cavity, jaws, and associated structures.

Pediatric Otolaryngology – Our state-of-the-art service provides for management of otolaryngological problems of childhood.

General Otolaryngology Services – We treat common disorders of the ear, nose, and throat.

Thyroid and Parathyroid Surgery – We believe that a team approach involving an experienced surgeon, a dedicated endocrinologist, and a team of physicians trained in nuclear medicine is of critical importance for the treatment of thyroid cancers.

THE MOUNT SINAI HOSPITAL

One of the oldest and most respected departments in the nation, Mount Sinai's Department of Otolaryngology is consistently ranked among the top in the nation.

The *U.S. News & World Report* ranked Mount Sinai's Department of Otolaryngology *#1 in New York City* and *#16 in the nation.*

In its Special Issue of "The Best Hospitals in New York," *New York Magazine* said of Mount Sinai's otolaryngology department:

"...the leading hospital in this area is Mount Sinai, home to one of the oldest and busiest otolaryngology departments in the country. Sinai handles virtually every subspecialty in otolaryngology with finesse."

In the **Department of Otolaryngology** at **The Mount Sinai Medical Center,** all physicians are board certified specialists dedicated to healing disorders of the ear, nose, throat, head, and neck and are members of the Mount Sinai School of Medicine.

***

The Grabscheid Voice Center offers the highest level of medical care for the professional voice, along with a profound understanding of the special medical, psychological, and professional needs of singers, actors, and lecturers.

DEPARTMENT OF OTOLARYNGOLOGY
THE NEW YORK EYE & EAR INFIRMARY

NY Eye & Ear Infirmary

Affiliated Teaching
Hospital of New York
Medical College

310 East 14th Street (corner Second Avenue)
New York, NY 10003
212-979-4000 • FAX: 212-228-0664
Physician Referral: 1-800-449-HOPE (4673)
website: www.nyee.edu

Continuum Health Partners, Inc.

PROVIDING EXCEPTIONAL CARE OF THE EAR, NOSE, THROAT, AND HEAD & NECK

Established in 1820 the Department of Otolaryngology/Head & Neck Surgery is the first training program in this specialty in the Western Hemisphere. Over nearly two centuries the department has evolved to be an international referral center for the medical and surgical treatment of diseases of the ear, nose, and throat.

OUTSTANDING SERVICES AVAILABLE ARE:

Facial Plastic Surgery: In-office or ambulatory procedures utilizing computer imaging, new techniques and materials produce outstanding results with minimal incisions, rapid recovery and a natural, youthful appearance.

Head and Neck Oncology: A multi-disciplinary team including board certified surgeons, medical & radiation oncologists, nutritionists and rehabilitation specialists insure rapid recovery from complex, life saving surgical procedures and return to daily activities.

Thyroid Center: A newly established center has concentrated on streamlining the diagnosis of thyroid diseases and cancers. A highly skilled team of surgeons, endocrinologists and radiologists manage the patient's care.

Center for Voice Disorders: Combines the expertise of physicians, speech pathologists and a voice physiologist to diagnose and treat voice problems – not only for performing artists but also for teachers, stockbrokers, receptionists, salespeople – anyone for whom voice is an important part of life.

Otology & Neuro-otology: Specializing in the care of chronic ear disease including hearing loss, cochlear implantation, dizziness, tinnitus, intra cranial tumors and facial nerve disorders. Our advanced otologic and vestibular diagnostic labs assist our physicians in treatment.

Pediatric Otolaryngology: Treating children has long been a priority at the Infirmary. Pediatric care ranges from middle ear infection, tonsil and adenoid disease and neck masses to complicated sinus and airway diseases.

Rhinology and Sinus Surgery: Internationally known specialists utilize minimally invasive techniques to treat disorders from sinusitis to intra-cranial tumors.

CLINICAL SERVICES

Facial Plastic & Reconstructive Surgery

Head & Neck Oncology
  Thyroid Center

General Otolaryngology

Laryngology
  Swallowing Disorders
  Voice & Vocal Dynamics

Otology & Neuro-otology
  Cochlear Implantation

Pediatric Otolaryngology

Rhinology & Sinus Surgery

FACILITIES

Ambulatory Care Services
  Faculty Practice
  Teaching Practice

Hearing Aid Dispensary

HOLA: Bilingual Program

Vestibular Rehabilitation

Voice Center

ABOUT THE NEW YORK EYE AND EAR INFIRMARY

The Infirmary is the nation's oldest, continuously operating specialty hospital and one of the most experienced in terms of the number of patients it treats and complexity of its cases. Each year the Otolaryngology department performs more than 6,000 surgeries and sees more than 60,000 visits from outpatients.

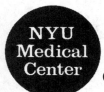

NYU Medical Center

550 First Avenue (at 31st Street)
New York, NY 10016
Physician Referral: (888) 7-NYU-MED
(888-769-8633) www.nyumedicalcenter.org

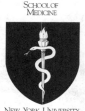

SCHOOL OF
MEDICINE

NEW YORK UNIVERSITY

OTOLARYNGOLOGY
(EAR, NOSE AND THROAT)

Treating the full spectrum of ear, nose, throat, head and neck disorders, the Department of Otolaryngology at NYU Medical Center provides state-of-the-art patient care and research through the following programs:

Cochlear Implants – the first center in the U.S. to use a multichannel cochlear implant in a profoundly deaf adult, in 1984. Since then we have implanted more than 700 adults and children from the age of 6 months to 85 years.

Sinus and Nasal Disorders – comprehensive diagnosis and minimally invasive treatment of sinus and nasal disorders.

Facial Plastic Surgery – plastic and reconstructive surgery for a variety of problems, including nasal obstruction, facial trauma, defects left after removing skin and other facial cancers, facial paralysis and spasm, congenital malformations.

Head and Neck Surgery – minimally invasive surgery to remove cancers of the head and neck with as little disturbance to everyday function as possible.

Sleep Apnea – repairing the collapse of soft tissue that leads to snoring and sleep apnea (a dangerous condition in which snorers stop breathing repeatedly during the night, taxing the heart and leaving the snorer unrested).

Skull Base Surgery – minimally invasive treatment of complex skull base tumors.

Swallowing Disorders – the only center of its kind in New York City, providing comprehensive diagnosis, treatment and therapy for swallowing disorders.

Voice Center – state-of-the-art biofeedback and therapy to rectify problems in speech.

Advanced Otologic Medicine & Surgery – treating patients with disorders of the ear and conditions that affect hearing, balance and facial nerve function.

NYU MEDICAL CENTER

The cochlear implant program at NYU Medical Center is one of the nation's finest. Since it set the standard in 1984 by implanting a profoundly deaf adult, the Division has been the site of numerous studies and research trials that will continue to improve the technologies available.

Adults and children travel from all over the world to get their cochlear implant at NYU Medical Center. Currently, NYU Medical Center is the only center performing bilateral implants under a special protocol designed to investigate the best method of programming devices, so that patients receive maximum benefits.

Physician Referral
(888) 7-NYU-MED
(888-769-8633)
www.nyumedicalcenter.org

Vanderbilt Bill Wilkerson Center
for Otolaryngology and Communication Sciences

Vanderbilt University Medical Center
S-2100 Medical Center North   Nashville, TN 37232
Tel. 615.936.5000 Fax. 615.936.5013
www.vanderbiltbillwilkersoncenter.com

Comprehensive Care

The Vanderbilt Bill Wilkerson Center offers one of the most comprehensive clinical, educational and research programs for communication and oto-laryngologic disorders in the nation. The mission of the Center is to bring together physicians, therapists, nurses, and researchers in equal partnership to provide a broad range of care to patients.

Patient Services

Patient services of the Vanderbilt Bill Wilkerson Center include complete medical and surgical manage-ment of otolaryngologic and head and neck diseases and disorders, as well as audiology, speech-language pathology, and comprehensive rehabilitation for acquired brain injury. These include deafness, autism, head and neck cancer, accidental brain injury, vocal disorders, sinus diseases, speech and language delays, balance disorders, and other debilitating conditions of the head, neck, ear, nose, and throat.

Research Programs

The research programs of the Vanderbilt Bill Wilkerson Center encompass a wide variety of top-ics in the areas of hearing science, language, speech production and perception, and human performance.

Within each of these areas, work focuses on both applied and basic issues.

Diagnostic and Research Facilities

The Vanderbilt Bill Wilkerson Center has over a dozen research laboratories, including an anechoic chamber, a hearing aid research laboratory, three auditory research laboratories, two speech science lab-oratories, two language science laboratories, vestibular research laboratory, voice center laboratory, neuro-physiology laboratory, fluency laboratory, and a computer network center.

The Center is equipped for comprehensive diagnostic audio-vestibular assessment, instrument-ation for recording sensory evoked responses, laryngeal videostroboscopy, oto-acoustic emissions, and electro-nystagmography. Research facilities include a neurophysiology laboratory for basic investigation of auditory, facial nerve, and laryngeal physiology.

PHYSICIAN LISTINGS

New England

Cheney, Mack Lowell MD (Oto) - *Spec Exp:* Facial Reconstruction; Cosmetic Surgery-Face; Facial Paralysis; **Hospital:** Mass Eye & Ear Infirmary; **Address:** Facial Plastic Surgery Unit, 243 Charles St, Boston, MA 02114; **Phone:** (617) 573-3709; **Board Cert:** Otolaryngology 1987; **Med School:** Univ Miss 1982; **Resid:** Surgery, Tulane Univ, New Orleans, LA 1983-1987; **Fellow:** Plastic Surgery, Harvard Med Sch, Boston, MA 1987; **Fac Appt:** Assoc Prof Otolaryngology, Harvard Med Sch

Fabian, Richard MD (Oto) - *Spec Exp:* Head & Neck Cancer; **Hospital:** Mass Eye & Ear Infirmary; **Address:** 243 Charles St, Boston, MA 02114; **Phone:** (617) 573-4084; **Board Cert:** Otolaryngology 1972; **Med School:** Tufts Univ 1966; **Resid:** Otolarynological Rhinoplasty, Mass Genl Hosp, Boston, MA 1968-1971; Surgery, Kings Co Hosp - SUNY Brooklyn, Brooklyn, NY 1967-1968; **Fac Appt:** Assoc Prof Otolaryngology, Harvard Med Sch

Kveton, John MD (Oto) - *Spec Exp:* Ear Disorders; Cochlear Implants; Acoustic Nerve Tumors; **Hospital:** Yale - New Haven Hosp; **Address:** 46 Prince St, Ste 601, New Haven, CT 06519-1634; **Phone:** (203) 752-1726; **Board Cert:** Otolaryngology 1982; **Med School:** St Louis Univ 1978; **Resid:** Otolaryngology, Yale-New Haven Hosp, New Haven, CT 1978-1982; **Fellow:** Otolaryngology, The Otology Group, Nashville, TN 1982-1983; **Fac Appt:** Prof Otolaryngology, Yale Univ

Metson, Ralph MD (Oto) - *Spec Exp:* Endoscopic Sinus Surgery; Facial Plastic Surgery; **Hospital:** Mass Eye & Ear Infirmary; **Address:** Zero Emerson Pl, Ste 2D, Boston, MA 02114; **Phone:** (617) 227-4366; **Board Cert:** Otolaryngology 1985; **Med School:** UCSD 1979; **Resid:** Otolaryngology, UCLA Med Ctr, Los Angeles, CA 1981-1985; **Fac Appt:** Assoc Clin Prof Otolaryngology, Harvard Med Sch

Nadol, Joseph MD (Oto) - *Spec Exp:* Ear Disorders/Surgery; Hearing Disorders; **Hospital:** Mass Eye & Ear Infirmary; **Address:** Mass Eye & Ear, 243 Charles St, Boston, MA 02114; **Phone:** (617) 573-3632; **Board Cert:** Otolaryngology 1975; **Med School:** Johns Hopkins Univ 1970; **Resid:** Surgery, Beth Israel Hosp, Boston, MA 1971-1972; Otolaryngology, Mass EE Infirm, Boston, MA 1972-1975; **Fac Appt:** Prof Otolaryngology, Harvard Med Sch

Poe, Dennis MD (Oto) - *Spec Exp:* Neuro-Otology; Cochlear Implants; Skull Base Surgery; **Hospital:** Mass Eye & Ear Infirmary; **Address:** Zero Emerson Pl, Boston, MA 02114; **Phone:** (617) 636-5498; **Board Cert:** Otolaryngology 1987; **Med School:** SUNY Syracuse 1982; **Resid:** Surgery, Univ Mass Med Ctr, Worcester 1982-1983; Otolaryngology, Univ Chicago Med Ctr 1983-1987; **Fellow:** Neurological Otology, Otology Grp, Nashville, TN 1987-1988; **Fac Appt:** Asst Clin Prof Otolaryngology, Harvard Med Sch

Sasaki, Clarence T MD (Oto) - *Spec Exp:* Head & Neck Cancer; Voice/Swallowing Disorders; **Hospital:** Yale - New Haven Hosp; **Address:** 333 Cedar St, Box 208041, New Haven, CT 06520-8041; **Phone:** (203) 785-2592; **Board Cert:** Otolaryngology 1973; **Med School:** Yale Univ 1966; **Resid:** Surgery, Dartmouth-Mary Hitchcock Hosp, Hanover, NH 1967-1968; Otolaryngology, Yale Sch Med, New Haven, CT 1970-1973; **Fellow:** Head and Neck Surgery, Univ of Milan, Italy 1978; Skull Base Surgery, Univ Zurich, Switzerland 1982; **Fac Appt:** Prof Otolaryngology, Yale Univ

Vining, Eugenia MD (Oto) - *Spec Exp:* Sinus Disorders/Surgery; **Hospital:** Yale - New Haven Hosp; **Address:** 46 Prince St, Ste 601, New Haven, CT 06519; **Phone:** (203) 752-1726; **Board Cert:** Otolaryngology 1993; **Med School:** Yale Univ 1987; **Resid:** Otolaryngology, Yale-New Haven Hosp, New Haven, CT 1988-1991; Otolaryngology, Yale-New Haven Hosp, New Haven, CT 1991-1992; **Fellow:** Sinus Surgery, Univ Penn Med Ctr, Philadelphia, PA 1992-1993

Zeitels, Steven MD (Oto) - *Spec Exp:* Laryngeal Disorders; Voice Disorders; Head & Neck Surgery; **Hospital:** Mass Eye & Ear Infirmary; **Address:** Mass Eye & Ear Infirm, Dept Oto, 243 Charles St, rm 712F, Boston, MA 02114; **Phone:** (617) 573-3557; **Board Cert:** Otolaryngology 1988; **Med School:** Boston Univ 1982; **Resid:** Surgery, Univ Hosp-Boston City Hosp, Boston, MA 1982-1983; Otolaryngology, Boston Univ-Tufts Univ, Boston, MA 1983-1987; **Fellow:** Head and Neck Surgery, Boston VA Med Ctr-Boston Univ, Boston, MA 1987-1988; **Fac Appt:** Assoc Prof Otolaryngology, Harvard Med Sch

Mid Atlantic

Abramson, Allan MD (Oto) - *Spec Exp:* Throat Tumors; Head & Neck Surgery; **Hospital:** Long Island Jewish Med Ctr; **Address:** LIJ Med Ctr, Dept Otolaryngology, 270-05 76th Ave, New Hyde Park, NY 11040; **Phone:** (516) 470-7555; **Board Cert:** Otolaryngology 1972; **Med School:** SUNY Downstate 1967; **Resid:** Surgery, Long Island Jewish Med Ctr, New Hyde Park, NY 1968-1969; Otolaryngology, Mount Sinai Med Ctr, New York, NY 1969-1972; **Fac Appt:** Prof Otolaryngology, Albert Einstein Coll Med

April, Max MD (Oto) - *Spec Exp:* Pediatric Otolaryngology; Pediatric Sinus Disorders; **Hospital:** Lenox Hill Hosp (page 64); **Address:** New York Otolaryngology Institute, 186 E 76th St Fl 2, New York, NY 10021; **Phone:** (212) 327-3000; **Board Cert:** Otolaryngology 1990; **Med School:** Boston Univ 1985; **Resid:** Otolaryngology, Boston Univ Med, Boston, MA 1985-1990; **Fellow:** Pediatric Otolaryngology, Johns Hopkins, Baltimore, MD 1990-1991

Arriaga, Moises Alberto MD (Oto) - *Spec Exp:* Neuro-Otolaryngology; **Hospital:** Allegheny General Hosp; **Address:** Pittsburgh Ear Assoc, 420 E North Ave, Ste 402, Pittsburgh, PA 15212; **Phone:** (412) 359-6690; **Board Cert:** Otolaryngology 1990; **Med School:** Brown Univ 1985; **Resid:** Otolaryngology, Univ Pittsburgh, Pittsburgh, PA 1986-1990; **Fellow:** Neurological Otology, House Ear Clin, Los Angeles, CA 1990-1991

Aviv, Jonathan MD (Oto) - *Spec Exp:* Voice Disorders; Swallowing Disorders; **Hospital:** NY Presby Hosp - Columbia Presby Med Ctr (page 70); **Address:** 16 E 60th St, Ste 360, New York, NY 10022-1002; **Phone:** (212) 326-8475; **Board Cert:** Otolaryngology 1990; **Med School:** Columbia P&S 1985; **Resid:** Surgery, Mount Sinai Med Ctr, New York, NY 1986-1987; Otolaryngology, Mount Sinai Med Ctr, New York, NY 1987-1990; **Fellow:** Otolaryngology, Mount Sinai Med Ctr, New York, NY 1990-1991; **Fac Appt:** Prof Otolaryngology, Columbia P&S

Blitzer, Andrew MD (Oto) - *Spec Exp:* Voice/Swallowing Disorders; Pain-Oromandibular & Facial; Nasal & Sinus Surgery; **Hospital:** St Luke's - Roosevelt Hosp Ctr - Roosevelt Div (page 58); **Address:** 425 W 59th St, Fl 10, New York, NY 10019-1128; **Phone:** (212) 262-9500; **Board Cert:** Otolaryngology 1977; **Med School:** Mount Sinai Sch Med 1973; **Resid:** Surgery, Beth Israel Med Ctr, New York, NY 1973-1974; Otolaryngology, Mount Sinai Hosp Med Ctr, New York, NY 1974-1977; **Fac Appt:** Prof Otolaryngology, Columbia P&S

Brookler, Kenneth MD (Oto) - *Spec Exp:* Dizziness; Hearing Loss/Tinnitus; Meniere's Disease; **Hospital:** Lenox Hill Hosp (page 64); **Address:** 111 E 77th St, New York, NY 10021-1892; **Phone:** (212) 861-6900; **Board Cert:** Otolaryngology 1968; **Med School:** Canada 1962; **Resid:** Surgery, Deer Lodge Hospital, Winnipeg, Canada 1963-1964; Otolaryngology, Mayo Clinic, Rochester, MN 1964-1967; **Fellow:** Neurological Otology, Mayo Clinic, Rochester, MN 1968

Carrau, Ricardo L. MD (Oto) - *Spec Exp:* Skull Base Surgery; Swallowing Disorders; **Hospital:** UPMC - Presbyterian Univ Hosp; **Address:** Univ Pittsburgh Med Ctr, 200 Lothrop St, Ste 300, Pittsburg, PA 15213-2546; **Phone:** (412) 647-2100; **Board Cert:** Otolaryngology 1987; **Med School:** Univ Puerto Rico 1981; **Resid:** Surgery, University Hosp, San Juan, Puerto Rico 1984-1987; Head and Neck Surgery, University Hosp, San Juan, Puerto Rico 1982-1984; **Fellow:** Head and Neck Surgery, University Pittsburgh, Pittsburgh, PA 1989-1990; **Fac Appt:** Asst Prof Otolaryngology, Univ Pittsburgh

Close, Lanny Garth MD (Oto) - *Spec Exp:* Skull Base Surgery; Head & Neck Cancer; Sinus Disorders/Surgery; **Hospital:** NY Presby Hosp - Columbia Presby Med Ctr (page 70); **Address:** 16 E 60th St, Ste 360, New York, NY 10022-1002; **Phone:** (212) 326-8475; **Board Cert:** Otolaryngology 1977; **Med School:** Baylor Coll Med 1972; **Resid:** Surgery, Johns Hopkins, Baltimore, MD 1972-1974; Otolaryngology, Baylor Affil Hosp, Houston, TX 1974-1977; **Fellow:** Otolaryngology, MD Anderson, Houston, TX 1978-1979; **Fac Appt:** Prof Otolaryngology, Columbia P&S

Cohen, Noel L MD (Oto) - *Spec Exp:* Cochlear Implants; Acoustic Nerve Tumors; **Hospital:** NYU Med Ctr (page 71); **Address:** 530 1st Ave, Fl 3C, New York, NY 10016; **Phone:** (212) 263-7373; **Board Cert:** Otolaryngology 1963; **Med School:** Netherlands 1957; **Resid:** Otolaryngology, NYU Med Ctr, New York, NY 1959-1962; **Fac Appt:** Clin Prof Otolaryngology, NYU Sch Med

Costantino, Peter D MD (Oto) - *Spec Exp:* Skull Base Surgery; Craniofacial Surgery; Reconstructive Surgery-Face & Skull; **Hospital:** St Luke's - Roosevelt Hosp Ctr - Roosevelt Div (page 58); **Address:** 425 W 59th St Fl 10, New York, NY 10019; **Phone:** (212) 523-7791; **Board Cert:** Otolaryngology 1990; **Med School:** Northwestern Univ 1984; **Resid:** Surgery, Northwestern Meml Hosp, Chicago, IL 1985-1986; Otolaryngology, Northwestern Meml Hosp, Chicago, IL 1986-1989; **Fellow:** Head and Neck Surgery, Northwestern Meml Hosp, Chicago, IL 1989-1990; Skull Base Surgery, Univ Pittsburgh, Pittsburgh, PA 1990-1991; **Fac Appt:** Prof Otolaryngology

Cummings, Charles MD (Oto) - *Spec Exp:* Head & Neck Surgery; Laryngeal Disorders; **Hospital:** Johns Hopkins Hosp - Baltimore; **Address:** Johns Hopkins U-Dept. Oto HNS, 601 N Caroline St, Baltimore, MD 21205-2000; **Phone:** (410) 955-7400; **Board Cert:** Otolaryngology 1968; **Med School:** Univ VA Sch Med 1961; **Resid:** Surgery, Univ Va Hosp, Charlottesville, VA 1963-1965; Otolaryngology, Mass Genl Hosp, Boston, MA 1965-1968; **Fac Appt:** Prof Otolaryngology, Johns Hopkins Univ

Davidson, Bruce J MD (Oto) - *Spec Exp:* Head & Neck Cancer; Thyroid Disorders; **Hospital:** Georgetown Univ Hosp; **Address:** GUMC, Dept Oto/HNS, 3800 Reservoir Rd NW, Bldg 1 Gorman, Washington, DC 20007; **Phone:** (202) 687-8186; **Board Cert:** Otolaryngology 1993; **Med School:** W VA Univ 1987; **Resid:** Otolaryngology, Georgetown, Washington, DC 1988-1992; **Fellow:** Otolaryngology, Memorial Sloan Kettering, New York, NY 1992-1994; **Fac Appt:** Asst Prof Otolaryngology, Georgetown Univ

Edelstein, David MD (Oto) - *Spec Exp:* Sinus Disorders/Surgery; Endoscopic Sinus Surgery; **Hospital:** Manhattan Eye, Ear & Throat Hosp; **Address:** 1421 3rd Ave, New York, NY 10028; **Phone:** (212) 452-1500; **Board Cert:** Otolaryngology 1985; **Med School:** Boston Univ 1980; **Resid:** Otolaryngology, Mount Sinai Hosp, New York, NY 1980-1984; **Fac Appt:** Clin Prof Otolaryngology, Cornell Univ-Weill Med Coll

Fried, Marvin MD (Oto) - *Spec Exp:* Endoscopic Sinus Surgery; Head & Neck Tumors; **Hospital:** Montefiore Med Ctr (page 67); **Address:** Montefiore Med Ctr, Dept Otolaryngology, 111 E 210th St, Bronx, NY 10467; **Phone:** (718) 920-2991; **Board Cert:** Otolaryngology 1975; **Med School:** Tufts Univ 1969; **Resid:** Otolaryngology, Jewish Hosp, St Louis, MI 1970-1975; **Fellow:** Stroke, Washington Univ, St Louis, MI 1975-1976; **Fac Appt:** Prof Otolaryngology, Albert Einstein Coll Med

Glasgold, Alvin MD (Oto) - *Spec Exp:* Cosmetic Surgery-Face; **Hospital:** Robert Wood Johnson Univ Hosp @ New Brunswick; **Address:** 31 River Rd, Highland Park, NJ 08904; **Phone:** (732) 846-6540; **Board Cert:** Otolaryngology 1967; **Med School:** NY Med Coll 1961; **Resid:** Surgery, Bronx VA Hosp, Bronx, NY 1962-1963; Otolaryngology, Bronx VA Hosp, Bronx, NY 1963-1966; **Fac Appt:** Clin Prof Otolaryngology, UMDNJ-RW Johnson Med Sch

Har-El, Gady MD (Oto) - *Spec Exp:* Head & Neck Cancer; Sinus & Skull Base Surgery; **Hospital:** Long Island Coll Hosp (page 58); **Address:** 134 Atlantic Ave, Brooklyn, NY 11201; **Phone:** (718) 780-1498; **Board Cert:** Otolaryngology 1992; **Med School:** Israel 1982; **Resid:** Otolaryngology, SUNY Downstate, Brooklyn, NY 1986-1991; **Fac Appt:** Prof Otolaryngology, SUNY Hlth Sci Ctr

Hayden, Richard Earle MD (Oto) - *Spec Exp:* Head & Neck Surgery; **Hospital:** Hahnemann Univ Hosp; **Address:** Med Coll Penn - Hahnemann Univ, 2 Logan Sq, Ste 1815, Philadelphia, PA 19103-2722; **Phone:** (215) 665-8140; **Board Cert:** Otolaryngology 1978; **Med School:** McGill Univ 1974; **Resid:** Otolaryngology, Univ Toronto, Toronto, Canada 1975-1978; **Fellow:** Head and Neck Surgery, MD Anderson Hosp, Houston, TX 1978-1979; Radiation Oncology, Princess Margaret Hosp, Toronto, Canada 1979-1980; **Fac Appt:** Prof Otolaryngology, Hahnemann Univ

Hurst, Michael K MD (Oto) - *Spec Exp:* Nasal Allergy; **Hospital:** WV Univ Hosp - Ruby Memorial; **Address:** ENT Clinic, 1188 Pineview Dr, Morgantown, WV 26505; **Phone:** (304) 599-3959; **Board Cert:** Otolaryngology 1994; **Med School:** Marshall Univ 1988; **Resid:** Otolaryngology, W Va Sch Med Hosps, Morgantown, WV 1989-1993; **Fac Appt:** Asst Prof Otolaryngology, W VA Sch Osteo Med

Johnson, Jonas Talmadge MD (Oto) - *Spec Exp:* Head & Neck Surgery; Head & Neck Cancer; Snoring/Sleep Apnea; **Hospital:** UPMC - Presbyterian Univ Hosp; **Address:** Eye and Ear Inst, 200 Lothrop St, Ste 300, Pittsburgh, PA 15213; **Phone:** (412) 647-2100; **Board Cert:** Otolaryngology 1977; **Med School:** SUNY Syracuse 1972; **Resid:** Surgery, Med Ctr VA, Richmond, VA 1973-1974; Otolaryngology, SUNY Hlth Sci Ctr, Syracuse, NY 1974-1977; **Fac Appt:** Prof Otolaryngology, Univ Pittsburgh

Josephson, Jordan S MD (Oto) - *Spec Exp:* Sinus Surgery-Endoscopic; Snoring & Hoarseness; Rhinoplasty; **Hospital:** Manhattan Eye, Ear & Throat Hosp; **Address:** 111 E 77th St, New York, NY 10021-1802; **Phone:** (212) 717-1773; **Board Cert:** Otolaryngology 1988; **Med School:** SUNY Hlth Sci Ctr 1983; **Resid:** Otolaryngology, Long Island Jewish Med Ctr, New Hyde Park, NY 1984-1988; **Fellow:** Sinus Surgery, Johns Hopkins Med Ctr, Baltimore, MD 1988-1989

Kennedy, David MD (Oto) - *Spec Exp:* Endoscopic Sinus Surgery; Skull Base Tumors; **Hospital:** Hosp Univ Penn (page 78); **Address:** Univ Penn, Dept Oto/HNS, 3400 Spruce St, Philadelphia, PA 19104; **Phone:** (215) 662-2777; **Board Cert:** Otolaryngology 1978; **Med School:** Ireland 1972; **Resid:** Surgery, Johns Hopkins Hosp, Baltimore, MD 1973-1974; Otolaryngology, Johns Hopkins Hosp, Baltimore, MD 1974-1978; **Fac Appt:** Prof Otolaryngology, Univ Penn

Koch, Wayne Martin MD (Oto) - *Spec Exp:* Head & Neck Cancer; Sinus Cancer; **Hospital:** Johns Hopkins Hosp - Baltimore; **Address:** Johns Hopkins Hosp, Dept Otolaryngology, Box 41402, Baltimore, MD 21203-6402; **Phone:** (410) 955-4906; **Board Cert:** Otolaryngology 1987; **Med School:** Univ Pittsburgh 1982; **Resid:** Otolaryngology, Tufts-Boston U., Boston, MA 1983-1987; **Fellow:** Surgical Oncology, Johns HopkinsHosp, Baltimore, MD 1987-1989; **Fac Appt:** Assoc Prof Otolaryngology, Johns Hopkins Univ

Lawson, William MD (Oto) - *Spec Exp:* Sinus Disorders/Surgery; Cosmetic Surgery-Face; **Hospital:** Mount Sinai Hosp (page 68); **Address:** 5 E 98th St Fl 8, Fl 8, New York, NY 10029-6501; **Phone:** (212) 241-9410; **Board Cert:** Otolaryngology 1974; **Med School:** NYU Sch Med 1965; **Resid:** Surgery, Bronx VA Hosp, Bronx, NY 1966-1967; Otolaryngology, Mount Sinai Hosp, New York, NY 1970-1973; **Fellow:** Otolaryngology, Mount Sinai Hosp, New York, NY 1969-1970; **Fac Appt:** Prof Otolaryngology, Mount Sinai Sch Med

Linstrom, Christopher MD (Oto) - *Spec Exp:* Hearing Loss; Acoustic Nerve Tumors; Encephalocele; **Hospital:** New York Eye & Ear Infirm (page 69); **Address:** 310 E 14th St, New York, NY 10003; **Phone:** (212) 979-4200; **Board Cert:** Otolaryngology 1987; **Med School:** Canada 1982; **Resid:** Otolaryngology, NY-Cornell Med Ctr, New York, NY 1984-1987; **Fellow:** Otology & Neurotology, Michigan Ear Inst, Farmington Hills, MI 1987-1989; **Fac Appt:** Asst Prof Otolaryngology, NY Med Coll

Minor, Lloyd B MD (Oto) - *Spec Exp:* Balance Disorders; Neuro-otology; **Hospital:** Johns Hopkins Hosp - Baltimore; **Address:** Johns Hopkins Outpatient Ctr, 601 N Caroline St, rm 6255, Baltimore, MD 21287; **Phone:** (410) 955-3403; **Board Cert:** Otolaryngology 1993; **Med School:** Brown Univ 1982; **Resid:** Otolaryngology, Univ Chicago Hosps, Chicago, IL 1988-1992; **Fellow:** Otolaryngology, Ear Foundation/Baptist Hosp, Nashville, TN 1992-1993; **Fac Appt:** Prof Otolaryngology, Johns Hopkins Univ

Myers, Eugene MD (Oto) - *Spec Exp:* Head & Neck Surgery; Head & Neck Cancer; **Hospital:** UPMC - Presbyterian Univ Hosp; **Address:** Dept Otolaryngology, 200 Lothrop St Bldg EEI Fl 3rd - Ste 300, Pittsburgh, PA 15213; **Phone:** (412) 647-2100; **Board Cert:** Otolaryngology 1966; **Med School:** Temple Univ 1960; **Resid:** Surgery, VA Hosp, Boston, MA 1961-1962; Otolaryngology, Mass EE Infirm, Boston, MA 1962-1965; **Fellow:** Otolaryngology, Harvard Med School, Boston, MA 1964-1965; Otolaryngology, St Vincent's Hosp, New York, NY 1967-1968; **Fac Appt:** Prof Otolaryngology, Univ Pittsburgh

Niparko, John MD (Oto) - *Spec Exp:* Ear Disorders/Surgery; Neuro-Otology; **Hospital:** Johns Hopkins Hosp - Baltimore; **Address:** Johns Hopkins Hosp, Dept Otolaryngology, 601 N Caroline St, Ste 6223, Baltimore, MD 21287-6214; **Phone:** (410) 955-2689; **Board Cert:** Otolaryngology 1986; **Med School:** Univ Mich Med Sch 1980; **Resid:** Otolaryngology, Univ Mich, Ann Arbor, MI 1982-1986; Surgery, William Beaumont Hosp., Royal Oak, MI 1980-1982; **Fellow:** Otolaryngology, Univ Mich, Ann Arbor, MI 1986; **Fac Appt:** Prof Otolaryngology, Johns Hopkins Univ

Papel, Ira David MD (Oto) - *Spec Exp:* Cosmetic Surgery-Face; Nasal Reconstruction; Skin Cancer/Skin Reconstructive Surgery; **Hospital:** Johns Hopkins Hosp - Baltimore; **Address:** Facial Plastic Surgicenter, 21 Crossroads Dr, Owing Mills, MD 21117-5441; **Phone:** (410) 363-6677; **Board Cert:** Otolaryngology 1986; **Med School:** Boston Univ 1981; **Resid:** Otolaryngology, Johns Hopkins Hosp, Baltimore, MD 1982-1986; **Fellow:** Facial Plastic Surgery, UCSF Med Ctr, San Francisco, CA 1986-1987; **Fac Appt:** Assoc Prof Otolaryngology, Johns Hopkins Univ

Parisier, Simon MD (Oto) - *Spec Exp:* Cochlear Implants; Hearing Loss; Ear Infections; **Hospital:** Lenox Hill Hosp (page 64); **Address:** 210 E 64th St Fl 3, New York, NY 10021-7400; **Phone:** (212) 535-6400; **Board Cert:** Otolaryngology 1967; **Med School:** Boston Univ 1961; **Resid:** Otolaryngology, Mount Sinai, New York, NY 1962-1966; **Fac Appt:** Clin Prof Otolaryngology, NY Coll Osteo Med

Pastorek, Norman MD (Oto) - *Spec Exp:* Cosmetic Surgery-Face; Rhinoplasty/Facelift; Cosmetic Eye Lid Surgery; **Hospital:** NY Presby Hosp - NY Weill Cornell Med Ctr (page 70); **Address:** 12 E 88th St, New York, NY 10128-0535; **Phone:** (212) 987-4700; **Board Cert:** Otolaryngology 1970; **Med School:** Univ IL Coll Med 1964; **Resid:** Surgery, VA Hosp, Hines, IL 1966-1967; Otolaryngology, U Illinois Med Ctr, Chicago, IL 1967-1969; **Fac Appt:** Clin Prof Otolaryngology, Cornell Univ-Weill Med Coll

Persky, Mark MD (Oto) - *Spec Exp:* Head & Neck Cancer; Skull Base Tumors; **Hospital:** Beth Israel Med Ctr - Singer Div (page 58); **Address:** 10 Union Square East, Ste 4J, New York, NY 10003-3314; **Phone:** (212) 844-8648; **Board Cert:** Otolaryngology 1976; **Med School:** SUNY Syracuse 1972; **Resid:** Otolaryngology, Bellevue Hosp, New York, NY 1973-1976; **Fellow:** Head and Neck Surgery, Beth Israel Med Ctr, New York, NY 1976-1977; **Fac Appt:** Clin Prof Otolaryngology, Albert Einstein Coll Med

Picken, Catherine A MD (Oto) - *Spec Exp:* Head & Neck Reconstruction; Thyroid Disorders; Sinus Disorders/Surgery; **Hospital:** Georgetown Univ Hosp; **Address:** 3800 Reservoir Rd NW, Washington, DC 20007-2113; **Phone:** (202) 687-8186; **Board Cert:** Otolaryngology 1989; **Med School:** Northwestern Univ 1979; **Resid:** Surgery, Northwestern Meml Hosp, Chicago, IL 1980-1981; Otolaryngology, Georgetown Univ, Washington, DC 1985-1989; **Fellow:** Surgery, Natl Heart Lung Blood Inst, Bethesda, MD 1981-1983; **Fac Appt:** Assoc Prof Otolaryngology, Georgetown Univ

Quatela, Vito Charles MD (Oto) - *Spec Exp:* Cosmetic Surgery-Face; Rhinoplasty; Forehead Lift-Endoscpic; **Hospital:** Strong Memorial Hosp - URMC; **Address:** University of Rochester, 973 East Ave, Ste 100, Rochester, NY 14607; **Phone:** (716) 244-1000; **Board Cert:** Otolaryngology 1985; **Med School:** Northwestern Univ 1979; **Resid:** Surgery, Med Ctr Hosp Vermont, Burlington 1980-1981; Orthopaedic Surgery, Northwestern Univ, Chicago, IL 1982-1985; **Fellow:** Facial Plastic Surgery, Tulane Univ, New Orleans, LA 1985-1986; Facial Plastic Surgery, Oregon Hlth Science Univ, Portland 1986-1987; **Fac Appt:** Assoc Clin Prof Otolaryngology, Univ Rochester

Romo III, Thomas MD (Oto) - *Spec Exp:* Cosmetic Surgery-Face; Rhinoplasty; Ear Reconstruction/Microtia; **Hospital:** Lenox Hill Hosp (page 64); **Address:** 135 E 74th St, New York, NY 10021; **Phone:** (212) 288-1500; **Board Cert:** Otolaryngology 1985; **Med School:** Baylor Coll Med 1979; **Resid:** Plastic Surgery, New York Eye & Ear, New York, NY 1984-1985; Otolaryngology, New York Eye & Ear, New York, NY 1982-1984; **Fellow:** Plastic Surgery, Tampa General, Tampa, FL 1985

Sataloff, Robert MD (Oto) - *Spec Exp:* Laryngeal Disorders; Voice Disorders; **Hospital:** Thomas Jefferson Univ Hosp; **Address:** 1721 Pine Street, Philadelphia, PA 19103-6701; **Phone:** (215) 545-3322; **Board Cert:** Otolaryngology 1980; **Med School:** Jefferson Med Coll 1975; **Resid:** Otolaryngology, Unvi Mich Hosp, Ann Harbor, MI 1976-1980; **Fellow:** Otolaryngology, Univ Mich Hosp, Ann Harbor, MI 1980-1981; **Fac Appt:** Prof Otolaryngology, Jefferson Med Coll

Schaefer, Steven D MD (Oto) - *Spec Exp:* Sinus Disorders/Surgery; Head & Neck Surgery; Endoscopic Surgery; **Hospital:** New York Eye & Ear Infirm (page 69); **Address:** 310 E 14th St, New York, NY 10003-4201; **Phone:** (212) 979-4200; **Board Cert:** Otolaryngology 1978; **Med School:** UC Irvine 1972; **Resid:** Surgery, UCLA Med Ctr, Los Angeles, CA 1972-1974; Otolaryngology, Stanford Med Ctr, Stanford, CA 1973-1974; **Fac Appt:** Prof Otolaryngology, NY Med Coll

Urken, Mark MD (Oto) - *Spec Exp:* Microvascular Reconstruction; Head & Neck Surgery; Head & Neck Cancer; **Hospital:** Mount Sinai Hosp (page 68); **Address:** 5 E 98th St, Ste 8, New York, NY 10029-6501; **Phone:** (212) 241-9410; **Board Cert:** Otolaryngology 1986; **Med School:** Univ VA Sch Med 1981; **Resid:** Otolaryngology, Mount Sinai Hosp, New York, NY 1983-1986; **Fellow:** Plastic Surgery, Mercy Hospital, Pittsburgh, PA 1986-1987; **Fac Appt:** Assoc Prof Otolaryngology, Mount Sinai Sch Med

Ward, Robert MD (Oto) - *Spec Exp:* Pediatric Otolaryngology; Sinus Disorders/Surgery; **Hospital:** NY Presby Hosp - NY Weill Cornell Med Ctr (page 70); **Address:** 186 E 76th St Fl 2, New York, NY 10021; **Phone:** (212) 327-3000; **Board Cert:** Otolaryngology 1986; **Med School:** Cornell Univ-Weill Med Coll 1981; **Resid:** Surgery, New York Hosp, New York, NY 1982-1983; Otolaryngology, New York Hosp, New York, NY 1983-1986; **Fellow:** Pediatric Otolaryngology, Chldns Hosp, Boston, MA 1986; **Fac Appt:** Assoc Clin Prof Otolaryngology, Cornell Univ-Weill Med Coll

Wazen, Jack MD (Oto) - *Spec Exp:* Skull Base Surgery; Meniere's Disease; Acoustic Nerve Tumors; **Hospital:** NY Presby Hosp - Columbia Presby Med Ctr (page 70); **Address:** 111 E 77th St, New York, NY 10021-1802; **Phone:** (212) 249-3232; **Board Cert:** Otolaryngology 1983; **Med School:** Lebanon 1978; **Resid:** Surgery, St Lukes Hosp, New York, NY 1979-1980; Otolaryngology, Columbia Presby Hosp, New York, NY 1980-1983; **Fellow:** Neurological Otology, Ear Rsch Fdn, Sarasota, FL 1983-1984; **Fac Appt:** Assoc Clin Prof Otolaryngology, Columbia P&S

Weber, Randal Scott MD (Oto) - *Spec Exp:* Thyroid Disorders; Thyroid & Parathyroid Surgery; Skull Base Tumors; **Hospital:** Hosp Univ Penn (page 78); **Address:** Hosp Univ Penn, Dept Otolayngology, 3400 Spruce St, 5-Ravdin, Philadelphia, PA 19104; **Phone:** (215) 662-2777; **Board Cert:** Otolaryngology 1985; **Med School:** Univ Tenn Coll Med, Memphis 1976; **Resid:** Surgery, Baylor Coll Med, Houston, TX 1981-1982; Otolaryngology, Baylor Coll Med, Houston, TX 1982-1985; **Fellow:** Head and Neck Surgery, Univ TX MD Anderson Cancer Ctr, Houston, TX 1985-1986; **Fac Appt:** Prof Otolaryngology, Univ Penn

Weinstein, Gregory MD (Oto) - *Spec Exp:* Head & Neck Cancer; Larygeal Cancer-Organ Preservation; **Hospital:** Hosp Univ Penn (page 78); **Address:** Hosp of Univ Penn, Dept Oto, 3400 Spruce St, Bldg Ravdin 5, Philadelphia, PA 19104; **Phone:** (215) 349-5390; **Board Cert:** Otolaryngology 1990; **Med School:** NY Med Coll 1985; **Resid:** Otolaryngology, St Vincent's Hosp, New York, NY 1985-1986; Otolaryngology, Univ Iowa Hosp, Iowa City, IA 1986-1990; **Fellow:** Head and Neck Oncology, Sacramento, CA 1990-1991; **Fac Appt:** Assoc Prof Otolaryngology, Univ Penn

Woo, Peak MD (Oto) - *Spec Exp:* Voice Disorders; Laryngeal Disorders; Laryngeal Cancer; **Hospital:** Mount Sinai Hosp (page 68); **Address:** 5 E 98th St Fl 1, New York, NY 10029-6501; **Phone:** (212) 241-9425; **Board Cert:** Otolaryngology 1983; **Med School:** Boston Univ 1978; **Resid:** Otolaryngology, Boston Univ, Boston, MA 1979-1983; **Fac Appt:** Prof Otolaryngology, Mount Sinai Sch Med

Zalzal, George MD (Oto) - *Spec Exp:* Airway Disorders; Laryngeal & Tracheal Disorders; Ear Disorders/Surgery; **Hospital:** Chldns Natl Med Ctr - DC; **Address:** 111 Michigan Ave NW, Washington, DC 20010; **Phone:** (202) 884-2159; **Board Cert:** Otolaryngology 1996; **Med School:** Lebanon 1979; **Resid:** American Univ Hosp, Beirut, Lebanon 1979-1983; **Fellow:** Pediatric Otolaryngology, Univ Cincinnati, Cincinnati, OH 1983-1985; **Fac Appt:** Prof Pediatric Otolaryngology, Geo Wash Univ

549

Southeast

Antonelli, Patrick MD (Oto) - ***Spec Exp:*** *Hearing Disorders; Ear Disorders/Surgery;* **Hospital:** Shands Hlthcre at Univ of FL (page 73); **Address:** 1600 SW Archer Rd, Box 100264, Gainesville, FL 32610; **Phone:** (352) 392-4061; **Board Cert:** Otolaryngology 1994; **Med School:** Univ Minn 1988; **Resid:** Surgery, Hannepin Co Med Ctr, Minneapolis, MN 1986-1989; Otolaryngology, Univ of Minnesota, Minneapolis, MN 1989-1993; **Fellow:** Neurological Otology, Michigan Ear Inst, Farmington, MI 1993-1994; **Fac Appt:** Assoc Prof Otolaryngology, Univ Fla Coll Med

Balkany, Thomas Jay MD (Oto) - ***Spec Exp:*** *Deafness & Ear Disorders; Neuro-Otology; Cochlear Implants;* **Hospital:** Univ of Miami - Jackson Meml Hosp; **Address:** Univ of Miami Ear Inst, ACC East Bldg, 1666 NW 10th Ave, Ste 316, Miami, FL 33136-1015; **Phone:** (305) 585-7129; **Board Cert:** Otolaryngology 1977; **Med School:** Univ Miami Sch Med 1972; **Resid:** Surgery, St Joseph Hosp, Denver, CO 1973-1974; Otolaryngology, Colo Med Ctr, Denver, CO 1974-1977; **Fellow:** Otolaryngology, House Ear Inst, Los Angeles, CA 1978; **Fac Appt:** Clin Prof Otolaryngology, Univ Miami Sch Med

Becker, Ferdinand Francis MD (Oto) - ***Spec Exp:*** *Cosmetic Surgery-Face;* **Hospital:** Indian River Mem Hosp; **Address:** 5070 N A1a, Ste A, Vero Beach, FL 32963-1229; **Phone:** (561) 234-3700; **Board Cert:** Otolaryngology 1972; **Med School:** Tulane Univ 1965; **Resid:** Surgery, Charity Hosp, New Orleans, LA 1968-1969; Otolaryngology, Charity Hosp, New Orleans, LA 1969-1972; **Fac Appt:** Asst Clin Prof Otolaryngology, Univ Fla Coll Med

Burkey, Brian MD (Oto) - ***Spec Exp:*** *Parotid Gland Tumors; Head & Neck Cancer;* **Hospital:** Vanderbilt Univ Med Ctr (page 80); **Address:** Vanderbilt Univ, Dept Oto, S-2100 MCN, Nashville, TN 37232-2559; **Phone:** (615) 322-7267; **Board Cert:** Otolaryngology 1992; **Med School:** Univ VA Sch Med 1986; **Resid:** Otolaryngology, Univ Mich, Ann Arbor, MI 1987-1991; **Fellow:** Microsurgery, Ohio State Univ, Columbus, OH 1991; **Fac Appt:** Assoc Prof Otolaryngology, Vanderbilt Univ

Cassisi, Nicholas J MD (Oto) - ***Spec Exp:*** *Head & Neck Cancer; Voice Disorders;* **Hospital:** Shands Hlthcre at Univ of FL (page 73); **Address:** Shands Healthcare at Univ FL, 1600 SW Archer Rd, Box 100264, Gainesville, FL 32610; **Phone:** (352) 392-4461; **Board Cert:** Otolaryngology 1971; **Med School:** Univ Miami Sch Med 1965; **Resid:** Surgery, Jackson Memorial Hosp, Miami, FL 1966-1967; Otolaryngology, Barnes Hosp - Washington U, Seattle, WA 1968-1971; **Fac Appt:** Prof Otolaryngology, Univ Fla Coll Med

Courey, Mark Sam MD (Oto) - ***Spec Exp:*** *Laryngeal Disorders;* **Hospital:** Vanderbilt Univ Med Ctr (page 80); **Address:** Vanderbilt Voice Ctr, 1500 21st Ave S, Nashville, TN 37212; **Phone:** (615) 343-7464; **Board Cert:** Otolaryngology 1993; **Med School:** SUNY Buffalo 1987; **Resid:** Otolaryngology, SUNY-Buffalo, Buffalo, NY 1989-1992; **Fellow:** Otolaryngology, Vanderbilt Univ, Nashville, TN 1992-1993; **Fac Appt:** Assoc Prof Otolaryngology, Vanderbilt Univ

Farmer, Joseph MD (Oto) - ***Spec Exp:*** *Ear Disorders/Surgery; Hearing Disorders; Balance Disorders;* **Hospital:** Duke Univ Med Ctr (page 60); **Address:** Duke Univ Med Ctr, Box 3805, Durham, NC 27710; **Phone:** (919) 684-6357; **Board Cert:** Otolaryngology 1971; **Med School:** Duke Univ 1962; **Resid:** Surgical Oncology, Natl Cancer Inst, Bethesda, MD 1965-1967; Otolaryngology, Duke Univ Med Ctr, Durham, NC 1967-1970; **Fellow:** Thoracic Surgery, Duke Univ Med Ctr, Durham, NC 1964; **Fac Appt:** Prof Otolaryngology, Duke Univ

Farrior, Edward MD (Oto) - ***Spec Exp:*** *Cosmetic Surgery-Face;* **Hospital:** Tampa Genl Hosp; **Address:** 2908 W Azeele St, Tampa, FL 33609-3109; **Phone:** (813) 875-3223; **Board Cert:** Otolaryngology 1987; **Med School:** Univ VA Sch Med 1982; **Resid:** Otolaryngology, Univ Mich Hosps, Ann Arbor, MI 1983-1987; **Fellow:** Facial Plastic Surgery, Tampa Genl Hosp, Tampa, Fl 1987-1988; **Fac Appt:** Assoc Clin Prof Surgery, Univ Fla Coll Med

Farrior, Joseph Brown MD (Oto) - *Spec Exp:* Ear Disorders/Surgery; **Hospital:** St Joseph's Hosp - Tampa; **Address:** 509 W Bay St, Tampa, FL 33606; **Phone:** (800) 342-3277; **Board Cert:** Otolaryngology 1981; **Med School:** Emory Univ 1975; **Resid:** Surgery, Johns Hopkins Hosp, Baltimore, MD 1976-1977; Otolaryngology, Johns Hopkins HOsp, Baltimore, MD 1977-1981; **Fellow:** Otolaryngology, Farrior Clin/St Josephs Hosp, Tampa, FL 1979-1980; **Fac Appt:** Assoc Clin Prof Otolaryngology, Univ S Fla Coll Med

Goodwin, W Jarrard MD (Oto) - *Spec Exp:* Head & Neck Cancer; **Hospital:** Univ of Miami & Clinics/Sylvestor Comp Cancer Ctr; **Address:** Dept Otolaryngology, 1475 NW 12th Ave, Ste 4037, Miami, FL 33136-1015; **Phone:** (305) 243-4387; **Board Cert:** Otolaryngology 1978; **Med School:** Albany Med Coll 1972; **Resid:** Surgery, Univ Miami/Jackson Hosp Meml Hosp, Miami, FL 1972-1973; Otolaryngology, Univ Miami/Jackson Hosp, Miami, FL 1974-1977; **Fellow:** Surgery, MD Anderson Hosp, Houston, TX 1979-1980; **Fac Appt:** Prof Otolaryngology, Univ Miami Sch Med

Grobman, Lawrence R MD (Oto) - *Spec Exp:* Cochlear Implants; Otosclerosis; Deafness-Genetic; **Hospital:** Mercy Hosp - Miami, FL; **Address:** 3661 S Miami Ave, Ste 409, Miami, FL 33133-4236; **Phone:** (305) 854-5971; **Board Cert:** Otolaryngology 1986; **Med School:** Univ Miami Sch Med 1980; **Resid:** Surgery, U Miami Med Ctr, Miami, FL 1981-1982; Otolaryngology, U Miami Med Ctr, Miami, FL 1982-1985; **Fellow:** Otology & Neurotology, U Zurich Med Ctr, Zurich, Switzerland 1985-1986; **Fac Appt:** Assoc Prof Otolaryngology, Univ Miami Sch Med

Koufman, James Alan MD (Oto) - *Spec Exp:* Voice Disorders; Laryngeal Disorders; **Hospital:** Wake Forest Univ Baptist Med Ctr (page 81); **Address:** Wake Forest Univ Baptist Med Ctr, Dept Oto, Medical Center Blvd, Winston Salem, NC 27157; **Phone:** (336) 716-4161; **Board Cert:** Otolaryngology 1978; **Med School:** Boston Univ 1973; **Resid:** Surgery, Hartford Hosp, Hartford, CT 1974-1975; Otolaryngology, Boston Univ Med Ctr, Boston, MA 1975-1978; **Fac Appt:** Prof Surgery, Wake Forest Univ Sch Med

Kuhn, Frederick MD (Oto) - *Spec Exp:* Nasal & Sinus Disorders; Endoscopic Sinus Surgery; Head & Neck Surgery; **Hospital:** Meml Med Ctr - Savannah; **Address:** Georgia Nasal & Sinus Inst, 4750 Waters Ave, Ste 112, Savannah, GA 31404; **Phone:** (912) 355-1070; **Board Cert:** Otolaryngology 1972; **Med School:** Univ Okla Coll Med 1966; **Resid:** Surgery, Univ Oklahoma Teaching Hosp, Oklahoma City, OK 1966-1967; Surgery, St Luke's Hosp, St Louis, MO 1967-1968; **Fellow:** Otolaryngology, Barnes Hosp/Wash Univ, St Louis, MO 1968-1972; **Fac Appt:** Prof Otolaryngology

Lambert, Paul R MD (Oto) - *Spec Exp:* Neuro-Otology; **Hospital:** Med Univ Hosp Authority; **Address:** MUSC, Dep Otolaryngology, 150 Ashley Ave, Box 250582, Charleston, SC 29425; **Phone:** (843) 792-3531; **Board Cert:** Otolaryngology 1981; **Med School:** Duke Univ 1976; **Resid:** Surgery, UCLA Med Ctr, Los Angeles, CA 1977-1978; Otolaryngology, UCLA Med Ctr, Los Angeles, CA 1978-1981; **Fellow:** Neurological Otology, Otologic Med Group, Los Angeles, CA 1981-1982; **Fac Appt:** Prof Otolaryngology, Med Univ SC

Levine, Paul MD (Oto) - *Spec Exp:* Head & Neck Cancer; Head & Neck Reconstruction; **Hospital:** Univ of VA Hlth Sys (page 79); **Address:** UVA Health Systems, Dept Otolaryngology, PO Box 800713, Charlottesville, VA 22908; **Phone:** (804) 924-5593; **Board Cert:** Otolaryngology 1978; **Med School:** Albany Med Coll 1973; **Resid:** Otolaryngology, Yale-New Haven Hosp, New Haven, CT 1974-1977; **Fellow:** Head and Neck Surgery, Stanford Med Ctr, Stanford, CA 1977-1978; **Fac Appt:** Prof Otolaryngology, Univ VA Sch Med

Mattox, Douglas MD (Oto) - *Spec Exp:* Neuro-Otology; **Hospital:** Emory Univ Hosp; **Address:** Dept Otolaryngology, 1365-A Clifton Rd NE, Atlanta, GA 30322; **Phone:** (404) 778-3381; **Board Cert:** Otolaryngology 1977; **Med School:** Yale Univ 1973; **Resid:** Otolaryngology, Stanford Univ Hosp, Stanford, CA 1974-1977; **Fac Appt:** Prof Otolaryngology, Emory Univ

McGuirt, W Fredrick MD (Oto) - *Spec Exp:* Head & Neck Cancer; Laryngeal Disorders; **Hospital:** Wake Forest Univ Baptist Med Ctr (page 81); **Address:** Wake Forest Baptist Med Ctr-Dept Otolaryngology, Medical Center Blvd, Winston Salem, NC 27157; **Phone:** (336) 716-4161; **Board Cert:** Otolaryngology 1976; **Med School:** Wake Forest Univ Sch Med 1968; **Resid:** Otolaryngology, Iowa Hosp, Iowa City, IA 1972-1976; Surgery, NC Bapt Hosp, Winston Salem, NC 1969-1970

Netterville, James MD (Oto) - *Spec Exp:* Head & Neck Surgery; **Hospital:** Vanderbilt Univ Med Ctr (page 80); **Address:** Vanderbilt Univ Med Ctr, Dept Oto, 1301 22nd Ave S, Ste 2900, Nashville, TN 37232; **Phone:** (615) 322-6180; **Board Cert:** Otolaryngology 1985; **Med School:** Univ Tenn Coll Med, Memphis 1980; **Resid:** Surgery, Methodist Hosp, Memphis, TN 1981-1982; Otolaryngology, Univ Tenn, Memphis, TN 1982-1985; **Fellow:** Surgical Oncology, Univ Iowa, Iowa City, IA 1985-1986; **Fac Appt:** Assoc Prof Otolaryngology, Vanderbilt Univ

Orobello Jr, Peter W MD (Oto) - *Spec Exp:* Otolaryngology-Pediatric; **Hospital:** All Children's Hosp; **Address:** 801 6th St S, St Petersburg, FL 33701-4816; **Phone:** (727) 892-4305; **Board Cert:** Otolaryngology 1988; **Med School:** Univ Cincinnati 1983; **Resid:** Surgery, Univ Cincinnati, Cincinnati, OH 1984; Otolaryngology, Univ Cincinnati, Cincinnati, OH 1984-1988; **Fellow:** Pediatric Otolaryngology, Johns Hopkins Univ, Baltimore, MD 1989; **Fac Appt:** Asst Clin Prof Pediatrics, Univ S Fla Coll Med

Pearson, Bruce MD (Oto) - *Spec Exp:* Laryngeal Cancer; Head & Neck Surgery; **Hospital:** St Luke's Hosp; **Address:** 4500 San Pablo Rd, Jacksonville, FL 32224-1865; **Phone:** (904) 953-2217; **Board Cert:** Otolaryngology 1975; **Med School:** Univ Toronto 1966; **Resid:** Otolaryngology, Univ Toronto, Toronto, Canada 1967-1971; Head and Neck Surgery, Royal National, London, England 1972; **Fellow:** Head and Neck Surgery, Mayo Clinic, Rochester, MN 1973; **Fac Appt:** Prof Otolaryngology, Mayo Med Sch

Peters, Glenn Eidson MD (Oto) - *Spec Exp:* Head & Neck Cancer; Skull Base Surgery; **Hospital:** Univ of Ala Hosp at Birmingham; **Address:** UAB Medical Center, Head and Neck Surgery Clinic, 1501 5 Ave S, Birmingham, AL 35233; **Phone:** (205) 934-9766; **Board Cert:** Otolaryngology 1985; **Med School:** Louisiana State Univ 1980; **Resid:** Surgery, Bapt Med Ctr, Birmingham, AL 1981-1982; Otolaryngology, Univ Ala, Birmingham, AL 1982-1984; **Fellow:** Medical Oncology, Johns Hopkins Hosp, Baltimore, MD 1986-1987

Pillsbury, Harold Crockett MD (Oto) - *Spec Exp:* Cochlear Implants; **Hospital:** Univ of NC Hosp (page 77); **Address:** 610 Burnett-Womack Bldg, Box CB7070, Chapel Hill, NC 27599-7070; **Phone:** (919) 966-8926; **Board Cert:** Otolaryngology 1978; **Med School:** Geo Wash Univ 1972; **Resid:** Surgery, Univ NC, Chapel Hill, NC 1973-1976; Otolaryngology, NC Meml Hosp, Chapel Hill, NC 1973-1976; **Fac Appt:** Prof Otolaryngology, Univ NC Sch Med

Postma, Gregory N MD (Oto) - *Spec Exp:* Voice Disorders; **Hospital:** Wake Forest Univ Baptist Med Ctr (page 81); **Address:** Wake Forest Univ Sch Med-Dept Oto, Med Ctr Blvd, Winston Salem, NC 27157; **Phone:** (336) 716-4161; **Board Cert:** Otolaryngology 1994; **Med School:** Hahnemann Univ 1984; **Resid:** Otolaryngology, Oakland Naval Hosp, Oakland, CA 1989-1992; Otolaryngology, Univ NC, Chapel Hill, NC 1992-1993; **Fellow:** Otolaryngology, Vanderbilt Univ, Nashvile, TN 1995-1996; **Fac Appt:** Asst Prof Otolaryngology, Wake Forest Univ Sch Med

Robbins, Thomas MD (Oto) - *Spec Exp:* Head & Neck Surgery; **Hospital:** Shands Hlthcre at Univ of FL (page 73); **Address:** Univ Florida, Dept Oto, 1600 SW Archer Rd, Bldg M - rm 228, Box 100264, Gainesville, FL 32610; **Phone:** (352) 392-4461; **Board Cert:** Otolaryngology 1981; **Med School:** Dalhousie Univ 1973; **Resid:** Surgery, Dalhousie Univ, Halifax, Canada 1978-1979; Otolaryngology, Univ Toronto, Toronto, Canada 1979-1981; **Fellow:** Head and Neck Surgery, Inst Laryngology & Otology, London, England 1981-1982; Head and Neck Surgery, MD Anderson, Houston, TX 1982-1982; **Fac Appt:** Prof Otolaryngology, Univ Fla Coll Med

Sillers, Michael MD (Oto) - *Spec Exp:* Nasal & Sinus Disorders; Sinus Disorders/Surgery; **Hospital:** Univ of Ala Hosp at Birmingham; **Address:** UAB Med Ctr, Head and Neck Surg Clin, 1501 5th Ave S, Birmingham, AL 35233; **Phone:** (205) 934-9779; **Board Cert:** Otolaryngology 1994; **Med School:** Univ Ala 1988; **Resid:** Otolaryngology, Univ of Alabama, Birmingham, AL 1989-1993; **Fellow:** Sinus Surgery, Med Coll Ga, Augusta, GA 1993-1994; **Fac Appt:** Asst Prof Surgery, Univ Ala

Silverstein, Herbert MD (Oto) - *Spec Exp:* Ear Disorders/Surgery; Meniere's Disease; **Hospital:** Sarasota Mem Hosp; **Address:** 1961 Floyd St, Ste A, Sarasota, FL 34239-2931; **Phone:** (941) 366-9222; **Board Cert:** Otolaryngology 1967; **Med School:** Temple Univ 1961; **Resid:** Surgery, Univ Penn, Philadelphia, PA 1961-1963; Otolaryngology, Mass EE Infirm, Boston, MA 1963-1966; **Fac Appt:** Clin Prof Surgery, Univ S Fla Coll Med

Spektor, Zorik MD (Oto) - *Spec Exp:* Otolaryngology - General; **Hospital:** St Mary's Med Ctr - W Palm Bch; **Address:** St. Mary's Med Ctr Bldg Ranes Pavilion - Ste 202, 5325 Greenwood Ave, West Palm Beach, FL 33407; **Phone:** (561) 736-8141; **Board Cert:** Otolaryngology 1995; **Med School:** Albany Med Coll 1986; **Resid:** Otolaryngology, Univ Conn Hlth Ctr, Farmington, CT 1987-1991; **Fellow:** Surgery, Le Bonheur Chldns Med Ctr, Memphis, TN 1994-1995

Stringer, Scott Pearson MD (Oto) - *Spec Exp:* Head & Neck Cancer; Nasal & Sinus Disorders; Maxillofacial Surgery; **Hospital:** Univ Hosps & Clins - Mississippi; **Address:** Univ Mississippi Med Ctr, Dept Surg, Div Oto, 2500 N State St, Jackson, MS 39216; **Phone:** (601) 984-5167; **Board Cert:** Otolaryngology 1987; **Med School:** Univ Tex SW, Dallas 1982; **Resid:** Otolaryngology, Univ Tex SW Med Ctr, Dallas, TX 1984-1987; Surgery, Univ Tex SW Med Ctr, Dallas, TX 1982-1984; **Fac Appt:** Prof Otolaryngology, Univ Fla Coll Med

Tucci, Debara Lyn MD (Oto) - *Spec Exp:* Skull Base Surgery; Middle Ear Disorders; **Hospital:** Duke Univ Med Ctr (page 60); **Address:** Duke Univ Med Ctr, Box 3805, Durham, NC 27710; **Phone:** (919) 684-6968; **Board Cert:** Otolaryngology 1990; **Med School:** Univ VA Sch Med 1985; **Resid:** Otolaryngology, Univ Va Hlth Sci Ctr, Charlottesville, VA 1986-1990; **Fellow:** Otology & Neurotology, Univ Mich Med Ctr, Ann Arbor, MI 1990-1992; **Fac Appt:** Assoc Prof Surgery, Duke Univ

Valentino, Joseph MD (Oto) - *Spec Exp:* Head & Neck Cancer; **Hospital:** Univ Kentucky Med Ctr; **Address:** 740 S Limestone St, rm B-317, Lexington, KY 40536-0284; **Phone:** (859) 257-5405; **Board Cert:** Otolaryngology 1993; **Med School:** UMDNJ-RW Johnson Med Sch 1987; **Resid:** Otolaryngology, Univ Minn, Minneapolis, MN 1988-1992; **Fellow:** Otolaryngology, Univ Iowa Coll Med, Iowa City, IA 1992-1993; **Fac Appt:** Asst Prof Otolaryngology, Univ KY Coll Med

Weissler, Mark Christian MD (Oto) - *Spec Exp:* Head & Neck Cancer; Voice Disorders; **Hospital:** Univ of NC Hosp (page 77); **Address:** 610 Burnett-Womack Bldg, Chapel Hill, NC 27599-7070; **Phone:** (919) 966-3341; **Board Cert:** Otolaryngology 1985; **Med School:** Boston Univ 1980; **Resid:** Surgery, Mass Genl Hosp, Boston, MA 1980-1982; Otolaryngology, Mass Eye & Ear Infirm, Boston, MA 1982-1985; **Fellow:** Otolaryngology, Univ Cincinnati, Cincinnati, OH 1985-1986; **Fac Appt:** Prof Surgery, Univ NC Sch Med

Woodson, Gayle Ellen MD (Oto) - *Spec Exp:* Voice Disorders; **Hospital:** Shands Hlthcre at Univ of FL (page 73); **Address:** Shands Healthcare at Univ Florida, 1600 SW Archer Rd, rm M228, Gainesville, FL 32610; **Phone:** (352) 392-4461; **Board Cert:** Otolaryngology 1981; **Med School:** Baylor Coll Med **Resid:** Surgery, Johns Hopkins Hosp, Baltimore, MD 1977-1978; Otolaryngology, Baylor Coll Med, Houston, TX 1978-1981; **Fellow:** Otolaryngology, London, Engalnd, London, England 1981-1982; **Fac Appt:** Prof Otolaryngology, Univ Fla Coll Med

Midwest

Baim, Howard MD (Oto) - *Spec Exp:* Head & Neck Surgery; Head & Neck Tumors; Sinus Disorders; **Hospital:** Advocate IL Masonic Med Ctr; **Address:** 2532 N Lincoln Ave, Chicago, IL 60614-1712; **Phone:** (773) 883-1177; **Board Cert:** Otolaryngology 1978; **Med School:** Univ IL Coll Med 1973; **Resid:** Otolaryngology, IL Met Grp Hosps, Chicago, IL 1973-1975; Surgery, IL EE Infirmary, Chicago, IL 1975-1978; **Fac Appt:** Asst Clin Prof Otolaryngology, Univ IL Coll Med

Baker, Shan Ray MD (Oto) - *Spec Exp:* Cosmetic Surgery-Face & Neck; Facial Cosmetic Surgery; Reconstructive Surgery; **Hospital:** Univ of MI Hlth Ctr; **Address:** Center for Facial & Cosmetic Surgery, 19900 Haggerty Rd, Ste 103, Livonia, MI 48152-1054; **Phone:** (734) 432-7823; **Board Cert:** Otolaryngology 1977; **Med School:** Univ Iowa Coll Med 1971; **Resid:** Otolaryngology Head & Neck, Univ Iowa Hosps, Iowa City, IA 1973-1977; Surgery, Univ California San Diego Med Ctr, San Diego, CA 1971-1973; **Fac Appt:** Prof Otolaryngology, Univ Mich Med Sch

Benninger, Michael S MD (Oto) - *Spec Exp:* Vocal Cord Disorders; Nasal & Sinus Disorders; **Hospital:** Henry Ford Hosp; **Address:** 2799 W Grand Blvd , Fl 8 - rm k807, Detroit, MI 48202; **Phone:** (313) 916-3275; **Board Cert:** Otolaryngology 1988; **Med School:** Case West Res Univ 1983; **Resid:** Surgery, Cleveland Clin Fdn, Cleveland, OH 1983-1985; Otolaryngology, Cleveland Clin Fdn, Cleveland, OH 1985-1988; **Fac Appt:** Prof Otolaryngology, Case West Res Univ

Branham, Gregory H MD (Oto) - *Spec Exp:* Facial Plastic Surgery; **Hospital:** St Louis Univ Hospital; **Address:** 3660 Vista St, Ste 312, Saint Louis, MO 63110; **Phone:** (314) 577-6110; **Board Cert:** Otolaryngology 1989; **Med School:** USC Sch Med 1983; **Resid:** Otolaryngology, St Louis Univ Hosp, Saint Louis, MO 1985-1989; **Fellow:** Facial Plastic Surgery, Washington Univ, St Louis, MO 1989-1990; **Fac Appt:** Assoc Prof Otolaryngology, St Louis Univ

Caldarelli, David D MD (Oto) - *Spec Exp:* Larynx & Vocal Cord Surgery; Meniere's Disease; **Hospital:** Rush-Presby - St Luke's Med Ctr (page 72); **Address:** 1725 W Harrison St, Ste 308, Chicago, IL 60612-3814; **Phone:** (312) 733-4341; **Board Cert:** Otolaryngology 1970; **Med School:** Univ Hlth Sci/Chicago Med Sch 1965; **Resid:** Surgery, Presby-St Lukes Hosp, Chicago, IL 1966-1967; Otolaryngology, Univ Illinois Eye/Ear Infirm, Chicago, IL 1967-1970; **Fac Appt:** Prof Otolaryngology, Rush Med Coll

Chernoff, William Gregory MD (Oto) - *Spec Exp:* Facial Plastic/Reconstructive Surgery; Ear, Nose & Throat; Laser Surgery; **Hospital:** Methodist Hosp - Indianapolis (page 66); **Address:** 9002 N Meridian St, Ste 205, Indianapolis, IN 46260; **Phone:** (317) 573-8899; **Board Cert:** Otolaryngology 1994; **Med School:** Canada 1986; **Resid:** Otolaryngology, Univ of Western Ontario, London, Canada 1987-1992; **Fellow:** Head and Neck Surgery, Methodist Hosp of Indiana, Indianapolis, ID 1992-1993; **Fac Appt:** Asst Prof Otolaryngology, Indiana Univ

Christiansen, Thomas MD (Oto) - *Spec Exp:* Ear, Nose & Throat; **Hospital:** Fairview-Univ Med Ctr - Univ Campus; **Address:** ENT Specialty Care of MN, 2211 Park Ave S, Minneapolis, MN 55404; **Phone:** (612) 871-1144; **Board Cert:** Otolaryngology 1973; **Med School:** Univ IL Coll Med 1968; **Resid:** Otolaryngology, Univ of MN Hosp, Minneapolis, MN 1969-1974; **Fac Appt:** Asst Clin Prof Otolaryngology, Univ Minn

Corey, Jacquelynne P MD (Oto) - *Spec Exp:* Nasal & Sinus Disorders; Allergy; Voice Disorders; **Hospital:** Univ of Chicago Hosps (page 76); **Address:** Univ of Chicago Hosps, 5841 S Maryland St, MC-1035, Chicago, IL 60637; **Phone:** (773) 702-1865; **Board Cert:** Otolaryngology 1985; **Med School:** Univ IL Coll Med 1979; **Resid:** Otolaryngology, Rush Presby-St Lukes Med Ctr, Chicago, IL 1979-1984; **Fac Appt:** Assoc Prof Surgery, Univ Chicago-Pritzker Sch Med

Ford, Charles N MD (Oto) - *Spec Exp:* Voice Disorders; Laryngeal Endoscopic Surgery; **Hospital:** Univ WI Hosp & Clins; **Address:** Univ of WI Hosp & Clinics, 600 Highland Avenue-K4-714, Madison, WI 53792; **Phone:** (608) 263-0192; **Board Cert:** Otolaryngology 1971; **Med School:** Univ Louisville Sch Med 1965; **Resid:** Otolaryngology, Henry Ford Hosp, Detroit, MI 1966-1970

Friedman, Michael MD (Oto) - *Spec Exp:* Sleep Disorders/Apnea; Snoring-Surgery; Sinus Disorders/Surgery; **Hospital:** Rush-Presby - St Luke's Med Ctr (page 72); **Address:** 30 N Michigan St, Ste 1107, Chicago, IL 60602; **Phone:** (312) 236-3642; **Board Cert:** Otolaryngology 1977; **Med School:** Univ IL Coll Med 1972; **Resid:** Surgery, Illinois Med Ctr, Chicago, IL 1973-1974; Otolaryngology, Univ IL Med Ctr, Chicago, IL 1974-1977; **Fac Appt:** Prof Otolaryngology, Rush Med Coll

Funk, Gerry Franklin MD (Oto) - *Spec Exp:* Head & Neck Trauma; **Hospital:** Univ of IA Hosp and Clinics; **Address:** Dept Otolaryngology, Div Head & Neck Surgery, 200 Hawkins Dr, Iowa City, IA 52242; **Phone:** (319) 356-2201; **Board Cert:** Otolaryngology 1992; **Med School:** Univ Chicago-Pritzker Sch Med 1986; **Resid:** Otolaryngology, LAC - USC Med Ctr, Los Angeles, CA; **Fellow:** Head and Neck Surgery, Univ Iowa Hosp, Iowa City, IA; **Fac Appt:** Asst Prof Otolaryngology, Univ Iowa Coll Med

Gantz, Bruce MD (Oto) - *Spec Exp:* Ear Disorders/Surgery; Neuro-Otology; **Hospital:** Univ of IA Hosp and Clinics; **Address:** Dept Otolaryngology, 200 200 Hawkins Drive, rm 21200-PFP, Iowa City, IA 52242; **Phone:** (319) 356-2173; **Board Cert:** Otolaryngology 1980; **Med School:** Univ Iowa Coll Med 1974; **Resid:** Otolaryngology, Univ Iowa Hosps, Iowa City, IA 1976-1980; **Fellow:** Otolaryngology, Univ Iowa Hosps, Iowa City, IA 1975-1976; Neurology, Univ Zurich, Zurich, Switzerland 1981-1982

Gluckman, Jack L MD (Oto) - *Spec Exp:* Head & Neck Cancer; Head & Neck Surgery; **Hospital:** Univ Hosp - Cincinnati; **Address:** Dept Otolaryngology, Box 670528, Cincinnati, OH 45267-0001; **Phone:** (513) 558-4152; **Board Cert:** Otolaryngology 1990; **Med School:** South Africa 1967; **Resid:** Surgery, St James Hosp, London, England 1969-1971; Otolaryngology, Groote Schuur Hosp, Capetown, South Africa 1971-1974; **Fellow:** Otolaryngology, Univ Cincinnati Med Ctr, Cincinnati, OH 1977-1979; **Fac Appt:** Prof Otolaryngology, Univ Cincinnati

Goebel, Joel Alan MD (Oto) - *Spec Exp:* Dizziness; Hearing Disorders; **Hospital:** Barnes-Jewish Hosp (page 55); **Address:** Barnes Jewish Hosp South, 517 S Euclid, Fl 8th, St. Louis, MO 63110; **Phone:** (314) 362-7509; **Board Cert:** Otolaryngology 1985; **Med School:** Washington Univ, St Louis 1980; **Resid:** Otolaryngology, Barnes Hosp/Wash Univ, St Louis, MO 1981-1985; **Fac Appt:** Assoc Prof Otolaryngology, Washington Univ, St Louis

Hamaker, Ronald MD (Oto) - *Spec Exp:* Head & Neck Cancer; Ear, Nose & Throat; **Hospital:** Methodist Hosp - Indianapolis (page 66); **Address:** 7440 N Shadeland Ave, Ste 107, Indianapolis, IN 46250; **Phone:** (317) 926-1056; **Board Cert:** Otolaryngology 1971; **Med School:** Wayne State Univ 1965; **Resid:** Surgery, Butterworth Hosp, Grand Rapids, MI 1966-1967; Otolaryngology, Wayne St Univ, Detroit, MI 1967-1970; **Fellow:** Head and Neck Surgery, New York, NY 1972-1973; **Fac Appt:** Assoc Clin Prof Orthopaedic Surgery, Indiana Univ

Haughey, Bruce MD (Oto) - *Spec Exp:* Cosmetic Surgery-Face; Head & Neck Cancer; **Hospital:** Barnes-Jewish Hosp (page 55); **Address:** Barnes Jewish Hospital South, 8th Fl, 660 S Euclid Ave, Box 8115, St Louis, MO 63110; **Phone:** (314) 362-7509; **Board Cert:** Otolaryngology 1984; **Med School:** New Zealand 1976; **Resid:** Surgery, Univ Auckland, Auckland, NZ 1977-1980; Otolaryngology, Univ Iowa, Iowa City, IA 1981-1984; **Fac Appt:** Assoc Prof Otolaryngology, St Louis Univ

Hilger, Peter A MD (Oto) - *Spec Exp:* Facial Head & Neck Surgery; **Hospital:** Regions Hosp - St Paul; **Address:** Centennial Lakes Med Bldg, Ste 410, 7373 France Ave S, Edina, MN 55435; **Phone:** (952) 844-0404; **Board Cert:** Otolaryngology 1979; **Med School:** Univ Minn 1974; **Resid:** Surgery, Univ Minnesota Hosp, Minneapolis, MN 1974-1975; Otolaryngology, Univ Minnesota Hosp, Minneapolis, MN 1975-1979; **Fellow:** Plastic Surgery, Mass Eye & Ear Infirm, Boston, MA 1979-1980; **Fac Appt:** Asst Prof Otolaryngology, Univ Minn

Jones, Paul John MD (Oto) - *Spec Exp:* Otolaryngology - General; **Hospital:** Rush-Presby - St Luke's Med Ctr (page 72); **Address:** 25 E Washington St, Ste 820, Chicago, IL 60602-1708; **Phone:** (312) 553-0152; **Board Cert:** Otolaryngology 1989; **Med School:** Rush Med Coll 1983; **Resid:** Otolaryngology, Rush Presby St Lukes Med Ctr, Chicago, IL 1984-1988; **Fac Appt:** Asst Prof Otolaryngology, Rush Med Coll

Kartush, Jack MD (Oto) - *Spec Exp:* Ear Disorders/Surgery; **Hospital:** Providence Hosp - Southfield; **Address:** Mich Ear Inst, 3055 Northwest Hwy, Farmington Hills, MI 48334; **Phone:** (248) 476-4622; **Board Cert:** Otolaryngology 1984; **Med School:** Univ Mich Med Sch 1978; **Resid:** Otolaryngology, U Mich., Ann Arbor, MI 1980-1984; **Fellow:** Otolaryngology, U Mich., Ann Arbor, MI 1984-1985; **Fac Appt:** Assoc Clin Prof Otolaryngology, Wayne State Univ

Kern, Robert MD (Oto) - *Spec Exp:* Head & Neck Cancer; Sinusitis; Rhinoplasty; **Hospital:** Northwestern Meml Hosp; **Address:** 675 N St Clair St, Ste 15-200, Chicago, IL 60611; **Phone:** (312) 695-8182; **Board Cert:** Otolaryngology 1990; **Med School:** Jefferson Med Coll 1985; **Resid:** Otolaryngology, Wayne State Affil Hosp, Detroit, MI 1986-1990; **Fellow:** Research, Natl Inst Hlth, Bethesda, MD 1990-1991; **Fac Appt:** Assoc Prof Otolaryngology, Northwestern Univ

Lanza, Donald MD (Oto) - *Spec Exp:* Skull Base Tumors; Sinus Disorders/Surgery; Rhinitis; **Hospital:** Cleveland Clin Fdn (page 57); **Address:** 9500 Euclid Ave/Desk A71, Cleveland, OH 44195-0001; **Phone:** (216) 444-4939; **Board Cert:** Otolaryngology 1990; **Med School:** SUNY Hlth Sci Ctr 1985; **Resid:** Surgery, Albany Med Ctr, Albany, NY 1986-1987; Otolaryngology, Albany Med Ctr, Albany, NY 1987-1990; **Fellow:** Johns Hopkins Univ, Baltimore, MD 1990-1991; Univ Of Penn, Philadelphia, PA 1991

Leonetti, John MD (Oto) - *Spec Exp:* Skull Base Surgery; **Hospital:** Loyola Univ Med Ctr; **Address:** 2160 S First Ave Bldg 105 - Ste 1870, Maywood, IL 60153; **Phone:** (708) 216-9183; **Board Cert:** Otolaryngology 1987; **Med School:** Loyola Univ-Stritch Sch Med 1982; **Resid:** Otolaryngology, Fell-House Ear Inst, Los Angeles, CA 1987; Otolaryngology, Loyola U-Stritch Sch Med., Maywood, IL 1983-1987; **Fellow:** Neurological Otology, Barnes Hosp, St Louis, MO 1987-1988; **Fac Appt:** Assoc Prof Otolaryngology, Loyola Univ-Stritch Sch Med

Mangat, Devinder Singh MD (Oto) - *Spec Exp:* Cosmetic Surgery-Face; **Hospital:** Christ Hospital; **Address:** 8400 Montgomery Rd, Ste 230, Cincinnati, OH 45236; **Phone:** (513) 984-3223; **Board Cert:** Otolaryngology 1978; **Med School:** Univ KY Coll Med 1973; **Resid:** Otolaryngology, U Okla Hlth Scis Ctr, Oklahoma City, OK 1975-1978; **Fac Appt:** Assoc Prof Otolaryngology, Univ Cincinnati

Miyamoto, Richard MD (Oto) - *Spec Exp:* Neuro-Otology; Acoustic Nerve Tumors; Middle Ear Disorders; **Hospital:** IN Univ Hosp (page 63); **Address:** 702 Barnhill Drive, Ste 0860, Indianapolis, IN 46202-5128; **Phone:** (317) 274-3556; **Board Cert:** Otolaryngology 1975; **Med School:** Univ Mich Med Sch 1970; **Resid:** Surgery, Butterworth Hosp, Grand Rapids, MI 1971-1972; Otolarynological Rhinoplasty, Indiana Univ Hosps, Indianapolis, IN 1972-1975; **Fellow:** Otolaryngology, Otologic Med Grp, Los Angeles, CA 1977-1978; **Fac Appt:** Prof Otolaryngology, Indiana Univ

Naclerio, Robert MD (Oto) - *Spec Exp:* Allergy; Otolaryngology-Pediatric; **Hospital:** Univ of Chicago Hosps (page 76); **Address:** Univ Chicago Hosps, 5841 S Maryland Ave , MC-1035, Chicago, IL 60637; **Phone:** (773) 702-0080; **Board Cert:** Otolaryngology 1983; **Med School:** Baylor Coll Med 1976; **Resid:** Surgery, Johns Hopkins Hosp, Baltimore, MD 1977-1978; Otolaryngology, Baylor Coll Med, Houston, TX 1978-1980; **Fellow:** Clinical Immunology, Johns Hopkins Hosp, Baltimore, MD 1980-1982; **Fac Appt:** Prof Otolaryngology, Univ Chicago-Pritzker Sch Med

Paparella, Michael MD (Oto) - *Spec Exp:* Hearing Disorders; Neurotology; Meniere's Disease; **Hospital:** Fairview-Univ Med Ctr - Riverside Campus; **Address:** MN EH&N Clinic, 701 25th Avenue S #200, Minneapolis, MN 55454-1443; **Phone:** (612) 339-2836; **Board Cert:** Otolaryngology 1963; **Med School:** Univ Mich Med Sch 1957; **Resid:** Otolaryngology, Henry Ford Hosp, Detroit, MI 1958-1961; **Fac Appt:** Clin Prof Otolaryngology, Univ Minn

Pelzer, Harold J MD/DDS (Oto) - *Spec Exp:* Head & Neck Cancer; Swallowing Disorders; **Hospital:** Northwestern Meml Hosp; **Address:** 675 N St Claire, Ste 15-200, Chicago, IL 60611; **Phone:** (312) 695-8182; **Board Cert:** Otolaryngology 1985; **Med School:** Northwestern Univ 1979; **Resid:** Surgery, Northwestern Meml Hosp, Chicago, IL 1981-1983; **Fellow:** Otolaryngology, Northwestern Meml Hosp, Chicago, IL 1984-1985; **Fac Appt:** Asst Prof Otolaryngology, Northwestern Univ

Pensak, Myles MD (Oto) - *Spec Exp:* Skull Base Tumors; Facial Paralysis; Vertigo; **Hospital:** Univ Hosp - Cincinnati; **Address:** Univ Cincinnati Dept Oto/HNS, PO Box 670528, Cincinnati, OH 45267-0528; **Phone:** (513) 475-8427; **Board Cert:** Otolaryngology 1983; **Med School:** NY Med Coll 1978; **Resid:** Surgery, Upstate Med Ctr, Syracuse, NY 1978-1980; Otolaryngology, Yale Univ, New Haven, CT 1980-1983; **Fellow:** Otolaryngology, Ear Foundation, Nashville, TN 1983-1984; **Fac Appt:** Prof Otolaryngology, Univ Cincinnati

Piccirillo, Jay MD (Oto) - *Spec Exp:* Sleep Disorders/Apnea; Sinus Disorders/Surgery; **Hospital:** Barnes-Jewish Hosp (page 55); **Address:** 660 S Euclid Ave, Box 8115, St Louis, MO 63110; **Phone:** (314) 362-7509; **Board Cert:** Otolaryngology 1990; **Med School:** Univ VT Coll Med 1985; **Resid:** Otolaryngology, Albany Med Ctr, Albany, NY 1987-1990; **Fellow:** Yale Univ, New Haven, CT 1990-1992; **Fac Appt:** Asst Prof Otolaryngology, Washington Univ, St Louis

Schuller, David MD (Oto) - *Spec Exp:* Head & Neck Cancer; Head & Neck Surgery; **Hospital:** Arthur G James Cancer Hosp & Research Inst; **Address:** 456 W 10th Ave, Ste 4110, Columbus, OH 43210-1240; **Phone:** (614) 293-8074; **Board Cert:** Otolaryngology 1975; **Med School:** Ohio State Univ 1970; **Resid:** Otolaryngology, OH State Univ Affil Hosps, Columbus, OH 1971-1975; Surgery, Univ Hosps Cleveland, Cleveland, OH 1972-1973; **Fellow:** Head and Neck Surgery, Pack Med Fdn; Head and Neck Oncology, Univ Iowa, Iowa City, IA 1975-1976

Siegel, Gordon J MD (Oto) - *Spec Exp:* Head & Neck Cancer; Nasal & Sinus Disorders; **Hospital:** Northwestern Meml Hosp; **Address:** 3 E Huron St Fl 1, Chicago, IL 60611; **Phone:** (312) 988-7777; **Board Cert:** Otolaryngology 1984; **Med School:** Univ Hlth Sci/Chicago Med Sch 1978; **Resid:** Otolaryngology, Northwestern Univ, Chicago, IL 1979-1982

Stankiewicz, James MD (Oto) - *Spec Exp:* Endoscopic Sinus Surgery; Rhinosinusitis; Nasal & Sinus Disorders; **Hospital:** Loyola Univ Med Ctr; **Address:** Loyola Univ Med Ctr, Dept Oto, 2160 S First Ave, Maywood, IL 60153; **Phone:** (708) 216-8563; **Board Cert:** Otolaryngology 1978; **Med School:** Univ Chicago-Pritzker Sch Med 1974; **Resid:** Otolaryngology, Univ Chicago Hosp, Chicago, IL 1975-1978; **Fac Appt:** Prof Otolaryngology, Loyola Univ-Stritch Sch Med

Strome, Marshall MD (Oto) - *Spec Exp:* Sleep Disorders; Voice Disorders; Head & Neck Cancer; **Hospital:** Cleveland Clin Fdn (page 57); **Address:** Cleveland Clinic Fdn, 9500 Euclid Ave, Ste A71, Cleveland, OH 44195; **Phone:** (216) 444-6686; **Board Cert:** Otolaryngology 1970; **Med School:** Univ Mich Med Sch 1964; **Resid:** Otorhinolaryngology, Univ Mich, Ann Arbor, MI 1966-1970; Surgery, Harper Hosp, Detroit, MI 1965-1966; **Fac Appt:** Prof Otolaryngology, Ohio State Univ

Szachowicz II, Edward H MD (Oto) - *Spec Exp:* Cosmetic Surgery-Face; Rhinoplasty; **Hospital:** Abbott - Northwestern Hosp; **Address:** 7373 France Ave S, Ste 310, Edina, MN 55435-4538; **Phone:** (952) 835-5665; **Board Cert:** Otolaryngology 1984; **Med School:** Univ IL Coll Med 1979; **Resid:** Surgery, Fairview Univ Med Ctr, Minneapolis, MN 1979-1980; Otolaryngology, Fairview Univ Med Ctr, Minneapolis, MN 1980-1984; **Fellow:** Facial Plastic Surgery, Fairview Univ Med Ctr, Minneapolis, MN 1985-1986; **Fac Appt:** Asst Clin Prof Otolaryngology, Univ Minn

Telian, Steven Allen MD (Oto) - *Spec Exp:* Cochlear Implants; Ear Disorders/Surgery; Acoustic Neuroma Hearing Preservation; **Hospital:** Univ Mich Med Ctr, Dept Oto-HNS, 1500 E Med Ctr Dr, Taubman Ctr, Ann Arbor, MI 48109-0312; **Phone:** (734) 936-8006; **Board Cert:** Otolaryngology 1985; **Med School:** Univ Penn 1980; **Resid:** Otolaryngology, Univ Penn, Philadelphia, PA 1982-1985; **Fellow:** Otology, Univ Mich Med Ctr, Ann Arbor, MI 1985-1986; **Fac Appt:** Prof Otolaryngology, Univ Mich Med Sch

Toriumi, Dean MD (Oto) - *Spec Exp:* Rhinoplasty; Cosmetic Surgery-Face; **Hospital:** Univ of IL at Chicago Med Ctr; **Address:** 1855 W Taylor St, rm 242, MC 648, Chicago, IL 60612; **Phone:** (312) 996-8897; **Board Cert:** Otolaryngology 1988; **Med School:** Rush Med Coll 1981; **Resid:** Surgery, Univ Illinois Med Ctr, Chicago, IL 1983-1985; Otolaryngology, Northwestern Univ Med Sch, Chicago, IL 1985-1987; **Fellow:** Facial Plastic Surgery, Tulane Med Sch, New Orleans, LA 1988; Facial Plastic Surgery, Virginia Mason Med Ctr, Seattle, WA 1989; **Fac Appt:** Assoc Prof Otolaryngology, Univ IL Coll Med

Wackym, Phillip MD (Oto) - *Spec Exp:* Cochlear Implants; Acoustic Nerve Tumors; Head & Neck Surgery; **Hospital:** Froedtert Meml Lutheran Hosp; **Address:** 9200 W Wisconsin Ave, Milwaukee, WI 53226; **Phone:** (414) 805-3666; **Board Cert:** Otolaryngology 1992; **Med School:** Vanderbilt Univ 1985; **Resid:** Neurological Surgery, UCLA Med Ctr, Los Angeles, CA 1985-1987; Head and Neck Surgery, UCLA Med Ctr, Los Angeles, CA 1987-1991; **Fellow:** Otology & Neurotology, Univ Iowa, Iowa City, IA 1991-1992; Neurological Science, UCLA Medical Center, Los Angeles, CA 1992-1995; **Fac Appt:** Prof Otolaryngology, Med Coll Wisc

Wiet, Richar James MD (Oto) - *Spec Exp:* Acoustic Nerve Tumors; Otosclerosis/ Hearing Loss; **Hospital:** Evanston Hosp; **Address:** 1000 Central St, Ste 610, Evanston, IL 60201; **Phone:** (847) 570-1360; **Board Cert:** Otolaryngology 1976; **Med School:** Loyola Univ-Stritch Sch Med 1971; **Resid:** Otolaryngology, Cincinnati Med Ctr, Cincinnati, OH 1972-1976; **Fellow:** Otolaryngology, Univ Zurich/Ear Foundation, Nashville, TN 1978-1979; **Fac Appt:** Clin Prof Otolaryngology, Northwestern Univ

Wolf, Gregory MD (Oto) - *Spec Exp:* Cosmetic Surgery-Face; Laryngeal Cancer; **Hospital:** Univ of MI Hlth Ctr; **Address:** Dept Otolaryngology, 1500 E Med Ctr Dr, Bldg Taubman Ctr - rm 1904, Ann Arbor, MI 48109; **Phone:** (734) 936-8029; **Board Cert:** Otolaryngology 1978; **Med School:** Univ Mich Med Sch 1973; **Resid:** Otolaryngology, SUNY Upstate Med Ctr, Syracuse, NY 1975-1978; Surgery, Georgetown Univ Hosp, Washington, DC 1973-1975; **Fac Appt:** Prof Otolaryngology, Univ Mich Med Sch

Woodson, B Tucker MD (Oto) - *Spec Exp:* Sleep Disorders/Apnea; **Hospital:** Froedtert Meml Lutheran Hosp; **Address:** Froedtert Meml Lutheran Hosp, 9200 W Wisconsin Ave, Milwaukee, WI 53226-3522; **Phone:** (414) 454-7667; **Board Cert:** Otolaryngology 1988; **Med School:** Univ MO-Columbia Sch Med 1983; **Resid:** Surgery, Henry Ford Hosp, Detroit, MI 1983-1984; Otolaryngology, Henry Ford Hosp, Detroit, MI 1984-1988; **Fac Appt:** Assoc Prof Otolaryngology, Med Coll Wisc

Great Plains and Mountains

Davis, R Kim MD (Oto) - *Spec Exp:* Laser Surgery-Larynx; Thyroid & Parathyroid Surgery; **Hospital:** Univ Utah Hosp and Clin; **Address:** 50 N Medical Center Dr, rm 3C 134, Salt Lake City, UT 84132; **Phone:** (801) 581-7514; **Board Cert:** Otolaryngology 1979; **Med School:** Univ Utah 1975; **Resid:** Otolaryngology, Madigan AMC 1976-1979; Surgery, Madigan AMC 1975-1976; **Fellow:** Medical Oncology, Boston Univ, Boston, MA 1979-1980; **Fac Appt:** Prof Surgery, Univ Utah

Denenberg, Steven M MD (Oto) - *Spec Exp:* Cosmetic Surgery-Face; Rhinoplasty; **Hospital:** Nebraska Meth Hosp; **Address:** 7640 Pacific St, Omaha, NE 68114-5421; **Phone:** (402) 391-7640; **Board Cert:** Otolaryngology 1984; **Med School:** Univ Nebr Coll Med 1980; **Resid:** Otolaryngology, Stanford univ, Palo Alto, CA 1981-1984; **Fellow:** Facial Plastic Surgery, McCollough Center, Birmingham, AL 1984-1985; **Fac Appt:** Asst Clin Prof Otolaryngology, Univ Nebr Coll Med

Jenkins, Herman A. MD (Oto) - *Spec Exp:* Ear Disorders/Surgery; Neuro-Otology; Acoustic Nerve Tumors; **Hospital:** Univ Colo HSC - Denver; **Address:** Univ of Colorado Hlth & Sci Ctr, Dept Otolaryngology, 4200 E 9th Ave, rm B205, Denver, CO 80262; **Phone:** (303) 372-3180; **Board Cert:** Otolaryngology 1977; **Med School:** Vanderbilt Univ 1970; **Resid:** Surgery, UCLA, Los Angeles, CA 1971-1972; Otolaryngology, UCLA, Los Angeles, CA 1974-1977; **Fellow:** Neurology, U Hosp, Zurich Switzerland 1979-1980; **Fac Appt:** Prof Univ Colo

Leopold, Donald Arthur MD (Oto) - *Spec Exp:* Olfactory Disorders; Sinus Disorders/Surgery; **Hospital:** Nebraska Hlth Sys; **Address:** Univ Nebr, Dept Oto-Head & Neck Surg, 981225 Nebraska Med Ctr, Omaha, NE 68198-1225; **Phone:** (402) 559-8007; **Board Cert:** Otolaryngology 1978; **Med School:** Ohio State Univ 1973; **Resid:** Surgery, St Luke's Med Ctr, New York, NY 1973-1974; Otolaryngology, Univ Iowa, Iowa City, IA 1974-1978; **Fac Appt:** Prof Otolaryngology, Univ Nebr Coll Med

Southwest

Alford, Bobby R MD (Oto) - *Spec Exp:* Neurovestibular Disease; Thyroid Surgery; **Hospital:** Methodist Hosp - Houston; **Address:** Neurosensory Ctr, 6501 Fannin, Ste NA-102, Houston, TX 77030; **Phone:** (713) 798-5906; **Board Cert:** Otolaryngology 1962; **Med School:** Baylor Coll Med 1956; **Resid:** Otolaryngology, Baylor Univ, Houston, TX 1957-1960; **Fellow:** Neurological Physiology, Johns Hopkins Med Sch, Baltimore, MD; **Fac Appt:** Prof Otolaryngology, Baylor Coll Med

Bailey, Byron J MD (Oto) - *Spec Exp:* Head & Neck Surgery; **Hospital:** Univ of TX Med Brch Hosps at Galveston; **Address:** Univ of Tex Medical Branch, Dept Oto, 301 University Blvd, Galveston, TX 77555-0521; **Phone:** (409) 772-2704; **Board Cert:** Otolaryngology 1965; **Med School:** Univ Okla Coll Med 1959; **Resid:** Surgery, UCLA Med Ctr, Los Angeles, CA 1960-1961; Head and Neck Surgery, UCLA Med Ctr, Los angeles, CA 1961-1964; **Fac Appt:** Prof Otolaryngology, Univ Tex Med Br, Galveston

Bower, Charles MD (Oto) - *Spec Exp:* Airway Disorders; Sleep Disorders/Apnea; Sinus Disorders/Surgery; **Hospital:** UAMS; **Address:** Dept Ped Oto, 800 Marshall St, Little Rock, AR 72202-3510; **Phone:** (501) 320-1047; **Board Cert:** Otolaryngology 1990; **Med School:** Univ Ark 1985; **Resid:** Otolaryngology, Univ Arkansas for Med Scis, Little Rock, AR 1986-1991; **Fellow:** Pediatric Otolaryngology, Chldns Hosp, Cincinnati, OH 1991-1992; **Fac Appt:** Assoc Prof Otolaryngology, Univ Ark

Clayman, Gary Lee MD (Oto) - *Spec Exp:* Thyroid Surgery; Salivary Gland Surgery; Head & Neck Cancer; **Hospital:** Univ of TX MD Anderson Cancer Ctr, The; **Address:** Univ TX/MD Anderson Cancer Center, 1515 Holcombe Blvd, Box 441, Houston, TX 77030-4009; **Phone:** (713) 792-8837; **Board Cert:** Otolaryngology 1992; **Med School:** NE Ohio Univ 1986; **Resid:** Surgery, Hennepin Co Med Ctr, Minneapolis, MN 1986-1987; Otolaryngology, Univ Minn, Minneapolis, MN 1987-1991; **Fellow:** Head and Neck Surgery, MD Anderson Cancer Ctr, Houston, TX 1991-1993; **Fac Appt:** Prof Otolaryngology, Univ Tex, Houston

Daspit, C Phillip MD (Oto) - *Spec Exp:* Hearing Loss & Balance Disorders; Skull Base Surgery; Cochlear Implants; **Hospital:** St Joseph's Hosp & Med Ctr - Phoenix; **Address:** 22222 W Thomas Rd, Ste 114, Phoenix, AZ 85013; **Phone:** (602) 279-5444; **Board Cert:** Otolaryngology 1977; **Med School:** Louisiana State Univ 1968; **Resid:** Surgery, UCSF Med Ctr, San Francisco, CA 1972-1973; Otolaryngology, Ft Miley VA Hosp, San Francisco, CA 1974-1977; **Fellow:** Otology & Neurotology, House Ear Institute, Los Angeles, CA 1977-1978; Skull Base Surgery, House Ear Institute, Los Angeles, CA 1977-1978; **Fac Appt:** Clin Prof Surgery, Univ Ariz Coll Med

Donovan, Donald Thomas MD (Oto) - *Spec Exp:* Head & Neck Cancer; Voice Disorders; Thyroid Disorders; **Hospital:** Methodist Hosp - Houston; **Address:** 6550 Fannin St, Ste 1701, Houston, TX 77030; **Phone:** (713) 798-3380; **Board Cert:** Otolaryngology 1981; **Med School:** Baylor Coll Med 1976; **Resid:** Surgery, Baylor Affil Hosps, Houston, TX 1977-1978; Otolaryngology, Baylor Affil Hosps, Houston, TX 1978-1981; **Fellow:** Head and Neck Surgery, Colum-Presby Med Ctr, New York, NY 1981-1982; **Fac Appt:** Assoc Prof Otolaryngology, Baylor Coll Med

Friedman, Ellen MD (Oto) - *Spec Exp:* Otolaryngology - General; **Hospital:** TX Chldns Hosp - Houston; **Address:** 6701 Fannon St, Houston, TX 77030; **Phone:** (832) 822-3250; **Board Cert:** Otolaryngology 1981; **Med School:** Albert Einstein Coll Med 1975; **Resid:** Surgery, Montefiore Hosp, New York, NY 1975-1976; Otolaryngology, Wash Hosp Ctr, Washington, DC 1976-1979; **Fellow:** Pediatric Otolaryngology, Boston Chldns Hosp, Boston, MA; **Fac Appt:** Prof Otolaryngology, Baylor Coll Med

Gianoli, Gerard MD (Oto) - *Spec Exp:* Otolaryngology - General; **Hospital:** North Oaks Med Ctr; **Address:** 17050 Medical Center Drive, Ste 315, Baton Rouge, LA 70816; **Phone:** (225) 293-6973; **Board Cert:** Otolaryngology 1993; **Med School:** Tulane Univ 1986; **Resid:** Pediatrics, Tulane Univ, New Orleans, LA 1987-1988; Otolaryngology Head & Neck, Tulane Univ, New Orleans, LA 1988-1992; **Fellow:** Skull Base Surgery, Michigan Ear Inst, Farmington Hills, MI

Goepfert, Helmuth MD (Oto) - *Spec Exp:* Head & Neck Surgery; Head & Neck Cancer; **Hospital:** Univ of TX MD Anderson Cancer Ctr, The; **Address:** 1515 Holcombe Blvd, Box 441, Houston, TX 77030-4009; **Phone:** (713) 792-6925; **Board Cert:** Otolaryngology 1974; **Med School:** Chile 1961; **Resid:** Otolaryngology, Baylor Coll Med, Houston, TX 1971-1974; Medical Oncology, UCLA, Los Angeles, CA 1964-1966; **Fellow:** Surgery, Univ Tex MD Anderson, Houston, TX 1966-1968; **Fac Appt:** Prof Otolaryngology, Univ Tex, Houston

Hanna, Ehab MD (Oto) - *Spec Exp:* Skull Base Surgery; Head & Neck Cancer; **Hospital:** UAMS; **Address:** Univ Arkansas for Medical Sciences, 4301 W Markham St, , Ste 543, Little Rock, AR 72205-7199; **Phone:** (501) 686-5140; **Board Cert:** Otolaryngology 1994; **Med School:** Egypt 1982; **Resid:** Otolaryngology, Cleveland Clinic, Cleveland, OH 1988-1989; Otolaryngology, Cleveland Clinic, Cleveland, OH 1990-1993; **Fellow:** Otolaryngology, Univ Pittsburgh Med Ctr, Pittsburgh, PA 1993-1994; **Fac Appt:** Asst Prof Otolaryngology, Univ Ark

Hansen, Lori Eldean MD (Oto) - *Spec Exp:* Cosmetic Surgery-Face; **Hospital:** Mercy Hlth Ctr - Oklahoma City; **Address:** 11011 Hefner Point Dr, Oklahoma City, OK 73120; **Phone:** (405) 752-0606; **Board Cert:** Otolaryngology 1985; **Med School:** Univ Okla Coll Med 1979; **Resid:** Otolaryngology, Univ Ala Hosp, Birmingham, AL 1980-1981; Otolaryngology, Univ Ok Hlth Scis Ctr, Oklahoma City, OK 1981-1984; **Fellow:** Plastic Surgery, Lasky Clinic, Beverly Hills, CA 1984-1985

Johnson Jr, Calvin M MD (Oto) - *Spec Exp:* Ear & Nasal Disorders/Surgery; Cosmetic Surgery-Face; **Hospital:** Meml Med Ctr - Baptist Campus; **Address:** Hedgewood Surg Ctr, 2427 St Charles Ave, New Orleans, LA 70130; **Phone:** (504) 895-7642; **Board Cert:** Otolaryngology 1974; **Med School:** Tulane Univ 1967; **Resid:** Surgery, Tulane Univ Sch Med, New Orleans, LA 1970-1971; Otolaryngology, Tulane Univ Sch Med, New Orleans, LA 1971-1974; **Fellow:** Facial Plastic Surgery, Amer Academy Facial Plastic & Recon Surg, Los Angeles, CA 1974-1975

Medina, Jesus MD (Oto) - *Spec Exp:* Head & Neck Cancer; **Hospital:** Univ OK Hlth Sci Ctr; **Address:** Univ Oklahoma Hlth Sci Ctr, Dept Otolaryngology, PO Box 26901, WP 1360, Oklahoma City, OK 73190; **Phone:** (405) 271-5504; **Board Cert:** Otolaryngology 1980; **Med School:** Peru 1973; **Resid:** Surgery, Wayne St Univ Affil Hosp, Detroit, MI 1975-1977; Otolaryngology, Wayne St Univ Affil Hosp, Detroit, MI 1977-1980; **Fellow:** Surgery, Univ Tex Sys Cancer Ctrs, Houston, TX 1980-1981; **Fac Appt:** Prof Otolaryngology, Univ Okla Coll Med

Otto, Randal A MD (Oto) - *Spec Exp:* Head & Neck Cancer; **Hospital:** Univ of Texas Hlth & Sci Ctr; **Address:** 7703 Floyd Curl Drive, MS 777, San Antonio, TX 78229-3900; **Phone:** (210) 567-6488; **Board Cert:** Otolaryngology 1987; **Med School:** Univ MO-Columbia Sch Med 1981; **Resid:** Pathology, Queens Med Ctr, Honolulu, HI 1981-1982; Otolaryngology, Univ Missouri, Colombia, MO 1982-1987; **Fac Appt:** Prof Otolaryngology, Univ Tex, San Antonio

Roland, Peter S MD (Oto) - *Spec Exp:* Ear Disorders/Surgery; Skull Base Surgery; Neurotology; **Hospital:** Zale Lipshy Univ Hosp; **Address:** Univ Tex SW Med Ctr, 5323 Harry Hines Blvd, Dallas, TX 75390-9035; **Phone:** (214) 648-3071; **Board Cert:** Otolaryngology 1981; **Med School:** Univ Tex Med Br, Galveston 1976; **Resid:** Otolaryngology, Hershey Med Ctr, Hershey, PA 1976-1979; **Fellow:** Skull Base Surgery, E.A.R. Institute, Nashville, TN 1984-1985; **Fac Appt:** Prof Otolaryngology, Univ Tex SW, Dallas

Suen, James MD (Oto) - *Spec Exp:* Head & Neck Cancer; Vascular Lesions-Head & Neck; Laryngeal Disorders; **Hospital:** UAMS; **Address:** Univ Hosp Arkansas Med Scis, 4301 W Markham St, Bldg 543, Little Rock, AR 72205; **Phone:** (501) 686-5140; **Board Cert:** Otolaryngology 1973; **Med School:** Univ Ark 1966; **Resid:** Surgery, Univ Arkansas Med Ctr, Little Rock, AR 1969-1970; Otolaryngology, Univ Arkansas Med Ctr, Little Rock, AR 1970-1973; **Fellow:** Surgery, Univ Texas-M D Anderson Hosp, Houston, TX 1973-1974; **Fac Appt:** Prof Otolaryngology, Univ Ark

Waner, Milton MD (Oto) - *Spec Exp:* Vascular Malformations; Hemangioma; **Hospital:** Arkansas Chldns Hosp; **Address:** 800 Marshall St, Little Rock, AR 72202; **Phone:** (501) 320-7546; **Med School:** South Africa 1977; **Resid:** Otolaryngology, Univ Witwatersrand, Johannesburg, South Africa; **Fellow:** Otolaryngology, Univ Cincinnatti Med Ctr, Cincinnatti, OH 1984-1985; **Fac Appt:** Prof Otolaryngology, Univ Ark

West Coast and Pacific

Berke, Gerald Spencer MD (Oto) - *Spec Exp:* Head & Neck Surgery; Voice Disorders; **Hospital:** UCLA Med Ctr; **Address:** 200 UCLA Med Plaza, Ste 550, Los Angeles, CA 90095; **Phone:** (310) 825-5179; **Board Cert:** Otolaryngology 1984; **Med School:** USC Sch Med 1978; **Resid:** Otolaryngology, LAC-USC Med Ctr, Los Angeles, CA 1978-1979; **Fellow:** Head and Neck Surgery, UCLA Med Ctr, Los Angeles, CA 1980-1984

Brackmann, Derald E MD (Oto) - *Spec Exp:* Ear Disorders-Surgery; Facial Nerve Disorders; Acoustic Neuromas; **Hospital:** St Vincent's Med Ctr - Los Angeles; **Address:** House Ear Clin Inc, 2100 W 3rd St, Fl 1st, Los Angeles, CA 90057-1902; **Phone:** (213) 483-9930; **Board Cert:** Otolaryngology 1971; **Med School:** Univ IL Coll Med 1962; **Resid:** Otolaryngology, LAC/USC Med Ctr, Los Angeles, CA 1966-1970; **Fellow:** Otology & Neurotology, House Ear Clinic, Los Angeles, CA 1970-1971; **Fac Appt:** Clin Prof Otolaryngology, USC Sch Med

Calcaterra, Thomas Charles MD (Oto) - *Spec Exp:* Head & Neck Cancer; Sinus Disorders/Surgery; **Hospital:** UCLA Med Ctr; **Address:** 10833 Le Conte Ave Bldg CHS - rm 62-158, Los Angeles, CA 90095-1624; **Phone:** (310) 825-6740; **Board Cert:** Otolaryngology 1969; **Med School:** Univ Mich Med Sch 1962; **Resid:** Surgery, Wadsworth VA Hosp, Los Angeles, CA 1965-1966; Otolaryngology, Washington Univ, St Louis, MO 1966-1969; **Fac Appt:** Prof Otolaryngology, UCLA

Cook, Ted MD (Oto) - *Spec Exp:* Cosmetic & Reconstructive Surgery-Face; **Hospital:** OR Hlth Sci Univ Hosp and Clinics; **Address:** Oregon Hlth and Sci Univ, 3181 SW Sam Jackson Park Rd, Portland, OR 97201-3079; **Phone:** (503) 494-5678; **Board Cert:** Otolaryngology 1973; **Med School:** Baylor Coll Med 1964; **Resid:** Surgery, Baylor Hosp, Houston, TX 1969-1970; Otolarynological Rhinoplasty, Baylor Hosp, Houston, TX 1970-1973; **Fellow:** Facial Plastic Surgery, Tampa General Hosp, Tampa, FL 1973; Facial Plastic Surgery, Melrose-Wakefield Hosp, Boston, MA 1975; **Fac Appt:** Prof Otolaryngology, Oregon Hlth Scis Univ

De la Cruz, Antonio MD (Oto) - *Spec Exp:* Head & Neck Surgery; Acoustic Nerve Tumors; Otosclerosis/Stapedotomy; **Hospital:** St Vincent's Med Ctr - Los Angeles; **Address:** 2100 W 3rd St Fl 1, Los Angeles, CA 90057; **Phone:** (213) 483-9930; **Board Cert:** Otolaryngology 1973; **Med School:** Costa Rica 1967; **Resid:** Otolaryngology, Univ Miami Med Ctr, Miami, FL 1970-1973; Surgery, Univ Costa Rica Hosp, Costa Rica 1968; **Fellow:** Otolaryngology, House Ear Clinic, Los Angeles, CA 1974; **Fac Appt:** Clin Prof Otolaryngology, USC Sch Med

Donald, Paul MD (Oto) - *Spec Exp:* Skull Base Surgery; Head & Neck Cancer; Ear, Nose & Throat; **Hospital:** Univ CA - Davis Med Ctr; **Address:** 2521 Stockton Blvd, rm 7200, Sacramento, CA 95817; **Phone:** (916) 734-2832; **Board Cert:** Otolaryngology 1973; **Med School:** Univ British Columbia Fac Med 1964; **Resid:** Surgery, St Paul's Hosp, Vancouver, Canada 1968-1969; Otolaryngology, Univ Iowa Hosp, Iowa City, IA 1969-1973; **Fac Appt:** Prof Otolaryngology, UC Davis

Eisele, David MD (Oto) - *Spec Exp:* Salivary Gland Tumors; Head & Neck Cancer; **Hospital:** UCSF Med Ctr; **Address:** UCSF, Dept Otolaryngology, 400 Parnassus Ave, Ste A 730, San Francisco, CA 94143-0342; **Phone:** (415) 502-0498; **Board Cert:** Otolaryngology 1988; **Med School:** Cornell Univ-Weill Med Coll 1982; **Resid:** Surgery, Univ Wash, Seattle, WA 1982-1984; Otolaryngology Head & Neck, Univ Wash, Seattle, WA 1984-1988; **Fac Appt:** Prof Otolaryngology, UCSF

Fee Jr, Willard E MD (Oto) - *Spec Exp:* ENT Cancer; Surgical Oncology; Head & Neck Surgery; **Hospital:** Stanford Med Ctr; **Address:** Bldg Edwards - rm R135-ENT, 300 Pasteur, Stanford, CA 94305; **Phone:** (650) 723-5281; **Board Cert:** Otolaryngology 1974; **Med School:** Univ Colo 1969; **Resid:** Surgery, Wadsworth VA Hosp, Los Angeles, CA 1970-1971; Otolaryngology, UCLA Med Ctr, Los Angeles, CA 1971-1974; **Fac Appt:** Prof Surgery, Stanford Univ

Geller, Kenneth Allen MD (Oto) - *Spec Exp:* Airway Disorders; Sinus Surgery-Pediatric; Head & Neck Cancer-Pediatric; **Hospital:** Chldns Hosp - Los Angeles; **Address:** Chldns Hosp, Dept Oto, 4650 Sunset Blvd, MS 58, Los Angeles, CA 90027; **Phone:** (323) 669-4145; **Board Cert:** Otolaryngology 1978; **Med School:** USC Sch Med 1972; **Resid:** Surgery, Wadsworth VA Hospital, Los Angeles, CA 1973-1975; Otolaryngology, UCLA Hlth Scis Ctr, Los Angeles, CA 1975-1978; **Fellow:** Pediatric Otolaryngology, Chldn's Hosp, Los Angeles, CA 1978-1979; **Fac Appt:** Assoc Clin Prof Otolaryngology, USC Sch Med

Jackler, Robert K MD (Oto) - *Spec Exp:* Neuro-Otology; Skull Base Surgery; Ear Tumors; **Hospital:** UCSF Med Ctr; **Address:** 400 Parnassus Ave, Ste 730, San Francisco, CA 94117; **Phone:** (415) 353-2757; **Board Cert:** Otolaryngology 1984; **Med School:** Boston Univ 1979; **Resid:** Otolaryngology, UCSF, San Francisco, CA 1980-1984; **Fellow:** Otolaryngology, Oto Med Grp, Los Angeles, CA 1985; **Fac Appt:** Prof Otolaryngology, UCSF

Kamer, Frank M MD (Oto) - *Spec Exp:* Rhinoplasty; Cosmetic Surgery-Face; **Hospital:** Cedars-Sinai Med Ctr; **Address:** 201 S Lasky Dr, Beverly Hills, CA 90212-3647; **Phone:** (310) 556-8155; **Board Cert:** Otolaryngology 1971; **Med School:** Albert Einstein Coll Med 1963; **Resid:** Surgery, Long Is Jewish Hosp, Long Island, NY 1964-1965; Otolaryngology, Mt Sinai Hosp, New York, NY 1968-1970; **Fac Appt:** Prof Otolaryngology, UCLA

Keller, Gregory Steele MD (Oto) - *Spec Exp:* Cosmetic Surgery-Face; **Hospital:** Goleta Vly Cottage Hosp; **Address:** 222 W Pueblo St, Santa Barbara, CA 93105-3878; **Phone:** (805) 687-6408; **Board Cert:** Otolaryngology 1976; **Med School:** Univ IL Coll Med 1971; **Resid:** Otolaryngology, Univ IL, Chicago, IL 1973-1976; Surgery, Cottage Hosp, Santa Barbara, CA 1972-1973; **Fac Appt:** Asst Clin Prof Surgery, UCLA

Larrabee Jr., Wayne F. MD (Oto) - *Spec Exp:* Cosmetic Surgery-Face; Eyelid Surgery; Rhinoplasty & Nasal Surgery; **Hospital:** Swedish Med Ctr; **Address:** Facial Plas Surg, 600 Broadway Ste 280, Seattle, WA 98122-5371; **Phone:** (206) 386-3550; **Board Cert:** Otolaryngology 1979; **Med School:** Tulane Univ 1971; **Resid:** Surgery, Charity Hosp/Tulane Univ Med Ctr, New Orleans, LA 1975-1976; Otolaryngology, Tulane Univ Med Ctr, New Orleans, LA 1976-1979; **Fac Appt:** Clin Prof Otolaryngology, Univ Wash

Perkins, Rodney MD (Oto) - *Spec Exp:* Neuro-Otology; Laser Stapedotomy; **Hospital:** Stanford Med Ctr; **Address:** 801 Welch Rd, Palo Alto, CA 94304; **Phone:** (650) 494-1000; **Board Cert:** Otolaryngology; **Med School:** Indiana Univ 1961; **Resid:** Otolaryngology, Parkland Meml Hosp, Dallas, TX 1961-1962; Otolaryngology, Stanford Univ Hosp, Stanford, CA 1963-1967; **Fellow:** Otolaryngology, Natl Inst Hlth, Bethesda, MD; **Fac Appt:** Clin Prof Surgery, Stanford Univ

OTOLARYNGOLOGY

Powell, Nelson B MD/DDS (Oto) - *Spec Exp:* Sleep Disorders/Apnea; Maxillofacial Surgery; **Hospital:** Stanford Med Ctr; **Address:** 750 Welch Rd, Ste 317, Palo Alto, CA 94304; **Phone:** (650) 328-0511; **Board Cert:** Otolaryngology 1984; **Med School:** Univ Wash 1979; **Resid:** Surgery, Stanford Univ Hosp & Clinics, Stanford, CA 1979-1980; Otolaryngology, Stanford Univ Hosp, Stanford, CA 1980-1983; **Fac Appt:** Clin Prof Surgery, Stanford Univ

Rice, Dale MD (Oto) - *Spec Exp:* Head & Neck Cancer; Endoscopic Sinus Surgery; **Hospital:** USC Univ Hosp - R K Eamer Med Plz; **Address:** USC Keck School of Medicine, 1200 N State St, Box 795, Los Angeles, CA 90033; **Phone:** (323) 442-5790; **Board Cert:** Otolaryngology 1976; **Med School:** Univ Mich Med Sch 1968; **Resid:** Otolaryngology, Univ Mich Med Ctr, Ann Arbor, MI 1972-1976; Surgery, Univ Mich Med Ctr, Ann Arbor, MI 1969-1970; **Fac Appt:** Prof Otolaryngology, USC Sch Med

Sinha, Uttam Kumar MD (Oto) - *Spec Exp:* Head & Neck Cancer; Voice Disorders; **Hospital:** USC Univ Hosp - R K Eamer Med Plz; **Address:** 1200 N State St, Box 795, Los Angeles, CA 90033; **Phone:** (323) 226-7315; **Board Cert:** Otolaryngology 1998; **Med School:** India 1985; **Resid:** LAC-USC Med Ctr, Los Angeles, CA 1991-1995; **Fellow:** Mount Sinai Med Sch, New York, NY 1986-1988; LAC-USC Med Ctr, Los Angeles, CA 1988-1990; **Fac Appt:** Asst Prof Otolaryngology, USC Sch Med

Weymuller, Ernest MD (Oto) - *Spec Exp:* Head & Neck Cancer; Sinus Disorders/Surgery; **Hospital:** Univ WA Med Ctr; **Address:** 1959 NE Pacific St, Box 356515, Seattle, WA 98195; **Phone:** (206) 543-5230; **Board Cert:** Otolaryngology 1973; **Med School:** Harvard Med Sch 1966; **Resid:** Otolaryngology, Mass Eye and Ear Infirm, Boston, MA 1970-1973; Surgery, Vanderbilt Univ Hosp, Nashville, TN 1967-1968; **Fac Appt:** Prof Otolaryngology, Univ Wash

Pain Management

(Subspecialty of ANESTHESIOLOGY, NEUROLOGY, PHYSICAL MEDICINE AND REHABILITATION or PSYCHIATRY)

Some physicians who have their primary board certification in anesthesiology, neurology, physical medicine and rehabilitation, or psychiatry have completed additional training and passed an examination in the subspecialty called pain management. These doctors provide a high level of care, either as a primary physician or consultant, for patients experiencing problems with acute, chronic and/or cancer pain in both hospital and ambulatory settings.

For more information about the main specialties of these physicians, see **Anesthesiology** *(see page 1019)*, **Neurology** *(see page 423)*, **Physical Medicine and Rehabilitation** *(see page 673)* or **Pyschiatry** *(see page 711)*.

Training required: Number of years required for primary specialty *plus* additional training and examination

PHYSICIAN LISTINGS

New England

Acquadro, Martin A MD/DMD (PM) - *Spec Exp:* Pain-Neuropathic; Pain-Chronic; Pain-Cancer; **Hospital:** MA Genl Hosp; **Address:** Mass Genl Hosp, Pain Clinic - ACC324, 15 Parkman St, Boston, MA 02114; **Phone:** (617) 726-8810; **Board Cert:** Anesthesiology 1989, Internal Medicine 1990, Pain Management 1998; **Med School:** Boston Univ 1983; **Resid:** Internal Medicine, Carney Hosp, Boston, MA 1983-1985; Anesthesiology, Mass Genl Hosp, Boston, MA 1986-1988; **Fellow:** Pain Management, Mass Genl Hosp, Boston, MA 1987-1988; **Fac Appt:** Assoc Clin Prof Anesthesiology, Harvard Med Sch

Berde, Charles Benjamin MD (PM) - *Spec Exp:* Pain Management-Pediatric; Critical Care; **Hospital:** Children's Hospital - Boston; **Address:** Dept Anesthesiology, 333 Longwood Ave, Fl 5, Boston, MA 02115; **Phone:** (617) 355-6995; **Board Cert:** Pediatric Critical Care Medicine 1999, Pain Management 1993; **Med School:** Stanford Univ 1980; **Resid:** Pediatrics, Chldns Hosp, Boston, MA 1981-1983; Anesthesiology, Mass Genl Hosp, Boston, MA 1983-1985; **Fellow:** Pediatric Anesthesiology, Chldns Hosp, Boston, MA 1985; **Fac Appt:** Prof Pediatrics, Harvard Med Sch

Carr, Daniel B MD (PM) - *Spec Exp:* Pain-Neuropathic; Pain-Chronic; Headache; **Hospital:** New England Med Ctr - Boston; **Address:** New England Med Ctr, Dept Pain Management, 750 Washington St, Box NEMC298, Boston, MA 02111; **Phone:** (617) 636-6208; **Board Cert:** Internal Medicine 1979, Endocrinology 1981, Anesthesiology 1989, Pain Management 1993; **Med School:** Columbia P&S 1976; **Resid:** Internal Medicine, Columbia-Presby Med Ctr, New York, NY 1977-1979; Anesthesiology, Mass Genl Hosp, Boston, MA 1984-1986; **Fellow:** Endocrinology, Mass Genl Hosp, Boston, MA 1979-1981; **Fac Appt:** Prof Anesthesiology, Tufts Univ

Mid Atlantic

Dubois, Michel MD (PM) - *Spec Exp:* Pain-Back & Neck; Pain-Neuropathic; Pain-Chronic; **Hospital:** NYU Med Ctr (page 71); **Address:** 530 1st Ave Bldg Skirb Fl 9 - Ste T, New York, NY 10016-6402; **Phone:** (212) 263-7316; **Board Cert:** Pain Management 1993, Anesthesiology 1985; **Med School:** France 1974; **Resid:** Anesthesiology, Georgetown Univ Hosp, Washington, DC 1978-1980; London Hosp, London 1974-1976; **Fellow:** Pain Management, Georgetown Univ Hosp, Washington, DC 1983; **Fac Appt:** Prof Anesthesiology, NYU Sch Med

Foley, Kathleen M MD (PM) - *Spec Exp:* Palliative Care; Pain-Cancer; **Hospital:** Mem Sloan Kettering Cancer Ctr; **Address:** 1275 York Ave, Box 52, New York, NY 10021-6007; **Phone:** (212) 639-7050; **Board Cert:** Neurology 1977; **Med School:** Cornell Univ-Weill Med Coll 1969; **Resid:** Neurology, NY Hosp-Cornell, New York, NY 1969-1970; **Fellow:** Clinical Genetics, NY Hosp-Cornell, New York, NY 1970-1971; **Fac Appt:** Prof Neurology, Cornell Univ-Weill Med Coll

Hendler, Nelson H MD (PM) - *Spec Exp:* Electrical Injuries; Lightning Electrocution; **Hospital:** Johns Hopkins Hosp - Baltimore; **Address:** Mensana Clinic, 1718 Greenspring Valley Rd, Stevenson, MD 21153-9999; **Phone:** (410) 653-2403; **Board Cert:** Psychiatry 1977; **Med School:** Univ MD Sch Med 1972; **Resid:** Psychiatry, Johns Hopkins Hosp, Baltimore, MD 1972-1975; **Fellow:** Neurological Physiology, Univ MD Graduate Sch, Baltimore, MD; **Fac Appt:** Asst Prof Neurological Surgery, Johns Hopkins Univ

Jain, Subhash MD (PM) - *Spec Exp:* Pain-Cancer; Pain-Pelvic; Reflex Sympathetic Dystrophy(RSD); **Hospital:** Mem Sloan Kettering Cancer Ctr; **Address:** 1275 York Ave, New York, NY 10021; **Phone:** (212) 639-6851; **Board Cert:** Anesthesiology 1994, Pain Management 1998; **Med School:** India 1968; **Resid:** Surgery, St Vincent Med Ctr, Staten Island, NY 1976-1977; Anesthesiology, NY Hosp-Cornell Med Ctr, New York, NY 1977-1979; **Fellow:** Pain Management, NY Hosp-Cornell Med Ctr, New York, NY 1979-1980; **Fac Appt:** Assoc Prof Pain Management, Cornell Univ-Weill Med Coll

Kreitzer, Joel MD (PM) - *Spec Exp:* Pain-Back; Pain-Cancer; **Hospital:** Mount Sinai Hosp (page 68); **Address:** Pain Management Service, 5 E 98th St, Fl 6, Box 1192, New York, NY 10029; **Phone:** (212) 241-6372; **Board Cert:** Anesthesiology 1990, Pain Management 1993; **Med School:** Albert Einstein Coll Med 1985; **Resid:** Anesthesiology, Mount Sinai, New York, NY 1986-1989; **Fellow:** Pain Management, Mount Sinai, New York, NY 1988-1989; **Fac Appt:** Assoc Clin Prof Anesthesiology, Mount Sinai Sch Med

Lema, Mark J MD/PhD (PM) - *Spec Exp:* Pain-Cancer; Palliative Care; Neuropathic Pain; **Hospital:** Roswell Park Cancer Inst; **Address:** Carlton & Elm Streets, Buffalo, NY 14263-0001; **Phone:** (716) 845-3240; **Board Cert:** Anesthesiology 1987, Pain Management 1994; **Med School:** SUNY Downstate 1982; **Resid:** Anesthesiology, Brigham & Women's Hosp, Boston, MA 1983-1984; **Fellow:** Physiology, SUNY Buffalo Genl Hosp, Buffalo, NY 1974-1978; **Fac Appt:** Prof Anesthesiology, SUNY Buffalo

Ngeow, Jeffrey MD (PM) - *Spec Exp:* Pain-Musculoskeletal; Acupuncture; **Hospital:** Hosp For Special Surgery (page 62); **Address:** 535 E 70th St, New York, NY 10021; **Phone:** (212) 606-1059; **Board Cert:** Anesthesiology 1980, Pain Management 1994; **Med School:** England 1971; **Resid:** Anesthesiology, Peter Bent Brigham Hosp., Boston, MA 1975-1977; **Fellow:** Pain Management, Tufts NE Med Ctr, Boston, MA 1977-1978; **Fac Appt:** Assoc Clin Prof Anesthesiology, Cornell Univ-Weill Med Coll

Payne, Richard MD (PM) - *Spec Exp:* Palliative Care; **Hospital:** Mem Sloan Kettering Cancer Ctr; **Address:** 1275 York Ave, Ste C723, New York, NY 10021; **Phone:** (212) 639-8031; **Board Cert:** Neurology 1984; **Med School:** Harvard Med Sch 1977; **Resid:** Neurology, NY Hosp-Cornell Med Ctr, New York, NY 1979-1982; **Fellow:** Medical Oncology, Meml Sloan Kettering Cancer Ctr, New York, NY 1982-1984; **Fac Appt:** Prof Neurology, Cornell Univ-Weill Med Coll

Portenoy, Russell MD (PM) - *Spec Exp:* Pain Management; Palliative Care; **Hospital:** Beth Israel Med Ctr - Petrie Division (page 58); **Address:** Beth Israel Med Ctr, Dept Pain Med & Palliative Care, First Ave at 16th St, New York, NY 10003; **Phone:** (212) 844-1505; **Board Cert:** Neurology 1985; **Med School:** Univ MD Sch Med 1980; **Resid:** Neurology, Albert Einstein, Bronx, NY 1981-1984; **Fellow:** Pain Management, Meml Sloan-Kettering, New York, NY 1984-1985; **Fac Appt:** Prof Neurology, Albert Einstein Coll Med

Raja, Srinivasa MD (PM) - *Spec Exp:* Pain-Sympathetic; **Hospital:** Johns Hopkins Hosp - Baltimore; **Address:** Osler 292, 600 N Wolfe St, Baltimore, MD 21287; **Phone:** (410) 955-1822; **Board Cert:** Pain Management 1993, Anesthesiology 1982; **Med School:** India 1974; **Resid:** Anesthesiology, Univ of Washington, Seattle, WA 1977-1979; **Fellow:** Pain Management, Univ of Virginia, Charlottesville, VA 1979-1981; **Fac Appt:** Prof Anesthesiology, Johns Hopkins Univ

Rosner, Howard L MD (PM) - *Spec Exp:* Reflex Sympathetic Dystrophy(RSD); **Hospital:** NY Presby Hosp - NY Weill Cornell Med Ctr (page 70); **Address:** 525 E 68th St, Fl Sub Bsmnt - Ste M0026, New York, NY 10021; **Phone:** (212) 746-2960; **Board Cert:** Anesthesiology 1989, Pain Management 1993; **Med School:** Univ Miami Sch Med 1980; **Resid:** Anesthesiology, Mass General Hosp, Boston, MA 1980-1983; **Fellow:** Pain Management, Columbia-Presbyterian Medical Center, New York, NY; **Fac Appt:** Assoc Prof Anesthesiology, Cornell Univ-Weill Med Coll

Sarno, John E MD (PM) - *Spec Exp:* Pain-Mind/Body Disorder; **Hospital:** Rusk Inst of Rehab Med (page 71); **Address:** Rusk Institute, Ground Floor, 400 E 34th St, rm 30, New York, NY 10016-4901; **Phone:** (212) 263-6035; **Board Cert:** Physical Medicine & Rehabilitation 1965; **Med School:** Columbia P&S 1950; **Resid:** Physical Medicine & Rehabilitation, NYU Med Ctr, New York, NY 1951-1952; Pediatrics, Babies Hosp/Columbia-Presby Med Ctr, New York, NY 1960-1961; **Fellow:** Physical Medicine & Rehabilitation, NYU Med Ct, New York, NY 1961-1963; **Fac Appt:** Clin Prof Physical Medicine & Rehabilitation, NYU Sch Med

Staats, Peter MD (PM) - *Spec Exp:* Pain-Cancer; **Hospital:** Johns Hopkins Hosp - Baltimore; **Address:** 601 N Caroline St, Ste 3062, Baltimore, MD 21287; **Phone:** (410) 955-7246; **Board Cert:** Pain Management 1994, Anesthesiology 1994; **Med School:** Univ Mich Med Sch 1989; **Resid:** Anesthesiology, Johns Hopkins Hosp, Baltimore, MD 1990-1993; **Fellow:** Anesthesiology, Johns Hopkins Hosp, Baltimore, MD 1993-1994; **Fac Appt:** Asst Prof Anesthesiology, Johns Hopkins Univ

Weinberger, Michael MD (PM) - *Spec Exp:* Pain-Cancer; Pain-Back; **Hospital:** NY Presby Hosp - Columbia Presby Med Ctr (page 70); **Address:** 622 W 168th St, rm 500, New York, NY 10032; **Phone:** (212) 305-7114; **Board Cert:** Anesthesiology 1990, Pain Management 1991; **Med School:** Columbia P&S 1983; **Resid:** Internal Medicine, St Vincent's Hosp & Med Ctr, New York, NY 1983-1986; Anesthesiology, Columbia-Presby, New York, NY 1986-1989; **Fellow:** Pain Management, Memorial Sloan Kettering, New York, NY 1990

Southeast

Berger, Jerry J MD (PM) - *Spec Exp:* Pain Management - General; **Hospital:** Shands Hlthcre at Univ of FL (page 73); **Address:** 1600 SW Archer Rd, Shands at U FL-AnesPreOp, Gainesville, FL 32610; **Phone:** (352) 395-9763; **Board Cert:** Anesthesiology 1981, Pain Management 1993; **Med School:** Duke Univ 1977; **Resid:** Anesthesiology, Shands-Univ Florida, Gainesville, FL 1978-1980; **Fellow:** Pain Management, Shands-Univ Florida, Gainesville, FL 1980-1981; **Fac Appt:** Asst Prof Anesthesiology, Univ Fla Coll Med

Midwest

Benzon, Honorio T MD (PM) - *Spec Exp:* Pain-Back; Complex Regional Pain Syndrome-CRPS; Myofacial Pain Syndrome; **Hospital:** Northwestern Meml Hosp; **Address:** 675 N Saint Clair St, Fl 20 - Ste 20-100, Chicago, IL 60611-3015; **Phone:** (312) 695-2500; **Board Cert:** Anesthesiology 1995, Pain Management 1993; **Med School:** Philippines 1971; **Resid:** Anesthesiology, Cincinnati Med Ctr, Cincinnati, OH 1973-1975; Anesthesiology, Northwestern Meml Hosp, Chicago, IL 1975-1976; **Fellow:** Pain Management, Brigham & Womens, Boston, MA 1985-1986; **Fac Appt:** Prof Anesthesiology, Northwestern Univ

Green, Carmen R MD (PM) - *Spec Exp:* Pain Management; **Hospital:** Univ of MI Hlth Ctr; **Address:** Univ Mich Med Ctr, Multidisciplinary Pain Ctr, 1500 E Medical Center Drive, rm 1G323, Ann Arbor, MI 48109; **Phone:** (734) 763-5459; **Board Cert:** Anesthesiology 1996, Pain Management 1998; **Med School:** Mich State Univ 1988; **Fellow:** Anesthesiology, U Mich Medical Ctr, Ann Haror, MI 1993

Harden, R Norman MD (PM) - *Spec Exp:* Pain Management-Back & Headache; Reflex Sympathetic Dystrophy(RSD); Fibromyalgia; **Hospital:** Rehab Inst - Chicago; **Address:** 1030 N Clark St, Ste 320, Chicago, IL 60610; **Phone:** (312) 238-7800; **Med School:** Med Coll GA 1984; **Resid:** Neurology, Univ South Carolina, Columbia, SC 1984-1985; **Fellow:** Pain Management, Rehab Inst - Georgia, Atlanta, GA 1989; **Fac Appt:** Asst Prof Physical Medicine & Rehabilitation, Northwestern Univ

Mullin, Vildan MD (PM) - *Spec Exp:* Pain Management; **Hospital:** Univ of MI Hlth Ctr; **Address:** Med Inn - Pain Center, 1500 E Med Ctr Drive, rm 1H247, Box 0048, Ann Arbor, MI 48109; **Phone:** (734) 936-4280; **Board Cert:** Anesthesiology 1987, Pain Management 1993; **Med School:** Turkey 1972; **Resid:** Anesthesiology, Univ Michigan, Ann Arbor, MI 1976-1978; Surgery, Sinai Hosp, Detroit, MI 1975-1976; **Fellow:** Pain Management, Univ Virginia, Charlottesville, VA 1978-1979; **Fac Appt:** Assoc Prof Pain Management, Univ Mich Med Sch

Robbins, Lawrence D MD (PM) - *Spec Exp:* Headache; Migraine; **Hospital:** Highland Park Hosp; **Address:** 1535 Lake Cook Rd, Ste 506, Northbrook, IL 60062-1451; **Phone:** (847) 480-9399; **Board Cert:** Pain Management 1995; **Med School:** Univ IL Coll Med 1981; **Resid:** Neurology, Univ of Illinois, Chicago, IL 1982-1985; **Fellow:** Pain Management, Diamond Headache Clinic, Chicago, IL 1985-1986; **Fac Appt:** Asst Prof Neurology, Rush Med Coll

Swarm, Robert A MD (PM) - *Spec Exp:* Pain-Acute; Pain-Chronic; Pain-Cancer; **Hospital:** Barnes-Jewish Hosp (page 55); **Address:** Pain Mngmt Ctr, 4921 Parkview Pl, 10th Fl - Ctr for Advanced Med, St Louis, MO 63110; **Phone:** (314) 362-8820; **Board Cert:** Anesthesiology 1990, Pain Management 1993; **Med School:** Washington Univ, St Louis 1983; **Resid:** Surgery, Barnes Hosp-Washington Univ, St Louis, MO 1983-1986; Anesthesiology, Barnes Hosp-Washington Univ, St Louis, MO 1986-1989; **Fellow:** Pain Management, Univ Sydney Hosp, Sydney, Australia 1991; **Fac Appt:** Assoc Prof Anesthesiology, Washington Univ, St Louis

Weisman, Steven Jay MD (PM) - *Spec Exp:* Pain Management-Pediatric; Palliative Care-Pediatric; Anesthesiology-Pediatric; **Hospital:** Chldrns Hosp - Wisconsin; **Address:** Children's Hosp - Wisc, 9000 W Wisconsin Ave, Milwaukee, WI 53226; **Phone:** (414) 266-2775; **Board Cert:** Pediatric Hematology-Oncology 1984, Anesthesiology 1996; **Med School:** Albert Einstein Coll Med 1978; **Resid:** Pediatrics, Chldns Hosp, Philadelphia, PA 1978-1981; Anesthesiology, UCONN Hlth Ctr, Farmington, CT 1992-1994; **Fellow:** Pediatric Hematology-Oncology, Indiana Univ Sch Med, Indianapolis, IN 1981-1984; **Fac Appt:** Prof Anesthesiology, Med Coll Wisc

Great Plains and Mountains

Ashburn, Michael MD (PM) - *Spec Exp:* Pain Management; Palliative Care; **Hospital:** Univ Utah Hosp and Clin; **Address:** U Utah Hosps & Clinics-Pain Mgmt Ctr, 546 Chipeta Way , Ste G-200, Salt Lake City, UT; **Phone:** (801) 581-7246; **Board Cert:** Anesthesiology 1988, Pain Management 1993; **Med School:** Univ S Ala Coll Med 1984; **Resid:** Anesthesiology, U South Ala, Mobile, AL 1984-1987; **Fellow:** Pain Management, U Utah, Salt Lake City, UT 1987-1988; **Fac Appt:** Prof Pain Management, Univ Utah

Waldman, Steven D MD (PM) - *Spec Exp:* Pain-Neuropathic; **Address:** The Headache & Pain Ctr, 4801 College Blvd, Leawood, KS 66211; **Phone:** (913) 491-6451; **Board Cert:** Anesthesiology 1983, Pain Management 1993; **Med School:** Univ MO-Kansas City 1977; **Resid:** Anesthesiology, Mayo Clinic, Rochester, MN 1978-1980; **Fac Appt:** Clin Prof Anesthesiology, Univ MO-Kansas City

Southwest

Abram, Stephen Edward MD (PM) - *Spec Exp:* Critical Care; **Hospital:** Univ NM Hosp; **Address:** Univ New Mexico, Dept Anes & Critical Care, 2701 Frontier NE, Albuquerque, NM 87131-5216; **Phone:** (505) 272-2730; **Board Cert:** Anatomic Pathology 1976, Pain Management 1993; **Med School:** Jefferson Med Coll 1970; **Resid:** Anesthesiology, Mary Hitchcock Meml Hosp, Lebanon, NH 1971-1973; **Fac Appt:** Prof Anesthesiology, Univ New Mexico

Racz, Gabor MD (PM) - *Spec Exp:* Pain Management; Reflex Symapathetic Dystrophy (RSD); Pain-Back & Neck; **Hospital:** Univ Med Ctr - Lubbock; **Address:** 3601 4th St, rm 1C282, Lubbock, TX 79430; **Phone:** (806) 743-3112; **Board Cert:** Anesthesiology 1993, Pain Management 1993; **Med School:** England 1962; **Resid:** Anesthesiology, SUNY Upstate Med Ctr, Syracuse, NY 1966; **Fac Appt:** Prof Anesthesiology, Texas Tech Univ

Ramamurthy, Somayaji MD (PM) - *Spec Exp: Pain-Back; Pain-Chronic;* **Hospital:** Univ of Texas Hlth & Sci Ctr; **Address:** Univ Texas Hlth Sci Ctr, Dept Anes, 7703 Floyd Curl Drive, MC 7838, San Antonio, TX 78229-3900; **Phone:** (210) 567-4543; **Board Cert:** Pain Management 1993, Anesthesiology 1972; **Med School:** India 1965; **Resid:** Anesthesiology, Cook Co Hosp, San Antonio, TX 1968-1970; **Fac Appt:** Prof Anesthesiology, Univ Tex, San Antonio

Rogers, James N MD (PM) - *Spec Exp: Pain-Chronic; Pain-Acute;* **Hospital:** Univ of Texas Hlth & Sci Ctr; **Address:** Univ Rexas Hlth Sci Ctr, Dept Anes, 7703 Floyd Curl Drive, MC 7838, San Antonio, TX 78229-3900; **Phone:** (210) 567-4543; **Board Cert:** Pain Management 1994, Anesthesiology 1993; **Med School:** Univ Ariz Coll Med 1987; **Resid:** Anesthesiology, Bexar Co Hosp, San Antonio, TX 1988-1991; **Fellow:** Pain Management, Bexar Co Hosp, San Antonio, TX 1991-1992; **Fac Appt:** Prof Anesthesiology, Univ Tex, San Antonio

Walsh, Nicolas E MD (PM) - *Spec Exp: Pain Management; Pain-Amputee; Trauma;* **Hospital:** Univ of Texas Hlth & Sci Ctr; **Address:** Univ Texas Hlth Sci Ctr, Rehab Med, 7703 Floyd Curl Drive, San Antonio, TX 78229-3900; **Phone:** (210) 567-5350; **Board Cert:** Physical Medicine & Rehabilitation 1983, Pain Management 2000; **Med School:** Univ Colo 1979; **Resid:** Physical Medicine & Rehabilitation, Univ Tex Hlth Sci Ctr, San Antonio, TX 1979-1982; **Fac Appt:** Prof Physical Medicine & Rehabilitation, Univ Tex, San Antonio

West Coast and Pacific

Du Pen, Stuart L MD (PM) - *Spec Exp: Pain-Cancer; Pain-Chronic;* **Hospital:** Swedish Med Ctr; **Address:** 747 Broadway 6 W, Seattle, WA 98122; **Phone:** (206) 386-2013; **Board Cert:** Anesthesiology 1972, Pain Management 1993; **Med School:** St Louis Univ 1967; **Resid:** Anesthesiology, VA Mason Clin, Seattle, WA 1968-1971; **Fac Appt:** Assoc Clin Prof Anesthesiology, Univ Wash

Ferrante, F Michael MD (PM) - *Spec Exp: Pain Management - General;* **Hospital:** UCLA Med Ctr; **Address:** UCLA Pain Program, 200 Medical Plaza, Ste 660, Los Angeles, CA 90095; **Phone:** (310) 794-1841; **Board Cert:** Anesthesiology 1987, Pain Management 1993, Internal Medicine 1985; **Med School:** NY Med Coll 1980; **Resid:** Internal Medicine, Emroy Univ Affil Hosp, Atlanta, GA 1981-1983; Anesthesiology, Emroy Univ Affil Hosp, Atlanta, GA 1984-1986; **Fellow:** Infectious Disease, Barnes Hosp-Wash Univ, St Louis, MO 1983-1984; Pain Management, Brigham-Women's Hosp, Boston, MA 1986-1987; **Fac Appt:** Clin Prof Anesthesiology, UCLA

Fitzgibbon, Dermot Richard MD (PM) - *Spec Exp: Pain Management-Pre Operative; Pain-Cancer;* **Hospital:** Univ WA Med Ctr; **Address:** Dept Anesthesiology, 1959 NE Pacific St, Box 356540, Seattle, WA 98195; **Phone:** (206) 598-4260; **Board Cert:** Pain Management 1998, Anesthesiology 1996; **Med School:** Ireland 1983; **Resid:** Anesthesiology, St Vincent's Hosp, Dublin, Ireland 1985-1992; Anesthesiology, Univ Wash, Seattle, WA 1994-1995; **Fellow:** Pain Management, Univ Wash-Pain Mngmt Clinic, Seattle, WA 1992

Prager, Joshua Philip MD (PM) - *Spec Exp: Internal Medicine;* **Hospital:** UCLA Med Ctr; **Address:** 100 UCLA Med Plaza, Ste 760, Los Angeles, CA 90095; **Phone:** (310) 264-7246; **Board Cert:** Anesthesiology 1987, Pain Management 1993; **Med School:** Stanford Univ 1981; **Resid:** Internal Medicine, UCLA Med Ctr, Los Angeles, CA 1982-1984; Anesthesiology, Mass Genl Hosp, Boston, MA 1984-1986; **Fac Appt:** Assoc Prof Anesthesiology, UCLA

Ready, L Brian MD (PM) - *Spec Exp: Pain Management-Cancer;* **Hospital:** Tacoma Gen Hosp; **Address:** 316 Martin Luther King Jr Way, Ste 103, Tacoma, WA 98415; **Phone:** (253) 403-1375; **Board Cert:** Anesthesiology; **Med School:** Canada 1967; **Resid:** Anesthesiology, Univ WA Med Ctr, Seattle, WA 1973-1975

Rowbotham, Michael Charles MD (PM) - *Spec Exp:* *Reflex Sympathetic Dystrophy(RSD); Pain-Nerve Injury; Herpetic Neuralgia;* **Hospital:** UCSF - Mount Zion Med Ctr; **Address:** 2255 Post St, San Francisco, CA 94115; **Phone:** (415) 885-7246; **Board Cert:** Neurology 1989; **Med School:** UCSF 1979; **Resid:** Neurology, Boston Univ, Boston, MD 1984-1986; Neurology, UCSF, San Francisco, CA 1986-1987; **Fellow:** Neurological Pharmacology, UCSF, San Francisco, CA 1979-1980; Pain Management, UCSF, San Francisco, CA 1987-1989; **Fac Appt:** Assoc Prof Neurology, UCSF

PATHOLOGY

A pathologist deals with the causes and nature of disease and contributes to diagnosis, prognosis and treatment through knowledge gained by the laboratory application of the biologic, chemical and physical sciences.

A pathologist uses information gathered from the microscopic examination of tissue specimens, cells and body fluids, and from clinical laboratory tests on body fluids and secretions for the diagnosis, exclusion and monitoring of disease.

Training required: Five to seven years

Certification in the following subspecialty requires additional training and examination.

Dermatopathology: A dermatopathologist has the expertise to diagnose and monitor diseases of the skin including infectious, immunologic, degenerative and neoplastic diseases. This entails the examination and interpretation of specially prepared tissue sections, cellular scrapings and smears of skin lesions by means of routine and special (electron and flourescent) microscopes.

PHYSICIAN LISTINGS

Pathology

New England

Bhan, Atul Kumar MD (Path) - *Spec Exp: Immunopathology; Liver Disease;* **Hospital:** MA Genl Hosp; **Address:** Mass Genl Hosp, 55 Fruit St, Bldg WARRE - Fl 501, Boston, MA 02114-2620; **Phone:** (617) 726-2588; **Board Cert:** Anatomic Pathology 1976, Immunopathology 1985; **Med School:** India 1965; **Resid:** Pathology, Boston Univ Hosp, Boston, MA 1970-1971; Pathology, Chldns Univ Hosp, Boston, MA 1971-1974; **Fac Appt:** Prof Pathology, Harvard Med Sch

Carter, Darryl MD (Path) - *Spec Exp: Breast Cancer;* **Hospital:** Yale - New Haven Hosp; **Address:** PO Box 208070, New Haven, CT 06520-8070; **Phone:** (203) 785-2786; **Board Cert:** Anatomic Pathology 1969; **Med School:** Johns Hopkins Univ 1961; **Resid:** Pathology, Johns Hopkins Hosp, Baltimore, MD 1965-1968; Surgery, Ohio State Univ, Columbus, OH 1962-1963; **Fellow:** Pathology, Meml Hosp Cancer, New York, NY 1968-1969; **Fac Appt:** Prof Pathology, Yale Univ

Cole, Solon R MD (Path) - *Spec Exp: Lung Disease;* **Hospital:** Hartford Hosp; **Address:** 80 Seymour St, rm 354, Hartford, CT 06102; **Phone:** (860) 545-2866; **Board Cert:** Anatomic Pathology 1971; **Med School:** Tulane Univ 1962; **Resid:** Anatomic Pathology, Boston City Hosp, Boston, MA 1964-1967; **Fellow:** Pulmonary Pathology, AFIP, Washington, DC 1970-1972; Electron Microscopy, Harvard Med Sch, Boston, MA 1967-1969; **Fac Appt:** Assoc Prof Pathology, Univ Conn

Connolly, James Leo MD (Path) - *Spec Exp: Breast Pathology;* **Hospital:** Beth Israel Deaconess Med Ctr - Boston; **Address:** Beth Israel, Dept Pathology, 330 Brookline Ave, rm ES 112, Boston, MA 02215-5400; **Phone:** (617) 667-4344; **Board Cert:** Anatomic Pathology 1980; **Med School:** Vanderbilt Univ 1974; **Resid:** Anatomic Pathology, Beth Israel Hospital, Boston, MA 1974-1978; **Fac Appt:** Prof Pathology, Harvard Med Sch

Fletcher, Christopher MD (Path) - *Spec Exp: Soft-Tissue Tumors/Sarcomas; Surgical Pathology;* **Hospital:** Brigham & Women's Hosp; **Address:** Dept Path-75 Francis St, Boston, MA 02115; **Phone:** (617) 732-8558; **Board Cert:** Pathology 1988; **Med School:** England 1981; **Resid:** Pathology, St Thomas Hosp, London, England 1982-1985; **Fellow:** Pathology, St Thomas Hosp, London, England 1985; **Fac Appt:** Prof Pathology, Harvard Med Sch

Harris, Nancy L MD (Path) - *Spec Exp: Lymphoma; Hematopathology;* **Hospital:** MA Genl Hosp; **Address:** 55 Fruit St, Warren Bldg 2, Boston, MA 02114; **Phone:** (617) 726-5155; **Board Cert:** Anatomic Pathology 1978, Clinical Pathology 1978; **Med School:** Stanford Univ 1970; **Resid:** Pathology, Beth Israel Hosp, Boston, MA 1974-1978; **Fellow:** Hematology, Mass Genl Hosp, Boston, MA 1978-1980; **Fac Appt:** Prof Pathology, Harvard Med Sch

Mark, Eugene J. MD (Path) - *Spec Exp: Lung Disease; Cardiac Pathology;* **Hospital:** MA Genl Hosp; **Address:** Mass Genl Hospital, 55 Fruit St, Bldg Warren 246, Boston, MA 02114; **Phone:** (617) 726-8891; **Board Cert:** Anatomic Pathology 1973, Dermatopathology 1975; **Med School:** Harvard Med Sch 1967; **Resid:** Pathology, Mass Genl Hosp., Boston, MA 1968-1972; Pathology, Mass Genl Hosp., Boston, MA 1974-1979; **Fellow:** Pathology, Dantonsspital, Winterhur 1965-1966; **Fac Appt:** Assoc Prof Pathology, Harvard Med Sch

Schnitt, Stuart MD (Path) - *Spec Exp: Breast Pathology;* **Hospital:** Beth Israel Deaconess Med Ctr - Boston; **Address:** Beth Israel Deaconess Med Ctr, Dept Pathology, 330 Brookline Ave, Boston, MA 02215-5400; **Phone:** (617) 667-4344; **Med School:** Albany Med Coll 1979

Young, Robert Henry MD (Path) - *Spec Exp:* Breast Pathology; **Hospital:** MA Genl Hosp; **Address:** 55 Fruit St, Warren Bldg 215, Boston, MA 02114; **Phone:** (617) 726-8892; **Board Cert:** Anatomic Pathology 1980; **Med School:** Ireland 1974; **Resid:** Pathology, Mas Genl Hosp, Boston, MA 1977-1979; Pathology, Dublin Univ, Dublin, Ireland 1975-1977; **Fac Appt:** Assoc Prof Pathology, Harvard Med Sch

Mid Atlantic

Burger, Peter MD (Path) - *Spec Exp:* Brain Tumors; **Hospital:** Johns Hopkins Hosp - Baltimore; **Address:** 600 N Wolfe St, Pathology 710, Baltimore, MD 21287; **Phone:** (410) 955-8378; **Board Cert:** Anatomic Pathology 1976, Neuropathology 1976; **Med School:** Northwestern Univ 1966; **Resid:** Anatomic Pathology, Duke U Med Ctr, Durham, NC 1969-1973; **Fellow:** Neuropathology, Duke U Med Ctr, Durham, NC 1969-1973

Dorfman, Howard MD (Path) - *Spec Exp:* Bone Tumor Pathology; Soft Tissue Tumors; Joint Pathology; **Hospital:** Montefiore Med Ctr (page 67); **Address:** Orthopaedic Pathology Div, 111 E 210th St, Bronx, NY 10467-2401; **Phone:** (718) 920-5622; **Board Cert:** Pathology 1958; **Med School:** SUNY Downstate 1951; **Resid:** Pathology, Mt Sinai Hosp, New York, NY 1952-1953; Pathology, Columbia-Presby Med Ctr, New York, NY 1956-1958; **Fellow:** Pathology, Mt Sinai Med Ctr, New York, NY 1953-1954; **Fac Appt:** Prof Pathology, Albert Einstein Coll Med

Epstein, Jonathan MD (Path) - *Spec Exp:* Urologic Pathology; **Hospital:** Johns Hopkins Hosp - Baltimore; **Address:** 401 N Broadway, rm 2242, Baltimore, MD 21231; **Phone:** (410) 955-3580; **Board Cert:** Pathology 1986; **Med School:** Boston Univ 1981; **Resid:** Pathology, Johns Hopkins, Baltimore, MD 1984-1985; **Fellow:** Pathology, Meml Sloan Kettering Canc. C., New York, NY 1983-1984; **Fac Appt:** Prof Pathology, Johns Hopkins Univ

Frizzera, Glauco MD (Path) - *Spec Exp:* Hematopathology; Lymph Node Pathology; Bone Marrow Pathology; **Hospital:** NY Presby Hosp - NY Weill Cornell Med Ctr (page 70); **Address:** 525 E 68th St Bldg Starr - Ste 737-A, New York, NY 10021; **Phone:** (212) 746-6401; **Board Cert:** Anatomic Pathology 1997; **Med School:** Italy 1964; **Resid:** Pathology, Univ Bologna, Bologna, Italy 1965-1969; **Fellow:** Hematology, Univ Chicago, Chicago, IL 1972-1974; **Fac Appt:** Prof Pathology, Cornell Univ-Weill Med Coll

Hruban, Ralph H MD (Path) - *Spec Exp:* Gastrointestinal Pathology; **Hospital:** Johns Hopkins Hosp - Baltimore; **Address:** Johns Hopkins Hosp, Dept Pathology, 401 N Broadway Bldg Weinberg - rm 2242, Baltimore, MD 21231; **Phone:** (410) 955-9132; **Board Cert:** Anatomic Pathology 1990; **Med School:** Johns Hopkins Univ 1985; **Resid:** Pathology, Johns Hopkins Hosp, Baltimore, MD 1986-1990; **Fellow:** Meml Sloan Kettering Cancer Ctr, New York, NY 1988-1989; **Fac Appt:** Prof Pathology, Johns Hopkins Univ

Huvos, Andrew G MD (Path) - *Spec Exp:* Bone Pathology; Head & Neck Pathology; **Hospital:** Mem Sloan Kettering Cancer Ctr; **Address:** 1275 York Ave, Dept Path, New York, NY 10021-6007; **Phone:** (212) 639-5905; **Board Cert:** Anatomic Pathology 1998; **Med School:** Germany 1963; **Resid:** Pathology, Meml Sloan Kettering Cancer Ctr, New York, NY 1967-1969; **Fellow:** Surgical Pathology, Columbia Presby Med Ctr, New York, NY 1966-1967; **Fac Appt:** Prof Pathology, Cornell Univ-Weill Med Coll

Ishak, Kamal G. MD (Path) - *Spec Exp:* Liver Pathology; **Hospital:** Armed Forces Inst of Path; **Address:** Armed Forces Institute of Pathology, 6825 16th St NW, Bldg 54 - rm 3107, Washington, DC 20306-0004; **Phone:** (202) 782-1707; **Board Cert:** Anatomic Pathology 1961, Clinical Pathology 1962; **Med School:** Egypt 1951; **Resid:** Anatomic Pathology, Baptist Meml Hosp, San Antonio, TX 1957-1959; Clinical Pathology, Baylor Univ Med Ctr, Dallas, TX 1959-1961; **Fellow:** Pathology, US Naval Rsch Unit, Cairo, Egypt 1955-1956

Jaffe, Elaine Sarkin MD (Path) - *Spec Exp:* Lymphoma; Hematopathology; **Hospital:** Natl Inst of Hlth - Clin Ctr; **Address:** Natl Cancer Inst. NIH-Lab Path., Bldg 10 - rm 2N202 MSC 1500, Bethesda, MD 20892-0001; **Phone:** (301) 496-0183; **Board Cert:** Anatomic Pathology 1974; **Med School:** Univ Penn 1969; **Resid:** Pathology, Clin Ctr/NIH, Bethesda, MD 1970-1972; **Fellow:** Hematology, Natl Cancer Inst, Bethesda, MD 1972-1974; Pathology, Natl Cancer Inst, Bethesda, MD 1972-1974; **Fac Appt:** Clin Prof Pathology, Geo Wash Univ

Katzenstein, Anna-Luise A. MD (Path) - *Spec Exp:* Pulmonary Pathology; Interstitial Lung Disease; Vasculitis; **Hospital:** Crouse Hosp; **Address:** Crouse Hosp, 736 Irving Ave, Fl 9, Syracuse, NY 13210-1690; **Phone:** (315) 470-7396; **Board Cert:** Anatomic Pathology 1976; **Med School:** Johns Hopkins Univ 1971; **Resid:** Pathology, Univ Hospital, San Diego, CA 1972-1975; **Fellow:** Surgical Pathology, Barnes Hosp-Wash Univ, St Louis, MO 1976-1977; **Fac Appt:** Prof Pathology, SUNY Syracuse

Knowles, Daniel MD (Path) - *Spec Exp:* Lymph Node Pathology; Bone Marrow Pathology; **Hospital:** NY Presby Hosp - NY Weill Cornell Med Ctr (page 70); **Address:** Cornell-Weill Medical College , Dept Pathology, 1300 York Ave, New York, NY 10021-4805; **Phone:** (212) 746-6464; **Board Cert:** Pathology 1978, Immunopathology 1984; **Med School:** Univ Chicago-Pritzker Sch Med 1973; **Resid:** Anatomic Pathology, Columbia-Presby Med Ctr, New York, NY 1974-1975; Anatomic Pathology, Columbia-Presby Med Ctr, New York, NY 1977-1978; **Fellow:** Immunopathology, Rockefeller Univ, New York, NY 1975-1977; **Fac Appt:** Prof Pathology, Cornell Univ-Weill Med Coll

Kurman, Robert J MD (Path) - *Spec Exp:* Gynecologic Pathology; **Hospital:** Johns Hopkins Hosp - Baltimore; **Address:** Johns Hopkins Hosp, 401 N Broadway Bldg Weinberg - rm 2242, Baltimore, MD 21231-2410; **Phone:** (410) 955-0471; **Board Cert:** Anatomic Pathology 1972, Obstetrics & Gynecology 1980; **Med School:** SUNY Syracuse 1968; **Resid:** Pathology, Peter Bent Brigham Hosp, Boston, MA 1969-1971; Pathology, Mass Genl Hosp, Boston, MA 1971-1972; **Fellow:** Obstetrics & Gynecology, Harvard Univ Hosp, Boston, MA 1972-1973; **Fac Appt:** Prof Pathology, Johns Hopkins Univ

McCormick, Steven MD (Path) - *Spec Exp:* Ophthalmic Pathology; **Hospital:** New York Eye & Ear Infirm (page 69); **Address:** 310 E 14th St, New York, NY 10003; **Phone:** (212) 979-4156; **Board Cert:** Anatomic Pathology 1988; **Med School:** W VA Univ 1984; **Resid:** Anatomic Pathology, W VA Univ Hosp, Morgantown, WV 1984-1988; **Fellow:** Ophthalmological Pathology, W Va Univ Hosp, Morgantown, WV 1987-1988; **Fac Appt:** Assoc Prof Pathology, NY Med Coll

McNutt, N Scott MD (Path) - *Spec Exp:* Skin Pathology; **Hospital:** NY Presby Hosp - NY Weill Cornell Med Ctr (page 70); **Address:** 525 E 68th St, Ste F309, New York, NY 10021-4873; **Phone:** (212) 746-6434; **Board Cert:** Anatomic Pathology 1973, Dermatopathology 1979; **Med School:** Harvard Med Sch 1966; **Resid:** Pathology, Mass Genl Hosp, Boston, MA 1968-1970; **Fellow:** Pathology, Mass Genl Hosp, Boston, MA 1970-1972; **Fac Appt:** Prof Pathology, Cornell Univ-Weill Med Coll

Rosen, Paul Peter MD (Path) - *Spec Exp:* Breast Pathology; **Hospital:** NY Presby Hosp - NY Weill Cornell Med Ctr (page 70); **Address:** New York Presbyterian, Dept Pathology, 525 E 68th St, Ste C410, New York, NY 10021-4870; **Phone:** (212) 746-6482; **Board Cert:** Anatomic Pathology 1998; **Med School:** Columbia P&S 1964; **Resid:** Pathology, Presby Hosp, New York, NY 1965-1966; Pathology, VA Hosp, New York, NY 1966-1968; **Fellow:** Pathology, Meml Hosp, New York, NY 1968-1970; **Fac Appt:** Prof Pathology, Cornell Univ-Weill Med Coll

Sanchez, Miguel MD (Path) - *Spec Exp:* Breast Cancer; **Hospital:** Englewood Hosp & Med Ctr; **Address:** Englewood Hosp & Med Ctr, Dept Pathology, 350 Engle St, Englewood, NJ 07631-1898; **Phone:** (201) 894-3423; **Board Cert:** Cytopathology 1991, Clinical Pathology 1979, Anatomic Pathology 1975; **Med School:** Spain 1969; **Resid:** Pathology, Englewood Hosp, Englewood, NJ 1971-1972; Pathology, Temple University, Philadelphia, NY 1972-1973; **Fellow:** Pathology, Meml Sloan Kettering Cancer Ctr, New York, NY 1973-1974; **Fac Appt:** Assoc Prof Pathology, Mount Sinai Sch Med

Schiller, Alan MD (Path) - *Spec Exp:* Bone & Joint Pathology; Soft Tissue Pathology; Autopsy Pathology; **Hospital:** Mount Sinai Hosp (page 68); **Address:** 1 Gustave Levy Pl, Box 1194, Dept Pathology, New York, NY 10029-6500; **Phone:** (212) 241-8014; **Board Cert:** Anatomic Pathology 1973; **Med School:** Univ Hlth Sci/Chicago Med Sch 1967; **Resid:** Pathology, Mass Genl Hosp, Boston, MA 1968-1972; **Fac Appt:** Prof Pathology, Mount Sinai Sch Med

Schlaepfer, William W MD (Path) - *Spec Exp:* Neurofilament Metabolism; Neuro-Pathology; **Hospital:** Hosp Univ Penn (page 78); **Address:** 609 Stellar Chance Lab, 422 Curie Blvd, Philadelphia, PA 19104-6100; **Phone:** (215) 662-7372; **Board Cert:** Anatomic Pathology 1964, Neuropathology 1964; **Med School:** Yale Univ 1958; **Resid:** Pathology, Grace-New Haven Comm Hosp, New Haven, CT 1959-1961

Swerdlow, Steven Howard MD (Path) - *Spec Exp:* Lymphoma; Hematopatholgy; **Hospital:** UPMC - Presbyterian Univ Hosp; **Address:** UPMC-Presby, Div Hematopathology, 200 Lothrop St, rm C606, Box PUH, Pittsburgh, PA 15213; **Phone:** (412) 647-5191; **Board Cert:** Anatomic Pathology 1979; **Med School:** Harvard Med Sch 1975; **Resid:** Pathology, Beth Israel Hosp., Boston, MA 1976-1979; **Fellow:** Hematopathology, Vanderbilt Univ, Nashville, TN 1979-1981; Hematopathology, St Bartholmew's Hosp, London, UK 1981-1983; **Fac Appt:** Prof Pathology, Univ Pittsburgh

Woodruff, James M. MD (Path) - *Spec Exp:* Soft Tissue Tumors; **Hospital:** Mem Sloan Kettering Cancer Ctr; **Address:** 1275 York Ave Fl 6, Box 36, New York, NY 10021; **Phone:** (212) 639-5905; **Board Cert:** Anatomic Pathology 1970; **Med School:** Temple Univ 1963; **Resid:** Anatomic Pathology, Cornell Med Ctr, New York, NY 1964-1966; Clinical Pathology, Colorado Med Ctr, Denver, CO 1968-1970; **Fellow:** Surgical Pathology, NY Meml Cancer Ctr, New York, NY 1970-1971; **Fac Appt:** Prof Pathology, Cornell Univ-Weill Med Coll

Yousem, Samuel A. MD (Path) - *Spec Exp:* Lung Disease; **Hospital:** UPMC - Presbyterian Univ Hosp; **Address:** Dept Pathology, A-610, 200 Lothrop St, Pittsburgh, PA 15213; **Phone:** (412) 647-6193; **Board Cert:** Anatomic Pathology 1985; **Med School:** Univ MD Sch Med 1981; **Resid:** Pathology, Stanford Univ Med Ctr, Palo Alto, CA 1982-1983; **Fellow:** Pathology, Stanford Univ Med Ctr, Palo Alto, CA 1983-1984; **Fac Appt:** Prof Pathology, Univ Pittsburgh

Southeast

Banks, Peter MD (Path) - *Spec Exp:* Hematopathology; Lymphoma; **Hospital:** Carolinas Med Ctr; **Address:** Dept Pathology, 1000 Blythe Blvd, 4th Fl Lab, Charlotte, NC 28203; **Phone:** (704) 355-3467; **Board Cert:** Anatomic Pathology 1997; **Med School:** Harvard Med Sch 1971; **Resid:** Pathology, Natl Cancer Inst, Bethesda, MD 1972-1974; Duke U Med Ctr, Durham, NC 1974-1975; **Fellow:** Anatomic Pathology, U Minn Med Ctr, Minneapolis, MN 1975-1976; **Fac Appt:** Prof Pathology, Univ NC Sch Med

Bostwick, David MD (Path) - *Spec Exp:* Urologic Pathology; Gastrointestinal Pathology; **Address:** 2807 N Parham Rd, Ste 114, Richmond, VA 23294; **Phone:** (804) 288-6564; **Board Cert:** Pathology 1985; **Med School:** Univ MD Sch Med 1979; **Resid:** Pathology, Stanford Univ, Stanford, CA 1979-1981; **Fellow:** Pathology, Stanford Univ, Stanford, CA 1981-1984; **Fac Appt:** Clin Prof Pathology, Univ VA Sch Med

Braylan, Raul MD (Path) - *Spec Exp:* Lymphoma; Leukemia-Pathology; **Hospital:** Shands Hlthcre at Univ of FL (page 73); **Address:** Dept Pathology, Box 100275, Gainesville, FL 32610; **Phone:** (352) 392-3477; **Board Cert:** Pathology 1972; **Med School:** Argentina 1960; **Resid:** Pathology, Meml Hosp Cancer, New York, NY 1967-1968; Pathology, Einstein Affil Hosps, New York, NY 1965-1967; **Fellow:** Pathology, Natl Cancer Ctr, Bethesda, MD 1973-1977; Pathology, Univ Chicago, Chicago, IL 1971-1973; **Fac Appt:** Prof Pathology, Univ Fla Coll Med

Hardt, Nancy S MD (Path) - *Spec Exp:* Breast Pathology; Women's Health; Gynecologic Pathology; **Hospital:** Shands Hlthcre at Univ of FL (page 73); **Address:** Shands Healthcare at Univ Florida, Dept Pathology, Gainesville, FL 32610; **Phone:** (352) 392-3741; **Board Cert:** Anatomic Pathology 1989, Obstetrics & Gynecology 1998; **Med School:** Louisiana State Univ 1970; **Resid:** Obstetrics & Gynecology, Univ Kentucky, KY; Pathology, Shands Hosp, Gainesville, FL; **Fellow:** Gynecologic Pathology, Shands Hosp, Gainesville, FL; **Fac Appt:** Asst Prof Pathology, Univ Fla Coll Med

Kao, Kuo-Jang MD/PhD (Path) - *Spec Exp:* Bleeding/Coagulation Disorders; Transfusion Medicine; Paternity Testing; **Hospital:** Shands Hlthcre at Univ of FL (page 73); **Address:** Dept Pathology, Box 100275, Gainesville, FL 32610-0275; **Phone:** (352) 392-7841; **Board Cert:** Pathology 1983; **Med School:** Taiwan 1974; **Resid:** Pathology, Duke Univ Med Ctr, Durham, NC 1981-1983; **Fac Appt:** Prof Pathology, Univ Fla Coll Med

McCurly, Thomas L MD (Path) - *Spec Exp:* Hematopathology; Lymphoma; **Hospital:** Vanderbilt Univ Med Ctr (page 80); **Address:** Vanderbilt Univ Hosp, Dept Pathology, 21st & Garland Ave, Nashville, TN 37232; **Phone:** (615) 343-9167; **Board Cert:** Anatomic & Clinical Pathology 1981, Immunopathology 1986, Hematology 1999; **Med School:** Vanderbilt Univ 1974; **Resid:** Internal Medicine, UCSF Med Ctr, San Francisco, CA 1975-1976; Pathology, Vanderbilt Univ Med Ctr, Nashville, TN 1977-1981; **Fellow:** Hematopathology, Vanderbilt Univ Med Ctr, Nashville, TN 1981-1984; **Fac Appt:** Assoc Prof Pathology, Vanderbilt Univ

Mills, Stacey E MD (Path) - *Spec Exp:* Breast Pathology; Otolaryngologic Pathology; **Hospital:** Univ of VA Hlth Sys (page 79); **Address:** UVA Health System, Dept Pathology, PO Box 800214, Charlottesville, VA 22908; **Phone:** (804) 982-4406; **Board Cert:** Pathology 1981; **Med School:** Univ VA Sch Med 1977; **Resid:** Pathology, UVA Med Ctr, Charlottesville, VA 1977-1980; **Fac Appt:** Prof Pathology, Univ VA Sch Med

Norenberg, Michael D MD (Path) - *Spec Exp:* Liver Metabolic Disorders; Parkinson's Disease; **Hospital:** Univ of Miami - Jackson Meml Hosp; **Address:** Jackson Meml Hosp, Dept Pathology, 1611 NW 12th Ave, Miami, FL 33136; **Phone:** (305) 585-7049; **Board Cert:** Pathology 1972, Neuropathology 1974; **Med School:** Univ Rochester 1965; **Resid:** Pathology, Strong Meml Hosp, Rochester, MN 1966-1970; **Fellow:** Neuropathology, Strong Meml Hosp, Rochester, MN 1970-1972; **Fac Appt:** Prof Pathology, Univ Miami Sch Med

Page, David L MD (Path) - *Spec Exp:* Breast Cancer; Skin Cancer; **Hospital:** Vanderbilt Univ Med Ctr (page 80); **Address:** Vanderbilt Univ, MCN, 1161 21st Ave S, rm C 3909, Nashville, TN 37232-2561; **Phone:** (615) 322-3759; **Board Cert:** Anatomic Pathology 1972, Dermatopathology 1974; **Med School:** Johns Hopkins Univ 1966; **Resid:** Pathology, Mass Genl Hosp, Boston, MA 1967-1969; Pathology, Johns Hopkins Hosp, Baltimore, MD 1971-1972; **Fac Appt:** Prof Pathology, Vanderbilt Univ

Petito, Carol MD (Path) - *Spec Exp:* Neuro-Pathology; **Hospital:** Univ of Miami - Jackson Meml Hosp; **Address:** 1550 NW 10th Ave, Bldg Pap - Fl 4 - rm 417, Miami, FL 33136; **Phone:** (305) 243-3584; **Board Cert:** Anatomic Pathology 1973, Neuropathology 1973; **Med School:** Columbia P&S 1967; **Resid:** Pathology, NY Hosp-Cornell Med Ctr, New York, NY 1968-1970; Neuropathology, Armed Forces Inst, Washington, DC 1971; **Fac Appt:** Prof Pathology, Cornell Univ-Weill Med Coll

Sewell, Charles W MD (Path) - *Spec Exp:* Breast Pathology; Surgical Pathology; **Hospital:** Emory Univ Hosp; **Address:** Emory Univ Hosp, Dept Pathology, 1364 Clifton Rd NE, rm H187, Atlanta, GA 30322; **Phone:** (404) 712-7003; **Board Cert:** Anatomic Pathology 1974, Clinical Pathology 1974; **Resid:** Pathology, Emory Univ Hosp, Atlanta, GA 1970-1974; **Fac Appt:** Prof Emeritus Pain Management

Weiss, Sharon MD (Path) - *Spec Exp:* Soft Tissue Pathology; Surgical Pathology; Sarcomas; **Hospital:** Emory Univ Hosp; **Address:** Emory Univ Hosp, Dept Path, 1364 Clifton Rd NE, Fl H180, Atlanta, GA 30322-1061; **Phone:** (404) 712-0708; **Board Cert:** Anatomic Pathology 1974; **Med School:** Johns Hopkins Univ 1971; **Resid:** Pathology, Johns Hopkins Hosp, Baltimore, MD 1972-1975; **Fac Appt:** Prof Pathology, Emory Univ

Midwest

Appelman, Henry MD (Path) - *Spec Exp:* Gastrointestinal Pathology; **Hospital:** Univ of MI Hlth Ctr; **Address:** Dept of Pathology, 1500 E Medical Center Drive, Ann Arbor, MI 48109-0054; **Phone:** (734) 936-6770; **Board Cert:** Anatomic Pathology 1966, Clinical Pathology 1966; **Med School:** Univ Mich Med Sch 1961; **Resid:** Pathology, Univ of Michigan Hlth Care Ctr, Ann Arbor, MI 1962-1966; **Fac Appt:** Prof Pathology, Univ Mich Med Sch

Hart, William MD (Path) - *Spec Exp:* Gynecologic Pathology; **Hospital:** Cleveland Clin Fdn (page 57); **Address:** 9500 Euclid Ave, MS L21, Cleveland, OH 44195; **Phone:** (216) 444-2840; **Board Cert:** Anatomic Pathology 1970; **Med School:** Univ Mich Med Sch 1965; **Resid:** Anatomic Pathology, Univ Mich Med Ctr, Ann Arbor, MI 1966-1970; **Fac Appt:** Prof Pathology, Ohio State Univ

Scheithauer, Bernd MD (Path) - *Spec Exp:* Brain Tumors; Pituitary Disorders; Neuro-Pathology; **Hospital:** Mayo Med Ctr & Clin - Rochester, MN; **Address:** 200 1st St SW, Rochester, MN 55905-0001; **Phone:** (507) 284-8350; **Board Cert:** Anatomic Pathology 1979, Neuropathology 1979; **Med School:** Loma Linda Univ 1973; **Resid:** Anatomic Pathology, Stanford Med Ctr, CA 1974-1976; Neuropathology, Stanford Med Ctr, CA 1976-1978; **Fac Appt:** Prof Pathology, Mayo Med Sch

Unni, K Krishnan MD (Path) - *Spec Exp:* Bone Tumor Pathology; Surgical Pathology; **Hospital:** Mayo Med Ctr & Clin - Rochester, MN; **Address:** Mayo Clinic, Dept Pathology, 200 1st St SW, Rochester, MN 55905; **Phone:** (507) 284-1193; **Board Cert:** Anatomic Pathology 1969; **Med School:** India 1962; **Resid:** Pathology, Mayo Grad Sch, Rochester, MN 1967-1970; **Fellow:** Pathology, Mayo Clinic, Rochester, MN 1973-1974; **Fac Appt:** Prof Pathology, Mayo Med Sch

Great Plains and Mountains

Weisenburger, Dennis MD (Path) - *Spec Exp:* Hematopathology; Lymphoma; **Hospital:** Nebraska Hlth Sys; **Address:** Univ Nebr Med Ctr, Dept Path, 983135 Nebraska Medical Center, Omaha, NE 68198-3135; **Phone:** (402) 559-7688; **Board Cert:** Pathology 1979; **Med School:** Univ Minn 1974; **Resid:** Anatomic Pathology, Iowa Hosp, Iowa City, IA 1975-1978; **Fellow:** Hematology, City of Hope Natl Med Ctr, Duarte, CA 1979-1980; **Fac Appt:** Prof Pathology, Univ Nebr Coll Med

Southwest

Colby, Thomas V MD (Path) - *Spec Exp:* Pulmonary Pathology; Surgical Pathology; **Hospital:** Mayo Clin Hosp - Scottsdale; **Address:** Mayo Med Ctr & Clinic, 13400 E Shea Blvd, Scottsdale, AZ 85259; **Phone:** (480) 301-6550; **Board Cert:** Anatomic Pathology 1978; **Med School:** Univ Mich Med Sch 1974; **Resid:** Anatomic Pathology, Stanford Univ Hosp, Stanford, CA; **Fellow:** Surgical Pathology, Stanford Univ Hosp, Stanford, CA; **Fac Appt:** Prof Pathology, Mayo Med Sch

Grogan, Thomas MD (Path) - *Spec Exp:* *Immunopathology; Lymphoma;* **Hospital:** Univ Med Ctr; **Address:** Arizona Hlth Sci Ctr, Dept Pathology, 1501 N Campbell Ave, rm 5212, Tucson, AZ 85724; **Phone:** (520) 626-2212; **Board Cert:** Anatomic Pathology 1976; **Med School:** Geo Wash Univ 1971; **Resid:** Pathology, Letterman Army Med Ctr, San Francisco, CA 1972-1976; **Fellow:** Immunopathology, Stanford Univ Sch Med, Stanford, CA 1978-1979; **Fac Appt:** Prof Pathology, Univ Ariz Coll Med

Kinney, Marsha C MD (Path) - *Spec Exp:* *Hematopathology; Lymphoma;* **Hospital:** Univ of Texas Hlth & Sci Ctr; **Address:** Univ Texas Hlth & Sci Ctr, Dept Pathology, 7703 Floyd Curl Drive, San Antonio, TX 78229; **Phone:** (210) 567-4098; **Board Cert:** Anatomic & Clinical Pathology 1985, Hematology 1998; **Med School:** Univ Tex SW, Dallas 1981; **Resid:** Pathology, Vanderbilt Univ Med Ctr, Nashville, TN 1981-1985; **Fellow:** Hematopathology, Vanderbilt Univ Med Ctr, Nashville, TN 1985-1988

Logrono, Roberto MD (Path) - *Spec Exp:* *Pancreatic Masses; Lymph Node Pathology; Gastrointestinal Submucosal Masses;* **Hospital:** Univ of TX Med Brch Hosps at Galveston; **Address:** Univ Texas Medical Br, Dept Pathology, 9300 John Sealy Annex, 301 University Blvd, Galveston, TX 77555-0548; **Phone:** (409) 772-5896; **Board Cert:** Anatomic Pathology 1991, Cytopathology 1995; **Med School:** Dominican Republic 1982; **Resid:** Anatomic Pathology, St Barnabas Med Ctr, Livingston, NJ 1986-1991; **Fellow:** Cytopathology, Univ Wisconsin MedCtr, Madison, WI 1994-1995; **Fac Appt:** Assoc Prof Pathology, Univ Tex Med Br, Galveston

Reed, Richard J MD (Path) - *Spec Exp:* *Dermatopathology;* **Address:** 234 Loyola Ave, Ste 302, New Orleans, LA 70115; **Phone:** (504) 581-2888; **Board Cert:** Anatomic Pathology 1961, Dermatopathology 1974; **Med School:** Tulane Univ 1952; **Resid:** Anatomic Pathology, Tulane Univ Sch Med, New Orleans, LA 1957-1960; **Fellow:** Surgical Pathology, Barnes Hosp, St Louis, MO 1960-1961; **Fac Appt:** Prof Emeritus Pathology, Tulane Univ

Roberts, William C MD (Path) - *Spec Exp:* *Preventive Cardiology; Cardiac Pathology;* **Hospital:** Baylor Univ Medical Ctr; **Address:** Baylor Heart & Vascular Institute, 3500 Gaston Ave, Dallas, TX 75246-2096; **Phone:** (214) 820-7500; **Board Cert:** Anatomic Pathology 1965; **Med School:** Emory Univ 1958; **Resid:** Anatomic Pathology, Natl Heart Inst-NIH, Bethesda, MD 1959-1962; Internal Medicine, Johns Hopkins Hosp, Baltimore, MD 1962-1963; **Fellow:** Cardiology (Cardiovascular Disease), Natl Heart Inst-NIH, Bethesda, MD 1963-1964

Thor, Ann D MD (Path) - *Spec Exp:* *Breast Cancer; Gynecologic Cancer;* **Hospital:** Univ OK Hlth Sci Ctr; **Address:** Univ Oklahoma Hlth Sci Ctr, BMSB 451, 940 Stanton L Young Blvd, Oklahoma City, OK 73104; **Phone:** (405) 271-2422; **Board Cert:** Anatomic Pathology 1987, Cytopathology 1989; **Med School:** Vanderbilt Univ 1981; **Resid:** Pathology, Vanderbilt Univ, Nashville, TN 1981-1983; **Fellow:** Immunopathology, Natl Cancer Inst, Bethesda, MD 1983-1986; Gynecologic Pathology, Mass Genl Hosp, Boston, MA 1987-1990; **Fac Appt:** Prof Pathology, Univ Okla Coll Med

Walker, David H MD (Path) - *Spec Exp:* *Infectious Disease; Tropical Diseases; Ehrlichiosis;* **Hospital:** Univ of TX Med Brch Hosps at Galveston; **Address:** UT Med Br Galveston, Dept Path, 301 University Blvd, MC-0609, Galveston, TX 77555-0609; **Phone:** (409) 772-9998; **Board Cert:** Anatomic & Clinical Pathology 1974; **Med School:** Vanderbilt Univ 1969; **Resid:** Anatomic Pathology, Peter Bent Brigham Hosp, Boston, MA 1970-1973; **Fellow:** Pathology, Harvard/Boston Hosps, Boston, MA 1971-1973; **Fac Appt:** Prof Pathology, Univ Tex Med Br, Galveston

Wheeler, Thomas M MD (Path) - *Spec Exp:* Thyroid Disorders; **Hospital:** Methodist Hosp - Houston; **Address:** Methodist Hosp, 6565 Fannin St, rm M227A, MS 205, Houston, TX 77030; **Phone:** (713) 394-6475; **Board Cert:** Anatomic & Clinical Pathology 1999, Cytopathology 1990; **Med School:** Baylor Coll Med 1977; **Resid:** Pathology, Baylor Coll Med, Houston, TX 1977-1981; **Fac Appt:** Prof Pathology, Baylor Coll Med

West Coast and Pacific

Bollen, Andrew W MD (Path) - *Spec Exp:* Neuropathology; Brain Tumors; Brain Infections; **Hospital:** UCSF Med Ctr; **Address:** Dept of Neuropathology, 513 Parnassus Ave, rm HSW430, San Francisco, CA 94143-0511; **Phone:** (415) 476-5236; **Board Cert:** Clinical Pathology 1993, Anatomic Pathology 1992, Neuropathology 1992; **Med School:** UCSD 1985; **Resid:** Anatomic Pathology, Univ California San Fran Med Ctr, San Francisco, CA 1985-1991; **Fellow:** Neuropathology, Univ California San Fran Med Ctr, San Francisco, CA 1988-1989; **Fac Appt:** Prof Pathology, UCSF

Chandrasoma, Parakrama T MD (Path) - *Spec Exp:* Gastrointestinal Pathology; Neuro-Pathology; **Hospital:** LAC & USC Med Ctr; **Address:** 1200 N State St, rm 16-905, Los Angeles, CA 90033; **Phone:** (323) 226-4600; **Board Cert:** Anatomic Pathology 1982; **Med School:** Sri Lanka 1971; **Resid:** Anatomic Pathology, Univ Sri Lanka, Colombo, Sri Lanka 1973-1978; Anatomic Pathology, Los Angeles County-USC Med Ctr, Los Angeles, CA 1978-1982; **Fac Appt:** Prof Pathology, USC Sch Med

Cochran, Alistair J MD (Path) - *Spec Exp:* Melanoma-Sentinel Node; Dermatopathology; **Hospital:** UCLA Med Ctr; **Address:** UCLA Med Ctr, Dept Path & Med, 10833 Le Conte Ave, rm 13-145CHS, Box 951732, Los Angeles, CA 90095-1713; **Phone:** (310) 825-8182; **Med School:** Scotland 1966; **Resid:** Dermatopathology, Western Infirmary, Glasgow, UK 1962-1968; **Fellow:** Immunology, Karolinska Inst, Stockholm,Sweden 1968-1970; **Fac Appt:** Prof Pathology, UCLA

Cote, Richard MD (Path) - *Spec Exp:* Sentinel Node Pathology; Bladder Cancer; **Hospital:** USC Norris Cancer Comp Ctr; **Address:** 1441 Eastlake Ave, rm 2424, Los Angeles, CA 90033; **Phone:** (323) 865-3270; **Board Cert:** Anatomic Pathology 1987; **Med School:** Univ Chicago-Pritzker Sch Med 1980; **Resid:** Pathology, NY Hosp-Cornell Med Ctr, New York, NY 1985-1987; **Fellow:** Pathology, Meml Sloan-Kettering Cancer Ctr, New York, NY 1987-1989; **Fac Appt:** Prof Pathology, USC Sch Med

Dubeau, Louis MD (Path) - *Spec Exp:* Ovarian Cancer; Breast Cancer; **Hospital:** USC Norris Cancer Comp Ctr; **Address:** USC Norris Cancer Ctr, Dept Pathology, 1441 Eastlake Ave, Los Angeles, CA 90033-1048; **Phone:** (323) 865-0720; **Board Cert:** Anatomic Pathology 1984; **Med School:** McGill Univ 1979; **Resid:** Anatomic Pathology, McGill Univ Med Ctr, Montreal, Canada 1980-1984; **Fac Appt:** Assoc Prof Pathology, USC Sch Med

Ferrell, Linda MD (Path) - *Spec Exp:* Liver Disease; **Hospital:** UCSF Med Ctr; **Address:** UCSF Med Ctr, Dept Pathology, 505 Parnassus Ave, rm M590, San Francisco, CA 94143-0102; **Phone:** (415) 353-1090; **Board Cert:** Anatomic Pathology 1982; **Med School:** Univ Kans 1977; **Resid:** Anatomic Pathology, UCSF, San Francisco, CA 1980-1981; Anatomic Pathology, Univ Kansas Med Ctr, Kansas City, KS 1978-1979; **Fac Appt:** Prof Anatomic Pathology, UCSF

Govindarajan, Sugantha MD (Path) - *Spec Exp:* Liver Pathology; **Hospital:** Rancho Los Amigos Natl Rehab Ctr; **Address:** Rancho Los Amigos Natl Rehab Ctr, Dept Pathology, 7601 E Imperial Hwy, Bldg JPI - rm B170, Downey, CA 90242; **Phone:** (562) 401-8994; **Board Cert:** Anatomic Pathology 1976; **Med School:** India 1969; **Resid:** Pathology, St Lukes Hosp, Cleveland, OH 1972-1976; **Fellow:** Pathology, Cleveland Clinic, Cleveland, OH 1976-1977; **Fac Appt:** Prof Pathology, USC Sch Med

Hendrickson, Michael MD (Path) - *Spec Exp: Gynecologic Pathology;* **Hospital:** Stanford Med Ctr; **Address:** Dept Path, 300 Pasteur Drive, Stanford, CA 94305-5324; **Phone:** (650) 498-6460; **Board Cert:** Anatomic Pathology 1975; **Med School:** Stanford Univ 1971; **Resid:** Anatomic Pathology, Stanford Univ Med Sch, Stanford, CA 1972-1974; **Fac Appt:** Prof Pathology, Stanford Univ

Kanel, Gary Craig MD (Path) - *Spec Exp: Liver Disease;* **Hospital:** Rancho Los Amigos Natl Rehab Ctr; **Address:** 7601 E Imperial Hwy, Bldg JPI - Ste B170, Downey, CA 90242; **Phone:** (562) 401-8994; **Board Cert:** Pathology 1979; **Med School:** Tufts Univ 1974; **Resid:** Pathology, Tufts-New England Med Ctr, Boston, MA 1975-1976; Pathology, Univ Chicago Hosp, Chicago, IL 1976-1977; **Fellow:** Pathology, Tufts-New England Med Ctr, Boston, MA 1977-1979; **Fac Appt:** Prof Pathology, USC Sch Med

Kempson, Richard MD (Path) - *Spec Exp: Breast Pathology; Gynecologic Pathology;* **Hospital:** Stanford Med Ctr; **Address:** 300 Pasteur Drive, Ste H2110, Stanford, CA 94305-5243; **Phone:** (650) 723-7211; **Board Cert:** Anatomic Pathology 1963; **Med School:** Tulane Univ 1955; **Resid:** Surgical Pathology, Barnes Hosp, St Louis, MO 1962-1963; **Fellow:** Anatomic Pathology, Tulane Univ Med Ctr, New Orleans, LA 1959-1962; **Fac Appt:** Prof Pathology, Stanford Univ

Lewin, Klaus J MD (Path) - *Spec Exp: Liver Disease; Gastrointestinal Pathology; Pancreatic Pathology;* **Hospital:** UCLA Med Ctr; **Address:** UCLA Hlth Scis Ctr, Dept Path, 10833 Le Conte Ave, Los Angeles, CA 90095-1732; **Phone:** (310) 825-9377; **Board Cert:** Anatomic Pathology 1973; **Med School:** England 1959; **Resid:** Pathology, Westminister Med Sch, London, England 1962-1968; **Fac Appt:** Prof Pathology, UCLA

Nathwani, Bharat N MD (Path) - *Spec Exp: Lymphoma;* **Hospital:** LAC & USC Med Ctr; **Address:** LAC+USC Med Ctr, Dept Pathology, 1200 N State St, rm 2422, Los Angeles, CA 90033-4526; **Phone:** (323) 226-7064; **Board Cert:** Pathology 1977; **Med School:** India 1969; **Resid:** Pathology, JJ Group-Grant Med Ctr, Columbus, OH 1969-1972; Pathology, Rush-Presbyterian-St Luke's Med Ctr, Chicago, IL 1974; **Fellow:** Hematopathology, City Hope Natl Med Ctr, Duarte, CA 1975; **Fac Appt:** Prof Pathology, USC Sch Med

Turner, Roderick Randolph MD (Path) - *Spec Exp: Sentinel Node Pathology; Breast Cancer; Melanoma;* **Hospital:** St John's Hlth Ctr; **Address:** St John's Health Center, Dept Pathology, 1328 22nd St, Santa Monica, CA 90404-2032; **Phone:** (310) 829-8101; **Board Cert:** Hematology 1991, Anatomic Pathology 1985; **Med School:** UCLA 1979; **Resid:** Anatomic Pathology, UCLA, Los Angeles, CA 1983-1985; Anatomic Pathology, Stanford Univ, Stanford, CA 1979-1982; **Fellow:** Pathology, Stanford Univ, Stanford, CA 1982-1983; **Fac Appt:** Asst Clin Prof Pathology, USC Sch Med

Warnke, Roger Allen MD (Path) - *Spec Exp: Lymphoma; Hemopathology;* **Hospital:** Stanford Med Ctr; **Address:** Stanford Univ, Dept Pathology, 300 Pasteur, Ste L235, Stanford, CA 94304; **Phone:** (650) 725-5167; **Board Cert:** Anatomic Pathology 1975; **Med School:** Washington Univ, St Louis 1971; **Resid:** Pathology, Stanford Med Ctr, Stanford, CA 1972-1973; **Fellow:** Surgical Pathology, Stanford Med Ctr, Stanford, CA 1973-1975; **Fac Appt:** Prof Pathology, Stanford Univ

Weiss, Lawrence M MD (Path) - *Spec Exp: Lymphoma; Surgical Pathology; Adrenal Pathology;* **Hospital:** City of Hope Natl Med Ctr & Beckman Rsch; **Address:** City of Hope Natl Med Ctr, Div Pathology, 1500 E Duarte Rd, Duarte, CA 91010-0269; **Phone:** (626) 359-8111; **Board Cert:** Anatomic Pathology 1985; **Med School:** Univ MD Sch Med 1981; **Resid:** Pathology, Brigham & Women's Hosp, Boston, MA 1981-1983; **Fellow:** Pathology, Stanford Univ Hosp, Stanford, CA 1983-1984

PEDIATRICS

A pediatrician is concerned with the physical, emotional and social health of children from birth to young adulthood. Care encompasses a broad spectrum of health services ranging from preventive healthcare to the diagnosis and treatment of acute and chronic diseases.

A pediatrician deals with biological, social and environmental influences on the developing child, and with the impact of disease and dysfunction on development.

Training required: Three years

Pediatric Allergy and Immunology: An allergist-immunologist is trained in evaluation, physical and laboratory diagnosis and management of disorders involving the immune system. Selected examples of such conditions include asthma, anaphylaxis, rhinitis, eczema and adverse reactions to drugs, foods and insect stings as well as immune deficiency diseases (both acquired and congenital), defects in host defense and problems related to autoimmune disease, organ transplantation or malignancies of the immune system. As our understanding of the immune system develops, the scope of this specialty is widening.

Training programs are available at some medical centers to provide individuals with expertise in both allergy/immunology and pediatric pulmonology. Such individuals are candidates for dual certification.

Training required: Prior certification in pediatrics *plus* two years in allergy/immunology

Certification in one of the following subspecialties requires additional training and examination.

Pediatric Cardiology: A pediatric cardiologist provides comprehensive care to patients with cardiovascular problems. This specialist is skilled in selecting, performing and evaluating the structural and functional assessment of the heart and blood vessels and the clinical evaluation of cardiovascular disease.

Pediatric Endocrinology: A pediatrician who provides expert care to infants, children and adolescents who have diseases that result from an abnormality in the endocrine glands (glands which secrete hormones). These diseases include diabetes mellitus, growth failure, unusual size for age, early or late pubertal development, birth defects, the genital region and disorders of the thyroid, the adrenal and pituitary glands.

Pediatric Gastroenterology: A pediatrician who specializes in the diagnosis and treatment of diseases of the digestive systems of infants, children and adolescents. This specialist treats conditions such as abdominal pain, ulcers, diarrhea, cancer and jaundice and performs complex diagnostic and therapeutic procedures using lighted scopes to see internal organs.

Pediatric Hematology-Oncology: A pediatrician trained in the combination of pediatrics, hematology and oncology to recognize and manage pediatric blood disorders and cancerous diseases.

Pediatric Infectious Diseases: A pediatrician trained to care for children in the diagnosis, treatment and prevention of infectious diseases. This specialist can apply specific knowledge to affect a better outcome for pediatric infections with complicated courses, underlying diseases that predispose to unusual or severe

586

infections, unclear diagnoses, uncommon diseases and complex or investigational treatments.

Pediatric Nephrology: A pediatrician who deals with the normal and abnormal development and maturation of the kidney and urinary tract, the mechanisms by which the kidney can be damaged, the evaluation and treatment of renal diseases, fluid and electrolyte abnormalities, hypertension and renal replacement therapy.

Pediatric Otolaryngology: A pediatric otolaryngologist has special expertise in the management of infants and children with disorders that include congenital and acquired conditions involving the aerodigestive tract, nose and paranasal sinuses, the ear and other areas of the head and neck. The pediatric otolaryngologist has special skills in the diagnosis, treatment and management of childhood disorders of voice, speech, language and hearing.

Pediatric Pulmonology: A pediatrician dedicated to the prevention and treatment of all respiratory diseases affecting infants, children and young adults. This specialist is knowledgeable about the growth and development of the lung, assessment of respiratory function in infants and children and experienced in a variety of invasive and noninvasive diagnostic techniques.

Pediatric Rheumatology: A pediatrician who treats diseases of joints, muscle, bones and tendons. A pediatric rheumatologist diagnoses and treats arthritis, back pain, muscle strains, common athletic injuries and ìcollagenî diseases.

Pediatric Surgery: A surgeon with expertise in the management of surgical conditions in premature and newborn infants, children and adolescents.

RILEY HOSPITAL FOR CHILDREN

A Part of Clarian Health Partners

702 Barnhill Road
Indianapolis, Indiana 46202
317-962-2000

www.rileyhospital.org   www.clarian.org

COMPREHENSIVE CARE FOR CHILDREN

Riley Hospital for Children is Indiana's first and only comprehensive hospital dedicated exclusively to the care of children. Opened in 1924, it is today among the largest children's hospitals in the nation and the leader for pediatric care in the state and the region. Each year Riley serves over 150,000 inpatients and outpatients from across Indiana, the nation and the world.

OUTSTANDING STAFF AND FACILITIES

With 262 beds, Riley is one of the nation's most extensive children's hospitals. Riley-based IU School of Medicine physicians and surgeons, along with Riley nurses and staff, provide in-patient care for more than 7,500 patients a year. Facilities include the $55 million Riley Outpatient Center, a 255,000 square-foot, multi-level facility that combines virtually all outpatient services under one roof. Riley is 17th nationally in NIH funding for pediatric centers and is rated by Arbor Associates as the best performer in overall satisfaction among outpatients. The extracorporeal membrane oxygenation (ECMO) survival rate at Riley exceeds national benchmarks, and the hospital has the Midwest's best five-year survival rate across five forms of childhood cancer.

EXTENSIVE SERVICES AND SPECIALTIES

Riley Hospital's partnership with Clarian Health and its strong affiliation with the Indiana University School of Medicine give it the resources to provide a wide range of care. Riley provides one of the most comprehensive neonatal systems and the largest pediatric sleep disorder center in the nation. Riley also serves as a major educational facility for professionals serving children's health needs and as a specialty referral center with many unduplicated life-saving services for newborns, infants, children and adolescents. Riley doctors are leaders in the treatment of children with heart disorders, and Riley is the only center for pediatric heart transplantation in the state.

INNOVATIONS IN PEDIATRIC CARE

Together with the IU School of Medicine, Riley is considered among the top research centers in the country. Riley Hospital has pioneered several crucial medical techniques, including transplants, extracorporeal membrane oxygenation (ECMO) and gene therapy.

Riley contains the largest and most advanced group of medical specialties of any children's hospital in the nation. Each year, Riley doctors perform more than 10,000 in- and outpatient surgeries, including pediatric heart and liver transplants.

Additionally, Riley Hospital offers Indiana's only pediatric centers for burns, kidney dialysis, cystic fibrosis, spina bifida, craniofacial abnormalities, sleep abnormalities and many others. Riley also operates Indiana's first children's emergency department and the state's only Level I Regional Pediatric Trauma Center as designated by the American College of Surgeons.

CHILDREN'S HOSPITAL OF MICHIGAN

3901 Beaubien • Detroit, Michigan 48201
1-888-DMC-2500 • www.chmkids.org

Rated Best In the Midwest!

STATE'S ONLY FREESTANDING HOSPITAL DEDICATED TO CHILDREN

Children's Hospital of Michigan is the only hospital in the state exclusively dedicated to caring for children. Specialists in pediatric medicine and surgery offer a wide range of distinctive specialties including cardiology, ear, nose and throat, metabolic disorders, oncology, allergies, neurology, orthopedics and surgery. The hospital has the most kid-friendly emergency room in the state, treating over 60,000 kids a year and has Michigan's only pediatric trauma center.

BEST IN THE MIDWEST

The hospital was named as one of the best children's hospitals in the country by *Child* magazine. The publication called attention to the hospital's neurosurgery, bleeding disorders programs and cancer-survival rates.

SPECIALISTS IN TREATING CHILDREN

The hospital is staffed by more than 200 pediatricians, 600 pediatric nurses, 125 pediatric specialists and over 1,000 specially trained employees. Children's Hospital of Michigan is an international leader in pediatric neurosurgery, and a national leader in pediatric heart, kidney and bone marrow transplantation. It is the state leader in the treatment and education of children with asthma.

A LEADER IN RESEARCH

The Children's Research Center of Michigan is focused on treatments and cures for devastating pediatric diseases like HIV, sickle cell anemia, cerebral palsy and cancer. Staffed by internationally recognized researchers and scientists, the center is equipped with state-of-the-art laboratories and draws upon the research-rich environment of Wayne State University School of Medicine.

SPECIAL PROGRAMS AND SERVICES

- Home of Michigan's only burn center dedicated exclusively to children.

- Michigan's only Level I trauma center for children.

- One of only two Regional Poison Control Centers in Michigan.

- Home of the world's only Positron Emission Tomography Center dedicated to children.

- Training ground for more Michigan pediatricians than any other hospital in the state.

- First hospital in the nation to implement computer assisted robot-enhanced surgical system for pediatric patients.

Children's Hospital of Michigan
Detroit Medical Center / Wayne State University

INFANTS AND CHILDREN'S HOSPITAL
MAIMONIDES MEDICAL CENTER

4802 Tenth Avenue • Brooklyn, NY 11219
Phone (718) 283-7500   Fax (718) 283-7005
www.maimonidesmed.org

Led by Steven Shelov, MD—author of several best-selling books on child-rearing—Maimonides Medical Center's Infants and Children's Hospital of Brooklyn provides the best primary and specialty care a child could ever need. Serving one of the largest pediatric populations in New York City, Maimonides has made a commitment to caring for babies, children, adolescents and their families.

Caring for many young patients is simply a matter of preventing illness, facilitating healthy growth or addressing common childhood diseases. For others, however, the problems are more complicated. It is for the benefit of these children that Maimonides provides a full complement of specialists trained to deal with nearly every manner of childhood disorder, no matter how rare or complex.

Dr. Shelov has helped recruit many oustanding physicians in the following pediatric specialties:

- Adolescent Medicine
- Allergy
- Anesthesiology
- Behavioral and
  Developmental Pediatrics
- Cardiology
- Critical Care Medicine
- Dentistry and Dental Surgery
- Emergency Medicine
- Endocrinology
- Gastroenterology
- Genetics
- Hematology/Oncology
- Immunology
- Infectious Disease
- Neonatology
- Nephrology
- Neurology
- Ophthalmology
- Orthopaedic Surgery
- Otolaryngology
- Plastic Surgery
- Psychiatry/Psychology
- Pulmonology
- Radiology
- Rheumatology
- Surgery
- Urology

INFANTS AND CHILDREN'S HOSPITAL

The physicians at Infants and Children's Hospital work in some of the most advanced medical environments in the New York region. In recent years, Maimonides Medical Center has renovated and expanded its pediatric emergency room, opened the Norma Sutton Center for Neonatology, and dedicated a new pediatric critical care unit. Pediatric services also are available at outpatient sites throughout Brooklyn.

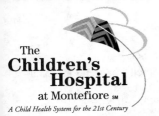

The
Children's
Hospital
at Montefiore ℠
A Child Health System for the 21st Century

3415 BAINBRIDGE AVENUE
BRONX, NY 10467
1-800-MD-MONTE
WWW.MONTEFIORE.ORG

WE'VE CREATED A NEW KIND OF CHILDREN'S HOSPITAL

At **The Children's Hospital at Montefiore**, we've created a pediatric facility unlike any other in the United States or the world. Staffed by our nationally-renowned pediatricians and designed around a philosophy of family-centered care, our 106-bed hospital provides the highest quality care.

Our mission is to provide the children of the Bronx, Southern Westchester County and surrounding communities with the finest, most accessible healthcare services and in doing so, provide a healthcare system that will be a national model for 21st century child health services, teaching, research and policy.

We take into account every aspect of the child's physical, emotional and family life – and we will continue to apply all our human and technological resources to provide the very highest quality care. We encourage families to get involved in their child's care – to partner with our doctors here and at the renowned Albert Einstein College of Medicine to develop the perfect care plan for their child.

The Carl Sagan Discovery Program, the nation's first science education program incorporated in a pediatric hospital, focuses on learning, discovery and inspiration of interactivity. It is our aim to create a new role for children's hospitals, one where we not only save lives, but hopefully transform children forever by leading them on a path of lifelong health and learning. In doing so, we have the medical and educational resources necessary for children to discover both themselves and the world around them.

Physician Referral: Please call 1-800-MD-MONTE

DEDICATED TO CHILDREN AND THEIR FAMILIES

◆ **Pediatric Emergency Department** – a state-of-the-art emergency facility exclusively for treating children.

◆ **Pediatric Critical Care Unit**

◆ **Private Patient Rooms**

◆ **The Day Hospital** – a family-friendly environment for children having tests taking longer than a doctor's visit can accommodate, yet don't require admission.

◆ **Horizon Program for Communication Disorders** – for children with speech, hearing and language disorders.

◆ **Computer Technology Stations** in each room as well as throughout the hospital.

◆ **The Novartis Center for International Child Health** – treating critically ill children from around the world who do not have the specific medical expertise in their countries.

◆ **The Suzanne Pincus Family Learning Place** – a resource for children and families seeking information about their health and treatment.

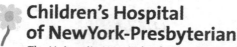

Children's Hospital of NewYork-Presbyterian
The University Hospitals of Columbia and Cornell

Morgan Stanley Children's Hospital
of NewYork-Presbyterian
Columbia Presbyterian Medical Center
3959 Broadway
New York, NY 10032

NewYork Weill Cornell Children's Hospital
of NewYork-Presbyterian
NewYork Weill Cornell Medical Center
525 East 68th Street
New York, NY 10021

Sponsorship: Voluntary Not-for-Profit
Beds: 387
Accreditation: Joint Commission on Accreditation of Healthcare Organizations (JCAHO)

OVERVIEW:

The Children's Hospital of NewYork-Presbyterian brings together the outstanding pediatric services and resources of the Morgan Stanley Children's Hospital and the NewYork Weill Cornell Children's Hospital to create one of the largest, most comprehensive children's hospital in the world.

With more than 1,000 pediatricians and medical and surgical subspecialists on staff, and teams of specially trained pediatric health professionals, the Children's Hospital of NewYork-Presbyterian provides the highest level of care from infancy to adolescence. The Hospital's expertise in addressing simple and complex medical conditions and the psychological and emotional issues that accompany them is unparalleled. The Hospital offers:

- Adolescent Medicine
- Allergy
- Anesthesiology and Pain Management
- Cardiology
- Child Development and Behavioral Medicine
- Critical Care
- Dermatology
- Diabetes and Endocrinology
- Gastroenterology
- Genetics
- Hematology
- Infectious Disease
- Neonatal-Perinatal Medicine
- Nephrology
- Neurology
- Neurosurgery
- Oncology
- Primary Care
- Psychiatry and Mental Health
- Rheumatology
- Laboratory and Radiology Diagnostic Services
- Pediatric Emergency Care in emergency medicine, burn and trauma
- Surgical Services in cardiac, dental, oral and maxillo-facial, general neurosurgery, ophthalmology, orthopedics, otolaryngology, plastic surgery, transplantation and urology

CHILDREN'S HOSPITAL HIGHLIGHTS INCLUDE:

- One of the country's largest and most successful pediatric cardiology and cardiac surgery programs.

- Only provider in the region to offer three major transplant surgeries – heart, liver and kidney.

- One of three Level 1-designated Pediatric Trauma Centers in New York State and only one in New York City.

- Nationally recognized pediatric oncologists. Bone marrow transplantation program is one of the largest in the nation.

- Sophisticated neonatal intensive care that sets standards nationwide.

- Referral center and regional resource for hospitals needing expertise of our pediatric intensive care units. Seriously ill children can be transferred to Children's Hospital of NewYork-Presbyterian through the Pediatric Critical Care Transport Program.

Physician Referral: For a physician referral or to learn more about the Children's Hospital of NewYork-Presbyterian, call **1-800-245-KIDS** (1-800-245-5437) or visit our Web site at **www.nypchildren.org**.

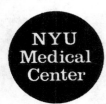

550 First Avenue (at 31st Street)
New York, NY 10016
Physician Referral: (866) CHILD-NYU
(866-244-5369) www.nyuchildrens.org

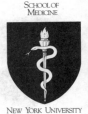

NYU CHILDREN'S HEALTH

NYU Medical Center's Children's Health Team is comprised of some of the best clinical specialists in the country. Among the programs they offer are:

Apnea/SIDS Program –identifying and treating of infants with apnea and infants who are are at increased risk for SIDS

Center for Child and Adolescent Sports Medicine – developmentally sensitive and comprehensive evaluation and treatment of sports-related injuries in children

NYU- Hospital for Joint Diseases Center for Children – holistic outpatient treatment of children and adolescents with a wide range of orthopaedic and neurological conditions

Child Study Center – advancing the field of mental health for children and adolescents through evidence-based practice, science, and education

Cochlear Implant Program – restoring hearing to profoundly deaf children

Craniofacial Program – treating facial deformities discovered at birth

Epilepsy Program – state-of-the-art evaluation and multidisciplinary treatment of children with epilepsy

Familial Dysautonomia Program – the only center in the U.S. providing care to individuals affected with this genetic disorder

Hassenfeld Children's Center – comprehensive outpatient care for children with cancer and blood disorders

Headache Center – thorough diagnosis and evaluation to help pediatric patients manage frequency and severity of chronic headaches

Hemangiomas and Vascular Malformation Program – multidisciplinary care for children with hemangiomas and vascular malformations

Orthopaedic Immediate Care Center at the Hospital for Joint Diseases – evaluation and treatment of urgent pediatric and adult orthopaedic problems, such as fractures

Pediatric Rehabilitation Service – multi-disciplinary pediatric rehabilitation for a variety of congenital and acquired disabilities on an inpatient and outpatient basis

Preschool and Early Intervention Program – individualized educational and early intervention services for children under five

Stem Cell Transplant Program – Using stem cell transplant to treat brain and other solid tumors, under the auspices of the Hassenfeld Children's Center, which was the site of much of the original stem cell harvest and transplantation research.

NYU MEDICAL CENTER

Children's Services at NYU Medical Center provides comprehensive, family-centered care for children with all types of conditions. Specialized care for children are provided in the following areas:

- Adolescent Medicine
- Allergy
- Anesthesia
- Cardiology
- Cardio-Vascular Surgery
- Critical Care
- Dermatology
- Developmental Pediatrics
- Dysautonomia
- Emergency Medicine
- Endocrinology
- Epilepsy
- Gastroenterology
- Genetics
- Hematology
- Infectious Diseases
- Neonatology
- Nephrology
- Neurology
- Neurosurgery
- Oncology
- Ophthamology
- Orthopaedics
- Otolaryngology
- Pediatrics
- Plastic Surgery/ Cranial Facial
- Psychiatry
- Pulmonology
- Radiology
- Rehabilitation Medicine
- Rheumatology
- Surgery
- Urology

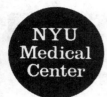

550 First Avenue (at 31st Street)
New York, NY 10016
Physician Referral: (866) CHILD-NYU
(866-244-5369) www.nyuchildrens.org

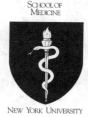

NEW YORK UNIVERSITY

NYU CHILDREN'S HEALTH

NYU Medical Center's Children's Health Team is comprised of some of the best clinical specialists in the country. Among the programs they offer are:

Apnea/SIDS Program –identifying and treating of infants with apnea and infants who are are at increased risk for SIDS

Center for Child and Adolescent Sports Medicine – developmentally sensitive and comprehensive evaluation and treatment of sports-related injuries in children

NYU- Hospital for Joint Diseases Center for Children – holistic outpatient treatment of children and adolescents with a wide range of orthopaedic and neurological conditions

Child Study Center – advancing the field of mental health for children and adolescents through evidence-based practice, science, and education

Cochlear Implant Program – restoring hearing to profoundly deaf children

Craniofacial Program – treating facial deformities discovered at birth

Epilepsy Program – state-of-the-art evaluation and multidisciplinary treatment of children with epilepsy

Familial Dysautonomia Program – the only center in the U.S. providing care to individuals affected with this genetic disorder

Hassenfeld Children's Center – comprehensive outpatient care for children with cancer and blood disorders

Headache Center – thorough diagnosis and evaluation to help pediatric patients manage frequency and severity of chronic headaches

Hemangiomas and Vascular Malformation Program – multidisciplinary care for children with hemangiomas and vascular malformations

Orthopaedic Immediate Care Center at the Hospital for Joint Diseases Orthopaedic Institute – evaluation and treatment of urgent pediatric and adult orthopaedic problems, such as fractures

Pediatric Rehabilitation Service – multi-disciplinary pediatric rehabilitation for a variety of congenital and acquired disabilities on an inpatient and outpatient basis

Preschool and Early Intervention Program – individualized educational and early intervention services for children under five

Stem Cell Transplant Program – Using stem cell transplant to treat brain and other solid tumors, under the auspices of the Hassenfeld Children's Center, which was the site of much of the original stem cell harvest and transplantation research.

PEDIATRIC ALLERGY AND IMMUNOLOGY

NYU Children's Health provides family-centered care for pediatric allergy problems within the setting of a world-class academic medical center. Our allergy specialists work side-by-side with physicians from many other medical specialties and have ready access to their expertise, to optimize your child's treatment. Together, these teams will work with you to determine the therapy or combination of therapies that is right for you and your child.

NYU Medical Center also enjoys a strong history in pediatric immunology. Perhaps its most important achievement is the discovery of a vaccine for rubella. But that is by no means its only achievement. With a superb clinical faculty and staff that is highly committed to basic science and clinical research, NYU Medical Center continues to conduct research that positively and directly impacts on children's health.

Physician Referral
(866) CHILD-NYU
(866-244-5369)
www.nyuchildrens.org

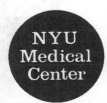

NYU Medical Center

550 First Avenue (at 31st Street)
New York, NY 10016
Physician Referral: (866) CHILD-NYU
(866-244-5369)   www.nyuchildrens.org

SCHOOL OF
MEDICINE

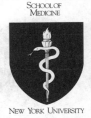

NEW YORK UNIVERSITY

PEDIATRIC CARDIOLOGY

NYU's Pediatric Cardiology Program is motivated by an academic approach to patient care. A leader for more than three decades, the Pediatric Cardiology Program remains at the forefront of innovation in both research and clinical care. It is also an outstanding training ground for future pediatricians dedicated to the heart health of children.

There is a long list of recent advances that are benefiting infants, children, and young adults with a wide range of heart problems. First, a growing emphasis on minimally invasive surgical techniques allows for quicker recoveries and shorter hospital stays. Various clinical sub-disciplines further support the Pediatric Cardiology Program, including:

Cardiothoracic Surgery – corrective procedures for all types of congenital and acquired heart disease.

Pediatric Cardiac Critical Care – intensive care for children with heart disease, provided capably and compassionately by a staff of pediatric cardiologists, neonatologists, cardiac anesthesiologists, respiratory therapists, and pediatric intensive care nurses.

Pediatric Non-Invasive Cardiac Imaging – the use of echocardiography and magnetic resonance imaging (MRI) to diagnose and monitor a wide range of cardiac abnormalities.

Pediatric Cardiac Electrophysiology – a wide array of diagnostic and therapeutic services, including arrhythmia detection and pacemaker placement.

Pediatric Interventional Cardiac Catheterization – the treatment of serious heart conditions in a nonsurgical setting, sometimes used in combination with open-heart surgery.

Pediatric Cardiopulmonary Exercise Laboratory – assesses the cardiorespiratory response of exercise in children as young as three and four years old. The Lab features some of the most sophisticated equipment in the region for measuring oxygen consumption, cardiac output, and lung capacity.

NYU MEDICAL CENTER

At NYU, a child's heart health is a family affair.

The Pediatric Cardiology staff at NYU is vigilant in helping children stay in contact with their parents during a stay at the Medical Center.

Whenever possible, parents are welcome to stay overnight in their child's room on the pediatric floor. Social workers and child life experts are always on hand to give families the information and support they need to cope with their child's disease during and after their hospital stay.

Physician Referral
(866) CHILD-NYU
(866-244-5369)
www.nyuchildrens.org

NYU Medical Center

550 First Avenue (at 31st Street)
New York, NY 10016
Physician Referral: (866) CHILD-NYU
(866-244-5369)   www.nyuchildrens.org

SCHOOL OF
MEDICINE

NEW YORK UNIVERSITY

PEDIATRIC CRITICAL CARE

When children experience medical problems, they deserve the most compassionate, state-of-the-art medical care possible. Yet, pediatric patients have needs, medical and emotional, that are unique and different from those of adults. To better meet these needs, Tisch Hospital at NYU Medical Center has recently completed a major expansion and improvement of its Pediatric Intensive Care Unit (PICU).

In most hospitals, pediatric patients recover in specialized areas annexed to the adult units for their particular ailment. For example, children recovering from neurosurgery would have awakened in a pediatric section of the neurosurgery unit to find a crowded and noisy recovery room that did not cater to their unique physical and emotional needs. At NYU, they recover in an environment developed especially for them, with a multidisciplinary staff assembled just for them.

The PICU at NYU Medical Center has the added advantage of being a real resource to referring physicians, providing them with the technology, expertise and time-saving procedures that can help them save lives.

At NYU Medical Center, parents are viewed as integral members of the healthcare team because each child's recovery is strongly influenced by continued family involvement. In recognition of this, each room has a roll-away sofa or chair so one parent can spend the night in close proximity to the child for the duration of their stay. In addition, there is a special family room that was created to give families a quiet place to gather together. Of course, the PICU staff also strives to keep children in contact with their parents and to keep parents informed throughout their child's stay.

NYU MEDICAL CENTER

Understanding that healthcare concerns and pediatric emergencies may occur at any time, the PICU staff is available around the clock to provide a second opinion, consult on a specific case, or help expedite a patients' admission. Social services are also available, and there is an on-site pharmacy within the unit.

The new PICU has been equipped with state-of-the-art monitors, dialysis machines, ventilators, and an isolation room. Special capabilities are available to monitor patients who have had surgery for epilepsy.

For children who stay in the PICU for more than a week, physician and occupational therapists will help develop a post-discharge rehabilitation plan. In addition, PICU patients are assigned a social worker, when necessary, to provide referrals for home care and other services.

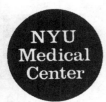

SCHOOL OF
MEDICINE

NYU Medical Center

550 First Avenue (at 31st Street)
New York, NY 10016
Physician Referral: (866) CHILD-NYU
(866-244-5369)   www.nyuchildrens.org

NEW YORK UNIVERSITY

PEDIATRIC GASTROENTEROLOGY

The Section of Gastroenterology in the Department of Pediatrics at NYU Medical Center is dedicated to providing the highest quality medical care and state-of-the-art techniques in the evaluation and management of gastrointestinal, liver, and nutritional disorders from infancy to young adulthood. With access to the latest in endoscopic procedures performed at one of the country's leading academic hospitals, patients can receive comprehensive and multidisciplinary treatments for a vast range of conditions. Below are just some of the disorders NYU's pediatric gastroenterologists evaluate and treat.

- Abdominal pain
- Celiac sprue
- Congenital bowel dysfunction
- Congenital liver disorders and chronic liver disease
- Constipation/Encopresis
- Diarrhea
- Feeding problems in infants
- Failure to thrive
- Food allergy
- Lactose intolerance
- Gastrointestinal bleeding
- Gastroesophageal reflux
- Hepatitis
- Malabsorption
- Pancreatitis
- Peptic disease
- Ulcerative colitis and Crohn's disease
- Vomiting

Among common disorders are chronic abdominal pain, diarrhea, constipation, and vomiting. Most children will occasionally experience one or more of these symptoms during their childhood years. Some children, however, develop recurrent symptoms, which interrupt their normal life, inhibit their development, disrupt their school performance and affect their emotional well being and self-esteem. It is these children who often need the pediatric gastroenterologist's expertise to pinpoint the problem and determine the most effective therapy. At NYU Medical Center, a whole range of therapeutic services is available, as well as access to clinical rehabilitation and some of the country's finest surgeons.

NYU MEDICAL CENTER

Some Services Provided by The Section of Gastroenterology in the Department of Pediatrics at NYU Hospitals Center:

- Endoscopic feeding tube placement (PEG, PEJ)
- Foreign body retrieval from esophagus and stomach
- Endoscopic treatment of strictures of the esophagus
- Endoscopic therapy of achalasia
- Treatment of gastrointestinal hemorrhage
- Nutrition support and parenteral nutrition
- Liver and small bowel biopsy
- Liver transplantation
- Feeding therapy
- Rectal suction biopsy for Hirschprung's disease
- PH probe testing for GE reflux
- ERCP (Endoscopic retrograde cholangiopancreatography)
- Diagnostic endoscopy of upper and lower bowel:
  - Esophagogastroduodenoscopy
  - Colonoscopy
- Flexible sigmoidoscopy

NYU Medical Center

SCHOOL OF MEDICINE

550 First Avenue (at 31st Street)
New York, NY 10016
Physician Referral: (866) CHILD-NYU
(866-244-5369) www.nyuchildrens.org

NEW YORK UNIVERSITY

PEDIATRIC HEMATOLOGY PROGRAM

For decades, children with chronic blood diseases have come to NYU Medical Center's Pediatric Hematology Program for comprehensive medical care, including a full range of psychosocial support services to meet every need. Members of the program's expert staff are guided by a patient- and family-centered approach to care, with all the advantages of a leading academic medical center at their fingertips.

The Program addresses the needs of patients with red blood cell disorders, including a variety of anemias and thalassemias – problems of hemoglobin metabolism – as well as vascular problems and malformations, coagulation disorders, and numerous other hemostatic abnormalities.

Patients requiring hospitalization are treated on the pediatric floor of Tisch Hospital, where they benefit from its advanced diagnostic and therapeutic expertise and the support of all pediatric subspecialties. Families are actively encouraged to become knowledgeable about their children's disease and its management. Our multidisciplinary team works closely with the patient's primary care physician to coordinate both medical and psychosocial care.

PSYCHOSOCIAL SERVICES

To help children and families cope with their disease and to prevent later psychological trauma, our behavioral health professionals are committed to a holistic approach to patient care. Among the services we provide are art therapy, relaxation training, play therapy, psychiatric evaluation, neuropsychological assessment, individual and group counseling, and patient education.

THE PEDIATRIC SPECIAL HEMATOLOGY LABORATORY

As a service to clinicians, the Pediatric Special Hematology Laboratory provides comprehensive hemostasis and red cell testing. Tests have been adapted so that small quantities of blood can be drawn from pediatric patients. The Laboratory's repertoire of test procedures is routinely upgraded to incorporate the latest developments in the field. It strives to provide fast, precise test information that leads to effective treatments while maintaining rigorous quality control standards.

NYU MEDICAL CENTER

Children with cancer or chronic blood diseases receive comprehensive outpatient care at the Steven D. Hassenfeld Center for Children with Cancer and Blood Disorders – a pediatric day hospital at NYU that provides fully coordinated care at a state-of-the-art facility. The medical team works hand in hand with a behavioral science team consisting of a full-time psychologist, social worker, and child life specialist. Most therapies and procedures are performed on an ambulatory basis. In addition to examining rooms and doctors' offices, the Center comprises the day hospital, an on-site laboratory, and a playroom.

Physician Referral
(866) CHILD-NYU
(866-244-5369)
www.nyuchildrens.org

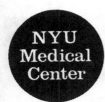

550 First Avenue (at 31st Street)
New York, NY 10016
Physician Referral: (888) 7-NYU-MED
(888-769-8633) www.nyumedicalcenter.org

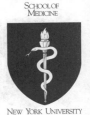

SCHOOL OF
MEDICINE

NEW YORK UNIVERSITY

PEDIATRIC INFECTIOUS DISEASES

PEDIATRIC INFECTIOUS DISEASES CLINIC

One major provider of health care services for mothers and children with HIV infection in Manhattan is the **Pediatric Infectious Diseases (PID) Family Clinic at Bellevue Hospital**, which follows over 300 families, including more than 120 children who are HIV-positive. Initiated in 1982 with the aid of private philanthropy and now funded in large part by federal support, this program has made major contributions to the understanding of the transmission of HIV from mothers to children and has contributed to their improved care and longevity.

The PID multidisciplinary health care team maintains a close relationship with patients and follows them closely, providing the majority of medical and psychosocial care for HIV-infected children on an outpatient basis. Thus far, the team has proved successful, as indicated by the average daily census of less than one HIV-infected child.

ADOLESCENT HIV CLINIC

The **Bellevue Adolescent Clinic** provides free, confidential HIV testing, pre- and post-test counseling, complete medical evaluations, comprehensive medical care, and referral to clinical trials for HIV-positive teens. NYU Medical Center was recently designated a Reaching for Excellence in Adolescent Care and Health (REACH) site, an NIH/HRSA-funded project. REACH's primary goal is to increase understanding of the natural history of HIV in teens.

DAY HOSPITAL PROGRAM

In addition to the outpatient program, children requiring intravenous infusions during the course of their illness are seen in the **Pediatric AIDS Day Hospital**. Candidates for infusion include patients receiving intravenous gammaglobulin or those with vomiting, diarrhea and/or decreased oral intake who would benefit from intravenous hydration. While these children do not routinely require hospitalization, they do require 4-6 hour periods of observation with adequate nursing and physician supervision. The Pediatric AIDS Day Hospital provides the medical, nursing, psychological, and social support services these patients require, maintaining an organized and efficient delivery of care, as well as providing a facility in which innovative treatments can be developed and implemented. Pediatric patients can also use the new Day Hospital for non-acute care outside of regular clinic hours.

NYU MEDICAL CENTER

Medical services are provided for the children by Pediatric Infectious Disease attendings, post-doctoral fellows, a pediatrician, with a dermatologist and a pedodontist available on call. Psychologists provide developmental testing. Medical care for parents is provided in the same clinic by adult infectious diseases specialists and an obstetrician/ gynecologist, who see parents while their children are being seen. In addition to nursing, staff also include public health advisors who screen mothers for risk factors, counsel, and initiate testing, as well as provide follow-up for mothers in prenatal care; a counselor who makes home visits, provides emotional support, and aids in the follow-up effort; and a full range of clinical social work and child life services.

Since 1988, the Division has been funded as an AIDS clinical trials unit by the National Institutes of Health, one of thirty units in the United States named to study the effectiveness and safety of medications used to treat HIV disease.

The Division has an interest in a variety of infections, including:

- Human Immunodeficiency Virus (HIV) infection
- Cytomegalovirus infection
- Tuberculosis
- Pneumocystis Carinii infection
- Measles virus infection
- Hepatitis B and C infections
- Pneumococcal infections

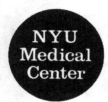

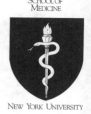

NYU Medical Center

550 First Avenue (at 31st Street)
New York, NY 10016
Physician Referral: (866) CHILD-NYU
(866-244-5369)   www.nyuchildrens.org

NEW YORK UNIVERSITY

PEDIATRIC NEPHROLOGY

The kidneys are a vital organ system in the body, and taking care of a child's kidneys and renal tract is of great importance to his or her growth into adulthood. In addition to clearing the blood of metabolic waste products, the kidneys perform vital support services to other systems. They help bone marrow produce red blood cells, and they are critical in producing the active form of Vitamin D that helps a child's bones grow strong.

NYU Medical Center prides itself in its ability to provide full, comprehensive care to pediatric patients with renal disease. Its physicians provide an expert, nondiscriminatory approach to treatment, regardless of a patient's age, race, sex, or insurance coverage. Furthermore, through the AT&T Language Line Services, the pediatric nephrology team is able to communicate with any patient, tearing down the often-frustrating language barrier. It also has several staff members that speak fluent Spanish.

Along with the diagnosis and treatment of these conditions, NYU Medical Center is dedicated to taking care of children with acute and chronic renal failure, and has an active program for treating children with end stage renal disease with dialysis and renal transplantation. Services offered include diagnostic evaluation, ongoing treatment, renal biopsy, hemodialysis, and peritoneal dialysis. And thanks to a desire to be on the forefront of technology, NYU Medical Center has for over a decade led the charge towards living donor transplantation and minimally invasive procedures.

NYU offers living donor kidney transplantation to patients with end stage renal failure, and thanks to new surgical techniques including minimally invasive kidney extraction, family members and other donors to donate a kidney to a loved one in need has become easier. Hospitalization lasts 1-2 days, and most donors return to normal activity in around one or two weeks, which means a faster return to daily activites after the surgery.

NYU MEDICAL CENTER

NYU Medical Center provides services to patients with the complete spectrum of kidney diseases and related problems, and the multidisciplinary team also is involved in ongoing clinical and basic scientific research, bringing the latest in research from the lab bench to the bedside. Medical consultation and evaluation for children with renal disease, electrolyte disorders, and hypertension is available.

Physician Referral
(866) CHILD-NYU

(866-244-5369)

www.nyuchildrens.org

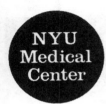

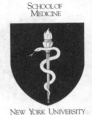

SCHOOL OF
MEDICINE

NEW YORK UNIVERSITY

NYU Medical Center

550 First Avenue (at 31st Street)
New York, NY 10016
Physician Referral: (866) CHILD-NYU
(866-244-5369)   www.nyuchildrens.org

PEDIATRIC PULMONOLOGY

On the forefront of technology, NYU pediatric lung care specialists utilize minimally invasive techniques, providing complete pediatric general surgical and thoracic services for infants, children and adolescents. This includes surgery for congenital and acquired problems, surgery in premature infants, tumor surgery, surgery on the lungs, esophageal surgery and repair of chest wall deformities. With over a decade of experience in using minimally invasive techniques to treat these problems and state-of-the-art instruments and techniques, the team of pediatricians can perform these procedures with minimal discomfort, little scarring, and limited hospitalization. Consultation requests for conditions prenatally diagnosed are welcome.

Because NYU Medical Center is committed to comprehensive care through an interdisciplinary approach, its pediatric lung specialists are able to join forces with other centers, departments, and divisions within the medical center. Pulmonary care at the NYU Infant Apnea/SIDS Program of Neonatology, within the Department Pediatrics, for example, is specially designed and dedicated to the identification and treatment of infants with apnea and infants who at are at an increased risk for sudden infant death syndrome (SIDS). The program consists of physicians and nurses specially trained in this area, and it provides testing and treatment for apnea and identification of high risk infants. Physicians and nurses also supply extensive education to the surrounding community and around-the-clock support to families of high risk infants.

NYU MEDICAL CENTER

The Infant Apnea program is only one of many pediatric pulmonary services offered. Among other areas of comprehensive diagnostic and therapeutic care for children with a wide range of respiratory conditions and disorders includes the following:

- Asthma
- Airway abnormalities
- Bronchopulmonary Dysplasia (BPD)
- Lung diseases in children with developmental delay and orthopedic conditions
- Gastroesophageal Reflux Disease (GERD)
- Neuromuscular diseases
- Apnea and sleep disorders
- Sinus problems

Physician Referral
(866) CHILD-NYU

(866-244-5369)

www.nyuchildrens.org

NYU Medical Center

SCHOOL OF MEDICINE

550 First Avenue (at 31st Street)
New York, NY 10016
Physician Referral: (888) 7-NYU-MED
(888-769-8633)   www.nyumedicalcenter.org

NEW YORK UNIVERSITY

PEDIATRIC RHEUMATOLOGY

Causes of Arthritis in Children

Arthritis is the term used to describe inflammation and swelling of the tissues in a joint. Perhaps surprisingly, viruses are the most common cause of arthritis in children. This type of arthritis is usually temporary and passes quickly without permanent damage. However, a bacterial joint infection is a more urgent matter. Called septic arthritis, this painful condition requires urgent care to prevent the spread of infection and the possibility of permanent damage to the joint. At its first sign, NYU's expert medical staff are quick to take steps to fight the infection at its source. Normally, septic arthritis is completely cured with antibiotics.

Juvenile Idiopathic Arthritis

An umbrella term for several different patterns of arthritis in children, Juvenile Idiopathic Arthritis (JIA) refers to arthritic disorders caused by an autoimmune reaction. Autoimmune disease occurs when the body begins to attack its own tissues as if they were foreign substances. NYU's pediatric rheumatologists are expert in diagnosing and treating at least seven different types of JIA. These are diagnosed by putting together a total picture that includes the age of the child and the presence of associated arthritis in the family. The physician also considers which joints have been tender and swollen and for how long, and which laboratory tests are abnormal.

Although JIA is not curable at present, rheumatologists have learned that aggressive, early treatment with methotrexate and injections of corticosteroids into the joints can usually prevent significant damage. The increased use of methotrexate in combination with newly discovered biologic agents, such as Etanercept and Infliximab, gives even greater reason for optimism. Juvenile arthritis, once a crippler of children, is fast becoming a highly manageable disease.

REASONS FOR OPTIMISM

Rheumatic disease in children can differ in origin from the same condition in adults, and there are differences in how they are treated. NYU Medical Center houses a program in Pediatric Rheumatology that is uniquely tailored to the needs of young patients with inflammatory and non-inflammatory disorders of the muscle, connective tissue, blood vessels, and skin. At NYU, children's physical and psychological development are important contributing factors in the total treatment equation.

NYU's outstanding specialists give children the compassionate care they need — easing their painful symptoms and helping them manage their disease over the long term.

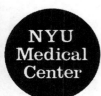

NYU
Medical
Center

550 First Avenue (at 31st Street)
New York, NY 10016
Physician Referral: (888) 7-NYU-MED
(888-769-8633) www.nyumedicalcenter.org

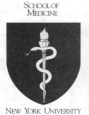

SCHOOL OF
MEDICINE

NEW YORK UNIVERSITY

PEDIATRIC SURGERY

When it comes to surgery, children are not just smaller versions of adults. NYU Medical Center provides comprehensive pediatric surgical care that starts even before the child is admitted and may continue long after patient discharge. In addition to its top-quality surgeons and surgical nurses, the Medical Center offers a wide array of Child Life Services to help children and their families become familiar with the hospital environment and allay fears that often accompany a hospital stay.

Surgical Expertise

Besides general surgical services, NYU is renowned for its achievements in the full spectrum of pediatric surgical specialties, including transplant, neurosurgery, thoracic surgery, cancer surgery, abdominal surgery, and reconstructive surgery, among others With more than a decade of experience using minimally invasive techniques to treat a broad range of medical problems, NYU surgeons strive to cut pain and scarring down to size and keep children as safe and comfortable as humanly possible. Shorter hospital stays and faster recovery – both benefits associated with minimally invasive surgery – mean that children can return home and resume their lives far sooner than in the recent past.

Child Life Services

The pediatric unit at Tisch Hospital is home to a Child Life Program that focuses on creating a supportive environment for children undergoing surgery. The Program comprises many small services that add up to a total approach to caring for the whole child and supporting families in the process. Just a few examples of these services are:

- **Pre-Admission Orientation and Information** – Informational packets are available for families through pre-admission testing and doctors' offices. Parents and their children are also encouraged to attend an orientation session with a member of the Child Life staff.
- **Therapeutic Play** – To help children face the challenges they may encounter during their hospital stay, therapists use arts and crafts, music, horticulture, games, and cooking.
- **Pediatric Library and Computer Center** – A great variety of children's books, videos, and audiotapes are available in the pediatric library, which also houses two computers with Internet access.
- **Teen Esteem Workshop Series** – In cooperation with the Social Work Department, this workshop series was developed to address the special needs of teenagers who are living with chronic or life-threatening illnesses.

NYU MEDICAL CENTER

Warmth, contact, and caring make all the difference in the world when a youngster is recovering from surgery. At every point, Child Life staff and volunteers reach out to each child in many different ways. Too sick to visit the playroom? A volunteer will make an individual bedside visit to make sure the young patient's needs are being met. Just a little bit lonely? Foster grandparents are on hand to comfort, console, and entertain children whose parents may be unable to be present during the day. And since everyone knows happiness is a warm puppy, a group of specially trained dogs and their owners volunteer regularly for special visits with eligible children.

Physician Referral
(888) 7-NYU-MED
(888-769-8633)
www.nyumedicalcenter.org

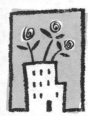

THE UNIVERSITY OF CHICAGO CHILDREN'S HOSPITAL

5839 S. Maryland Avenue
Chicago, Illinois 60637-1470
For help finding a physician: 1-888-UCH-0200

AT THE FOREFRONT OF KIDS' MEDICINE

Staffed by more than 100 faculty physicians, the University of Chicago Children's Hospital is dedicated to helping children with medical problems ranging from the routine to the complex. It is a place where patient care, teaching, and research come together to find cures for childhood illnesses.

At the hospital and through its outpatient clinics, pediatricians provide advanced therapies to children and teens in virtually all clinical areas, including allergy, arthritis, asthma, cancer, cardiology, child development, diabetes, ear/nose/throat, emergency medicine, gastroenterology, genetics, gynecology, infectious disease, neonatology, neurology, orthopaedics, psychiatry, and surgery.

WORLD-RENOWNED SPECIALTY EXPERTISE

Critically ill or injured children are cared for in the state-of-the-art Frankel Pediatric Intensive Care Unit. This 22-bed facility treats children with multiple traumas; complex medical problems; major surgery, including cardiac and neurosurgery; renal failure; and transplants. In addition, a 53-bassinet neonatal intensive care unit provides premature and critically ill infants with the most advanced medical care and life support systems available.

Our pediatric liver transplantation program is one of the largest in the country and was the first living-donor program in the world. In 1989, we performed the first successful liver transplant from a living donor.

Our pediatric cancer program offers virtually every available form of therapy, both conventional and investigational, for a child afflicted with cancer. The program is a principal member of the Children's Cancer Study Group, an international consortium of cancer research hospitals that participate in trials and exchange information on the latest advances in diagnosis and treatment. We also perform bone marrow transplants for virtually all indications, from leukemia and solid tumors to inborn errors of metabolism.

TAILORED TO THE NEEDS OF CHILDREN

Our physicians are particularly sensitive to the special physical and emotional needs of children and their families. Our staff is dedicated to teaching children about their illnesses and medical procedures, as well as helping children and families to cope with the stress of a child's illness.

To Find a University of Chicago Pediatrician, Call 1-888-UCH-0200
Visit our web site: www.uchospitals.edu

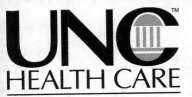

North Carolina Children's Hospital
The University of North Carolina Health Care System
101 Manning Drive Chapel Hill, NC 27514

www.unchealthcare.org

NORTH CAROLINA CHILDREN'S HOSPITAL

The North Carolina Children's Hospital, part of UNC Hospitals and UNC Health Care, is a new, 136-bed facility opened to patients in 2002. It is a state-of-the-art hospital with complete inpatient and outpatient services.

A MULTIDISCLIPINARY APPROACH

A full panel of pediatric and pediatric surgical subspecialists is on staff to care for routine and complex illnesses and provide preventive care. A multidisciplinary approach is taken to patient care with teams of physicians, specialized nurses and other support personnel.

FAMILY-CENTERED CARE

Our goal is to provide family-centered, child-focused care in an environment designed to promote healing of our patients and comfort for their families. The hospital has all private rooms for patients, state-of-the-art critical care facilities for newborns, infants, children and adolescents, and a multidisciplinary outpatient clinic.

REFERRALS FOR SPECIALIZED CARE

The primary focus of medical care in the North Carolina Children's Hospital is on complex diagnostic and management problems in children of all ages and serving as a primary referral hospital for North Carolina and surrounding states. A growing number of referrals for specialized care are coming from across the United States and other countries.

To request an appointment, call (919) 966-7890.

A TRIPLE MISSION

Our staff is engaged in the triple mission of patient care, education of future health care providers and research into children's health and diseases. We provide state-of-the-art care by applying the latest in research and technology to each child's health care needs while focusing on the needs of the child and his or her family.

WESTCHESTER MEDICAL CENTER
WORLD-CLASS MEDICINE THAT'S NOT A WORLD AWAY.®

Valhalla Campus • Valhalla, NY 10595 • (914) 493-7530

Website: www.worldclassmedicine.com

OVERVIEW

Our Children's Hospital echoes the many specialized services available at Westchester Medical Center. Whatever the medical problem facing the family, the Children's Hospital is second to none. The 109-bed Children's Hospital provides the highest level of pediatric care in all medical and surgical specialties with more than 350 health professionals dedicated specifically to children's healthcare. Each year 20,000 infants and children benefit from the specialized staff and treatment available at the Children's Hospital.

As part of a large university medical center, the Children's Hospital has the region's only Pediatric Intensive Care and Level IV (highest level) Neonatal Intensive Care Units, the region's only Cystic Fibrosis Center, Children's Cancer Center and pediatric bone marrow transplant program. The Medical Center also has the only Pediatric Trauma Center in the region. The Children's Hospital has the region's largest pediatric cardiology and only pediatric cardiac surgery programs, and offers pediatric neurosurgery, pediatric oncology and pediatric corneal, kidney and liver transplant.

Beyond special and advanced medical care, the Children's Hospital also provides emotional care for the child and the family. Our nurses and Child Life specialists take the lead in making each child's stay as "normal" as possible. Working with children before and after surgery and treatment, the Children's Hospital recognizes that family, play and laughter are an important part of a child's recovery. Visitors to the Children's Hospital are often surprised to see young patients bicycling through the halls. We're not.

A member of the National Association of Children's Hospitals and Related Institutions (NACHRI), the Children's Hospital works closely with the National Institutes of Health, receiving special trusts and grants to study pediatric cardiovascular disease, kidney disease, cystic fibrosis and other life-threatening problems. Doctors at the Children's Hospital also participate in the Rotarian Gift of Life heart surgery program, saving the lives of children from around the world.

Our Neonatal Intensive Care Unit takes care of the region's smallest and sickest newborns. Twenty-five years ago, only 5 percent of premature babies survived. Today, with weights measured in ounces instead of pounds, more than 75 percent survive and lead healthy lives.

CHILDREN'S HOSPITAL

The Children's Hospital at Westchester Medical Center provides the highest level of pediatric care in all medical and surgical specialties, including:

- Adolescent Medicine
- Cardiology
- Critical Care Medicine
- Developmental Pediatrics
- Emergency Medicine
- Endocrinology
- Gastroenterology
- General Pediatrics
- Hematology/Oncology
- Immunology/Infectious Diseases
- Medical Genetics
- Neonatology
- Nephrology
- Neurology
- Orthopaedics
- Plastic Surgery
- Psychology
- Pulmonology
- Rheumatology
- Surgery

1-866-WMC-PEDS
Call for a physician referral or a specialty office near you.

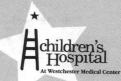

children's Hospital
At Westchester Medical Center

Physician Listings

Physician Listings

PEDIATRICS

New England

Rappaport, Leonard MD (Ped) - *Spec Exp:* Developmental & Behavioral Disorders; **Hospital:** Children's Hospital - Boston; **Address:** 319 Longwood Ave Fl 4, Boston, MA 02115; **Phone:** (617) 277-7320; **Board Cert:** Pediatrics 1983; **Med School:** Yale Univ 1977; **Resid:** Pediatrics, Chldns Hosp, Boston, MA 1978-1980; **Fellow:** Developmental Pediatrics, Chldns Hosp, Boston, MA 1980-1982; **Fac Appt:** Asst Prof Pediatrics, Harvard Med Sch

Shaywitz, Sally Epstein MD (Ped) - *Spec Exp:* Learning Disorders; Dyslexia; **Hospital:** Yale - New Haven Hosp; **Address:** Dept Pediatrics, 333 Cedar St, rm LMP-3089, New Haven, CT 06520; **Phone:** (203) 785-4641; **Board Cert:** Pediatrics 1971; **Med School:** Albert Einstein Coll Med 1966; **Resid:** Pediatrics, Albert Einstein Coll Med, Bronx, NY 1968-1970; **Fellow:** Pediatrics, Bronx Muni Hosp Ctr, Bronx, NY 1967-1968; Behavioral Pediatrics, Albert Einstein Coll Med, Bronx, NY 1968-1970; **Fac Appt:** Prof Pediatrics, Yale Univ

Mid Atlantic

Cohen, Herbert J MD (Ped) - *Spec Exp:* Developmental & Behavioral Disorders; Developmental Disorders; Developmental Delay; **Hospital:** Montefiore Med Ctr - Weiler-Einstein Div (page 67); **Address:** Children's Evaluation Rehab Ctr, 1410 Pelham Pkwy S, Bronx, NY 10461-1116; **Phone:** (718) 430-8522; **Board Cert:** Pediatrics 1964; **Med School:** SUNY Hlth Sci Ctr 1959; **Resid:** Pediatrics, NY Hosp-Cornell Med Ctr, New York, NY 1960-1962; **Fellow:** Developmental Pediatrics, Albert Einstein, Bronx, NY 1964-1966; **Fac Appt:** Prof Pediatrics, Albert Einstein Coll Med

Hofkosh, Dena MD (Ped) - *Spec Exp:* Developmental & Behavioral Disorders; **Hospital:** Chldn's Hosp of Pittsbrgh; **Address:** Chldns Hosp - Child Development Unit, 3705 Fifth Ave, Pittsburgh, PA 15213; **Phone:** (412) 692-5560; **Board Cert:** Pediatrics 1984; **Med School:** NYU Sch Med 1979; **Resid:** Pediatrics, Univ Pitts Med Ctr, Pittsburgh, PA 1979-1984

Ludwig, Stephen MD (Ped) - *Spec Exp:* Child Abuse; Emergency Medicine; **Hospital:** Chldn's Hosp of Philadelphia; **Address:** Chldns Hosp - Philadelphia, 34th St and Civic Center Blvd, rm 9557, Philadelphia, PA 19104; **Phone:** (215) 590-2162; **Board Cert:** Pediatrics 1992, Pediatric Emergency Medicine 2000; **Med School:** Temple Univ 1971; **Resid:** Pediatrics, Chldns Hosp Natl Med Ctr, Washington, DC 1972-1974; **Fac Appt:** Prof Pediatrics, Univ Penn

Pasquariello Jr, Patrick S MD (Ped) - *Spec Exp:* Chronic Fatigue Syndrome; Failure to Thrive; Spina Bifida; **Hospital:** Chldn's Hosp of Philadelphia; **Address:** Children's Hospital, 3400 Civic Center Blvd, Philadelphia, PA 19104-4303; **Phone:** (215) 590-2164; **Board Cert:** Pediatrics 1963; **Med School:** Jefferson Med Coll 1956; **Resid:** Pediatrics, Chldns Hosp, Philadelphia, PA 1961-1963; **Fac Appt:** Prof Pediatrics, Univ Penn

Peebles, Paul T MD (Ped) - *Spec Exp:* Pediatric Hematology-Oncology; Behavioral Disorders; **Hospital:** Chldns Natl Med Ctr - DC; **Address:** Pediatric Care Ctr, 5612 Spruce Tree Ave, Bethesda, MD 20814; **Phone:** (301) 564-5880; **Board Cert:** Pediatrics 1973, Pediatric Hematology-Oncology 1978; **Med School:** Case West Res Univ 1967; **Resid:** Pediatric Surgery, Chldn's Hosp Med Ctr, Boston, MA 1968-1970; **Fellow:** Pediatric Hematology-Oncology, Natl Inst Hlth, Bethesda, MD 1976-1978; **Fac Appt:** Asst Prof Pediatrics, Johns Hopkins Univ

Regan, Joan MD (Ped) - *Spec Exp:* Neonatal-Perinatal Medicine; Infection in Newborn; **Hospital:** NY Presby Hosp - Columbia Presby Med Ctr (page 70); **Address:** 3959 Broadway Bldg PH 4W - rm 474, New York, NY 10032-3702; **Phone:** (212) 305-0955; **Board Cert:** Pediatrics 1979; **Med School:** Univ MO-Columbia Sch Med **Resid:** Pediatrics, Montefiore Med Ctr, New York, NY 1976; **Fellow:** Neonatal-Perinatal Medicine, Columbia Univ, New York, NY 1976-1978; **Fac Appt:** Asst Prof Pediatrics, Columbia P&S

Southeast

Hall, Bryan Davis MD (Ped) - *Spec Exp:* Clinical Genetics-Birth Defects; Dysmorphology; **Hospital:** Univ Kentucky Med Ctr; **Address:** Dept Pediatrics, Kentucky Clinic, Lexington, KY 40536-0284; **Phone:** (859) 257-5559; **Board Cert:** Pediatrics 1970; **Med School:** Univ Louisville Sch Med 1965; **Resid:** Pediatrics, St Hosp Sick Chldn, London, England 1966-1967; Pediatrics, Chldns Hosp, Louisville, KY 1967-1968; **Fellow:** Clinical Genetics, Univ Wash, Seattle, WA 1970-1972; **Fac Appt:** Prof Pediatrics, Univ KY Coll Med

Levine, Melvin David MD (Ped) - *Spec Exp:* Learning Disorders; Developmental Disorders; **Hospital:** Univ of NC Hosp (page 77); **Address:** Ctr for Stdy of Dev & Lrng, 400 Roberson St, Carrboro, NC 27510; **Phone:** (919) 966-1020; **Board Cert:** Pediatrics 1971; **Med School:** Harvard Med Sch 1966; **Resid:** Pediatrics, Chldns Hosp, Boston, MA 1967-1969; **Fac Appt:** Prof Pediatrics, Univ NC Sch Med

Lohr, Jacob MD (Ped) - *Spec Exp:* Infectious Disease; Urinary Tract Infection; **Hospital:** Univ of NC Hosp (page 77); **Address:** 50021 Brogden, Chapel Hill, NC 27514-8589; **Phone:** (919) 966-2674; **Board Cert:** Pediatrics 1999; **Med School:** Univ NC Sch Med 1967; **Resid:** Pediatrics, Univ Virginia Hosp, Charlottesville, VA 1968-1970; **Fac Appt:** Prof Pediatrics, Univ NC Sch Med

Underwood, Louis MD (Ped) - *Spec Exp:* Endocrinology; Growth/Development Disorders; **Hospital:** Univ of NC Hosp (page 77); **Address:** 361 Medical Science Research Bldg, Chapel Hill, NC 27599; **Phone:** (919) 966-4435; **Board Cert:** Pediatrics 1993, Pediatric Endocrinology 1993; **Med School:** Vanderbilt Univ 1961; **Resid:** Pediatrics, Vanderbilt Univ Hosp, Nashville, TN 1962-1963; Pediatrics, North Carolina Mem Hosp, Chapel Hill, NC 1963-1964; **Fellow:** Pediatric Endocrinology, Univ North Carolina, Chapel Hill, NC 1967-1970; **Fac Appt:** Prof Pediatrics, Univ NC Sch Med

Midwest

Berman, Brian MD (Ped) - *Spec Exp:* Sickle Cell Anemia; Thrombocytopenia; Anemia; **Hospital:** Rainbow Babies & Chldns Hosp; **Address:** Rainbow Babies & Chldn's Hosp, 11100 Euclid Ave, Cleveland, OH 44106-6019; **Phone:** (216) 844-3752; **Board Cert:** Pediatrics 1989, Pediatric Hematology-Oncology 1989; **Med School:** Temple Univ 1975; **Resid:** Pediatrics, St Chris Hosp Chldn, Philadelphia, PA 1976-1978; **Fellow:** Pediatric Hematology-Oncology, Yale, New Haven, CT 1978-1980; **Fac Appt:** Prof Pediatrics, Case West Res Univ

Jacob, Molly MD (Ped) - *Spec Exp:* Asthma; ADD/ADHD; **Hospital:** Children's Mem Hosp; **Address:** 4315 N Lincoln Ave, Fl 1, Chicago, IL 60618-1711; **Phone:** (773) 528-3403; **Board Cert:** Pediatrics 1980; **Med School:** India 1968; **Resid:** Pediatrics, Ill Masonic Med Ctr, Chicago, IL 1975-1979; **Fellow:** Ambulatory Pediatrics, Ill Masonic Med Ctr, Chicago, IL 1978-1979; **Fac Appt:** Asst Clin Prof Pediatrics, Univ IL Coll Med

Lantos, John MD (Ped) - *Spec Exp:* Chronic Disease; Palliative Care; Ethics; **Hospital:** La Rabida Children's Hosp; **Address:** East 65th Street at Lake Michigan, Chicago, IL 60649; **Phone:** (773) 363-6700; **Board Cert:** Pediatrics 1986; **Med School:** Univ Pittsburgh 1981; **Resid:** Pediatrics, Chldrns Natl Med Ctr, Washington, DC 1982-1984; **Fellow:** Clinical Ethics, Univ Chicago, Chicago, IL 1986; **Fac Appt:** Assoc Prof Pediatrics, Univ Chicago-Pritzker Sch Med

Mendelsohn, Janis MD (Ped) - *Spec Exp:* Pediatrics - General; **Hospital:** Univ of Chicago Hosps (page 76); **Address:** 800 E 55th St, Chicago, IL 60615; **Phone:** (773) 702-0660; **Board Cert:** Pediatrics 1973; **Med School:** Univ Tenn Coll Med, Memphis 1967; **Resid:** Pediatrics, Chldns Meml Hosp, Chicago, IL 1969-1971; **Fac Appt:** Assoc Prof Pediatrics, Univ Chicago-Pritzker Sch Med

Southwest

Boyd, Robert MD (Ped) - *Spec Exp:* Pediatrics - General; **Hospital:** TX Chldns Hosp - Houston; **Address:** Houston Pediatric Associates, 4110 Bellaire Blvd, Houston, TX 77025-1099; **Phone:** (713) 666-1953; **Board Cert:** Pediatrics 1987; **Med School:** Univ Kans 1969; **Resid:** Pediatrics, Baylor Coll Med, Houston, TX 1969-1972; **Fac Appt:** Assoc Clin Prof Pediatrics, Baylor Coll Med

Drutz, Jan Edwin MD (Ped) - *Spec Exp:* Pediatrics - General; **Hospital:** TX Chldns Hosp - Houston, Ben Taub General Hosp; **Address:** Clinical Care Center D1540.00, 6621 Fannin St, Houston, TX 77030; **Phone:** (832) 822-3441; **Board Cert:** Pediatrics 1989; **Med School:** Univ Louisville Sch Med 1968; **Resid:** Pediatrics, Baylor Affil Hosps, Houston, TX 1969-1971; **Fac Appt:** Assoc Prof Pediatrics, Baylor Coll Med

West Coast and Pacific

Berkowitz, Carol D MD (Ped) - *Spec Exp:* Behavioral Pediatrics; Child Abuse; **Hospital:** UCLA Med Ctr; **Address:** Harbor-UCLA Med Ctr, 1000 W Carson St, Box 437, Torrance, CA 90509; **Phone:** (310) 222-3091; **Board Cert:** Pediatrics 1980, Pediatric Emergency Medicine 1998; **Med School:** Columbia P&S 1969; **Resid:** Pediatrics, Roosevelt Hosp, New York, NY 1970-1972; **Fac Appt:** Clin Prof Pediatrics, UCLA

Jones, Kenneth L MD (Ped) - *Spec Exp:* Clinical Genetics-Dysmorphology; **Hospital:** UCSD Healthcare; **Address:** 200 W Arbor Drive, San Diego, CA 92103-8446; **Phone:** (619) 543-2040; **Board Cert:** Pediatrics 1971; **Med School:** Hahnemann Univ 1966; **Resid:** Pediatrics, Chldns Ortho Hosp, Seattle, WA 1967-1969; Pediatrics, Chldns Ortho Hosp, Seattle, WA 1971-1972; **Fac Appt:** Prof Pediatrics, UCSD

McCabe, Edward MD (Ped) - *Spec Exp:* Neonatal Genetics; **Hospital:** UCLA Med Ctr; **Address:** UCLA Sch Med, Dept Ped, 10833 LeConte Ave Bldg MDCC - rm 22-412, Los Angeles, CA 90095-1752; **Phone:** (310) 825-5095; **Board Cert:** Pediatrics 1979, Clinical Genetics 1982; **Med School:** USC Sch Med 1974; **Resid:** Pediatrics, Univ Minn Hosp, Minneapolis, MN 1975-1976; **Fellow:** Pediatric Metabolism, Univ Colo Hosp, Denver, CO 1976-1978; **Fac Appt:** Prof Pediatrics, UCLA

Miller, Carol A MD (Ped) - *Spec Exp:* Neonatology; **Hospital:** UCSF Med Ctr; **Address:** 400 Parnassus Ave Fl 2, U Calif Med Ctr, San Francisco, CA 94122; **Phone:** (415) 353-2364; **Board Cert:** Pediatrics 1981; **Med School:** Stanford Univ 1975; **Resid:** Pediatrics, Mt Zion Hosp, San Francisco, CA 1975-1977; **Fellow:** Neonatology, Mt Zion Hosp, San Francisco, CA 1977-1979; **Fac Appt:** Clin Prof Pediatrics, UCSF

PEDIATRICS

West Coast and Pacific

Pantell, Robert H MD (Ped) - *Spec Exp:* Febrile Infants; **Hospital:** UCSF Med Ctr; **Address:** 400 Parnassus Ave, Box 0374, San Francisco, CA 94122-2721; **Phone:** (415) 353-2000; **Board Cert:** Pediatrics 1974; **Med School:** Boston Univ 1969; **Resid:** Pediatrics, NC Meml Hosp, Chapel Hill, NC 1970-1972; **Fellow:** Pediatrics, Stanford Univ Hosp, Stanford, CA 1974-1977; **Fac Appt:** Prof Pediatrics, UCSF

Zeltzer, Lonnie Kaye MD (Ped) - *Spec Exp:* Pain Management; Adolescent Medicine; **Hospital:** UCLA Med Ctr; **Address:** Pediatric Pain Program, 10833 Le Conte Ave Bldg MDCC - rm 22-464, Los Angeles, CA 90095; **Phone:** (310) 825-0731; **Board Cert:** Pediatrics 1976; **Med School:** Univ Cincinnati 1970; **Resid:** Pediatrics, Univ Ariz Hosp, Tucson, AZ 1971-1973; **Fellow:** Adolescent Medicine, Chldns Hosp, Los Angeles, CA 1975-1976; **Fac Appt:** Prof Pediatrics, UCLA

PEDIATRIC ALLERGY & IMMUNOLOGY

Mid Atlantic

Eggleston, Peyton Archer MD (PA&I) - *Spec Exp:* Allergy; **Hospital:** Johns Hopkins Hosp - Baltimore; **Address:** Johns Hopkins Hosp, Div Immun-Ped, 600 N Wolfe St, Ste CMSC 1102, Baltimore, MD 21287; **Phone:** (410) 955-5883; **Board Cert:** Allergy & Immunology 1974, Pediatrics 1992; **Med School:** Univ VA Sch Med 1965; **Resid:** Pediatrics, Univ Wash, Seattle, WA 1968-1970; **Fellow:** Allergy & Immunology, Univ Wash, Seattle, WA 1970-1972; **Fac Appt:** Prof Pediatrics, Johns Hopkins Univ

Sampson, Hugh MD (PA&I) - *Spec Exp:* Food Allergy; Atopic Dermatitis; Asthma; **Hospital:** Mount Sinai Hosp (page 68); **Address:** Mt Sinai Sch Med, Dept Peds, 1 Gustave Levy Pl, Box 1198, New York, NY 10029-6500; **Phone:** (212) 241-5548; **Board Cert:** Pediatrics 1980, Allergy & Immunology 1981; **Med School:** SUNY Buffalo 1975; **Resid:** Pediatrics, Childns Meml Hosp-NW Univ, Chicago, IL 1976-1979; **Fellow:** Allergy & Immunology, Duke Univ Med Ctr, Durham, NC 1978-1980; **Fac Appt:** Prof Pediatrics, Mount Sinai Sch Med

Schuberth, Kenneth Charles MD (PA&I) - *Spec Exp:* Allergy; **Hospital:** Johns Hopkins Hosp - Baltimore; **Address:** 10807 Falls Rd, Ste 200, Lutherville, MD 21093; **Phone:** (410) 427-1604; **Board Cert:** Allergy & Immunology 1983, Pediatrics 1979; **Med School:** Johns Hopkins Univ 1973; **Resid:** Pediatrics, Johns Hopkins, Baltimore, MD 1974-1978; **Fellow:** Allergy & Immunology, Johns Hopkins, Baltimore, MD 1978-1980; **Fac Appt:** Assoc Prof Pediatrics, Johns Hopkins Univ

Skoner, David Peter MD (PA&I) - *Spec Exp:* Rhinitis; Asthma; Allergy; **Hospital:** Chldn's Hosp of Pittsbrgh; **Address:** Dept Allergy & Immunology, 3705 5th Ave, rm 4B-320, Pittsburgh, PA 15213; **Phone:** (412) 692-6850; **Board Cert:** Pediatrics 1985, Allergy & Immunology 1985; **Med School:** Temple Univ 1980; **Resid:** Pediatrics, Chldns Hosp, Cincinnati, OH 1981-1983; **Fellow:** Allergy & Immunology, Chldns Hosp, Pittsburgh, PA 1983-1985

Sly, Ridge Michael MD (PA&I) - *Spec Exp:* Asthma; Allergy; Atopic Dermatitis; **Hospital:** Chldns Natl Med Ctr - DC; **Address:** Children's Natl Med Ctr, 111 Michigan Ave NW, Washington, DC 20010-2970; **Phone:** (202) 884-2033; **Board Cert:** Pediatrics 1980, Allergy & Immunology 1987; **Med School:** Washington Univ, St Louis 1960; **Resid:** Pediatrics, St Louis Chldns Hosp, St Louis, MI 1960-1962; Pediatrics, Univ KY Med Ctr, Lexington, KY 1962-1963; **Fellow:** Pediatric Allergy & Immunology, UCLA, Los Angeles, CA 1965-1967; **Fac Appt:** Prof Pediatrics, Geo Wash Univ

Winkelstein, Jerry Allen MD (PA&I) - *Spec Exp:* Immune Deficiency; **Hospital:** Johns Hopkins Hosp - Baltimore; **Address:** Johns Hopkins Hosp, Dept Ped, 600 N Wolfe St, Baltimore, MD 21287-0001; **Phone:** (410) 955-5883; **Board Cert:** Pediatrics 1972; **Med School:** Albert Einstein Coll Med 1965; **Resid:** Pediatrics, Johns Hopkins Hosp, Baltimore, MD 1966-1968; Pediatrics, Johns Hopkins Hosp, Baltimore, MD 1971-1972; **Fellow:** Immunology, Johns Hopkins Hosp, Baltimore, MD 1970-1973; **Fac Appt:** Prof Pediatrics, Johns Hopkins Univ

Wood, Robert Alan MD (PA&I) - *Spec Exp:* Food Allergy; Asthma; **Hospital:** Johns Hopkins Hosp - Baltimore; **Address:** 10807 Falls Rd, Ste 200, Lutherville, MD 21093; **Phone:** (410) 321-9393; **Board Cert:** Allergy & Immunology 1997, Pediatrics 1987; **Med School:** Univ Rochester 1982; **Resid:** Pediatrics, Johns Hopkins Hosp, Baltimore, MD 1983-1985; **Fellow:** Allergy & Immunology, Johns Hopkins Hosp, Baltimore, MD 1986-1988; **Fac Appt:** Assoc Prof Pediatrics, Johns Hopkins Univ

Southeast

Barrett, Douglas John MD (PA&I) - *Spec Exp:* IVIG Infusion; Immune Deficiency; **Hospital:** Shands Hlthcre at Univ of FL (page 73); **Address:** 1600 SW Archer Rd, rm R-1-118, Gainesville, FL 32610; **Phone:** (352) 846-1327; **Board Cert:** Allergy & Immunology 1981, Pediatrics 1979; **Med School:** Univ S Fla Coll Med 1974; **Resid:** Pediatrics, SUNY, Syracuse, NY 1975-1977; **Fac Appt:** Prof Pediatric Allergy & Immunology, Univ Fla Coll Med

Buckley, Rebecca Hatcher MD (PA&I) - *Spec Exp:* Immune Deficiency; Allergy; **Hospital:** Duke Univ Med Ctr (page 60); **Address:** Duke Univ Sch of Med, Box 2898, Durham, NC 27710-2898; **Phone:** (919) 684-2922; **Board Cert:** Pediatrics 1963, Allergy & Immunology 1977, Clinical & Laboratory Immunology 1986; **Med School:** Univ NC Sch Med 1958; **Resid:** Pediatrics, Duke Univ Med Ctr, Durham, NC 1959-1961; **Fellow:** Pediatric Allergy & Immunology, Duke Univ Med Ctr, Durham, NC 1961-1963; **Fac Appt:** Prof Pediatric Allergy & Immunology, Duke Univ

Hemstreet, Mary Pat MD (PA&I) - *Spec Exp:* Asthma; **Hospital:** Children's Hospital - Birmingham; **Address:** Children's Hosp, Dept Pediatric Allergy, 1600 7th Ave S, Ste ACC614, Birmingham, AL 35233-1711; **Phone:** (205) 939-9586; **Board Cert:** Pediatrics 1973, Allergy & Immunology 1974; **Med School:** Temple Univ 1968; **Resid:** Pediatrics, Univ Okla Med Ctr, Oklahoma City, OK 1969-1970; Pediatrics, DukeMed Ctr, Durham, NC 1970-1971; **Fellow:** Pediatric Allergy & Immunology, Duke Med Ctr, Durham, NC 1971-1973

Midwest

Berger, Melvin MD/PhD (PA&I) - *Spec Exp:* Immune Deficiency; Asthma & Allergy; Adult Allergy & Immunology; **Hospital:** Rainbow Babies & Chldns Hosp; **Address:** 11100 Euclid Ave Bldg RB&C - rm 586, Cleveland, OH 44106-1736; **Phone:** (216) 844-3237; **Board Cert:** Pediatrics 1981, Allergy & Immunology 1981; **Med School:** Case West Res Univ 1976; **Resid:** Pediatrics, Children's Hosp Med Ctr, Boston, MA 1976-1978; **Fellow:** Allergy & Immunology, Natl Inst Allergy & Infect Dis (NIH), Bethesda, MD 1978-1981; **Fac Appt:** Prof Pediatrics, Case West Res Univ

Blum, Paul MD (PA&I) - *Spec Exp:* Asthma; **Hospital:** Fairview-Univ Med Ctr - Univ Campus; **Address:** Southdale Pediatrics, 3955 Park Lawn Ave, Ste 120, Edina, MN 55435; **Phone:** (952) 831-4454; **Board Cert:** Pediatrics 1973, Allergy & Immunology 1981; **Med School:** Univ Minn 1968; **Resid:** Pediatrics, Univ Minnesota Hosp, Minneapolis, MN 1969-1971; **Fellow:** Allergy & Immunology, UCLA Med Ctr, Los Angeles, CA 1978-1980; **Fac Appt:** Asst Clin Prof Pediatrics, Univ Minn

Evans III, Richard MD (PA&I) - *Spec Exp:* Asthma; Food Allergy; Drug allergy; **Hospital:** Children's Mem Hosp; **Address:** Children's Memorial Medical Ctr, 2300 N Childrens Plaza, Box 60, Chicago, IL 60614-3318; **Phone:** (773) 880-3562; **Board Cert:** Allergy & Immunology 1972, Pediatrics 1967; **Med School:** Univ Colo 1961; **Resid:** Pediatrics, Wm Beaumont Genl Hosp, El Paso, TX 1962-1964; **Fellow:** Allergy & Immunology, Walter Reed, Washington, DC 1969-1970; Allergy & Immunology, Buffalo Chldns Hosp, Buffalo, NY 1970-1971; **Fac Appt:** Prof Pediatric Allergy & Immunology, Northwestern Univ

Gewurz, Anita MD (PA&I) - *Spec Exp:* Asthma; Allergy; Immune Deficiency; **Hospital:** Rush-Presby - St Luke's Med Ctr (page 72); **Address:** Univ Consultants, 1725 W Harrison St, Ste 207, Chicago, IL 60612-3817; **Phone:** (312) 942-6296; **Board Cert:** Pediatrics 1976, Allergy & Immunology 1977; **Med School:** Albany Med Coll 1970; **Resid:** Pediatrics, Univ Illinois, Chicago, IL 1972-1973; Allergy & Immunology, Rush-Presby-St Lukes Hosp, Chicago, IL 1974-1976; **Fellow:** Allergy & Immunology, Grant Hosp, Chicago, IL 1976-1977; Allergy & Immunology, Northwestern Univ Med Sch, Chicago, IL 1983-1985; **Fac Appt:** Assoc Prof Allergy & Immunology, Rush Med Coll

Lemanske Jr, Robert F MD (PA&I) - *Spec Exp:* *Asthma;* **Hospital:** Univ WI Hosp & Clins; **Address:** 600 Highland Ave, rm K4/916-9988, Madison, WI 53792; **Phone:** (608) 263-6180; **Board Cert:** Allergy & Immunology 1981, Pediatrics 1980; **Med School:** Univ Wisc 1975; **Resid:** Pediatrics, Univ Wisc Hosp, Madison, WI 1976-1978; **Fac Appt:** Prof Medicine, Univ Wisc

Pongracic, Jacqueline MD (PA&I) - *Spec Exp:* *Latex Allergy; Asthma; Food Allergy;* **Hospital:** Children's Mem Hosp; **Address:** 2300 Children's Plaza, Box 60, Chicago, IL 60614; **Phone:** (773) 880-4233; **Board Cert:** Allergy & Immunology 1991, Internal Medicine 1988; **Med School:** Northwestern Univ 1985; **Resid:** Internal Medicine, North Shore Univ Hosp, Manhasset, NY 1985-1988; **Fellow:** Allergy & Immunology, Johns Hopkins Univ Med Sch, Baltimore, MD 1988-1991; **Fac Appt:** Asst Prof Pediatrics, Northwestern Univ

Strunk, Robert MD (PA&I) - *Spec Exp:* *Asthma;* **Hospital:** St Louis Children's Hospital; **Address:** One Children's Place, Ste 5S30, St Louis, MO 63110-1002; **Phone:** (314) 454-2694; **Board Cert:** Pediatric Allergy & Immunology 1987, Pediatrics 1974; **Med School:** Northwestern Univ 1968; **Resid:** Pediatrics, Cincinnati Chldns Hosp, Cincinnati, OH 1969-1970; **Fellow:** Pediatric Allergy & Immunology, Boston Chldns Hosp, Boston, MA 1972-1974; **Fac Appt:** Prof Pediatrics, Washington Univ, St Louis

Wolf, Raoul MD (PA&I) - *Spec Exp:* *Asthma; Allergy;* **Hospital:** Univ of Chicago Hosps (page 76); **Address:** Dept Allergy, E 65th St at Lake Michigan, Chicago, IL 60649; **Phone:** (773) 753-8637; **Board Cert:** Allergy & Immunology 1983, Pediatrics 1980; **Med School:** South Africa 1969; **Resid:** Pediatrics, Baragwanath Hosp, Johannesburg, South Africa 1970-1973; Pediatrics, Transvaal Meml Hosp Chldn, Johannesburg, South Africa 1973-1976; **Fellow:** Allergy & Immunology, Chldns Hosp Med Ctr, Boston, MA 1976-1979; **Fac Appt:** Assoc Clin Prof Pediatrics, Univ Chicago-Pritzker Sch Med

Great Plains and Mountains

Gelfand, Erwin MD (PA&I) - *Spec Exp:* *Immune Deficiency; Asthma; Allergy;* **Hospital:** Natl Jewish Med & Rsrch Ctr; **Address:** National Jewish Med & Research Ctr, 1400 Jackson St, Denver, CO 80206; **Phone:** (303) 398-1196; **Board Cert:** Pediatrics 1972, Allergy & Immunology 1979; **Med School:** McGill Univ 1966; **Resid:** Pediatrics, Montreal Children's Hosp, Montreal, Canada 1967-1968; Pediatrics, Children's Hosp Med Ctr, Boston, MA 1968-1969; **Fellow:** Allergy & Immunology, Children's Hosp Med Ctr, Boston, MA 1969-1971; **Fac Appt:** Prof Pediatrics, Univ Colo

Leung, Donald MD/PhD (PA&I) - *Spec Exp:* *Atopic Dermatitis; Kawasaki Disease;* **Hospital:** Natl Jewish Med & Rsrch Ctr; **Address:** 1400 Jackson St, Bldg K - Ste 926l, Denver, CO 80206; **Phone:** (303) 398-1379; **Board Cert:** Pediatrics 1982, Allergy & Immunology 1983; **Med School:** Univ Chicago-Pritzker Sch Med 1977; **Resid:** Pediatrics, Chldns Hosp, Boston, MA 1978-1979; **Fellow:** Pediatrics, Harvard Med Sch, Boston, MA 1977-1979; Allergy & Immunology, Chldns Hosp, Boston, MA 1979-1981; **Fac Appt:** Prof Pediatrics, Univ Colo

Southwest

Mazow, Jack Bernard MD (PA&I) - *Spec Exp:* *Pediatric Allergy & Immunology - General;* **Hospital:** TX Chldns Hosp - Houston; **Address:** 6621 Fannin St, Ste A380, MC 1-3291, Houston, TX 77030; **Phone:** (832) 824-1319; **Board Cert:** Internal Medicine 1974, Allergy & Immunology 1989; **Med School:** Univ Tex, Houston 1947; **Resid:** Internal Medicine, Jefferson Davis Hosp, Houston, TX 1948-1949; Internal Medicine, VA Hosp-Baylor, Houston, TX 1949-1954; **Fellow:** Allergy & Immunology, SUNY Affil Hosp, Buffalo, NY 1962-1964; **Fac Appt:** Clin Prof Medicine, Univ Tex, Houston

Shearer, William T MD (PA&I) - Spec Exp: *AIDS/HIV; Immune Deficiency;* **Hospital:** TX Chldns Hosp - Houston; **Address:** Texas Chldns Hosp-Allergy & Immun Service, 6621 Fannin, MC-1-3291, Houston, TX 77030-2399; **Phone:** (832) 824-1274; **Board Cert:** Pediatrics 1986, Allergy & Immunology 1989, Clinical & Laboratory Immunology 1986; **Med School:** Washington Univ, St Louis 1970; **Resid:** Pediatrics, Chldns Hosp-Wash Univ, St Louis, MO 1971-1972; **Fellow:** Allergy & Immunology, Barnes Hosp-Wash Univ, St Louis, MO 1972-1974; **Fac Appt:** Prof Pediatrics, Baylor Coll Med

West Coast and Pacific

Bahna, Sami Labib MD (PA&I) - Spec Exp: *Food Allergy; Asthma;* **Address:** 7471 N Fresno St, Fresno, CA 93720; **Phone:** (559) 436-4500; **Board Cert:** Allergy & Immunology 1981, Pediatrics 1980; **Med School:** Egypt 1964; **Resid:** Pediatrics, Univ Maryland, Baltimore, MD 1974-1975; **Fellow:** Allergy & Immunology, Harbor-UCLA Med Ctr, Torrance, CA 1976-1978; **Fac Appt:** Prof Pediatrics, Univ S Fla Coll Med

Church, Joseph August MD (PA&I) - Spec Exp: *AIDS/HIV; Immune Deficiency;* **Hospital:** Chldns Hosp - Los Angeles; **Address:** 4661 W Sunset Blvd, Box 54700, MS 75, Los Angeles, CA 90054; **Phone:** (323) 669-2501; **Board Cert:** Pediatrics 1977, Allergy & Immunology 1977; **Med School:** UMDNJ-NJ Med Sch, Newark 1972; **Resid:** Pediatrics, Chldns Hosp/Natl Med Ctr, Washington, DC 1973-1974; **Fellow:** Allergy & Immunology, Georgetown Med Ctr, Washington, DC 1974-1976; **Fac Appt:** Prof Pediatrics, USC Sch Med

Epstein, Stuart Zane MD (PA&I) - Spec Exp: *Pediatric Asthma & Allergy; Allergy/Food Allergy;* **Hospital:** Cedars-Sinai Med Ctr; **Address:** 9735 Wilshire Blvd, Bldg 121, Beverly Hills, CA 90212-2101; **Phone:** (310) 274-6853; **Board Cert:** Allergy & Immunology 1999, Pediatrics 1998; **Med School:** Univ IL Coll Med 1978; **Resid:** Pediatrics, Cedars Sinai Med Ctr, Los Angeles, CA 1979-1980; **Fellow:** Pediatrics, USC Med Ctr, Los Angeles, CA 1981-1982; Pediatrics, Univ CA Irvine, Orange, CA 1980-1981; **Fac Appt:** Assoc Clin Prof Pediatrics, UCLA

Fanous, Yvonne F MD (PA&I) - Spec Exp: *Asthma & Allergy; Cystic Fibrosis; Immune Deficiency;* **Hospital:** Loma Linda Univ Med Ctr; **Address:** 11370 Anderson St, Ste B-100, Loma Linda, CA 92354; **Phone:** (909) 558-2387; **Board Cert:** Allergy & Immunology 1985, Pediatrics 1981; **Med School:** Egypt 1973; **Resid:** Pediatrics, Loma Linda Univ, Loma Linda, CA 1980-1981; Pediatrics, Texas Tech Hosp, El Paso, TX 1978-1980; **Fellow:** Allergy & Immunology, Univ CA, Irvine, CA 1981-1983; **Fac Appt:** Assoc Prof Pediatric Allergy & Immunology, Loma Linda Univ

Ostrom, Nancy Kay MD (PA&I) - Spec Exp: *Asthma & Allergy;* **Hospital:** Children's Hosp and Hlth Ctr - San Diego; **Address:** 9610 Granite Ridge Drive, Ste B, San Diego, CA 92123; **Phone:** (858) 268-2368; **Board Cert:** Pediatrics 1984, Allergy & Immunology 1987; **Med School:** Mayo Med Sch 1980; **Resid:** Pediatrics, Mayo Grad Sch Med, Rochester 1981-1983; **Fellow:** Allergy & Immunology, Mayo Grad Sch Med, Rochester 1983-1985; **Fac Appt:** Asst Clin Prof Pediatric Allergy & Immunology, UCSD

Stiehm, E Richard MD (PA&I) - Spec Exp: *AIDS/HIV; Immune Deficiency;* **Hospital:** UCLA Med Ctr; **Address:** UCLA Children's Hosp, 22-387 MDCC, 10833 Le Conte Ave, Los Angeles, CA 90095; **Phone:** (310) 825-6481; **Board Cert:** Pediatrics 1964, Allergy & Immunology 1974; **Med School:** Univ Wisc 1957; **Resid:** Pediatrics, Babies Hosp, New York, NY 1961-1963; **Fellow:** Allergy & Immunology, Univ Wisc, Madison, WI 1958-1959; Allergy & Immunology, Univ CA, San Francisco, CA 1963-1965; **Fac Appt:** Prof Pediatrics, UCLA

Umetsu, Dale T MD/PhD (PA&I) - *Spec Exp:* Asthma; Immune Deficiency; **Hospital:** Stanford Med Ctr; **Address:** Stanford Med Ctr, Dept Peds-Div A&I, 300 Pasteur, rm G309, Stanford, CA 94305-5208; **Phone:** (650) 723-5227; **Board Cert:** Pediatrics 1984, Allergy & Immunology 1985; **Med School:** NYU Sch Med 1979; **Resid:** Pediatrics, Chldns Hosp/Harvard Med Sch, Boston, MA 1980-1982; **Fellow:** Allergy & Immunology, Chldns Hosp/Harvard Med Sch, Boston, MA 1982-1984; **Fac Appt:** Prof Pediatrics, Stanford Univ

Wara, Diane W MD (PA&I) - *Spec Exp:* AIDS/HIV; Immune Deficiency; **Hospital:** UCSF Med Ctr; **Address:** 505 Parnassus Ave, Box 0105, San Francisco, CA 94143; **Phone:** (415) 476-2865; **Board Cert:** Pediatrics 1974, Allergy & Immunology 1975; **Med School:** UC Irvine 1969; **Resid:** Pediatrics, UCSF Med Ctr, San Francisco, CA 1970-1972; **Fellow:** Immunology, UCSF Med Ctr, San Francisco, CA 1972-1975; **Fac Appt:** Prof Pediatrics, UCSF

PEDIATRIC CARDIOLOGY

New England

Lock, James E MD (PCd) - *Spec Exp:* Interventional Cardiology; Angioplasty-Pulmonary Artery; **Hospital:** Children's Hospital - Boston; **Address:** Chldns Hosp, Dept Cardiology, 300 Longwood Ave, Boston, MA 02115-5724; **Phone:** (617) 355-7313; **Board Cert:** Pediatrics 1978, Pediatric Cardiology 1981; **Med School:** Stanford Univ 1973; **Resid:** Pediatrics, Univ Minn Hosp, Minneapolis, MN 1974-1975; Pediatric Cardiology, Univ Minn Hosp, Minneapolis, MN 1975-1977; **Fellow:** Cardiology (Cardiovascular Disease), Hosp Sick Chldn, Toronto,Canada 1977-1979; **Fac Appt:** Prof Pediatrics, Harvard Med Sch

Newburger, Jane MD (PCd) - *Spec Exp:* Cholesterol/Lipid Disorders; Heart Disease-Congenital; Kawasaki Disease; **Hospital:** Children's Hospital - Boston; **Address:** Children's Hospital - Pediatric Cardiology - Bader Building, 300 Longwood Ave, Boston, MA 02115; **Phone:** (617) 355-5427; **Board Cert:** Pediatrics 1979, Pediatric Cardiology 1983; **Med School:** Harvard Med Sch 1974; **Resid:** Pediatrics, Chldns Hosp Med Ctr, Boston, MA 1975-1976; **Fellow:** Pediatric Cardiology, Chldns Hosp Med Ctr, Boston, MA 1976-1979; **Fac Appt:** Assoc Prof Pediatrics, Harvard Med Sch

Perry, Stanton Bruce MD (PCd) - *Spec Exp:* Interventional Cardiology; **Hospital:** Children's Hospital - Boston; **Address:** Boston Children's Hosp, Dept Cardiology, 300 Longwood Ave, Boston, MA 02115; **Phone:** (617) 355-4278; **Board Cert:** Pediatrics 1986, Pediatric Cardiology 1988; **Med School:** Iceland 1978; **Resid:** Pediatrics, St Louis Chldns Hosp, St Louis, MO 1980-1983; **Fellow:** Pediatric Cardiology, Chldns Hosp, Boston, MA 1983-1984; **Fac Appt:** Asst Prof Pediatrics, Harvard Med Sch

Walsh, Edward Patrick MD (PCd) - *Spec Exp:* Cardiac Electrophysiology; Arrhythmias; **Hospital:** Children's Hospital - Boston; **Address:** 300 Longwood Ave, Bader#2, Boston, MA 02115; **Phone:** (617) 355-6328; **Board Cert:** Pediatric Cardiology 1985, Pediatrics 1985; **Med School:** Univ Penn 1979; **Resid:** Pediatrics, Chldns Hosp, Philadelphia, PA 1980-1982; **Fellow:** Pediatric Cardiology, Chldns Hosp, Boston, MA 1982-1985; **Fac Appt:** Assoc Prof Pediatrics, Harvard Med Sch

Mid Atlantic

Beerman, Lee MD (PCd) - *Spec Exp:* Congenital Heart Disease; Arrhythmias; **Hospital:** Chldn's Hosp of Pittsbrgh; **Address:** Chldns Hosp Pittsburgh - Heart Ctr, 3705 5th Ave, Pittsburgh, PA 15213; **Phone:** (412) 692-5540; **Board Cert:** Pediatrics 1979, Pediatric Cardiology 1979; **Med School:** Univ Pittsburgh 1974; **Resid:** Pediatrics, Children's Hospital of Philadelphia, Philadelphia, PA 1974-1977; **Fellow:** Pediatric Cardiology, Children's Hospital of Pittsburgh, Pittsburgh, PA 1977-1979; **Fac Appt:** Prof Pediatrics, Univ Pittsburgh

Brenner, Joel I MD (PCd) - *Spec Exp:* Heart Disease-Congenital; **Hospital:** Johns Hopkins Hosp - Baltimore; **Address:** 600 N Wolfe St, Brady 522, Baltimore, MD 21287; **Phone:** (410) 955-5910; **Board Cert:** Pediatrics 1975, Pediatric Cardiology 1977; **Med School:** NY Med Coll 1970; **Resid:** Pediatrics, New York Hospital, New York, NY 1971-1972; **Fellow:** Pediatric Cardiology, Yale New Haven 1972-1974; **Fac Appt:** Assoc Prof Pediatrics, Johns Hopkins Univ

Gersony, Welton Mark MD (PCd) - *Spec Exp:* *Heart Disease-Congenital;* **Hospital:** NY Presby Hosp - Columbia Presby Med Ctr (page 70); **Address:** Babies Hospital, 3959 Broadway, 2nd Fl N, rm 263, New York, NY 10032; **Phone:** (212) 305-3262; **Board Cert:** Pediatrics 1963, Pediatric Cardiology 1966; **Med School:** SUNY Hlth Sci Ctr 1958; **Resid:** Pediatrics, Babies Chldns Hosp, Cleveland, OH 1959-1961; **Fellow:** Pediatric Cardiology, Harvard Chldns Hosp, Boston, MA 1963-1965; **Fac Appt:** Prof Pediatrics, Columbia P&S

Gewitz, Michael MD (PCd) - *Spec Exp:* *Neonatal Cardiology; Kawasaki Disease; Echocardiography;* **Hospital:** Westchester Med Ctr (page 82); **Address:** New York Medical College/Westchester Med Ctr, Rte 100, Munger Pavillion, Ste 618, Valhalla, NY 10595; **Phone:** (914) 594-4370; **Board Cert:** Pediatrics 1979, Pediatric Cardiology 1981; **Med School:** Hahnemann Univ 1974; **Resid:** Pediatrics, Children's Hosp, Philadelphia, PA 1974-1976; Pediatrics, Hosp Sick Children, London England 1976-1977; **Fellow:** Pediatric Cardiology, Yale-New Haven, New Haven, CT 1977-1979; **Fac Appt:** Prof Pediatric Cardiology, NY Med Coll

Hellenbrand, William E MD (PCd) - *Spec Exp:* *Interventional Cardiology;* **Hospital:** NY Presby Hosp - Columbia Presby Med Ctr (page 70); **Address:** 3959 Broadway, Ste 255, New York, NY 10032; **Phone:** (212) 305-8509; **Board Cert:** Pediatric Cardiology 1977, Pediatrics 1975; **Med School:** SUNY Downstate 1970; **Resid:** Pediatrics, Yale-New Haven, New Haven, CT 1970-1972; **Fellow:** Pediatric Cardiology, Yale-New Haven, New Haven, CT 1972-1973; Pediatric Cardiology, Yale-New Haven, New Haven, CT 1975-1976; **Fac Appt:** Prof Pediatrics, Yale Univ

Kan, Jean MD (PCd) - *Spec Exp:* *Angioplasty;* **Hospital:** Johns Hopkins Hosp - Baltimore; **Address:** Johns Hopkins Hosp, Ped Dept, 600 N Wolfe St, Bldg Brady 5, Baltimore, MD 21287; **Phone:** (410) 955-3665; **Board Cert:** Pediatrics 1974, Pediatric Cardiology 1977; **Med School:** Case West Res Univ 1969; **Resid:** Pediatrics, Johns Hopkins Hosp, Baltimore, MD 1976; Pediatrics, Yale New Haven Hosp, New Haven, CT

Parness, Ira MD (PCd) - *Spec Exp:* *Echocardiography; Birth Defects-Cardiac; Echocardiography-Fetal;* **Hospital:** Mount Sinai Hosp (page 68); **Address:** 1 Gustave Levy Pl, Box 1201, New York, NY 10029-6500; **Phone:** (212) 241-8662; **Board Cert:** Pediatrics 1984, Pediatric Cardiology 1985; **Med School:** SUNY Hlth Sci Ctr 1979; **Resid:** Pediatrics, Brookdale Hosp, Brooklyn, NY 1979-1982; **Fellow:** Pediatric Cardiology, Children's Hosp, Boston, MA 1982-1985; **Fac Appt:** Assoc Prof Pediatrics, Mount Sinai Sch Med

Walsh, Christine A MD (PCd) - *Spec Exp:* *Arrhythmias; Heart Disease-Congenital;* **Hospital:** Montefiore Med Ctr (page 67); **Address:** 111 E 210th St, Bronx, NY 10467-2401; **Phone:** (718) 920-4793; **Board Cert:** Pediatric Cardiology 1983, Pediatric Critical Care Medicine 1987; **Med School:** Yale Univ 1973; **Resid:** Pediatrics, Columbia-Presby, New York, NY 1973-1976; **Fellow:** Pediatric Cardiology, Columbia-Presby, New York, NY 1976-1980; **Fac Appt:** Prof Pediatrics, Albert Einstein Coll Med

Southeast

Bayron, Harry MD (PCd) - *Spec Exp:* *Heart Murmurs; Heart Failure;* **Hospital:** St Mary's Med Ctr - W Palm Bch; **Address:** 5325 Greenwood Ave, Ste 302, West Palm Beach, FL 33407; **Phone:** (561) 844-9858; **Board Cert:** Pediatric Cardiology 1992, Pediatrics 1986; **Med School:** Univ Puerto Rico 1978; **Resid:** Pediatrics, Univ Conn, Farmington, CT 1979-1982; **Fellow:** Pediatric Cardiology, Univ Miami Jackson Meml Hosp, Miami, FL 1982-1985

Boucek, Robert MD (PCd) - *Spec Exp:* Heart Disease-Congenital; Cardiomyopathy; Transplant Medicine-Heart; **Hospital:** All Children's Hosp; **Address:** 880 6th St S, Ste 280, St Petersburg, FL 33701; **Phone:** (727) 892-4200; **Board Cert:** Pediatrics 1975; **Med School:** Tulane Univ 1969; **Resid:** Pediatrics, Duke Univ, Durham, NC 1969-1971; **Fellow:** Pediatric Cardiology, Vanderbilt Med Ctr, Nashville, TN 1973-1976; **Fac Appt:** Prof Pediatrics, Univ S Fla Coll Med

Colvin, Edward V MD (PCd) - *Spec Exp:* Heart Disease-Congenital; Fetal Echogram; Transplant Medicine-Heart; **Hospital:** Univ of Ala Hosp at Birmingham; **Address:** Hillman Bldg 320, 620 20th St S, Birmingham, AL 35233; **Phone:** (201) 934-3460; **Board Cert:** Pediatrics 1982, Pediatric Cardiology 1985; **Med School:** Univ Ala 1977; **Resid:** Pediatrics, Chldns Hosp, Birmingham, AL 1977-1980; **Fellow:** Pediatric Cardiology, Baylor Coll Med, Houston, TX 1980-1983; **Fac Appt:** Prof Pediatrics, Univ Ala

Fricker, Frederick Jay MD (PCd) - *Spec Exp:* Transplant Medicine-Heart; **Hospital:** Shands Hlthcre at Univ of FL (page 73); **Address:** 1600 SW Archer Rd, Box 100296, Gainesville, FL 32610-0296; **Phone:** (352) 392-6431; **Board Cert:** Pediatrics 1975, Pediatric Cardiology 1981; **Med School:** Loyola Univ-Stritch Sch Med 1970; **Resid:** Pediatrics, Children's Hosp, Pittsburgh, PA 1971-1973; **Fellow:** Pediatric Cardiology, Children's Hosp, Pittsburgh, PA 1975-1977; **Fac Appt:** Prof Pediatrics, Univ Fla Coll Med

O'Laughlin, Martin P MD (PCd) - *Spec Exp:* Cardiac Catheterization; **Hospital:** Duke Univ Med Ctr (page 60); **Address:** Duke Univ Med Ctr, Ste 7607DHN, Box 3090, Durham, NC 27710; **Phone:** (919) 684-3574; **Board Cert:** Pediatrics 1985, Pediatric Cardiology 1996; **Med School:** Columbia P&S 1980; **Resid:** Pediatrics, Baylor Coll Med, Houston, TX 1980-1983; Pediatrics, Baylor Coll Med, Houston, TX 1983-1984; **Fellow:** Pediatric Cardiology, Baylor Coll Med, Houston, TX 1984-1987; **Fac Appt:** Assoc Prof Pediatrics, Duke Univ

Sanders, Stephen Pruett MD (PCd) - *Spec Exp:* Echocardiography; Fetal Cardiology; **Hospital:** Duke Univ Med Ctr (page 60); **Address:** Duke Univ Med Ctr, Ste 7617DHN, Box 3090, Durham, NC 27710; **Phone:** (919) 681-2916; **Board Cert:** Pediatrics 1980, Pediatric Cardiology 1981; **Med School:** Univ Louisville Sch Med 1975; **Resid:** Pediatrics, Univ Oregon Hlth Sci Ctr, Portland, OR 1976-1978; Pediatrics; **Fellow:** Pediatric Cardiology, Children's Hosp, Boston, MA 1978-1981; **Fac Appt:** Prof Pediatrics, Duke Univ

Tamer, Dolores MD (PCd) - *Spec Exp:* Kawasaki Disease; **Hospital:** Univ of Miami - Jackson Meml Hosp; **Address:** Univ Miami-Jackson Mem Hosp, PO Box 016960 (R76), Miami, FL 33101; **Phone:** (305) 585-6683; **Board Cert:** Pediatrics 1966, Pediatric Cardiology 1967; **Med School:** SUNY Buffalo 1961; **Resid:** Pediatrics, Chldns Hosp, Philadelphia, PA 1962-1963; Pediatrics, Chldns Hosp, Buffalo, NY 1963-1964; **Fellow:** Pediatrics, Chldns Hosp, Buffalo, NY 1964-1965; **Fac Appt:** Prof Pediatrics, Univ Miami Sch Med

Wolff, Grace Susan MD (PCd) - *Spec Exp:* Arrhythmias; Cardiac Electrophysiology; **Hospital:** Univ of Miami - Jackson Meml Hosp; **Address:** 1475 NW 12th Ave, Miami, FL 33101; **Phone:** (305) 585-6683; **Board Cert:** Pediatrics 1971, Pediatric Cardiology 1973; **Med School:** Med Coll Wisc 1965; **Resid:** Pediatrics, Colum-Presby Med Ctr, New York, NY 1967-1969; **Fellow:** Pediatric Cardiology, Children's Hosp, Boston, MA 1969-1971; **Fac Appt:** Prof Pediatric Cardiology, Univ Miami Sch Med

Young, Ming-Lon MD (PCd) - *Spec Exp:* *Cardiac Electrophysiology; Arrhythmias;* **Hospital:** Univ of Miami - Jackson Meml Hosp; **Address:** Univ Miami, Dept Ped, Box 016960 (R-76), Miami, FL 33101; **Phone:** (305) 585-6683; **Board Cert:** Pediatric Cardiology 1985, Pediatrics 1985; **Med School:** Taiwan 1976; **Resid:** Pediatrics, St Agnes Hosp, Baltimore, MD 1979-1981; Preventive Medicine, Johns Hopkins Univ, Baltimore, MD 1978-1979; **Fellow:** Pediatric Cardiology, Univ Miami Project to Cure Paralysis, Miami, FL 1981-1985; **Fac Appt:** Prof Pediatrics, Univ Miami Sch Med

Midwest

Agarwala, Brojendra MD (PCd) - *Spec Exp:* *Pediatric Cardiology;* **Hospital:** Univ of Chicago Hosps (page 76); **Address:** 5839 S Maryland St, Chicago, IL 60637; **Phone:** (773) 702-6172; **Board Cert:** Pediatrics 1970, Pediatric Cardiology 1978; **Med School:** India 1965; **Resid:** Pediatrics, St Vincent Hosp Med Ctr, New York, NY 1967-1969; **Fellow:** Pediatric Cardiology, NYU Med Ctr, New York, NY 1969-1972; **Fac Appt:** Prof Pediatrics, Univ Chicago-Pritzker Sch Med

Beekman, Robert H MD (PCd) - *Spec Exp:* *Interventional Cardiology; Cardiac Catheterization;* **Hospital:** Cincinnati Chldns Hosp Med Ctr; **Address:** Children's Hosp, Div Cardiology, 3333 Burnet Ave Bldg C, MS 2003, Cincinnati, OH 45229-3039; **Phone:** (513) 636-7072; **Board Cert:** Pediatrics 1981, Pediatric Cardiology 1983; **Med School:** Duke Univ 1976; **Resid:** Pediatrics, UCLA Med Ctr, Los Angeles, CA 1977-1979; **Fellow:** Pediatric Cardiology, Univ Mich Hosp, Ann Arbor, MI 1979-1982; **Fac Appt:** Prof Pediatrics, Univ Cincinnati

Caldwell, Randall MD (PCd) - *Spec Exp:* *Transplant Medicine-Heart; Echocardiography;* **Hospital:** Riley Chldrn's Hosp (page 588); **Address:** 702 Barnhill Drive, Ste RR104, Indianapolis, IN 46202; **Phone:** (317) 274-8906; **Board Cert:** Pediatric Cardiology 1978, Pediatrics 1976; **Med School:** Indiana Univ 1971; **Resid:** Pediatrics, Ind Med Ctr, Indianapolis, IN 1972-1975; **Fellow:** Pediatric Cardiology, Ind Med Ctr, Indianapolis, IN 1975-1978; **Fac Appt:** Prof Pediatric Cardiology, Indiana Univ

Cutilletta, Anthony F MD (PCd) - *Spec Exp:* *Angioplasty; Cardiomyopathy;* **Hospital:** Rush-Presby - St Luke's Med Ctr (page 72); **Address:** 1725 W Harrison, Ste 710, Chicago, IL 60612; **Phone:** (312) 942-6003; **Board Cert:** Pediatrics 1973, Pediatric Cardiology 1973; **Med School:** Univ Chicago-Pritzker Sch Med 1968; **Resid:** Pediatrics, Wyler Chldns Hosp, Chicago, IL 1969-1970; **Fellow:** Pediatric Cardiology, Wyler Chldns Hosp, Chicago, IL 1970-1972; **Fac Appt:** Prof Pediatrics, Rush Med Coll

Dick, Macdonald MD (PCd) - *Spec Exp:* *Cardiac Electrophysiology;* **Hospital:** Motts Chldns Hosp; **Address:** Motts Children's Hosp, L1242 Womens, 1500 E Medical Ctr Drive, Ann Arbor, MI 48109; **Phone:** (734) 936-7418; **Board Cert:** Pediatrics 1972, Pediatric Cardiology 1979; **Med School:** Univ VA Sch Med 1967; **Resid:** Pediatrics, Univ Va Hosp, Charlottesville, VA 1968-1971; **Fellow:** Pediatric Cardiology, Chldn's Hosp Med Ctr, Boston, MA 1971-1974; **Fac Appt:** Prof Pediatrics, Univ Mich Med Sch

Driscoll, David J MD (PCd) - *Spec Exp:* *Exercise Physiology; Klippel-Trenaunay Syndrome; Cardiomyopathy;* **Hospital:** Mayo Med Ctr & Clin - Rochester, MN; **Address:** Mayo Clinic - Pediatric Cardiology, 200 1st St SW, Rochester, MN 55905; **Phone:** (507) 284-3297; **Board Cert:** Pediatrics 1976, Pediatric Cardiology 1999; **Med School:** Marquette Sch Med 1970; **Resid:** Pediatrics, Milwaukee Chldns Hosp, Milwaukee, WI 1971-1972; Pediatrics, Milwaukee Chldns Hosp, Milwaukee, WI 1974-1975; **Fellow:** Pediatric Cardiology, Baylor Coll Med, Houston, TX 1975-1978; **Fac Appt:** Prof Pediatrics, Mayo Med Sch

Epstein, Michael MD (PCd) - *Spec Exp:* Heart Disease-Congenital; **Hospital:** Chldns Hosp of Michigan (page 59); **Address:** Chldns Hosp Mich, Dept Cardiology, 3901 Beaubien Blvd, Fl 2nd, Detroit, MI 48201; **Phone:** (313) 745-5956; **Board Cert:** Pediatrics 1976, Pediatric Cardiology 1981; **Med School:** Univ Tex Med Br, Galveston 1971; **Resid:** Pediatrics, Univ Ariz Hlth Sci Ctr, Tucson, AZ 1971-1974; **Fellow:** Pediatric Cardiology, Univ MN Hosp, Minneapolis, MN 1976-1979; **Fac Appt:** Prof Pediatrics, Wayne State Univ

Hijazi, Ziyad M MD (PCd) - *Spec Exp:* Interventional Cardiology; Heart Disease-Congenital; **Hospital:** Univ of Chicago Hosps (page 76); **Address:** Univ Chicago Chldns Hosp/Dept Ped Cardio, 5841 S Maryland Ave, rm C104, MC-4051, Chicago, IL 60637; **Phone:** (773) 702-6172; **Board Cert:** Pediatrics 1991, Pediatric Cardiology 1992; **Med School:** Jordan 1982; **Resid:** Pediatrics, Yale-New Haven Hosp, New Haven, CT 1987-1988; **Fellow:** Pediatric Cardiology, Yale-New Haven Hosp, New Haven, CT 1988-1991; **Fac Appt:** Prof Pediatrics, Univ Chicago-Pritzker Sch Med

Liebman, Jerome MD (PCd) - *Spec Exp:* Cholesterol/Lipid Disorders; Heart Disease-Congenital; **Hospital:** Rainbow Babies & Chldns Hosp; **Address:** Dept Ped Cardiology, 11100 Euclid Ave, Cleveland, OH 44106-6011; **Phone:** (216) 844-3528; **Board Cert:** Pediatric Cardiology 1962, Pediatrics 1959; **Med School:** Harvard Med Sch 1955; **Resid:** Pediatrics, Babies & Chldns Hosp, Cleveland, OH 1955-1957; **Fellow:** Pediatric Cardiology, Harvard Med Sch, Boston, MA 1957-1959; **Fac Appt:** Prof Pediatrics, Case West Res Univ

Moodie, Douglas MD (PCd) - *Spec Exp:* Marfan's Syndrome; Heart Disease-Congenital; **Hospital:** Cleveland Clin Fdn (page 57); **Address:** Cleveland Clinic Foundation, 9500 Euclid Ave, MC-A120, Cleveland, OH 44195; **Phone:** (216) 444-6717; **Board Cert:** Pediatrics 1977, Pediatric Cardiology 1977; **Med School:** Med Coll Wisc 1972; **Resid:** Pediatrics, Mayo Med Clinic, Rochester, MN 1974-1977; **Fellow:** Pediatric Cardiology, Mayo Med Clinic, Rochester, MN 1973-1974

Porter, Co-burn Joseph MD (PCd) - *Spec Exp:* Arrhythmias; Arrhythmias-Fetal; Transplant Medicine-Heart; **Hospital:** St Mary's Hosp - Rochester, MN; **Address:** Mayo Med Ctr, Dept Ped Cardiology, 200 1st St SW, Rochester, MN 55905; **Phone:** (507) 284-3297; **Board Cert:** Pediatrics 1977, Pediatric Cardiology 1983; **Med School:** Creighton Univ 1972; **Resid:** Pediatrics, Univ Colo Hlth Sci Ctr, Denver, CO 1973-1975; **Fellow:** Pediatric Cardiology, Baylor Coll Med, Houston, TX 1975-1977; Pediatric Cardiology, Baylor Coll Med, Houston, TX 1980-1981; **Fac Appt:** Prof Pediatrics, Mayo Med Sch

Rocchini, Albert P MD (PCd) - *Spec Exp:* Interventional Cardiology; Heart Disease-Congenital; **Hospital:** Univ of MI Hlth Ctr; **Address:** L1242 Women's Hosp, Dept Ped Card, Box 0204, 1500 E Med Ctr Drive, Ann Arbor, MI 48109; **Phone:** (734) 764-5176; **Board Cert:** Pediatric Cardiology 1989, Pediatrics 1989; **Med School:** Univ Pittsburgh 1972; **Resid:** Pediatrics, Univ Mich Med, Ann Arbor, MI 1973-1974; **Fellow:** Pediatric Cardiology, Children's Hosp, Boston, MA 1974-1977; **Fac Appt:** Prof Pediatric Cardiology, Northwestern Univ

Rosenthal, Amnon MD (PCd) - *Spec Exp:* Heart Disease-Congenital; **Hospital:** Univ of MI Hlth Ctr; **Address:** Univ Mich-Mott Children's Hosp, 1500 E Medical Ctr Dr, Ann Arbor, MI 48109-0204; **Phone:** (734) 764-5176; **Board Cert:** Pediatric Cardiology 1986, Pediatrics 1986; **Med School:** Albany Med Coll 1959; **Resid:** Pediatrics, Boston Chldns Hosp., Boston, MA 1960-1962; **Fellow:** Cardiology (Cardiovascular Disease), Boston Chldns Hosp., Boston, MA 1965-1968; **Fac Appt:** Prof Pediatrics, Univ Mich Med Sch

Sodt, Peter MD (PCd) - *Spec Exp:* Birth Defects-Cardiac; Arrhythmias; **Hospital:** St Alexius Med Ctr; **Address:** 1575 N Barrington Rd, Ste 430, Hoffman Estates, IL 60194; **Phone:** (847) 884-1212; **Board Cert:** Pediatric Cardiology 1995, Pediatrics 1986; **Med School:** Northwestern Univ 1980; **Resid:** Pediatrics, Oregon Hlth Scis Univ, Portland, OR 1981-1984; **Fellow:** Pediatric Cardiology, Univ Chicago, Chicago, IL 1984-1986; **Fac Appt:** Asst Clin Prof Pediatrics, Loyola Univ-Stritch Sch Med

Great Plains and Mountains

Boucek, Mark M. MD (PCd) - *Spec Exp:* Transplant Medicine-Heart; Cardiac Catheterization; **Hospital:** Chldn's Hosp - Denver; **Address:** Dept Ped Cardiology, 1056 E 19th Ave, Denver, CO 80218-1007; **Phone:** (303) 837-2940; **Board Cert:** Pediatrics 1982, Pediatric Cardiology 1983; **Med School:** Univ Miami Sch Med 1977; **Resid:** Pediatrics, Vanderbilt Univ Hosp, Nashville, TN 1978-1979; **Fellow:** Pediatric Cardiology, Univ Utah Hlth Sci Ctr, Salt Lake City, UT 1979-1981; **Fac Appt:** Prof Pediatrics, Loma Linda Univ

Minich, Lois LuAnn MD (PCd) - *Spec Exp:* Echocardiography; **Hospital:** Primary Children's Med Ctr; **Address:** Primary Chidren's Med Ctr, Dept Pediatric Cardiology, 100 North Medical Drive, Ste 1500, Salt Lake City, UT 84113; **Phone:** (801) 588-2600; **Board Cert:** Pediatrics 2000, Pediatric Cardiology 2000; **Med School:** W VA Univ 1986

Southwest

Bricker, John Timothy MD (PCd) - *Spec Exp:* Preventive Cardiology; Transplant Medicine-Heart; **Hospital:** TX Chldns Hosp - Houston; **Address:** 6621 Fannin St, MC 19345-C, Houston, TX 77030; **Phone:** (832) 826-5677; **Board Cert:** Pediatrics 1981, Pediatric Cardiology 1997, Pediatric Critical Care Medicine 1998; **Med School:** Ohio State Univ 1976; **Resid:** Pediatrics, Texas Chlds Hosp, Houston, TX 1976-1980; **Fellow:** Pediatric Cardiology, Texas Chlds Hosp, Houston, TX 1980-1983; **Fac Appt:** Prof Pediatrics, Baylor Coll Med

Dreyer, William Jeffrey MD (PCd) - *Spec Exp:* Heart Disease-Congenital; Transplant Medicine-Cardiac; Cardiomyopathy; **Hospital:** TX Chldns Hosp - Houston; **Address:** Texas Children's Hosp, 6621 Fannin St, MC 19345-C, Houston, TX 77030; **Phone:** (832) 826-5600; **Board Cert:** Pediatrics 1987, Pediatric Cardiology 2005; **Med School:** Univ Fla Coll Med 1981; **Resid:** Pediatrics, Univ CA, San Francisco, CA 1982-1984; **Fellow:** Pediatric Cardiology, Baylor Coll Med, Houston, TX 1984-1988; **Fac Appt:** Assoc Prof Pediatrics, Baylor Coll Med

Friedman, Richard Alan MD (PCd) - *Spec Exp:* Cardiac Electrophysiology; **Hospital:** TX Chldns Hosp - Houston; **Address:** Texas Children's Hospital, 6621 Fannin St, MC 19345-C, Houston, TX 77030; **Phone:** (832) 826-5600; **Board Cert:** Pediatrics 1986, Pediatric Cardiology 1996; **Med School:** Univ Pittsburgh 1980; **Resid:** Pediatrics, Baylor Affil Hosps, Houston, TX 1980-1983; **Fellow:** Pediatric Cardiology, Baylor Affil Hosps, Houston, TX 1983-1985

Gillette, Paul Crawford MD (PCd) - *Spec Exp:* Arrhythmias; **Hospital:** Cook Children's Med Ctr; **Address:** Pediatric Cardiology, 901 7th Ave, Ste 310, Fort Worth, TX 76104; **Phone:** (817) 810-2140; **Board Cert:** Pediatrics 1974, Pediatric Cardiology 1975; **Med School:** Med Univ SC 1969; **Resid:** Pediatrics, Baylor Coll Med, Houston, TX 1971-1972; **Fellow:** Pediatric Cardiology, Baylor Coll Med, Houston, TX 1972-1974

Mahony, Lynn MD (PCd) - *Spec Exp:* Heart Disease-Congenital; **Hospital:** Chldns Med Ctr of Dallas; **Address:** 1935 Motor St, Dallas, TX 75235; **Phone:** (214) 456-2333; **Board Cert:** Pediatrics 1979, Pediatric Cardiology 1987; **Med School:** Stanford Univ 1975; **Resid:** Pediatrics, Stanford Univ, Stanford, CA 1976-1978; **Fellow:** Pediatric Cardiology, UCSF, San Francisco, CA 1978; **Fac Appt:** Assoc Prof Pediatrics, Univ Tex SW, Dallas

Mullins, Charles MD (PCd) - *Spec Exp:* Heart Disease-Congenital; **Hospital:** TX Chldns Hosp - Houston; **Address:** Texas Children's Hospital, 6621 Fannin St, MC 19345C, Houston, TX 77030-2399; **Phone:** (832) 826-5600; **Board Cert:** Pediatric Surgery 1986, Pediatric Cardiology 1986; **Med School:** Geo Wash Univ 1958; **Resid:** Pediatrics, Walter Reed Genl Hosp, Washington, DC 1959-1961; Cardiology (Cardiovascular Disease), Walter Reed Genl Hosp, Washington, DC 1961-1962; **Fellow:** Cardiology (Cardiovascular Disease), Walter Reed Genl Hosp, Washington, DC 1962-1963; **Fac Appt:** Prof Pediatrics, Baylor Coll Med

Rogers Jr, James Henry MD (PCd) - *Spec Exp:* Heart Disease-Congenital; **Hospital:** Univ Hosp-San Antonio; **Address:** Univ Tex Hlth Sci Ctr, Dept Ped, 7730 Floyd Curl Dr, San Antonio, TX 78229-3900; **Phone:** (210) 341-7722; **Board Cert:** Pediatrics 1976, Pediatric Cardiology 1977; **Med School:** Med Coll GA 1971; **Resid:** Pediatrics, Wilford Hall USAF Med Ctr, San Antonio, TX 1972-1974; **Fellow:** Pediatric Cardiology, Med Coll GA, Augusta, GA 1974-1976; **Fac Appt:** Clin Prof Pediatrics, Univ Tex, San Antonio

West Coast and Pacific

Bernstein, Daniel MD (PCd) - *Spec Exp:* Transplant Medicine-Heart; Cardiomyopathy; **Hospital:** Stanford Med Ctr; **Address:** Lucile Packard Chldns Hosp, Div Ped Card, 750 Welch Rd, Ste 305, Palo Alto, CA 94304-5731; **Phone:** (650) 723-7913; **Board Cert:** Pediatrics 1984, Pediatric Cardiology 1985; **Med School:** NYU Sch Med 1978; **Resid:** Pediatrics, Montefiore Hosp-Einstein, Bronx, NY 1978-1982; **Fellow:** Pediatric Cardiology, UCSF, San Francisco, CA 1983-1986; **Fac Appt:** Assoc Prof Pediatric Cardiology, Stanford Univ

Hohn, Arno R MD (PCd) - *Spec Exp:* Hypertension; Preventive Cardiology; **Hospital:** Chldns Hosp - Los Angeles; **Address:** Childrens Hospital LA, 4650 Sunset Blvd, MS 34, Los Angeles, CA 90027; **Phone:** (323) 669-2535; **Board Cert:** Pediatrics 1963, Pediatric Cardiology 1965; **Med School:** NY Med Coll 1956; **Resid:** Pediatrics, Buffalo Childrens Hosp, Buffalo, NY 1957-1958; Pediatrics, Childrens Hosp, Philadelphia, PA 1961-1962; **Fellow:** Pediatric Cardiology, Buffalo Childrens Hosp, Buffalo, NY 1962-1963; Pediatric Cardiology, Buffalo Childrens Hosp, Buffalo, NY 1958-1959; **Fac Appt:** Prof Pediatrics, USC Sch Med

Pitlick, Paul T MD (PCd) - *Spec Exp:* Interventional Cardiology; **Hospital:** Stanford Med Ctr; **Address:** 750 Welch Rd, Ste 305, Palo Alto, CA 94304; **Phone:** (650) 723-7913; **Board Cert:** Pediatrics 1975, Pediatric Cardiology 1978; **Med School:** St Louis Univ 1970; **Resid:** Pediatrics, Univ Hosp, San Diego, CA 1971-1972; **Fellow:** Pediatric Cardiology, Univ Hosp, San Diego, CA 1972-1976; **Fac Appt:** Assoc Prof Pediatrics, Stanford Univ

Takahashi, Masato MD (PCd) - *Spec Exp:* Kawasaki Disease; Cardiac Catheterization; **Hospital:** Chldns Hosp - Los Angeles; **Address:** Children's Hosp-LA, Dept Cardiology, 4650 Sunset Blvd, MS 34, Los Angeles, CA 90027-6062; **Phone:** (323) 669-4634; **Board Cert:** Pediatrics 1966, Pediatric Cardiology 1992; **Med School:** Indiana Univ 1960; **Resid:** Pediatrics, Ind Med Ctr, Indianapolis, IN 1961-1963; **Fellow:** Pediatric Cardiology, UCLA Med Ctr, Los Angeles, CA 1964-1967; **Fac Appt:** Prof Pediatrics, USC Sch Med

Teitel, David F MD (PCd) - *Spec Exp:* Pediatric Cardiology - General; **Hospital:** UCSF Med Ctr; **Address:** UCSF, Dept Ped Cardiology, 521 Parnassus St, rm C346, San Francisco, CA 94143; **Phone:** (415) 476-1040; **Board Cert:** Pediatrics 1980, Pediatric Cardiology 1997; **Med School:** Univ Toronto 1975; **Resid:** Pediatrics, Children's Hosp, Montreal, Canada 1980; **Fellow:** Pediatric Cardiology, UCSF Med Ctr, San Francisco, CA 1980-1982; **Fac Appt:** Prof Pediatrics, UCSF

PEDIATRIC CRITICAL CARE MEDICINE

New England

Fleisher, Gary Robert MD (PCCM) - *Spec Exp:* *Trauma;* **Hospital:** Children's Hospital - Boston; **Address:** 300 Longwood Ave, Boston, MA 02115-5724; **Phone:** (617) 355-6000; **Board Cert:** Pediatric Emergency Medicine 1999, Pediatric Infectious Disease 1999; **Med School:** Jefferson Med Coll 1973; **Resid:** Pediatrics, Chldns Hosp, Philadelphia, PA 1974-1976; Pediatrics, Chldns Hosp, Philadelphia, PA 1976-1977; **Fellow:** Infectious Disease, Chldns Hosp, Philadelphia, PA 1977-1979; **Fac Appt:** Prof Pediatrics, Harvard Med Sch

Lister, George MD (PCCM) - *Spec Exp:* *Pediatric Critical Care Medicine - General;* **Hospital:** Yale - New Haven Hosp; **Address:** Yale Univ. Sch Med-Peds, 333 Cedar St., New Haven, CT 06520-8064; **Phone:** (203) 785-4651; **Board Cert:** Pediatric Critical Care Medicine 1996, Pediatrics 1992; **Med School:** Yale Univ 1973; **Resid:** Pediatrics, Yale-New Haven Hosp., New Haven, CT 1974-1975; **Fellow:** Pediatric Critical Care Medicine, Univ California, CA 1975-1978; **Fac Appt:** Prof Pediatrics, Yale Univ

Mid Atlantic

Fuhrman, Bradley P MD (PCCM) - *Spec Exp:* *Liquid Ventilation;* **Hospital:** Chldn's Hosp of Buffalo; **Address:** Chldns Hosp Buffalo, Dept Ped Critical Care, 219 Bryant St, Buffalo, NY 14222-2006; **Phone:** (716) 878-7442; **Board Cert:** Pediatrics 1976, Neonatal-Perinatal Medicine 1979, Pediatric Cardiology 1979, Pediatric Critical Care Medicine 1996; **Med School:** NYU Sch Med 1971; **Resid:** Pediatrics, Univ Minnesota, Minneapolis, MN 1972-1973; **Fellow:** Pediatric Cardiology, Univ Minnesota, Minneapolis, MN 1973-1974; Neonatal-Perinatal Medicine, Univ Minnesota, Minneapolis, MN 1976-1979; **Fac Appt:** Prof Pediatrics, SUNY Buffalo

Holbrook, Peter MD (PCCM) - *Spec Exp:* *Pediatric Critical Care Medicine - General;* **Hospital:** Chldns Natl Med Ctr - DC; **Address:** Chldns Natl Med Ctr, 111 Michigan Ave NW, Washington, DC 20010-2916; **Phone:** (202) 884-3256; **Board Cert:** Pediatrics 1975, Pediatric Critical Care Medicine 1987; **Med School:** Penn State Univ-Hershey Med Ctr 1970; **Resid:** Pediatrics, Johns Hopkins Hosp, Baltimore, MD 1971-1972; **Fellow:** Pediatric Critical Care Medicine, Univ Pittsburgh, Pittsburgh, PA 1972-1973; **Fac Appt:** Prof Pediatrics, Geo Wash Univ

Kochanek, Patrick MD (PCCM) - *Spec Exp:* *Head Injury;* **Hospital:** Chldn's Hosp of Pittsbrgh; **Address:** Safar Ctr for Resuscitation Research, 3434 5th Ave, Ste 201, Pittsburgh, PA 15260; **Phone:** (412) 383-1900; **Board Cert:** Pediatrics 1985, Pediatric Critical Care Medicine 1987; **Med School:** Univ Chicago-Pritzker Sch Med 1980; **Resid:** Pediatrics, UC San Diego, San Diego, CA 1981-1983; **Fellow:** Pediatric Critical Care Medicine, Chldns Hosp, Washington, DC 1983-1986; **Fac Appt:** Assoc Prof Critical Care Medicine, Univ Pittsburgh

Nichols, David Gregory MD (PCCM) - *Spec Exp:* *Respiratory Failure; Mechanical Ventilation;* **Hospital:** Johns Hopkins Hosp - Baltimore; **Address:** Johns Hopkins Univ Hosp, 600 N Wolfe St, Bldg Blalock - rm 912, Baltimore, MD 21287-4912; **Phone:** (410) 955-6412; **Board Cert:** Pediatrics 1982, Pediatric Critical Care Medicine 1996; **Med School:** Mount Sinai Sch Med 1977; **Resid:** Pediatrics, Chldns Hosp, Philadelphia, PA 1978-1980; Anesthesiology, Hosp Univ Penn, Philadelphia, PA 1981-1983; **Fellow:** Anesthesiology, Chldns Hosp, Philadelphia, PA 1983; **Fac Appt:** Prof Pediatrics, Johns Hopkins Univ

Thompson, Ann Ellen MD (PCCM) - *Spec Exp:* Mechanical Ventilation; Critical Care; Respiratory Failure; **Hospital:** Chldn's Hosp of Pittsbrgh; **Address:** Dept Pediatric Critical Care, 3705 Fifth Ave Bldg Main Tower - rm 6840, Pittsburgh, PA 15213-2524; **Phone:** (412) 692-5164; **Board Cert:** Pediatric Critical Care Medicine 1996, Pediatrics 1992, Anesthesiology 1980; **Med School:** Tufts Univ 1974; **Resid:** Pediatrics, Chldns Hosp, Philadelphia, PA 1976-1977; Anesthesiology, Hosp Penn, Philadelphia, PA 1977-1980; **Fellow:** Pediatric Anatomy, Chldns Hosp, Philadelphia, PA 1979; **Fac Appt:** Prof Anesthesiology, Univ Pittsburgh

Midwest

Latson, Larry Allen MD (PCCM) - *Spec Exp:* Heart Disease-Congenital; Interventional Cardiology; **Hospital:** Cleveland Clin Fdn (page 57); **Address:** 9500 Euclid Ave/Desk M41, Cleveland, OH 44195; **Phone:** (216) 445-6532; **Board Cert:** Pediatric Cardiology 1983, Pediatric Critical Care Medicine 1992; **Med School:** Baylor Coll Med 1976; **Resid:** Pediatrics, Baylor Coll Med, Houston, TX 1976-1978; **Fellow:** Pediatric Cardiology, Baylor Coll Med, Houston, TX 1978-1981

Perez Fontan, J Julio MD (PCCM) - *Spec Exp:* Respiratory Failure; **Hospital:** St Louis Children's Hospital; **Address:** 1 Children's Pl, Ste 5S20, St Louis, MO 63110; **Phone:** (314) 454-2527; **Board Cert:** Pediatrics 1987, Pediatric Critical Care Medicine 1996; **Med School:** Spain 1977; **Resid:** Pediatrics, Chldns Hosp/Univ Barcelona 1979-1981; **Fellow:** Critical Care Medicine, UCSF, San Francisco, CA 1981-1984; **Fac Appt:** Prof Pediatrics, Washington Univ, St Louis

Sarnaik, Ashok P MD (PCCM) - *Spec Exp:* Critical Care; Perinatal Medicine; **Hospital:** Chldns Hosp of Michigan (page 59); **Address:** Critical Care Medicine, 3901 Beaubien, Detroit, MI 48201-2119; **Phone:** (313) 745-5629; **Board Cert:** Pediatric Critical Care Medicine 1996, Neonatal-Perinatal Medicine 1979; **Med School:** India 1969; **Resid:** Pediatrics, Chldns Hosp Mich, Detroit, MI 1971-1974; Critical Care Medicine, JJ Hosp-Bombay Univ, Bombay, India 1970-1971; **Fellow:** Neonatal-Perinatal Medicine, Chldns Hosp Mich, Detroit, MI 1974-1975; **Fac Appt:** Prof Pediatrics, Wayne State Univ

Southwest

Anand, Kanwaljeet Singh MD/PhD (PCCM) - *Spec Exp:* Pain Management; Critical Care; **Hospital:** Arkansas Chldns Hosp; **Address:** Arkansas Childrens Hosp, Div CCM, 800 Marshall Street, Bldg Sturg - rm 431, Little Rock, AR 72202-3591; **Phone:** (501) 320-1008; **Board Cert:** Pediatrics 1991, Critical Care Medicine 1994; **Med School:** India 1981; **Resid:** Pediatrics, Children's Hosp, Boston, MA 1988-1991; Pediatric Critical Care Medicine, Mass Genl Hosp, Boston, MA 1991-1993; **Fellow:** Neonatal-Perinatal Medicine, John Radcliffe Hosp, Headington, Oxford, U.K. 1982-1985; Anesthesiology, Children's Hosp, Boston, MA 1985-1988; **Fac Appt:** Prof Pediatrics, Univ Ark

West Coast and Pacific

Brill, Judith Eileen MD (PCCM) - *Spec Exp:* Pediatric Critical Care Medicine - General; **Hospital:** UCLA Med Ctr; **Address:** 10833 Le Conte Ave Bldg MDCC - rm 1294, Los Angeles, CA 90095; **Phone:** (310) 825-9124; **Board Cert:** Anesthesiology 1986, Pediatrics 1982; **Med School:** Harvard Med Sch 1977; **Resid:** Pediatrics, Chldns Hosp Med Ctr, Boston, MA 1978-1979; Pediatrics, UCLA, Los Angeles, CA 1980-1981; **Fellow:** Anesthesiology, Mass Genl Hosp, Boston, MA 1979-1982; **Fac Appt:** Prof Medicine, UCLA

Zimmerman, Jerry John MD (PCCM) - *Spec Exp:* *Inflammation in Critical Illness; Sepsis & Septic Shock;* **Hospital:** Chldns Hosp and Regl Med Ctr - Seattle; **Address:** Children's Hosp & Regl Med Ctr, G-906 CH-05, 4800 Sandpoint Way NE, Seattle, WA 98105; **Phone:** (206) 527-3862; **Board Cert:** Pediatrics 1984, Pediatric Critical Care Medicine 1987; **Med School:** Univ Wisc 1979; **Resid:** Pediatrics, Univ Wisc, Madison, WI 1980-1982; **Fellow:** Pediatric Critical Care Medicine, Chldns Natl Med Ctr, Washintgon, DC 1982-1984; **Fac Appt:** Prof Pediatrics, Univ Wash

PEDIATRIC ENDOCRINOLOGY

New England

Casella, Samuel Joseph MD (PEn) - *Spec Exp:* Thyroid Disorders; Growth/Development Disorders; **Hospital:** Dartmouth - Hitchcock Med Ctr; **Address:** 1 Medical Center Drive, Lebanon, NH 03756; **Phone:** (603) 650-5487; **Board Cert:** Pediatric Endocrinology 1986, Pediatrics 1985; **Med School:** SUNY Syracuse 1981; **Resid:** Pediatrics, Upstate Med Ctr, Syracuse, NY 1981-1984; **Fellow:** Pediatric Endocrinology, NC Meml Hosp-Univ NC, Chapel Hill, NC 1984-1986; **Fac Appt:** Assoc Prof Pediatrics, Johns Hopkins Univ

Levitsky, Lynne Lipton MD (PEn) - *Spec Exp:* Diabetes; Growth/Development Disorders; Cushing's Syndrome; **Hospital:** MA Genl Hosp; **Address:** Mass Genl Hosp, Dept Endo, 55 Fruit St, Boston, MA 02114; **Phone:** (617) 726-2909; **Board Cert:** Pediatrics 1971, Pediatric Endocrinology 1978; **Med School:** Yale Univ 1966; **Resid:** Pediatrics, Albert Einstein Coll Med, Bronx, NY 1966-1967; Pediatrics, Children's Hosp, Philadelphia, PA 1967-1968; **Fellow:** Pediatric Endocrinology, Univ Maryland Hosp, Baltimore, MD 1968-1970; **Fac Appt:** Assoc Prof Pediatrics, Harvard Med Sch

Tamborlane, William V MD (PEn) - *Spec Exp:* Diabetes; **Hospital:** Yale - New Haven Hosp; **Address:** Yale Sch Med, 333 Cedar St, New Haven, CT 06510-3289; **Phone:** (203) 785-4648; **Board Cert:** Pediatrics 1978, Pediatric Endocrinology 1986; **Med School:** Georgetown Univ 1972; **Resid:** Pediatrics, Georgetown U Hosp, Washington, DC 1972-1975; **Fellow:** Pediatric Endocrinology, Yale U Sch Med, New Haven, CT 1975-1977; **Fac Appt:** Prof Pediatrics, Yale Univ

Mid Atlantic

Becker, Dorothy J MD (PEn) - *Spec Exp:* Diabetes; **Hospital:** Chldn's Hosp of Pittsbrgh; **Address:** Children's Hosp-Pitts, Div EDM, 3705 5th Ave, Pittsburgh, PA 15213; **Phone:** (412) 692-5172; **Board Cert:** Pediatrics 1978, Pediatric Endocrinology 1978; **Med School:** Univ Pittsburgh 1964; **Resid:** Endocrinology, Diabetes & Metabolism, Univ Capetown, South Africa 1972-1974; Pediatrics, Univ Capetown, South Africa 1970-1972; **Fellow:** Pediatric Endocrinology, Univ Pittsburgh, Pittsburgh, PA 1974-1976; **Fac Appt:** Prof Pediatrics, Univ Pittsburgh

Chrousos, George MD (PEn) - *Spec Exp:* Stress Disorders; **Hospital:** Natl Inst of Hlth - Clin Ctr; **Address:** 10 Centre Drive, Bldg 10, Ste 9D42, Bethesda, MD 20892-1583; **Phone:** (301) 496-5800; **Board Cert:** Pediatrics 1980, Pediatric Endocrinology 1980; **Med School:** Greece 1975; **Resid:** Pediatrics, NYU Med Ctr, New York, NY 1976-1978; **Fellow:** Endocrinology, Natl Inst Hlth, Bethesda, MD 1978-1980

Levine, Lenore MD (PEn) - *Spec Exp:* Sexual Development; Growth Disorders; Adrenal Disorders; **Hospital:** NY Presby Hosp - Columbia Presby Med Ctr (page 70); **Address:** 630 W 168th St, rm PHE522, New York, NY 10032-3702; **Phone:** (212) 305-6559; **Board Cert:** Pediatrics 1993, Pediatric Endocrinology 1993; **Med School:** NYU Sch Med 1958; **Resid:** Pediatrics, Bellevue Hosp Ctr, New York, NY 1958-1960; **Fellow:** Pediatrics, NY Hosp, New York, NY 1960-1961; Pediatric Endocrinology, NY Hosp, New York, NY 1967-1969; **Fac Appt:** Prof Pediatrics, Columbia P&S

Moshang Jr., Thomas MD (PEn) - *Spec Exp:* Growth/Development Disorders; **Hospital:** Chldn's Hosp of Philadelphia; **Address:** Children's Hospital of Philadelphia - Div Endocrinology, 34th St and Civic Center Blvd, rm 8216, Philadelphia, PA 19104; **Phone:** (215) 590-3174; **Board Cert:** Pediatrics 1967, Pediatric Endocrinology 1978; **Med School:** Univ MD Sch Med 1962; **Resid:** Pediatrics, Childrens Hosp, Philadelphia, PA 1963-1965; **Fellow:** Pediatric Endocrinology, Childrens Hosp, Philadelphia, PA 1967-1970; **Fac Appt:** Prof Pediatrics, Univ Penn

New, Maria Iandolo MD (PEn) - *Spec Exp:* Diabetes; Adrenal Disorders; Growth/Development Disorders; **Hospital:** NY Presby Hosp - NY Weill Cornell Med Ctr (page 70); **Address:** 525 E 68th St, Ste M622, New York, NY 10021; **Phone:** (212) 746-3450; **Board Cert:** Pediatrics 1960; **Med School:** Univ Penn 1954; **Resid:** Pediatrics, NY Hosp, New York, NY 1955-1957; **Fellow:** Pediatric Endocrinology, NY Hosp, New York, NY 1957-1958; Endocrinology, Diabetes & Metabolism, NY Hosp, New York, NY 1961-1964; **Fac Appt:** Prof Pediatrics, Cornell Univ-Weill Med Coll

Oberfield, Sharon MD (PEn) - *Spec Exp:* Adrenal Disorders; Thyroid Disorders; Growth & Pubertal Disorders; **Hospital:** NY Presby Hosp - Columbia Presby Med Ctr (page 70); **Address:** 630 W 168th St, Bldg PHE522, New York, NY 10032-3702; **Phone:** (212) 305-6559; **Board Cert:** Pediatrics 2000, Pediatric Endocrinology 2000; **Med School:** Cornell Univ-Weill Med Coll 1974; **Resid:** Pediatrics, NY Hosp-Cornell, New York, NY 1974-1976; **Fellow:** Pediatric Endocrinology, NY Hosp-Cornell, New York, NY 1976-1979; **Fac Appt:** Prof Pediatric Endocrinology, Columbia P&S

Plotnick, Leslie Parker MD (PEn) - *Spec Exp:* Diabetes; **Hospital:** Johns Hopkins Hosp - Baltimore; **Address:** 600 N Wolfe St Bldg Park - rm 211, Baltimore, MD 21287-2520; **Phone:** (410) 955-6463; **Board Cert:** Pediatric Endocrinology 1978, Pediatrics 1975; **Med School:** Univ MD Sch Med 1970; **Resid:** Pediatrics, Johns Hopkins Hosp, Baltimore, MD 1971-1972; **Fellow:** Pediatric Endocrinology, Johns Hopkins Hosp, Baltimore, MD 1972-1974; **Fac Appt:** Assoc Prof Pediatrics, Johns Hopkins Univ

Slonim, Alfred MD (PEn) - *Spec Exp:* Muscular Disorders-Metabolic; Inflammatory Bowel Disease/Crohn's; **Hospital:** N Shore Univ Hosp at Manhasset; **Address:** 1165 Northern Blvd Fl 4, Manhasset, NY 11030-3801; **Phone:** (516) 869-3390; **Board Cert:** Pediatrics 1978, Pediatric Endocrinology 1986; **Med School:** Australia 1958; **Resid:** Pediatrics, Royal Chlds Hosp, Melbourne, Australia 1961-1963; **Fellow:** Pediatrics, Royal Chlds Hosp, Melbourne, Australia 1964-1965; **Fac Appt:** Assoc Prof Pediatrics, NYU Sch Med

Sperling, Mark Alexander MD (PEn) - *Spec Exp:* Diabetes; Growth/Development Disorders; Hypoglycemia; **Hospital:** Chldn's Hosp of Pittsbrgh; **Address:** Chldns Hosp-Pittsburgh, Dept Endo, 3705 Fifth Ave, DeSot Bldg, Fl 4A - Ste 400, Pittsburgh, PA 15213-2524; **Phone:** (412) 692-5172; **Board Cert:** Pediatrics 1986, Pediatric Endocrinology 1986; **Med School:** Australia 1962; **Resid:** Internal Medicine, Prince Henry Hosp, Melbourne, Australia 1963-1964; Pediatrics, Royal Chldns Hosp, Melbourne, Australia 1964-1968; **Fellow:** Pediatric Endocrinology, Chldns Hosp, Pittsburgh, PA 1968-1970; **Fac Appt:** Prof Pediatrics, Univ Pittsburgh

Stanley, CHarles A MD (PEn) - *Spec Exp:* Hyperinsulinism-Congenital; **Hospital:** Chldn's Hosp of Philadelphia; **Address:** Children's Hospital of Philadelphia, Div Endocrinology, 34th & Civic Ctr Blvd, 802 ARC, Philadelphia, PA 19104; **Phone:** (215) 590-3420; **Board Cert:** Pediatrics 1976, Pediatric Endocrinology 1978; **Med School:** Univ VA Sch Med 1970; **Resid:** Pediatrics, Chldrns Hosp, Philadelphia, PA 1970-1972; **Fellow:** Pediatric Endocrinology, Chldrns Hosp, Philadelphia, PA 1972-1976; **Fac Appt:** Prof Pediatrics, Univ Penn

Southeast

Cleveland, William MD (PEn) - *Spec Exp:* Pediatric Endocrinology - General; **Hospital:** Univ of Miami - Jackson Meml Hosp; **Address:** 1601 NW 12th Ave, Miami, FL 33136; **Phone:** (305) 243-6936; **Board Cert:** Pediatrics 1957, Pediatric Endocrinology 1978; **Med School:** Meharry Med Coll 1950; **Resid:** Pediatrics, Vanderbilt Univ, Nashville, TN 1951-1952; Pediatrics, Childrens Hosp, St Louis, MO 1955-1956; **Fellow:** Pediatric Endocrinology, Johns Hopkins Hosp, Baltimore, MD 1958-1960; **Fac Appt:** Prof Pediatric Endocrinology, Univ Miami Sch Med

PEDIATRIC ENDOCRINOLOGY

Southeast

Diamond, Frank MD (PEn) - *Spec Exp:* Pediatric Endocrinology - General; **Hospital:** All Children's Hosp; **Address:** 880 6th St South, Ste 120, St Petersburg, FL 33701; **Phone:** (727) 892-4237; **Board Cert:** Pediatrics 1979, Pediatric Endocrinology 1980; **Med School:** Penn State Univ-Hershey Med Ctr 1974; **Resid:** Pediatrics, Childrens Hosp-Univ Alabama, Birmingham, AL 1975-1976; **Fellow:** Pediatric Endocrinology, Childrens Hosp-Univ Penn, Philadelphia, PA 1976-1978; **Fac Appt:** Asst Clin Prof Pediatrics, Univ S Fla Coll Med

Freemark, Michael Scott MD (PEn) - *Spec Exp:* Thyroid Disorders; Growth/Development Disorders; Diabetes; **Hospital:** Duke Univ Med Ctr (page 60); **Address:** Duke Univ Med Ctr, Erwin Rd, Bldg Bell - rm 314, Box 3080, Durham, NC 27710; **Phone:** (919) 684-3772; **Board Cert:** Pediatrics 1980, Pediatric Endocrinology 1984; **Med School:** Duke Univ 1976; **Resid:** Pediatrics, Duke Univ Med Ctr, Durham, NC 1976-1979; **Fellow:** Pediatric Endocrinology, Duke Univ Med Ctr, Durham, NC 1980-1984; Pediatric Endocrinology, Hospital Necker Enfants Malades, Paris, France 1993; **Fac Appt:** Assoc Prof Pediatrics, Duke Univ

Friedman, Nancy Eisenberg MD (PEn) - *Spec Exp:* Calcium Disorders; Bone Disorders-Metabolic; Growth/Development Disorders; **Hospital:** Duke Univ Med Ctr (page 60); **Address:** Duke Univ Med Ctr, Div Endocrinology, PO Box 3080, Durham, NC 27710; **Phone:** (919) 684-3772; **Board Cert:** Pediatrics 1979, Pediatric Endocrinology 1995; **Med School:** Med Coll VA 1975; **Resid:** Pediatrics, Chldns Hosp Med Ctr, Cincinnati, OH 1975-1977; Pediatrics, Chldns Meml Hosp, Chicago, IL 1977-1978; **Fellow:** Endocrinology, Diabetes & Metabolism, Michael Reese Hosp, Chicago, IL 1978-1980; **Fac Appt:** Asst Clin Prof Pediatrics, Duke Univ

Schwartz, Robert P MD (PEn) - *Spec Exp:* Pediatric Endocrinology - General; **Hospital:** Wake Forest Univ Baptist Med Ctr (page 81); **Address:** Wake Forest Univ Sch of Med - Dept Ped, Med Ctr Blvd, Winston-Salem, NC 27157; **Phone:** (336) 716-4126; **Board Cert:** Pediatric Endocrinology 1986, Pediatrics 1994; **Med School:** Univ Fla Coll Med 1968; **Resid:** Pediatrics, Charlotte Meml Hosp, Charlotte, NC 1969-1970; Pediatrics, Duke Med Ctr, Durham, NC 1971; **Fellow:** Pediatric Endocrinology, Duke Med Ctr, Durham, NC 1970-1971; Pediatric Endocrinology, Duke Med Ctr, Durham, NC 1973-1974; **Fac Appt:** Assoc Prof Pediatrics, Wake Forest Univ Sch Med

Silverstein, Janet H MD (PEn) - *Spec Exp:* Diabetes; Growth/Development Disorders; **Hospital:** Shands Hlthcre at Univ of FL (page 73); **Address:** Univ Florida - Shands Hlthcare, 1600 SW Archer Rd, Box 100296, Gainesville, FL 32610; **Phone:** (352) 334-1390; **Board Cert:** Pediatrics 1975, Pediatric Endocrinology 1978; **Med School:** Univ Penn 1970; **Resid:** Pediatrics, Children's Hosp, Philadelphia, PA 1970-1972; Pediatrics, Children's Hosp, Philadelphia, PA 1974-1975; **Fellow:** Pediatric Endocrinology, Duke Univ Med Ctr, Durham, NC 1975-1977; **Fac Appt:** Prof Pediatric Endocrinology, Univ Fla Coll Med

Midwest

Allen, David Bruce MD (PEn) - *Spec Exp:* Diabetes; **Hospital:** Univ WI Hosp & Clins; **Address:** 600 Highland Ave, rm H4-4, Madison, WI 53792; **Phone:** (608) 263-6420; **Board Cert:** Pediatric Endocrinology 1997, Pediatrics 1986; **Med School:** Duke Univ 1980; **Resid:** Pediatrics, Univ Wisc Hosp, Madison, WI 1982-1985; **Fellow:** Pediatric Endocrinology, Univ Wisc Hosp, Madison, WI 1985-1988; **Fac Appt:** Assoc Prof Pediatrics, Univ Wisc

Dahms, William MD (PEn) - *Spec Exp:* Diabetes; Growth/Development Disorders; **Hospital:** Rainbow Babies & Chldns Hosp; **Address:** 11100 Euclid Ave, Ste 737, Dept Peds, Diabetes Endocrine Metabolism Div, Cleveland, OH 44106; **Phone:** (216) 844-3661; **Board Cert:** Pediatrics 1974, Pediatric Endocrinology 1983; **Med School:** Univ Wash 1969; **Resid:** Pediatrics, Cornell Med Ctr, New York, NY 1969-1973; **Fellow:** Pediatric Endocrinology, ULCA-Harbor Genl Hosp, Los Angeles, CA 1973-1975; **Fac Appt:** Prof Pediatrics, Case West Res Univ

632

Foster, Carol M MD (PEn) - *Spec Exp:* Diabetes; Growth/Development Disorders; Pubertal Disorders; **Hospital:** Motts Chldns Hosp; **Address:** A Alfred Taubman Hlth Care Ctr, Dept Endocrinology, 1500 E Medical Center Dr, 1st Fl, Reception Area D, Rm D1205, Ann Arbor, MI 48109-0718; **Phone:** (734) 764-5175; **Board Cert:** Pediatrics 1983, Pediatric Endocrinology 1983; **Med School:** Washington Univ, St Louis 1978; **Resid:** Pediatrics, Univ Utah Hlth Scis Ctr, Salt Lake City, UT 1979-1981; **Fellow:** Pediatric Endocrinology, Natl Inst Hlth, Bethesda, MD 1981-1984; **Fac Appt:** Prof Pediatrics, Univ Mich Med Sch

Gutai, James MD (PEn) - *Spec Exp:* Pediatric Endocrinology - General; **Hospital:** Chldns Hosp of Michigan (page 59); **Address:** Wayne State Univ , Morris J Hood Comp Diabetes Ctr, Univ Hlth Ctr, 4201 St Antoine, Rm 9A11, Detroit, MI 48201; **Phone:** (313) 577-0133; **Board Cert:** Pediatrics 1977, Pediatric Endocrinology 1980; **Med School:** Temple Univ 1970; **Resid:** Pediatrics, Johns Hopkins Hosp, Baltimore, MD 1975-1976; **Fellow:** Pediatric Endocrinology, Johns Hopkins Hosp, Baltimore, MD 1973-1976; **Fac Appt:** Prof Pediatrics, Wayne State Univ

Levy, Richard Alshuler MD (PEn) - *Spec Exp:* Adrenal Disorders; Pituitary Disorders; Thyroid Disorders; **Hospital:** Rush-Presby - St Luke's Med Ctr (page 72); **Address:** 1725 W Harrison St, Ste 328, Chicago, IL 60612-3863; **Phone:** (312) 942-8989; **Board Cert:** Endocrinology 1985, Pediatric Endocrinology 1986; **Med School:** Louisiana State Univ 1971; **Resid:** Internal Medicine, Univ Mass Med, Worchester, MA 1975-1977; Pediatrics, Beth Israel, New York, NY 1977-1978; **Fellow:** Endocrinology, Diabetes & Metabolism, Barnes Hosp, St Louis, MO 1979-1982; **Fac Appt:** Asst Prof Medicine, Rush Med Coll

Maurer, William MD (PEn) - *Spec Exp:* Growth/Development Disorders; Thyroid Disorders; Diabetes; **Hospital:** St Francis Hosp - Evanston; **Address:** 320 E Armstrong Ave, Peoria, IL 61603; **Phone:** (309) 624-9680; **Board Cert:** Pediatrics 1971, Pediatric Endocrinology 1978; **Med School:** Ohio State Univ 1966; **Resid:** Pediatrics, Columbus Children's Hosp, Columbus, OH 1966-1968; **Fellow:** Pediatric Endocrinology, Columbus Children's Hosp, Columbus, OH 1968-1970; Pediatric Endocrinology, Duke Univ Med Ctr, Durham, NC 1972-1975

Rogers, Douglas G MD (PEn) - *Spec Exp:* Diabetes; Growth/Development Disorders; Thyroid Disorders; **Hospital:** Cleveland Clin Fdn (page 57); **Address:** Department of Pediatric Endocrinology, 9500 Euclid Ave, Box A120, Cleveland, OH 44195-0001; **Phone:** (216) 445-8048; **Board Cert:** Pediatrics 1984, Pediatric Endocrinology 1986; **Med School:** Univ Hlth Sci/Chicago Med Sch 1978; **Resid:** Pediatrics, Cardinal Glennon Chldns Hosp, St Louis, MO 1978-1981; **Fellow:** Endocrinology, Diabetes & Metabolism, St Louis Chldns Hosp, St Louis, MO 1983-1985

Rosenfield, Robert L MD (PEn) - *Spec Exp:* Polycystic Ovary Disease; Pubertal Disorders; Menstrual Disorders; **Hospital:** Univ of Chicago Hosps (page 76); **Address:** Univ Chicago Chldns Hosp/Dept of Ped Endo, 5841 S Maryland Ave, MC-5303, Chicago, IL 60637-1463; **Phone:** (773) 702-6169; **Board Cert:** Pediatrics 1986, Pediatric Endocrinology 1986; **Med School:** Northwestern Univ 1960; **Resid:** Pediatrics, Children's Hosp, Philadelphia, PA 1961-1963; **Fellow:** Pediatric Endocrinology, Children's Hosp, Philadelphia, PA 1965-1968; **Fac Appt:** Prof Pediatrics, Univ Chicago-Pritzker Sch Med

White, Neil H MD (PEn) - *Spec Exp:* Pediatric Endocrinology - General; **Hospital:** St Louis Children's Hospital; **Address:** One Chldns Pl, Ste 4S30, Box CB8116, St Louis, MO 63110; **Phone:** (314) 454-6051; **Board Cert:** Pediatrics 1981, Pediatric Endocrinology 1983; **Med School:** Albert Einstein Coll Med 1975; **Resid:** Pediatrics, St Louis Chldns Hosp, St Louis, MO 1976-1977; **Fellow:** Endocrinology, Diabetes & Metabolism, Washington Univ, St Louis, MO 1977-1979; **Fac Appt:** Assoc Prof Pediatrics, Univ Mich Med Sch

Zimmerman, Donald MD (PEn) - *Spec Exp:* Growth/Development Disorders; Thyroid Cancer; Hyperthyroidism; **Hospital:** Mayo Med Ctr & Clin - Rochester, MN; **Address:** Dept Peds, 200 1st St SW, Rochester, MN 55905; **Phone:** (507) 284-2091; **Board Cert:** Internal Medicine 1977, Endocrinology 1979, Pediatrics 1983, Pediatric Endocrinology 1983; **Med School:** Univ IL Coll Med 1974; **Resid:** Internal Medicine, Johns Hopkins Hosp, Baltimore, MD 1975-1977; Pediatrics, Mayo Grad Sch Med, Rochester, MN 1980-1981; **Fellow:** Endocrinology, Diabetes & Metabolism, Mayo Grad Sch Med, Rochester, MN 1977-1980; **Fac Appt:** Prof Pediatrics, Mayo Med Sch

Great Plains and Mountains

Kappy, Michael Steven MD/PhD (PEn) - *Spec Exp:* Growth/Development Disorders; Thyroid Disorders; Pubertal Disorders; **Hospital:** Chldn's Hosp - Denver; **Address:** Children's Hospital, Dept Ped Endocrinology, 1056 E 19th Ave, Box 265, Denver, CO 80218; **Phone:** (303) 861-6061; **Board Cert:** Pediatrics 1973, Pediatric Endocrinology 1980; **Med School:** Univ Wisc 1967; **Resid:** Pediatrics, Univ Colorado Med Ctr, Boulder, CO 1967-1968; Pediatrics, Univ Colorado Med Ctr, Boulder, CO 1970-1972; **Fellow:** Pediatric Endocrinology, Johns Hopkins Hosp, Baltimore, MD 1978-1980; **Fac Appt:** Prof Pediatrics, Univ Colo

Klingensmith, Georgeanna MD (PEn) - *Spec Exp:* Diabetes; **Hospital:** Univ Colo HSC - Denver; **Address:** Barbara Davis Ctr for Childhood Diabetes, 4200 E Ninth Ave, Box B-140, Denver, CO 80262; **Phone:** (303) 315-8796; **Board Cert:** Pediatrics 1976, Pediatric Endocrinology 1978; **Med School:** Duke Univ 1971; **Resid:** Pediatrics, Chldns Hosp, St Louis, MO 1972-1973; **Fellow:** Pediatric Endocrinology, Johns Hopkins Hosp, Batimore, MD 1974-1976; **Fac Appt:** Prof Pediatrics, Univ Colo

Southwest

Kirkland III, John Lindsey MD (PEn) - *Spec Exp:* Endochrinology-Pediatric; **Hospital:** TX Chldns Hosp - Houston; **Address:** Texas Chldns Hosp, Endo Clinic, 6621 Fannin St, Houston, TX 77030; **Phone:** (832) 822-3670; **Board Cert:** Pediatrics 1973, Pediatric Endocrinology 1978; **Med School:** Univ NC Sch Med 1968; **Resid:** Pediatrics, Baylor, Houston, TX 1969-1970; Pediatrics, Guys Hosp, London,England 1970; **Fellow:** Pediatric Endocrinology, Baylor, Houston, TX 1971-1973; **Fac Appt:** Prof Pediatrics, Baylor Coll Med

West Coast and Pacific

Geffner, Mitchell Eugene MD (PEn) - *Spec Exp:* Growth/Development Disorders; Pubertal Disorders; **Hospital:** Chldns Hosp - Los Angeles; **Address:** Div Endocrinology, 4650 Sunset Blvd, MS 61, Los Angeles, CA 90027; **Phone:** (323) 669-4606; **Board Cert:** Pediatric Endocrinology 1983, Pediatrics 1980; **Med School:** Albert Einstein Coll Med 1975; **Resid:** Pediatrics, LAC-USC Med Ctr, Los Angeles, CA 1975-1979; **Fellow:** Pediatric Endocrinology, UCLA, Los Angeles, CA 1979; **Fac Appt:** Prof Pediatric Endocrinology, UCLA

Kaufman, Francine R MD (PEn) - *Spec Exp:* Diabetes; Growth/Development Disorders; **Hospital:** Chldns Hosp - Los Angeles; **Address:** Children's Hospital - Div of Endocrinology, 4650 W Sunset Blvd, Los Angeles, CA 90027-6062; **Phone:** (323) 669-4606; **Board Cert:** Pediatrics 1980, Pediatric Endocrinology 1983; **Med School:** Univ Hlth Sci/Chicago Med Sch 1976; **Resid:** Pediatrics, Chldn's Hosp, Los Angeles, CA 1976-1978; **Fellow:** Pediatric Endocrinology, Chldn's Hosp, Los Angeles, CA 1978-1980; **Fac Appt:** Prof Pediatrics, USC Sch Med

Wilson, Darrell Mealer MD (PEn) - *Spec Exp:* Endocrinology; Diabetes; **Hospital:** Stanford Med Ctr; **Address:** Stanford Med Ctr, 300 Pasteur Bldg Grant - rm S-302, Stanford, CA 94305-5208; **Phone:** (650) 723-5791; **Board Cert:** Pediatrics 1982, Pediatric Endocrinology 1995; **Med School:** UCSD 1977; **Resid:** Pediatrics, Stanford Med Ctr, Stanford, CA 1978-1980; **Fellow:** Endocrinology, Diabetes & Metabolism, Stanford Med Ctr, Stanford, CA 1980-1984; **Fac Appt:** Assoc Prof Pediatrics, Stanford Univ

PEDIATRIC GASTROENTEROLOGY

New England

Kleinman, Ronald Ellis MD (PGe) - *Spec Exp:* Transplant Medicine-Liver; Nutrition; **Hospital:** MA Genl Hosp; **Address:** 55 Fruit St Bldg Vincent - Ste 107, Boston, MA 02114; **Phone:** (617) 726-2930; **Board Cert:** Pediatrics 1992, Pediatric Gastroenterology 1998; **Med School:** NY Med Coll 1972; **Resid:** Pediatrics, Albert Einstein Coll Med, Bronx, NY 1973-1977; **Fellow:** Pediatric Gastroenterology, Mass Genl Hosp, Boston, MA 1977-1980

Mid Atlantic

Hillemeier, A Craig MD (PGe) - *Spec Exp:* Gastroesophageal Reflux; Inflammatory Bowel Disease/Crohn's; **Hospital:** Hershey Med Ctr - Univ Hosp; **Address:** 500 University Drive, Milton S. Hershey Med Ctr, Dept Ped, MC H085, Hershey, PA 17033-0850; **Phone:** (717) 531-6700; **Board Cert:** Pediatrics 1981, Pediatric Gastroenterology 1998; **Med School:** Loyola Univ-Stritch Sch Med 1976; **Resid:** Pediatrics, Loyola Univ Stritch, Maywood, IL 1976-1978; **Fellow:** Pediatric Gastroenterology, Yale New Haven Med Ctr, New Haven, CT 1978-1982; **Fac Appt:** Prof Pediatrics, Univ Mich Med Sch

Levy, Joseph MD (PGe) - *Spec Exp:* Inflammatory Bowel Disease/Crohn's; Ulcerative Colitis; Gastroesophageal Reflux (GERD); **Hospital:** NY Presby Hosp - Columbia Presby Med Ctr (page 70); **Address:** 3959 Broadway Bldg BHN - rm 726, New York, NY 10032; **Phone:** (212) 305-5693; **Board Cert:** Pediatrics 1979, Pediatric Gastroenterology 1990; **Med School:** Israel 1973; **Resid:** Pediatrics, Beth Israel Med Ctr, New York, NY 1975-1977; **Fellow:** Pediatric Gastroenterology, Columbia-Presby Med Ctr, New York, NY 1977-1979; **Fac Appt:** Clin Prof Pediatrics, Columbia P&S

Mones, Richard MD (PGe) - *Spec Exp:* Inflammatory Bowel Disease/Crohn's; **Hospital:** NY Presby Hosp - Columbia Presby Med Ctr (page 70); **Address:** 205 W End Ave, Ste 8C, New York, NY 10023; **Phone:** (212) 362-6275; **Board Cert:** Pediatrics 1977, Pediatric Gastroenterology 1997; **Med School:** NY Med Coll 1971; **Resid:** Pediatrics, Columbia-Presby, New York, NY 1971-1973; Pediatrics, Columbia-Presby, New York, NY 1975-1977; **Fellow:** Pediatrics, Columbia-Presby, New York, NY; **Fac Appt:** Assoc Clin Prof Pediatrics, Columbia P&S

Newman, Leonard MD (PGe) - *Spec Exp:* Pediatric Gastroenterology - General; **Hospital:** Westchester Med Ctr (page 82); **Address:** NY Med College, Dept Ped, Munger Pavillion - rm 123, Valhalla, NY 10595; **Phone:** (914) 594-4280; **Board Cert:** Pediatrics 1975, Pediatric Gastroenterology 1990; **Med School:** NY Med Coll 1970; **Resid:** Pediatrics, Univ of Calif, San Diego, CA 1971-1972; Pediatrics, NY Med Coll, New York, NY 1972-1973; **Fellow:** Gastroenterology, Albert Einstein, Bronx, NY 1973-1974; **Fac Appt:** Prof Pediatrics, NY Med Coll

Oliva-Hemker, Maria Magdalena MD (PGe) - *Spec Exp:* Inflammatory Bowel Disease/Crohn's; **Hospital:** Johns Hopkins Hosp - Baltimore; **Address:** Johns Hopkins Hosp, 600 N Wolfe St, Bldg Brady - Fl 320, Baltimore, MD 21287; **Phone:** (410) 955-8769; **Board Cert:** Pediatric Gastroenterology 2000, Pediatrics 1990; **Med School:** Johns Hopkins Univ 1986; **Resid:** Pediatrics, Johns Hopkins Hosp, Baltimore, MD 1986-1989; **Fellow:** Gastroenterology, Johns Hopkins Hosp, Baltimore, MD 1989-1992

Schwarz, Kathleen MD (PGe) - *Spec Exp:* Hepatitis C; Hepatitis B; **Hospital:** Johns Hopkins Hosp - Baltimore; **Address:** Johns Hopkins Hosp, Div Pediatric Gastro, 600 N Wolfe St Bldg Brady - Ste 320, Baltimore, MD 21287; **Phone:** (410) 955-8769; **Board Cert:** Pediatric Gastroenterology 1998, Pediatrics 1977; **Med School:** Washington Univ, St Louis 1972; **Resid:** Pediatric Surgery, St Louis Chldrns Hosp, St Louis, MO 1972-1974; **Fac Appt:** Assoc Prof Pediatrics, Johns Hopkins Univ

Schwarz, Steven M MD (PGe) - *Spec Exp:* Gastroesophageal Reflux; Nutritional and Feeding Disorders; Endoscopy-Pediatric; **Hospital:** Long Island Coll Hosp (page 58); **Address:** LI Coll Hosp - Dept of Pediatrics, 339 Hicks St, Brooklyn, NY 11201-5514; **Phone:** (718) 780-1146; **Board Cert:** Pediatrics 1979, Pediatric Gastroenterology 1997; **Med School:** Columbia P&S 1974; **Resid:** Pediatrics, Columbia-Presby Med Ctr, New York, NY 1974-1977; **Fellow:** Pediatric Gastroenterology, Stanford Med Ctr, Stanford, CA 1977-1978; Pediatric Gastroenterology, Columbia-Presby Med Ctr, New York, NY 1978-1980; **Fac Appt:** Prof Pediatrics, SUNY Downstate

Southeast

Novak, Donald A MD (PGe) - *Spec Exp:* Liver Disease; **Hospital:** Shands Hlthcre at Univ of FL (page 73); **Address:** Shands at U F, Dept PedGastro, 1600 SW Archer Rd, Box 100296, Gainesville, FL 32610-0296; **Phone:** (352) 392-6410; **Board Cert:** Pediatrics 1987, Pediatric Gastroenterology 1990; **Med School:** Univ S Fla Coll Med 1981; **Resid:** Pediatrics, Univ South Fla, Tampa, FL 1982-1984; **Fellow:** Pediatric Gastroenterology, Childrens Hosp, Cincinnati, OH 1984-1987; **Fac Appt:** Prof Pediatrics, Univ Fla Coll Med

Rhoads, Jon Marc MD (PGe) - *Spec Exp:* Pediatric Gastroenterology - General; **Hospital:** Univ of NC Hosp (page 77); **Address:** Univ NC-Dept Ped, Box CB7220, Chapel Hill, NC 27599-7220; **Phone:** (919) 966-1343; **Board Cert:** Pediatrics 1986, Pediatric Gastroenterology 1998; **Med School:** Johns Hopkins Univ 1980; **Resid:** Pediatric Surgery, UCLA Med Ctr, Los Angeles, CA 1981-1983; **Fellow:** Pediatrics, Hosp for Sick Chldn, Toronto, Canada 1983-1986; **Fac Appt:** Prof Pediatrics, Univ NC Sch Med

Thompson, John MD (PGe) - *Spec Exp:* Inflammatory Bowel Disease/Crohn's; Short Bowel Syndrome; Ulcerative Colitis; **Hospital:** Univ of Miami - Jackson Meml Hosp; **Address:** Jackson Meml Hosp, Dept Ped, Div GE & Nutrition, 1601 NW 12th Ave, rm 3005A, MC-CD 6001, Miami, FL 33136; **Phone:** (305) 243-6426; **Board Cert:** Pediatric Gastroenterology 1998, Pediatrics 1983; **Med School:** Loyola Univ-Stritch Sch Med 1977; **Resid:** Pediatrics, Wylers Chldns Hosp-Univ Chicago, Chicago, IL 1978-1980; **Fellow:** Pediatric Gastroenterology, Babies Hosp-Columbia Univ, New York, NY 1982-1984; **Fac Appt:** Assoc Prof Pediatrics, Univ Miami Sch Med

Treem, William R MD (PGe) - *Spec Exp:* Liver Disease; Inflammatory Bowel Disease/Crohn's; **Hospital:** Duke Univ Med Ctr (page 60); **Address:** Duke Univ Med Ctr, Box 3009, Durham, NC 27710; **Phone:** (919) 684-5068; **Board Cert:** Pediatrics 1981, Pediatric Gastroenterology 1997; **Med School:** Stanford Univ 1977; **Resid:** Pediatrics, Children's Hosp, Boston, MA 1977-1980; **Fellow:** Pediatric Gastroenterology, Children's Hosp, Philadelphia, PA 1982-1985; **Fac Appt:** Prof Pediatrics, Duke Univ

Ulshen, Martin H MD (PGe) - *Spec Exp:* Intestinal Disease; Liver Disease; **Hospital:** Duke Univ Med Ctr (page 60); **Address:** Duke Univ Med Ctr, Box 3009, Durham, NC 27710; **Phone:** (919) 684-5068; **Board Cert:** Pediatrics 1993, Pediatric Gastroenterology 1998; **Med School:** Univ Rochester 1969; **Resid:** Pediatrics, Univ North Carolina Hosps, Chapel Hill, NC 1969-1970; Pediatrics, Univ Colorado, Denver, CO 1972-1974; **Fellow:** Pediatric Gastroenterology, Univ Colorado, Denver, CO 1974-1975; Pediatric Gastroenterology, Chldns Hosp, Boston, MA 1975-1977; **Fac Appt:** Prof Pediatrics, Duke Univ

Midwest

Berman, James MD (PGe) - *Spec Exp:* Inflammatory Bowel Disease/Crohn's; Feeding & Nutrition; Ulcerative Colitis; **Hospital:** Loyola Univ Med Ctr; **Address:** Loyola Univ Med Ctr, Dept Ped Gastroenterology, 2160 S 1st Ave Bldg 105 - rm 3346, Maywood, IL 60153; **Phone:** (708) 327-9073; **Board Cert:** Pediatrics 1986, Pediatric Gastroenterology 1997; **Med School:** Univ Pittsburgh 1981; **Resid:** Pediatrics, Chldns Hosp, Pittsburgh, PA 1981-1984; **Fellow:** Pediatric Gastroenterology, Chldns Hosp, Boston, MA 1984-1987; **Fac Appt:** Asst Clin Prof Pediatrics, Loyola Univ-Stritch Sch Med

El-Youssef, Mounif MD (PGe) - *Spec Exp:* Liver Disease; **Hospital:** Mayo Med Ctr & Clin - Rochester, MN; **Address:** Div of Pediatric Gastroenterology, 200 1st St SW, 41402, Rochester, MN 55905; **Phone:** (507) 284-2141; **Board Cert:** Pediatric Gastroenterology 1990, Pediatrics 1989; **Med School:** Belgium 1982; **Resid:** Pediatrics, Cleveland Clinic, Cleveland, OH 1985-1987; **Fellow:** Pediatric Gastroenterology, Harvard Med Sch, Cambridge, MA 1987-1990

Gunasekaran, T S MD (PGe) - *Spec Exp:* Pediatric Gastroenterology - General; **Hospital:** Advocate Lutheran Gen Hosp; **Address:** Lutheran Genl Chldns Hosp, Dept Ped Gastro, 1675 Dempster St, Park Ridge, IL 60068; **Phone:** (847) 723-7700; **Board Cert:** Pediatrics 2000, Pediatric Gastroenterology 2000; **Med School:** India 1977; **Resid:** Pediatrics, India 1977-1982; Pediatrics, United Kingdom 1983-1987; **Fellow:** Pediatric Gastroenterology, BC Childrens Hosp, Vancouver, Canada 1991-1992; **Fac Appt:** Assoc Clin Prof Pediatrics, Loyola Univ-Stritch Sch Med

Kirschner, Barbara S MD (PGe) - *Spec Exp:* Ulcerative Colitis; Abdominal Pain-Recurrent; Inflammatory Bowel Disease/Crohn's; **Hospital:** Univ of Chicago Hosps (page 76); **Address:** 5839 S Maryland Ave, Ste C-474, MC 4065, Chicago, IL 60637; **Phone:** (773) 702-6418; **Board Cert:** Pediatrics 1977, Pediatric Gastroenterology 1999; **Med School:** Med Coll PA Hahnemann 1967; **Resid:** Pediatrics, Univ of Chicago, Chicago, IL 1967-1970; **Fellow:** Pediatric Gastroenterology, Univ of Chicago, Chicago, IL 1975-1977; **Fac Appt:** Prof Pediatrics, Univ Chicago-Pritzker Sch Med

Rothbaum, Robert Jay MD (PGe) - *Spec Exp:* Inflammatory Bowel Disease/Crohn's; **Hospital:** St Louis Children's Hospital; **Address:** 1 Children's Pl, Ste 11E10, St Louis, MO 63110; **Phone:** (314) 454-6173; **Board Cert:** Pediatrics 1981, Pediatric Gastroenterology 2004; **Med School:** Univ Chicago-Pritzker Sch Med 1976; **Resid:** Pediatrics, Chldns Hosp Med Ctr, St Louis, MO 1977-1978; **Fellow:** Ambulatory Pediatrics, Chldns Hosp Med Ctr, St Louis, MO 1978-1979; Pediatric Gastroenterology, Chldns Hosp Med Ctr, Cincinnati, OH 1979-1982; **Fac Appt:** Prof Pediatrics, Washington Univ, St Louis

Whitington, Peter MD (PGe) - *Spec Exp:* Transplant Medicine-Liver; Liver Disease; **Hospital:** Children's Mem Hosp; **Address:** Div Pediatric Gastroenterology, 2300 Children's Plaza, Box 57, Chicago, IL 60614; **Phone:** (773) 880-4643; **Board Cert:** Pediatric Gastroenterology 1998, Pediatrics 1977; **Med School:** Univ Tenn Coll Med, Memphis 1971; **Resid:** Pediatrics, Univ Tenn Hosp, Memphis, TN 1971-1974; **Fellow:** Gastroenterology, Johns Hopkins Hosp, Baltimore, MD 1975-1977; Gastroenterology, Univ Wisconsin, Madison, WI 1977-1978; **Fac Appt:** Prof Pediatrics, Northwestern Univ

Wyllie, Robert MD (PGe) - *Spec Exp:* Inflammatory Bowel Disease/Crohn's; Esophageal Disorders; **Hospital:** Cleveland Clin Fdn (page 57); **Address:** 9500 Euclid Ave, Desk A111, Cleveland, OH 44195; **Phone:** (216) 444-2237; **Board Cert:** Pediatrics 1982, Pediatric Gastroenterology 1997; **Med School:** Indiana Univ 1976; **Resid:** Pediatrics, Indiana Univ Med Ctr, Indianapolis, IN 1977-1979; **Fellow:** Pediatric Gastroenterology, Indiana Univ Med Ctr, Indianapolis, IN 1979-1980

Southwest

Klish, William John MD (PGe) - *Spec Exp:* Pediatric Gastroenterology - General; **Hospital:** TX Chldns Hosp - Houston; **Address:** 6701 Fannin St, Ste 1000, Houston, TX 77030-2303; **Phone:** (832) 822-3600; **Board Cert:** Pediatrics 1992, Pediatric Gastroenterology 1998; **Med School:** Univ Wisc 1967; **Resid:** Pediatrics, Baylor Sch Med, Houston, TX 1970-1972; **Fellow:** Nutrition, Baylor Sch Med, Houston, TX 1972-1974; **Fac Appt:** Prof Pediatrics, Baylor Coll Med

West Coast and Pacific

Christie, Dennis MD (PGe) - *Spec Exp:* Gastroenterology; **Hospital:** Chldns Hosp and Regl Med Ctr - Seattle; **Address:** Chldns Hosp Med Ctr, Div GE, 4800 Sand Point Way NE, Box C-5371, Seattle, WA 98105; **Phone:** (206) 526-2521; **Board Cert:** Pediatric Gastroenterology 1998, Pediatrics 1992; **Med School:** Northwestern Univ 1968; **Resid:** Pediatrics, Univ Washington, Seattle, WA 1969-1971; **Fellow:** Pediatric Gastroenterology, UCLA Ctr Hlth & Sci, Los Angeles, CA 1974-1976; **Fac Appt:** Assoc Prof Pediatrics, Univ Wash

Heyman, Melvin Bernard MD (PGe) - *Spec Exp:* Inflammatory Bowel Disease/Crohn's; Short Bowel Syndrome; Gastroesophageal Reflux; **Hospital:** UCSF Med Ctr; **Address:** UCSF, Dept Ped Gastro, 500 Parnassus Ave, Box 0136, San Francisco, CA 94143-0136; **Phone:** (415) 476-5892; **Board Cert:** Pediatrics 1981, Pediatric Gastroenterology 1998; **Med School:** UCLA 1976; **Resid:** Pediatrics, LA Co-USC Med Ctr, Loa Angeles, CA 1976-1979; **Fellow:** Gastroenterology, UCLA Med Ctr, Los Angeles, CA 1979-1981; **Fac Appt:** Prof Pediatrics, UCSF

McDiarmid, Suzanne V MD (PGe) - *Spec Exp:* Transplant Medicine-Liver; Transplant Medicine-Intestine; Transplant Immunology; **Hospital:** UCLA Med Ctr; **Address:** UCLA Med Ctr, 200 Medical Plaza, Ste 265, Los Angeles, CA 90024; **Phone:** (310) 206-6134; **Board Cert:** Pediatrics 1984, Pediatric Gastroenterology 2000; **Med School:** New Zealand 1976; **Resid:** Pediatrics, UCLA Med Center, Los Angeles, CA 1977-1980; **Fac Appt:** Clin Prof Pediatrics, UCLA

PEDIATRIC HEMATOLOGY-ONCOLOGY

New England

Weinstein, Howard MD (PHO) - *Spec Exp:* Bone Marrow Transplant; Leukemia; Lymphoma; **Hospital:** MA Genl Hosp; **Address:** 55 Fruit St, WAC-712, Boston, MA 02114; **Phone:** (617) 724-3315; **Board Cert:** Pediatrics 1977; **Med School:** Univ MD Sch Med 1972; **Resid:** Pediatrics, Mass Genl Hosp, Boston, MA 1974

Mid Atlantic

Brodeur, Garrett MD (PHO) - *Spec Exp:* Neuroblastoma; **Hospital:** Chldn's Hosp of Philadelphia; **Address:** Children's Hospital of Philadelphia, 3615 Civic Center Blvd Bldg 9 Abramson Research Center, Philadelphia, PA 19104; **Phone:** (215) 590-2817; **Board Cert:** Pediatrics 1980, Pediatric Hematology-Oncology 1980; **Med School:** Washington Univ, St Louis 1975; **Resid:** Pediatrics, St Louis Childrns Hosp, St Louis, MO 1976-1977; **Fellow:** Pediatric Hematology-Oncology, St Jude Childrns Rsch Hosp, Memphis, TN 1977-1979; **Fac Appt:** Prof Pediatrics, Univ Penn

Bussel, James MD (PHO) - *Spec Exp:* Platelet Disorders; Immune Deficiency; Bleeding/Coagulation Disorders; **Hospital:** NY Presby Hosp - NY Weill Cornell Med Ctr (page 70); **Address:** 525 E 68th St, Ste P-695, New York, NY 10021; **Phone:** (212) 746-3474; **Board Cert:** Pediatrics 1979, Pediatric Hematology-Oncology 1981; **Med School:** Columbia P&S 1975; **Resid:** Pediatrics, Chldrns Hosp, Cincinnati, OH 1975-1978; **Fellow:** Pediatric Hematology-Oncology, New York Hosp, New York, NY 1978-1981; **Fac Appt:** Prof Pediatric Hematology-Oncology, Cornell Univ-Weill Med Coll

Cairo, Mitchell S MD (PHO) - *Spec Exp:* Bone Marrow Transplant; Leukemia; Lymphoma; **Hospital:** NY Presby Hosp - Columbia Presby Med Ctr (page 70); **Address:** Babies & Chldns Hosp, Columbia Presby, 161 Fort Washington Ave, rm 754, New York, NY 10032-1551; **Phone:** (212) 305-8316; **Board Cert:** Pediatrics 1980, Pediatric Hematology-Oncology 1982; **Med School:** UCSF 1976; **Resid:** Pediatrics, UCLA Med Ctr, Los Angeles, CA 1976-1978; **Fellow:** Pediatric Hematology-Oncology, Indiana Univ Med Ctr, Indianapolis, IN 1979-1981; **Fac Appt:** Prof Pediatrics, Columbia P&S

Civin, Curt Ingraham MD (PHO) - *Spec Exp:* Pediatric Hematology-Oncology - General; **Hospital:** Johns Hopkins Hosp - Baltimore; **Address:** 1650 Orleans St, Ste 2M44, Baltimore, MD 21231; **Phone:** (410) 955-8816; **Board Cert:** Pediatrics 1979, Pediatric Hematology-Oncology 1980; **Med School:** Harvard Med Sch 1974; **Resid:** Pediatrics, Chldns Hosp, Boston, MA 1974-1975; Pediatrics, Chldns Hosp, Boston, MA 1975-1976; **Fellow:** Pediatric Hematology-Oncology, Natl Cancer Inst, Bethesda, MD 1976-1979; **Fac Appt:** Prof Medical Oncology, Johns Hopkins Univ

Dover, George Joseph MD (PHO) - *Spec Exp:* Sickle Cell Disease; **Hospital:** Johns Hopkins Hosp - Baltimore; **Address:** 600 N Wolfe St, Ste CMSC - rm 2-116, Baltimore, MD 21287; **Phone:** (410) 955-5976; **Board Cert:** Pediatric Hematology-Oncology 1978, Pediatrics 1976; **Med School:** Louisiana State Univ 1972; **Resid:** Pediatrics, Johns Hopkins Hosp, Baltimore, MD 1973-1975; **Fellow:** Pediatric Hematology-Oncology, Johns Hopkins Hosp, Baltimore, MD 1975-1977; **Fac Appt:** Prof Medicine, Johns Hopkins Univ

Garvin, James MD/PhD (PHO) - *Spec Exp:* Bone Marrow Transplant; Brain Tumors; **Hospital:** NY Presby Hosp - Columbia Presby Med Ctr (page 70); **Address:** 161 Fort Washington Ave, rm 718, New York, NY 10032; **Phone:** (212) 305-9770; **Board Cert:** Pediatrics 1982, Pediatric Hematology-Oncology 1984; **Med School:** Jefferson Med Coll 1976; **Resid:** Pediatrics, Chldns Hosp, Philadelphia, PA 1976-1978; Pediatrics, Middlesex Hosp, London, England 1978-1979; **Fellow:** Pediatric Hematology-Oncology, Chldns Hosp, Boston, MA 1979-1982; **Fac Appt:** Clin Prof Pediatrics, Columbia P&S

Green, Daniel M MD (PHO) - *Spec Exp:* Wilms' Tumor; **Hospital:** Roswell Park Cancer Inst; **Address:** Roswell Park Cancer Inst, Dept Pediatrics, Elm & Carlton Sts, Buffalo, NY 14263; **Phone:** (716) 845-2334; **Board Cert:** Pediatrics 1978, Pediatric Hematology-Oncology 1997; **Med School:** St Louis Univ 1973; **Resid:** Pediatrics, Boston City Hosp, Boston, MA 1973-1975; **Fellow:** Pediatric Hematology-Oncology, Chldn's Hosp Med Ctr, Boston, MA 1975-1978; **Fac Appt:** Prof Pediatrics, SUNY Buffalo

Helman, Lee Jay MD (PHO) - *Spec Exp:* Solid Tumors; **Hospital:** Natl Inst of Hlth - Clin Ctr; **Address:** National Cancer Inst, NIH, 10 Center Drive Bldg 10 - rm 13N 240, Bethesda, MD 20892-1880; **Phone:** (301) 496-4257; **Board Cert:** Internal Medicine 1983, Medical Oncology 1985; **Med School:** Univ MD Sch Med 1980; **Resid:** Internal Medicine, Barnes Hosp., St. Louis, MO 1981-1983; **Fellow:** Oncology, Natl Insts Hlth, Bethesda, MD 1983-1986

Keller Jr, Frank G MD (PHO) - *Spec Exp:* Pediatric Hematology-Oncology - General; **Hospital:** WV Univ Hosp - Ruby Memorial; **Address:** Dept Pediatric Hematology/Oncology, One Medical Center Drive, Box 9214, Morgantown, WV 26506; **Phone:** (304) 293-1217; **Board Cert:** Pediatric Hematology-Oncology 1994, Pediatrics 1990; **Med School:** Univ NC Sch Med 1986; **Resid:** Pediatrics, Vanderbilt Univ Med Ctr, Nashville, TN 1986-1990; **Fellow:** Pediatric Hematology-Oncology, Duke Univ Med Ctr, Durham, NC 1990-1993

Kushner, Brian MD (PHO) - *Spec Exp:* Neuroblastoma; Bone Marrow Transplant; Immunotherapy; **Hospital:** Mem Sloan Kettering Cancer Ctr; **Address:** 1275 York Ave, rm H1113, New York, NY 10021-6007; **Phone:** (212) 639-6793; **Board Cert:** Pediatric Hematology-Oncology 1987, Pediatrics 1983; **Med School:** Johns Hopkins Univ 1976; **Resid:** Pediatrics, Columbia-Presbyterian Med Ctr, New York, NY 1977-1978; Pediatrics, NY Hosp, New York, NY 1978-1979; **Fellow:** Pediatric Hematology-Oncology, Boston Childrens Hosp, Boston, MA 1979-1980; Pediatric Hematology-Oncology, Meml Sloan Kettering Cancer Ctr, NY, NY 1983-1986; **Fac Appt:** Assoc Prof Pediatrics, Cornell Univ-Weill Med Coll

Meek, Rita MD (PHO) - *Spec Exp:* Pediatric Hematology-Oncology - General; **Hospital:** Alfred I Dupont Hosp for Children; **Address:** 1600 Rockland Rd, Wilmington, DE 19899; **Phone:** (302) 651-5500; **Board Cert:** Pediatrics 1979, Pediatric Hematology-Oncology 1980; **Med School:** Geo Wash Univ 1974; **Resid:** Pediatrics, Chldns Hosp Natl Med Ctr, Washington, DC 1975-1977; **Fellow:** Pediatric Hematology-Oncology, Chldns Hosp Natl Med Ctr, Washington, DC 1977-1979; **Fac Appt:** Assoc Clin Prof Pediatrics, Jefferson Med Coll

Meyers, Paul MD (PHO) - *Spec Exp:* Solid Tumors; Bone Tumors; **Hospital:** Mem Sloan Kettering Cancer Ctr; **Address:** 1275 York Ave, Box 411, New York, NY 10021-6007; **Phone:** (212) 639-5952; **Board Cert:** Pediatrics 1978, Pediatric Hematology-Oncology 1978; **Med School:** Mount Sinai Sch Med 1973; **Resid:** Pediatrics, Mount Sinai, New York, NY 1973-1976; **Fellow:** Pediatric Hematology-Oncology, NY Hosp-Cornell, New York, NY 1976-1979; **Fac Appt:** Assoc Clin Prof Pediatrics, Cornell Univ-Weill Med Coll

O'Reilly, Richard MD (PHO) - *Spec Exp:* Bone Marrow Transplant; **Hospital:** Mem Sloan Kettering Cancer Ctr; **Address:** 1275 York Ave, rm H1409, New York, NY 10021; **Phone:** (212) 639-5957; **Board Cert:** Pediatric Hematology-Oncology 1973, Pediatrics 1974; **Med School:** Univ Rochester 1968; **Resid:** Pediatrics, Chldrns Hosp, Boston, MA 1971-1972; **Fellow:** Infectious Disease, Chldrns Hosp, Boston, MA 1972-1973

Reaman, Gregory MD (PHO) - *Spec Exp:* Leukemia; Oncology; **Hospital:** Chldns Natl Med Ctr - DC; **Address:** 111 Michigan Ave NW, Washington, DC 20010-2916; **Phone:** (202) 884-2147; **Board Cert:** Pediatric Hematology-Oncology, Pediatrics; **Med School:** Loyola Univ-Stritch Sch Med 1973; **Resid:** Hematology, Montreal Chldrns Hosp-McGill, Montreal, Canada 1974-1975; Pediatrics, Montreal Chldrns Hosp-McGill, Montreal, Canada 1975-1976; **Fellow:** Pediatric Neuro-Oncology, Natl Cancer Inst, Bethesda, MD 1976-1979; **Fac Appt:** Prof Pediatrics, Geo Wash Univ

Schwartz, Cindy Lee MD (PHO) - *Spec Exp:* Hodgkin's Disease; Osteosarcoma; Consequences of Cancer Therapy; **Hospital:** Johns Hopkins Hosp - Baltimore; **Address:** Johns Hopkins Hosp, 601 N Wolfe St, rm CMSC-800, Baltimore, MD 21287-0004; **Phone:** (410) 955-2457; **Board Cert:** Pediatrics 1985, Pediatric Hematology-Oncology 1994; **Med School:** Brown Univ 1979; **Resid:** Pediatrics, Johns Hopkins Hosp, Baltimore, MD 1979-1982; **Fellow:** Pediatric Hematology-Oncology, Johns Hopkins Hosp, Baltimore, MD 1982-1985; **Fac Appt:** Assoc Prof Pediatrics, Johns Hopkins Univ

Steinherz, Peter G MD (PHO) - *Spec Exp:* Burkett's Lymphoma; Leukemia; **Hospital:** Mem Sloan Kettering Cancer Ctr; **Address:** 1275 York Ave, MSKCC - Pediatric Cardiology Dept, New York, NY 10021; **Phone:** (212) 639-7951; **Board Cert:** Pediatrics 1973, Pediatric Hematology-Oncology 1978; **Med School:** Albert Einstein Coll Med 1968; **Resid:** Pediatrics, NY Cornell Med Ctr, New York, NY 1969-1971; **Fellow:** Pediatric Hematology-Oncology, NY Cornell Med Ctr, New York, NY 1973-1975; **Fac Appt:** Prof Pediatrics, Cornell Univ-Weill Med Coll

Weiner, Michael MD (PHO) - *Spec Exp:* Hodgkin's Disease; Lymphoma; Leukemia; **Hospital:** NY Presby Hosp - Columbia Presby Med Ctr (page 70); **Address:** 161 Fort Washington Ave, Irving Pavilion-FL 7, New York, NY 10032-3710; **Phone:** (212) 305-9770; **Board Cert:** Pediatrics 1980, Pediatric Hematology-Oncology 1980; **Med School:** SUNY Hlth Sci Ctr 1972; **Resid:** Pediatrics, Montefiore Med Ctr, Bronx, NY 1973-1974; **Fellow:** Pediatric Hematology-Oncology, NYU Med Ctr, New York, NY 1974-1976; Pediatric Hematology-Oncology, Johns Hopkins Univ Hosp, Baltimore, MD 1977-1977; **Fac Appt:** Prof Pediatrics, Columbia P&S

Southeast

Barbosa, Jerry L MD (PHO) - *Spec Exp:* Oncology; **Hospital:** All Children's Hosp; **Address:** Dept Pediatric Hematology-Oncology, 880 6th St S, Ste 140, St Petersburg, FL 33701; **Phone:** (727) 892-4175; **Board Cert:** Pediatric Hematology-Oncology 1978, Pediatrics 1976; **Med School:** Spain 1969; **Resid:** Pediatrics, RI Hosp-Brown Univ, Providence, RI 1972-1974; **Fellow:** Pediatric Hematology-Oncology, Med Coll VA, Richmond, VA 1974-1976; **Fac Appt:** Assoc Clin Prof Pediatric Hematology-Oncology, Univ S Fla Coll Med

Falletta, John MD (PHO) - *Spec Exp:* Hematology; **Hospital:** Duke Univ Med Ctr (page 60); **Address:** Duke Univ Med Center, Box 2916, Durham, NC 27710-2916; **Phone:** (919) 684-3401; **Board Cert:** Pediatrics 1972, Pediatric Hematology-Oncology 1974; **Med School:** Univ Kans 1966; **Resid:** Pediatrics, Baylor, Houston, TX 1969-1971; Pediatrics, Texas Childns Hosp, Houston, TX 1971; **Fellow:** Pediatric Hematology-Oncology, Baylor, Houston, TX 1971-1973; **Fac Appt:** Prof Pediatric Hematology-Oncology, Duke Univ

Graham-Pole, John R MD (PHO) - *Spec Exp:* Bone Marrow Trasplant; **Hospital:** Shands Hlthcre at Univ of FL (page 73); **Address:** Dept Ped Hematology-Oncology, 1600 SW Archer Rd, rm M401, Gainesville, FL 32610-0296; **Phone:** (352) 392-5633; **Board Cert:** Pediatrics 1983, Pediatric Hematology-Oncology 1987; **Med School:** England 1966; **Resid:** Pediatrics, Hosp Sick Chldn, London, England 1968; Pediatrics, Royal Hosp Sick Chldn, London, England 1970; **Fellow:** Pediatric Hematology-Oncology, Royal Hosp for Sick Chldn, Glasgow, England 1971; **Fac Appt:** Prof Pediatrics, Univ Fla Coll Med

Pegelow Jr, Charles Henry MD (PHO) - *Spec Exp:* Sickle Cell Disease; Bleeding/Coagulation Disorders; **Hospital:** Univ of Miami - Jackson Meml Hosp; **Address:** Univ Miami Sch of Med - Dept Ped (R131), 1611 NW 12th East Tower Ave, rm 6006, Miami, FL 33136; **Phone:** (305) 585-6042; **Board Cert:** Pediatrics 1989, Pediatric Hematology-Oncology 1989; **Med School:** Univ Minn 1970; **Resid:** Pediatrics, LA County - USC Med Ctr, Los Angeles, CA 1971-1973; **Fellow:** Pediatric Hematology-Oncology, LA County - USC Med Ctr, Los Angeles, CA 1973-1974; **Fac Appt:** Prof Pediatrics, Univ Miami Sch Med

Rosoff, Phillip Martin MD (PHO) - *Spec Exp:* Cancer Survivors; Down Syndrome; Leukemia; **Hospital:** Duke Univ Med Ctr (page 60); **Address:** Duke University, Box 2916, Durham, NC 27710; **Phone:** (919) 684-6946; **Board Cert:** Pediatrics 1984, Pediatric Hematology-Oncology 1994; **Med School:** Case West Res Univ 1978; **Resid:** Pediatrics, Children's Hosp, Boston, MA 1978-1980; **Fellow:** Pediatric Hematology-Oncology, Children's Hosp, Boston, MA 1980-1984; **Fac Appt:** Assoc Prof Pediatric Hematology-Oncology, Duke Univ

Wang, Winfred C MD (PHO) - *Spec Exp:* Sickle Cell Disease; Bone Marrow Failure Disorders; **Hospital:** St Jude Children's Research Hosp; **Address:** St Jude Chldn Research Hosp, 332 N Lauderdale St, rm R6010, Memphis, TN 38105; **Phone:** (901) 495-3497; **Board Cert:** Pediatrics 1972, Pediatric Hematology-Oncology 1974; **Med School:** Univ Chicago-Pritzker Sch Med 1967; **Resid:** Pediatrics, Montefiore Med Ctr, Bronx, NY 1968-1969; Pediatrics, Kauikeolani Chldn's Hosp, Honolulu, HI 1969-1970; **Fellow:** Pediatric Hematology-Oncology, Univ California, San Fransisco, CA 1973-1975; **Fac Appt:** Prof Pediatrics, Univ Tenn Coll Med, Memphis

Midwest

Abella, Esteban MD (PHO) - *Spec Exp:* Bone Marrow Transplant; Aplastic Anemia; Neuroblastoma; **Hospital:** Chldns Hosp of Michigan (page 59); **Address:** 3901 Breubein Blvd Fl 2 - Ste M28, Div of PedHem, Detroit, MI 48201; **Phone:** (313) 745-5515; **Board Cert:** Pediatric Hematology-Oncology 2001, Pediatrics 1998; **Med School:** Dominican Republic 1985; **Resid:** Pediatrics, Children's Hospital of MI, Detroit, MI 1985-1988; **Fellow:** Pediatric Hematology-Oncology, Children's Hospital of MI, Detroit, MI 1988-1991; **Fac Appt:** Assoc Prof Pediatric Hematology-Oncology, Wayne State Univ

Castle, Valerie MD (PHO) - *Spec Exp:* Neuroblastoma; Bleeding/Coagulation Disorders; **Hospital:** Univ of MI Hlth Ctr; **Address:** 1500 E Med Center Drive, Ste 4303, Box 0938, Ann Arbor, MI 48109; **Phone:** (734) 936-9814; **Board Cert:** Pediatrics 1992, Pediatric Hematology-Oncology 1998; **Med School:** McMaster Univ 1983; **Resid:** Pediatrics, McMaster Univ Med Ctr, Hamilton, ON 1984-1986; **Fellow:** Pediatric Hematology-Oncology, Univ Mich Hosp, Ann Arbor, MI 1986-1989; **Fac Appt:** Assoc Prof Pediatrics, Univ Mich Med Sch

Ferrara, James MD (PHO) - *Spec Exp:* Bone Marrow Transplant; Graft vs Host Disease; **Hospital:** Univ of MI Hlth Ctr; **Address:** 1500 E Med Center Drive, Ste 6308, Ann Arbor, MI 48109-0942; **Phone:** (734) 936-4015; **Board Cert:** Pediatrics 1997; **Med School:** Georgetown Univ 1980; **Resid:** Pediatrics, Chldns Hosp, Boston, MA; **Fellow:** Pediatric Hematology-Oncology, Chldns Hosp, Boston, MA; **Fac Appt:** Prof Pediatrics, Univ Mich Med Sch

Nachman, James MD (PHO) - *Spec Exp:* Leukemia; Osteogenic Sarcomas; Hodgkin's Disease; **Hospital:** Univ of Chicago Hosps (page 76); **Address:** 5841 S Maryland Ave, MC-4060, Chicago, IL 60637; **Phone:** (773) 702-6808; **Board Cert:** Pediatrics 1979, Pediatric Hematology-Oncology 1980; **Med School:** Johns Hopkins Univ 1974; **Resid:** Pediatrics, Chldns Meml Hosp, Chicago, IL 1975-1977; Pediatrics, Fell-Wylers Chldns Hosp, Chicago, IL 1979-1980; **Fellow:** Pediatric Hematology-Oncology, Chldns Meml Hosp, Chicago, IL 1977-1979; **Fac Appt:** Prof Pediatric Surgery, Univ Chicago-Pritzker Sch Med

Puccetti, Diane MD (PHO) - *Spec Exp:* Brain Tumors; Neuro-Oncology; **Hospital:** Univ WI Hosp & Clins; **Address:** 600 Highland Ave, rm H6/411, Madison, WI 53792; **Phone:** (608) 263-6420; **Board Cert:** Pediatric Hematology-Oncology 2000, Pediatrics 1989; **Med School:** Med Coll OH 1985; **Resid:** Pediatrics, UC-Irvine, Orange, CA 1985-1986; Pediatrics, Med Coll Ohio, Toledo, OH 1986-1988; **Fellow:** Pediatric Hematology-Oncology, Riley Hosp for Chldn, Indianapolis, IN 1988-1991; **Fac Appt:** Asst Clin Prof Pediatrics, Univ Wisc

Salvi, Sharad MD (PHO) - *Spec Exp:* Leukemia; Blood Disorders; **Hospital:** Advocate Christ Med Ctr; **Address:** Hope Children's Hosp, 4440 W 95th St, rm 4091, Oak Lawn, IL 60453-2600; **Phone:** (708) 346-4094; **Board Cert:** Pediatrics 1982, Pediatric Hematology-Oncology 1982; **Med School:** India 1974; **Resid:** Pediatrics, Lincoln Meml Hosp, Bronx, NY 1977-1979; **Fellow:** Pediatric Hematology-Oncology, Children's Hosp/Roswell Park Meml Cancer Inst, Buffalo, NY 1979-1981

Sondel, Paul M MD (PHO) - *Spec Exp:* Immunotherapy; Oncology-Pediatric; **Hospital:** Univ WI Hosp & Clins; **Address:** Univ Wisc Clinics, 600 Highland Ave, K4/448 Clinical Sci Ctr, Madison, WI 53792; **Phone:** (608) 263-6420; **Board Cert:** Pediatrics 1981; **Med School:** Harvard Med Sch 1977; **Resid:** Pediatrics, Univ Wisc Hosp, Madison, WI 1978-1980; **Fellow:** Research, Sidney Farber Cancer Inst/Harvard, Boston, MA 1975-1977; **Fac Appt:** Prof Pediatrics, Univ Wisc

Valentino, Leonard A MD (PHO) - *Spec Exp:* Hematology; Bleeding/Coagulation Disorders; Thrombotic Disorders; **Hospital:** Rush-Presby - St Luke's Med Ctr (page 72); **Address:** 1725 W Harrison St, Ste 710, Chicago, IL 60612-3828; **Phone:** (312) 942-5983; **Board Cert:** Pediatrics 1988, Pediatric Hematology-Oncology 1998; **Med School:** Creighton Univ 1984; **Resid:** Pediatrics, Univ Illinios Med Ctr, Chicago, IL 1984-1987; **Fellow:** Pediatric Hematology-Oncology, UCLA Med Ctr, Los Angeles, CA 1987-1990; **Fac Appt:** Assoc Prof Pediatrics, Rush Med Coll

Great Plains and Mountains

Carroll, William L MD (PHO) (relocated to New York, NY)- *Spec Exp:* Pediatric Hematology-Oncology - General; **Hospital:** Mount Sinai Hosp (page 68); **Address:** Mount Sinai Hosp, Div Pediatric Hem/Onc, 1 Gustave L. Levy Pl, Box 1208, New York, NY 10029; **Phone:** (212) 241-7022; **Board Cert:** Pediatrics 1984, Pediatric Hematology-Oncology 1987; **Med School:** UC Irvine 1978; **Resid:** Pediatrics, Chldns Hosp, Cincinnati, OH 1978-1979; Pediatrics, Chldns Hosp, Cincinnati, OH 1979-1981; **Fellow:** Pediatric Hematology-Oncology, Stanford Univ, Stanford, CA 1982-1984; Pediatric Hematology-Oncology, Stanford Univ, Stanford, CA 1984-1987; **Fac Appt:** Prof Pediatrics, Mount Sinai Sch Med

Manco-Johnson, Marilyn MD (PHO) - *Spec Exp:* Hemophilia; Thrombophilia; **Hospital:** Univ Colo HSC - Denver; **Address:** Univ Colorado Hlth Sci Ctr, Hemophilia Ctr, Box 6507, MS F416, Aurora, CO 80045-0507; **Phone:** (303) 724-0365; **Board Cert:** Pediatrics 1979, Pediatric Hematology-Oncology 1980; **Med School:** Jefferson Med Coll 1974; **Resid:** Pediatrics, Univ Colo Affil Hosps, Denver, CO 1975-1977; **Fellow:** Pediatric Hematology-Oncology, Chldn's Hosp/Colo Med Ctr, Denver, CO 1978-1981; **Fac Appt:** Prof Pediatrics, Univ Colo

Odom, Lorrie Furman MD (PHO) - **Spec Exp:** *Leukemia; Solid Tumors;* **Hospital:** Chldn's Hosp - Denver; **Address:** Children's Hosp Cancer Ctr, 1056 E 19th Ave, Ste 4HC3, Box B115, Denver, CO 80218-1007; **Phone:** (303) 861-6740; **Board Cert:** Pediatrics 1974, Pediatric Hematology-Oncology 1976; **Resid:** Pediatrics, Chldns Hosp, Boston, MA 1969-1970; Pediatrics, Chldrns Hosp, Boston, MA 1970-1972; **Fellow:** Pediatric Hematology-Oncology, Dana-Farber Cancer Inst, Boston, MA 1972-1974; Pediatric Hematology-Oncology, Univ Colo Med Ctr, Denver, CO 1974-1975; **Fac Appt:** Prof Pediatrics

Southwest

Berg, Stacey MD (PHO) - **Spec Exp:** *Pediatric Hematology-Oncology - General;* **Hospital:** TX Chldns Hosp - Houston; **Address:** Pediatric Hematology-Oncology, 6621 Fannin St, MC 3-3320, Houston, TX 77030; **Phone:** (832) 824-4588; **Board Cert:** Pediatrics 2000, Pediatric Hematology-Oncology 2000; **Med School:** Univ Pittsburgh 1985; **Resid:** Pediatrics, Chldns Hosp, Pittsburgh, PA 1985-1988; **Fellow:** Pediatric Hematology-Oncology, Natl Inst Hlth, Bethesda, MD 1988-1991

Bleyer, W Archie MD (PHO) - **Spec Exp:** *Adolescent/Young Adult Oncology; Brain & Spinal Cord Tumors;* **Hospital:** Univ of TX MD Anderson Cancer Ctr, The; **Address:** Univ Texas/MD Anderson Cancer Ctr, 1515 Holcombe Blvd, Houston, TX 77030-4009; **Phone:** (713) 792-6603; **Board Cert:** Pediatrics 1986, Pediatric Hematology-Oncology 1986; **Med School:** Univ Rochester 1969; **Resid:** Pediatrics, Univ Washington, Seattle, Wa 1970-1971; Pediatric Hematology-Oncology, Natl Cancer Inst, Bethesda, MD 1971-1974; **Fellow:** Pediatric Hematology-Oncology, Univ Washington, Seattle, WA 1974-1975; Radiation Oncology, Univ Washington, Seattle, WA 1984; **Fac Appt:** Prof Pediatrics, Univ Tex, Houston

Graham, Michael L MD (PHO) - **Spec Exp:** *Bone Marrow Transplant;* **Hospital:** Univ Med Ctr; **Address:** Univ Arizona Hlth Scis, 1501 N Campbell Ave, rm 3336, Box 245073, Tucson, AZ 85724; **Phone:** (520) 626-6527; **Board Cert:** Pediatrics 1980, Pediatric Hematology-Oncology 1984; **Med School:** Brown Univ 1975; **Resid:** Pediatrics, Johns Hopkins Hosp, Baltimore, MD 1975-1978; Pediatric Hematology-Oncology, Johns Hopkins Hosp, Baltimore, MD 1979-1980; **Fellow:** Medical Oncology, Yale-New Haven Hosp, New Haven, CT 1980-1982; **Fac Appt:** Assoc Prof Pediatric Hematology-Oncology, Univ Ariz Coll Med

West Coast and Pacific

Feig, Stephen A MD (PHO) - **Spec Exp:** *Anemia; Bone Marrow Transplant;* **Hospital:** UCLA Med Ctr; **Address:** Department of Pediatrics, 10833 Le Conte Ave, rm A2-410 MDCC, Los Angeles, CA 90024; **Phone:** (310) 825-6708; **Board Cert:** Pediatric Hematology-Oncology 1974, Pediatrics 1968; **Med School:** Columbia P&S 1963; **Resid:** Pediatrics, Mt Sinai Hospital, New York, NY 1963-1966; **Fellow:** Pediatric Hematology-Oncology, Children's Hospital, Boston, MA 1968-1972; **Fac Appt:** Prof Pediatrics, UCLA

Glader, Bertil E MD (PHO) - **Spec Exp:** *Genetic Blood Disorders;* **Hospital:** Stanford Med Ctr; **Address:** Dept Pediatric Hem-Onc, 300 Pasteur Dr, rm H-314B, Stanford, CA 94305-5208; **Phone:** (650) 497-8953; **Board Cert:** Pediatric Hematology-Oncology 1994, Hematology 1983; **Med School:** Northwestern Univ 1968; **Resid:** Pediatrics, Chldns Hosp Med Ctr, Boston, MA 1972-1973; **Fellow:** Hematology, Chldns Hosp Med Ctr, Boston, MA 1973-1975; **Fac Appt:** Prof Pediatrics, Stanford Univ

Matthay, Katherine K MD (PHO) - ***Spec Exp:*** *Neuroblastoma; Bone Marrow & Stem Cell Transplant; Retinoblastoma;* **Hospital:** UCSF Med Ctr; **Address:** UCSF, Dept Ped Onc, 505 Parnassus Ave, Box 0106, San Francisco, CA 94143; **Phone:** (415) 476-0603; **Board Cert:** Pediatrics 1979, Pediatric Hematology-Oncology 1980; **Med School:** Univ Penn 1973; **Resid:** Pediatrics, Univ Colorado, Denver, CO 1974-1976; **Fellow:** Pediatric Hematology-Oncology, UCSF, San Francisco, CA 1977-1979; **Fac Appt:** Prof Pediatrics, UCSF

Siegel, Stuart E MD (PHO) - ***Spec Exp:*** *Leukemias & Solid Tumors; Infections in Pediatric Cancer; Psychosocial Aspects of Pediatric Cancer;* **Hospital:** Chldns Hosp - Los Angeles; **Address:** Children's Hospital, 4650 Sunset Blvd, MS 54, Los Angeles, CA 90027-6016; **Phone:** (323) 669-2205; **Board Cert:** Pediatrics 1973, Pediatric Hematology-Oncology 1976; **Med School:** Boston Univ 1967; **Resid:** Pediatrics, Univ Minnesota Hosps, Minneapolis, MN 1968-1969; **Fellow:** Pediatric Hematology-Oncology, Natl Cancer Inst, Bethesda, MD 1969-1972; **Fac Appt:** Prof Pediatrics, USC Sch Med

PEDIATRIC INFECTIOUS DISEASE

New England

Andiman, Warren A MD (PInf) - *Spec Exp:* AIDS/HIV; **Hospital:** Yale - New Haven Hosp; **Address:** 333 Cedar St, rm 418 LSOG, Box 278064, New Haven, CT 06510-3289; **Phone:** (203) 785-4730; **Board Cert:** Pediatrics 1975; **Med School:** Albert Einstein Coll Med 1969; **Resid:** Pediatrics, Babies Hosp-Col Presby, New York, NY 1969-1971; **Fellow:** Pediatric Infectious Disease, Yale Univ Sch Med, New Haven, CT 1971-1973; **Fac Appt:** Prof Pediatrics, Yale Univ

Durbin, William Applebee MD (PInf) - *Spec Exp:* Pediatric Infectious Disease - General; **Hospital:** U Mass Meml Hlth Care - Worcester; **Address:** 55 Lake Ave N, Worcester, MA 01655; **Phone:** (508) 856-2650; **Board Cert:** Pediatrics 1978, Pediatric Infectious Disease 2001; **Med School:** Columbia P&S 1972; **Resid:** Pediatrics, Boston Chlns Hosp, Boston, MA 1975-1977; **Fellow:** Infectious Disease, Boston Chldns Hosp/beth Israel, Boston, MA 1977-1979; **Fac Appt:** Prof Pediatrics, Univ Mass Sch Med

Shapiro, Eugene D MD (PInf) - *Spec Exp:* Lyme Disease; **Hospital:** Yale - New Haven Hosp; **Address:** Dept Pediatrics, 333 Cedar St, New Haven, CT 06520; **Phone:** (203) 688-4518; **Board Cert:** Pediatric Infectious Disease 1994, Pediatrics 1980; **Med School:** UCSF 1976; **Resid:** Pediatrics, Chldns Hosp, Pittsburgh, PA 1976-1979; **Fellow:** Pediatric Infectious Disease, Chldns Hosp, Pittsburgh, PA 1979-1981; Research, Yale Univ, New Haven, CT 1981-1983; **Fac Appt:** Assoc Prof Pediatrics, Yale Univ

Mid Atlantic

Borkowsky, William MD (PInf) - *Spec Exp:* AIDS/HIV; **Hospital:** NYU Med Ctr (page 71); **Address:** 550 1st Ave Fl 8W - rm 51, New York, NY 10016; **Phone:** (212) 263-6513; **Board Cert:** Pediatrics 1979, Infectious Disease 1979; **Med School:** NYU Sch Med 1979; **Resid:** Pediatrics, Bellevue Hosp, New York, NY 1972-1975; **Fellow:** Infectious Disease, NYU Sch of Med, New York, NY 1975-1978; **Fac Appt:** Prof Pediatrics, NYU Sch Med

Gershon, Anne MD (PInf) - *Spec Exp:* Herpes; Meningitis; **Hospital:** NY Presby Hosp - Columbia Presby Med Ctr (page 70); **Address:** 650 W 168th St, Ste BB4-427, New York, NY 10032; **Phone:** (212) 305-9445; **Board Cert:** Pediatric Infectious Disease 1994, Pediatrics 1992; **Med School:** Cornell Univ-Weill Med Coll 1964; **Resid:** Pediatrics, NY Hosp-Cornell, New York, NY 1966-1968; **Fellow:** Infectious Disease, New York Univ, New York, NY 1968-1970; Infectious Disease, Oxford Univ, Oxford, England; **Fac Appt:** Prof Pediatrics, Columbia P&S

Krilov, Leonard MD (PInf) - *Spec Exp:* Infections-Respiratory; Infections in Int'l Adopted Children; Chronic Fatigue Syndrome; **Hospital:** Winthrop - Univ Hosp; **Address:** 222 Station Plaza North, Ste 611A, Mineola, NY 11501; **Phone:** (516) 663-9570; **Board Cert:** Pediatrics 2001, Pediatric Infectious Disease 2001; **Med School:** Columbia P&S 1978; **Resid:** Pediatrics, Johns Hopkins Hosp, Baltimore, MD 1978-1981; **Fellow:** Pediatric Infectious Disease, Children's Hosp, Boston, MA 1981-1984

Long, Sarah S MD (PInf) - *Spec Exp:* Whooping Cough; **Hospital:** St Christopher's Hosp for Children; **Address:** St Christopher's Hosp for Chldrn, Erie Ave @ Front St, Ste 1112, Philadelphia, PA 19134; **Phone:** (215) 427-5204; **Board Cert:** Pediatrics 1993, Pediatric Infectious Disease 2001; **Med School:** Jefferson Med Coll 1970; **Resid:** Pediatrics, St Chris Hosp Chldn, Philadelphia, PA 1971-1973; **Fellow:** Pediatric Infectious Disease, Temple Univ Sch Med, Philadelphia, PA 1973-1975; **Fac Appt:** Prof Pediatrics, Hahnemann Univ

PEDIATRIC INFECTIOUS DISEASE *Mid Atlantic*

Munoz, Jose Luis MD (PInf) - *Spec Exp:* Lyme Disease; Immune Deficiency; Pediatric HIV Infection; **Hospital:** Westchester Med Ctr (page 82); **Address:** NY Med Coll, Pediatric Infectious Disease, Munger Pavillion, Valhalla, NY 10595; **Phone:** (914) 493-8333; **Board Cert:** Pediatrics 1989, Pediatric Infectious Disease 1994; **Med School:** Yale Univ 1978; **Resid:** Pediatrics, Yale New Haven Hosp, New Haven, CT 1979-1981; **Fellow:** Infectious Disease, Univ Rochester, Rochester, NY 1981-1984; **Fac Appt:** Assoc Prof Pediatric Infectious Disease, NY Med Coll

Rennels, Margaret MD (PInf) - *Spec Exp:* Immunizations/Vaccines; **Hospital:** University of MD Med Sys; **Address:** Univ Maryland Sch of Med, Dept Pediatrics, 22 S Greene St, rm N-5-W-70, Baltimore, MD 21201; **Phone:** (410) 328-6919; **Board Cert:** Pediatric Infectious Disease 1994, Pediatrics 1979; **Med School:** Univ MD Sch Med 1973; **Resid:** Pediatrics, Univ Maryland Hosp, Baltimore, MD 1974-1977; **Fellow:** Infectious Disease, Univ Maryland Hosp, Baltimore, MD 1977-1979; **Fac Appt:** Prof Pediatrics, Univ MD Sch Med

Saiman, Lisa MD (PInf) - *Spec Exp:* Cystic Fibrosis Infection; Fungal Infection; Hospital Epidemiology; **Hospital:** NY Presby Hosp - Columbia Presby Med Ctr (page 70); **Address:** 650 W 168th St, Ste 429, New York, NY 10032-3702; **Phone:** (212) 305-7935; **Board Cert:** Pediatrics 1987, Pediatric Infectious Disease 2002; **Med School:** Albert Einstein Coll Med 1983; **Resid:** Pediatrics, Babies Hosp, New York, NY 1983-1986; **Fellow:** Infectious Disease, Babies Hosp, New York, NY

Singh, Nalini MD (PInf) - *Spec Exp:* Infectious Disease; **Hospital:** Chldns Natl Med Ctr - DC; **Address:** 111 Michigan Ave NW, Washington, DC 20010; **Phone:** (202) 884-6150; **Board Cert:** Pediatrics 1982, Pediatric Infectious Disease 1997; **Med School:** India 1973; **Resid:** Pediatrics, Univ Mass Med Ctr, Worcester, MA 1976-1979; **Fellow:** Infectious Disease, Natl Inst Med Sci, Bethesda, MD 1979-1981; **Fac Appt:** Assoc Prof Infectious Disease, Geo Wash Univ

Wald, Ellen MD (PInf) - *Spec Exp:* Urinary Tract Infections; Infection-Respiratory; Meningitis; **Hospital:** Chldn's Hosp of Pittsbrgh; **Address:** Chldns Hosp of Pittsburgh, 3705 Fifth Ave, Pittsburgh, PA 15213; **Phone:** (412) 692-5105; **Board Cert:** Pediatrics 1973, Pediatric Infectious Disease 1994; **Med School:** SUNY Downstate 1968; **Resid:** Pediatrics, Kings Co Hosp, Brooklyn, NY 1969-1971; **Fellow:** Infectious Disease, Univ MD Hosp, Baltimore, MD 1973; **Fac Appt:** Prof Pediatrics, Univ Pittsburgh

Southeast

Clements III, Dennis Alfred MD/PhD (PInf) - *Spec Exp:* Vaccine Preventable Diseases; **Hospital:** Duke Univ Med Ctr (page 60); **Address:** Duke Univ Med Center, Box 3810, Durham, NC 27710; **Phone:** (919) 613-7651; **Board Cert:** Pediatrics 1978, Pediatric Infectious Disease 2004; **Med School:** Univ Rochester 1973; **Resid:** Pediatrics, Duke Univ Med Ctr, Durham, NC 1974-1976; **Fellow:** Pediatric Infectious Disease, Duke Univ Med Ctr, Durham, NC 1986-1988; **Fac Appt:** Assoc Prof Pediatrics, Duke Univ

Emmanuel, Patricia MD (PInf) - *Spec Exp:* Infections in Immune Deficient; **Hospital:** Tampa Genl Hosp; **Address:** 17 Davis Blvd, Ste 200, Tampa, FL 33606; **Phone:** (813) 259-8800; **Board Cert:** Pediatrics 1998, Pediatric Infectious Disease 1994; **Med School:** Univ Fla Coll Med 1986; **Resid:** Pediatrics, Univ So Fla, Tampa, FL 1986-1989; **Fellow:** Infectious Disease, Univ So Fla, Tampa, FL 1990-1993; **Fac Appt:** Asst Prof Pediatrics, Univ S Fla Coll Med

Givner, Laurence Bruce MD (PInf) - *Spec Exp:* Streptococcal Infections; Rocky Mountain Spotted Fever; **Hospital:** Wake Forest Univ Baptist Med Ctr (page 81); **Address:** Wake Forest Univ Sch Medicine, Dept. Pediatrics, 1 Medical Center Blvd, Winston Salem, NC 27157-0001; **Phone:** (336) 716-6568; **Board Cert:** Pediatrics 1984, Pediatric Infectious Disease 2001; **Med School:** Univ MD Sch Med 1978; **Resid:** Pediatrics, Univ Maryland, Baltimore, MD 1979-1982; **Fellow:** Infectious Disease, Baylor Coll Med, Houston, TX 1982-1984; **Fac Appt:** Prof Pediatrics, Wake Forest Univ Sch Med

Gorensek, Margaret MD (PInf) - *Spec Exp:* Infectious Disease; AIDS/HIV; Chronic Fatigue Syndrome; **Hospital:** Cleveland Clin FL; **Address:** Cleveland Clinic Florida, 2950 Cleveland Clinic Blvd, Weston, FL 33331; **Phone:** (954) 978-5165; **Board Cert:** Pediatrics 1986, Infectious Disease 1988, Internal Medicine 1985, Pediatric Infectious Disease 1994; **Med School:** Case West Res Univ 1981; **Resid:** Pediatrics, Cleveland Clinic, Cleveland, OH 1981-1985; **Fellow:** Infectious Disease, Cleveland Clinic, Cleveland, OH 1985-1987; **Fac Appt:** Asst Clin Prof Medicine, Univ Miami Sch Med

Ingram, David MD (PInf) - *Spec Exp:* Infectious Disease; **Hospital:** WakeMed New Bern; **Address:** 3024 New Bern Ave, Ste 307, Raleigh, NC 27610-1215; **Phone:** (919) 350-7846; **Board Cert:** Pediatrics 1980, Pediatric Infectious Disease 1994; **Med School:** Yale Univ 1967; **Resid:** Pediatrics, Yale-New Haven Hosp, New Haven, CT 1968-1971; **Fellow:** Pediatric Infectious Disease, Chldns Hosp Med Ctr, Boston, MA 1971-1973; **Fac Appt:** Prof Pediatrics, Univ NC Sch Med

McKinney Jr, Ross E MD (PInf) - *Spec Exp:* Infections in Immune Deficient; **Hospital:** Duke Univ Med Ctr (page 60); **Address:** Duke Univ Med Ctr, Box 3461, Durham, NC 27710-0001; **Phone:** (919) 684-6335; **Board Cert:** Pediatrics 1983, Pediatric Infectious Disease 1994; **Med School:** Univ Rochester 1979; **Resid:** Pediatrics, Duke Univ Med Ctr, Durham, NC 1982-1985; **Fellow:** Pediatric Infectious Disease, Duke Univ Med Ctr, Durham, NC 1979-1982; **Fac Appt:** Assoc Prof Pediatrics, Duke Univ

Mitchell, Charles MD (PInf) - *Spec Exp:* AIDS/HIV; Viral Infections; **Hospital:** Univ of Miami - Jackson Meml Hosp; **Address:** Jackson Meml, Dept Ped Inf Disease, 1550 NW 10th Ave, Ste 201, Miami, FL 33136; **Phone:** (305) 243-2755; **Board Cert:** Pediatric Infectious Disease 1994, Pediatrics 1986; **Med School:** Univ Tex Med Br, Galveston 1977; **Resid:** Pediatrics, Univ Minn Hosp, Minneapolis, MN; **Fellow:** Pediatric Infectious Disease, Univ Minn Hosp, Minneapolis, MN; **Fac Appt:** Asst Prof Pediatrics, Univ Miami Sch Med

Scott, Gwendolyn MD (PInf) - *Spec Exp:* AIDS/HIV; **Hospital:** Univ of Miami - Jackson Meml Hosp; **Address:** Univ Miami Sch Med, Dept Pediatric Infectious Disease, Div Inf Dis/Immun, Box 016960 (D4-4), Miami, FL 33101; **Phone:** (305) 243-6676; **Board Cert:** Pediatrics 1978, Pediatric Infectious Disease 1994; **Med School:** UCSF 1972; **Resid:** Pediatrics, San Fran Genl Hosp, San Francisco, CA 1972-1973; Pediatrics, Univ MD Hosp, Baltimore, MD 1974-1975; **Fellow:** Pediatric Infectious Disease, Univ Miami Project to Cure Paralysis, Miami, FL 1976-1978; **Fac Appt:** Prof Pediatrics, Univ Miami Sch Med

Midwest

Kleiman, Martin MD (PInf) - *Spec Exp:* Pediatric Infectious Disease - General; **Hospital:** Riley Chldrn's Hosp (page 588); **Address:** 702 Barnhill Drive, Ste 5487, Indianapolis, IN 46202-5128; **Phone:** (317) 274-5000; **Board Cert:** Pediatrics 1973, Pediatric Infectious Disease 1994; **Med School:** SUNY Syracuse 1968; **Resid:** Pediatrics, Upstate Med Ctr, Syracuse, NY 1969-1971; **Fellow:** Infectious Disease, Johns Hopkins Hosp, Baltimore, MD 1973-1976; **Fac Appt:** Prof Pediatrics, Indiana Univ

PEDIATRIC INFECTIOUS DISEASE

Shackelford, Penelope Greta MD (PInf) - *Spec Exp:* Pediatric Infectious Disease - General; **Hospital:** St Louis Children's Hospital; **Address:** 1 Children's Pl, Box 8116, St Louis, MO 63110; **Phone:** (314) 454-6050; **Board Cert:** Pediatric Infectious Disease 2001, Pediatrics 1973; **Med School:** Washington Univ, St Louis 1968; **Resid:** Pediatrics, St Louis Chldns Hosp, St Louis, MO 1969-1971; **Fellow:** Infectious Disease, St Louis Chldns Hosp, St Louis, MO 1970-1972; **Fac Appt:** Prof Pediatrics, Washington Univ, St Louis

Southwest

Baker, Carol MD (PInf) - *Spec Exp:* Infection-B Strep; Neonatal Infections; **Hospital:** TX Chldns Hosp - Houston; **Address:** Texas Children's Hospital, 6621 Fannin, MC-3-2371, Houston, TX 77030-2399; **Phone:** (713) 798-4790; **Board Cert:** Pediatrics 1973, Pediatric Infectious Disease 1994; **Med School:** Baylor Coll Med 1968; **Resid:** Pediatrics, Baylor Coll Med, Houston, TX 1969-1971; **Fellow:** Infectious Disease, Baylor Coll Med, Houston, TX 1971-1973; Infectious Disease, Boston City Hosp/Harvard Med Sch, Boston, MA 1973-1974; **Fac Appt:** Prof Pediatrics, Baylor Coll Med

Jacobs, Richard F MD (PInf) - *Spec Exp:* Tuberculosis; Virus Infections; Antiviral Therapy; **Hospital:** Arkansas Chldns Hosp; **Address:** 800 Marshall St, Little Rock, AR 72202-3591; **Phone:** (501) 320-1416; **Board Cert:** Pediatrics 1982, Pediatric Infectious Disease 2001; **Med School:** Univ Ark 1977; **Resid:** Pediatrics, Ark Chldns Hosp, Little Rock, AR 1977-1980; **Fellow:** Infectious Disease, Univ Wash, Seattle, WA 1980-1982; **Fac Appt:** Prof Pediatrics, Univ Ark

Jenson, Hal B MD (PInf) - *Spec Exp:* Infectious Disease; Viral Infections; Epstein-Barr Virus; **Hospital:** Univ of Texas Hlth & Sci Ctr; **Address:** 7703 Floyd Curl Dr., Dept. of Pediatrics, San Antonio, TX 78229-3900; **Phone:** (210) 567-5301; **Board Cert:** Pediatric Infectious Disease 1994, Pediatrics 1985; **Med School:** Geo Wash Univ 1979; **Resid:** Pediatrics, Rainbow Babies-Chldns Hosp., Cleveland, OH 1979-1983; **Fellow:** Pediatric Infectious Disease, Yale U. Sch. Med., New Haven, CT 1983-1985; **Fac Appt:** Prof Pediatrics, Univ Tex, San Antonio

Kaplan, Sheldon MD (PInf) - *Spec Exp:* Pneumococcal Infections; **Hospital:** TX Chldns Hosp - Houston; **Address:** Texas Chldrns Hosp, Div Ped Inf Dis, 6621 Fannin St, Ste 1150, MC-3-2371, Houston, TX 77030; **Phone:** (832) 824-4330; **Board Cert:** Pediatrics 1978, Pediatric Infectious Disease 1994; **Med School:** Univ MO-Columbia Sch Med 1973; **Resid:** Pediatrics, St Louis Chldns Hosp, St Louis, MO 1973-1975; **Fellow:** Pediatric Infectious Disease, St Louis Chldns Hosp, St Louis, MO 1975-1977; **Fac Appt:** Prof Pediatrics, Baylor Coll Med

Kline, Mark MD (PInf) - *Spec Exp:* AIDS/HIV; **Hospital:** TX Chldns Hosp - Houston; **Address:** Baylor Coll of Med, Dept Peds, 1 Baylor Plaza, MC-1-4000, Houston, TX 77030-3411; **Phone:** (832) 824-1038; **Board Cert:** Pediatrics 1987, Pediatric Infectious Disease 1994; **Med School:** Baylor Coll Med 1981; **Resid:** Pediatrics, Baylor Coll Med, Houston, TX 1981-1985; **Fellow:** Pediatric Infectious Disease, Baylor Coll Med, Houston, TX 1985-1987; **Fac Appt:** Prof Pediatrics, Baylor Coll Med

Waagner, David MD (PInf) - *Spec Exp:* Pediatric Infectious Disease - General; **Hospital:** Univ Med Ctr - Lubbock; **Address:** 3601 4th St, rm 4b104, Lubbock, TX 79430-0001; **Phone:** (806) 743-7337; **Board Cert:** Pediatrics 1998, Pediatric Infectious Disease 1994; **Med School:** Texas Tech Univ 1984; **Resid:** Pediatrics, Lubbock Genl Hosp/Tex Tech, Lubbock, TX 1984-1987; **Fellow:** Pediatric Infectious Disease, Univ Tex Med Ctr, Dallas, TX 1987-1989; **Fac Appt:** Assoc Prof Pediatrics, Texas Tech Univ

West Coast and Pacific

Bradley, John S MD (PInf) - *Spec Exp:* Meningococcemia; Brain Infections; Meningitis; **Hospital:** Children's Hosp and Hlth Ctr - San Diego; **Address:** 3020 Children's Way, MC 5041, San Diego, CA 92123; **Phone:** (858) 495-7785; **Board Cert:** Pediatrics 1981, Pediatric Infectious Disease 1994; **Med School:** UC Davis 1976; **Resid:** Pediatrics, UC - Davis, Sacramento, CA; **Fellow:** Pediatric Infectious Disease, Stanford Univ, Stanford, CA; **Fac Appt:** Assoc Clin Prof Pediatrics, UCSD

Bryson, Yvonne Joyce MD (PInf) - *Spec Exp:* AIDS/HIV; Herpes Simplex; **Hospital:** UCLA Med Ctr; **Address:** 10833 Le Conte Ave Bldg MDCC - rm 222-42, Los Angeles, CA 90095-1752; **Phone:** (310) 825-5235; **Board Cert:** Pediatrics 1976; **Med School:** Univ Tex SW, Dallas 1970; **Resid:** Pediatrics, UCSD Med Ctr, San Diego, CA 1971-1974; Pediatrics, UCSD Med Ctr, San Diego, CA 1974-1974; **Fellow:** Infectious Disease, UCSD Med Ctr, San Diego, CA 1974-1976; **Fac Appt:** Prof Pediatric Infectious Disease, UCLA

Cherry, James Donald MD (PInf) - *Spec Exp:* Vaccines; **Hospital:** Chldns Hosp - Los Angeles; **Address:** UCLA, Dept Ped rm 22-442 MDCC, 10833 Le Conte Ave, Los Angeles, CA 90095-1752; **Phone:** (310) 825-5226; **Board Cert:** Pediatrics 1962, Pediatric Infectious Disease 2001; **Med School:** Univ VT Coll Med 1957; **Resid:** Pediatrics, Boston City Hosp, Boston, MA 1958-1959; Pediatrics, Kings Co Hosp, Brooklyn, NY 1959-1960; **Fellow:** Internal Medicine, Boston, Boston, MA 1961-1962; **Fac Appt:** Prof Pediatrics, UCLA

Mason, Wilbert Henry MD (PInf) - *Spec Exp:* Kawasaki Disease; **Hospital:** Chldns Hosp - Los Angeles; **Address:** Children's Hospital, 4650 Sunset Blvd, MS 51, Los Angeles, CA 90027-6062; **Phone:** (323) 669-2509; **Board Cert:** Pediatrics 1975, Pediatric Infectious Disease 1994; **Med School:** UC Irvine 1970; **Resid:** Childrens Hosp, Los Angeles, CA 1971-1973; **Fellow:** Infectious Disease, Childrens Hospital, Los Angeles, CA 1973-1974; **Fac Appt:** Assoc Clin Prof Pediatrics, USC Sch Med

PEDIATRIC NEPHROLOGY

New England

Harmon, William E MD (PNep) - *Spec Exp:* Pediatric Nephrology - General; **Hospital:** Children's Hospital - Boston; **Address:** 300 Longwood Ave, Ste HU319, Boston, MA 02115; **Phone:** (617) 355-6129; **Board Cert:** Pediatrics 1976, Pediatric Critical Care Medicine 1998; **Med School:** Case West Res Univ 1971; **Resid:** Pediatrics, Childrens Hosp Med Ctr, Boston, MA 1972-1976; **Fellow:** Pediatric Nephrology, Childrens Hosp Med Ctr, Boston, MA 1976-1979; **Fac Appt:** Assoc Prof Pediatrics, Harvard Med Sch

Mid Atlantic

Dabbagh, Shermine MD (PNep) - *Spec Exp:* Kidney Disease; Kidney Failure-Chronic; Transplant-Kidney; **Hospital:** Alfred I Dupont Hosp for Children; **Address:** Dept Peds, Div Nephrology, 1600 Rockland Rd, Wilmington, DE 19899; **Phone:** (302) 651-4200; **Board Cert:** Pediatrics 1985, Pediatric Nephrology 1985; **Med School:** Lebanon 1979; **Resid:** Pediatrics, Univ Virginia, Charlottesville, VA 1979-1981; **Fellow:** Pediatric Nephrology, Univ Wisconsin, Madison, WI 1981-1984

Fivush, Barbara A MD (PNep) - *Spec Exp:* Pediatric Nephrology - General; **Hospital:** Johns Hopkins Hosp - Baltimore; **Address:** Johns Hopkins Hosp-Div. Nephrology, 600 N Wolfe St Bldg Park - rm 335, Baltimore, MD 21205-2104; **Phone:** (410) 955-2467; **Med School:** Boston Univ 1978; **Resid:** Pediatrics, Johns Hopkins Hosp, Baltimore, MD 1979-1981; **Fellow:** Pediatric Nephrology, Johns Hopkins Hosp, Baltimore, MD 1981-1983; Pediatric Nephrology, Childns Hosp-Natl Med Ctr, Washington, DC 1983-1984; **Fac Appt:** Assoc Prof Pediatrics, Johns Hopkins Univ

Kaplan, Bernard S MD (PNep) - *Spec Exp:* Hemolytic Uremic Syndrome; Polycystic Kidney Disease; **Hospital:** Chldn's Hosp of Philadelphia; **Address:** Children's Hosp-Philadelphia, Dept Nephrology, 34th St & Civic Blvd, rm 2143, Philadelphia, PA 19104; **Phone:** (215) 590-2449; **Board Cert:** Pediatrics 1972, Pediatric Nephrology 1974; **Med School:** South Africa 1964; **Resid:** Pediatrics, South Africa 1967-1970; **Fellow:** Nephrology, Montreal Chldns Hosp, Canada 1970-1972; **Fac Appt:** Prof Pediatrics, Univ Penn

Nash, Martin MD (PNep) - *Spec Exp:* Nephrotic Syndrome; Renal Failure; **Hospital:** NY Presby Hosp - Columbia Presby Med Ctr (page 70); **Address:** Babies & Childrens Hosp of New York, 3959 Broadway, rm 701, New York, NY 10032-1537; **Phone:** (212) 305-5825; **Board Cert:** Pediatrics 1969, Nephrology 1974; **Med School:** Duke Univ 1964; **Resid:** Internal Medicine, Georgetown Univ Hosp, Washington, DC 1964-1965; Pediatrics, Columbia-Presbyterian Hosp, New York, NY 1965-1967; **Fellow:** Pediatric Nephrology, Albert Einstein Coll Med, Bronx, NY 1969-1971; **Fac Appt:** Clin Prof Pediatrics, Columbia P&S

Roskes, Saul David MD (PNep) - *Spec Exp:* Pediatric Nephrology - General; **Hospital:** Johns Hopkins Hosp - Baltimore; **Address:** 10807 Falls Rd, Ste 200, Lutherville, MD 21093; **Phone:** (410) 321-9393; **Board Cert:** Pediatric Nephrology 1976, Pediatrics 1970; **Med School:** Johns Hopkins Univ 1963; **Resid:** Pediatrics, Bronx Muni Hosp Ctr., New York, NY 1964-1965; Pediatrics, Johns Hopkins Hosp, Baltimore, MD 1967-1968; **Fac Appt:** Assoc Prof Pediatrics, Johns Hopkins Univ

Southeast

Bunchman, Timothy E MD (PNep) - *Spec Exp:* Lupus/SLE; **Hospital:** Univ of Ala Hosp at Birmingham; **Address:** Univ Alabama-Birmingham, 1600 7th Ave S, Birmingham, AL 35233-0011; **Phone:** (205) 939-9141; **Board Cert:** Pediatrics 1986, Pediatric Nephrology 1996; **Med School:** Loyola Univ-Stritch Sch Med 1981; **Resid:** Pediatrics, St Louis Univ, St Louis, MO 1982-1984; Internal Medicine, St Louis Univ, St Louis, MO; **Fellow:** Pediatric Nephrology, Mayo Clinic, Rochester, MN 1985-1986; Pediatric Nephrology, Univ Minn, Minneapolis, MN 1986-1987; **Fac Appt:** Prof Pediatrics, Univ Ala

Chandar, Jayanthi MD (PNep) - *Spec Exp:* Pediatric Nephrology - General; **Hospital:** Univ of Miami - Jackson Meml Hosp; **Address:** Jackson Memorial Hosp, Div Ped Nephrology, Box 016960, MS M714, Miami, FL 33163; **Phone:** (305) 585-6726; **Board Cert:** Pediatric Nephrology 1995, Pediatrics 1998; **Med School:** India 1983; **Resid:** Pediatrics, Jackson Memorial Hosp, Miami, FL 1985-1987; **Fellow:** Pediatric Nephrology, Jackson Memorial Hosp, Miami, FL 1991; **Fac Appt:** Asst Prof Pediatrics, India

Fennell III, Robert Samuel MD (PNep) - *Spec Exp:* Transplant Medicine-Kidney; Kidney Failure-Chronic; **Hospital:** Shands Hlthcre at Univ of FL (page 73); **Address:** Shands Healthcare at Univ Florida, PO Box 100296, Gainesville, FL 32610-0296; **Phone:** (352) 392-4434; **Board Cert:** Pediatrics 1974, Pediatric Nephrology 2000; **Med School:** Univ Fla Coll Med 1964; **Resid:** Pediatrics, Shands Teaching Hosp, Gainesville, FL 1969-1971; **Fellow:** Pediatric Nephrology, Shands Teaching Hosp, Gainesville, FL 1972-1973; **Fac Appt:** Prof Pediatrics, Univ Fla Coll Med

Garin, Eduardo Humberto MD (PNep) - *Spec Exp:* Pediatric Nephrology - General; **Hospital:** Tampa Genl Hosp; **Address:** 17 Davis Blvd, Ste 200, Tampa, FL 33606-3438; **Phone:** (813) 259-8763; **Board Cert:** Pediatrics 1976, Pediatric Nephrology 1976; **Med School:** Chile 1970; **Resid:** Pediatrics, Univ Hosp and Clinics, Colombia, MO 1972-1973; **Fellow:** Pediatric Nephrology, Shands Hosp Univ FL, Gainesville, FL 1973-1975; **Fac Appt:** Prof Pediatrics, Univ S Fla Coll Med

Richard, George MD (PNep) - *Spec Exp:* Hypertension; Kidney Disease; Pediatric Nephrology; **Hospital:** Shands Hlthcre at Univ of FL (page 73); **Address:** Shands Healthcare at Univ Fla, 1600 SW Archer Rd, rm HD214, Box 100296, Gainesville, FL 32610-0296; **Phone:** (352) 392-4434; **Board Cert:** Pediatrics 1967, Pediatric Nephrology 1974; **Med School:** Univ Pittsburgh 1961; **Resid:** Pediatrics, Chldn's Hosp, Pittsburgh, PA 1964-1967; **Fellow:** Nephrology, Univ Florida, Gainesville, FL 1967-1968; **Fac Appt:** Prof Pediatrics, Univ Fla Coll Med

Zilleruelo, Gaston E MD (PNep) - *Spec Exp:* Transplant Medicine-Kidney; Nephrotic Syndrome; Genitourinary-Congenital Anomaly; **Hospital:** Univ of Miami - Jackson Meml Hosp; **Address:** Jackson Meml Hosp, Dept Ped Nephrology, 1601 NW 12th Ave, Box 16960(M714), Miami, FL 33101-6960; **Phone:** (305) 585-6726; **Board Cert:** Pediatrics 1979, Pediatric Nephrology 1979; **Med School:** Chile 1969; **Resid:** Pediatrics, L Calvo-Mackenna Chldns Hosp, Santiago, Chile 1969-1972; Pediatrics, Jackson Meml Hosp, Miami, FL 1976-1977; **Fellow:** Pediatric Nephrology, Jackson Meml Hosp, Miami, FL 1976-1978; **Fac Appt:** Prof Pediatrics, Univ Miami Sch Med

Midwest

Andreoli, Sharon MD (PNep) - *Spec Exp:* Kidney Disease; **Hospital:** Riley Chldrn's Hosp (page 588); **Address:** 699 West Drive, rm 213, Indianapolis, IN 46202; **Phone:** (317) 274-2563; **Board Cert:** Pediatrics 1983, Pediatric Nephrology 1985; **Med School:** Indiana Univ 1978; **Resid:** Pediatrics, James W Riley Hosp, Indianapolis, IN 1978-1981; **Fellow:** Pediatric Nephrology, Univ Minnesota, Minneapolis, MN 1981; Pediatric Nephrology, James W Riley Hosp/Indiana Univ, Indianapolis, IN 1982-1984; **Fac Appt:** Prof Pediatrics, Indiana Univ

Avner, Ellis D MD (PNep) - *Spec Exp:* Polycystic Kidney Disease; **Hospital:** Rainbow Babies & Chldns Hosp; **Address:** Rainbow Babies & Chldrn's Hosp, 11100 Euclid Ave, Cleveland, OH 44106; **Phone:** (216) 844-3884; **Board Cert:** Pediatric Nephrology 1982, Pediatrics 1980; **Med School:** Univ Penn 1975; **Resid:** Pediatrics, Chldn's Hosp, Boston, MA 1976-1978; **Fellow:** Pediatric Nephrology, Chldrn's Hosp, Boston, MA 1978-1980; **Fac Appt:** Prof Pediatrics, Case West Res Univ

Bergstein, Jerry MD (PNep) - *Spec Exp:* Dialysis-Peritoneal; Kidney Disease; Hypertension; **Hospital:** Riley Chldrn's Hosp (page 588); **Address:** 702 Barnhill Drive, Indianapolis, IN 46202-5200; **Phone:** (317) 274-2563; **Board Cert:** Pediatrics 1971, Pediatric Nephrology 1974; **Med School:** Univ Minn 1965; **Resid:** Pediatrics, Fairview Univ Med Ctr, Minneapolis, MN 1966-1967; Pediatrics, Fairview Univ Med Ctr, Minneapolis, MN 1969-1970; **Fellow:** Pediatric Nephrology, Fairview Univ Med Ctr, Minneapolis, MN 1970-1973; **Fac Appt:** Prof Pediatric Nephrology, Indiana Univ

Cohn, Richard MD (PNep) - *Spec Exp:* Transplant Medicine-Kidney; Nephrotic Syndrome; **Hospital:** Children's Mem Hosp; **Address:** 2300 Children's Plaza, Box 37, Chicago, IL 60614-3394; **Phone:** (773) 880-4326; **Board Cert:** Pediatrics 1978, Pediatric Nephrology 1979; **Med School:** Albert Einstein Coll Med 1972; **Resid:** Pediatrics, Johns Hopkins, Baltimore, MD 1972-1975; **Fellow:** Pediatric Nephrology, Univ Minnesota, Minneapolis, MN 1975-1978; **Fac Appt:** Assoc Prof Pediatrics, Northwestern Univ

Davis, Ira D MD (PNep) - *Spec Exp:* Kidney Development; Kidney Failure-Chronic; **Hospital:** Rainbow Babies & Chldns Hosp; **Address:** Rainbow Babies & Chldns Hosp, Div Ped Nep, 11100 Euclid Ave, Ste 740, Cleveland, OH 44106; **Phone:** (216) 844-1389; **Board Cert:** Pediatrics 1999, Pediatric Nephrology 1999; **Med School:** Univ Minn 1980; **Resid:** Pediatrics, Univ Hosps Cleveland, Cleveland, OH 1984-1987; **Fellow:** Pediatric Nephrology, Univ Minn Hosps, Minneapolis, MN 1987-1990; **Fac Appt:** Assoc Prof Pediatrics, Case West Res Univ

Friedman, Aaron MD (PNep) - *Spec Exp:* Hypertension; Transplant Medicine-Kidney; **Hospital:** Chldrns Hosp - Wisconsin; **Address:** Univ Wisconsin Chldns Hosp, 600 Highland Ave Ave, Box 4108, Madison, WI 53792; **Phone:** (608) 263-6420; **Board Cert:** Pediatrics 1979, Pediatric Nephrology 1996; **Med School:** SUNY Syracuse 1974; **Resid:** Pediatrics, Univ Wisconsin, Madison, WI 1975-1976; **Fellow:** Pediatric Nephrology, Univ Wisconsin, Madison, WI 1976-1980; **Fac Appt:** Prof Pediatrics, Univ Wisc

Kashtan, Clifford MD (PNep) - *Spec Exp:* Transplant Medicine-Kidney; Genetic Kidney Disease; **Hospital:** Fairview-Univ Med Ctr - Univ Campus; **Address:** U Minnesota Physicians, Dept Ped Nephrology, 420 Delaware St SE, Minneapolis, MN 55455; **Phone:** (612) 626-2922; **Board Cert:** Pediatrics 1983, Pediatric Nephrology 1996; **Med School:** Wayne State Univ 1978; **Resid:** Pediatrics, City Hospital, Boston, MA 1979-1981; **Fellow:** Pediatric Nephrology, Mass Genl Hosp, Boston, MA 1983-1984; Pediatric Nephrology, Univ Minnesota Hosp, Minneapolis, MN 1984-1987; **Fac Appt:** Prof Pediatric Nephrology, Univ Minn

Langman, Craig MD (PNep) - *Spec Exp:* Kidney Stones; Osteoporosis-Juvenile; Oxalosis; **Hospital:** Children's Mem Hosp; **Address:** Children's Meml Hosp, 2300 N Children's Plaza, Box 37, Chicago, IL 60614-3394; **Phone:** (773) 880-4326; **Board Cert:** Pediatrics 1982, Pediatric Nephrology 1982; **Med School:** Hahnemann Univ 1977; **Resid:** Pediatrics, Chldns Hosp, Philadelphia, PA 1977-1979; **Fellow:** Pediatric Nephrology, Chldns Hosp, Philadelphia, PA 1979-1981; **Fac Appt:** Prof Pediatrics, Northwestern Univ

Nevins, Thomas E MD (PNep) - *Spec Exp:* Kidney Failure-Chronic; Transplant Medicine-Kidney; Hypertension; **Hospital:** Fairview-Univ Med Ctr - Univ Campus; **Address:** Fairview Univ Med Ctr, Dept Peds, 420 Delaware St SE, MC 491, Minneapolis, MN 55455-0374; **Phone:** (612) 626-2922; **Board Cert:** Pediatrics 1975, Pediatric Nephrology 1979; **Med School:** Washington Univ, St Louis 1969; **Resid:** Pediatrics, Minnesota Hosps, Minneapolis, MN 1970-1972; **Fellow:** Nephrology, Minnesota Hosps, Minneapolis, MN 1974-1978; **Fac Appt:** Prof Pediatrics, Univ Minn

Warady, Bradley MD (PNep) - *Spec Exp:* Peritoneal Dialysis; Transplant Medicine-Kidney; **Hospital:** Chldns Mercy Hosps & Clinics; **Address:** Dept Pediatric Nephrology, 2401 Gillham Rd, Kansas City, MO 64108; **Phone:** (816) 234-3010; **Board Cert:** Pediatrics 1984, Pediatric Nephrology 1985; **Med School:** Univ IL Coll Med 1979; **Resid:** Pediatrics, Chldns Mercy Hosp, Kansas City, MO 1979-1982; **Fellow:** Pediatric Nephrology, Colorado Univ Med Ctr, Denver, CO 1982-1984

West Coast and Pacific

Alexander, Steven R MD (PNep) - *Spec Exp:* Kidney Failure; Transplant Medicine-Kidney; Nephrotic Syndrome; **Hospital:** Stanford Med Ctr; **Address:** Lucile Packard Chldn's Hosp, 300 Pasteur Drive, rm G306, Stanford, CA 94305-5208; **Phone:** (650) 723-7903; **Board Cert:** Pediatrics 1986, Pediatric Nephrology 1986; **Med School:** Baylor Coll Med 1971; **Resid:** Pediatrics, Baylor Affil Hosps, Houston, TX 1974-1976; **Fellow:** Pediatric Nephrology, Baylor Affil Hosps, Houston, TX 1976-1978; **Fac Appt:** Prof Pediatrics, Stanford Univ

Ettenger, Robert Bruce MD (PNep) - *Spec Exp:* Transplant Medicine-Kidney; **Hospital:** UCLA Med Ctr; **Address:** UCLA Children's Hosp, Dept Ped Nephrology, 10833 Le Conte Ave, Box 951752, Los Angeles, CA 90095; **Phone:** (310) 206-6987; **Board Cert:** Pediatrics 1986, Pediatric Nephrology 1986; **Med School:** Univ Penn 1968; **Resid:** Pediatrics, St Christophers Hosp Chldn, Philadelphia, PA 1969-1971; **Fellow:** Pediatric Nephrology, Chldns Hosp, Los Angeles, CA 1973-1975; **Fac Appt:** Prof Pediatrics, UCLA

McDonald, Ruth A MD (PNep) - *Spec Exp:* Transplant Medicine-Kidney; **Hospital:** Chldns Hosp and Regl Med Ctr - Seattle; **Address:** 4800 Sand Point Way NE, MS CH-46, Seattle, WA 98105; **Phone:** (206) 526-2524; **Board Cert:** Pediatrics 1997, Pediatric Nephrology 2004; **Med School:** Univ Minn 1987; **Resid:** Pediatrics, Chldns Hosp & Med Ctr, Seattle, WA 1988-1990; **Fellow:** Pediatric Nephrology, Chldns Hosp & Med Ctr, Seattle, WA 1990-1993; **Fac Appt:** Assoc Prof Pediatrics, Univ Wash

Stapleton, F Bruder MD (PNep) - *Spec Exp:* Kidney Stones; **Hospital:** Chldns Hosp and Regl Med Ctr - Seattle; **Address:** 4800 Sand Point Way NE, MS CH-65, Seattle, WA 98105; **Phone:** (206) 526-2150; **Board Cert:** Pediatrics 1989, Pediatric Nephrology 1997; **Med School:** Univ Kans 1972; **Resid:** Pediatrics, Univ Washington Med Ctr, Seattle, WA 1972-1974; **Fellow:** Pediatric Nephrology, Univ Kansas Med Ctr, Kansas City, KS 1975-1977; **Fac Appt:** Prof Pediatrics, Univ Wash

Watkins, Sandra MD (PNep) - *Spec Exp:* Kidney Failure-Chronic; Hemolytic Uremic Syndrome; **Hospital:** Chldns Hosp and Regl Med Ctr - Seattle; **Address:** 4800 Sand Point Way NE, MC CH-46, Seattle, WA 98105; **Phone:** (206) 526-2524; **Board Cert:** Pediatrics 1987, Pediatric Nephrology 1988; **Med School:** Univ Tex, Houston 1981; **Resid:** Pediatrics, Univ WA Chldns Hosp, Seattle, WA 1982-1984; **Fellow:** Nephrology, Univ WA Sch Med, Seattle, WA 1984-1986; **Fac Appt:** Asst Prof Pediatric Nephrology, Univ Wash

PEDIATRIC OTOLARYNGOLOGY

New England

Eavey, Roland Douglas MD (PO) - *Spec Exp:* Microtia Reconstruction; Ear Disorders/Surgery; **Hospital:** Mass Eye & Ear Infirmary; **Address:** 243 Charles St, Boston, MA 02114; **Phone:** (617) 573-3190; **Board Cert:** Pediatrics 1982, Otolaryngology 1981; **Med School:** Univ Penn 1975; **Resid:** Pediatrics, Chldns Hoso, Los Angeles, CA 1976-1977; Surgery, Kaiser Hosp, San Francisco, CA 1977-1978; **Fellow:** Otolaryngology, Mass EE Infirm, Boston, MA 1978-1981; **Fac Appt:** Assoc Prof Otolaryngology, Harvard Med Sch

Grundfast, Kenneth MD (PO) - *Spec Exp:* Pediatric Otolaryngology - General; **Hospital:** Boston Med Ctr; **Address:** 88 E Newton St, Ste D616, Boston, MA 02118-2393; **Phone:** (617) 638-7934; **Board Cert:** Otolaryngology 1977; **Med School:** SUNY Syracuse 1969; **Resid:** Surgery, Sibley Meml Hosp, Washington, DC 1973-1974; Otolaryngology, Boston-Affil Hosps, Boston, MA 1974-1977; **Fellow:** Pediatric Otolaryngology, Chldns Hosp, Pittsburgh, PA 1977-1978

Healy, Gerald MD (PO) - *Spec Exp:* Pediatric Otolaryngology - General; **Hospital:** Children's Hospital - Boston; **Address:** 300 Longwood Ave, Fegan Bldg- Fl 9, Boston, MA 02115; **Phone:** (617) 355-6417; **Board Cert:** Otolaryngology 1972; **Med School:** Boston Univ 1967; **Resid:** Surgery, Univ Boston Hosps, Boston, MA 1968-1969; Otolaryngology, Univ Boston Hosps, Boston, MA 1969-1972; **Fac Appt:** Prof Otolaryngology, Harvard Med Sch

Mid Atlantic

Bluestone, Charles D MD (PO) - *Spec Exp:* Pediatric Otolaryngology - General; **Hospital:** Chldn's Hosp of Pittsbrgh; **Address:** Chldn Hosp, Dept Otolaryngology, 3705 5th Ave, Pittsburgh, PA 15213-2524; **Phone:** (412) 692-5902; **Board Cert:** Otolaryngology 1963; **Med School:** Univ Pittsburgh 1958; **Resid:** Otolaryngology, Eye and Ear Infirmary, Chicago, IL 1959-1962; **Fac Appt:** Prof Otolaryngology, Univ Pittsburgh

Goldsmith, Ari MD (PO) - *Spec Exp:* Airways Disorders; Otitis Media; **Hospital:** Long Island Coll Hosp (page 58); **Address:** University Otolaryngologists, 134 Atlantic Ave, Brooklyn, NY 11201; **Phone:** (718) 780-1498; **Board Cert:** Otolaryngology 1994; **Med School:** Albert Einstein Coll Med 1988; **Resid:** Otolaryngology, Long Island Jewish Hosp, New Hyde Park, NY 1989-1993; **Fellow:** Pediatric Otolaryngology, Children's Hospital/Harvard, Boston, MA 1993-1994; **Fac Appt:** Prof Otolaryngology, SUNY Hlth Sci Ctr

Jones, Jacqueline MD (PO) - *Spec Exp:* Pediatric Otolaryngology - General; **Hospital:** NY Presby Hosp - NY Weill Cornell Med Ctr (page 70); **Address:** 520 E 70th St, Ste 541, New York, NY 10021; **Phone:** (212) 746-2236; **Board Cert:** Otolaryngology 1989; **Med School:** Cornell Univ-Weill Med Coll 1984; **Resid:** Otolaryngology, Hosp-Univ of Penn, Philadelphia, PA 1984-1989; **Fellow:** Pediatric Otolaryngology, Children's Hosp, Boston, MA 1989-1990; **Fac Appt:** Assoc Prof Cornell Univ-Weill Med Coll

Milmoe, Gregory J MD (PO) - *Spec Exp:* Sinus Disorders/Surgery; Airway Disorders; **Hospital:** Georgetown Univ Hosp; **Address:** 3800 Reservoir Rd, Gorman Bldg, Fl 1, Washington, DC 20007; **Phone:** (202) 687-8186; **Board Cert:** Otolaryngology 1981; **Med School:** Univ Chicago-Pritzker Sch Med 1973; **Resid:** Surgery, Hosp of Univ Penn, Philadelphia, PA 1975-1976; Otolaryngology, Yale Univ Hosp, Philadelphia, PA 1976-1979; **Fellow:** Pediatric Otolaryngology, Chldrns Hosp, Pittsburgh, PA 1979-1980; **Fac Appt:** Assoc Prof Otolaryngology, Georgetown Univ

Potsic, William Paul MD (PO) - *Spec Exp:* *Ear Disorders/Surgery; Ear Tumors; Hearing Disorders;* **Hospital:** Chldn's Hosp of Philadelphia; **Address:** Childrens Hosp-Philadelphia, 34 Civic Center Blvd, Bldg Wood - Fl 1, Philadelphia, PA 19104-4303; **Phone:** (215) 590-3450; **Board Cert:** Otolaryngology 1974; **Med School:** Emory Univ 1969; **Resid:** Otolaryngology, Univ Chicago, Chicago, IL 1969-1974; **Fac Appt:** Prof Otolaryngology, Univ Penn

Rosenfeld, Richard M MD (PO) - *Spec Exp:* *Sinus Disorders/Surgery; Head & Neck Surgery;* **Hospital:** Long Island Coll Hosp (page 58); **Address:** Univ Otolaryngologists, 134 Atlantic Ave, Brooklyn, NY 11201; **Phone:** (718) 780-1498; **Board Cert:** Otolaryngology 1989; **Med School:** SUNY Buffalo 1984; **Resid:** Otolaryngology, Mount Sinai Med Ctr, New York, NY 1984-1989; **Fellow:** Pediatric Otolaryngology, Chldrn's Hosp, Pittsburgh, PA 1989-1991; **Fac Appt:** Prof Otolaryngology, SUNY Downstate

Tunkel, David Eric MD (PO) - *Spec Exp:* *Head & Neck Surgery;* **Hospital:** Johns Hopkins Hosp - Baltimore; **Address:** 601 N Caroline St, rm 6231, Baltimore, MD 21287; **Phone:** (410) 955-1559; **Board Cert:** Otolaryngology 1990; **Med School:** Johns Hopkins Univ 1984; **Resid:** Surgery, Johns Hopkins Hosp, Baltimore, MD 1984-1986; Otolaryngology, Johns Hopkins Hosp, Baltimore, MD 1986-1990; **Fellow:** Pediatric Otolaryngology, Chldns Natl Med Ctr, Washington, DC 1990-1991; **Fac Appt:** Assoc Prof Otolaryngology, Johns Hopkins Univ

Southeast

Drake, Amelia MD (PO) - *Spec Exp:* *Pediatric Surgery; Head & Neck Surgery;* **Hospital:** Univ of NC Hosp (page 77); **Address:** 610 Burnett Wolmack Bldg, CB#7070, Chapel Hill, NC 27599; **Phone:** (919) 966-8926; **Board Cert:** Otolaryngology 1987; **Med School:** Univ NC Sch Med 1981; **Resid:** Otolaryngology, Univ MI Hosps; Surgery, Univ MI Hosps

Gross, Charles MD (PO) - *Spec Exp:* *Sinus Disorders/Surgery; Otolaryngology-Pediatric;* **Hospital:** Univ of VA Hlth Sys (page 79); **Address:** UVA Health System, P. O. Box 800713, Charlottesville, VA 22908-0713; **Phone:** (804) 924-5934; **Board Cert:** Pediatric Otolaryngology 1967; **Med School:** Univ VA Sch Med 1961; **Resid:** Otolaryngology, Mass EE Infirm, Boston, MA 1963-1966; Surgery, Beckley Meml Hosp 1962-1963; **Fac Appt:** Prof Otolaryngology, Univ VA Sch Med

Midwest

Belenky, Walter MD (PO) - *Spec Exp:* *Otolaryngology; Cochlear Implants;* **Hospital:** Chldns Hosp of Michigan (page 59); **Address:** Dept of Ped Oto, 3901 Beaubien, Detroit, MI 48201; **Phone:** (313) 745-9048; **Board Cert:** Otolaryngology 1970; **Med School:** Univ Mich Med Sch 1963; **Resid:** Surgery, William Beaumont Hosps, Royal Oak, MI 1964-1965; Otolaryngology, Wayne Affil Hosp, Detroit, MI 1965-1968

Cotton, Robin MD (PO) - *Spec Exp:* *Tracheal Reconstruction; Head & Neck Surgery;* **Hospital:** Cincinnati Chldns Hosp Med Ctr; **Address:** 3333 Burnet Ave, Cincinnati, OH 45229-2883; **Phone:** (513) 636-4355; **Board Cert:** Otolaryngology 1972; **Med School:** England 1965; **Resid:** Otolaryngology, Univ Birmingham, Birmingham, AL 1966-1968; Otolaryngology, Univ Toronto, Toronto, Canada 1968-1972; **Fellow:** Otolaryngology, Univ Toronto, Toronto, Canada 1971-1973; **Fac Appt:** Prof Otolaryngology, Univ Cincinnati

PEDIATRIC OTOLARYNGOLOGY

Holinger, Lauren D. MD (PO) - *Spec Exp:* Airway Disorders; Swallowing Disorders; Aspiration; **Hospital:** Children's Mem Hosp; **Address:** Childrens Meml Hosp, 2300 N Childrens Plaza, Box 25, Chicago, IL 60614-3394; **Phone:** (773) 880-4457; **Board Cert:** Otolaryngology 1975; **Med School:** Univ Hlth Sci/Chicago Med Sch 1971; **Resid:** Surgery, Univ Colorado Affil Hosp, Denver, CO 1971-1972; Otolaryngology, Univ Colorado Affil Hosp, Denver, CO 1972-1975; **Fellow:** Pediatric Otolaryngology, Childrens Meml Hosp, Chicago, IL 1975-1976; **Fac Appt:** Prof Otolaryngology, Northwestern Univ

Katz, Robert L MD (PO) - *Spec Exp:* Ear Infections & Hearing Problems; Sinus Disorders/Surgery; **Hospital:** Cleveland Clin Fdn (page 57); **Address:** 29800 Bainbridge Rd, Solon, OH 44139; **Phone:** (440) 519-6950; **Board Cert:** Otolaryngology 1968; **Med School:** Case West Res Univ 1963; **Resid:** Surgery, Mount Sinai Hosp, Cleveland, OH 1963-1965; Otolaryngology, Mass EE Infirm, Boston, MA 1965-1968; **Fac Appt:** Clin Prof Otolaryngology, Ohio State Univ

Lusk, Rodney MD (PO) - *Spec Exp:* Cochlear Implants; Sinus Disorders/Surgery; Sleep Disorders/Apnea; **Hospital:** St Louis Children's Hospital; **Address:** 1 Children's Place, Fl 3, St. Louis, MO 63110-1077; **Phone:** (314) 454-6162; **Board Cert:** Otolaryngology 1982; **Med School:** Univ MO-Columbia Sch Med 1977; **Resid:** Head and Neck Surgery, Univ. Iowa Hosp/Clinic, Iowa City, IA 1978-1982; **Fellow:** Otolaryngology, Childrens hospital, Pittsburgh, PA 1982-1983; **Fac Appt:** Assoc Prof Pediatrics, Washington Univ, St Louis

Miller, Robert P MD (PO) - *Spec Exp:* Ear Disorders/Surgery; Airway Disorders; **Hospital:** Advocate Lutheran Gen Hosp; **Address:** 8780 Golf Rd, Ste 200, Niles, IL 60714; **Phone:** (847) 674-5585; **Board Cert:** Otolaryngology 1978; **Med School:** Loyola Univ-Stritch Sch Med 1974; **Resid:** Otolaryngology, Univ Ill Hosps, Chicago, IL 1975-1978; **Fellow:** Pediatric Otolaryngology, Chldns Hosp Med Ctr, Cincinnati, OH 1986-1987; **Fac Appt:** Asst Clin Prof Otolaryngology, Univ IL Coll Med

Southwest

Duncan III, Newton Oran MD (PO) - *Spec Exp:* Otolaryngology-Pediatric; Head & Neck Surgery-Pediatric; Airway Disorders; **Hospital:** TX Chldns Hosp - Houston; **Address:** 6550 Fannin St, Ste 2001, Houston, TX 77030; **Phone:** (713) 796-2001; **Board Cert:** Otolaryngology 1986; **Med School:** Baylor Coll Med 1978; **Resid:** Surgery, Baylor Coll Med, Houston, TX 1982-1983; Otolaryngology, Baylor Coll Med, Houston, TX 1983-1986; **Fellow:** Pediatric Otolaryngology, Univ Wash, Seattle, WA 1990-1991; Pediatric Otolaryngology, Royal Alexandra Hosp Chld, Sydney, Australia 1991-1992; **Fac Appt:** Asst Clin Prof Otolaryngology, Baylor Coll Med

West Coast and Pacific

Crockett, Dennis M MD (PO) - *Spec Exp:* Airway Disorders; **Hospital:** Chldns Hosp - Los Angeles; **Address:** 4650 Sunset Blvd, MS 58, Los Angeles, CA 90027; **Phone:** (323) 669-2145; **Board Cert:** Otolaryngology 1985; **Med School:** USC Sch Med 1979; **Resid:** Otolaryngology, LA Co-USC Med Ctr, Los Angeles, CA 1980-1984; **Fellow:** Pediatrics, Boston Chldns Hosp, Boston, MA 1984-1985; **Fac Appt:** Assoc Prof Otolaryngology, USC Sch Med

Inglis, Andrew MD (PO) - *Spec Exp:* Airway Disorders; Voice Disorders; **Hospital:** Chldns Hosp and Regl Med Ctr - Seattle; **Address:** Children's Hospital & Regional Medical Center, 4800 Sand Point Way NE, Seattle, WA 98105-3916; **Phone:** (206) 526-2105; **Board Cert:** Otolaryngology 1987; **Med School:** Med Coll PA Hahnemann 1981; **Resid:** Surgery, Virginia Mason Hosp, Seattle, WA 1982-1983; Otolaryngology, Univ Washington, Seattle, WA 1983-1987; **Fellow:** Pediatric Otolaryngology, Alexandria Hosp Chldn 1986-1987; **Fac Appt:** Assoc Prof Otolaryngology, Univ Wash

Richardson, Mark A MD (PO) - *Spec Exp:* Sinus Disorders; Airway Reconstruction; Lymphatic Malformations-Head & Neck; **Hospital:** Doernbecher Chldns Hosp; **Address:** Dept Oto/HNS, 3181 SW Sam Jackson Park Rd, Portland, OR 97201-3098; **Phone:** (503) 494-0062; **Board Cert:** Otolaryngology 1979; **Med School:** Med Univ SC 1975; **Resid:** Otolaryngology, Med Univ Hosp, Charleston, SC 1976-1979; **Fellow:** Pediatric Otolaryngology, Chldns Hosp Med Ctr, Cincinnati, OH 1979-1980; **Fac Appt:** Prof Otolaryngology, Oregon Hlth Scis Univ

PEDIATRIC PULMONOLOGY

New England

Lapey, Allen MD (PPul) - *Spec Exp:* Cystic Fibrosis; Asthma; Food Allergy; **Hospital:** MA Genl Hosp; **Address:** 15 Parkman St Bldg WAC - rm 707, Boston, MA 02114; **Phone:** (617) 726-8707; **Board Cert:** Pediatric Pulmonology 1996, Allergy & Immunology 1978; **Med School:** Univ Rochester 1966; **Resid:** Pediatrics, Chldns Hosp Med Ctr., Boston, MA 1967-1968; **Fellow:** Pediatric Pulmonology, Mass Genl Hosp., Boston, MA 1970-1972; Allergy & Immunology, Mass Genl Hosp., Boston, MA 1970-1972; **Fac Appt:** Asst Clin Prof Pediatrics, Harvard Med Sch

Mid Atlantic

Loughlin, Gerald M MD (PPul) - *Spec Exp:* Asthma; Sleep & Breathing Disorders; Chronic Lung Disease; **Hospital:** Johns Hopkins Hosp - Baltimore; **Address:** Johns Hopkins Hosp- Dept. Ped, 600 N Wolfe St, Bldg Park - rm 316, Baltimore, MD 21287-2533; **Phone:** (410) 955-2035; **Board Cert:** Pediatric Pulmonology 1996, Pediatrics 1993; **Med School:** Univ Rochester 1973; **Resid:** Pediatrics, U Ariz Med Ctr, Tucson, AZ 1973-1975; **Fellow:** Pediatric Pulmonology, U Ariz Med Ctr, Tucson, AZ 1975-1977; **Fac Appt:** Prof Pediatrics, Johns Hopkins Univ

Mellins, Robert MD (PPul) - *Spec Exp:* Asthma; Pneumonia; **Hospital:** NY Presby Hosp - Columbia Presby Med Ctr (page 70); **Address:** 3959 Broadway Fl 7, New York, NY 10032-1537; **Phone:** (212) 305-5122; **Board Cert:** Pediatrics 1958, Pediatric Pulmonology 1995; **Med School:** Johns Hopkins Univ 1952; **Resid:** Pediatrics, NY Hosp, New York, NY 1955-1956; Pediatrics, Columbia Presby Med Ctr, New York, NY 1956-1957; **Fellow:** Pulmonary Disease, Columbia Presby Med Ctr, New York, NY 1961-1964; **Fac Appt:** Prof Pediatrics, Columbia P&S

Quittell, Lynne MD (PPul) - *Spec Exp:* Cystic Fibrosis; Asthma; **Hospital:** NY Presby Hosp - Columbia Presby Med Ctr (page 70); **Address:** 3959 Broadway, rm 7 South, New York, NY 10032-1551; **Phone:** (212) 305-5122; **Board Cert:** Pediatrics 1986, Pediatric Pulmonology 1996; **Med School:** Israel 1981; **Resid:** Pediatrics, Schneider Chldn's Hosp, New Hyde Park, NY 1981-1984; **Fellow:** Pediatric Pulmonology, St Christopher Med Ctr, Philadelphia, PA 1984-1988; **Fac Appt:** Assoc Prof Pediatrics, Columbia P&S

Zeitlin, Pamela Leslie MD (PPul) - *Spec Exp:* Cystic Fibrosis; **Hospital:** Johns Hopkins Hosp - Baltimore; **Address:** 600 N Wolfe St Bldg Park - rm 316, Baltimore, MD 21287-2533; **Phone:** (410) 955-2035; **Board Cert:** Pediatric Pulmonology 2000, Pediatrics 1988; **Med School:** Yale Univ 1983; **Resid:** Pediatrics, Johns Hopkins Hosp, Baltimore, MD 1983-1986; **Fellow:** Pediatric Pulmonology, Johns Hopkins Hosp, Baltimore, MD 1986-1989; **Fac Appt:** Assoc Prof Pediatrics, Johns Hopkins Univ

Southeast

Murphy, Thomas M M MD (PPul) - *Spec Exp:* Cystic Fibrosis; Bronchopulmonary Dysplasia; Pneumonia-Chronic; **Hospital:** Duke Univ Med Ctr (page 60); **Address:** Duke Univ Med Ctr, Box 2994, Durham, NC 27710; **Phone:** (919) 684-3364; **Board Cert:** Internal Medicine 1976, Pediatric Pulmonology 1989; **Med School:** Univ Rochester 1973; **Resid:** Internal Medicine, Georgetown Univ Hosp, Washington, DC 1973-1976; **Fellow:** Pediatric Pulmonology, Georgetown Univ Hosp, Washington, DC 1976-1978; **Fac Appt:** Assoc Prof Pediatrics, Duke Univ

Sallent, Jorge MD (PPul) - *Spec Exp:* Pediatric Pulmonology - General; **Hospital:** St Mary's Med Ctr - W Palm Bch; **Address:** Pediatric Respiratory Ctr, 5325 Greenwood Avenue Ste 301, West Palm Beach, FL 33407-2452; **Phone:** (561) 863-0105; **Board Cert:** Pediatrics 1984, Pediatric Pulmonology 1996; **Med School:** Dominican Republic 1978; **Resid:** Pediatrics, Orlando Regional Med Ctr, Orlando, FL 1980-1983; **Fellow:** Pediatric Pulmonology, Univ Florida, Gainesville, FL 1985-1986; **Fac Appt:** Asst Prof Pediatrics, Univ Fla Coll Med

Sherman, James MD (PPul) - *Spec Exp:* Cystic Fibrosis; **Hospital:** Shands Hlthcre at Univ of FL (page 73); **Address:** Medical Plaza, 2000 SW Archer Rd, Fl 2, Gainesville, FL 32608; **Phone:** (352) 392-4458; **Board Cert:** Pediatrics 1981, Pediatric Pulmonology 1996; **Med School:** Univ S Fla Coll Med 1975; **Resid:** Pediatrics, SUNY Upstate Med Ctr, Syracuse, NY 1976-1977; Pediatrics, Tampa Genl Hosp- Univ So Florida, Tampa, FL 1977-1978; **Fellow:** Pediatric Pulmonology, Rainbow Babies & Children's Hosp, Cleveland, OH 1978-1981; **Fac Appt:** Prof Pediatrics, Univ Fla Coll Med

Midwest

Kim, Young-Jee MD (PPul) - *Spec Exp:* Asthma; Bronchopulmonary Dysplasia; Home Ventilator; **Hospital:** Univ of Chicago Hosps (page 76); **Address:** Univ Chicago, Dept Peds, Sect Pulm Biology/Crit Care, 5841 S Maryland Ave, MC-4064, Chicago, IL 60637; **Phone:** (773) 702-6178; **Board Cert:** Pediatrics 1995, Pediatric Pulmonology 1998; **Med School:** South Korea 1986; **Resid:** Pediatrics, Duke Univ Med Ctr, Durham, NC 1992-1995; **Fellow:** Pediatric Pulmonology, Yale Univ Med Sch, New Haven, CT 1988-1991; Pediatric Pulmonology, Riley Hosp for Childrn, Indianapolis, IN 1995-1998; **Fac Appt:** Asst Prof Pediatric Pulmonology, Univ Chicago-Pritzker Sch Med

Kurachek, Stephen Charles MD (PPul) - *Spec Exp:* Critical Care; Asthma; **Hospital:** Chldns Hosp and Clinics - Minneapolis; **Address:** Chldrns Respiratory and Crit Care Specialists, 2545 Chicago Ave S, Ste 617, Minneapolis, MN 55404; **Phone:** (612) 863-3226; **Board Cert:** Pediatric Pulmonology 1995, Pediatric Critical Care Medicine 1995; **Med School:** Univ Miami Sch Med 1978; **Resid:** Pediatrics, Univ Hosp, Ann Arbor, MI 1979-1981; **Fellow:** Pulmonary Disease, Boston Chldns Hosp, Boston, MA 1981-1984; **Fac Appt:** Asst Clin Prof Pediatrics, Univ Minn

Stern, Robert C MD (PPul) - *Spec Exp:* Cystic Fibrosis; Lung Disease; **Hospital:** Rainbow Babies & Chldns Hosp; **Address:** 11100 Euclid Ave, Div of Ped Pulmonary Disease, Cleveland, OH 44106; **Phone:** (216) 844-3267; **Board Cert:** Pediatrics 1968, Pediatric Pulmonology 1994; **Med School:** Albert Einstein Coll Med 1963; **Resid:** Pediatrics, Univ Hosp, Cleveland, OH 1964-1965; Pediatrics, Municipal Hosp Ctr, Bronx, NY 1965-1966; **Fellow:** Pediatric Pulmonology, Univ Hosp, Cleveland, OH 1968; **Fac Appt:** Prof Pediatrics, Case West Res Univ

Great Plains and Mountains

Accurso, Frank J MD (PPul) - *Spec Exp:* Cystic Fibrosis; **Hospital:** Chldn's Hosp - Denver; **Address:** Chldns Hosp, 1056 E 19th Ave, rm B-395, Denver, CO 80218-1007; **Phone:** (303) 837-2522; **Board Cert:** Pediatrics 1980, Pediatric Critical Care Medicine 1996; **Med School:** Albert Einstein Coll Med 1974; **Resid:** Pediatrics, Univ Colo Hlth Sci Ctr, Denver, CO 1978-1980; **Fellow:** Pulmonary Disease, Univ Colo Hlth Sci Ctr, Denver, CO 1975-1977; **Fac Appt:** Prof Pediatrics, Univ Colo

Larsen, Gary MD (PPul) - *Spec Exp:* Lung Disease; **Hospital:** Natl Jewish Med & Rsrch Ctr; **Address:** Natl Jewish Med & Rsrch Ctr, 1400 Jackson St, Denver, CO 80206-2761; **Phone:** (303) 398-1617; **Board Cert:** Pediatric Pulmonology 1996, Pediatrics 1976; **Med School:** Columbia P&S 1971; **Resid:** Pediatrics, Univ Colorado, Denver, CO 1972-1974; **Fellow:** Pediatric Pulmonology, Univ Colorado, Denver, CO 1976-1978; **Fac Appt:** Prof Pediatrics, Univ Colo

Southwest

Fan, Leland Lane MD (PPul) - *Spec Exp:* Interstitial Lung Disease; **Hospital:** TX Chldns Hosp - Houston; **Address:** Tex Chldns Hosp Feigin Ctr, 6621 Fannin , Ste CC-1040, Houston, TX 77030; **Phone:** (832) 822-3300; **Board Cert:** Pediatrics 1978, Pediatric Pulmonology 1996, Pediatric Critical Care Medicine 1996; **Med School:** Baylor Coll Med 1973; **Resid:** Pediatrics, UCSF Med Ctr, San Francisco, CA 1974-1975; Pediatrics, Univ Colo Hlth Sci Ctr, Denver, CO 1975-1976; **Fellow:** Pediatric Critical Care Medicine, Univ Colo Hlth Sci Ctr, Denver, CO 1976-1978; **Fac Appt:** Prof Pediatrics, Baylor Coll Med

Morgan, Wayne J MD (PPul) - *Spec Exp:* Cystic Fibrosis; **Hospital:** Univ Med Ctr; **Address:** U Ariz Hlth Sci Ctr-Ped Pulm, 1501 N Campbell Ave, Box 24-5073, Tucson, AZ 85724; **Phone:** (520) 626-6412; **Board Cert:** Pediatrics 1982, Pediatric Pulmonology 1996; **Med School:** McGill Univ 1976; **Resid:** Pediatrics, Montreal Chldns Hosp., Montreal, CN 1977-1980; **Fellow:** Pediatric Pulmonology, Univ Ariz, Tucson, AZ 1980-1982; **Fac Appt:** Assoc Prof Pediatric Pulmonology, Univ Ariz Coll Med

Warren, Robert Hughes MD (PPul) - *Spec Exp:* Assisted Breathing; Muscular Dystrophy; **Hospital:** Arkansas Chldns Hosp; **Address:** Arkansas Chldns Hosp, Dept Pul, 800 Marshall St, MS 512-17, Little Rock, AR 72202; **Phone:** (501) 320-1006; **Board Cert:** Pediatrics 1973, Pediatric Pulmonology 1996; **Med School:** Univ Ark 1967; **Resid:** Pediatrics, LSU Med Ctr, Shreveport, LA 1968-1971; **Fellow:** Pediatric Pulmonology, Tulane Univ Sch Med, New Orleans, LA 1973; **Fac Appt:** Assoc Prof Pediatrics, Univ Ark

West Coast and Pacific

Platzker, Arnold CG MD (PPul) - *Spec Exp:* Asthma; Bronchopulmonary Dysplasia; **Hospital:** Chldns Hosp - Los Angeles; **Address:** 4650 Sunset Blvd, Box 83, Los Angeles, CA 90027; **Phone:** (323) 669-2101; **Board Cert:** Pediatrics 1967, Neonatal-Perinatal Medicine 1975; **Med School:** Tufts Univ 1962; **Resid:** Pediatrics, City Hosp, Boston, MA 1962-1964; Pediatrics, Stanford Univ, Palo Alto, CA 1964-1966; **Fellow:** Pediatric Pulmonology, Univ Calif Med Ctr, San Francisco, CA 1968-1971; **Fac Appt:** Prof Pediatrics, UCLA

Ramsey, Bonnie W MD (PPul) - *Spec Exp:* Cystic Fibrosis; **Hospital:** Chldns Hosp and Regl Med Ctr - Seattle; **Address:** 4800 Sand Point Way NE, Box C5371, MS CL-11, Seattle, WA 98105; **Phone:** (206) 527-5725; **Board Cert:** Pediatrics 1981, Pediatric Pulmonology 2006; **Med School:** Harvard Med Sch 1976; **Resid:** Pediatrics, Chldns Hosp, Boston, MA 1977-1978; Pediatrics, Chldns Hosp, Boston, MA 1978-1979; **Fellow:** Pediatric Critical Care Medicine, Chldns Hosp, Seattle, WA 1979-1981; **Fac Appt:** Prof Pediatrics, Univ Wash

Redding, Gregory MD (PPul) - *Spec Exp:* Asthma; Ventilator Dependent Children; Infection-Respiratory; **Hospital:** Chldns Hosp and Regl Med Ctr - Seattle; **Address:** 4800 Sand Point Way NE, MS CH-65, Seattle, WA 98105; **Phone:** (206) 526-2174; **Board Cert:** Pediatrics 1993, Pediatric Pulmonology 1996; **Med School:** Stanford Univ 1974; **Resid:** Pediatrics, Harbor-UCLA Affil Hosps, Los Angeles, CA 1974-1977; **Fellow:** Pediatric Pulmonology, Univ Colo Affil Hosps, Denver, CO 1977-1980; **Fac Appt:** Prof Pediatrics, Univ Wash

PEDIATRIC RHEUMATOLOGY

New England

McCarthy, Paul L MD (PRhu) - *Spec Exp:* Arthritis; Juvenile Arthritis; **Hospital:** Yale - New Haven Hosp; **Address:** Yale School of Medicine, 333 Cedar St, Box 208064, New Haven, CT 06520; **Phone:** (203) 785-2475; **Board Cert:** Pediatric Rheumatology 1992, Rheumatology 1974; **Med School:** Georgetown Univ 1969; **Resid:** Pediatrics, Children's Hosp, Buffalo, NY 1970-1972; **Fellow:** Pediatrics, Children's Hosp, Boston, MA 1972-1974; **Fac Appt:** Prof Pediatrics, Yale Univ

Mid Atlantic

Haines, Kathleen MD (PRhu) - *Spec Exp:* Pediatric Rheumatology - General; **Hospital:** Hosp For Joint Diseases (page 61); **Address:** 305 2nd Ave St, Ste 16, New York, NY 10003; **Phone:** (212) 598-6516; **Board Cert:** Pediatric Rheumatology 2000, Clinical & Laboratory Immunology 1994, Allergy & Immunology 1981, Pediatrics 1980; **Med School:** Albert Einstein Coll Med 1975; **Resid:** Pediatrics, NY Hosp, New York, NY 1975-1977; **Fellow:** Allergy & Immunology, NY Hosp, New York, NY 1977-1980; Rheumatology, NYU Med Sch, New York, NY 1980-1982; **Fac Appt:** Assoc Prof Pediatrics, NYU Sch Med

Ilowite, Norman T MD (PRhu) - *Spec Exp:* Rheumatoid Arthritis-Juvenile; Lyme Disease; **Hospital:** Schneider's Chldns Hosp; **Address:** 269-01 76th Ave, rm CH 197, New Hyde Park, NY 11040; **Phone:** (718) 470-3530; **Board Cert:** Pediatric Rheumatology 2000, Clinical & Laboratory Immunology 1990, Pediatrics 1985; **Med School:** SUNY Downstate 1979; **Resid:** Pediatrics, Children's Hosp Natl Med Ctr, Washington, DC 1979-1982; **Fellow:** Pediatric Rheumatology, Univ WA Med Ctr, Seattle, WA 1982-1984; **Fac Appt:** Assoc Prof Pediatrics, Albert Einstein Coll Med

Lehman, Thomas MD (PRhu) - *Spec Exp:* Arthritis; Kawasaki Disease; Lupus/SLE; **Hospital:** Hosp For Special Surgery (page 62); **Address:** 535 E 70th St, New York, NY 10021-4872; **Phone:** (212) 606-1151; **Board Cert:** Pediatrics 1979, Pediatric Rheumatology 1999; **Med School:** Jefferson Med Coll 1974; **Resid:** Pediatrics, Chldns Hosp, Los Angeles, CA 1974-1976; Pediatrics, UCSF Med Ctr, San Francisco, CA 1976-1977; **Fellow:** Pediatric Rheumatology, Chldns Hosp, Los Angeles, CA 1977-1979; Rheumatology, Nat Inst Hlth, Bethesda, MD 1981-1983; **Fac Appt:** Clin Prof Pediatrics, Cornell Univ-Weill Med Coll

Sills, Edward M MD (PRhu) - *Spec Exp:* Juvenile Arthritis; Lupus/SLE; Dermatomyositis; **Hospital:** Johns Hopkins Hosp - Baltimore; **Address:** 600 N Wolfe St, rm Park 321, Baltimore, MD 21287-2534; **Phone:** (410) 955-6145; **Board Cert:** Pediatric Rheumatology 1999, Pediatrics 1968; **Med School:** NYU Sch Med 1963; **Resid:** Pediatrics, Bronx Muni Hosp, New York, NY 1963-1967; **Fac Appt:** Assoc Prof Pediatrics, Johns Hopkins Univ

Southeast

Kredich, Deborah Welt MD (PRhu) - *Spec Exp:* Connective Tissue Disorders; **Hospital:** Duke Univ Med Ctr (page 60); **Address:** Duke Univ Med Ctr, Box 3127, Durham, NC 27710; **Phone:** (919) 684-2356; **Board Cert:** Pediatrics 1992, Pediatric Rheumatology 2000; **Med School:** Univ Mich Med Sch 1962; **Resid:** Pediatrics, Duke Univ Med Ctr, Durham, NC 1969-1971; Pediatrics, Duke Univ Med Ctr, Durham, NC 1963-1964; **Fac Appt:** Assoc Prof Pediatrics, Duke Univ

PEDIATRIC RHEUMATOLOGY

Schanberg, Laura Eve MD (PRhu) - **Spec Exp:** *Rrheumatic Diseases of Childhood; Fibromyalgia;* **Hospital:** Duke Univ Med Ctr (page 60); **Address:** 3212 Erwing Rd, Durham, NC 27710; **Phone:** (919) 684-6575; **Board Cert:** Pediatric Rheumatology 2000, Pediatrics 2000; **Med School:** Duke Univ 1984; **Resid:** Pediatrics, Duke Univ Med Ctr, Durham, NC 1984-1987; **Fellow:** Pediatric Rheumatology, Duke Univ Med Ctr, Durham, NC 1987-1991; **Fac Appt:** Asst Prof Pediatrics, Duke Univ

Sleasman, John W MD (PRhu) - **Spec Exp:** *Infectious Disease;* **Hospital:** Shands Hlthcre at Univ of FL (page 73); **Address:** Univ FL Sch Med, Dept Peds, 1600 SW Archer Rd, Gainesville, FL 32610; **Phone:** (352) 392-2961; **Board Cert:** Pediatrics 1988, Pediatric Rheumatology 1994; **Med School:** Univ Tenn Coll Med, Memphis 1981; **Resid:** Pediatrics, Shands Hosp, Gainesville, FL 1982-1984; **Fellow:** Pediatric Infectious Disease, Shands Hosp, Gainesville, FL 1985-1987; Immunology, Dana Farber Canc Inst, Boston, MA 1987-1988; **Fac Appt:** Assoc Prof Pediatrics, Univ Fla Coll Med

Midwest

Passo, Murray Howard MD (PRhu) - **Spec Exp:** *Pediatric Rheumatology - General;* **Hospital:** Cincinnati Chldns Hosp Med Ctr; **Address:** 3333 Burnett Ave, Cincinnati, OH 45229; **Phone:** (513) 636-4676; **Board Cert:** Pediatrics 1979, Pediatric Rheumatology 2000; **Med School:** Indiana Univ 1974; **Resid:** Pediatrics, Riley Chldns Hosp, Indianapolis, IN 1975-1977; **Fellow:** Rheumatology, Ind Univ Hosps, Indianapolis, IN 1977-1979

Wagner-Weiner, Linda MD (PRhu) - **Spec Exp:** *Lupus/SLE; Arthritis-Juvenile;* **Hospital:** Univ of Chicago Hosps (page 76); **Address:** La Rabida Chldns Hosp, East 65th Street at Lake Michigan, Chicago, IL 60649; **Phone:** (773) 753-8644; **Board Cert:** Pediatric Rheumatology 1999, Pediatrics 1984; **Med School:** Rush Med Coll 1979; **Resid:** Pediatrics, Univ Chicago Hosps, Chicago, IL 1979-1982; **Fellow:** Pediatric Rheumatology, Univ Chicago/La Rabida Chldns Hosp, Chicago, IL 1982-1984; **Fac Appt:** Asst Prof Pediatrics, Univ Chicago-Pritzker Sch Med

Southwest

Myones, Barry Lee MD (PRhu) - **Spec Exp:** *Vasculitis; Kawasaki Disease; Juvenile Dermatomyositis, Sclerdoma;* **Hospital:** TX Chldns Hosp - Houston; **Address:** Texas Chldns Hosp, Ped Rheum Ctr, 6621 Fannin St, MC 3-2290, Houston, TX 77030; **Phone:** (832) 824-3830; **Board Cert:** Pediatrics 1983, Pediatric Rheumatology 2000; **Med School:** Albany Med Coll 1977; **Resid:** Pediatrics, Duke University Med Ctr, Durham, NC 1978-1980; **Fellow:** Pediatric Rheumatology, Chldns Hosp-Stanford, Palo Alto, CA 1981-1983; Rheumatology, Univ North Carolina, Chapel Hill, NC 1983-1988; **Fac Appt:** Assoc Clin Prof Pediatrics, Baylor Coll Med

Warren, Robert Wells MD (PRhu) - **Spec Exp:** *Rheumatoid Arthritis-Juvenile; Lupus/SLE;* **Hospital:** TX Chldns Hosp - Houston; **Address:** Texas Chldns Hosp/Ped Rheumatology, 6621 Fannin St, Ste 940, MC-3-2290, Houston, TX 77030; **Phone:** (832) 824-3830; **Board Cert:** Pediatrics 1983, Aerospace Medicine 1983, Pediatric Rheumatology 2000; **Med School:** Washington Univ, St Louis 1978; **Resid:** Pediatrics, Duke Univ Med Ctr, Durham, NC 1978-1980; **Fellow:** Rheumatology, Duke Univ Med Ctr, Durham, NC 1980-1982; Rheumatology, Duke Univ Med Ctr, Durham, NC 1982-1983; **Fac Appt:** Assoc Prof Pediatric Rheumatology, Baylor Coll Med

Wilking, Andrew MD (PRhu) - **Spec Exp:** *Pediatric Rheumatology - General;* **Hospital:** TX Chldns Hosp - Houston; **Address:** 6621 Fannin St, MC 3-2290, Houston, TX 77030; **Phone:** (832) 824-3826; **Board Cert:** Pediatrics 1985; **Med School:** Columbia P&S 1978; **Resid:** Pediatrics, Babies Hosp, New York, NY 1979-1981; **Fellow:** Pediatric Rheumatology, Tex Chldns Hosp, Houston, TX 1981-1983; **Fac Appt:** Assoc Prof Pediatrics, Baylor Coll Med

West Coast and Pacific

Bernstein, Bram Henry MD (PRhu) - *Spec Exp:* *Reheumatic Diseases of Childhood;* **Hospital:** Chldns Hosp - Los Angeles; **Address:** 4650 W Sunset Blvd, Chldns Hosp Los Angeles M/S 60, Los Angeles, CA 90027-6062; **Phone:** (323) 669-2119; **Board Cert:** Pediatrics 1969, Pediatric Rheumatology 1998; **Med School:** McGill Univ 1964; **Resid:** Pediatrics, Chldns Hosp, Los Angeles, CA 1965-1967; Rheumatology, Chldns Hosp, Los Angeles, CA 1967-1968; **Fellow:** Rheumatology, Vancouver Genl Hosp, Canada 1968-1970; **Fac Appt:** Clin Prof Pediatrics, Univ SC Sch Med

Emery, Helen Margaret MD (PRhu) - *Spec Exp:* *Rheumatic Diseases of Childhood;* **Hospital:** UCSF Med Ctr; **Address:** 533 Parnassus Ave, Box 0107, San Francisco, CA 94143; **Phone:** (415) 476-1736; **Board Cert:** Pediatric Rheumatology 2000, Pediatrics 1992; **Med School:** Australia 1971; **Resid:** Pediatrics, Chldns Or Hosp-Univ Wash, Washington, DC 1973-1975; **Fellow:** Pediatric Rheumatology, Chldns Or Hosp-Univ Wash, Washington, DC 1975-1977; **Fac Appt:** Clin Prof Pediatrics, UCSF

Sherry, David MD (PRhu) - *Spec Exp:* *Reflex Sympathetic Dystrophy(RSD);* **Hospital:** Chldns Hosp and Regl Med Ctr - Seattle; **Address:** 4800 Sand Point Way NE, MS CH-73, Seattle, WA 98105-5371; **Phone:** (206) 526-2057; **Board Cert:** Pediatrics 1981, Pediatric Rheumatology 1992; **Med School:** Texas Tech Univ 1977; **Resid:** Pediatrics, Duke Univ Med Ctr, Durham, NC 1977-1980; **Fellow:** Pediatric Rheumatology, Univ British Columbia, Vancouver, Canada 1980-1982; **Fac Appt:** Assoc Prof Pediatrics, Univ Wash

PEDIATRIC SURGERY

New England

Mayer, John MD (PS) - *Spec Exp:* Cardiac Surgery; **Hospital:** Children's Hospital - Boston; **Address:** Children's Hospital Dept. Cardiac Surgery, 300 Longwood Ave, Boston, MA 02115; **Phone:** (617) 355-8258; **Board Cert:** Thoracic Surgery 1994; **Med School:** Yale Univ 1972; **Resid:** Surgery, University Minn, Minneapolis, MN 1973-1979; **Fellow:** Cardiothoracic Surgery, University Minn, Minnepolis, MN 1979-1981; **Fac Appt:** Prof Surgery, Harvard Med Sch

Ziegler, Moritz M MD (PS) - *Spec Exp:* Cancer & General Surgery; **Hospital:** Children's Hospital - Boston; **Address:** 300 Longwood Ave, Boston, MA 02115; **Phone:** (617) 355-2469; **Board Cert:** Pediatric Surgery 1995, Surgical Critical Care 1990, Surgery 1975; **Med School:** Univ Mich Med Sch 1968; **Resid:** Surgery, Univ Penn Hosp, Philadelphia, PA 1969-1975; Pediatric Surgery, Chldns Hosp, Philadelphia, PA 1975-1977; **Fellow:** Medical Oncology, Amer Oncologic Hosp, Philadelphia, PA 1975; **Fac Appt:** Prof Surgery, Harvard Med Sch

Mid Atlantic

Adkins, John C MD (PS) - *Spec Exp:* Neonatal Surgery-Gastrointestinal; **Hospital:** Chldn's Hosp of Pittsbrgh; **Address:** Children's Hospital - Pittsburgh, 3705 5th Ave Fl 4A - rm 480, Pittsburgh, PA 15213; **Phone:** (412) 359-5222; **Board Cert:** Surgery 1974, Pediatric Surgery 1993; **Med School:** Johns Hopkins Univ 1965; **Resid:** Surgery, Duke Med Ctr, Durham, NC 1966-1967; Surgery, Pittsburgh Med Ctr, Pittsburgh, PA 1970-1973; **Fellow:** Pediatric Surgery, Chldns Hosp, Pittsburgh, PA 1973-1974; **Fac Appt:** Asst Prof Pediatrics, Univ Pittsburgh

Adzick, Nick Scott MD (PS) - *Spec Exp:* Fetal Surgery; **Hospital:** Chldn's Hosp of Philadelphia; **Address:** Chldns Hosp-Philadelphia, Wood Bldg, 34th and Civic Ctr Blvd, Fl 5, Philadelphia, PA 19104-4399; **Phone:** (215) 590-2727; **Board Cert:** Surgery 1997, Surgical Critical Care 1991, Pediatric Surgery 1999; **Med School:** Harvard Med Sch 1979; **Resid:** Surgery, Mass Genl Hosp, Boston, MA 1985-1986; Pediatric Surgery, Chldns Hosp, Boston, MA 1986-1988; **Fac Appt:** Prof Surgery, UCSF

Colombani, Paul M MD (PS) - *Spec Exp:* Pediatric Surgery - General; **Hospital:** Johns Hopkins Hosp - Baltimore; **Address:** 600 N Wolfe St, Box CMSC 7-113, Baltimore, MD 21287; **Phone:** (410) 955-2717; **Board Cert:** Surgery 1993, Pediatric Surgery 1993; **Med School:** Univ KY Coll Med 1976; **Resid:** Surgery, Geo Wash Univ Hosp, Washington, DC 1977-1981; **Fellow:** Pediatric Surgery, Johns Hopkins Hosp, Baltimore, MD 1981-1983; **Fac Appt:** Prof Surgery, Johns Hopkins Univ

Ginsburg, Howard MD (PS) - *Spec Exp:* Neonatal Surgery; Tumor Surgery; Urology-Pediatric; **Hospital:** NYU Med Ctr (page 71); **Address:** 530 1st Ave, Ste 10W, New York, NY 10016-6497; **Phone:** (212) 263-7391; **Board Cert:** Surgery 1978, Pediatric Surgery 1991; **Med School:** Univ Cincinnati 1972; **Resid:** Surgery, NYU-Bellvue Hosp, New York, NY 1972-1977; Pediatric Surgery, Colum-Presby Med Ctr, New York, NY 1977-1979; **Fellow:** Pediatric Surgery, Mass General Hosp, Boston, MA 1979-1980; **Fac Appt:** Assoc Prof Surgery, NYU Sch Med

Harris, Burton H MD (PS) - *Spec Exp:* Pediatric Surgery - General; **Hospital:** Montefiore Med Ctr (page 67); **Address:** Children's Hosp at Montefiore, Dept Ped Surgery, 111 E 210th St, Bronx, NY 10467; **Phone:** (718) 920-6643; **Board Cert:** Surgery 1973, Pediatric Surgery 1995; **Med School:** SUNY Downstate 1965; **Resid:** Surgery, SUNY-Kings Co Hosp, Brooklyn, NY 1966-1969; Pediatric Surgery, SUNY-Kings Co Hosp, Brooklyn, NY 1969-1972; **Fac Appt:** Prof Surgery, Albert Einstein Coll Med

La Quaglia, Michael MD (PS) - *Spec Exp:* Cancer Surgery; Neuroblastoma; Liver Tumors; **Hospital:** Mem Sloan Kettering Cancer Ctr; **Address:** 1275 York Ave, Ste 1176, New York, NY 10021-6007; **Phone:** (212) 639-7002; **Board Cert:** Pediatric Surgery 1985; **Med School:** UMDNJ-NJ Med Sch, Newark 1976; **Resid:** Surgery, Mass Genl Hosp, Boston, MA 1977-1983; **Fellow:** Cardiothoracic Surgery, Broadgreen Ctr, Liverpool, England 1982; Pediatric Surgery, Children's Hosp, Boston, MA 1984-1985; **Fac Appt:** Prof Pediatric Surgery, Cornell Univ-Weill Med Coll

Lehman, Wallace B MD (PS) - *Spec Exp:* Hip/Leg/Feet Orthopedic Surgery; Limb Lengthening & Reconstruction; Blount's Disease & Bone Deformities; **Hospital:** Hosp For Joint Diseases (page 61); **Address:** Hosp Joint Diseases, Dept Ped Orth Surg, 301 E 17th St, Ste 413, New York, NY 10003; **Phone:** (212) 598-6403; **Board Cert:** Orthopaedic Surgery 1966; **Med School:** SUNY Hlth Sci Ctr 1958; **Resid:** Orthopaedic Surgery, Hosp Joint Diseases, New York, NY 1958-1963; **Fac Appt:** Clin Prof Orthopaedic Surgery, NYU Sch Med

Paidas, Charles Nicholas MD (PS) - *Spec Exp:* Tumor Surgery; Chest Wall Deformities; **Hospital:** Johns Hopkins Hosp - Baltimore; **Address:** Johns Hopkins Hosp, Dept Ped Surg, 600 N Wolfe St, Bldg CMSC - rm 7-116, Baltimore, MD 21287; **Phone:** (410) 955-2960; **Board Cert:** Pediatric Surgery 1992, Surgical Critical Care 1992; **Med School:** NY Med Coll 1981; **Resid:** Surgery, NY Med Coll Affil Hosps, Westchester, NY 1982-1987; **Fellow:** Pediatric Surgery, Johns Hopkins Hosp, Baltimore, MD 1987-1991; **Fac Appt:** Assoc Prof Surgery, Johns Hopkins Univ

Quaegebeur, Jan Modest MD (PS) - *Spec Exp:* Arterial Switch; Heart Valve Surgery; Cardiac Surgery; **Hospital:** NY Presby Hosp - Columbia Presby Med Ctr (page 70); **Address:** 3959 Broadway, Ste BN 276, New York, NY 10032; **Phone:** (212) 305-5975; **Med School:** Belgium 1969; **Resid:** Surgery, St Michel Clinic, Brussels, Belgium 1969-1973; **Fellow:** Thoracic Surgery, Baylor Coll Med, Houston, TX 1973-1974; Thoracic Surgery, Univ Hosp, Leiden, Belgium 1974-1978; **Fac Appt:** Prof Surgery, Columbia P&S

Shlasko, Edward MD (PS) - *Spec Exp:* Laparoscopic Surgery; Pediatric Oncology; Robotic Surgery; **Hospital:** Maimonides Med Ctr (page 65); **Address:** Pediatric Surgery, 921 49th St, Brooklyn, NY 11219; **Phone:** (718) 283-7384; **Board Cert:** Surgery 1992, Pediatric Surgery 1994; **Med School:** Columbia P&S 1985; **Resid:** Surgery, Mount Sinai Medical Ctr, New York, NY 1985-1991; Pediatric Surgery, SUNY-HSCB, Brooklyn, NY 1991-1993; **Fac Appt:** Asst Prof Pediatric Surgery, Mount Sinai Sch Med

Spray, Thomas L MD (PS) - *Spec Exp:* Cardiac Surgery; Transplant-Heart & Lung; Ross Procedure; **Hospital:** Chldn's Hosp of Philadelphia; **Address:** 34th St & Civic Center Blvd, Ste 8527, Philadelphia, PA 19104; **Phone:** (215) 590-2708; **Board Cert:** Thoracic Surgery 1985, Surgery 1983; **Med School:** Duke Univ 1973; **Resid:** Surgery, Duke Univ Med Ctr, Durham, NC 1973-1975; Thoracic Surgery, Duke Univ Med Ctr, Durham, NC 1977-1980; **Fac Appt:** Prof Surgery, Univ Penn

Stolar, Charles J MD (PS) - *Spec Exp:* Surgical Oncology; Neonatal Surgery; **Hospital:** NY Presby Hosp - Columbia Presby Med Ctr (page 70); **Address:** 3959 Broadway, Fl 2 - rm 212 North, New York, NY 10032; **Phone:** (212) 305-2305; **Board Cert:** Surgery 1991, Pediatric Surgery 1995; **Med School:** Georgetown Univ 1974; **Resid:** Surgery, U IL Med Ctr, Chicago, IL 1974-1980; **Fellow:** Pediatric Surgery, Children's Hosp, Washington, DC 1980-1982; **Fac Appt:** Prof Surgery, Columbia P&S

Stylianos, Steven MD (PS) - *Spec Exp:* Trauma; Plastic Surgery; **Hospital:** NY Presby Hosp - Columbia Presby Med Ctr (page 70); **Address:** 3959 Broadway, rm 205, New York, NY 10032-1551; **Phone:** (212) 305-8861; **Board Cert:** Surgery 1989, Pediatric Surgery 1994, Surgical Critical Care 1990; **Med School:** NYU Sch Med 1983; **Resid:** Surgery, Columbia Presby Med Ctr, New York, NY 1983-1988; Pediatric Surgery, Chldns Hosp, Boston, MA 1990-1992; **Fellow:** Pediatric Trauma, New England Med Ctr, Boston, MA 1988-1990; **Fac Appt:** Assoc Prof Pediatric Surgery, Columbia P&S

Velcek, Francisca MD (PS) - *Spec Exp:* Anorectal Disorders; **Hospital:** Lenox Hill Hosp (page 64); **Address:** 965 5th Ave, New York, NY 10021; **Phone:** (212) 744-9396; **Board Cert:** Surgery 1974, Pediatric Surgery 1997; **Med School:** Philippines 1966; **Resid:** Surgery, St Clares Hosp, New York, NY 1966-1971; **Fellow:** Pediatric Surgery, SUNY Hosp, Brooklyn, NY 1973-1975; SUNY Hosp, Brooklyn, NY 1972-1973; **Fac Appt:** Prof Surgery, SUNY Hlth Sci Ctr

Wiener, Eugene MD (PS) - *Spec Exp:* Cancer Surgery; **Hospital:** Chldn's Hosp of Pittsbrgh; **Address:** Chldns Hosp, Dept Ped Surgery, 3705 5th Ave, Pittsburgh, PA 15213; **Phone:** (412) 692-7280; **Board Cert:** Pediatric Surgery 1995, Surgery 1973; **Med School:** Med Coll VA 1964; **Resid:** Surgery, Med Coll VA Hosps, Richmond, VA 1965-1971; **Fac Appt:** Prof Surgery, Univ Pittsburgh

Southeast

Drucker, David E MD (PS) - *Spec Exp:* Pediatric Surgery - General; **Hospital:** Mem Reg Hosp - Hollywood; **Address:** 1150 N 35th Ave, Ste 555, Hollywood, FL 33021-5431; **Phone:** (954) 981-0072; **Board Cert:** Pediatric Surgery 1999, Surgical Critical Care 1992; **Med School:** Univ Hlth Sci/Chicago Med Sch 1978; **Resid:** Surgery, Med Coll VA Hosps, Richmond, VA 1983-1988; **Fellow:** Pediatric Surgery, Chldns Hosp, Detroit, MI 1988-1990

Georgeson, Keith E MD (PS) - *Spec Exp:* Hirschsprung's Disease; Laparoscopic Surgery; Gastroesophageal Reflux; **Hospital:** Children's Hospital - Birmingham; **Address:** Chlds Hosp of Alabama, Dept Ped Surgery, 1600 7th Ave S, Ste ACC300, Birmingham, AL 35233-1711; **Phone:** (205) 939-9688; **Board Cert:** Surgery 1992, Pediatric Surgery 1995; **Med School:** Loma Linda Univ 1969; **Resid:** Surgery, Loma Linda Univ Med Ctr, Loma Linda, CA 1970-1973; Pediatric Surgery, Chldn's Hosp of Mich, Detroit, MI 1973-1975; **Fac Appt:** Prof Surgery, Univ Ala

Lobe, Thom E MD (PS) - *Spec Exp:* Minimally Invasive Surgery; **Hospital:** Le Bonheur Chldns Med Ctr; **Address:** Le Bonheur Chldn's Med Ctr, 777 Washington Ave, Ste 230, Memphis, TN 38105; **Phone:** (901) 572-3031; **Board Cert:** Surgery 1989, Pediatric Surgery 1989; **Med School:** Univ MD Sch Med 1975; **Resid:** Surgery, Ohio State Univ Med Ctr, Columbus, OH 1975-1979; Pediatric Surgery, Chldn's Hosp, Columbus, OH 1979-1981; **Fac Appt:** Prof Pediatric Surgery, Univ Tenn Coll Med, Memphis

Nakayama, Don Ken MD (PS) - *Spec Exp:* Neonatal Surgery; Minimally Invasive Surgery; **Hospital:** Univ of NC Hosp (page 77); **Address:** 3010 Old Clinic Bldg, Box CB7210, Chapel Hill, NC 27599-7210; **Phone:** (919) 966-4643; **Board Cert:** Pediatric Surgery 1998, Surgery 1994; **Med School:** UCSF 1978; **Resid:** Surgery, UCSF Hosps, San Francisco, CA 1978-1984; **Fellow:** Pediatric Surgery, Chldns Hosp, Philadelphia, PA 1984-1986; **Fac Appt:** Prof Surgery, Univ NC Sch Med

Neblett, Wallace W MD (PS) - *Spec Exp:* Thyroid Surgery; Pancreatic Disease; Inflammatory Bowel Disease/Crohn's; **Hospital:** Vanderbilt Univ Med Ctr (page 80); **Address:** Vanderbilt Univ Med Ctr, Dept Ped Surg, 1211 21st Ave S, Ste 338, Nashville, TN 37232-1586; **Phone:** (615) 936-1050; **Board Cert:** Pediatric Surgery 1991; **Med School:** Vanderbilt Univ **Resid:** Surgery, Vanderbilt Univ Med Ctr, Nashville, TN 1973-1977; Pediatric Surgery, Chldns Hosp Med Ctr, Cincinnati, OH 1978-1980; **Fac Appt:** Prof Surgery, Vanderbilt Univ

Rodgers, Bradley Moreland MD (PS) - *Spec Exp:* Thoracic Surgery; **Hospital:** Univ of VA Hlth Sys (page 79); **Address:** UVA Health System, Dept Surgery, PO Box 800709, Charlottesville, VA 22908; **Phone:** (804) 924-2673; **Board Cert:** Surgery 1997, Pediatric Surgery 1995, Thoracic Surgery 1975; **Med School:** Johns Hopkins Univ 1966; **Resid:** Surgery, Duke Univ Med Ctr, Durham, NC 1967-1968; Surgery, Duke Univ Med Ctr, Durham, NC 1970-1973; **Fellow:** Pediatric Surgery, Chldns Hosp, Montreal, CN 1973-1974; **Fac Appt:** Prof Pediatric Surgery, Univ VA Sch Med

Toufanian, Ahmad MD (PS) - *Spec Exp:* Hernia; **Hospital:** St Mary's Med Ctr - W Palm Bch; **Address:** 1500 N Dixie Hwy, Ste 202, West Palm Beach, FL 33401-2716; **Phone:** (561) 655-6800; **Board Cert:** Surgery 1983; **Med School:** Iran 1971; **Resid:** Pediatric Surgery, Chldns Hosp, Columbus, OH 1977-1978; Pediatric Surgery, Univ Miami Project to Cure Paralysis, Miami, FL 1978-1980; **Fellow:** Pediatric Surgery, Univ Miami Project to Cure Paralysis, Miami, FL 1978-1980

Weinberger, Malvin MD (PS) - *Spec Exp:* Neonatal Surgery; Trauma; Cancer in Children; **Hospital:** Miami Children's Hosp; **Address:** 3200 SW 60th Ct, Miami, FL 33155-4070; **Phone:** (305) 662-8320; **Board Cert:** Surgery 1970, Pediatric Surgery 1995; **Med School:** Temple Univ 1962; **Resid:** Surgery, Temple Univ Hlth Scis Ctr, Philadelphia, PA 1965-1969; Pediatric Surgery, Columbus Chldns Hosp/Ohio St U, Columbus, OH 1969-1971; **Fac Appt:** Assoc Clin Prof Surgery, Univ Miami Sch Med

Midwest

Aiken, John Judson MD (PS) - *Spec Exp:* Tumor Surgery-Pediatric; **Hospital:** Chldrns Hosp - Wisconsin; **Address:** 9000 W Wisconsin Ave, MS 402, Milwaukee, WI 53226; **Phone:** (414) 266-6550; **Board Cert:** Pediatric Surgery 2000, Surgery 1995; **Med School:** Univ Cincinnati 1984; **Resid:** Surgery, Mass Genl Hosp, Cambridge, MA 1985-1991; **Fellow:** Pediatric Surgery, Chldns Hosp, Cincinnati, OH; **Fac Appt:** Asst Prof Surgery, Med Coll Wisc

Alexander, Frederick MD (PS) - *Spec Exp:* Transplant-Small Bowel; Solid Tumors; Congenital Gastrointestinal Anomalies; **Hospital:** Cleveland Clin Fdn (page 57); **Address:** Cleveland Clinic, Dept Pediatric Surgery, 9500 Euclid Ave, M14, Cleveland, OH 44195; **Phone:** (216) 445-6846; **Board Cert:** Pediatric Surgery 1999, Surgery 2001; **Med School:** Columbia P&S 1976; **Resid:** Surgery, Brigham-Womens Hosp, Boston, MA 1977-1984; **Fellow:** Pediatric Surgery, Chldns Hosp, Cincinnati, OH 1984-1986; **Fac Appt:** Assoc Prof Pediatric Surgery, Ohio State Univ

Bove, Edward MD (PS) - *Spec Exp:* Cardiothoracic Surgery; Hypoplastic Left Heart Syndrome; **Hospital:** Univ of MI Hlth Ctr; **Address:** 1500 E Med Center Dri, Bldg Mott - Ste F7830, Ann Arbor, MI 48109-0223; **Phone:** (734) 763-7354; **Board Cert:** Thoracic Surgery 1998, Surgery 1978; **Med School:** Albany Med Coll 1972; **Resid:** Surgery, Univ Mich Med Ctr, Ann Arbor, MI 1973-1976; Thoracic Surgery, Univ Mich Med Ctr, Ann Arbor, MI 1977-1979; **Fellow:** Pediatric Cardiac Surgery, Hosp Sick Chldn, London, England 1979-1980; **Fac Appt:** Prof Surgery, Univ Mich Med Sch

Cohen, Roger David MD (PS) - *Spec Exp:* Thoracic Surgery; Laparoscopic Surgery; **Hospital:** Chldrns Hosp - Wisconsin; **Address:** 9000 W Wisconsin Ave, Ste 403, Milwaukee, WI 53226; **Phone:** (414) 266-6550; **Board Cert:** Pediatric Surgery 1995, Thoracic Surgery 1972; **Med School:** Columbia P&S 1963; **Resid:** Surgery, Presbyterian Hosp, New York, NY 1964-1969; Surgery, Chldns Meml Hosp, Chicago, IL 1969-1971; **Fac Appt:** Prof Surgery, Med Coll Wisc

PEDIATRIC SURGERY

Midwest

Coran, Arnold G MD (PS) - *Spec Exp:* Ulcerative Colitis; Hirschsprung's Disease; **Hospital:** Motts Chldns Hosp; **Address:** 1500 E Med Center Drive, Ste F3970, Box 0245, Ann Arbor, MI 48109-0245; **Phone:** (734) 764-4151; **Board Cert:** Surgery 1969, Thoracic Surgery 1970, Surgical Critical Care 1987, Pediatric Surgery 1993; **Med School:** Harvard Med Sch 1963; **Resid:** Surgery, Peter Bent Brigham Hosp, Boston, MA 1964-1968; Surgery, Children's Hosp, Boston, MA 1964-1968; **Fellow:** Neonatal Metabolism, Univ of Oslo, Oslo, Norway 1969; **Fac Appt:** Prof Surgery, Univ Mich Med Sch

Grosfeld, Jay L MD (PS) - *Spec Exp:* Cancer Surgery; **Hospital:** Riley Chldrn's Hosp (page 588); **Address:** 702 Barnhill Drive, Ste 2500, Indianapolis, IN 46202-5200; **Phone:** (317) 274-4682; **Board Cert:** Surgery 1989, Pediatric Surgery 1982; **Med School:** NYU Sch Med 1961; **Resid:** Surgery, Bellevue-NYU Hosp, New York, NY 1962-1966; Pediatric Surgery, Ohio State Univ, Columbus, OH 1968-1970; **Fellow:** Pediatric Hematology-Oncology, Childrens Hosp, Columbus, OH 1968-1970; **Fac Appt:** Prof Surgery, Indiana Univ

Oldham, Keith T MD (PS) - *Spec Exp:* Neonatal Surgery; Cardiothoracic Surgery; **Hospital:** Chldrns Hosp - Wisconsin; **Address:** 9000 W Wisconsin Ave, MS 402, Milwaukee, WI 53226; **Phone:** (414) 266-6557; **Board Cert:** Surgery 1995, Pediatric Surgery 1991; **Med School:** Med Coll VA 1976; **Resid:** Surgery, Univ Wash Med Ctr, Seattle, WA 1977-1981; **Fellow:** Pediatric Surgery, Univ Cincinnati Chldns Hosp, Cincinnati, OH 1981-1983; **Fac Appt:** Prof Pediatric Surgery, Med Coll Wisc

Reynolds, Marleta MD (PS) - *Spec Exp:* Critical Care; Trauma; **Hospital:** Children's Mem Hosp; **Address:** Dept Pediatric Surgery, 2300 Children's Plaza, Chicago, IL 60614; **Phone:** (773) 880-4292; **Board Cert:** Thoracic Surgery 1995, Pediatric Surgery 1986; **Med School:** Tulane Univ 1976; **Resid:** Surgery, Tulane Univ Affil Hosp, New Orleans, LA 1977-1981; Pediatric Surgery, Chldns Meml Hosp, Chicago, IL 1981-1983; **Fellow:** Cardiothoracic Surgery, Northwestern Univ, Chicago, IL 1983-1985; **Fac Appt:** Asst Prof Surgery, Northwestern Univ

Sato, Thomas Tad MD (PS) - *Spec Exp:* Neonatal Surgery; Congenital Defect Repair; Laparoscopy & Thoracostomy; **Hospital:** Chldrns Hosp - Wisconsin; **Address:** 9000 W Wisconsin Ave, MS 403, Milwaukee, WI 53226; **Phone:** (414) 266-6550; **Board Cert:** Pediatric Surgery 1998, Surgery 1996; **Med School:** USC Sch Med 1988; **Resid:** Surgery, Univ Wash Med Ctr, Seattle, WA 1988-1995; **Fellow:** Surgery, Harborview Med Ctr, Seattle, WA 1991-1993; Pediatric Surgery, Chldns Natl Med Ctr, Washington, DC 1995-1997; **Fac Appt:** Asst Prof Pediatric Surgery, Med Coll Wisc

West Coast and Pacific

Anderson, Kathryn D MD (PS) - *Spec Exp:* Esophageal Surgery; **Hospital:** Chldns Hosp - Los Angeles; **Address:** Chldns Hosp - Los Angeles, Dept Ped Surgery, 4650 Sunset Blvd, MS 72, Los Angeles, CA 90027; **Phone:** (323) 669-2104; **Board Cert:** Surgery 1971, Pediatric Surgery 1993; **Med School:** Harvard Med Sch 1964; **Resid:** Surgery, Georgetown Univ Hosp, Washington, DC 1965-1969; **Fellow:** Pediatric Surgery, Chldns Natl Med Ctr, Washington, DC 1970-1972; **Fac Appt:** Prof Surgery, USC Sch Med

Atkinson, James B MD (PS) - *Spec Exp:* Pediatric Surgery - General; **Hospital:** UCLA Med Ctr; **Address:** 10833 LeConte Ave, Box 709818, Los Angeles, CA 90095-1749; **Phone:** (310) 206-2429; **Board Cert:** Surgery 1989, Pediatric Surgery 1993; **Med School:** Wake Forest Univ Sch Med 1976; **Resid:** Surgery, UCLA Med Ctr, Los Angeles, CA 1977-1981; **Fellow:** Pediatric Surgery, Chldns Hosp, Los Angeles, CA 1981-1983; **Fac Appt:** Prof Surgery, UCLA

Fonkalsrud, Eric W MD (PS) - *Spec Exp:* Chest Wall Deformities; Gastroesophageal Reflux; Colorectal Surgery; **Hospital:** UCLA Med Ctr; **Address:** UCLA Med Ctr, Dept Surg 72-126CHS, 10833 Le Conte Ave, Los Angeles, CA 90095-1749; **Phone:** (310) 825-6712; **Board Cert:** Pediatric Surgery 1984, Thoracic Surgery 1966; **Med School:** Johns Hopkins Univ 1957; **Resid:** Surgery, Johns Hopkins Hosp, Baltimore, MD 1957-1959; Thoracic Surgery, UCLA Med Ctr, Los Angeles, CA 1959-1963; **Fellow:** Pediatric Surgery, Columbus Chldns Hosp, Columbus, OH 1963-1965; **Fac Appt:** Prof Emeritus Surgery, UCLA

Harrison, Michael R MD (PS) - *Spec Exp:* Fetal Surgery; **Hospital:** UCSF Med Ctr; **Address:** 533 Parnassus Ave, Ste U149, Box 0712, San Francisco, CA 94143; **Phone:** (415) 476-2538; **Board Cert:** Surgical Critical Care 1991, Pediatric Surgery 1999; **Med School:** Harvard Med Sch 1969; **Resid:** Surgery, Mass Genl Hosp, Boston, MA 1970-1971; Surgery, Mass Genl Hosp, Boston, MA 1973-1975; **Fellow:** Pediatric Surgery, Rikshospitalet, Oslo, Norway 1975-1976; Pediatric Surgery, Chldns Hosp, Los Angeles, CA 1976-1978; **Fac Appt:** Prof Surgery, UCSF

Krummel, Thomas M. MD (PS) - *Spec Exp:* Minimally Invasive Surgery; Robotic Surgery; Fetal Surgery; **Hospital:** Stanford Med Ctr; **Address:** 701B Welch Rd, Ste 225, MC-5784, Stanford, CA 94305-5784; **Phone:** (650) 498-4292; **Board Cert:** Surgery 1994, Pediatric Surgery 1997; **Med School:** Univ Wisc 1977; **Resid:** Surgery, Med Coll Va Hosp, Richmond, VA 1978-1983; Pediatric Surgery, Chldns Hosp, Pittsburgh, PA 1983-1985; **Fellow:** Surgery, Med Coll Va Hosp, Richmond, VA 1979-1980; Fetal Surgery, UCSF Med Ctr, San Francisco, CA 1985; **Fac Appt:** Prof Surgery, Stanford Univ

Tapper, David MD (PS) - *Spec Exp:* Critical Care; Solid Tumors; Birth Defects; **Hospital:** Chldns Hosp and Regl Med Ctr - Seattle; **Address:** 4800 NE Sand Point Way, Box C5371, Seattle, WA 98105-3916; **Phone:** (206) 526-2039; **Board Cert:** Surgical Critical Care 1987, Surgery 1998, Pediatric Surgery 1999; **Med School:** Univ MD Sch Med 1970; **Resid:** Surgery, Moffitt Hosp, San Francisco, CA 1971-1977; **Fellow:** Pediatric Surgery, Chldns Hosp Med Ctr, Boston, MA 1977-1979; **Fac Appt:** Prof Surgery, Univ Wash

PHYSICAL MEDICINE & REHABILITATION

Physical medicine and rehabilitation, also referred to as rehabilitation medicine, is the medical specialty concerned with diagnosing, evaluating and treating patients with physical disabilities. These disabilities may arise from conditions affecting the musculoskeletal system such as neck and back pain, sports injuries, or other painful conditions affecting the limbs, for example carpal tunnel syndrome. Alternatively, the disabilities may result from neurological trauma or disease such as spinal cord injury, head injury or stroke.

A physician certified in physical medicine and rehabilitation is often called a physiatrist. The primary goal of the physiatrist is to achieve maximal restoration of physical, psychological, social and vocational function through comprehensive rehabilitation. Pain management is often an important part of the role of the physiatrist. For diagnosis and evaluation, a physiatrist may include the techniques of electromyography to supplement the standard history, physical, X-ray and laboratory examinations. The physiatrist has expertise in the appropriate use of therapeutic exercise, prosthetics (artificial limbs), orthotics and mechanical and electrical devices.

Training required: Four years *plus* one year clinical practice

REHABILITATION INSTITUTE OF MICHIGAN

261 Mack Boulevard • Detroit, Michigan 48201
1-888-DMC-2500 • www.RIMrehab.org

HELPING TO REBUILD LIVES

Rehabilitation Institute of Michigan (RIM) is a 94-bed specialty hospital dedicated to physical medicine and rehabilitation. A full spectrum of inpatient and outpatient services are available for spinal cord injuries, brain injuries, stroke, cerebral palsy, musculoskeletal disorders, low back problems, amputations, geriatric conditions, work-related injuries, sports injuries and other medical conditions requiring physical rehabilitation. The Rehabilitation Institute of Michigan also operates 12 state-of-the-art outpatient locations, making it one of the largest rehabilitation providers in the nation. The Institute is accredited by the Joint Commission on Accreditation of Healthcare Organizations (JCAHO) and the Commission on Accreditation of Rehabilitation Facilities (CARF).

INTERNATIONALLY RENOWNED STAFF

Rehabilitation Institute of Michigan's physicians are among the brightest in their field, publishing numerous professional articles each year and guest lecturing both nationally and internationally. Because the Institute's physicians are also faculty members at Wayne State University School of Medicine, they not only practice medicine, but they are on the forefront of advancing it by contributing to new scientific knowledge and discoveries. Other members of the rehabilitation team include specialists in physical and occupational therapy, rehabilitation nursing, speech-language pathology, respiratory therapy, therapeutic recreation, social work, orthotics, psychology/neuropsychology, and nutrition.

A LEADER IN RESEARCH & TREATMENT

During the last 10 years, Rehabilitation Institute of Michigan has been awarded $16 million in federal and private grants for rehabilitation research focusing on restoring function, improving quality of life and developing innovative therapeutic techniques. One example of the Institute's state-of-the-art capabilities is the Gait and Motion Analysis Laboratory, which focuses on improving skills such as walking or stair climbing, and improving sports related techniques through proper body mechanics.

DMC
Rehabilitation Institute of Michigan
Detroit Medical Center/Wayne State University

POINTS OF PRIDE

- Rehabilitation Institute was named as one of "America's Best Hospitals" by *U.S. News and World Report*.

- The Institute has earned the rare distinction of being one of 17 federally designated "model systems" of care for the treatment of traumatic brain injuries.

- The Institute treats more than 1,600 inpatients and conducts nearly 125,000 outpatient visits each year.

- The hospital treats more spinal cord injury patients than any other program in Michigan.

- The brain injury program at RIM was the first program of its kind established in the Midwest when it opened in 1979.

THE MOUNT SINAI HOSPITAL
REHABILITATION MEDICINE

One Gustave L. Levy Place (Fifth Avenue and 98th Street)
New York, NY 10029-6574   Phone: (212) 987-6043
Physician Referral: 1-800-MD-SINAI (637-4624)
www.mountsinai.org

The Mount Sinai Hospital's Department of Rehabilitation Medicine is a center for excellence in the delivery of complete care for people with disabilities. A wide range of comprehensive patient care services is available for individuals with spinal cord injuries, traumatic brain injuries, and neuromuscular, musculosketetal, and chronic conditions. It is CARF-accredited for its inpatient spinal cord injury, brain injury, and comprehensive rehabilitation medicine programs.

The Team-Oriented Approach
A team-oriented approach is pivotal to successful rehabilitation. The interdisciplinary team approach at Mount Sinai takes advantage of each discipline's expertise to provide quality coordinated care. Highly experienced professionals meet to evaluate thoroughly, develop, and implement an individualized treatment plan in partnership with the patient and his or her family.

The Rehabilitation Care Center team is led by Dr. Kristjan T. Ragnarsson, whose leadership and innovation have revolutionized the field of Rehabilitation Medicine. It includes a primary nurse and other nursing staff, physicians, surgeons, nurse practitioners, and professional staff in physical therapy, respiratory therapy, pharmacy, nutrition, social work, and radiology for:

- *Spinal Cord Injury Center*
  The Center provides comprehensive care to meet the diverse needs of persons with spinal cord injury (SCI).

- *Sports Therapy Center*
  The Center is a comprehensive physical and occupational therapy facility specializing in musculoskeletal exercise and sports-related conditions.

- *Community Integration of Individuals with Traumatic Brain Injury Research and Training Center*
  We work to improve the lives of individuals with TBI – in their home, work, school, and community life. The Center works to educate family members, people with TBI, service providers and researchers, and provides training and expertise to others.

THE MOUNT SINAI HOSPITAL

The Mount Sinai Hospital's Department of Rehabilitation Medicine consistently ranks among the top 15 rehabilitation centers in the nation by *U.S. News & World Report.*

It is designated by the National Institute on Disability Rehabilitation Research as a model system of care for spinal cord injury, and as a residency and training center for community integration after traumatic brain injury, the only such designated program in New York State.

Our Comprehensive Programs are as Follows:

Amputee Rehabilitation Program

"Do It" Program for Spinal Cord Patients

Neuromuscular Program

Psychological Services

Traumatic Brain Injury Rehabilitation Program

Vocational Rehabilitation Program

A Range Of Social Work Services

PHYSICIAN LISTINGS

New England

Frontera, Walter R MD/PhD (PMR) - *Spec Exp:* *Sports Medicine;* **Hospital:** Spauding Rehab Hosp; **Address:** Spaulding Rehab Hosp-Physical Med Rehab, 125 Nashua St, Boston, MA 02114-1101; **Phone:** (617) 573-7180; **Board Cert:** Physical Medicine & Rehabilitation 1985; **Med School:** Univ Puerto Rico 1979; **Resid:** Physical Medicine & Rehabilitation, U Hosp/U of Puerto Rico, San Juan, PR 1980-1983

Kerrigan, D Casey MD (PMR) - *Spec Exp:* *Gait Disorders;* **Hospital:** Spauding Rehab Hosp; **Address:** Spaulding Rehab Hosp-Physical Med Rehab, 125 Nashua St, Boston, MA 02114; **Phone:** (617) 573-2745; **Board Cert:** Physical Medicine & Rehabilitation 1992; **Med School:** Harvard Med Sch 1987; **Resid:** Physical Medicine & Rehabilitation, UCLA Med Ctr, Los Angeles, CA 1988-1991

Siebens, Hilary C MD (PMR) - *Spec Exp:* *Stroke Rehabilitation;* **Hospital:** Spauding Rehab Hosp; **Address:** Beacon Hill Senior Health, 100 Charles River Plaza, Boston, MA 02114; **Phone:** (617) 726-4600; **Board Cert:** Internal Medicine 1983, Physical Medicine & Rehabilitation 1988; **Med School:** Harvard Med Sch 1980; **Resid:** Internal Medicine, Johns Hopkins Hosp, Baltimore, MD 1980-1983; Physical Medicine & Rehabilitation, Tufts New England Med Ctr, Boston, MA 1985-1987; **Fellow:** Geriatric Medicine, Beth Israel Hosp/Harvard, Boston, MA 1983-1985; **Fac Appt:** Harvard Med Sch

Mid Atlantic

Ahn, Jung Hwan MD (PMR) - *Spec Exp:* *Spinal Cord Injury; Stroke Rehabilitation;* **Hospital:** NYU Med Ctr (page 71); **Address:** 400 E 34th St, rm 421, New York, NY 10016-4901; **Phone:** (212) 263-6122; **Board Cert:** Physical Medicine & Rehabilitation 1980, Spinal Cord Injury Medicine 1998; **Med School:** South Korea 1970; **Resid:** Obstetrics & Gynecology, Elmhurst City Hosp - Mt Sinai, New York, NY 1975-1976; Physical Medicine & Rehabilitation, NYU Med Ctr, New York, NY 1976-1979; **Fellow:** Spinal Cord Injury Medicine, NYU Med Ctr, New York, NY 1979-1980; **Fac Appt:** Assoc Clin Prof Physical Medicine & Rehabilitation, NYU Sch Med

Aseff, John Namer MD (PMR) - *Spec Exp:* *Electrodiagnosis; Pain-Soft Tissue;* **Hospital:** Natl Rehab Hosp; **Address:** National Rehabilitation Hosp, 102 Irving St NW, Washington, DC 20010; **Phone:** (202) 877-1916; **Board Cert:** Physical Medicine & Rehabilitation 1978; **Med School:** Ohio State Univ 1973; **Resid:** Surgery, Case Western Reserve Univ Hosps, Cleveland, OH 1973-1975; Physical Medicine & Rehabilitation, Ohio State Univ Hosps, Columbus, OH 1975-1977; **Fac Appt:** Assoc Clin Prof Physical Medicine & Rehabilitation, Georgetown Univ

Bach, John MD (PMR) - *Spec Exp:* *Mechanical Ventilation; Spinal Cord Injury; Neuromuscular Disorders;* **Hospital:** UMDNJ-Univ Hosp-Newark; **Address:** 150 Bergen St, Ste B403, Newark, NJ 07103-2425; **Phone:** (973) 972-7195; **Board Cert:** Physical Medicine & Rehabilitation 1986; **Med School:** UMDNJ-NJ Med Sch, Newark 1976; **Resid:** Physical Medicine & Rehabilitation, NYU Med Ctr, New York, NY 1977-1980; **Fellow:** Univ Hosp, Poitiers France 1981-1983; **Fac Appt:** Prof Physical Medicine & Rehabilitation, UMDNJ-NJ Med Sch, Newark

Ballard, Pamela H MD (PMR) - *Spec Exp:* *Spasticity Management; Neuromuscular Rehabilitation;* **Hospital:** Natl Rehab Hosp; **Address:** 102 Irving St NW, Ste 2164, Washington, DC 20010; **Phone:** (202) 877-1750; **Board Cert:** Physical Medicine & Rehabilitation 1991, Spinal Cord Injury Medicine 1999; **Med School:** Howard Univ 1986; **Resid:** Physical Medicine & Rehabilitation, Sinai Hosp, Baltimore, MD 1987-1990

De Lateur, Barbara J MD (PMR) - *Spec Exp:* Frailty; **Hospital:** Johns Hopkins Hosp - Baltimore; **Address:** 5601 Loch Raven Blvd, Ste 406, Baltimore, MD 21239-2905; **Phone:** (410) 532-4717; **Board Cert:** Physical Medicine & Rehabilitation 1970; **Med School:** Univ Wash 1963; **Resid:** Physical Medicine & Rehabilitation, Univ Wash Hosp, Seattle, WA 1964-1968; **Fac Appt:** Prof Physical Medicine & Rehabilitation, Johns Hopkins Univ

Dillingham, Timothy R MD (PMR) - *Spec Exp:* Physical Medicine & Rehabilitation - General; **Hospital:** Johns Hopkins Hosp - Baltimore; **Address:** 5601 Loch Raven Blvd, Ste 406, Baltimore, MD 21239; **Phone:** (410) 532-4702; **Board Cert:** Physical Medicine & Rehabilitation 1991; **Med School:** Univ Wash 1986; **Resid:** Physical Medicine & Rehabilitation, Univ Wash Affil, Seattle, WA 1987-1990

Ditunno, John F MD (PMR) - *Spec Exp:* Spinal Cord Injury; **Hospital:** Thomas Jefferson Univ Hosp; **Address:** 132 S 10th St, Bldg 375 Main, Philadelphia, PA 19107; **Phone:** (215) 955-5580; **Board Cert:** Physical Medicine & Rehabilitation 1968, Spinal Cord Injury Medicine 1998; **Med School:** Hahnemann Univ 1958; **Resid:** Physical Medicine & Rehabilitation, Abraham Jacobi Hosp, New York, NY 1963; Physical Medicine & Rehabilitation, U Penn Hospital, Philadelphia, PA 1964-1965; **Fac Appt:** Prof Physical Medicine & Rehabilitation, Jefferson Med Coll

Esquenazi, Alberto MD (PMR) - *Spec Exp:* Amputee Rehabilitation; Mobility Evaluation & Treatment; Polio Rehabilitation; **Hospital:** Moss Rehab Hosp; **Address:** Moss Rehab Hosp, 1200 W Tabor Rd, Philadelphia, PA 19141-3019; **Phone:** (215) 456-9470; **Board Cert:** Physical Medicine & Rehabilitation 1986; **Med School:** Mexico 1981; **Resid:** Physical Medicine & Rehabilitation, Temple Univ, Philadelphia, PA 1982-1985; **Fellow:** Gait Prostheses, Moss Rehab Hosp, Philadelphia, PA 1985-1986; **Fac Appt:** Assoc Prof Physical Medicine & Rehabilitation, Temple Univ

Feinberg, Joseph Hunt MD (PMR) - *Spec Exp:* Sports-Orthopedic Related Injuries; Spine & Nerve Injuries; **Hospital:** Hosp For Special Surgery (page 62); **Address:** 535 E 70th St, New York, NY 10021; **Phone:** (212) 606-1568; **Board Cert:** Physical Medicine & Rehabilitation 1991; **Med School:** Albany Med Coll 1983; **Resid:** Surgery, Mt Sinai Hosp, New York, NY 1984-1985; Physical Medicine & Rehabilitation, Rusk Inst Rehab, New York, NY 1987-1990; **Fellow:** Orthopaedic Pathology, Hosp Spec Surg, New York, NY 1985-1986; Orthopedic Biomechanics, Univ Iowa Hosp & Clins, Iowa City, IA 1986-1987; **Fac Appt:** Asst Prof Medicine, UMDNJ-NJ Med Sch, Newark

Francis, Kathleen MD (PMR) - *Spec Exp:* Lymphedema; Amyotrophic Lateral Sclerosis(ALS); Neurodegenerative Disease; **Hospital:** Kessler Inst for Rehab - W Orange; **Address:** Kessler Inst for Rehab, 1199 Pleasant Valley Way, West Orange, NJ 07052-1499; **Phone:** (973) 731-3600; **Board Cert:** Physical Medicine & Rehabilitation 1994; **Med School:** UMDNJ-NJ Med Sch, Newark 1989; **Resid:** Physical Medicine & Rehabilitation, UMDNJ-Kessler Inst Rehab, Newark, NJ 1990-1993; **Fac Appt:** Asst Clin Prof Physical Medicine & Rehabilitation, UMDNJ-NJ Med Sch, Newark

Kirshblum, Steven C MD (PMR) - *Spec Exp:* Spinal Cord Injury; **Hospital:** Kessler Inst for Rehab - East Orange; **Address:** 1199 Pleasant Valley Way, West Orange, NJ 07052; **Phone:** (973) 731-3600; **Board Cert:** Physical Medicine & Rehabilitation 1991, Spinal Cord Injury Medicine 1998; **Med School:** Univ Hlth Sci/Chicago Med Sch 1986; **Resid:** Physical Medicine & Rehabilitation, Mount Sinai Med Ctr, New York, NY 1987-1990; **Fac Appt:** Assoc Prof Physical Medicine & Rehabilitation, UMDNJ-NJ Med Sch, Newark

Lieberman, James MD (PMR) - *Spec Exp:* Physical Medicine & Rehabilitation - General; **Hospital:** NY Presby Hosp - Columbia Presby Med Ctr (page 70); **Address:** Rehabilitation Med Assoc, 630 W 168th St, Box 38, New York, NY 10032; **Phone:** (212) 305-4818; **Board Cert:** Neurology 1971, Physical Medicine & Rehabilitation 1981; **Med School:** UCSF 1963; **Resid:** Neurology, Univ Mich Med Ctr, Ann Arbor, MI 1964-1965; Neurology, Yale-New Haven Hosp, New Haven, CT 1965-1967; **Fellow:** Physical Medicine & Rehabilitation, UC Davis, Sacramento, CA 1978-1980; **Fac Appt:** Prof Physical Medicine & Rehabilitation, Columbia P&S

Lutz, Gregory MD (PMR) - *Spec Exp:* Spinal Rehabilitation; Sports Medicine; Pain-Lower Back (IDET procedure); **Hospital:** Hosp For Special Surgery (page 62); **Address:** 535 E 70th St, Hospital for Special Surgery, New York, NY 10021; **Phone:** (212) 606-1648; **Board Cert:** Physical Medicine & Rehabilitation 1993; **Med School:** Georgetown Univ 1988; **Resid:** Physical Medicine & Rehabilitation, Mayo Clinic, Rochester, MN 1989-1992; **Fellow:** Sports Medicine, Hosp For Spec Surg, New York, NY 1992-1993; **Fac Appt:** Asst Prof Physical Medicine & Rehabilitation, Cornell Univ-Weill Med Coll

Ma, Dong M MD (PMR) - *Spec Exp:* Electrodiagnosis; Electromyography; Musculoskeletal Disorders; **Hospital:** NYU Med Ctr (page 71); **Address:** 400 E 34th St, New York, NY 10016; **Phone:** (212) 263-6338; **Board Cert:** Physical Medicine & Rehabilitation 1979; **Med School:** South Korea 1968; **Resid:** Physical Medicine & Rehabilitation, NYU Med Ctr, New York, NY 1973-1975; **Fellow:** Physical Medicine & Rehabilitation, NYU Med Ctr, New York, NY 1976-1977; **Fac Appt:** Assoc Clin Prof Physical Medicine & Rehabilitation, NYU Sch Med

Mayer, Nathaniel MD (PMR) - *Spec Exp:* Motor Control Analysis; Spasticity Management; Brain Injury Rehabilitation; **Hospital:** Moss Rehab Hosp; **Address:** Moss Rehab Hosp, Drucker Brain Injury Ctr, 1200 W Tabor Rd, Philadelphia, PA 19141; **Phone:** (215) 456-9560; **Board Cert:** Physical Medicine & Rehabilitation 1976; **Med School:** Albert Einstein Coll Med 1968; **Resid:** Physical Medicine & Rehabilitation, Temple Hospital, Philadelphia, PA 1969-1973; **Fac Appt:** Prof Physical Medicine & Rehabilitation, Temple Univ

Munin, Michael Craig MD (PMR) - *Spec Exp:* Spasticity Management; Amputee Rehabilitation; Hip Surgery Rehabilitation; **Hospital:** UPMC - Presbyterian Univ Hosp; **Address:** Univ Pittsburgh Physicians- PM&R Assoc, 3471 Fifth Ave Lilliane S Kaufman Bldg Ste 1103, Pittsburgh, PA 15213; **Phone:** (412) 692-4400; **Board Cert:** Physical Medicine & Rehabilitation 1993; **Med School:** Jefferson Med Coll 1988; **Resid:** Physical Medicine & Rehabilitation, Thomas Jefferson Univ Hosp, Philadelphia, PA 1989-1992; **Fac Appt:** Assoc Prof Physical Medicine & Rehabilitation, Univ Pittsburgh

Myers, Stanley MD (PMR) - *Spec Exp:* Neuromuscular Diseases; Stroke Rehabilitation; **Hospital:** NY Presby Hosp - Columbia Presby Med Ctr (page 70); **Address:** 180 Fort Washington Ave, Ste 199 - rm 171, New York, NY 10032-3710; **Phone:** (212) 305-3344; **Board Cert:** Physical Medicine & Rehabilitation 1971; **Med School:** SUNY Hlth Sci Ctr 1961; **Resid:** Internal Medicine, Maimonides Medical Ctr, Brooklyn, NY 1962-1964; Physical Medicine & Rehabilitation, Columbia-Presby, New York, NY 1967-1969; **Fellow:** Neurological Muscular Disease, Maimonides Medical Ctr, Brooklyn, NY 1964-1965; **Fac Appt:** Prof Physical Medicine & Rehabilitation, Columbia P&S

Ragnarsson, Kristjan MD (PMR) - *Spec Exp:* Spinal Cord Injury; Brain Injury; Pain-Neck & Back; **Hospital:** Mount Sinai Hosp (page 68); **Address:** 5 E 98th St, New York, NY 10029; **Phone:** (212) 659-9370; **Board Cert:** Physical Medicine & Rehabilitation 1976; **Med School:** Iceland 1969; **Resid:** Physical Medicine & Rehabilitation, NYU Med Ctr, New York, NY 1971-1974; **Fellow:** Physical Medicine & Rehabilitation, NYU Med Ctr, New York, NY 1974-1975; **Fac Appt:** Prof Physical Medicine & Rehabilitation, Mount Sinai Sch Med

Staas Jr, William E MD (PMR) - *Spec Exp:* Spinal Cord Injury; **Hospital:** Magee Rehab Hosp; **Address:** Six Franklin Plaza, Ste 406, Philadelphia, PA 19102; **Phone:** (215) 587-3394; **Board Cert:** Spinal Cord Injury Medicine 1998, Physical Medicine & Rehabilitation 1970; **Med School:** Jefferson Med Coll 1962; **Resid:** Physical Medicine & Rehabilitation, Univ Penn Hosp, Philadelphia, PA 1965-1968; **Fac Appt:** Prof Physical Medicine & Rehabilitation, Jefferson Med Coll

Zafonte, Ross DO (PMR) - *Spec Exp:* Brain Injury Rehabilitation; Spinal Cord Injury; **Hospital:** UPMC - Presbyterian Univ Hosp; **Address:** Lillian Kaufman Bldg, 3471 Fifth Ave, Ste 901, Pittsburgh, PA 15213-3221; **Phone:** (412) 648-6979; **Board Cert:** Physical Medicine & Rehabilitation 1990; **Med School:** Nova SE Univ, Coll Osteo Med 1985; **Resid:** Physical Medicine & Rehabilitation, Mt Sinai Sch Med, New York, NY 1986-1989; **Fac Appt:** Prof Physical Medicine & Rehabilitation, Univ Pittsburgh

Southeast

Creamer, Michael DO (PMR) - *Spec Exp:* Spinal Cord Injury; **Hospital:** Florida Hosp; **Address:** 100 W Gore St, Ste 203, Orlando, FL 32806-1041; **Phone:** (407) 649-8707; **Board Cert:** Physical Medicine & Rehabilitation 1992, Spinal Cord Injury Medicine 1998; **Med School:** Chicago Coll Osteo Med 1987; **Resid:** Physical Medicine & Rehabilitation, Rehab Inst Chicago, Chicago, IL 1988-1991; **Fac Appt:** Asst Prof Physical Medicine & Rehabilitation, Southeastern Univ Coll Osteo Med

Jackson, Amie Brown MD (PMR) - *Spec Exp:* Spinal Cord Injury; **Hospital:** Univ of Ala Hosp at Birmingham; **Address:** 1717 6th Ave S, Birmingham, AL 35233-1801; **Phone:** (205) 934-4131; **Board Cert:** Physical Medicine & Rehabilitation 1990; **Med School:** Univ Ala 1984; **Resid:** Physical Medicine & Rehabilitation, Univ Alabama, Birmingham, AL 1984-1987; **Fac Appt:** Prof Physical Medicine & Rehabilitation, Univ Ala

Lipkin, David L MD (PMR) - *Spec Exp:* Geriatric Medicine; Pain-Back; Rheumatology; **Hospital:** Mount Sinai Med Ctr; **Address:** Assocs Rehab, Lowenstein Bldg, 4300 Alton Rd, Ste 137, Miami Beach, FL 33140-2800; **Phone:** (305) 674-2171; **Board Cert:** Physical Medicine & Rehabilitation 1971; **Med School:** Belgium 1964; **Resid:** Pediatrics, Jersey City Med Ctr, Jersey City, NJ 1964-1966; Physical Medicine & Rehabilitation, Bronx Muni Hosp, New York, NY 1966-1969; **Fellow:** Research, Natl Inst Hlth-Eins Coll Med, Bronx, NY 1966-1969; **Fac Appt:** Asst Prof Physical Medicine & Rehabilitation, Univ Miami Sch Med

Peppard, Terrence Richard MD (PMR) - *Spec Exp:* Physical Medicine & Rehabilitation - General; **Hospital:** Mercy Hosp - Miami, FL; **Address:** 3663 S Miami Ave, Miami, FL 33133; **Phone:** (305) 285-2966; **Board Cert:** Physical Medicine & Rehabilitation 1989; **Med School:** Univ Miami Sch Med 1984; **Resid:** Physical Medicine & Rehabilitation, NYU Med Ctr, New York, NY 1984-1987; **Fellow:** Neurological Muscular Disease, NYU Med Ctr, New York, NY 1987-1988

Midwest

Braddom, Randall L MD (PMR) - *Spec Exp:* Pain-Chronic; **Hospital:** IN Univ Hosp (page 63); **Address:** Indiana Univ Med Ctr, Dept Physical Medicine, 541 N Clinical Drive, rm 368, Indianapolis, IN 46202; **Phone:** (317) 278-0200; **Board Cert:** Physical Medicine & Rehabilitation 1974; **Med School:** Ohio State Univ 1968; **Resid:** Physical Medicine & Rehabilitation, Ohio State Univ Hosp, Columbus, OH 1970-1973; **Fac Appt:** Prof Physical Medicine & Rehabilitation, Indiana Univ

Chen, David MD (PMR) - *Spec Exp:* Spinal Cord Injury; **Hospital:** Rehab Inst - Chicago; **Address:** 345 E Superior St, Ste 1146, Chicago, IL 60611; **Phone:** (312) 238-0764; **Board Cert:** Physical Medicine & Rehabilitation 1992, Spinal Cord Injury Medicine 1998; **Med School:** Univ IL Coll Med 1987; **Resid:** Physical Medicine & Rehabilitation, Northwestern Med Sch, Chicago, IL 1988-1991; **Fac Appt:** Asst Prof Physical Medicine & Rehabilitation, Northwestern Univ

Clairmont, Albert MD (PMR) - *Spec Exp:* Pain Management; Spasticity Management; Electrodiagnosis; **Hospital:** Ohio St Univ Med Ctr; **Address:** 480 W 9th Ave, Columbus, OH 43210; **Phone:** (614) 293-4837; **Board Cert:** Physical Medicine & Rehabilitation 1985, Pediatrics 1985; **Med School:** Jamaica 1974; **Resid:** Pediatric Surgery, Columbus Chldns Hosp, Columbus, OH 1980-1981; Physical Medicine & Rehabilitation, Ohio St Univ Hosps, Columbus, OH 1981-1983; **Fac Appt:** Assoc Clin Prof Physical Medicine & Rehabilitation, Ohio State Univ

Colachis III, Samuel C MD (PMR) - *Spec Exp:* Spinal Cord Injury; Electrodiagnosis; **Hospital:** Ohio St Univ Med Ctr; **Address:** 1025 Dodd Hall, Columbus, OH 43210; **Phone:** (614) 293-4837; **Board Cert:** Physical Medicine & Rehabilitation 1988; **Med School:** USC Sch Med 1984; **Resid:** Physical Medicine & Rehabilitation, Ohio State Univ Hosps, Columbus, OH 1985-1987; **Fellow:** Electrodiagnosis, Ohio State Univ Hosps, Columbus, OH 1987-1988; **Fac Appt:** Assoc Prof Physical Medicine & Rehabilitation, Ohio State Univ

Gittler, Michelle MD (PMR) - *Spec Exp:* Spinal Cord Injury; Amputee Rehabilitation; **Hospital:** Schwab Rehab Hosp; **Address:** 1401 S California Blvd, Chicago, IL 60608; **Phone:** (773) 522-5853; **Board Cert:** Physical Medicine & Rehabilitation 1993, Spinal Cord Injury Medicine 1998; **Med School:** Univ IL Coll Med 1988; **Resid:** Physical Medicine & Rehabilitation, Rehab Inst Chicago, Chicago, IL 1989-1992; **Fac Appt:** Asst Clin Prof Physical Medicine & Rehabilitation, Univ Chicago-Pritzker Sch Med

Haig, Andrew MD (PMR) - *Spec Exp:* Sports Medicine; Pain-Back & Neck; Electrodiagnosis-EMG; **Hospital:** Univ of MI Hlth Ctr; **Address:** Univ Michigan Spine Program, 325 E Eisenhower Pkwy, Burlington Bldg, Fl 2, Ste 202, Ann Artbor, MI 48108; **Phone:** (888) 254-2225; **Board Cert:** Physical Medicine & Rehabilitation 1987; **Med School:** Med Coll Wisc 1983; **Resid:** Physical Medicine & Rehabilitation, Northwestern Univ, Chicago, IL 1984-1986; **Fac Appt:** Asst Prof Physical Medicine & Rehabilitation, Univ Mich Med Sch

La Ban, Myron M MD (PMR) - *Spec Exp:* Pain-Back; **Hospital:** William Beaumont Hosp; **Address:** 3535 W Thirteen Mile Rd, Ste 437, Royal Oak, MI 48073; **Phone:** (248) 288-2237

Leonard Jr., James A. MD (PMR) - *Spec Exp:* Amputee Rehabilitation; Electrodiagnosis; **Hospital:** Univ of MI Hlth Ctr; **Address:** Univ Hosp Dept. Physical Medicine & Rehabilitation, 1500 E Medical Center Drive, Ann Arbor, MI 48109-0718; **Phone:** (734) 936-7190; **Board Cert:** Physical Medicine & Rehabilitation 1977; **Med School:** Univ Mich Med Sch 1972; **Resid:** U Mich Med Ctr, Ann Arbor, MI 1972-1975; **Fac Appt:** Clin Prof Physical Medicine & Rehabilitation, Univ Mich Med Sch

Mason, Kristin MD (PMR) (relocated to Englewood, CO) - *Spec Exp:* Stroke Rehabilitation; Electrodiagnostics; Entrapment Neuropathy; **Hospital:** Swedish Med Ctr - Englewood; **Address:** Rehab Assoc of Colorado, 125 E Hampden Ave, Englewood, CO,80110; **Phone:** (303) 762-9297; **Board Cert:** Physical Medicine & Rehabilitation 1993; **Med School:** Baylor Coll Med 1988; **Resid:** Physical Medicine & Rehabilitation, Rehab Inst Chicago, Chicago, IL 1989-1992

681

Nobunaga, Austin MD (PMR) - *Spec Exp:* Spinal Cord Injury; Electrodiagnosis; **Hospital:** Univ Hosp - Cincinnati; **Address:** Univ Cincinnati Coll Med, Dept PM&R, 151 W Galbraith Rd, Cincinnati, OH 45216; **Phone:** (513) 948-2707; **Board Cert:** Physical Medicine & Rehabilitation 1990, Spinal Cord Injury Medicine 1999; **Med School:** Univ Mich Med Sch 1985; **Resid:** Physical Medicine & Rehabilitation, Rehab Inst Chicago, Chicago, IL 1986-1989

Press, Joel MD (PMR) - *Spec Exp:* Sports Medicine; Pain-Back; Musculoskeletal Injuries; **Hospital:** Rehab Inst - Chicago; **Address:** Rehab Institute, Dept Spine & Sport, 1030 N Clark St, Ste 500, Chicago, IL 60610; **Phone:** (312) 238-7767; **Board Cert:** Physical Medicine & Rehabilitation 1988; **Med School:** Univ IL Coll Med 1984; **Resid:** Physical Medicine & Rehabilitation, Northwestern Meml Hosp, Chicago, IL 1984-1988; **Fac Appt:** Assoc Clin Prof Medicine, Northwestern Univ

Roth, Elliot MD (PMR) - *Spec Exp:* Stroke Rehabilitation; Neuro-Rehabilitation; **Hospital:** Rehab Inst - Chicago; **Address:** 345 E Superior St, Ste 1576, Chicago, IL 60611; **Phone:** (312) 238-4637; **Board Cert:** Physical Medicine & Rehabilitation 1987; **Med School:** Northwestern Univ 1982; **Resid:** Physical Medicine & Rehabilitation, Northwestern Univ, Chicago, IL 1983-1985; **Fellow:** Physical Medicine & Rehabilitation, Rehab Inst- Chicago, Chicago, IL 1986; **Fac Appt:** Prof Physical Medicine & Rehabilitation, Northwestern Univ

Sisung, Charles MD (PMR) - *Spec Exp:* Rheumatic Diseases of Childhood; Trauma; Burns; **Hospital:** Rehab Inst - Chicago; **Address:** 345 E Superior St, rm 1158, Chicago, IL 60611; **Phone:** (312) 238-1246; **Board Cert:** Pediatrics 1997, Physical Medicine & Rehabilitation 1991; **Med School:** Univ Mich Med Sch 1981; **Resid:** Pediatrics, Univ Mich Med Ctr, Ann Arbor, MI 1981-1984; Physical Medicine & Rehabilitation, Schwab Rehab Hosp, Chicago, IL 1986-1989; **Fellow:** Pediatric Rheumatology, Univ Chicago Hosp, Chicago, IL 1989-1991; **Fac Appt:** Asst Prof Physical Medicine & Rehabilitation, Northwestern Univ

Sliwa, James A DO (PMR) - *Spec Exp:* Pain-Back; Multiple Sclerosis; Cancer Rehabilitation; **Hospital:** Rehab Inst - Chicago; **Address:** 345 E Superior St, Ste 1108, Chicago, IL 60611-3015; **Phone:** (312) 238-4093; **Board Cert:** Physical Medicine & Rehabilitation 1985; **Med School:** Chicago Coll Osteo Med 1980; **Resid:** Physical Medicine & Rehabilitation, Rehab Inst, Chicago, IL 1981-1984; **Fac Appt:** Physical Medicine & Rehabilitation, Northwestern Univ

Smith, Joanne MD (PMR) - *Spec Exp:* Pain - Pelvic; Pregnancy & Back/Hip/Pelvic pain; **Hospital:** Rehab Inst - Chicago; **Address:** 345 E Superior St, rm 1579, Chicago, IL 60611; **Phone:** (312) 238-0838; **Board Cert:** Physical Medicine & Rehabilitation 1993; **Med School:** Mich State Univ 1988; **Resid:** Physical Medicine & Rehabilitation, Northwestern Univ Med Sch, Chicago, IL 1989-1992; **Fac Appt:** Asst Prof Physical Medicine & Rehabilitation, Northwestern Univ

Volshteyn, Oksana MD (PMR) - *Spec Exp:* Spinal Cord Injury; **Hospital:** Barnes-Jewish Hosp (page 55); **Address:** 660 S Euclid Ave, Box CB8111, St Louis, MO 63110; **Phone:** (314) 454-7757; **Board Cert:** Physical Medicine & Rehabilitation 1986, Spinal Cord Injury Medicine 1999; **Med School:** Russia 1976; **Resid:** Physical Medicine & Rehabilitation, Barnes Jewish Hosp, St Louis, MO 1982-1985; **Fac Appt:** Asst Prof Neurology, Washington Univ, St Louis

Great Plains and Mountains

Lammertse, Daniel MD (PMR) - *Spec Exp:* Spinal Cord Injury; **Hospital:** Craig Hospital; **Address:** CNF Medical Group, 3425 S Clarkson St, Engelwood, CO 80110-2811; **Phone:** (303) 789-8220; **Board Cert:** Physical Medicine & Rehabilitation 1980, Spinal Cord Injury Medicine 1998; **Med School:** Ohio State Univ 1976; **Resid:** Physical Medicine & Rehabilitation, Ohio State Univ Hosp, Columbus, OH 1976-1979; **Fac Appt:** Asst Clin Prof Physical Medicine & Rehabilitation, Univ Colo

Matthews, Dennis Jerome MD (PMR) - *Spec Exp:* Brain Injury Rehabilitation; Musculoskeletal Disorders; Cerebral Palsy; **Hospital:** Chldn's Hosp - Denver; **Address:** Chldns Hosp - Denver, Rehabilitation, 1056 E 19th Ave, Denver, CO 80218-1007; **Phone:** (303) 861-6633; **Board Cert:** Physical Medicine & Rehabilitation 1979; **Med School:** Univ Colo 1975; **Resid:** Physical Medicine & Rehabilitation, Minn Hosps, Minneapolis, MN 1975-1978; **Fellow:** Research, Minn Hosps, Minneapolis, MN 1978; **Fac Appt:** Assoc Prof Physical Medicine & Rehabilitation, Univ Colo

Southwest

Barber, Douglas Byron MD (PMR) - *Spec Exp:* Spinal Cord Injury; **Hospital:** Univ Hlth Sys - San Antonio; **Address:** Univ Hlth Sci Ctr, Dept of Rehab Med, 7790, 7703 Floyd Curl Drive, San Antonio, TX 78229-3900; **Phone:** (210) 567-5351; **Board Cert:** Physical Medicine & Rehabilitation 1992, Spinal Cord Injury Medicine 1999; **Med School:** Univ Tex, Houston 1987; **Resid:** Physical Medicine & Rehabilitation, Univ TX Hlth Scis Ctr, San Antonio, TX 1988-1991; **Fac Appt:** Assoc Prof Physical Medicine & Rehabilitation, Univ Tex, San Antonio

Donovan, William Henry MD (PMR) - *Spec Exp:* Spinal Cord Injury; Amputee Rehabilitation; **Hospital:** TIRR; **Address:** 1333 Moursund St, Ste D-107, Houston, TX 77030-3405; **Phone:** (713) 797-5912; **Board Cert:** Physical Medicine & Rehabilitation 1975; **Med School:** Albany Med Coll 1966; **Resid:** Internal Medicine, Marquette Univ, Milwaukee, WI 1967-1968; Physical Medicine & Rehabilitation, Univ Wash, Seattle, WA 1970-1972; **Fac Appt:** Prof Physical Medicine & Rehabilitation, Univ Tex, Houston

Dumitru, Daniel MD (PMR) - *Spec Exp:* Electrodiagnosis; **Hospital:** Univ of Texas Hlth & Sci Ctr; **Address:** Univ Texas Hlth Sci Ctr, Dept Rehab Medicine, 7703 Floyd Curl Drive, San Antonio, TX 78229-3900; **Phone:** (210) 567-5347; **Board Cert:** Physical Medicine & Rehabilitation 1984; **Med School:** Univ Cincinnati 1980; **Resid:** Physical Medicine & Rehabilitation, VA Hosp, San Antonio, TX 1980-1983; **Fac Appt:** Prof Physical Medicine & Rehabilitation, Univ Tex, San Antonio

Francisco, Gerard E MD (PMR) - *Spec Exp:* Physical Medicine & Rehabilitation - General; **Hospital:** TIRR; **Address:** 1333 Moursund St, Ste D-108, Houston, TX 77030-3405; **Phone:** (713) 797-5246; **Board Cert:** Physical Medicine & Rehabilitation 1995; **Med School:** Philippines 1989; **Resid:** Physical Medicine & Rehabilitation, UMDNJ-Univ Hosp, Newark, NJ 1991-1994; **Fellow:** Physical Medicine & Rehabilitation, Baylor Coll Med, Houston, TX 1994-1995; **Fac Appt:** Asst Clin Prof Physical Medicine & Rehabilitation, Univ Tex, Houston

Ivanhoe, Cindy MD (PMR) - *Spec Exp:* Brain Injury Rehabilitation; **Hospital:** TIRR; **Address:** 1333 Moursund Ave, Houston, TX 77030-3405; **Phone:** (713) 797-5236; **Board Cert:** Physical Medicine & Rehabilitation 1993; **Med School:** Mexico 1984; **Resid:** Physical Medicine & Rehabilitation, U ILL Coll Med, Chicago, IL 1989-1992; **Fellow:** Baylor Coll Of Med, Houston, TX 1992-1993; **Fac Appt:** Asst Clin Prof Univ Tex, Houston

Kevorkian, Charles George MD (PMR) - *Spec Exp:* Stroke Rehabilitation; Neuromuscular Rehabilitation; Electrodiagnosis; **Hospital:** St Luke's Episcopal Hosp - Houston; **Address:** Baylor Coll Med, 6624 Fannin St, Ste 2330, Houston, TX 77030; **Phone:** (713) 798-4061; **Board Cert:** Physical Medicine & Rehabilitation 1980; **Med School:** Australia 1972; **Resid:** Physical Medicine & Rehabilitation, Prince Henry Hosp, Sydney, Australia 1975-1976; Physical Medicine & Rehabilitation, Mayo Clin, Rochester 1976-1979; **Fac Appt:** Assoc Prof Physical Medicine & Rehabilitation, Baylor Coll Med

King, John Chandler MD (PMR) - *Spec Exp: Stroke Rehabilitation;* **Hospital:** Univ of Texas Hlth & Sci Ctr; **Address:** Univ Tx Hlth Sci Ctr, Dept Rehab Med, 7703 Floyd Curl Dr, rm 615E, San Antonio, TX 78229-3900; **Phone:** (210) 567-5345; **Board Cert:** Physical Medicine & Rehabilitation 1987; **Med School:** Oral Roberts Sch Med 1983; **Resid:** Physical Medicine & Rehabilitation, Baylor Coll Med, Houston, TX 1984-1986; **Fac Appt:** Assoc Prof Physical Medicine & Rehabilitation, Univ Tex, San Antonio

Nelson, Maureen R MD (PMR) - *Spec Exp: Rehabilitation-Pediatric;* **Hospital:** TX Chldns Hosp - Houston; **Address:** 6621 Fannin St, MC WT21-329, Houston, TX 77030; **Phone:** (832) 826-6106; **Board Cert:** Physical Medicine & Rehabilitation 1990; **Med School:** Univ IL Coll Med 1985; **Resid:** Physical Medicine & Rehabilitation, Univ Tex Hlth Scis Ctr, San Antonio, TX 1986-1989; **Fellow:** Pediatric Sports Medicine, Alfred I Dupont Inst, Wilmington, DE 1989-1990; **Fac Appt:** Assoc Prof Physical Medicine & Rehabilitation, Baylor Coll Med

Parsons, Kenneth C. MD (PMR) - *Spec Exp: Spinal Cord Injury;* **Hospital:** TIRR; **Address:** Inst Rehab and Research, 1333 Moursund Ave, Houston, TX 77030-3405; **Phone:** (713) 797-5252; **Board Cert:** Physical Medicine & Rehabilitation 1977, Spinal Cord Injury Medicine 1998; **Med School:** Univ Mich Med Sch 1970; **Resid:** Physical Medicine & Rehabilitation, Univ Hosp, Ann Arbor, MI 1971-1976; **Fac Appt:** Asst Clin Prof Physical Medicine & Rehabilitation, Baylor Coll Med

West Coast and Pacific

Cardenas, Diana MD (PMR) - *Spec Exp: Spinal Cord Injury; Spina Bifida;* **Hospital:** Univ WA Med Ctr; **Address:** Univ Wash, Dept Rehab Med, Box 356490, Seattle, WA 98195; **Phone:** (206) 543-8171; **Board Cert:** Physical Medicine & Rehabilitation 1977; **Med School:** Univ Tex SW, Dallas 1973; **Resid:** Physical Medicine & Rehabilitation, Univ Wash Affil Hosp, Seattle, WA 1973-1976; **Fac Appt:** Prof Physical Medicine & Rehabilitation, Univ Wash

Jaffe, Kenneth M MD (PMR) - *Spec Exp: Brain/Spinal Cord Injury; Muscular Dystrophy; Arthrogryposis-Limb Deficiency;* **Hospital:** Chldns Hosp and Regl Med Ctr - Seattle; **Address:** 4800 Sand Point Way NE, MC CH71, Seattle, WA 98105; **Phone:** (206) 526-2114; **Board Cert:** Pediatrics 1980, Physical Medicine & Rehabilitation 1982; **Med School:** Harvard Med Sch 1975; **Resid:** Pediatrics, Univ Wash-Chldns Hosp, Seattle, WA 1975-1980; Physical Medicine & Rehabilitation, Univ Wash Affil Hosp, Seattle, WA 1980-1982

Kraft, George Howard MD (PMR) - *Spec Exp: Multiple Sclerosis; Spinal Cord Injury;* **Hospital:** Univ WA Med Ctr; **Address:** 1959 NE Pacific St, Box 356157, Seattle, WA 98195; **Phone:** (206) 598-4295; **Board Cert:** Physical Medicine & Rehabilitation 1969, Spinal Cord Injury Medicine 1998; **Med School:** Ohio State Univ 1963; **Resid:** Physical Medicine & Rehabilitation, UCSF-Moffitt Hosp, San Francisco, CA 1964-1965; Physical Medicine & Rehabilitation, Ohio State Univ Med Ctr, Columbus, OH 1965-1967; **Fac Appt:** Prof Physical Medicine & Rehabilitation, Univ Wash

Massagli, Teresa Luisa MD (PMR) - *Spec Exp: Spinal Cord Injury-Pediatric; Brain Injury Rehabiliation-Pediatric; Cerebral Palsy;* **Hospital:** Chldns Hosp and Regl Med Ctr - Seattle; **Address:** Chlds Hosp & Med Ctr, 4800 Sand Point Way NE, Box 5371, Seattle, WA 98105; **Phone:** (206) 526-2114; **Board Cert:** Physical Medicine & Rehabilitation 1989, Spinal Cord Injury Medicine 1998; **Med School:** Yale Univ 1982; **Resid:** Pediatrics, Yale New Haven Hosp, New Haven, CT 1982-1985; **Fellow:** Physical Medicine & Rehabilitation, Univ. Washington, Seattle, WA 1985-1988; **Fac Appt:** Assoc Prof Physical Medicine & Rehabilitation, Univ Wash

Robinson, Lawrence MD (PMR) - *Spec Exp:* *Electrodiagnosis; Electromyography; Botulinum Toxin Injections;* **Hospital:** Harborview Med Ctr; **Address:** Univ Washington Med Ctr-Haborview, Dept Rehab Med, 325 9th Ave, Box 359740, Seattle, WA 98104; **Phone:** (206) 731-3167; **Board Cert:** Physical Medicine & Rehabilitation 1987; **Med School:** Baylor Coll Med 1982; **Resid:** Physical Medicine & Rehabilitation, Northwestern Meml Hosp, Chicago, IL 1982-1985; **Fac Appt:** Prof Physical Medicine & Rehabilitation, Univ Wash

PLASTIC SURGERY

A plastic surgeon deals with the repair, reconstruction or replacement of physical defects of form or function involving the skin, musculoskeletal system, craniomaxillofacial structures, hand, extremities, breast and trunk and external genitalia. He/she uses aesthetic surgical principles not only to improve undesirable qualities of normal structures (commonly called "cosmetic surgery") but in all reconstructive procedures as well.

A plastic surgeon possesses special knowledge and skill in the design and surgery of grafts, flaps, free tissue transfer and replantation. Competence in the management of complex wounds, the use of implantable materials, and in tumor surgery is required.

Training required: Five to seven years

Certification in one of the following subspecialties requires additional training and examination.

Plastic Surgery within the Head and Neck: A plastic surgeon with additional training in plastic and reconstructive procedures within the head, face, neck and associated structures, including cutaneous head and neck oncology and reconstruction, management of maxillofacial trauma, soft tissue repair and neural surgery.

The field is diverse and involves a wide age range of patients, from the newborn to the aged. While both cosmetic and reconstructive surgery are practiced, there are many additional procedures which interface with them.

Surgery of the Hand (*see Hand Surgery page 273*)

PHYSICIAN LISTINGS

Plastic Surgery

New England

Ariyan, Stephan MD (PIS) - *Spec Exp:* Melanoma; Head & Neck Surgery; Reconstructive Surgery; **Hospital:** Yale - New Haven Hosp; **Address:** 60 Temple St, Ste 7C, New Haven, CT 06510-2716; **Phone:** (203) 786-3000; **Board Cert:** Plastic Surgery 1978; **Med School:** NY Med Coll 1966; **Resid:** Surgery, Yale Univ Hosp, New Haven, CT 1971-1975; Plastic Surgery, Yale Univ Hosp, New Haven, CT 1973-1976; **Fellow:** Surgical Oncology, Yale Univ Hosp, New Haven, CT 1970-1971; **Fac Appt:** Clin Prof Plastic Surgery, Yale Univ

Collins, Eva Dale MD (PIS) - *Spec Exp:* Breast Cancer; Reconstruction; **Hospital:** Dartmouth - Hitchcock Med Ctr; **Address:** One Medical Center Drive, Lebanon, NH 03756; **Phone:** (603) 650-7943; **Board Cert:** Plastic Surgery 1997; **Med School:** Emory Univ 1989; **Resid:** Plastic Surgery, Washinton Univ. Med Ctr, St. Louis, MO 1989-1994; **Fac Appt:** Asst Prof Plastic Surgery, Dartmouth Med Sch

Constantian, Mark B MD (PIS) - *Spec Exp:* Secondary Rhinoplasty; Rhinoplasty; Nasal Reconstruction; **Hospital:** St Joseph Hosp; **Address:** 19 Tyler St, Ste 302, Nashua, NH 03060-2951; **Phone:** (603) 880-7700; **Board Cert:** Plastic Surgery 1979; **Med School:** Univ VA Sch Med 1972; **Resid:** Surgery, Boston Med Ctr, Boston, MA 1972-1976; Surgery, NIGMS Academy Surg, Boston, MA 1973-1975; **Fellow:** Plastic Reconstructive Surgery, Medical Coll VA, Richmond, VA 1976-1978; **Fac Appt:** Asst Prof Surgery, Dartmouth Med Sch

Eriksson, Elof MD (PIS) - *Spec Exp:* Abdominal Plasty; Breast Reconstruction & Augmentation; Skin Laser Surgery; **Hospital:** Brigham & Women's Hosp; **Address:** 75 Francis St, Boston, MA 02115; **Phone:** (617) 732-5093; **Board Cert:** Plastic Surgery 1980, Surgery 1989; **Med School:** Sweden 1969; **Resid:** Surgery, Chicago Affil Hosps, Chicago, IL 1972-1977; **Fellow:** Plastic Surgery, Med Ctr Va, Charlottesville, VA 1977-1979; **Fac Appt:** Prof Plastic Surgery, Harvard Med Sch

Feldman, Joel MD (PIS) - *Spec Exp:* Cosmetic Surgery-Face; Reconstructive Surgery; **Hospital:** Mount Auburn Hosp; **Address:** 300 Mt Auburn St, Ste 304, Cambridge, MA 02238; **Phone:** (617) 661-5998; **Board Cert:** Surgery 1975, Plastic Surgery 1977; **Med School:** Harvard Med Sch 1969; **Resid:** Surgery, Mass Genl Hosp, Boston, MA 1970-1974; Plastic Surgery, Johns Hopkins Hosp, Baltimore, MD 1974-1976; **Fac Appt:** Asst Clin Prof Plastic Surgery, Harvard Med Sch

Gallico, G Gregory MD (PIS) - *Spec Exp:* Plastic Surgery - General; **Hospital:** MA Genl Hosp; **Address:** 275 Cambridge St, Ste 502, Boston, MA 02114; **Phone:** (617) 726-3440; **Board Cert:** Plastic Surgery 1982, Surgery 1981; **Med School:** Harvard Med Sch 1973; **Resid:** Surgery, Mass Genl Hosp, Boston, MA 1974-1980; Plastic Surgery, Mass Genl Hosp, Boston, MA 1980-1981; **Fellow:** Immunology, Oxford Univ Med Sch, Oxford, England 1975-1977; **Fac Appt:** Asst Prof Surgery, Harvard Med Sch

May Jr, James W MD (PIS) - *Spec Exp:* Cosmetic Surgery; Breast Reconstruction; Hand Surgery; **Hospital:** MA Genl Hosp; **Address:** 15 Parkman St Bldg Wang - rm ACC453, Boston, MA 02114; **Phone:** (617) 726-8220; **Board Cert:** Surgery 1975, Plastic Surgery 1977; **Med School:** Northwestern Univ 1969; **Resid:** Plastic Surgery, Mass Genl Hosp, Boston, MA 1970-1975; **Fellow:** Hand Surgery, Univ Louisville, Louisville, KY 1975; **Fac Appt:** Prof Surgery, Harvard Med Sch

Mulliken, John B. MD (PIS) - *Spec Exp:* Plastic Surgery-Pediatric; Cleft Palate/Lip; Vascular Malformations; **Hospital:** Children's Hospital - Boston; **Address:** 300 Longwood Ave Bldg Hunnewell-1, Boston, MA 02115-5724; **Phone:** (617) 355-7686; **Board Cert:** Surgery 1972, Plastic Surgery 1975; **Med School:** Columbia P&S 1964; **Resid:** Surgery, Mass Genl Hosp, Boston, MA 1965-1970; Plastic Surgery, Johns Hopkins Hosp, Baltimore, MD 1972-1974

PLASTIC SURGERY

Pribaz, Julian MD (PIS) - *Spec Exp:* Microsurgery; **Hospital:** Brigham & Women's Hosp; **Address:** Brigham & Women's Hosp, Dept Plastic Surg, 75 Francis St, Boston, MA 02115; **Phone:** (617) 732-6390; **Board Cert:** Plastic Surgery 1986, Hand Surgery 1990; **Med School:** Australia 1972; **Resid:** Surgery, St Vincent's Hosp, Melbourne, Austraila 1974-1976; Surgery, Geelong Hosp, Victoria, Austraila 1976-1977; **Fellow:** Plastic Surgery, Southern Ill Univ Sch Med, Springfield, IL 1980-1982; **Fac Appt:** Assoc Prof Surgery, Harvard Med Sch

Stahl, Richard S MD (PIS) - *Spec Exp:* Breast Reconstruction; Chest Wall Reconstruction; Abdominal Wall Reconstruction; **Hospital:** Yale - New Haven Hosp; **Address:** 5 Durham Rd, Guilford, CT 06437; **Phone:** (203) 458-4440; **Board Cert:** Surgery 1984, Plastic Surgery 1992; **Resid:** Surgery, Yale New Haven Hosp, New Haven, CT 1977-1981; Plastic Surgery, Emory Univ Med Ctr, Atlanta, GA 1981-1983; **Fac Appt:** Clin Prof Surgery

Sullivan, Patrick Kevin MD (PIS) - *Spec Exp:* Cosmetic Surgery-Face; Cosmetic Surgery-Breast; Rhinoplasty; **Hospital:** Rhode Island Hosp; **Address:** Rhode Island Hospital, 235 Plain St, Ste 502, Providence, RI 02905-3240; **Phone:** (401) 831-8300; **Board Cert:** Otolaryngology 1985, Plastic Surgery 1989; **Med School:** Mayo Med Sch 1979; **Resid:** Otolaryngology, Univ Colo Hlth Scis Ctr, Denver, CO 1981-1984; Plastic Surgery, Rhode Island Hosp, Providence, RI 1984-1986; **Fellow:** Craniofacial Surgery, Dr Paul Tessier & Dr Hugo Obwegeser, Paris, France-Zurich, Switzerland 1986-1987; **Fac Appt:** Asst Clin Prof Plastic Surgery, Brown Univ

Mid Atlantic

Aston, Sherrell MD (PIS) - *Spec Exp:* Cosmetic Surgery-Face; Rhinoplasty; **Hospital:** Manhattan Eye, Ear & Throat Hosp; **Address:** 728 Park Ave, New York, NY 10021; **Phone:** (212) 249-6000; **Board Cert:** Surgery 1974, Plastic Surgery 1978; **Med School:** Univ VA Sch Med 1968; **Resid:** Surgery, UCLA Med Ctr, Los Angeles, CA 1969-1973; Plastic Surgery, New York Univ, New York, NY 1973-1975; **Fellow:** Surgery, Johns Hopkins Hosp, Baltimore, MD 1970; **Fac Appt:** Assoc Prof Plastic Surgery, NYU Sch Med

Attinger, Chris MD (PIS) - *Spec Exp:* Lower Extremities Reconstruction; Diabetic Leg Reconstruction; **Hospital:** Georgetown Univ Hosp; **Address:** 3800 Reservoir Rd NW, Ste 1 Main West, Washington, DC 20007; **Phone:** (202) 784-5462; **Board Cert:** Plastic Surgery 1992; **Med School:** Yale Univ 1981; **Resid:** Surgery, Brigham & Women's Hosp, Boston, MA 1982-1986; Plastic Surgery, NYU Med Sch, New York, NY 1987-1989; **Fellow:** Vascular Surgery (General), Brigham & Women's Hosp, Boston, MA 1986-1987; Hand Surgery, NYU Med Sch, New York, NY 1989-1990; **Fac Appt:** Assoc Prof Surgery, Geo Wash Univ

Baker, Daniel MD (PIS) - *Spec Exp:* Cosmetic Surgery-Face; Reconstructive Plastic Surgery Face; Rhinoplasty; **Hospital:** Manhattan Eye, Ear & Throat Hosp; **Address:** 65 E 66th St, New York, NY 10021; **Phone:** (212) 734-9695; **Board Cert:** Plastic Surgery 1978; **Med School:** Columbia P&S 1968; **Resid:** Surgery, UC-San Francisco, San Francisco, CA 1973-1975; Plastic Surgery, NYU Med Ctr, New York, NY 1975-1977; **Fellow:** Head and Neck Surgery, NYU Med Ctr, New York, NY 1977-1978; **Fac Appt:** Assoc Prof Plastic Surgery, NYU Sch Med

Bartlett, Scott P MD (PIS) - *Spec Exp:* Craniofacial Surgery/Reconstruction; **Hospital:** Hosp Univ Penn (page 78); **Address:** Hosp Univ Penn, 10 Penn Tower, 3400 Spruce St, Philadelphia, PA 19104-4227; **Phone:** (215) 590-2209; **Board Cert:** Plastic Surgery 1987; **Med School:** Washington Univ, St Louis 1975; **Resid:** Surgery, Mass Genl Hosp, Boston, MA 1976-1983; Plastic Surgery, Mass Genl Hosp, Boston, MA 1983-1985; **Fellow:** Craniofacial Surgery, Univ Penn Hosp, Philadelphia, PA 1985-1986; **Fac Appt:** Assoc Prof Plastic Surgery, Univ Penn

Boyajian, Michael MD (PIS) - *Spec Exp:* Plastic Surgery-Pediatric; **Hospital:** Chldns Natl Med Ctr - DC; **Address:** Chldns Natl Med Ctr, 111 Michigan Ave NW, Ste 4W-100, Washington, DC 20010; **Phone:** (202) 884-2150; **Board Cert:** Surgery 1982, Plastic Surgery 1984; **Med School:** NYU Sch Med 1976; **Resid:** Surgery, Univ Colo Med Ctr, Denver, CO 1977-1979; Surgery, Univ Cincinnati Hosp, Cincinnati, OH 1979-1981; **Fellow:** Plastic Surgery, Brigham & Women's Hosp, Boston, MA 1981-1983; Craniofacial Surgery, Chldns Hosp, Boston, MA 1983; **Fac Appt:** Asst Prof Plastic Surgery, Geo Wash Univ

Bucky, Louis P MD (PIS) - *Spec Exp:* Cosmetic Surgery; Breast Reconstruction; **Hospital:** Pennsylvania Hosp (page 78); **Address:** Univ Penn Med Ctr, Div Plastic Surg, 230 W Washington Square, Ste 101, Philadelphia, PA 19106; **Phone:** (215) 829-6320; **Board Cert:** Surgery 1993, Plastic Surgery 1997; **Med School:** Harvard Med Sch 1986; **Resid:** Surgery, Mass Genl Hosp, Boston, MA 1987-1992; Plastic Surgery, Mass Genl Hosp, Boston, MA 1992-1994; **Fellow:** Microsurgery, Meml Sloan Kettering, New York, NY 1994-1995; Craniofacial Surgery, Miami Chldns Hosp, Miami, FL 1995; **Fac Appt:** Asst Prof Surgery, Univ Penn

Cutting, Court MD (PIS) - *Spec Exp:* Cleft Palate/Lip; Craniofacial Surgery/Reconstruction; **Hospital:** NYU Med Ctr (page 71); **Address:** 333 E 34th St, Ste 1K, New York, NY 10016-6481; **Phone:** (212) 263-5502; **Board Cert:** Otolaryngology 1980, Plastic Surgery 1986; **Med School:** Univ Chicago-Pritzker Sch Med 1975; **Resid:** Otolaryngology, Univ Iowa Hosps, Iowa City, IA 1976-1980; Plastic Surgery, NYU Med Ctr, New York, NY 1980-1983; **Fellow:** Craniofacial Surgery, NYU Med Ctr, New York, NY 1983-1984; **Fac Appt:** Assoc Prof Plastic Surgery, NYU Sch Med

Di Spaltro, Franklin MD (PIS) - *Spec Exp:* Plastic Surgery - General; **Hospital:** St Barnabas Med Ctr; **Address:** 101 Old Short Hills Rd, Ste 510, West Orange, NJ 07052; **Phone:** (973) 736-5907; **Board Cert:** Plastic Surgery 1975; **Med School:** NY Med Coll 1965; **Resid:** Surgery, Metropolitan Hosp Ctr, New York, NY 1966-1970; **Fellow:** Plastic Surgery, St Barnabas Med Ctr, Livingston, NJ 1970-1972; Plastic Surgery, Bellevue Hosp, New York, NY 1972-1973

Gold, Alan MD (PIS) - *Spec Exp:* Cosmetic Surgery; Reconstructive Surgery; **Hospital:** N Shore Univ Hosp at Manhasset; **Address:** 833 Northern Blvd, Ste 240, Great Neck, NY 11021; **Phone:** (516) 498-2800; **Board Cert:** Plastic Surgery 1979; **Med School:** SUNY Hlth Sci Ctr 1971; **Resid:** Surgery, North Shore Univ Hosp, Manhasset, NY 1972-1975; Plastic Surgery, Kings County-Suny Med Ctr, Brooklyn, NY 1976-1978; **Fellow:** Hand Surgery, Nassau County Med Ctr, East Meadow, NY 1975-1976; **Fac Appt:** Assoc Clin Prof Surgery, Cornell Univ-Weill Med Coll

Hidalgo, David MD (PIS) - *Spec Exp:* Breast Reconstruction; Reconstructive Microsurgery; Cosmetic Surgery-Face & Breast; **Hospital:** Manhattan Eye, Ear & Throat Hosp; **Address:** 655 Park Ave, Fl 1, New York, NY 10021; **Phone:** (212) 517-9777; **Board Cert:** Plastic Surgery 1987, Surgery 1984; **Med School:** Georgetown Univ 1978; **Resid:** Surgery, NYU, New York, NY 1978-1983; Plastic Surgery, NYU, New York, NY 1983-1985; **Fellow:** Surgery, NYU, New York, NY 1985-1986; **Fac Appt:** Assoc Prof Surgery, Cornell Univ-Weill Med Coll

Hoffman, Lloyd MD (PIS) - *Spec Exp:* Cosmetic Surgery; Burns; Breast Reconstruction; **Hospital:** NY Presby Hosp - NY Weill Cornell Med Ctr (page 70); **Address:** 50 E 69th St, New York, NY 10021; **Phone:** (212) 452-5125; **Board Cert:** Plastic Surgery 1989, Hand Surgery 1992; **Med School:** Northwestern Univ 1978; **Resid:** Surgery, NY Hosp-Cornell Med Ctr, New York, NY 1978-1983; Plastic Surgery, NYU Med Ctr, New York, NY 1983-1986; **Fellow:** Hand Surgery, NYU Med Ctr, New York, NY 1986-1987; **Fac Appt:** Assoc Prof Plastic Surgery, Cornell Univ-Weill Med Coll

Hurwitz, Dennis MD (PIS) - *Spec Exp:* Reconstructive & Cosmetic Breast Surgery; Cosmetic Surgery; Cleft Palate/Lip; **Hospital:** Magee Women's Hosp; **Address:** 3109 Forbes Ave Fl 5, Pittsburgh, PA 15213; **Phone:** (412) 802-6100; **Board Cert:** Surgery 1976, Plastic Surgery 1979; **Med School:** Univ MD Sch Med 1970; **Resid:** Surgery, Dartmouth Med Ctr, Lebanon, NH 1972-1975; Plastic Surgery, Univ Pitts Med Ctr, Pittsburgh, PA 1975-1977; **Fellow:** Craniofacial Surgery, Univ Mexico 1977; **Fac Appt:** Prof Surgery, Univ Pittsburgh

Jacobs, Elliot MD (PIS) - *Spec Exp:* Cosmetic Surgery; Gynecomastia; **Hospital:** New York Eye & Ear Infirm (page 69); **Address:** 815 Park Ave, New York, NY 10021; **Phone:** (212) 570-6080; **Board Cert:** Plastic Surgery 1982; **Med School:** Mount Sinai Sch Med 1970; **Resid:** Surgery, Mt Sinai Med Ctr, New York, NY 1970-1974; Plastic Surgery, Mt Sinai Med Ctr, New York, NY 1974-1977

Jelks, Glenn MD (PIS) - *Spec Exp:* Cosmetic Surgery-Eyelid; Cosmetic Surgery-Face; Rhinoplasty; **Hospital:** NYU Med Ctr (page 71); **Address:** 875 Park Ave, New York, NY 10021-0341; **Phone:** (212) 988-3303; **Board Cert:** Ophthalmology 1979, Plastic Surgery 1982; **Med School:** Mich State Univ 1973; **Resid:** Ophthalmology, UCLA Med Ctr, Los Angeles, CA 1975-1978; **Fellow:** Plastic Surgery, New York Univ, New York, NY 1978-1980; **Fac Appt:** Assoc Prof Plastic Surgery, NYU Sch Med

Klatsky, Stanley A MD (PIS) - *Spec Exp:* Cosmetic Surgery-Face; Eyelid Surgery; Cosmetic Surgery-Body; **Hospital:** Johns Hopkins Hosp - Baltimore; **Address:** 122 Slade Ave, Ste 100, Baltimore, MD 21208-4917; **Phone:** (410) 484-0400; **Board Cert:** Plastic Surgery 1970; **Med School:** Univ MD Sch Med 1962; **Resid:** Surgery, Sinai Hosp, Baltimore, MD 1962-1966; Plastic Surgery, Columbia-Presby Med Ctr, New York, NY 1966-1968; **Fac Appt:** Assoc Prof Surgery, Johns Hopkins Univ

Leipziger, Lyle S MD (PIS) - *Spec Exp:* Cosmetic Surgery-Face; **Hospital:** N Shore Univ Hosp at Manhasset; **Address:** 825 Northern Blvd Fl 3, Great Neck, NY 11021; **Phone:** (516) 465-8787; **Board Cert:** Plastic Surgery 1994; **Med School:** Cornell Univ-Weill Med Coll 1985; **Resid:** Plastic Surgery, NY Hosp-Cornell Med Ctr, New York, NY 1988-1990; **Fellow:** Craniofacial Surgery, Johns Hopkins Hosp, Baltimore, MD 1990-1991; **Fac Appt:** Asst Prof Surgery, Albert Einstein Coll Med

Little, John W MD (PIS) - *Spec Exp:* Cosmetic Surgery-Face; **Hospital:** Georgetown Univ Hosp; **Address:** 1145 19th St NW, Ste 802, Washington, DC 20036; **Phone:** (202) 467-6700; **Board Cert:** Surgery 1975, Plastic Surgery 1977; **Med School:** Harvard Med Sch 1969; **Resid:** Surgery, Univ Hosps-Case West Res, Cleveland, OH 1969-1974; Plastic Surgery, Univ Hosps-Case West Res, Cleveland, OH 1974-1975; **Fellow:** Plastic Surgery, Jackson Meml Hosp, Miami, FL 1976-1977; **Fac Appt:** Clin Prof Plastic Surgery, Georgetown Univ

Manson, Paul MD (PIS) - *Spec Exp:* Maxillofacial Surgery; Facial Trauma/Fractures; **Hospital:** Johns Hopkins Hosp - Baltimore; **Address:** 601 N Caroline St Bldg McElderry - rm 8152F, Baltimore, MD 21287-0980; **Phone:** (410) 955-9470; **Board Cert:** Plastic Surgery 1979; **Med School:** Northwestern Univ 1968; **Resid:** Surgery, New Eng Deaconess, Boston, MA 1968-1974; Plastic Surgery, Johns Hopkins Hosp, Baltimore, MD 1976-1978; **Fellow:** Surgery, Lahey Clinic, Boston, MA 1974-1975; **Fac Appt:** Prof Plastic Surgery, Johns Hopkins Univ

Matarasso, Alan MD (PIS) - *Spec Exp:* Cosmetic Surgery-Face; Eyelid Surgery; Rhinoplasty; **Hospital:** Manhattan Eye, Ear & Throat Hosp; **Address:** 1009 Park Ave, New York, NY 10028-0936; **Phone:** (212) 249-7500; **Board Cert:** Plastic Surgery 1986; **Med School:** Univ Miami Sch Med 1979; **Resid:** Surgery, Montefiore Med Ctr - Albert Einstein Coll Med, Bronx, NY 1979-1983; Plastic Surgery, Montefiore Med Ctr - Albert Einstein Coll Med, Bronx, NY 1983-1985; **Fellow:** Plastic Surgery, Manhattan EET Hosp, New York, NY 1985; **Fac Appt:** Assoc Clin Prof Plastic Surgery, Albert Einstein Coll Med

McCarthy, Joseph G MD (PIS) - *Spec Exp:* Craniofacial Surgery; Cosmetic Surgery-Face; Reconstructive Surgery-Face; **Hospital:** NYU Med Ctr (page 71); **Address:** 722 Park Ave, New York, NY 10021-4954; **Phone:** (212) 628-4420; **Board Cert:** Plastic Surgery 1974, Surgery 1972; **Med School:** Columbia P&S 1964; **Resid:** Surgery, Columbia-Presby Med Ctr, New York, NY 1967-1971; Plastic Surgery, NYU Med Ctr, New York, NY 1971-1973; **Fac Appt:** Prof Surgery, NYU Sch Med

Noone, R Barrett MD (PIS) - *Spec Exp:* Breast Reconstruction; **Hospital:** Bryn Mawr Hosp; **Address:** 888 Glenbrook Ave, Bryn Mawr, PA 19010-2506; **Phone:** (610) 527-4833; **Board Cert:** Surgery 1972, Plastic Surgery 1974; **Med School:** Univ Penn 1965; **Resid:** Surgery, Hosp Univ Penn, Philadelphia, PA 1966-1971; Plastic Surgery, Hosp Univ Penn, Philadelphia, PA 1971-1973; **Fac Appt:** Clin Prof Surgery, Univ Penn

Pitman, Gerald MD (PIS) - *Spec Exp:* Cosmetic Surgery-Face; Cosmetic Surgery-Liposuction; **Hospital:** Manhattan Eye, Ear & Throat Hosp; **Address:** 170 E 73rd St, New York, NY 10021; **Phone:** (212) 517-2600; **Board Cert:** Plastic Surgery 1978, Surgery 1976; **Med School:** Univ Penn 1968; **Resid:** Surgery, Columbia-Presby Hosp, New York, NY 1971-1975; Plastic Surgery, NYU Med Ctr, New York, NY 1975-1977; **Fellow:** Microsurgery, NYU Med Ctr, New York, NY 1980-1981; **Fac Appt:** Assoc Clin Prof Plastic Surgery, NYU Sch Med

Posnick, Jeffrey Craig MD/DMD (PIS) - *Spec Exp:* Cosmetic Surgery-Face; Craniofacial Surgery/Reconstruction; Maxillofacial Surgery; **Hospital:** Georgetown Univ Hosp; **Address:** Posnick Ctr for Plastic Surgery, 5530 Wisconsin Ave, Ste 1250, Chevy Chase, MD 20815; **Phone:** (301) 986-9475; **Board Cert:** Plastic Surgery 1988; **Med School:** Vanderbilt Univ 1979; **Resid:** Surgery, Eastern VA Med Sch, Norfolk, VA 1984-1986; Plastic Surgery, Mass Genl Hosp, Boston, MA 1981-1983; **Fellow:** Craniofacial Surgery, Univ Penn, Philadephia, PA 1983; Craniofacial Surgery, Vanderbilt Med Ctr, Nashville, TN 1979-1981; **Fac Appt:** Clin Prof Plastic Surgery, Georgetown Univ

Ramirez, Oscar M MD (PIS) - *Spec Exp:* Endoscopic Facelift (Scarless); **Hospital:** Greater Baltimore Med Ctr; **Address:** 2219 York Rd, Ste 100, Timonium, MD 21093; **Phone:** (410) 560-7090; **Board Cert:** Plastic Surgery 1985; **Med School:** Peru 1976; **Resid:** Surgery, Franklin Sq Hosp, Baltimore, MD 1977-1982; Plastic Surgery, Univ Pitts Affil Hosps, Pittsburgh, PA 1982-1984; **Fellow:** Craniofacial Surgery, Manuel Gea Gonzalez, Mexico City, Mexico 1984; **Fac Appt:** Asst Clin Prof Surgery, Johns Hopkins Univ

Slezak, Sheri MD (PIS) - *Spec Exp:* Breast Reconstruction; **Hospital:** University of MD Med Sys; **Address:** Univ Maryland Medical Systems, Dept Plastic Surgery, 22 S Greene St, rm S8D12, Baltimore, MD 21201-1544; **Phone:** (410) 328-2360; **Board Cert:** Plastic Surgery 1991; **Med School:** Harvard Med Sch 1980; **Resid:** Surgery, Columbia-Presby Med Ctr, New York, NY 1980-1985; Plastic Reconstructive Surgery, Johns Hopkins Hosp, Baltimore, MD 1985-1989; **Fac Appt:** Assoc Prof Plastic Surgery, Univ MD Sch Med

Spear, Scott L MD (PIS) - *Spec Exp:* Breast Reconstruction; Cosmetic Surgery-Face; **Hospital:** Georgetown Univ Hosp; **Address:** 3800 Reservoir Rd NW, Washington, DC 20007; **Phone:** (202) 687-8612; **Board Cert:** Surgery 1979, Plastic Surgery 1981; **Med School:** Univ Chicago-Pritzker Sch Med 1972; **Resid:** Surgery, Beth Israel Hosp, Boston, MA 1973-1978; Plastic Surgery, Univ Miami Hosps, Miami, FL 1978-1980; **Fac Appt:** Prof Plastic Surgery, Georgetown Univ

PLASTIC SURGERY

Spinelli, Henry M MD (PIS) - *Spec Exp:* Oculoplastic & Orbital Surgery; Craniofacial Surgery/Reconstruction; Cosmetic Surgery; **Hospital:** NY Presby Hosp - NY Weill Cornell Med Ctr (page 70); **Address:** 875 Fifth Ave, New York, NY 10021-4952; **Phone:** (212) 570-6235; **Board Cert:** Ophthalmology 1987, Plastic Surgery 1993; **Med School:** NYU Sch Med 1981; **Resid:** Surgery, Columbia-Presby, New York, NY 1985-1988; Plastic Surgery, NYU-Bellevue Hosp, New York, NY 1988-1990; **Fellow:** Craniofacial Surgery, NYU Med Ctr, New York, NY 1990-1991; Ophthalmology, Manhattan EET Hosp, New York, NY 1982-1985; **Fac Appt:** Assoc Prof Plastic Surgery, Cornell Univ-Weill Med Coll

Sultan, Mark MD (PIS) - *Spec Exp:* Breast Reconstruction; Cosmetic Surgery-Breast; Cosmetic Surgery-Face; **Hospital:** St Luke's - Roosevelt Hosp Ctr - Roosevelt Div (page 58); **Address:** 1100 Park Ave, New York, NY 10028; **Phone:** (212) 360-0700; **Board Cert:** Surgery 1988, Plastic Surgery 1992; **Med School:** Columbia P&S 1982; **Resid:** Surgery, Columbia-Presby Hosp, New York, NY 1982-1987; Plastic Surgery, Columbia-Presby Hosp, New York, NY 1987-1990; **Fellow:** Head and Neck Surgery, Emory Univ Hosp, Atlanta, GA 1988-1989; **Fac Appt:** Assoc Prof Surgery, Columbia P&S

Tabbal, Nicolas MD (PIS) - *Spec Exp:* Rhinoplasty; Prosthetic Nose; **Hospital:** Manhattan Eye, Ear & Throat Hosp; **Address:** 521 Park Ave, New York, NY 10021-8140; **Phone:** (212) 644-5800; **Board Cert:** Plastic Surgery 1980; **Med School:** Lebanon 1972; **Resid:** Surgery, Am Univ Med Ctr, Beirut, Lebanon 1972-1976; Plastic Surgery, Akron City Hosp, Akron, OH 1977-1979; **Fellow:** Surgery, Upstate Med Ctr, Syracuse, NY 1976-1977; Reconstructive Surgery, NYU Med Ctr, New York, NY 1979-1980; **Fac Appt:** Plastic Surgery, NYU Sch Med

Thorne, Charles MD (PIS) - *Spec Exp:* Ear Reconstruction; Cosmetic Surgery-Face & Breast; Cranial Plastic Surgery; **Hospital:** NYU Med Ctr (page 71); **Address:** 812 Park Ave, New York, NY 10021-2759; **Phone:** (212) 794-0044; **Board Cert:** Surgery 1987, Plastic Surgery 1991; **Med School:** UCLA 1981; **Resid:** Surgery, Mass Genl Hosp, Boston, MA 1981-1986; Plastic Surgery, NYU Med Ctr, New York, NY 1986-1988; **Fellow:** Craniofacial Surgery, NYU Med Ctr, New York, NY 1988-1989; **Fac Appt:** Assoc Prof Plastic Surgery, NYU Sch Med

Vander Kolk, Craig Alan MD (PIS) - *Spec Exp:* Craniofacial Surgery/Reconstruction; Cleft Palate/Lip; **Hospital:** Johns Hopkins Hosp - Baltimore; **Address:** Johns Hopkins Outpatient Ctr, 601 N Caroline St Fl 8, Baltimore, MD 21287; **Phone:** (410) 955-6897; **Board Cert:** Plastic Surgery 1989; **Med School:** Univ Mich Med Sch 1980; **Resid:** Surgery, Univ Mich Med Ctr, Ann Arbor, MI 1980-1983; Plastic Surgery, Univ Mich Med Ctr, Ann Arbor, MI 1983-1986; **Fellow:** Hand Surgery, St Vincents Hosp, Melbourne, Australia 1984-1985; Craniofacial Surgery, Chldns Hosp, Philadelphia, PA 1986-1987; **Fac Appt:** Assoc Prof Plastic Surgery, Johns Hopkins Univ

Whitaker, Linton A MD (PIS) - *Spec Exp:* Craniofacial Surgery/Reconstruction; Cosmetic Surgery-Face; **Hospital:** Hosp Univ Penn (page 78); **Address:** Univ Med Ctr-10 Penn Tower, 3400 Spruce St, Philadelphia, PA 19104; **Phone:** (215) 662-2048; **Board Cert:** Surgery 1970, Plastic Surgery 1978; **Med School:** Tulane Univ 1962; **Resid:** Surgery, Dartmouth Affl Hosp, Lebanon, NH 1965-1969; Plastic Surgery, Hosp Univ Penn, Philadelphia, PA 1969-1971; **Fac Appt:** Prof Plastic Surgery, Univ Penn

Wood-Smith, Donald MD (PIS) - *Spec Exp:* Cosmetic Surgery-Face; Rhinoplasty-Secondary; Maxillofacial Surgery; **Hospital:** New York Eye & Ear Infirm (page 69); **Address:** 830 Park Ave, New York, NY 10021-2757; **Phone:** (212) 744-2224; **Board Cert:** Plastic Surgery 1970; **Med School:** Australia 1954; **Resid:** Plastic Surgery, NYU Med Ctr, New York, NY 1961-1963; Surgery, Stanford Univ Hosp, Stanford, CA 1967-1968; **Fac Appt:** Prof Surgery, Columbia P&S

Southeast

Argenta, Louis Charles MD (PIS) - *Spec Exp:* Reconstructive Plastic Surgery; **Hospital:** Wake Forest Univ Baptist Med Ctr (page 81); **Address:** Wake Forest Univ Baptist Med Ctr, Dept Plastic Surgery, Medical Center Blvd, Winston Salem, NC 27157-1075; **Phone:** (336) 716-4416; **Board Cert:** Plastic Surgery 1982; **Med School:** Univ Mich Med Sch 1969; **Resid:** Surgery, Univ Mich, Ann Arbor, MI 1973-1977; Plastic Surgery, Univ Mich, Ann Arbor, MI 1977-1979; **Fellow:** Craniofacial Surgery, Hosp Foch, Paris, France 1982; **Fac Appt:** Prof Plastic Surgery, Wake Forest Univ Sch Med

Baker Jr, James L MD (PIS) - *Spec Exp:* Breast Augmentation; Liposuction; Cosmetic Surgery-Face; **Hospital:** Florida Hospital Orlando Apopka; **Address:** 400 W Morse Blvd, Ste 203, Winter Park, FL 32789-4280; **Phone:** (407) 644-5242; **Board Cert:** Plastic Surgery 1973; **Med School:** Holland 1964; **Resid:** Surgery, Monmouth Med Ctr, Long Branch, NJ 1965-1969; Plastic Surgery, Orlando Regional Med Ctr, Orlando, FL 1969-1971; **Fellow:** Hand Surgery, Harold Klinert-U, Louisville, KY 1971; **Fac Appt:** Clin Prof Plastic Surgery, Univ S Fla Coll Med

Baker Jr, Thomas J MD (PIS) - *Spec Exp:* Cosmetic Surgery; Skin Laser Surgery; Breast Surgery; **Hospital:** Mercy Hosp - Miami, FL; **Address:** 1501 S Miami Ave, Miami, FL 33129-1102; **Phone:** (305) 854-2424; **Board Cert:** Surgery 1958, Plastic Surgery 1959; **Med School:** Indiana Univ 1949; **Resid:** Surgery, Jackson Meml Hosp, Miami, FL 1951-1955; Plastic Surgery, Univ Texas Med Branch, Galveston, FL 1955-1957

Beasley, Michael MD (PIS) - *Spec Exp:* Breast Surgery; Cosmetic Surgery-Body; **Hospital:** Carolinas Med Ctr; **Address:** 2215 Randolph Rd, Charlotte, NC 28207; **Phone:** (704) 372-6846; **Board Cert:** Plastic Surgery 1989; **Med School:** Univ NC Sch Med 1980; **Resid:** Surgery, NC Meml Hosp, Chapel Hill, NC 1980-1985; Plastic Surgery, Emory U Hosp, Atlanta, GA 1985-1987; **Fellow:** Breast Surgery, St. Joseph Hospital, Atlanta, GA 1987; **Fac Appt:** Assoc Clin Prof Plastic Surgery, Univ NC Sch Med

Bermant, Michael A. MD (PIS) - *Spec Exp:* Gynecomastia; **Hospital:** CJW Med Ctr; **Address:** 11601 Ironbridge Rd, Ste 201, Ironbridge Med Park, Chester, VA 23831; **Phone:** (804) 748-7737; **Board Cert:** Plastic Surgery 1991; **Med School:** Northwestern Univ 1978; **Resid:** Surgery, St Vincents Hosp, New York, NY 1979-1982; Plastic Surgery, St Louis U Med Ctr, St Louis, MO 1982-1984; **Fellow:** Microsurgery, NYU, New York, NY 1985

Caffee, Henry Hollis MD (PIS) - *Spec Exp:* Breast Reconstruction; Microsurgery; Hand Surgery; **Hospital:** Shands Hlthcre at Univ of FL (page 73); **Address:** Shands Hlthcare at Univ FL, 1600 SW Archer Rd, Gainesville, FL 32610; **Phone:** (352) 395-6810; **Board Cert:** Plastic Surgery 1979, Hand Surgery 1997; **Med School:** Univ Fla Coll Med 1968; **Resid:** Surgery, Harbor Genl Hosp, Torrance, CA 1969-1975; Plastic Surgery, UCLA Med Ctr, Los Angeles, CA 1975-1977; **Fac Appt:** Prof Plastic Surgery, Univ Fla Coll Med

Carraway, James Howard MD (PIS) - *Spec Exp:* Oculoplastic Surgery; Cosmetic Surgery-Face; Eyelid Surgery; **Hospital:** Sentara Leigh Hosp; **Address:** Dept Plastic Surgery, 5589 Greenwich Rd, Ste 100, Virginia Beach, VA 23462; **Phone:** (757) 557-0300; **Board Cert:** Plastic Surgery 1974, Surgery 1972; **Med School:** Univ VA Sch Med 1962; **Resid:** Surgery, Norfolk Med Ctr, Norfolk, VA 1966-1970; Plastic Surgery, Eastern VA Med Ctr, Norfolk, VA 1971-1973; **Fellow:** Plastic Surgery, Glasgow Royal Infirmary, Glasgow,Scotland 1970; **Fac Appt:** Prof Plastic Surgery, Eastern VA Med Sch

Cruse, C Wayne MD (PIS) - *Spec Exp:* Burns; **Hospital:** Tampa Genl Hosp; **Address:** 12902 Magnolia Dr, Ste 4035, Tampa, FL 33612-9416; **Phone:** (813) 972-8410; **Board Cert:** Surgery 1978, Plastic Surgery 1981; **Med School:** Univ Louisville Sch Med 1972; **Resid:** Surgery, Univ S Fla Hosp, Tampa, FL 1973-1977; Plastic Surgery, Univ KY Hosp-Chandler Med Ctr, Lexington, KY 1977; **Fac Appt:** Prof Surgery, Univ S Fla Coll Med

Fisher, Jack MD (PIS) - *Spec Exp:* Breast Reconstruction; **Hospital:** Baptist Hosp; **Address:** Nashville Plas Surg Ltd, 2021 Church St, Ste 806, Nashville, TN 37203; **Phone:** (615) 284-8200; **Board Cert:** Plastic Surgery 1981; **Med School:** Emory Univ 1973; **Resid:** Surgery, Geo Wash Univ Hosp, Washington, DC 1974-1978; Plastic Surgery, Emory Univ Hosp, Atlanta, GA 1978-1980; **Fac Appt:** Asst Clin Prof Plastic Surgery, Vanderbilt Univ

Fix, R Jobe MD (PIS) - *Spec Exp:* Breast Reconstruction; Hand Surgery; Microsurgery; **Hospital:** Univ of Ala Hosp at Birmingham; **Address:** Div Plas Surg, 1813 6th Ave S, #Meb524, Birmingham, AL 35294-3295; **Phone:** (205) 934-3358; **Board Cert:** Surgery 1999, Hand Surgery 2001, Plastic Surgery 1991; **Med School:** Univ Nebr Coll Med 1982; **Resid:** Surgery, Valley Med Ctr, Fresno, CA 1982-1987; Plastic Surgery, Univ Ala Hosp, Birmingham, AL 1987-1989; **Fac Appt:** Prof Plastic Surgery, Univ Ala

Georgiade, Gregory MD (PIS) - *Spec Exp:* Breast Reconstruction; Cleft Palate/Lip; **Hospital:** Duke Univ Med Ctr (page 60); **Address:** Duke Univ Med Ctr, Box 3960, Durham, NC 27710-0001; **Phone:** (919) 684-3039; **Board Cert:** Plastic Surgery 1981, Surgery 1990; **Med School:** Duke Univ 1973; **Resid:** Surgery, Duke Univ Med Ctr, Durham, NC 1974-1978; Plastic Surgery, Duke Univ Med Ctr, Durham, NC 1979-1980; **Fac Appt:** Prof Surgery, Duke Univ

Gregory, Richard MD (PIS) - *Spec Exp:* Skin Laser Surgery; Cosmetic Surgery-Face; **Hospital:** Florida Hosp; **Address:** 400 Celebration Pl, Ste A320, Celebration, FL 34747; **Phone:** (407) 303-4250; **Board Cert:** Plastic Surgery 1981, Surgery 1979; **Med School:** Indiana Univ 1971; **Resid:** Surgery, Duke Univ Med Ctr, Durham, NC 1972-1977; Plastic Surgery, Duke Univ Med Ctr, Durham, NC 1977-1979; **Fellow:** Hand Surgery, Univ Louisville Hlth Sci Ctr, Louisville, KY 1978-1979; **Fac Appt:** Assoc Clin Prof Plastic Surgery, Univ S Fla Coll Med

Grotting, James MD (PIS) - *Spec Exp:* Cosmetic Surgery; Breast Reconstruction; **Hospital:** Healthsouth Med Ctr - Birmingham; **Address:** One Inverness Center Pkwy, Ste 100, Birmingham, AL 35242; **Phone:** (205) 930-1800; **Board Cert:** Plastic Surgery 1986, Hand Surgery 1989; **Med School:** Univ Minn 1978; **Resid:** Surgery, Univ Wash Affil Hosp, Seattle, WA 1979-1983; Plastic Surgery, UC-San Francisco, San Francisco, CA 1983-1985; **Fac Appt:** Asst Prof Plastic Surgery

Hagan, Kevin Francis MD (PIS) - *Spec Exp:* Reconstructive Surgery; **Hospital:** Vanderbilt Univ Med Ctr (page 80); **Address:** Vanderbilt Univ Med Ctr South, 2100 Pierce Ave, Ste 230, Nashville, TN 37232-3631; **Phone:** (615) 936-0160; **Board Cert:** Plastic Surgery 1983, Hand Surgery 1993; **Med School:** Johns Hopkins Univ 1974; **Resid:** Surgery, Med Coll VA Hosps, Richmond, VA 1975-1979; Plastic Surgery, UCSF Med Ctr, San Francisco, CA 1980-1982; **Fellow:** Microsurgery, Dr Harry Buncke Med Clinic, San Francisco, CA 1980; **Fac Appt:** Asst Prof Plastic Surgery, Vanderbilt Univ

Hester Jr, T Roderick MD (PIS) - *Spec Exp:* Cosmetic Surgery-Face; Breast Reconstruction; **Hospital:** Emory Univ Hosp; **Address:** 3200 Downwood Cir, Ste 640, Atlanta, GA 30327; **Phone:** (404) 351-0051; **Board Cert:** Plastic Surgery 1980, Surgery 1973; **Med School:** Emory Univ 1967; **Resid:** Surgery, Emory Affil Hosps, Atlanta, GA 1968-1972

Hunstad, Joseph P. MD (PIS) - *Spec Exp:* Cosmetic Surgery-Face & Body; **Hospital:** Unv Hosp-Charlotte, NC; **Address:** 8220 Univ Exec Park Drive, Ste 100, Charlotte, NC 28262; **Phone:** (704) 549-0500; **Board Cert:** Plastic Surgery 1989; **Med School:** Mich State Univ 1981; **Resid:** Surgery, Butterworth Hosp, Grand Rapids, MI 1982-1984; Plastic Surgery, Grand Rapids Area Med Ed Ct, Grand Rapids, MI 1984-1986; **Fellow:** Reconstructive Microsurgery, MECOM MicSurg Inst., Houston, TX 1986-1987

Levin, L Scott MD (PIS) - *Spec Exp:* Transplant-Toe to Hand; Reconstructive Microvascular Surgery; **Hospital:** Duke Univ Med Ctr (page 60); **Address:** Duke Univ Med Ctr Bldg Baker - rm 134, Box 3945, Durham, NC 27707; **Phone:** (919) 681-5079; **Board Cert:** Orthopaedic Surgery 1993, Hand Surgery 1994; **Med School:** Temple Univ 1982; **Resid:** Orthopaedic Surgery, Duke Univ Med Ctr, Durham, NC 1984-1988; Plastic Surgery, Duke Univ Med Ctr, Durham, NC 1988-1989; **Fac Appt:** Assoc Prof Surgery, Duke Univ

Mast, Bruce A MD (PIS) - *Spec Exp:* Breast Reconstruction; Wound Care; Microsurgery; **Hospital:** Shands Hlthcre at Univ of FL (page 73); **Address:** 1600 SW Archer Rd, Gainesville, FL 32610; **Phone:** (352) 846-0377; **Board Cert:** Surgery 1995, Plastic Surgery 1998; **Med School:** UMDNJ-RW Johnson Med Sch 1987; **Resid:** Surgery, Medical College of Virginia, Richmond, VA 1987-1993; Plastic Surgery, univ of Pittsburgh, Pittsburgh, PA 1993-1995; **Fac Appt:** Asst Prof Plastic Surgery, Univ S Fla Coll Med

Matthews, David MD (PIS) - *Spec Exp:* Craniofacial Surgery/Reconstruction; **Hospital:** Carolinas Med Ctr; **Address:** 2215 Randolph Rd, Charlotte, NC 28207-1523; **Phone:** (704) 372-6846; **Board Cert:** Plastic Surgery 1983, Surgery 1981; **Med School:** Univ Cincinnati 1974; **Resid:** Plastic Surgery, Univ of Penn Hosp, Philadelphia, PA 1980-1982; Surgery, Univ of Penn Hosp, Philadelphia, PA 1979-1980; **Fellow:** Royal Melbourne, Australia; **Fac Appt:** Assoc Clin Prof Plastic Surgery, Univ NC Sch Med

Maxwell, G Patrick MD (PIS) - *Spec Exp:* Breast Reconstruction; **Hospital:** Baptist Hosp; **Address:** 2021 Church St, Ste 806, Nashville, TN 37203; **Phone:** (615) 284-8200; **Board Cert:** Plastic Surgery 1981; **Med School:** Vanderbilt Univ 1972; **Resid:** Surgery, Johns Hopkins Hosp, Baltimore, MD 1973-1976; Plastic Surgery, Johns Hopkins Hosp, Baltimore, MD 1976-1979; **Fellow:** Microsurgery, Davies Med Ctr, San Francisco, CA 1975; **Fac Appt:** Asst Clin Prof Plastic Surgery, Vanderbilt Univ

McCraw, John MD (PIS) - *Spec Exp:* Breast Reconstruction; **Hospital:** Univ Hosps & Clins - Mississippi; **Address:** 2500 N State St, UMMC, Dept Surgery, Jackson, MS 32916-3600; **Phone:** (601) 984-5073; **Board Cert:** Surgery 1972, Plastic Surgery 1974; **Med School:** Univ MO-Columbia Sch Med 1966; **Resid:** Orthopaedic Surgery, Duke U Med Ctr, Durham, NC 1968-1969; Surgery, U Fla Med Ctr 1969-1971; **Fellow:** Plastic Surgery, U Fla/ Emory U 1971-1973; **Fac Appt:** Prof Plastic Surgery, Univ Miss

Mladick, Richard MD (PIS) - *Spec Exp:* Liposuction; Cosmetic Surgery-Face; Breast Augmentation; **Hospital:** Virginia Beach Gen Hosp; **Address:** Mladick Ctr Cosmetic Surg, 1037 First Colonial Rd, Virginia Beach, VA 23454; **Phone:** (757) 481-5151; **Board Cert:** Surgery 1965, Plastic Surgery 1969; **Med School:** Northwestern Univ 1959; **Resid:** Surgery, Cook Co Hosp, Chicago, IL 1960-1964; Plastic Surgery, Duke Med Ctr, Durham, NC 1964-1967; **Fac Appt:** Prof Plastic Surgery, Eastern VA Med Sch

Molnar, Joseph MD (PIS) - *Spec Exp:* Burns; Reconstructive Microvascular Surgery; **Hospital:** Wake Forest Univ Baptist Med Ctr (page 81); **Address:** Wake Forest Baptist Med Ctr, Medical Ctr Blvd, Winston Salem, NC 27157-1075; **Phone:** (336) 716-0432; **Board Cert:** Plastic Surgery 1996; **Med School:** Ohio State Univ 1977; **Resid:** Surgery, Univ Wash Med Ctr, Seattle, WA 1985-1989; Plastic Surgery, Med Coll VA, Richmond, VA 1990-1992; **Fellow:** Trauma, Mass Genl Hosp, Boston, MA 1979-1985; Hand Surgery, Med Coll Wisc, Milwaukee, WI 1992-1994; **Fac Appt:** Asst Prof Plastic Surgery, Wake Forest Univ Sch Med

Morgan, Raymond MD (PIS) - *Spec Exp:* Hand Surgery; **Hospital:** Univ of VA Hlth Sys (page 79); **Address:** Dept Plastic Surgery, PO Box 800376, Charlottesville, VA 22908; **Phone:** (804) 924-2413; **Board Cert:** Hand Surgery 1990, Plastic Surgery 1983; **Med School:** W VA Univ 1976; **Resid:** Surgery, Johns Hopkins Hosp, Baltimore, MD 1977-1980; Plastic Surgery, Johns Hopkins Hosp, Baltimore, MD 1980-1982; **Fellow:** Hand Surgery, Union Meml Hosp, Baltimore, MD; **Fac Appt:** Prof Plastic Surgery, Univ VA Sch Med

Mullin, Walter MD (PIS) - *Spec Exp:* Breast Reconstruction; Ear Reconstruction; Cosmetic Surgery-Face; **Hospital:** Cedars Med Ctr - Miami; **Address:** Plastic Surgery Ctr, 1444 NW 14th Ave, Miami, FL 33125-1645; **Phone:** (305) 325-1441; **Board Cert:** Plastic Surgery 1977; **Med School:** Univ Miami Sch Med 1969; **Resid:** Surgery, Jackson Meml Hosp, Miami, FL 1970-1973; Plastic Surgery, Jackson Meml Hosp, Miami, FL 1974-1976; **Fellow:** Plastic Surgery, Bangour Genl Hosp, Edinburgh, Scotland 1973-1974; **Fac Appt:** Assoc Clin Prof Plastic Surgery, Univ Miami Sch Med

Nahai, Foad MD (PIS) - *Spec Exp:* Cosmetic Surgery; Cosmetic Surgery-Face; Cosmetic Surgery-Liposuction; **Hospital:** St Joseph's Hosp - Atlanta; **Address:** 3200 Downwood Circle, Ste 640, Atlanta, GA 30327-1624; **Phone:** (404) 351-0051; **Board Cert:** Plastic Surgery 1980; **Med School:** England 1969; **Resid:** Surgery, Johns Hopkins Affil Hosps, Baltimore, MD 1970-1972; Surgery, Emory Univ Affil Hosps, Atlanta, GA 1972-1975; **Fellow:** Plastic Surgery, Emory Univ Affil Hosps, Atlanta, GA 1975-1978

Stuzin, James M MD (PIS) - *Spec Exp:* Cosmetic Surgery-Body; Breast Surgery; **Hospital:** Mercy Hosp - Miami, FL; **Address:** 1501 S Miami Ave, Miami, FL 33129-1102; **Phone:** (305) 854-2424; **Board Cert:** Plastic Surgery 1989; **Med School:** Univ Fla Coll Med 1978; **Resid:** Surgery, Univ Wash Affil Hosp, Seattle, WA 1979-1983; Plastic Surgery, NYU Med Ctr, New York, NY 1984-1986; **Fellow:** Craniofacial Surgery, UCLA Med Ctr, Los Angeles, CA 1987; **Fac Appt:** Asst Clin Prof Plastic Surgery, Univ Miami Sch Med

Tobin, Gordon R MD (PIS) - *Spec Exp:* Reconstructive Plastic Surgery; Transplant Surgery-Hand; **Hospital:** Univ Louisville Hosp; **Address:** University Surgical Associates, 601 S Floyd St, Ste 700, Louisville, KY 40202; **Phone:** (502) 583-8303; **Board Cert:** Plastic Surgery 1978; **Med School:** UCSF 1969; **Resid:** Surgery, Univ Ariz Affil Hosps, Tucson, AZ 1970-1975; Plastic Surgery, Univ Ariz Affil Hosps, Tucson, AZ 1975-1976; **Fellow:** Pediatric Plastic Surgery, Univ Miami, Miami, FL 1973; **Fac Appt:** Prof Surgery, Univ Louisville Sch Med

Vasconez, Luis O MD (PIS) - *Spec Exp:* Cosmetic Surgery-Face; Breast Reconstruction; **Hospital:** Univ of Ala Hosp at Birmingham; **Address:** 1813 6th Ave S Bldg MEB - rm 524, Birmingham, AL 35294; **Phone:** (205) 934-3245; **Board Cert:** Surgery 1970, Plastic Surgery 1971; **Med School:** Washington Univ, St Louis 1962; **Resid:** Surgery, Strong Meml Hosp, Rochester, NY 1963-1970; Plastic Surgery, Shands Hosp-Univ FL, Gainsville, FL 1966-1969; **Fac Appt:** Prof Surgery, Univ Ala

Wolfe, S Anthony MD (PlS) - *Spec Exp:* Craniofacial Surgery/Reconstruction; Maxillofacial Surgery; **Hospital:** Cedars Med Ctr - Miami; **Address:** Plastic Surgery Ctr, 1444 NW 14th Ave Fl 2, Miami, FL 33125-1645; **Phone:** (305) 325-1300; **Board Cert:** Surgery 1973, Plastic Surgery 1976; **Med School:** Harvard Med Sch 1965; **Resid:** Surgery, Peter Bent Brigham Hosp, Boston, MA 1968-1972; Plastic Surgery, Jackson Meml Hosp, Miami, FL 1972-1974; **Fac Appt:** Clin Prof Plastic Surgery, Univ Miami Sch Med

Midwest

Arnold, Phillip MD (PlS) - *Spec Exp:* Cosmetic Surgery-Face; Chemical Peel; **Hospital:** Mayo Med Ctr & Clin - Rochester, MN; **Address:** 200 SW First St, Rochester, MN 55905-0001; **Phone:** (507) 284-3214; **Board Cert:** Plastic Surgery 1977; **Med School:** Univ NC Sch Med 1967; **Resid:** Surgery, Univ NC Meml Hosp, Chapel Hill, NC 1968-1974; Plastic Surgery, Emory Univ Hosp, Atlanta, GA 1974-1976; **Fac Appt:** Prof Plastic Surgery, Mayo Med Sch

Bauer, Bruce MD (PlS) - *Spec Exp:* Cleft Palate/Lip; Giant Pigmented Nevi; Vascular Malformations; **Hospital:** Children's Mem Hosp; **Address:** Chldns Meml Hosp, 2300 Childrens Plaza, Box 41, Chicago, IL 60614-3394; **Phone:** (773) 880-4094; **Board Cert:** Plastic Surgery 1980; **Med School:** Northwestern Univ 1974; **Resid:** Surgery, Northwestern Meml Hosp, Chicago, IL 1975-1977; Plastic Surgery, Northwestestern Meml Hosp, Chicago, IL 1977-1979; **Fac Appt:** Assoc Prof Surgery, Northwestern Univ

Billmire, David A MD (PlS) - *Spec Exp:* Cleft Palate; Reconstructive Plastic Surgery; **Hospital:** Cincinnati Chldns Hosp Med Ctr; **Address:** 3333 Burnet Ave Fl 3 - rm OSB3, Cincinatti, OH 45229-3039; **Phone:** (513) 636-7181; **Board Cert:** Plastic Surgery 1985; **Med School:** Ohio State Univ 1975; **Resid:** Surgery, University Hosp, Cincinatti, OH 1976-1982; Plastic Reconstructive Surgery, University Hosp, Cincinatti, OH 1982-1984; **Fellow:** Craniofacial Surgery, Texas Craniofacial Fdn, Dallas, TX 1985; **Fac Appt:** Assoc Prof Surgery, Univ Cincinnati

Brandt, Keith MD (PlS) - *Spec Exp:* Breast Reconstruction; **Hospital:** Barnes-Jewish Hosp (page 55); **Address:** 660 S Euclid, Box 8238, St Louis, MO 63110; **Phone:** (314) 747-0541; **Board Cert:** Plastic Surgery 1995, Surgery 1999; **Med School:** Univ Tex, Houston 1983; **Resid:** Surgery, Baylor Univ Med Ctr, Dallas, TX 1984-1986; Surgery, Univ NE Med Ctr, Omaha, NB 1986-1989; **Fellow:** Hand Surgery, Wash Univ, St Louis, MO 1991-1992; **Fac Appt:** Assoc Prof Surgery, Washington Univ, St Louis

Burget, Gary C MD (PlS) - *Spec Exp:* Nasal Reconstruction; Cosmetic Surgery-Face; Reconstructive Surgery; **Hospital:** Saint Joseph Hosp; **Address:** 2913 N Commonwealth Ave, Ste 400, Chicago, IL 60657-6238; **Phone:** (773) 880-0062; **Board Cert:** Plastic Surgery 1980; **Med School:** Yale Univ 1967; **Resid:** Surgery, Jackson Meml Med Ctr, Miami, FL 1969-1972; Plastic Surgery, Jackson Meml Med Ctr, Miami, FL 1972-1974; **Fellow:** Pediatric Plastic Surgery, Chldns Meml Hosp, Chicago, IL 1985-1986; **Fac Appt:** Assoc Clin Prof Surgery, Univ Chicago-Pritzker Sch Med

Canady, John MD (PlS) - *Spec Exp:* Cleft Palate/Lip; Craniofacial Surgery; Pediatric Plastic Surgery; **Hospital:** Univ of IA Hosp and Clinics; **Address:** Univ Iowa Hosps and Clinics, Dept Plastic Surgery & Otolaryngology, 200 Hawkins Drive, Iowa City, IA 52242; **Phone:** (319) 356-2168; **Board Cert:** Otolaryngology 1988, Plastic Surgery 1992; **Med School:** Univ Iowa Coll Med 1983; **Resid:** Otolaryngology, Univ Iowa Med Ctr, Iowa City, IA 1984-1988; Plastic Surgery, Univ Kansas Med Ctr, Kansas City, KA 1988-1990; **Fac Appt:** Asst Prof Plastic Surgery, Univ Iowa Coll Med

Coleman, John MD (PlS) - *Spec Exp:* Cancer Reconstruction; Breast Reconstruction; Head & Neck Surgery; **Hospital:** IN Univ Hosp (page 63); **Address:** 545 Barnhill Dr, Emerson Hall 235, Indianapolis, IN 46202-5120; **Phone:** (317) 274-8106; **Board Cert:** Surgery 1998, Plastic Surgery 1981; **Med School:** Harvard Med Sch 1973; **Resid:** Surgery, Emory Univ Affil Hosp, Atlanta, GA 1974-1978; Plastic Surgery, Emory Univ Affil Hosp, Atlanta, GA 1978-1979; **Fellow:** Surgical Oncology, Univ MD Med Ctr, Baltimore, MD 1980; **Fac Appt:** Prof Surgery, Indiana Univ

Cram, Albert E MD (PlS) - *Spec Exp:* Breast Reconstruction; **Hospital:** Univ of IA Hosp and Clinics; **Address:** Univ Iowa Hosps and Clinics, Dept Plastic Surgery, 200 Hawkins Drive, Iowa City, IA 52242; **Phone:** (319) 356-2777; **Board Cert:** Plastic Surgery 1989; **Med School:** Univ Nebr Coll Med 1969; **Resid:** Sports Medicine, Univ Iowa Hosps, Iowa City, IA 1970-1974; Plastic Surgery, Univ Chicago Hosps, Chicago, IL 1985-1987; **Fac Appt:** Prof Emeritus Surgery, Univ Iowa Coll Med

Hammond, Dennis MD (PlS) - *Spec Exp:* Breast Surgery; **Hospital:** St. Mary's Mercy Med Ctr; **Address:** 4070 Lake Drive SE, Ste 202, 245 Cherry St, Ste 302, Grand Rapids, MI 49546; **Phone:** (616) 464-4420; **Board Cert:** Plastic Surgery 1994; **Med School:** Univ Mich Med Sch 1985; **Resid:** Plastic Surgery, Grand Rapids Med Edu & Res Ctr, Grand Rapids, MI

Luce, Edward MD (PlS) - *Spec Exp:* Reconstructive Surgery; **Hospital:** Rainbow Babies & Chldns Hosp; **Address:** 11100 Euclid Avenue, MS 5044, Cleveland, OH 44106; **Phone:** (216) 844-4780; **Board Cert:** Surgery 1972, Plastic Surgery 1974; **Med School:** Univ KY Coll Med 1965; **Resid:** Surgery, Barnes Hosp-Wash U, St Louis, MO 1966-1971; Plastic Surgery, Johns Hopkins Hosp, Baltimore, MD 1971-1973; **Fac Appt:** Prof Plastic Surgery, Univ KY Coll Med

Mackinnon, Susan MD (PlS) - *Spec Exp:* Peripheral Nerve Surgery; Nerve Transplantation; Hand Surgery; **Hospital:** Barnes-Jewish Hosp (page 55); **Address:** One Barnes-Jewish Hospital Plaza, St Louis, MO 63110; **Phone:** (314) 362-4587; **Board Cert:** Plastic Surgery 1980; **Med School:** Canada 1975; **Resid:** Surgery, Queens Univ-Kingston, Ontario, Canada 1975-1978; Plastic Surgery, Univ Toronto, Toronto, Canada 1978-1980; **Fellow:** Neurological Surgery, Univ Toronto, Toronto, Canada 1980-1981; Hand Surgery, Union Meml Hosp, Baltimore, MD 1981-1982; **Fac Appt:** Prof Surgery, Washington Univ, St Louis

Marsh, Jeffrey L MD (PlS) - *Spec Exp:* Cleft Palate/Lip; Craniofacial Surgery/Reconstruction; Pediatric Plastic Surgery; **Hospital:** St Louis Children's Hospital; **Address:** St Louis Chldns Hosp, One S Children's Pl, Box 8238, MS 2S86, St Louis, MO 63110-1077; **Phone:** (314) 454-6020; **Board Cert:** Plastic Surgery 1979, Surgery 1987; **Med School:** Johns Hopkins Univ 1970; **Resid:** Surgery, UCLA Med Ctr, Los Angeles, CA 1971-1975; Plastic Surgery, Univ Va Hosp, Charlottesville, VA 1975-1977; **Fellow:** Craniofacial Surgery, Cannisburn Hosp, Glasgow, Scotland 1977; Craniofacial Surgery, Clinic Belvedere Hosp, Foch, Paris 1977; **Fac Appt:** Prof Surgery, Washington Univ, St Louis

McKinney, Peter W MD (PlS) - *Spec Exp:* Cosmetic Surgery-Face; **Hospital:** Northwestern Meml Hosp; **Address:** 60 E Delaware Pl, Ste 1400, Chicago, IL 60611-1425; **Phone:** (312) 266-0300; **Board Cert:** Plastic Surgery 1968; **Med School:** McGill Univ 1960; **Resid:** Surgery, Bellevue Hosp Ctr, New York, NY 1961-1964; Plastic Surgery, NY Hosp-Cornell Med Ctr, New York, NY 1964-1967; **Fac Appt:** Prof Plastic Surgery, Northwestern Univ

Mustoe, Thomas MD (PlS) - *Spec Exp:* Facial Cosmetic Surgery; Breast Cosmetic Surgery; Breast Reconstruction; **Hospital:** Northwestern Meml Hosp; **Address:** NW Med Faculty Fdn-Plastic Surgery, 675 North St Clair St, Fl 19 - Ste 250, Chicago, IL 60611-5975; **Phone:** (312) 695-6022; **Board Cert:** Otolaryngology 1983, Plastic Surgery 1987; **Med School:** Harvard Med Sch 1978; **Resid:** Surgery, Brigham & Womens Hosp, Boston, MA 1979-1980; Otolaryngology, Mass Eye & Ear Infirmary, Boston, MA 1980-1983; **Fellow:** Plastic Surgery, Brigham & Womens Hosp, Boston, MA 1983-1985; **Fac Appt:** Prof Surgery, Northwestern Univ

Newman, M Haskell MD (PIS) - *Spec Exp:* Craniofacial Surgery/Reconstruction; **Hospital:** Univ of MI Hlth Ctr; **Address:** Mott Chldns Hosp, 1500 E Medical Center Drive, rm F7859, Ann Arbor, MI 48109-0219; **Phone:** (734) 763-8063; **Board Cert:** Otolaryngology 1969, Plastic Surgery 1978; **Med School:** Univ Tenn Coll Med, Memphis 1962; **Resid:** Otolaryngology, Univ Mich Hosps, Ann Arbor, MI 1963-1968; Plastic Surgery, Univ Mich Hosp, Ann Arbor, MI 1975-1977; **Fellow:** Craniofacial Surgery, Toronto Genl Hosp, Toronto, CN 1977; **Fac Appt:** Assoc Clin Prof Surgery, Univ Mich Med Sch

Polley, John MD (PIS) - *Spec Exp:* Craniomaxillofacial Surgery; Cosmetic Surgery; Pediatric Plastic Surgery; **Hospital:** Rush-Presby - St Luke's Med Ctr (page 72); **Address:** Rush/Presby-St Lukes Med Ctr, Div Plastic Surgery-Prof Bldg 1, 1725 W Harrison St, Ste 425, Chicago, IL 60612-3841; **Phone:** (312) 563-3000; **Board Cert:** Plastic Surgery 1992; **Med School:** Northwestern Univ 1983; **Resid:** Surgery, Mich State Univ, Grand Rapids, Lansing, MI 1983-1986; Plastic Surgery, Mich State Univ, Grand Rapids, Lansing, MI 1986-1988; **Fellow:** Craniofacial Surgery, Chang Gung Meml Hosp, Taipei, Taiwan 1988-1989; Pediatric Cranio-Maxillo-Facial Surgery, Hosp for Sick Chldn, Toronto, Canada 1989-1990; **Fac Appt:** Prof Plastic Surgery, Rush Med Coll

Puckett, Charles Linwood MD (PIS) - *Spec Exp:* Cosmetic & Reconstructive Surgery; Breast Surgery; **Hospital:** Univ of Missouri Hosp & Clinics; **Address:** 1 Hospital Drive, Ste M349, Columbia, MO 65212-5276; **Phone:** (573) 882-2275; **Board Cert:** Plastic Surgery 1977, Hand Surgery 1990; **Med School:** Wake Forest Univ Sch Med 1966; **Resid:** Surgery, Duke Univ Med Ctr, Durham, NC 1967-1971; Plastic Surgery, Duke Univ Med Ctr, Durham, NC 1973-1976; **Fac Appt:** Prof Plastic Surgery, Univ MO-Columbia Sch Med

Sanger, James MD (PIS) - *Spec Exp:* Reconstructive Surgery; Hand Surgery; **Hospital:** Froedtert Meml Lutheran Hosp; **Address:** Dept Plastic Surgery, 9200 W Wisconsin Ave, Milwaukee, WI 53226; **Phone:** (414) 805-3666; **Board Cert:** Hand Surgery 1999, Plastic Surgery 1982; **Med School:** Univ Wisc 1974; **Resid:** Surgery, LAC-Harbor UCLA Med Ctr, Torrance, CA 1974-1979; Plastic Surgery, Med Coll Wisc Affil Hosps, Milwaukee, WI 1979-1981; **Fellow:** Hand Surgery, Med Coll Wisc Affil Hosps, Milwaukee, WI 1981-1982; **Fac Appt:** Prof Surgery, Med Coll Wisc

Smith Jr., David J. MD (PIS) - *Spec Exp:* Breast Reconstruction; Burns; **Hospital:** Univ of MI Hlth Ctr; **Address:** 1500 E Medical Center Drive, Bldg Taubman HCC - rm 2130, University of Michigan Hospital Medical Center, Ann Arbor, MI 48109-0340; **Phone:** (734) 998-6022; **Board Cert:** Plastic Surgery 1981, Surgery 1979; **Resid:** Plastic Surgery, Ind U., Indianapolis, IN 1978-1980; Surgery, Emory U-Grady Hosp., Atlanta, GA 1974-1978; **Fellow:** Hand Surgery, U Louisville, Louisville, KY 1979; **Fac Appt:** Plastic Surgery, Univ Mich Med Sch

Vogt, Peter MD (PIS) - *Spec Exp:* Cosmetic Surgery; **Hospital:** Mercy Hosp - Coon Rapids; **Address:** 319 Barry Ave, Wayzata, MN 55391; **Phone:** (952) 473-1111; **Board Cert:** Plastic Surgery 1974; **Med School:** Canada 1965; **Resid:** Surgery, Montreal Genl Hosp, Montreal, Canada 1968-1970; Plastic Surgery, Winnipeg Hlth Scis Ctr, Mantoba, Canada 1971-1973

Walton Jr, Robert Lee MD (PIS) - *Spec Exp:* Cosmetic Surgery-Face; Nasal Reconstruction; Breast Reconstruction; **Hospital:** Univ of Chicago Hosps (page 76); **Address:** Dept Plas & Reconstruction Surg, 5841 S Maryland Ave, MS 6035, Chicago, IL 60637-1463; **Phone:** (773) 702-6302; **Board Cert:** Surgery 1989, Plastic Surgery 1980, Hand Surgery 2000; **Med School:** Univ Kans 1972; **Resid:** Surgery, Johns Hopkins Hosp, Baltimore, MD 1972-1974; Plastic Surgery, Yale-New Haven Hosp, New Haven, CT 1974-1978; **Fellow:** Hand Surgery, Hartford Hosp, Hartford, CT 1977-1978; **Fac Appt:** Prof Plastic Surgery, Univ Chicago-Pritzker Sch Med

Wilkins, Edwin G. MD (PIS) - *Spec Exp:* Breast Reconstruction; Lower Extremity Reconstruction; Microsurgery; **Hospital:** Univ of MI Hlth Ctr; **Address:** 1500 E Medical Center Dr., rm 2130, Box 0340, A. Alfred Taubman Health Care Ctr, Ann Arbor, MI 48109-0340; **Phone:** (734) 998-6022; **Board Cert:** Plastic Surgery 1991; **Med School:** Wake Forest Univ Sch Med 1981; **Resid:** Surgery, Charlotte Meml Hosp, Charlotte, NC 1982-1986; Plastic Surgery, Vanderbilt Univ Med Ctr, Nashville, TN 1986-1988; **Fellow:** Reconstructive Microsurgery, U Louisville Sch Med, Louisville, KY 1988-1989; **Fac Appt:** Assoc Prof Plastic Surgery, Univ Mich Med Sch

Yetman, Randall John MD (PIS) - *Spec Exp:* Breast Reconstruction; **Hospital:** Cleveland Clin Fdn (page 57); **Address:** 9500 Euclid Ave, rm A-60, Cleveland, OH 44195-0001; **Phone:** (216) 444-6908; **Board Cert:** Plastic Surgery 1984; **Med School:** Univ Miami Sch Med 1974; **Resid:** Plastic Surgery, NY Hosp-Cornell Med Ctr, New York, NY 1975-1979

Young, Vernon Leroy MD (PIS) - *Spec Exp:* Breast Augmentation; Skin Laser Surgery-Resurfacing; **Hospital:** Barnes-Jewish Hosp (page 55); **Address:** 1040 N Mason Rd, Ste 206, St Louis, MO 63141-6366; **Phone:** (314) 996-8050; **Board Cert:** Plastic Surgery 1981, Surgery 1988; **Med School:** Univ KY Coll Med 1970; **Resid:** Surgery, Univ KY Med Ctr, Lexington, KY 1973-1977; Plastic Surgery, Barnes Hosp-Wash Univ, St Louis, MO 1977-1979; **Fac Appt:** Prof Plastic Surgery, Washington Univ, St Louis

Zins, James MD (PIS) - *Spec Exp:* Cosmetic Surgery-Face; Maxillofacial Surgery; Craniofacial Surgery; **Hospital:** Cleveland Clin Fdn (page 57); **Address:** 9500 Euclid Ave, Desk A60, Cleveland, OH 44195; **Phone:** (216) 444-6901; **Board Cert:** Surgery 1981, Plastic Surgery 1985; **Med School:** Univ Penn 1974; **Resid:** Surgery, Hosp Univ Penn, Philadelphia, PA 1975-1980; Plastic Surgery, Hosp Univ Penn, Philadelphia, PA 1980-1982; **Fellow:** Craniofacial Surgery, Hosp Univ Penn, Philadelphia, PA 1977-1978; Maxillofacial Surgery, Hosp Sick Chldn, London, England 1982-1983

Great Plains and Mountains

Ketch, Lawrence Levant MD (PIS) - *Spec Exp:* Cosmetic Surgery-Face; Head & Neck Reconstruction; Cleft Palate/Lip; **Hospital:** Univ Colo HSC - Denver; **Address:** 4200 E 9th Ave, Box C309, Denver, CO 80262; **Phone:** (303) 372-3081; **Board Cert:** Plastic Surgery 1982, Surgery 1980; **Resid:** Surgery, Univ Colo Affil Hosp, Baltimore, MD 1975-1979; **Fellow:** Plastic Surgery, Univ Miami Project to Cure Paralysis, Miami, FL 1980-1981; **Fac Appt:** Assoc Prof Plastic Surgery

Knize, David Maurice MD (PIS) - *Spec Exp:* Cosmetic Surgery-Face; **Hospital:** Swedish Med Ctr - Englewood; **Address:** Knize Clin Plas Surg, 3701 S Clarkson St, Englewood, CO 80110; **Phone:** (303) 761-9990; **Board Cert:** Surgery 1971, Plastic Surgery 1975; **Med School:** Univ Tex SW, Dallas 1963; **Resid:** Surgery, Univ Colo Med Ctr, Denver, CO 1966-1969; Plastic Surgery, NYU Med Ctr, New York, NY 1971-1974; **Fac Appt:** Assoc Clin Prof Plastic Surgery, Univ Colo

Lockwood, Ted MD (PIS) - *Spec Exp:* Cosmetic Surgery-Body; **Hospital:** Overland Park Reg Med Ctr; **Address:** 10600 Quivira Rd, Ste 470, Overland Park, KS 66215-2377; **Phone:** (913) 894-1070; **Board Cert:** Plastic Surgery 1981; **Med School:** Univ Kans 1971; **Resid:** Surgery, Univ Texas Hlth Sci Ctrn, Dallas, TX 1972-1976; Plastic Surgery, Univ Penn, Philadelphia, PA 1978-1980; **Fac Appt:** Asst Clin Prof Surgery, Univ MO-Kansas City

Southwest

Barton Jr, Fritz MD (PIS) - *Spec Exp:* Cosmetic Surgery-Face; **Hospital:** Baylor Univ Medical Ctr; **Address:** 411 N Washington Ave, Ste 6000, Dallas, TX 75246-1713; **Phone:** (214) 821-9355; **Board Cert:** Surgery 1975, Plastic Surgery 1977; **Med School:** Univ Tex SW, Dallas 1967; **Resid:** Surgery, Parkland Meml Hosp, Dallas, TX 1970-1974; Plastic Surgery, NYU Med Ctr, New York, NY 1974-1976; **Fac Appt:** Prof Plastic Surgery, Univ Tex SW, Dallas

Biggs Jr, Thomas M MD (PIS) - *Spec Exp:* Cosmetic Surgery-Face; **Hospital:** Christus St Joseph's Hosp; **Address:** 1315 St Joseph Pkwy, Ste 900, Houston, TX 77002-8231; **Phone:** (713) 650-0800; **Board Cert:** Plastic Surgery 1978; **Med School:** Baylor Coll Med 1958; **Resid:** Surgery, Baylor Univ Affil Hosp, Houston, TX 1959-1962; Plastic Surgery, Baylor Univ Affil Hosp, Houston, TX 1963-1964; **Fac Appt:** Clin Prof Plastic Surgery, Baylor Coll Med

Burns, Alton Jay MD (PIS) - *Spec Exp:* Cosmetic Surgery; Skin Laser Surgery; **Hospital:** Baylor Univ Medical Ctr; **Address:** 411 N Washington St, Ste 6000, Dallas, TX 75246; **Phone:** (214) 823-1978; **Board Cert:** Surgery 1987, Plastic Surgery 1990; **Med School:** Univ Tex SW, Dallas 1981; **Resid:** Surgery, Univ Utah Hosp, Salt Lake City, UT 1982-1986; Plastic Surgery, Univ Texas SW Med Ctr, Dallas, TX 1986-1988; **Fellow:** Vascular Anomalies, Chldns Hosp, Boston, MA 1988; **Fac Appt:** Asst Prof Plastic Surgery, Univ Tex SW, Dallas

Byrd, Henry S MD (PIS) - *Spec Exp:* Cosmetic Surgery-Face; **Hospital:** Baylor Univ Medical Ctr; **Address:** 411 N Washington Ave, Ste 6000, Dallas, TX 75246-1713; **Phone:** (214) 821-9662; **Board Cert:** Surgery 1978, Plastic Surgery 1980; **Med School:** Univ Tex Med Br, Galveston 1972; **Resid:** Surgery, Univ Utah Med Ctr, Salt Lake City, UT 1973-1977; Plastic Surgery, Dallas Co Hosp-Parkland Meml, Dallas, TX 1977-1979; **Fac Appt:** Clin Prof Plastic Surgery, Univ Tex SW, Dallas

Colon, Gustavo MD (PIS) - *Spec Exp:* Cosmetic Surgery; **Hospital:** E Jefferson Genl Hosp; **Address:** 4204 Tueton St, Metairie, LA 70006; **Phone:** (504) 888-4297; **Board Cert:** Plastic Surgery 1978; **Med School:** Univ MD Sch Med 1964; **Resid:** Surgery, US Public Hlth Svc Hosp, New Orleans, LA 1965-1969; Plastic Surgery, Tulane Affil Prog, New Orleans, LA 1969-1971; **Fac Appt:** Prof Surgery, Tulane Univ

Gunter, Jack MD (PIS) - *Spec Exp:* Rhinoplasty; Rhinoplasty-Secondary Surgery; **Hospital:** Presby Hosp - Dallas; **Address:** 8315 Wallnut Hill Lane, Ste 225, Dallas, TX 75231-4218; **Phone:** (214) 369-8123; **Board Cert:** Otolaryngology 1969, Plastic Surgery 1981; **Med School:** Univ Okla Coll Med 1963; **Resid:** Surgery, U Ark Med Ctr, Little Rock, AR 1964-1965; Otolaryngology, Tulane U Hospital, New Orleans, LA 1965-1968; **Fellow:** Mercy Hospital, Pittsburgh, PA 1968-1969; Plastic Surgery, U Mich Hospital, Ann Arbor, MI 1978-1980; **Fac Appt:** Clin Prof Otolaryngology, Texas Tech Univ

Hamra, Sameer T MD (PIS) - *Spec Exp:* Cosmetic Surgery-Face; Rhinoplasty; **Hospital:** Mary Shiels Hosp; **Address:** 2731 Lemmon Ave E, Ste 306, Dallas, TX 75204; **Phone:** (214) 754-9001; **Board Cert:** Surgery 1970, Plastic Surgery 1977; **Med School:** Univ Okla Coll Med 1963; **Resid:** Plastic Surgery, NYU Med Ctr, New York, NY 1970-1973; Surgery, Univ Okla, Oklahoma City, OK 1964-1968; **Fellow:** Surgery, Univ Lausanne 1965-1966; **Fac Appt:** Asst Clin Prof Surgery, Univ Tex SW, Dallas

Kelly, John Michael MD (PIS) - *Spec Exp:* Cosmetic Surgery-Face; Breast Surgery; **Hospital:** Integris Baptist Med Ctr - OK; **Address:** 3301 NW 63rd St, Oklahoma City, OK 73116-3705; **Phone:** (405) 842-9732; **Board Cert:** Surgery 1970, Plastic Surgery 1978; **Med School:** Univ Ark 1963; **Resid:** Surgery, Univ Virginia Hosp, Charlottesville, VA 1964-1969; Plastic Surgery, Johns Hopkins Hosp, Baltimore, MD 1969-1971; **Fac Appt:** Clin Prof Surgery, Univ Okla Coll Med

Nath, Rahul Kamur MD (PIS) - *Spec Exp:* Brachial Plexus-Pediatric; **Hospital:** TX Chldns Hosp - Houston; **Address:** 11102 Bates Street, Ste 330, Houston, TX 77030; **Phone:** (832) 824-3193; **Board Cert:** Plastic Surgery 1998; **Med School:** Northwestern Univ 1988; **Resid:** Surgery, Northwestern Med Ctr., Chicago, IL 1989-1991; Plastic Surgery, Washington University, St. Louis, MO 1991-1994; **Fellow:** Washington University, St. Louis, MO 1995-1996; **Fac Appt:** Asst Prof Plastic Surgery, Baylor Coll Med

Rohrich, Rodney James MD (PIS) - *Spec Exp:* Nasal Surgery; Cosmetic Surgery-Face & Breast; Breast Reconstruction; **Hospital:** Zale Lipshy Univ Hosp; **Address:** Univ Texas SW Med Ctr, Plastic & Recon Surg, 5323 Harry Hines Blvd, Dallas, TX 75390-9132; **Phone:** (214) 648-3119; **Board Cert:** Plastic Surgery 1987, Hand Surgery 1990; **Med School:** Baylor Coll Med 1979; **Resid:** Plastic Surgery, Univ Mich Hosp, Ann Arbor, MI 1982-1985; Plastic Surgery, Radcliffe Infirm/Oxford, Oxford, England 1983; **Fellow:** Hand Surgery, Mass Genl Hosp-Harvard, Boston, MA 1986-1987; **Fac Appt:** Prof Plastic Surgery, Univ Tex SW, Dallas

Schnur, Paul MD (PIS) - *Spec Exp:* Hand Surgery; **Hospital:** Mayo Clin Hosp - Scottsdale; **Address:** Mayo Clinic Scottsdale, 13400 E Shea Blvd, Scottsdale, AZ 85259-5404; **Phone:** (480) 301-8139; **Board Cert:** Surgery 1971, Plastic Surgery 1973; **Med School:** Baylor Coll Med 1962; **Resid:** Surgery, Mayo Clin, Rochester, MN 1966-1970; Plastic Surgery, Mayo Clin, Rochester, MN 1970-1972; **Fac Appt:** Assoc Prof Plastic Surgery, Mayo Med Sch

Schusterman, Mark A MD (PIS) - *Spec Exp:* Breast Reconstruction; Cosmetic Surgery-Face; Cosmetic Surgery-Breast; **Hospital:** St Luke's Episcopal Hosp - Houston; **Address:** 7505 S Main St, Ste 200, Houston, TX 77030; **Phone:** (713) 794-0368; **Board Cert:** Surgery 1986, Plastic Surgery 1989; **Med School:** Univ Louisville Sch Med 1980; **Resid:** Surgery, Univ Hosp, Cincinnati, OH 1981-1985; Pediatric Surgery, Univ Pitts Med Ctr, Pittsburgh, PA 1985-1987; **Fellow:** Microsurgery, Univ Pitts Med Ctr, Pittsburgh, PA 1987-1988; **Fac Appt:** Clin Prof Plastic Surgery, Baylor Coll Med

Shenaq, Saleh MD (PIS) - *Spec Exp:* Microsurgery; Hand Surgery; **Hospital:** Methodist Hosp - Houston; **Address:** Baylor Coll Med, 6560 Fannin St, Scurlock Tower, Ste 800, Houston, TX 77030-2706; **Phone:** (713) 798-6141; **Board Cert:** Plastic Surgery 1983, Hand Surgery 1990; **Med School:** Egypt 1972; **Resid:** Surgery, Med Coll Ohio Hosp, Toledo, OH 1974-1979; Plastic Surgery, Univ Pitts Med Ctr, Pittsburgh, PA 1979-1981; **Fellow:** Hand Surgery, Univ Louisville Hosp, Louisville, KY 1981; **Fac Appt:** Prof Plastic Surgery, Baylor Coll Med

Tebbetts, John B MD (PIS) - *Spec Exp:* Cosmetic Surgery-Liposuction; Breast Augmentation; Rhinoplasty; **Hospital:** Mary Shiels Hosp; **Address:** 2801 Lemmon Ave, Ste 300, Dallas, TX 75204-2398; **Phone:** (214) 220-2712; **Board Cert:** Surgery 1978, Plastic Surgery 1980; **Med School:** Univ Tex Med Br, Galveston 1972; **Resid:** Surgery, Univ Utah Med Ctr, Salt Lake City, UT 1973-1977; Plastic Surgery, Dallas Co Hospital-Parkland Meml Hosp, Dallas, TX 1977-1979; **Fac Appt:** Asst Clin Prof Plastic Surgery, Univ Tex SW, Dallas

West Coast and Pacific

Berner, Carl Frederick MD (PIS) - *Spec Exp:* Cosmetic Surgery; **Hospital:** Overlake Hosp Med Ctr; **Address:** 1551 116th Ave NE, Bellevue, WA 98004; **Phone:** (425) 453-2161; **Board Cert:** Plastic Surgery 1974, Surgery 1967; **Med School:** Univ MD Sch Med 1961; **Resid:** Surgery, Univ MD Hosp, Baltimore, MD 1963-1966; Plastic Surgery, Univ Mich Med Ctr, Ann Arbor, MI 1969-1971; **Fac Appt:** Asst Clin Prof Surgery, Univ Wash

Brink, Robert Ross MD (PIS) - *Spec Exp:* Cosmetic Surgery; **Hospital:** Mills - Peninsula Hlth Ctr Hosp; **Address:** 66 Bovet Rd, Ste 101, San Mateo, CA 94402; **Phone:** (650) 570-6066; **Board Cert:** Plastic Surgery 1980, Surgery 1980; **Med School:** Univ Mich Med Sch 1970; **Resid:** Surgery, UC Davis Med Ctr, Sacramento, CA 1973-1977; Plastic Surgery, UCSF Med Ctr, San Francisco, CA 1977-1979

Brody, Garry S MD (PIS) - *Spec Exp:* Hand Surgery; **Hospital:** USC Univ Hosp - R K Eamer Med Ctr; **Address:** 1450 San Pablo St, Ste 2000, Los Angeles, CA 90033-1042; **Phone:** (323) 442-6462; **Board Cert:** Surgery 1963, Plastic Surgery 1967; **Med School:** Univ Alberta 1956; **Resid:** Surgery, Georetown Univ Hosp, Washington, DC 1959-1961; Plastic Surgery, Univ Pittsburgh, Pittsburgh, PA 1962-1964; **Fellow:** Surgery, McGill Univ, Montreal, Canada 1958-1959; **Fac Appt:** Clin Prof Plastic Surgery, USC Sch Med

Buncke Jr, Harry J MD (PIS) - *Spec Exp:* Microsurgery; Hand Surgery; **Hospital:** CA Pacific Med Ctr - Davies Campus; **Address:** Buncke Med Clin Inc, MOB Annex Ste 140, 45 Castro St, San Francisco, CA 94114; **Phone:** (415) 565-6136; **Board Cert:** Plastic Surgery 1978; **Med School:** NY Med Coll 1951; **Resid:** Surgery, Flower Fifth Ave Hosp, New York, NY 1952-1954; Plastic Surgery, Bronx VA Med Ctr, New York, NY 1954-1956; **Fellow:** Plastic Surgery, Queen Victoria Hosp, E Grinstead, England 1956-1957; **Fac Appt:** Assoc Clin Prof Plastic Surgery, Stanford Univ

Daniel, Rollin K MD (PIS) - *Spec Exp:* Cosmetic Surgery-Face; **Hospital:** Hoag Meml Hosp Presby; **Address:** 1441 Avocado Ave, Ste 308, Newport Beach, CA 92660; **Phone:** (949) 721-0494; **Board Cert:** Plastic Surgery 1977; **Med School:** Columbia P&S **Resid:** Plastic Surgery, McGill Univ Affil Hosps, Montreal, Canada 1973-1975; Hand Surgery, Univ Louisville Hosp, Louisville, KY 1975-1976; **Fellow:** Craniofacial Surgery, Toronto Genl Hosp, Toronto, Canada 1984

Flowers, Robert MD (PIS) - *Spec Exp:* Coronal Canthopexy; **Hospital:** Queen's Med Ctr - Honolulu; **Address:** 677 Ala Moana Blvd, Ste 1011, Honolulu, HI 96813; **Phone:** (808) 521-1999; **Board Cert:** Plastic Surgery 1971; **Med School:** Univ Ala 1960; **Resid:** Surgery, Cleveland Clinic, Cleveland, OH 1963-1966; Plastic Surgery, Cleveland Clinic, Cleveland, OH 1966-1968; **Fac Appt:** Asst Clin Prof Surgery, Univ Hawaii JA Burns Sch Med

Fodor, Peter Bela MD (PIS) - *Spec Exp:* Cosmetic Surgery; **Hospital:** Century City Hosp; **Address:** 2080 Century Park E, Ste 710, Los Angeles, CA 90067; **Phone:** (310) 203-9818; **Board Cert:** Plastic Surgery 1977; **Med School:** Univ Wisc 1966; **Resid:** Surgery, Columbia-Presbyterian Med Ctr, New York, NY 1967-1968; Plastic Surgery, St Luke's Hosp, New York, NY 1974-1976; **Fac Appt:** Asst Clin Prof Surgery, UCLA

Grossman, John A MD (PIS) - *Spec Exp:* Cosmetic Surgery; **Hospital:** Century City Hosp; **Address:** 416 N Bedford Drive, Ste 400, Beverly Hills, CA 90210-4346; **Phone:** (310) 557-2307; **Board Cert:** Plastic Surgery 1976, Surgery 1974; **Med School:** Cornell Univ-Weill Med Coll 1967; **Resid:** Surgery, Boston City Hosp, Boston, MA 1968-1973; Plastic Surgery, Univ Colo Hlth Scis Ctr, Denver, CO 1973-1975; **Fellow:** Surgery, Harvard Med Sch, Boston, MA 1971-1973

Gruss, Joseph MD (PIS) - *Spec Exp:* Maxillofacial & Craniofacial Surgery; Facial Trauma/Fractures; Cleft Palate/Lip; **Hospital:** Chldns Hosp and Regl Med Ctr - Seattle; **Address:** Childrens Hosp & Regional Med Ctr, 4800 Sand Point Way NE, Box 5371, MS CH-78, Seattle, WA 98105-3901; **Phone:** (206) 526-2039; **Med School:** South Africa 1969; **Resid:** Plastic Surgery, Toronto Western Hosp, Toronto, Canada 1976; Plastic Surgery, Hosp for Sick Children, Totonto, Canada 1976; **Fellow:** Surgical Oncology, Princess Margaret Hosp, Toronto, Canada 1977; Head and Neck Surgery, Princess Margaret Hosp, Toronto, Canada 1977; **Fac Appt:** Prof Plastic Surgery, Univ Wash

Hardesty, Robert MD (PIS) - *Spec Exp:* Facial Reconstruction; **Hospital:** Loma Linda Univ Med Ctr; **Address:** 11370 Anderson St, Ste 2100, Loma Linda, CA 92354; **Phone:** (909) 558-2822; **Board Cert:** Surgery 1984, Plastic Surgery 1989; **Med School:** Loma Linda Univ 1978; **Resid:** Surgery, Loma Linda Univ Med Ctr, Loma Linda, CA 1979-1983; Plastic Surgery, Univ Pittsburgh, Pittsburgh, PA 1984-1986; **Fellow:** Pediatric Plastic Surgery, Washington Univ Chldns Hosp, St Louis, MO 1986-1987

Hoefflin, Steven M MD (PIS) - *Spec Exp:* Cosmetic Surgery-Face; Reconstructive Surgery; **Hospital:** St John's Hlth Ctr; **Address:** 1530 Arizona Ave, Santa Monica, CA 90404-1234; **Phone:** (310) 451-4733; **Board Cert:** Plastic Surgery 1978; **Med School:** UCLA 1972; **Resid:** Surgery, UCLA Med Ctr, Los Angeles, CA 1973-1974; Plastic Surgery, UCLA Med Ctr, Los Angeles, CA 1976-1977; **Fac Appt:** Assoc Clin Prof Plastic Surgery, UCLA

Horowitz, Jed H MD (PIS) - *Spec Exp:* Breast Surgery; Cosmetic Surgery-Face; **Hospital:** Hoag Meml Hosp Presby; **Address:** 7677 Center Ave, Ste 401, Huntington Beach, CA 92647-3098; **Phone:** (714) 902-1100; **Board Cert:** Plastic Surgery 1986; **Med School:** SUNY Buffalo 1977; **Resid:** Surgery, Grady Meml Hosp/Emory Univ, Atlanta, GA 1978-1983; **Fellow:** Plastic Surgery, Univ Virginia, Charlottesville, VA 1983-1985; **Fac Appt:** Clin Prof Plastic Surgery, USC Sch Med

Jewell, Mark L MD (PIS) - *Spec Exp:* Hand Surgery; Burns; Breast Reconstruction; **Hospital:** Sacred Heart Med Ctr; **Address:** 630 E 13th St, Eugene, OR 97401; **Phone:** (541) 683-3234; **Board Cert:** Plastic Surgery 1981; **Resid:** Surgery, Los Angeles Co, Torrance, CA 1973-1976; Plastic Surgery, Erlanger Hosp, Chattanooga, TN 1977-1979; **Fellow:** Burn Surgery, USC med Ctr, Los Angeles, CA 1976-1977

Kawamoto Jr, Henry K MD (PIS) - *Spec Exp:* Cosmetic Surgery; Craniofacial Surgery/Reconstruction; Maxillofacial Surgery; **Hospital:** UCLA Med Ctr; **Address:** 1301 20th St, Ste 460, Santa Monica, CA 90404; **Phone:** (310) 829-0391; **Board Cert:** Surgery 1972, Plastic Surgery 1976; **Med School:** USC Sch Med 1964; **Resid:** Surgery, Columbia-Presby Med Ctr, New York, NY 1965-1971; Plastic Surgery, NYU Med Ctr, New York, NY 1971-1973; **Fellow:** Craniofacial Surgery, Dr Paul Tessier, Paris, France 1973-1974; **Fac Appt:** Assoc Clin Prof Plastic Surgery, UCLA

Koplin, Lawrence Mark MD (PIS) - *Spec Exp:* Cosmetic Surgery-Face; **Hospital:** Cedars-Sinai Med Ctr; **Address:** 436 N Bedford Dr, Ste 103, Beverly Hills, CA 90210-4310; **Phone:** (310) 277-3223; **Board Cert:** Surgery 1982, Plastic Surgery 1983; **Med School:** Baylor Coll Med 1976; **Resid:** Surgery, Kaiser Foundation Hosp, Los Angeles, CA 1978-1981; Plastic Surgery, St Joseph Hosp, Houston, TX 1981-1983

Leaf, Norman MD (PIS) - *Spec Exp:* Plastic Surgery - General; **Hospital:** Cedars-Sinai Med Ctr; **Address:** 436 N Bedford, Ste 103, Beverly Hills, CA 90210-4310; **Phone:** (310) 274-8001; **Board Cert:** Surgery 1973, Plastic Surgery 1974; **Med School:** Univ Chicago-Pritzker Sch Med 1966; **Resid:** Surgery, Univ Chicago Hosps, Chicago, IL 1967-1972; Plastic Surgery, Univ Chicago Hosps, Chicago, IL 1972-1973; **Fellow:** Research, Univ Chicago Hosp-US Pub Hlth Svc-NIH, Chicago, IL 1968-1969; **Fac Appt:** Asst Clin Prof Plastic Surgery, UCLA

Lesavoy, Malcolm A MD (PIS) - *Spec Exp:* Reconstructive Surgery; Cosmetic Surgery; **Hospital:** UCLA Med Ctr; **Address:** 16311 Ventura Blvd, Ste 550, Encino, CA 91436-4314; **Phone:** (818) 986-8270; **Board Cert:** Plastic Surgery 1977; **Med School:** Univ Hlth Sci/Chicago Med Sch 1969; **Resid:** Surgery, Univ Chicago Hosps, Chicago, IL 1969-1974; Plastic Surgery, Univ Miami Hosp/Clinics, Miami, FL 1974-1976; **Fac Appt:** Clin Prof Plastic Surgery, UCLA

Markowitz, Bernard Lloyd MD (PIS) - *Spec Exp:* Reconstructive Microvascular Surgery; Craniofacial Surgery/Reconstruction; Cosmetic Surgery; **Hospital:** UCLA Med Ctr; **Address:** 9675 Brighton Way, Ste 350, Beverly Hills, CA 90210; **Phone:** (310) 205-5557; **Board Cert:** Plastic Surgery 1989; **Med School:** NYU Sch Med 1979; **Resid:** Surgery, NYU Med Ctr, New York, NY 1979-1984; Plastic Surgery, NYU Med Ctr, New York, NY 1984-1986; **Fellow:** Maxillofacial Surgery, Johns Hopkins Hosp, Baltimore, MD 1986-1987; **Fac Appt:** Assoc Prof Plastic Surgery, UCLA

Marten, Timothy James MD (PIS) - *Spec Exp:* Cosmetic Surgery; Cosmetic Surgery-Face; **Hospital:** CA Pacific Med Ctr - Pacific Campus; **Address:** Marten Clinic of Plastic Surgery, 450 Sutter St, rm 826, San Francisco, CA 94108; **Phone:** (415) 677-9937; **Board Cert:** Plastic Surgery 1993; **Med School:** UC Davis 1982; **Resid:** Surgery, Kaiser Fdn Hosp, San Francisco, CA 1982-1987; Plastic Surgery, Univ Illinois Hosp, Chicago, IL 1987-1989; **Fellow:** Cosmetic Plastic Surgery, Connell Aesthetic Network, Santo Ana, CA 1989-1990

Mathes, Stephen MD (PIS) - *Spec Exp:* Breast Reconstruction; **Hospital:** UCSF Med Ctr; **Address:** 350 Parnassus Ave, Ste 509, San Francisco, CA 94117; **Phone:** (415) 476-3061; **Board Cert:** Surgery 1993, Plastic Surgery 1979; **Med School:** Louisiana State Univ 1968; **Resid:** Surgery, Emory Affil Hosp., Atlanta, GA 1972-1975; Plastic Surgery, Emory Affil Hosp, Atlanta, GA 1975-1977; **Fac Appt:** Prof Plastic Surgery, UCSF

Meltzer, Toby R MD (PIS) - *Spec Exp:* Transgender Surgery; Penile Inversion Technique; Breast Augmentation; **Hospital:** Eastmoreland Hosp; **Address:** Crown Plaza, Ste 1120, 1500 SW First Ave, Portland, OR 97201; **Phone:** (503) 525-9323; **Board Cert:** Plastic Surgery 1992, Surgery 1989; **Med School:** Louisiana State Univ 1983; **Resid:** Surgery, Charity Hosp of Louisiana, New Orleans, LA 1984-1988; Plastic Surgery, Univ Michigan, Ann Arbor, MI 1988-1990; **Fellow:** Burn Surgery, Wayne State Univ, Detroit, MI 1986-1987; **Fac Appt:** Asst Clin Prof Surgery, Oregon Hlth Scis Univ

Miller, Timothy Alden MD (PIS) - *Spec Exp:* Cosmetic Surgery-Face; Nasal & Eyelid Reconstruction; Skin Cancer; **Hospital:** UCLA Med Ctr; **Address:** UCLA Plastic Surgery, 200 UCLA Med Plaza, Ste 465, Los Angeles, CA 90095-8344; **Phone:** (310) 825-5644; **Board Cert:** Surgery 1971, Plastic Surgery 1973; **Med School:** UCLA 1963; **Resid:** Surgery, Johns Hopkins Hosp, Baltimore, MD 1967; Thoracic Surgery, UCLA Med Ctr, Los Angeles, CA 1967-1969; **Fellow:** Plastic Surgery, Univ Pittsburgh, Pittsburgh, PA 1970-1971; **Fac Appt:** Prof Surgery, UCLA

Owsley, John Q MD (PIS) - *Spec Exp:* Cosmetic Surgery-Face; Blepharoplasty; Rhinoplasty; **Hospital:** CA Pacific Med Ctr - Pacific Campus; **Address:** California Pacific Med Ctr-Davies Campus, 45 Castro St, Ste 111, San Francisco, CA 94114; **Phone:** (415) 861-8040; **Board Cert:** Plastic Surgery 1978; **Med School:** Vanderbilt Univ 1953; **Resid:** Surgery, UCSF Med Ctr, San Francisco, CA 1953-1958; Plastic Surgery, UCSF Med Ctr, San Francisco, CA 1958-1960; **Fac Appt:** Clin Prof Surgery, UCSF

Paul, Malcolm D MD (PIS) - *Spec Exp:* Cosmetic Surgery-Face; **Hospital:** Hoag Meml Hosp Presby; **Address:** 1401 Avocado Ave, Ste 810, Newport Beach, CA 92660-8708; **Phone:** (949) 760-5047; **Board Cert:** Plastic Surgery 1976; **Med School:** Univ MD Sch Med 1969; **Resid:** Surgery, Geo Wash Med Ctr, Washington, DC 1971-1973; Plastic Surgery, Geo Wash Med Ctr, Washington, DC 1973-1975; **Fac Appt:** Assoc Clin Prof Surgery, UC Irvine

Rand, Richard Pierce MD (PIS) - *Spec Exp:* Cosmetic Surgery; Breast Surgery; Breast Reconstruction; **Hospital:** Ovelake Hosp Med Ctr; **Address:** 1135 116th Ave NE, Ste 630, Bellevue, WA 98004; **Phone:** (425) 688-8828; **Board Cert:** Surgery 1998, Plastic Surgery 1991; **Med School:** Univ Mich Med Sch 1981; **Resid:** Surgery, New Eng Med Ctr, Boston, MA 1981-1986; Plastic Surgery, Emory Univ Hosp, Atlanta, GA 1986-1988; **Fellow:** Craniofacial Surgery, Univ Miami, Miami, FL 1989

Reinisch, John F MD (PIS) - *Spec Exp:* Ear Reconstruction; Cleft Palate/Lip; Craniofacial Surgery/Reconstruction; **Hospital:** Chldns Hosp - Los Angeles; **Address:** 4650 Sunset Blvd, MS 96, Los Angeles, CA 90027; **Phone:** (323) 669-4544; **Board Cert:** Plastic Surgery 1980; **Med School:** Harvard Med Sch 1970; **Resid:** Plastic Surgery, Univ VA Hosp, Richmond, VA 1976-1978; Surgery, Univ Mich Med Ctr, Ann Arbor, MI 1970-1975; **Fac Appt:** Prof Surgery, USC Sch Med

Ristow, Brunno MD (PIS) - *Spec Exp:* Cosmetic Surgery-Face; Facial Reconstruction; **Hospital:** CA Pacific Med Ctr - Pacific Campus; **Address:** 2100 Webster St, Ste 501, San Francisco, CA 94115-2381; **Phone:** (415) 202-1507; **Board Cert:** Plastic Surgery 1975; **Med School:** Brazil 1966; **Resid:** Surgery, NY Hosp-Cornell Med Ctr, New York, NY 1968-1971; Plastic Surgery, NYU Med Ctr, New York, NY 1971-1973; **Fellow:** Plastic Surgery, NYU Med Ctr, New York, NY 1968-1970

Romano, James John MD (PIS) - *Spec Exp:* Cosmetic Surgery; Breast Cosmetic Surgery; **Hospital:** St Mary's Med Ctr - San Fran; **Address:** 450 Sutter St, Ste 2600, San Francisco, CA 94108; **Phone:** (415) 981-3911; **Board Cert:** Surgery 1988, Plastic Surgery 1990; **Med School:** Eastern VA Med Sch 1980; **Resid:** Surgery, Georgetown Univ, Washington, DC 1982-1985; Plastic Surgery, Johns Hopkins Hosp, Baltimore, MD 1985-1988; **Fac Appt:** Asst Prof Plastic Surgery, USC Sch Med

Seyfer, Alan MD (PIS) - *Spec Exp:* Chest Wall Reconstruction; Cleft Palate/Lip; Hand Surgery; **Hospital:** OR Hlth Sci Univ Hosp and Clinics; **Address:** Dept Plastic Surgery, 3181 SW Sam Jackson Park Rd, MC L-352-A, Portland, OR 97201; **Phone:** (503) 494-7824; **Board Cert:** Hand Surgery 1989, Plastic Surgery 1982; **Med School:** Louisiana State Univ 1973; **Resid:** Surgery, Fitzsimons AMC, Denver, CO 1974-1978; Plastic Surgery, Walter Reed AMC, Washington, DC 1978-1981; **Fellow:** Hand Surgery, Duke U Med Ctr, Durham, NC 1980; **Fac Appt:** Prof Surgery, Oregon Hlth Scis Univ

Shaw, William Wei-Lien MD (PIS) - *Spec Exp:* Microsurgery; Breast Reconstruction; Cosmetic Surgery-Face; **Hospital:** UCLA Med Ctr; **Address:** 200 UCLA Medical Plaza, Ste 465, Los Angeles, CA 90095; **Phone:** (310) 206-7520; **Board Cert:** Plastic Surgery 1978; **Med School:** UCLA 1968; **Resid:** Surgery, UCLA Med Ctr, Los Angeles, CA 1969-1974; Plastic Surgery, NYU Med Ctr, New York, NY 1975-1977; **Fac Appt:** Prof Plastic Surgery, UCLA

Sheen, Jack MD (PIS) - *Spec Exp:* Rhinoplasty; Reconstructive Plastic Surgery; **Hospital:** St Francis Med Ctr of Santa Barbara; **Address:** 216 W Pueblo St., Ste A, Santa Barbara, CA 93105-3855; **Phone:** (805) 898-8888; **Board Cert:** Plastic Surgery 1968; **Med School:** Stanford Univ 1955; **Resid:** Surgery, Newton Wellesly Hosp, Newton Lwr Fls 1960-1962; Plastic Surgery, Cook Co Hosp, Chicago, IL 1962-1964; **Fac Appt:** Clin Prof Plastic Surgery, UCLA

Sherman, Randolph MD (PIS) - *Spec Exp:* Breast Reconstruction; Limb Surgery/Reconstruction; **Hospital:** USC Univ Hosp - R K Eamer Med Plz; **Address:** 1450 San Pablo St, Ste 2000, Los Angeles, CA 90033-4680; **Phone:** (323) 442-6482; **Board Cert:** Plastic Surgery 1986, Hand Surgery 1989; **Med School:** Univ MO-Columbia Sch Med 1977; **Resid:** Surgery, NY Upstate Med Ctr, Syracuse, NY 1981-1983; Surgery, State Univ of New York, Syracuse, NY 1981-1983; **Fellow:** Plastic Surgery, USC Med Ctr, Los Angeles, CA 1983-1985; **Fac Appt:** Prof Surgery, USC Sch Med

Singer, Robert MD (PIS) - *Spec Exp:* Reconstructive Surgery; **Hospital:** Scripps Meml Hosp - La Jolla; **Address:** 9834 Genesee Ave, Ste 100, La Jolla, CA 92037-1214; **Phone:** (858) 455-0290; **Board Cert:** Plastic Surgery 1977; **Med School:** SUNY Buffalo 1967; **Resid:** Surgery, Stanford Med Ctr, Palo Alto, CA 1968-1969; Physical Medicine & Rehabilitation, Vanderbilt Univ Hosp, Nashville, TN 1974-1976; **Fellow:** Neurological Surgery, Rigs Hosp-Kommunes Hosp, Copenhagen, Denmark; **Fac Appt:** Asst Clin Prof Plastic Surgery, UCSD

Stevenson, Thomas Ray MD (PIS) - *Spec Exp:* Reconstructive Surgery; Cosmetic Surgery; **Hospital:** Univ CA - Davis Med Ctr; **Address:** Univ Surg Assocs, 2825 J St, Ste 400, Sacramento, CA 95816; **Phone:** (916) 734-4323; **Board Cert:** Plastic Surgery 1983, Hand Surgery 1994; **Med School:** Univ Kans 1972; **Resid:** Surgery, Univ VA Hosp, Charlottesville, VA 1973-1978; Plastic Surgery, Emory Univ Hosp, Atlanta, GA 1980-1982; **Fac Appt:** Prof Plastic Surgery, UC Davis

Wells, James H MD (PIS) - *Spec Exp:* Cleft Palate/Lip; Breast Surgery; **Hospital:** Long Beach Meml Med Ctr; **Address:** 2880 Atlantic Ave, Ste 290, Long Beach, CA 90806-1716; **Phone:** (562) 95-6543; **Board Cert:** Plastic Surgery 1978; **Med School:** Univ Tex Med Br, Galveston 1966; **Resid:** urgery, Ochsner Fdn Hosp, New Orleans, LA 1967-1971; Plastic Surgery, Univ VA Hosp, Charlottesville, VA 1973-1975

arem, Harvey Alan MD (PIS) - *Spec Exp:* Breast Surgery; Cosmetic Surgery-Face; **Hospital:** St ohn's Hlth Ctr; **Address:** 1301 20th St, Ste 470, Santa Monica, CA 90404; **Phone:** (310) 315-0222; **oard Cert:** Plastic Surgery 1978, Surgery 1964; **Med School:** Columbia P&S 1957; **Resid:** Surgery, eter Bent Brigham Hosp, Boston, MA 1958-1961; Plastic Surgery, Johns Hopkins Hosp, Boston, MA 1964-1966; **Fellow:** Pathology, NYU Med Ctr, New York, NY 1963-1964; **Fac Appt:** Prof Emeritus lastic Surgery, UCLA

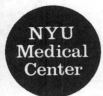

NYU Medical Center

550 First Avenue (at 31st Street)
New York, NY 10016
Physician Referral: (888) 7-NYU-MED
(888-769-8633)   www.nyumedicalcenter.org

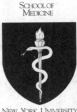

SCHOOL OF
MEDICINE

NEW YORK UNIVERSITY

PSYCHIATRY

In close collaboration with the NYU School of Medicine, which has one of the largest and most distinguished psychiatry faculties in the United States, the NYU Medical Center Department of Psychiatry offers these special services:

Behavioral Health Program - A full complement of inpatient and outpatient services

Silberstein Aging and Dementia Research Center - home to a 30-year longitudinal study of Alzheimer's disease with comprehensive psychosocial support for patients and caregivers

Electroconvulsant Therapy Center

Child Study Center - the first multi-specialty program in the New York area to offer complete child and adolescent psychiatric are fully integrated with scientific research and education. The NYU Child Study Center is home to several comprehensive programs including:

- Adolescent & Child Psychiatry Program
- Alcoholism and Drug Abuse Program
- Anxiety and Affective Disorders Service
- Attention Deficit Hyperactivity Disorder Program
- Family Studies Program
- Furman Diagnostic Service
- Human Sexuality and Sex Therapy
- Infancy and Early Childhood Development Program
- Institute for Children at Risk
- Institute for Learning and Academic Achievement
- NYU Summer Program for Kids with ADHD
- ParentCorps
- Parenting Institute
- Sex Therapy Clinic
- Young Adult Inpatient Program

The NYU Child Study Center's premiere clinicians implement the knowledge gained from research, resulting in care that incorporates the most up-to-date information about the causes, symptoms, and treatments of mental disorders. They are an important part of NYU Child Study Center's enriched environment for scientific research into the risks and causes of childhood mental disorders.

The NYU Child Study Center's educational outreach programs teach thousands of parents, educators, pediatricians and other mental health professionals about normal child development and how to promptly recognize and intervene when a child needs help.

A DRIVER OF CROSS-DISCIPLINARY CLINICAL EXCELLENCE

Today, radiology is playing an increasingly pivotal role in medical research. With an explosion of imaging technologies, researchers at NYU are making rapid strides in the understanding of complex diseases, able to visualize anatomical and metabolic changes in the body at the molecular level. No longer a merely supportive discipline, radiology has been transformed into a dynamic driver of medical knowledge itself. For example, the new imaging technologies allow physicians to observe minute changes in tumor activity during cancer treatment, adjust the dosage accordingly, and monitor the disease process with a depth and precision that would have been unimaginable ten years ago.

Physician Referral
(888) 7-NYU-MED
(888-769-8633)
www.nyumedicalcenter.org

PHYSICIAN LISTINGS

New England

Frances, Richard J MD (AdP) - *Spec Exp:* Alcoholism & Anxiety; Substance Abuse; Forensic Psychiatry; **Hospital:** Silver Hill Hosp; **Address:** 208 Valley Rd, New Canaan, CT 06840; **Phone:** (203) 966-3561; **Board Cert:** Addiction Psychiatry 1993, Psychiatry 1976; **Med School:** NYU Sch Med 1971; **Resid:** Psychiatry, Montefiore Med Ctr, Bronx, NY 1971-1974; **Fellow:** Psychoanalysis, NY Psyc Inst, New York, NY 1974-1976; **Fac Appt:** Clin Prof Psychiatry, NYU Sch Med

Kosten, Thomas MD (AdP) - *Spec Exp:* Cocaine Addiction; Alcohol Abuse; **Hospital:** VA Conn Hlthcre Sys; **Address:** 950 Campbell Ave, West Haven, CT 06516; **Phone:** (203) 932-5711; **Board Cert:** Addiction Psychiatry 1993, Psychiatry 1984; **Med School:** Cornell Univ-Weill Med Coll 1977; **Resid:** Psychiatry, Yale-New Haven Hosp, New Haven, CT 1978-1981; **Fellow:** Epidemiology, Yale-New Haven Hosp, New Haven, CT 1981-1983; **Fac Appt:** Assoc Prof Medicine, Yale Univ

Schottenfeld, Richard MD (AdP) - *Spec Exp:* Drug Abuse; **Hospital:** Yale - New Haven Hosp; **Address:** CMHC, 34 Park St, rm S-204, New Haven, CT 06519; **Phone:** (203) 974-7349; **Board Cert:** Addiction Psychiatry 1994, Psychiatry 1984; **Med School:** Yale Univ 1976; **Resid:** Psychiatry, Yale Psych Inst, New Haven, CT 1979-1982; **Fellow:** Epidemiology, Yale Univ, New Haven, CT 1982-1984; **Fac Appt:** Assoc Prof Psychiatry, Yale Univ

Mid Atlantic

Galanter, Marc MD (AdP) - *Spec Exp:* Alcohol Abuse; Drug Abuse; **Hospital:** NYU Med Ctr (page 71); **Address:** 285 Central Park West, New York, NY 10024-3006; **Phone:** (212) 877-4093; **Board Cert:** Psychiatry 1974, Addiction Psychiatry 1993; **Med School:** Albert Einstein Coll Med 1967; **Resid:** Psychiatry, UCLA Med Ctr, Los Angeles, CA 1967-1968; Psychiatry, Albert Einstein Med Ctr, Bronx, NY 1968-1971; **Fac Appt:** Prof Psychiatry, NYU Sch Med

Gorelick, David Alan MD (AdP) - *Spec Exp:* Addiction; **Hospital:** Natl Inst of Hlth - Clin Ctr; **Address:** Natl Inst on Drug Abuse, 5500 Nathan Shock Dr, Baltimore, MD 21224; **Phone:** (410) 550-1478; **Board Cert:** Psychiatry 1982, Addiction Psychiatry 1993; **Med School:** Albert Einstein Coll Med 1976; **Resid:** Psychiatry, UCLA-Neuropsyh Hosp, Los Angeles, CA 1977-1980; Brentwood VA Med Ctr, Los Angeles, CA 1980-1983; **Fac Appt:** Prof Psychiatry, Univ MD Sch Med

Kleber, Herbert MD (AdP) - *Spec Exp:* Addiction Psychiatry - General; **Hospital:** NY Presby Hosp - Columbia Presby Med Ctr (page 70); **Address:** 1051 Riverside Dr, New York, NY 10032; **Phone:** (212) 543-5570; **Med School:** Jefferson Med Coll 1960; **Resid:** Psychiatry, Yale-New Haven, New Haven, CT 1961-1964

Midwest

Compton III, Wilson M MD (AdP) - *Spec Exp:* Addiction Psychiatry - General; **Hospital:** Barnes-Jewish Hosp (page 55); **Address:** Washington Univ Sch Med, 40 N Kings Hwy, Ste 4, St Louis, MO 63108; **Phone:** (314) 286-2261; **Board Cert:** Psychiatry 1992, Addiction Psychiatry 1993; **Med School:** Washington Univ, St Louis 1986; **Resid:** Psychiatry, Barnes Hosp, St Louis, MO 1986-1990; **Fac Appt:** Assoc Prof Psychiatry, Washington Univ, St Louis

Miller, Norman S MD (AdP) - *Spec Exp:* Addiction/Substance Abuse; Opiate/Prescription Medicine Addiction; Medical Legal; **Hospital:** Sparrow Health System - St Lawrence; **Address:** Michigan State Univ, Dept Psychiatry, East Fee Hall, rm A227, East Lancing, IL 48824; **Phone:** (517) 355-8416; **Board Cert:** Psychiatry 1987, Neurology 1985, Addiction Psychiatry 1993, Forensic Psychiatry 1999; **Med School:** Howard Univ 1974; **Resid:** Psychiatry, Johns Hopkins Hosp, Baltimore, MD 1977-1978; Neurology, Univ Minn Med Ctr, Minneapolis, MN 1979-1982; **Fellow:** Clinical Pharmacology, Univ Minn Med Ctr, Minneapolis, MN 1982-1984; **Fac Appt:** Prof Psychiatry, Mich State Univ

Miller, Sheldon I MD (AdP) - *Spec Exp:* Addiction/Substance Abuse; **Hospital:** Northwestern Meml Hosp; **Address:** 222 E Superior St, Ste 240, Chicago, IL 60611; **Phone:** (312) 926-2323; **Board Cert:** Psychiatry 1972, Addiction Psychiatry 1993; **Med School:** Tufts Univ 1964; **Resid:** Psychiatry, Univ Hosp Cleveland, Cleveland, OH 1965-1968; **Fac Appt:** Prof Psychiatry, Northwestern Univ

Great Plains and Mountains

Crowley, Thomas J. MD (AdP) - *Spec Exp:* Addiction/Substance Abuse; Conduct Disorder; **Hospital:** Univ Colo HSC - Denver; **Address:** 4200 E 9th Ave, Box C268-35, Denver, CO 80220-3706; **Phone:** (303) 315-7573; **Board Cert:** Psychiatry 1971; **Med School:** Univ Minn 1962; **Resid:** Psychiatry, Univ Minnesota Hosp, Minneapolis, MN 1963-1966; **Fac Appt:** Prof Psychiatry, Univ Colo

West Coast and Pacific

Schuckit, Marc A MD (AdP) - *Spec Exp:* Alcohol Abuse; Psychopharmacology; **Hospital:** VA San Diego Hlthcre Sys; **Address:** VA San Diego Healthcare System, Dept Psyc (116A), 3350 La Jolla Village Dr, San Diego, CA 92161; **Phone:** (858) 552-8585; **Board Cert:** Psychiatry 1974; **Med School:** Washington Univ, St Louis 1968; **Resid:** Psychiatry, Washington Univ, St Louis, MO 1969-1971; Psychiatry, UC San Diego, San Diego, CA 1971-1972; **Fac Appt:** Prof Psychiatry, UCSD

Weinstock, Robert MD (AdP) - *Spec Exp:* Addiction Psychiatry - General; **Hospital:** Cedars-Sinai Med Ctr; **Address:** 1626 Westwood Blvd, Ste 105, Los Angeles, CA 90024; **Phone:** (310) 477-9933; **Board Cert:** Geriatric Psychiatry 1995, Addiction Psychiatry 1996; **Med School:** NYU Sch Med 1966; **Resid:** Psychiatry, McLean Hosp, Belmont, MA 1967-1970; Child & Adolescent Psychiatry, McLean Hosp, Belmont, MA 1970-1972; **Fellow:** Psychiatric Research, Boston Univ, Boston, MA 1972-1974; **Fac Appt:** Clin Prof Psychiatry, UCLA

CHILD & ADOLESCENT PSYCHIATRY

New England

Biederman, Joseph MD (ChAP) - *Spec Exp:* ADD/ADHD; Anxiety & Mood Disorders; Psychopharmacology; **Hospital:** MA Genl Hosp; **Address:** 15 Parkman St, WACC 725, Boston, MA 02114; **Phone:** (617) 726-1743; **Board Cert:** Psychiatry 1983, Child & Adolescent Psychiatry 1984; **Med School:** Brazil 1971; **Resid:** Psychiatry, Hadassah Univ Hosp, Jerusalem, Israel 1972-1977; Child & Adolescent Psychiatry, Harvard Chldns Hosp, Boston, MA 1977-1979; **Fellow:** Psychiatry, Mass Genl Hosp, Boston, MA 1979-1981; **Fac Appt:** Prof Psychiatry, Harvard Med Sch

Coyle, Joseph MD (ChAP) - *Spec Exp:* Mental Retardation; **Hospital:** McLean Hosp; **Address:** 15 Mill St, Belmont, MA 02478-1048; **Phone:** (617) 855-2101; **Board Cert:** Psychiatry 1980; **Med School:** Johns Hopkins Univ 1969; **Resid:** Psychiatry, Johns Hopkins Hosp, Baltimore, MD 1973-1976; **Fellow:** Psychiatry, NIMH, Bethesda, MD 1970-1973; **Fac Appt:** Prof Psychiatry, Harvard Med Sch

Fritz, Gregory K MD (ChAP) - *Spec Exp:* Asthma; **Hospital:** Rhode Island Hosp; **Address:** Rhode Island Hosp, 593 Eddy St, Providence, RI 02903; **Phone:** (401) 444-7573; **Board Cert:** Psychiatry 1977, Child & Adolescent Psychiatry 1978; **Med School:** Tufts Univ 1971; **Resid:** Psychiatry, San Mateo Co Hosp, CA 1972-1974; Child & Adolescent Psychiatry, Stanford Med Ctr, Stanford, CA 1974-1977; **Fac Appt:** Prof Psychiatry, Brown Univ

Herzog, David B MD (ChAP) - *Spec Exp:* Eating Disorders; Somatic Disorders-Adolescent; **Hospital:** MA Genl Hosp; **Address:** Mass Genl Hosp, 15 Parkman St, WACC 725, Boston, MA 02114; **Phone:** (617) 724-0799; **Board Cert:** Pediatrics 1980, Child & Adolescent Psychiatry 1986, Psychiatry 1982; **Med School:** Mexico 1973; **Resid:** Pediatrics, Univ Wisc, Madison, WI 1974-1975; Pediatrics, Boston City Hosp, Boston, MA 1975-1976; **Fellow:** Child & Adolescent Psychiatry, Chldns Hosp, Boston, MA 1976-1978; Psychiatry, Mass Genl Hosp, Boston, MA 1978-1980; **Fac Appt:** Prof Child & Adolescent Psychiatry, Harvard Med Sch

King, Bryan Harry MD (ChAP) - *Spec Exp:* Mental Retardation; Autism; **Hospital:** Dartmouth - Hitchcock Med Ctr; **Address:** One Medical Center, Lebanon, NH 00067-7923; **Phone:** (603) 650-7520; **Board Cert:** Psychiatry 1991, Child & Adolescent Psychiatry 1992; **Med School:** Med Coll Wisc 1983; **Resid:** Psychiatry, UCLA Neuropsych Inst, Los Angeles, CA 1984-1987; **Fellow:** Child & Adolescent Psychiatry, UCLA Neuropsych Inst, Los Angeles, CA 1987-1990; **Fac Appt:** Prof Psychiatry, Dartmouth Med Sch

King, Robert A. MD (ChAP) - *Spec Exp:* Tourette's Syndrome; Obsessive-Compulsive Disorder; Psychoanalysis; **Hospital:** Yale - New Haven Hosp; **Address:** 230 S Frontage Rd, Box 207900, New Haven, CT 06519-1124; **Phone:** (203) 785-5880; **Board Cert:** Psychiatry 1974, Child & Adolescent Psychiatry 1981; **Med School:** Harvard Med Sch 1968; **Resid:** Pediatrics, Children's Hosp Med Ctr, Boston, MA 1968-1969; Psychiatry, Mass Mental Health Ctr, Boston, MA 1969-1971; **Fellow:** Child Psychiatry, Children's Hosp Med Ctr, Boston, MA 1971-1972; Child Psychiatry, Children's Hosp Natl Med Ctr, Washington, DC 1972-1974; **Fac Appt:** Prof Psychiatry, Yale Univ

Leonard, Henrietta MD (ChAP) - *Spec Exp:* Neuro-Psychiatry; Movement Disorders; **Hospital:** Rhode Island Hosp; **Address:** Rhode Island Hosp, Dept Child Psyc, 593 Eddy St Bldg Potter Basement, Providence, RI 02903; **Phone:** (401) 444-8945; **Board Cert:** Psychiatry 1987, Child & Adolescent Psychiatry 1988; **Med School:** Geo Wash Univ 1982; **Resid:** Psychiatry, Geo Wash Med Ctr, Washington, DC 1982-1985; **Fellow:** Child & Adolescent Psychiatry, Chldns Hosp, Washington, DC 1985-1987; **Fac Appt:** Prof Psychiatry, Brown Univ

Nickman, Steven L MD (ChAP) - *Spec Exp:* Adoption; **Hospital:** MA Genl Hosp; **Address:** Mass Genl Hosp, 15 Parkman St, WACC 725, Boston, MA 02114; **Phone:** (617) 726-2724; **Board Cert:** Pediatrics 1971, Psychiatry 1977; **Med School:** Duke Univ 1964; **Resid:** Pediatrics, Montefiore Hosp, New York, NY 1965-1966; Psychiatry, Mass Genl Hosp, Boston, MA 1969-1971; **Fellow:** Child & Adolescent Psychiatry, Mass Genl Hosp, Boston, MA 1969-1973; **Fac Appt:** Asst Clin Prof Psychiatry, Harvard Med Sch

Spencer, Thomas MD (ChAP) - *Spec Exp:* ADD/ADHD; **Hospital:** MA Genl Hosp; **Address:** Mass Genl Hosp, 15 Parkman St, WACC 725, Boston, MA 02114; **Phone:** (617) 726-1731; **Board Cert:** Psychiatry 1984, Child & Adolescent Psychiatry 1993; **Med School:** Univ Wisc 1978; **Resid:** Psychiatry, New Eng Med Ctr, Boston, MA 1982; Child & Adolescent Psychiatry, Mass Genl Hosp, Boston, MA 1990; **Fac Appt:** Assoc Prof Psychiatry, Harvard Med Sch

Volkmar, Fred R MD (ChAP) - *Spec Exp:* Autism; Asperger's Syndrome; Mental Retardation; **Hospital:** Yale - New Haven Hosp; **Address:** Yale Child Study Ctr, 230 Frontage Rd S, Box 207900, New Haven, CT 06519-1124; **Phone:** (203) 785-2510; **Board Cert:** Psychiatry 1981, Child & Adolescent Psychiatry 1988; **Med School:** Stanford Univ 1976; **Resid:** Psychiatry, Stanford Univ, Stanford, CA 1978-1980; Child & Adolescent Psychiatry, Yale Univ Child Study Ctr, New Haven, CT 1980-1982; **Fac Appt:** Prof Child & Adolescent Psychiatry, Yale Univ

Wilens, Timothy MD (ChAP) - *Spec Exp:* ADD/ADHD; Bipolar/Mood Disorders; Addiction/Substance Abuse; **Hospital:** MA Genl Hosp; **Address:** Mass Genl Hosp, 15 Parkman St, WACC 725, Boston, MA 02114; **Phone:** (617) 726-1731; **Board Cert:** Psychiatry 1990, Child & Adolescent Psychiatry 1991, Addiction Psychiatry 1994; **Med School:** Univ Mich Med Sch 1985; **Resid:** Internal Medicine, Henry Ford Hosp, Detroit, MI 1985-1986; Psychiatry, Mass Genl Hosp, Boston, MA 1986-1988; **Fellow:** Child & Adolescent Psychiatry, Mass Genl Hosp, Boston, MA 1988-1990; **Fac Appt:** Assoc Prof Psychiatry, Harvard Med Sch

Mid Atlantic

Abright, Arthur Reese MD (ChAP) - *Spec Exp:* Depression and Bipolar Disorder; ADD/ADHD; Post Traumatic Stress Disorder; **Hospital:** St Vincent Cath Med Ctrs - Manhattan (page 75); **Address:** 144 W 12th St, New York, NY 10011; **Phone:** (212) 604-8213; **Board Cert:** Psychiatry 1978, Child & Adolescent Psychiatry 1981; **Med School:** Univ Tex SW, Dallas 1973; **Resid:** Psychiatry, St Vincent's Hosp, New York, NY 1973-1974; Psychiatry, NY Hosp-Cornell Med Ctr, New York, NY 1974-1977; **Fellow:** Child & Adolescent Psychiatry, NY Hosp-Cornell Med Ctr, New York, NY 1977-1979; **Fac Appt:** Assoc Prof Psychiatry, NY Med Coll

Bird, Hector MD (ChAP) - *Spec Exp:* ADD/ADHD; Depression; Personality Disorders; **Hospital:** NY Presby Hosp - Columbia Presby Med Ctr (page 70); **Address:** 145 Central Park West, Ste 1C, New York, NY 10023-2004; **Phone:** (212) 874-5311; **Board Cert:** Child & Adolescent Psychiatry 1977, Psychiatry 1975; **Med School:** Yale Univ 1965; **Resid:** Psychiatry, Columbia-Presbyterian, New York, NY 1968-1971; Child & Adolescent Psychiatry, Columbia-Presbyterian, New York, NY 1970-1972; **Fellow:** Psychoanalysis, WA White Institute, New York, NY 1972-1977; **Fac Appt:** Prof Psychiatry, Columbia P&S

Bogrov, Michael MD (ChAP) - *Spec Exp:* ADD/ADHD; Mood Disorders; **Hospital:** Sheppard Pratt Hlth Sys; **Address:** 6501 N Charles St, Baltimore, MD 21204-6819; **Phone:** (410) 938-4913; **Board Cert:** Psychiatry 1993, Child & Adolescent Psychiatry 1994; **Med School:** Emory Univ 1987; **Resid:** Psychiatry, Univ of Maryland, Baltimore, MD 1987-1990; Child & Adolescent Psychiatry, Johns Hopkins Hosp, Baltimore, MD 1990-1992; **Fac Appt:** Asst Prof Psychiatry, Johns Hopkins Univ

Campo, John V MD (ChAP) - *Spec Exp:* Psychosomatic Disorders; Psychiatry of Illness; **Hospital:** Western Psy Inst & Clin; **Address:** Western Psych Inst & Clinic, Dept Psychiatry, 3811 O'Hara St, Pittsburgh, PA 15213; **Phone:** (412) 624-5853; **Board Cert:** Psychiatry 1989, Child & Adolescent Psychiatry 1993; **Med School:** Univ Penn 1982; **Resid:** Pediatrics, Chldn's Hosp, Philadelphia, PA 1982-1985; Psychiatry, West Psych Inst Clin, Pittsburgh, PA 1985-1989; **Fac Appt:** Asst Prof Psychiatry, Univ Pittsburgh

Egan, James Harold MD (ChAP) - *Spec Exp:* Psychopharmocology; Psychotherapy; **Hospital:** Chldns Natl Med Ctr - DC; **Address:** 5480 Wisconsin Ave, Chevy Chase, MD 20815; **Phone:** (301) 913-5953; **Board Cert:** Psychiatry 1973, Child & Adolescent Psychiatry 1975; **Med School:** Columbia P&S 1964; **Resid:** Psychiatry, St Vincents Hosp, New York, NY 1967-1969; Child & Adolescent Psychiatry, St Lukes Hosp, New York, NY 1969-1971; **Fac Appt:** Clin Prof Pediatrics, Geo Wash Univ

Foley, Carmel MD (ChAP) - *Spec Exp:* Mood Disorders; **Hospital:** Schneider's Chldns Hosp; **Address:** Schneider Chldns Hosp, Div Child & Adolescent Psych, 269-01 76th Ave, rm 135, New Hyde Park, NY 11040; **Phone:** (718) 470-3510; **Board Cert:** Psychiatry 1979, Child & Adolescent Psychiatry 1981, Addiction Psychiatry 1997, Forensic Psychiatry 1999; **Med School:** Ireland 1972; **Resid:** Psychiatry, St Patrick's Hosp, Dublin, Ireland 1975-1976; Psychiatry, Lafayette Clinic, Detroit, MI 1976-1978; **Fellow:** Child & Adolescent Psychiatry, Lafayette Clinic, Detroit, MI 1977-1979; **Fac Appt:** Assoc Prof Psychiatry, Albert Einstein Coll Med

Fornari, Victor MD (ChAP) - *Spec Exp:* Eating Disorders; **Hospital:** N Shore Univ Hosp at Manhasset; **Address:** Dept Psychiatry, 400 Community Drive, Manhasset, NY 11030; **Phone:** (516) 562-3051; **Board Cert:** Child & Adolescent Psychiatry 1985, Psychiatry 1984; **Med School:** SUNY Downstate 1979; **Resid:** Psychiatry, Hosp Univ PA, Philadelphia, PA 1980-1982; **Fellow:** Child & Adolescent Psychiatry, LI Jewish Hosp, New Hyde Park, NY 1982-1984; **Fac Appt:** Assoc Prof Psychiatry, NYU Sch Med

Greenspan, Stanley MD (ChAP) - *Spec Exp:* Autism; Infant/Toddler Psychiatry; **Hospital:** G Washington Univ Hosp; **Address:** 7201 Glenbrook Rd, Bethesda, MD 20814-1242; **Phone:** (301) 657-2348; **Board Cert:** Psychiatry 1972; **Med School:** Yale Univ 1966; **Resid:** Psychiatry, Columbia-Presby Psych Inst, New York, NY 1967-1969; **Fellow:** Child & Adolescent Psychiatry, Childrens Hosp-NMC, Washington, DC 1969-1971; **Fac Appt:** Clin Prof Psychiatry, Geo Wash Univ

Hertzig, Margaret MD (ChAP) - *Spec Exp:* Developmental Disorders; ADD/ADHD; **Hospital:** NY Presby Hosp - NY Weill Cornell Med Ctr (page 70); **Address:** 525 E 68th St, Box 140, New York, NY 10021; **Phone:** (212) 746-5712; **Board Cert:** Psychiatry 1968, Child & Adolescent Psychiatry 1975; **Med School:** NYU Sch Med 1960; **Resid:** Pediatrics, Jewish Hosp, Brooklyn, NY 1961-1962; Psychiatry, Bellevue Psych Hosp, New York, NY 1962-1964; **Fellow:** Psychiatric Research, NYU Sch Med, New York, NY 1964-1966; **Fac Appt:** Prof Psychiatry, Cornell Univ-Weill Med Coll

Kestenbaum, Clarice J MD (ChAP) - *Spec Exp:* Anxiety Disorders; Dynamic Psychotherapy; **Hospital:** NY Presby Hosp - NY Weill Cornell Med Ctr (page 70); **Address:** 1051 Riverside Drive, Box 74, , New York, NY 10032; **Phone:** (212) 543-5333; **Board Cert:** Psychiatry 1971, Child & Adolescent Psychiatry 1975; **Med School:** USC Sch Med 1960; **Resid:** Psychiatry, Columbia Presby Med Ctr, New York, NY 1961-1963; Child & Adolescent Psychiatry, Columbia Presby Med Ctr, New York, NY 1963-1965; **Fac Appt:** Clin Prof Psychiatry, Columbia P&S

Koplewicz, Harold MD (ChAP) - *Spec Exp:* Anxiety Disorders; **Hospital:** NYU Med Ctr (page 71); **Address:** 550 1st Ave, New York, NY 10021; **Phone:** (212) 263-6205; **Board Cert:** Psychiatry 1983, Child & Adolescent Psychiatry 1984; **Med School:** Albert Einstein Coll Med 1978; **Resid:** Psychiatry, NY Hosp, White Plains, NY 1979-1981; Child & Adolescent Psychiatry, NYS Psyc Inst, New York, NY 1981-1983; **Fellow:** Psychiatric Research, NYS Psyc Inst, NY 1983-1985; **Fac Appt:** Prof Psychiatry, NYU Sch Med

Pruitt, David B. MD (ChAP) - *Spec Exp:* Child & Adolescent Psychiatry - General; **Hospital:** University of MD Med Sys; **Address:** U Maryland Sch Med, Div Child & Adol Psyc, 701 W Pratt St, Ste 429, Baltimore, MD 21201; **Phone:** (410) 328-3522; **Board Cert:** Child & Adolescent Psychiatry 1981, Psychiatry 1979; **Med School:** Univ Tex, Houston 1974; **Resid:** Psychiatry, Univ Penn, Philadelphia, PA 1975-1978; Child & Adolescent Psychiatry, Child Guidance Ctr, Philadelphia, PA 1977-1979; **Fac Appt:** Prof Child & Adolescent Psychiatry, Univ MD Sch Med

Rapoport, Judith MD (ChAP) - *Spec Exp:* Schizophrenia; Obsessive Compulsive Disorder; **Hospital:** Natl Inst of Hlth - Clin Ctr; **Address:** NIMH Bldg 10 - rm 3N202, 10 Center Drive, MS 1600, Bethesda, MD 20892-1600; **Phone:** (301) 496-6081; **Board Cert:** Psychiatry 1969, Child & Adolescent Psychiatry 1969; **Med School:** Harvard Med Sch 1959; **Resid:** Psychiatry, Mass Mental Hlth Ctr, Boston, MA 1960-1961; Psychiatry, St Elizabeth Hosp, Washington, DC 1961-1962; **Fellow:** Karolinska Inst, Stockholm, Sweden 1962-1964; Child & Adolescent Psychiatry, Childns Hosp, Washington, DC 1964-1966

Riddle, Mark A MD (ChAP) - *Spec Exp:* Psychopharmacology; **Hospital:** Johns Hopkins Hosp - Baltimore; **Address:** Johns Hopkins Hosp, CMSC 346, 600 N Wolfe St, Baltimore, MD 21287-3325; **Phone:** (410) 955-2320; **Board Cert:** Psychiatry 1982, Child & Adolescent Psychiatry 1986; **Med School:** Indiana Univ 1977; **Resid:** Psychiatry, Yale-New Haven Hosp, New Haven, CT 1978-1981; **Fellow:** Child & Adolescent Psychiatry, Yale Child Study Ctr, New Haven, CT 1981-1983; **Fac Appt:** Assoc Prof Child & Adolescent Psychiatry, Johns Hopkins Univ

Ryan, Neal David MD (ChAP) - *Spec Exp:* Mood Disorders; Depression; **Hospital:** UPMC - Presbyterian Univ Hosp; **Address:** Western Psyc Inst & Clin, 3811 O'Hara St, Pittsburgh, PA 15213-2593; **Phone:** (416) 624-1241; **Board Cert:** Psychiatry 1983, Child & Adolescent Psychiatry 1987; **Med School:** Yale Univ 1978; **Resid:** Psychiatry, NY State Psych-Columbia Univ, New York, NY 1979-1982; **Fellow:** Psychiatric Research, Columbia Univ, New York, NY 1981-1984; **Fac Appt:** Prof Psychiatry, Univ Pittsburgh

Walkup, John MD (ChAP) - *Spec Exp:* Child & Adolescent Psychiatry - General; **Hospital:** Johns Hopkins Hosp - Baltimore; **Address:** Johns Hopkins Hosp, Dept Child Psyc, 600 N Wolfe St, Bldg CMSC - rm 338, Baltimore, MD 21287; **Phone:** (410) 955-1925; **Board Cert:** Child & Adolescent Psychiatry 1992, Psychiatry 1987; **Med School:** Univ Minn 1982; **Resid:** Psychiatry, Yale Univ Med Sch, New Haven, CT 1983-1985; Child & Adolescent Psychiatry, Yale Chld Study Ctr, New Haven, CT 1985-1988; **Fac Appt:** Asst Prof Psychiatry, Johns Hopkins Univ

Wiener, Jerry M MD (ChAP) - *Spec Exp:* Psychiatry-Adolescent/College Age; Anxiety & Mood Disorders .; Psychotherapy & Psychoanalysis; **Hospital:** G Washington Univ Hosp; **Address:** George Washington Univ, 2150 Pennsylvania Ave NW, Washington, DC 20037-2396; **Phone:** (202) 994-8308; **Board Cert:** Psychiatry 1963, Child & Adolescent Psychiatry 1965; **Med School:** Baylor Coll Med 1956; **Resid:** Psychiatry, Mayo Clinic 1957-1961; Child & Adolescent Psychiatry, Mayo Clinic 1960-1961; **Fellow:** Child & Adolescent Psychiatry, Columbia-Presby Med Ctr 1961-1962; **Fac Appt:** Prof Emeritus Psychiatry, Geo Wash Univ

Southeast

Heston, Jerry D MD (ChAP) - *Spec Exp:* Child & Adolescent Psychiatry - *General;* **Hospital:** Le Bonheur Chldns Med Ctr; **Address:** Univ Tenn Hlth Sci Ctr, Div Child Psyc, 711 Jefferson Ave, Ste 137, Memphis, TN 38105; **Phone:** (901) 448-5944; **Board Cert:** Psychiatry 1988, Pediatrics 1997; **Med School:** Univ S Fla Coll Med 1981; **Resid:** Pediatrics, LeBonheur Chldns Hosp, Memphis, TN 1982-1984; Psychiatry, Univ Tennessee, Memphis, TN 1984-1986; **Fellow:** Child & Adolescent Psychiatry, Univ Tennessee, Memphis, TN 1986-1988; **Fac Appt:** Asst Prof Child & Adolescent Psychiatry, Univ Tenn Coll Med, Memphis

March, John MD (ChAP) - *Spec Exp:* Anxiety Disorders; Obsessive-Compulsive Disorder; **Hospital:** Duke Univ Med Ctr (page 60); **Address:** 718 Rutherford St, Box DUMC3527, Durham, NC 27710; **Phone:** (919) 416-2404; **Board Cert:** Psychiatry 1992, Child & Adolescent Psychiatry 1992, Family Practice 1987; **Med School:** UCLA 1978; **Resid:** Family Practice, Santa Monica Hosp Med Ctr, Santa Monica, CA 1978-1981; Psychiatry, Univ of Wisconsin Hosp, Milwaukee, WI 1986-1988; **Fellow:** Child & Adolescent Psychiatry, Univ of Wisconsin Hosp, Milwaukee, WI 1988-1990; **Fac Appt:** Prof Psychiatry, Duke Univ

Sexson, Sandra G B MD (ChAP) - *Spec Exp:* Transplant Patients; Death & Dying; **Hospital:** Emory Univ Hosp; **Address:** Emory West, Div Child & Adol Psyc, 1256 Briarcliff Rd, Ste 313S, Atlanta, GA 30306; **Phone:** (404) 727-3963; **Board Cert:** Child & Adolescent Psychiatry 1981, Psychiatry 1980; **Med School:** Univ Miss 1971; **Resid:** Psychiatry, Tex Hlth Sci Ctr, San Antonio, TX 1972-1974; Child & Adolescent Psychiatry, Washington Univ, St Louis, MO 1976-1978; **Fellow:** Child & Adolescent Psychiatry, Washington Univ, St Louis, MO 1976-1978; **Fac Appt:** Assoc Prof Psychiatry, Emory Univ

Tanguay, Peter MD (ChAP) - *Spec Exp:* Autism; Developmental Disorders; **Hospital:** Univ Louisville Hosp; **Address:** Bingham Child Guidance Center, Rm 228, 200 E Chestnut St, Louisville, KY 40202; **Phone:** (502) 852-1045; **Board Cert:** Child & Adolescent Psychiatry 1974, Psychiatry 1972; **Med School:** Univ Ottawa 1960; **Resid:** Psychiatry, UCLA Med Ctr, Los Angeles, CA 1961-1964; **Fellow:** Child & Adolescent Psychiatry, UCLA Med Ctr, Los Angeles, CA 1968-1970

Wright, Harry MD (ChAP) - *Spec Exp:* Infant/Toddler Psychiatry; Autism; Developmental Disorders; **Hospital:** William S Hall Psyc Inst; **Address:** 3555 Harden St, Columbia, SC 29203; **Phone:** (803) 434-4250; **Board Cert:** Psychiatry 1982, Child & Adolescent Psychiatry 1984; **Med School:** Univ Penn 1976; **Resid:** Psychiatry, William S Hall Psyc Inst, Columbia, SC 1978-1979; **Fellow:** Child & Adolescent Psychiatry, William S Hall Psyc Inst, Columbia, SC 1979-1981; **Fac Appt:** Prof Psychiatry, Univ SC Sch Med

Midwest

Alessi, Norman E MD (ChAP) - *Spec Exp:* Mood Disorders; Disorders of Aggression; **Hospital:** Univ of MI Hlth Ctr; **Address:** 1500 E Med Center Drive, Ann Arbor, MI 48109-0390; **Phone:** (734) 615-3490; **Board Cert:** Psychiatry 1982, Child & Adolescent Psychiatry 1985; **Med School:** Emory Univ 1976; **Resid:** Child & Adolescent Psychiatry, Univ Mich Med Ctr, Ann Arbor, MI 1980-1981; Psychiatry, Univ Mich Med Ctr, Ann Arbor, MI 1977-1980; **Fellow:** Child & Adolescent Psychiatry, Univ Mich Med Ctr, Ann Arbor, MI 1981-1983; **Fac Appt:** Assoc Prof Psychiatry, Univ Mich Med Sch

CHILD & ADOLESCENT PSYCHIATRY

Dulcan, Mina Karen MD (ChAP) - *Spec Exp:* ADD/ADHD; **Hospital:** Children's Mem Hosp; **Address:** Chldns Meml Hosp, Dept Psyc, 700 W Fullerton Ave, Box 10, Chicago, IL 60614; **Phone:** (773) 880-4811; **Board Cert:** Psychiatry 1978, Child & Adolescent Psychiatry 1979; **Med School:** Penn State Univ-Hershey Med Ctr 1974; **Resid:** Child & Adolescent Psychiatry, Univ Pittsburgh, Pittsburgh, PA 1974-1978; Psychiatry, Univ Pittsburgh, Pittsburgh, PA 1974-1977; **Fac Appt:** Prof Psychiatry, Northwestern Univ

Luby, Joan Lida MD (ChAP) - *Spec Exp:* Psychiatric Disorders of Young Children; Preschool Affective Disorders; Autism; **Hospital:** Barnes-Jewish Hosp (page 55); **Address:** Child & Adolescent Psyc Offices, Montclair Bldg, 24 S Kingshighway, St Louis, MO 63108-1301; **Phone:** (314) 286-2730; **Board Cert:** Psychiatry 1993, Child & Adolescent Psychiatry 1993; **Med School:** Wayne State Univ 1985; **Resid:** Psychiatry, Stanford Univ Sch Med, Palo Alto, CA 1986-1988; **Fellow:** Child & Adolescent Psychiatry, Stanford Univ Sch Med, Palo Alto, CA 1988-1990; **Fac Appt:** Asst Prof Psychiatry, Washington Univ, St Louis

Slomowitz, Marcia MD (ChAP) - *Spec Exp:* ADD/ADHD; Mood Disorders; **Hospital:** Northwestern Meml Hosp; **Address:** 333 N Michigan, Ste 1023, Chicago, IL 60601; **Phone:** (773) 391-4052; **Board Cert:** Child & Adolescent Psychiatry 1983, Psychiatry 1982; **Med School:** Univ Wisc 1977; **Resid:** Psychiatry, Univ Cincinnati, Cincinnati, OH 1978-1980; **Fellow:** Child & Adolescent Psychiatry, Univ Cincinnati, Cincinnati, OH 1980-1982; **Fac Appt:** Asst Prof Psychiatry, Northwestern Univ

Todd, Richard D MD/PhD (ChAP) - *Spec Exp:* Autism; **Hospital:** St Louis Children's Hospital; **Address:** 24 S Kings Hwy, St Louis, MO 63108; **Phone:** (314) 286-1740; **Board Cert:** Psychiatry 1988, Child & Adolescent Psychiatry 1989; **Med School:** Univ Tex, San Antonio 1981; **Resid:** Psychiatry, Stanford Med Sch, Palo Alto, CA 1982-1984; **Fellow:** Child Psychiatry, Washington Univ Sch Med, St Louis, MO 1984-1986; **Fac Appt:** Prof Child & Adolescent Psychiatry, Washington Univ, St Louis

Great Plains and Mountains

Bleiberg, Efrain MD (ChAP) - *Spec Exp:* Trauma Psychiatry; Personality Disorders; **Hospital:** Menninger Clinic; **Address:** Menninger Hosp & Clinic, 5800 SW 6th St, Box 829, Topeka, KS 66601-0829; **Phone:** (785) 350-5876; **Board Cert:** Psychiatry 1985, Child & Adolescent Psychiatry 1986; **Med School:** Mexico 1976; **Resid:** Psychiatry, Menninger Fdn, Topeka, KS 1977-1980; **Fellow:** Child & Adolescent Psychiatry, Menninger Fdn, Topeka, KS 1979-1981; **Fac Appt:** Prof Psychiatry, Univ Kans

Sokol, Mae Sandra MD (ChAP) - *Spec Exp:* Eating Disorders; Obesity; Activity Disorders; **Hospital:** Children's Mem Hosp - Omaha; **Address:** 916 S 96th St, Omaha, NE 68114; **Phone:** (888) 216-1860; **Board Cert:** Psychiatry 1986, Child & Adolescent Psychiatry 1987; **Med School:** Belgium 1980; **Resid:** Psychiatry, Bellevue Hosp-NYU Med Ctr, New York, NY 1981-1984; **Fellow:** Child & Adolescent Psychiatry, Bellevue Hosp-NYU Med Ctr, New York, NY 1984-1986; **Fac Appt:** Assoc Prof Psychiatry, Creighton Univ

Southwest

Drell, Martin J. MD (ChAP) - *Spec Exp:* Infant/Toddler Psychiatry; Family Therapy; **Hospital:** New Orleans Adol Hosp; **Address:** LSU Med Ctr, Child Psyc, 3rd Fl, 1542 Tulane Ave, New Orleans, LA 70112-2825; **Phone:** (504) 568-6350; **Board Cert:** Psychiatry 1982, Child & Adolescent Psychiatry 1982; **Med School:** Univ IL Coll Med 1974; **Resid:** Psychiatry, Cambridge Hospital, Cambridge, MA 1977-1979; **Fellow:** Child & Adolescent Psychiatry, Boston Childrens Hosp-JBGC, Boston, MA 1975-1977; **Fac Appt:** Prof Psychiatry, Louisiana State Univ

Emslie, Graham J MD (ChAP) - *Spec Exp:* Depression; **Hospital:** Chldns Med Ctr of Dallas; **Address:** Children's Med Ctr, Bank One Bldg -Dept Pediatric Psychiatry, 6300 Harry Hines Blvd, Ste 900, Dallas, TX 75235; **Phone:** (214) 456-5921; **Board Cert:** Psychiatry 1981; **Med School:** Scotland 1974; **Resid:** Psychiatry, Univ Rochester 1975-1978; Child & Adolescent Psychiatry, Stanford Med Ctr, Stanford, CA 1978-1981; **Fac Appt:** Prof Psychiatry, Univ Tex SW, Dallas

Sargent III, A John MD (ChAP) - *Spec Exp:* Eating Disorders; Suicide; Family Therapy; **Hospital:** Ben Taub General Hosp; **Address:** Baylor College of Medicine, Dept Psychiatry, One Baylor Plaza, Houston, TX 77030; **Phone:** (713) 798-7889; **Board Cert:** Pediatrics 1979, Child & Adolescent Psychiatry 1989; **Med School:** Univ Rochester 1973; **Resid:** Pediatrics, Univ Wisconsin Hosp, Madison, WI 1973-1977; Psychiatry, Hosp Univ Penn, Philadelphia, PA 1984-1987; **Fellow:** Pediatrics, Univ Wisconsin Hosp, Madison, WI 1975-1976; Child & Adolescent Psychiatry, Phila Child Guidance Ctr, Philadelphia, PA 1978-1980; **Fac Appt:** Prof Psychiatry, Baylor Coll Med

Zeanah Jr, Charles H MD (ChAP) - *Spec Exp:* Attachment Disorders; Abuse/Neglect; International Adoption; **Hospital:** Tulane Univ Med Ctr Hosp & Clinic; **Address:** Tulane U Sch Med, Dept Psych & Neurology, 1440 Canal St, Tidewater Bldg, TB52, New Orleans, LA 70112-2715; **Phone:** (504) 588-5405; **Board Cert:** Psychiatry 1983, Child & Adolescent Psychiatry 1983; **Med School:** Tulane Univ 1977; **Resid:** Psychiatry, Duke Univ, Durham, NC 1978-1980; Child & Adolescent Psychiatry, Stanford Univ, Palo Alto, CA 1980-1982; **Fellow:** Stanford Univ, Palo Alto, CA 1982-1984; **Fac Appt:** Prof Psychiatry, Tulane Univ

West Coast and Pacific

McCracken, James Thomas MD (ChAP) - *Spec Exp:* Obsessive Compulsive Disorder; Tourette's Syndrome; **Hospital:** UCLA Neuropsychiatric Hosp; **Address:** UCLA Neuropsychiatric Hospital, 760 Westwood Plaza, Los Angeles, CA 90024-1759; **Phone:** (310) 825-0470; **Board Cert:** Psychiatry 1986, Child & Adolescent Psychiatry 1988; **Med School:** Baylor Coll Med 1980; **Resid:** Psychiatry, Duke Univ Med Ctr, Durham, NC 1980-1984; **Fellow:** Child & Adolescent Psychiatry, UCLA Neuropsych Inst, Los Angeles, CA 1984; **Fac Appt:** Prof Psychiatry, UCLA

Ponton, Lynn Elisabeth MD (ChAP) - *Spec Exp:* Adolescent Risk-Taking; Eating Disorders; **Hospital:** UCSF Med Ctr; **Address:** 206 Edgewood Ave, San Francisco, CA 94117-3715; **Phone:** (415) 664-3039; **Board Cert:** Psychiatry 1985, Child & Adolescent Psychiatry 1985; **Med School:** Univ Wisc 1978; **Resid:** Psychiatry, Univ Penn, Philadelphia, PA 1979-1980; Psychiatry, UCSF Med Ctr, San Francisco, CA 1980-1981; **Fellow:** Child & Adolescent Psychiatry, UCSF Med Ctr, San Francisco, CA 1981-1983; **Fac Appt:** Prof Child & Adolescent Psychiatry, UCSF

Russak, Sidney MD (ChAP) - *Spec Exp:* Family Therapy; **Hospital:** LAC & USC Med Ctr; **Address:** 2020 Zonao Ave, Bldg IRD - Ste 106, Los Angeles, CA 90033; **Phone:** (323) 226-5288; **Board Cert:** Psychiatry 1974, Child & Adolescent Psychiatry 1975; **Med School:** UC Irvine 1962; **Resid:** Psychiatry, LAC-USC Med Ctr, Los Angeles, CA 1962-1965; Child & Adolescent Psychiatry, LAC-USC Med Ctr, Los Angeles, CA 1965-1967; **Fac Appt:** Asst Prof Psychiatry, USC Sch Med

Russell, Andrew Thomas MD (ChAP) - *Spec Exp:* ADD/ADHD; Schizophrenia; Depression; **Hospital:** UCLA Neuropsychiatric Hosp; **Address:** 760 Westwood Plaza, Los Angeles, CA 90024-8300; **Phone:** (310) 825-0389; **Board Cert:** Psychiatry 1980, Child & Adolescent Psychiatry 1988; **Med School:** Univ Colo 1970; **Resid:** Psychiatry, UCLA Med Ctr, Los Angeles, CA 1971-1973; **Fellow:** Child & Adolescent Psychiatry, UCLA Med Ctr, Los Angeles, CA 1973-1977; **Fac Appt:** Prof Psychiatry, UCLA

Steiner, Hans MD (ChAP) - *Spec Exp:* Disorders of Aggression; Eating Disorders; Trauma Psychiatry; **Hospital:** Stanford Med Ctr; **Address:** Division of Child Psych & Child Dev, 401 Quarry Rd, Stanford, CA 94305-5719; **Phone:** (650) 723-5446; **Board Cert:** Psychiatry 1979, Child & Adolescent Psychiatry 1981; **Med School:** Austria 1972; **Resid:** Psychiatry, SUNY Syracuse Med Ctr, Syracuse, NY 1973-1976; **Fellow:** Child & Adolescent Psychiatry, Univ Mich Hosps, Ann Arbor, MI 1976-1978; **Fac Appt:** Prof Psychiatry, Stanford Univ

Terr, Lenore Cagen MD (ChAP) - *Spec Exp:* Trauma Psychiatry; Forensic Psychiatry; **Hospital:** UCSF Med Ctr; **Address:** 450 Sutter St, Ste 2534, San Francisco, CA 94108-4204; **Phone:** (415) 433-7800; **Board Cert:** Psychiatry 1968, Child & Adolescent Psychiatry 1969; **Med School:** Univ Mich Med Sch 1961; **Resid:** Psychiatry, Univ Mich, Ann Arbor, MI 1962-1964; **Fellow:** Child & Adolescent Psychiatry, Univ Mich, Ann Arbor, MI 1964-1966; **Fac Appt:** Clin Prof Psychiatry, UCSF

Yates, Alayne MD (ChAP) - *Spec Exp:* Eating Disorders; **Hospital:** Kapiolani Med Ctr for Women & Chldn; **Address:** Kapiolani Med Ctr, 1319 Punahou St, Fl 6th, Honolulu, HI 96826-9931; **Phone:** (808) 945-1500; **Board Cert:** Psychiatry 1975, Child & Adolescent Psychiatry 1976; **Med School:** Univ IL Coll Med 1961; **Resid:** Pediatrics, Michael Reese Hosp, Chicago, IL 1962-1964; Child & Adolescent Psychiatry, UC Davis Affil Hosp, Sacramento, CA 1972-1973; **Fac Appt:** Prof Psychiatry, Univ Hawaii JA Burns Sch Med

GERIATRIC PSYCHIATRY

Mid Atlantic

Greenwald, Blaine MD (GerPsy) - *Spec Exp:* Depression; Dementia; **Hospital:** Long Island Jewish Med Ctr; **Address:** 75-59 263rd St, Glen Oaks, NY 11004; **Phone:** (718) 470-8159; **Board Cert:** Psychiatry 1983, Geriatric Psychiatry 1991; **Med School:** NY Med Coll 1978; **Resid:** Psychiatry, Mount Sinai Hosp, New York, NY 1979-1982; **Fellow:** Geriatric Psychiatry, Mount Sinai Hosp/Bronx VA, New York, NY 1982-1983; **Fac Appt:** Assoc Prof Psychiatry, Albert Einstein Coll Med

Katz, Ira Ralph MD (GerPsy) - *Spec Exp:* Geriatric Psychiatry - General; **Hospital:** Hosp Univ Penn (page 78); **Address:** Univ Penn, Geriatric Psyc Sect, 3600 Market St, rm 758, Philadelphia, PA 19104; **Phone:** (215) 349-8225; **Board Cert:** Psychiatry 1989, Geriatric Psychiatry 2001; **Med School:** Albert Einstein Coll Med 1973; **Resid:** Psychiatry, Bronx Muni Hosp Ctr, Bronx, NY 1975-1978; **Fellow:** Psychopharmacology, Albert Einstein Coll Med, Bronx, NY 1978-1979; **Fac Appt:** Prof Psychiatry, Univ Penn

Kennedy, Gary MD (GerPsy) - *Spec Exp:* Alzheimer's Disease; Dementia; Depression; **Hospital:** Montefiore Med Ctr (page 67); **Address:** 111 E 210th St, Dept Psyc & Behavioral Sci, Bronx, NY 10467-2401; **Phone:** (718) 920-4236; **Board Cert:** Psychiatry 1980, Geriatric Psychiatry 2001; **Med School:** Univ Tex, San Antonio 1975; **Resid:** Psychiatry, VA Hosp-Univ Texas, San Antonio, TX 1976-1979; **Fellow:** Geriatric Psychiatry, Montefiore Hosp, Bronx, NY 1981-1984; **Fac Appt:** Prof Psychiatry, Albert Einstein Coll Med

Klement, Maria MD (GerPsy) - *Spec Exp:* Dementia; **Hospital:** Sheppard Pratt Hlth Sys; **Address:** 6501 N Charles St, Baltimore, MD 21285; **Phone:** (410) 938-3000; **Board Cert:** Psychiatry 1972; **Med School:** Penn State Univ-Hershey Med Ctr 1959; **Resid:** Psychiatry, Philadelphia Genl Hosp, Philadelphia, PA 1960-1962; Psychiatry, Sheppeard Pratt Hosp, Towson, MD 1962-1963

Lyketsos, Constantine G MD (GerPsy) - *Spec Exp:* Alzheimer's Disease; Neuropsychiatry; Depression; **Hospital:** Johns Hopkins Hosp - Baltimore; **Address:** Johns Hopkins Hosp, Osler 320, 600 N Wolfe St, Baltimore, MD 21287; **Phone:** (410) 955-6158; **Board Cert:** Geriatric Psychiatry 1995, Psychiatry 1994; **Med School:** Washington Univ, St Louis 1988; **Resid:** Psychiatry, Johns Hopkins Hosp, Baltimore, MD 1989-1992; **Fellow:** Psychiatry, Johns Hopkins Hosp, Baltimore, MD 1992-1994; **Fac Appt:** Prof Psychiatry, Johns Hopkins Univ

Rabins, Peter MD (GerPsy) - *Spec Exp:* Geriatric Psychiatry - General; **Hospital:** Johns Hopkins Hosp - Baltimore; **Address:** Meyer Building, Rm 279, 600 N Wolfe St, Baltimore, MD 21287; **Phone:** (410) 955-6736; **Board Cert:** Geriatric Psychiatry 1991, Psychiatry 1980; **Med School:** Tulane Univ 1973; **Resid:** Psychiatry, Univ Oregon Hlth Scis Ctr, Portland, OR 1974-1977; **Fellow:** Neurology, Johns Hopkins Univ Sch Med, Baltimore, MD; **Fac Appt:** Prof Psychiatry, Johns Hopkins Univ

Reisberg, Barry MD (GerPsy) - *Spec Exp:* Alzheimer's Disease; Dementia; Depression; **Hospital:** NYU Med Ctr (page 71); **Address:** 550 1st Ave, Ste THN314, New York, NY 10016; **Phone:** (212) 263-8550; **Board Cert:** Psychiatry 1976, Geriatric Psychiatry 1991; **Med School:** NY Med Coll 1972; **Resid:** Psychiatry, NY Med-Metro Hosp, New York, NY 1972-1975; **Fellow:** U London, London, England 1975; **Fac Appt:** Prof Psychiatry, NYU Sch Med

Sunderland, Trey MD (GerPsy) - *Spec Exp:* Geriatric Psychiatry - General; **Hospital:** Natl Inst of Hlth - Clin Ctr; **Address:** Rm 3-N-218, MSC 1274, 10 Center Drive Bldg 10, Bethesda, MD 20892-1274; **Phone:** (301) 496-0948; **Board Cert:** Geriatric Psychiatry 1996, Psychiatry 1983; **Med School:** Geo Wash Univ 1978; **Resid:** Psychiatry, McLean Hosp, Belmont, MA 1979-1982; **Fellow:** Psychopharmacology, Natl Inst for Mental Hlth, Bethesda, MD 1982-1984

Southeast

Stein, Elliott MD (GerPsy) - *Spec Exp:* Geriatric Psychiatry - General; **Hospital:** Mount Sinai Med Ctr; **Address:** Mount Sinai Med Ctr, 4300 Alton Rd, Warner Bldg, Ste 360, Miami Beach, FL 33140; **Phone:** (305) 534-3636; **Board Cert:** Psychiatry 1979, Geriatric Psychiatry 1991; **Med School:** Univ Miami Sch Med 1973; **Resid:** Psychiatry, Herrick Meml Hosp, Berkerley, CA 1973-1976; **Fac Appt:** Adjct Prof Psychiatry, Univ Miami Sch Med

Midwest

Goldman, Samuel MD (GerPsy) - *Spec Exp:* Depression; Anxiety Disorders; Phobias; **Hospital:** Advocate Lutheran Gen Hosp; **Address:** Advocate Hlth Care, 401 S Milwaukee Ave, Ste 235, Wheeling, IL 60090; **Phone:** (312) 670-6444; **Board Cert:** Psychiatry 1982, Geriatric Psychiatry 1996; **Med School:** Univ Chicago-Pritzker Sch Med 1974; **Resid:** Psychiatry, Univ Chicago, Chicago, IL 1975-1978

Grossberg, George MD (GerPsy) - *Spec Exp:* Alzheimer's Disease; Depression; **Hospital:** St Louis Univ Hospital; **Address:** St Louis Univ Sch Med, Dept Psyc, 1221 S Grand Blvd, St Louis, MO 63104; **Phone:** (314) 577-8721; **Board Cert:** Psychiatry 1982, Geriatric Psychiatry 2001; **Med School:** St Louis Univ 1975; **Resid:** Psychiatry, St Louis Univ Med Ctr, St Louis, MO 1976-1979; **Fac Appt:** Prof Psychiatry, St Louis Univ

Isenberg, Keith Eugene MD (GerPsy) - *Spec Exp:* Alzheimer's Disease; Anxiety Disorders; **Hospital:** Barnes-Jewish Hosp (page 55); **Address:** 660 S Euclid Ave, Box 8134, St. Louis, MO 63110; **Phone:** (314) 362-1819; **Board Cert:** Geriatric Psychiatry 1994, Psychiatry 1984; **Med School:** Indiana Univ 1978; **Resid:** Psychiatry, Wash Univ/Barnes Hosp, St Louis, MO 1978-1982; **Fac Appt:** Psychiatry, Washington Univ, St Louis

Lazarus, Lawrence W MD (GerPsy) - *Spec Exp:* Obsessive-Compulsive Disorder; Anxiety Disorders; **Hospital:** Rush-Presby - St Luke's Med Ctr (page 72); **Address:** 2130 Lincoln Park W, Chicago, IL 60614; **Phone:** (773) 248-4948; **Board Cert:** Psychiatry 1974, Geriatric Psychiatry 1991; **Med School:** Hahnemann Univ 1967; **Resid:** Psychiatry, Michael Reese Hosp, Chicago, IL 1968-1971

Luchins, Daniel MD (GerPsy) - *Spec Exp:* Psychiatry-Geriatric; Mental Retardation; Dementia; **Hospital:** Univ of Chicago Hosps (page 76); **Address:** 5841 S Maryland Ave, MC 3077, Chicago, IL 60637-1463; **Phone:** (773) 702-9716; **Board Cert:** Psychiatry 1978, Geriatric Psychiatry 1992; **Med School:** Canada 1973; **Resid:** Psychiatry, Douglas Hosp, Montreal, Canada 1975; Psychiatry, St Mary's Hosp, Montreal, Canada 1976; **Fellow:** Psychiatry, Allan Meml Inst, Montreal, Canada 1976-1977; **Fac Appt:** Assoc Prof Psychiatry, Univ Chicago-Pritzker Sch Med

Mellow, Alan M. MD/PhD (GerPsy) - *Spec Exp:* Dementia; Depression; **Hospital:** Univ of MI Hlth Ctr; **Address:** University of Michigan Department of Psychiatry, 1500 E Med Ctr Drive, Ann Arbor, MI 48100-0704; **Phone:** (734) 930-5630; **Board Cert:** Psychiatry 1988, Geriatric Psychiatry 1991; **Med School:** Northwestern Univ 1981; **Resid:** Internal Medicine, Univ Chicago Hosp, Chicago, IL 1981-1982; Psychiatry, McLean Hosp-Harvard, Belmont, MA 1982-1985; **Fellow:** Psychiatry, Nat Inst Mental Health, Bethesda, MD 1985-1988; **Fac Appt:** Prof Psychiatry, Univ Mich Med Sch

West Coast and Pacific

Borson, Soo MD (GerPsy) - *Spec Exp:* Alzheimer's Disease; Psychiatry in Chronic Medical Illness; Psychiatry-Geriatric; **Hospital:** Univ WA Med Ctr; **Address:** 4245 Roosevelt Way NE, Box 354760, Seattle, WA 98105; **Phone:** (206) 598-8750; **Board Cert:** Psychiatry 1985, Geriatric Psychiatry 1991; **Med School:** Stanford Univ 1969; **Resid:** Psychiatry, Univ Wash, Seattle, WA 1977-1979; **Fellow:** Geriatric Psychiatry, Univ Wash, Seattle, WA 1979-1981; **Fac Appt:** Prof Psychiatry, Univ Wash

Friedman, Barry MD (GerPsy) - *Spec Exp:* Psychopharmacology; **Hospital:** Cedars-Sinai Med Ctr; **Address:** 435 N Bedford Dr, Ste 112, Beverly Hills, CA 90210; **Phone:** (310) 274-4372; **Board Cert:** Geriatric Psychiatry 1995, Psychiatry 1974; **Med School:** UCSF 1965; **Resid:** Neurology, UCLA, Los Angeles, CA 1968-1971; Psychiatry, UCLA, Los Angeles, CA 1968-1971; **Fac Appt:** Assoc Clin Prof Psychiatry, UCLA

Kramer, Barry Alan MD (GerPsy) - *Spec Exp:* Electroconvulsive Therapy (ECT); Depression; **Hospital:** Cedars-Sinai Med Ctr; **Address:** Cedars-Sinai Med Ctr, Dept Psyc, 8730 Alden Drive, rm W-223, Los Angeles, CA 90048; **Phone:** (310) 423-4014; **Board Cert:** Psychiatry 1978, Geriatric Psychiatry 1991; **Med School:** Hahnemann Univ 1974; **Resid:** Psychiatry, Montefiore Hosp& Medical Ctr, Bronx, NY 1974-1978; **Fellow:** Geriatric Psychiatry, UCLA-USC Long Term Gero Ctr, Los Angeles, CA 1985-1986

Leuchter, Andrew Francis MD (GerPsy) - *Spec Exp:* Depression; **Hospital:** UCLA Neuropsychiatric Hosp; **Address:** 760 Westwood Plaza, rm 37430, Los Angeles, CA 90024-8300; **Phone:** (310) 825-0207; **Board Cert:** Psychiatry 1986, Geriatric Psychiatry 1991; **Med School:** Baylor Coll Med 1980; **Resid:** Psychiatry, UCLA - NPI&H, Los Angeles, CA 1981-1984; **Fellow:** Geriatric Psychiatry, UCLA, Los Angeles, CA 1984-1986; **Fac Appt:** Assoc Prof Psychiatry, UCLA

Schneider, Lon S MD (GerPsy) - *Spec Exp:* Alzheimer's Disease; Depression; Psychopharmacology; **Hospital:** USC Univ Hosp - R K Eamer Med Plz; **Address:** 1975 Zonal Ave, Bldg KAM-400, , Los Angeles, CA 90033; **Phone:** (323) 442-3715; **Board Cert:** Psychiatry 1984, Geriatric Psychiatry 1991; **Med School:** Hahnemann Univ 1978; **Resid:** Psychiatry, USC Sch Med, Los Angeles, CA 1979-1982; **Fellow:** Geriatric Psychiatry, USC Sch Med, Los Angeles, CA 1982-1983; **Fac Appt:** Prof Geriatric Psychiatry, USC Sch Med

Small, Gary William MD (GerPsy) - *Spec Exp:* Dementia; **Hospital:** UCLA Med Ctr; **Address:** UCLA, Neuropsych Inst, 760 Westwood Plaza, 88-201 NPI, Los Angeles, CA 90024-1759; **Phone:** (310) 825-0291; **Board Cert:** Psychiatry 1983, Geriatric Psychiatry 1991; **Med School:** USC Sch Med 1977; **Resid:** Psychiatry, Mass Genl Hosp, Boston, MA 1978-1981; **Fellow:** Psychiatry, UCLA Med Ctr, Los Angeles, CA 1981-1983; **Fac Appt:** Prof Psychiatry, UCLA

Veith, Richard MD (GerPsy) - *Spec Exp:* Depression in Cardiovascular Disease; Elderly Cardiovascular Affects; **Hospital:** Univ WA Med Ctr; **Address:** BB-1644 UW Health Sciences Center, Box 356560, Seattle, WA 98195; **Phone:** (206) 543-3752; **Board Cert:** Psychiatry 1979, Geriatric Psychiatry 1991; **Med School:** Univ Wash 1973; **Resid:** Psychiatry, Univ Washington, Seattle, WA 1974-1977; **Fac Appt:** Prof Psychiatry, Univ Wash

PSYCHIATRY

Baldessarini, Ross MD (Psyc) - *Spec Exp:* Bipolar/Mood Disorders; Schizophrenia; Psychotic Disorders; **Hospital:** McLean Hosp; **Address:** McLean Hosp, Mailman Rsch Ctr, 115 Mill St, Belmont, MA 02478; **Phone:** (617) 855-3203; **Board Cert:** Psychiatry 1972; **Med School:** Johns Hopkins Univ 1963; **Resid:** Psychiatry, Johns Hopkins Hosp, Baltimore, MD 1966-1969; **Fellow:** Natl Inst Mental Hlth 1964-1966; **Fac Appt:** Prof Psychiatry, Harvard Med Sch

Bowers Jr, Malcolm B MD (Psyc) - *Spec Exp:* Schizophrenia; Psychopharmacology; **Hospital:** Yale - New Haven Hosp; **Address:** Yale Univ Hosp, Dept Psyc, 25 Park St, New Haven, CT 06519-1110; **Phone:** (203) 785-2121; **Board Cert:** Psychiatry 1970; **Med School:** Washington Univ, St Louis 1958; **Resid:** Psychiatry, Yale-New Haven Hosp, New Haven, CT 1962-1965; **Fellow:** Psychiatry, Yale-New Haven Hosp, New Haven, CT 1963-1964; **Fac Appt:** Prof Psychiatry, Yale Univ

Cohen, Bruce M MD (Psyc) - *Spec Exp:* Psychopharmacology; **Hospital:** McLean Hosp; **Address:** 115 Mill St, Belmont, MA 02478; **Phone:** (617) 855-3227; **Board Cert:** Psychiatry 1979; **Med School:** Case West Res Univ 1975; **Resid:** Psychiatry, McLean Hospital, Belmont, MA 1975-1978; **Fac Appt:** Prof Psychiatry, Harvard Med Sch

Herman, John Benjamin MD (Psyc) - *Spec Exp:* Psychiatry - General; **Hospital:** MA Genl Hosp; **Address:** 55 Fruit St, Bldg Bulfinch 351, Boston, MA 02114-3139; **Phone:** (617) 726-2972; **Board Cert:** Psychiatry 1987; **Med School:** Univ Wisc 1980; **Resid:** Psychiatry, Mass Genl Hosp., Boston, MA 1981-1984; **Fac Appt:** Asst Prof Psychiatry, Harvard Med Sch

Hobson, John Allan MD (Psyc) - *Spec Exp:* Sleep Disorders/Apnea; **Hospital:** MA Mental Hlth Ctr; **Address:** 74 Fenwood Rd, Boston, MA 02115-6106; **Phone:** (617) 734-9645; **Board Cert:** Psychiatry 1968; **Med School:** Harvard Med Sch 1959; **Resid:** Psychiatry, Mass Mental Hlth Ctr, Boston, MA 1960-1961; Psychiatry, NIMH, Bethesda, MD 1961-1963; **Fellow:** Clinical Neurophysiology, Univ Lyon, France 1963-1964; **Fac Appt:** Prof Psychiatry, Harvard Med Sch

Jenike, Michael Andrew MD (Psyc) - *Spec Exp:* Obsessive-Compulsive Disorder; Psychiatry-Geriatric; **Hospital:** MA Genl Hosp; **Address:** Obsessive Compulsive Disorders Unit, 149 13th St, CYN-149, Charlestown, MA 02129; **Phone:** (617) 726-2998; **Board Cert:** Psychiatry 1984; **Med School:** Univ Okla Coll Med 1978; **Resid:** Psychiatry, Mass Genl Hosp, Boston, MA 1979-1982; **Fellow:** Psychiatry, Harvard Med Sch, Cambridge, MA 1982; Psychiatry, Mass Genl Hosp, Boston, MA 1983; **Fac Appt:** Prof Psychiatry, Harvard Med Sch

McGlashan, Thomas MD (Psyc) - *Spec Exp:* Schizophrenia; Personality Disorders-Borderline; **Hospital:** Yale - New Haven Hosp; **Address:** Dept Psychiatry, 301 Cedar St Fl 2, New Haven, CT 06519; **Phone:** (203) 785-7210; **Board Cert:** Psychiatry 1973; **Med School:** Univ Penn 1967; **Resid:** Psychiatry, Mass Mental Hlth Ctr, Boston, MA 1968-1971; **Fac Appt:** Prof Psychiatry, Yale Univ

Nelson, J Craig MD (Psyc) - *Spec Exp:* Psychiatry-Geriatric; Psychopharmacology; Mood Disorders; **Hospital:** Yale - New Haven Hosp; **Address:** 20 York St, New Haven, CT 06504; **Phone:** (203) 688-9893; **Board Cert:** Geriatric Psychiatry 1992, Psychiatry 1974; **Med School:** Univ Wisc 1968; **Resid:** Psychiatry, Yale-New Haven Hosp, New Haven, CT 1969-1970; Psychiatry, Yale-New Haven Hosp, New Haven, CT 1973-1974; **Fac Appt:** Prof Psychiatry, Yale Univ

Pitman, Roger Keith MD (Psyc) - *Spec Exp:* Post-Traumatic Stress Disorder; **Hospital:** MA Genl Hosp; **Address:** Post-Traumatic Stress Disorder Research Lab, 13th St Bldg 149, Charlestown, MA 02129; **Phone:** (617) 726-5333; **Board Cert:** Psychiatry 1975; **Med School:** Univ VT Coll Med 1969; **Resid:** Psychiatry, Tufts Univ Hosp, Boston, MA 1970-1973; **Fellow:** Behavioral Neurology, Beth Israel Hosp/Harvard, Boston, MA 1985; **Fac Appt:** Asst Prof Psychiatry, Harvard Med Sch

Pope Jr, Harrison G MD (Psyc) - *Spec Exp:* Addiction/Substance Abuse; *Psychopharmacology;* **Hospital:** McLean Hosp; **Address:** McLean Hosp, Dept Psyc, 115 Mill St, Belmont, MA 02478; **Phone:** (617) 855-2911; **Board Cert:** Psychiatry 1980; **Med School:** Harvard Med Sch 1974; **Resid:** Psychiatry, McLean Hosp, Belmont, MA 1974-1977; **Fac Appt:** Prof Psychiatry, Harvard Med Sch

Rasmussen, Steven A MD (Psyc) - *Spec Exp:* Obsessive-Compulsive Disorder; **Hospital:** Butler Hosp; **Address:** Butler Hospital, 345 Blackstone Blvd, Providence, RI 02906-7010; **Phone:** (401) 455-6209; **Board Cert:** Psychiatry 1983; **Med School:** Brown Univ 1977; **Resid:** Psychiatry, Yale U, New Haven, CT 1977-1981; **Fac Appt:** Assoc Prof Psychiatry, Brown Univ

Rosenbaum, Jerrold Frank MD (Psyc) - *Spec Exp:* Anxiety & Mood Disorders; **Hospital:** MA Genl Hosp; **Address:** 15 Parkman St, Ste WAC 812, Boston, MA 02114; **Phone:** (617) 726-3482; **Board Cert:** Psychiatry 1978; **Med School:** Yale Univ 1973; **Resid:** Psychiatry, Mass Genl Hosp, Boston, MA 1974-1977; **Fac Appt:** Prof Psychiatry, Harvard Med Sch

van der Kolk, Bessel MD (Psyc) - *Spec Exp:* Post Traumatic Stress Disorder; Child Abuse; **Hospital:** Boston Med Ctr; **Address:** 16 Braddock Park, Boston, MA 02116-5804; **Phone:** (617) 247-3918; **Board Cert:** Psychiatry 1976; **Med School:** Univ Chicago-Pritzker Sch Med 1970; **Resid:** Psychiatry, Harvard Med Sch, Boston, MA 1971-1974; **Fac Appt:** Prof Psychiatry, Boston Univ

Yonkers, Kimberly A MD (Psyc) - *Spec Exp:* Anxiety & Mood Disorders; Premenstrual Dysphoric Disorder; **Hospital:** Yale - New Haven Hosp; **Address:** 142 Temple St, Ste 301, New Haven, CT 06510; **Phone:** (203) 764-6621; **Board Cert:** Psychiatry 1991; **Med School:** Columbia P&S 1986; **Resid:** Psychiatry, McLean Hosp- Harvard, Belmont, MA 1987-1990; **Fellow:** Psychiatry, McLean Hosp-Harvard, Belmont, MA 1990-1992; **Fac Appt:** Assoc Prof Psychiatry, Yale Univ

Mid Atlantic

Alexopoulos, George MD (Psyc) - *Spec Exp:* Psychiatry-Geriatric; Depression; *Psychopharmacology;* **Hospital:** NY Presby Hosp - NY Weill Cornell Med Ctr (page 70); **Address:** 21 Bloomingdale Rd, White Plains, NY 10605; **Phone:** (914) 997-5767; **Board Cert:** Psychiatry 1978, Geriatric Psychiatry 1992; **Med School:** Greece 1970; **Resid:** Psychiatry, UMDNJ Univ Hosp, Newark, NJ 1974-1976; Psychiatry, NY Hosp-Cornell Univ, White Plains, NY 1976-1977; **Fellow:** Biological Psychiatry, NY Hosp-Cornell Med Ctr, New York, NY 1977-1978; **Fac Appt:** Prof Psychiatry, Cornell Univ-Weill Med Coll

Boronow, John Joseph MD (Psyc) - *Spec Exp:* Psychotic Disorders; Schizophrenia; **Hospital:** Sheppard Pratt Hlth Sys; **Address:** 6501 N Charles St, Towson, MD 21204; **Phone:** (410) 938-4306; **Board Cert:** Psychiatry 1983; **Med School:** Yale Univ 1977; **Resid:** Psychiatry, NY Hosp-Cornell Med Ctr, New York, NY 1978-1981; **Fellow:** Psychopharmacology, Natl Inst Mntl Hlth, Bethesda, MD 1981-1983

Breitbart, William MD (Psyc) - *Spec Exp:* Pain-Cancer; AIDS/HIV; Palliative Care; **Hospital:** Mem Sloan Kettering Cancer Ctr; **Address:** Meml Sloan Kettering Cancer Ctr-Counseling Ctr, 1246 2nd Ave, New York, NY 10021-6804; **Phone:** (212) 639-4770; **Board Cert:** Internal Medicine 1982, Psychiatry 1986; **Med School:** Albert Einstein Coll Med 1978; **Resid:** Internal Medicine, Bronx Muni Hosp Ctr, Bronx, NY 1980-1982; Psychiatry, Bronx Muni Hosp Ctr, Bronx, NY 1982-1984; **Fellow:** Psychiatric Oncology, Meml Sloan Kettering Cancer Ctr, New York, NY 1984-1986; **Fac Appt:** Prof Psychiatry, Cornell Univ-Weill Med Coll

Cancro, Robert MD (Psyc) - *Spec Exp:* Schizophrenia; Depression; **Hospital:** NYU Med Ctr (page 71); **Address:** 550 1st Ave, New York, NY 10016-6402; **Phone:** (212) 263-6214; **Board Cert:** Psychiatry 1962; **Med School:** SUNY Hlth Sci Ctr 1955; **Resid:** Psychiatry, Kings County Hosp, Brooklyn, NY 1956-1959; **Fac Appt:** Prof Psychiatry, NYU Sch Med

Carpenter Jr, William T MD (Psyc) - *Spec Exp:* Schizophrenia; **Hospital:** Maryland Psyc Research Ctr; **Address:** Maryland Psychiatric Rsch Ctr, Univ MD Sch Med, Box 21247, Baltimore, MD 21228-0747; **Phone:** (410) 402-7101; **Board Cert:** Psychiatry 1972; **Med School:** Wake Forest Univ Sch Med 1962; **Resid:** Psychiatry, Strong Meml Hosp-Univ Roch, Rochester, NY 1963-1966; **Fac Appt:** Prof Psychiatry, Univ MD Sch Med

Davis, Kenneth MD (Psyc) - *Spec Exp:* Alzheimer's Disease; Schizophrenia; **Hospital:** Mount Sinai Hosp (page 68); **Address:** Mount Sinai Sch Med, Dept Psychiatry, 1 Gustave Levy Pl, New York, NY 10029-6504; **Phone:** (212) 659-8760; **Board Cert:** Psychiatry 1980; **Med School:** Mount Sinai Sch Med 1973; **Resid:** Psychiatry, Stanford Med Ctr, Stanford, CA 1973-1976; **Fac Appt:** Prof Psychiatry, Mount Sinai Sch Med

DePaulo, Jr, J Raymond MD (Psyc) - *Spec Exp:* Mood Disorders; Depression; **Hospital:** Johns Hopkins Hosp - Baltimore; **Address:** Johns Hopkins Hosp, Dept Psyc, 601 N Wolfe St, Bldg Meyer 3-181, Baltimore, MD 21287-7381; **Phone:** (410) 955-3246; **Board Cert:** Psychiatry 1977; **Med School:** Johns Hopkins Univ 1972; **Resid:** Psychiatry, Johns Hopkins, Baltimore, MD 1974-1977; **Fac Appt:** Prof Psychiatry, Johns Hopkins Univ

Eth, Spencer MD (Psyc) - *Spec Exp:* Forensic Psychiatry; Depression-Postpartum; **Hospital:** St Vincent Cath Med Ctrs - Manhattan (page 75); **Address:** 144 W 12th St, rm 174, New York, NY 10011-8202; **Phone:** (212) 604-8196; **Board Cert:** Psychiatry 1980, Forensic Psychiatry 1994; **Med School:** UCLA 1976; **Resid:** Psychiatry, NY Cornell Med Ctr, New York, NY 1976-1979; **Fellow:** Child & Adolescent Psychiatry, Cedars -Sinai Med Ctr, Los Angeles, CA 1979-1981; **Fac Appt:** Prof Psychiatry, NY Med Coll

Ganguli, Rohan MD (Psyc) - *Spec Exp:* Schizophrenia; **Hospital:** Western Psy Inst & Clin; **Address:** UPMC-Western Psyc Inst & Clin, 3811 O'Hara St, Pittsburgh, PA 15213; **Phone:** (412) 624-1103; **Board Cert:** Psychiatry 1980; **Med School:** India 1973; **Resid:** Psychiatry, Meml Univ, New Foundland, Canada 1975-1978; Psychiatry, Univ Pitts Med Ctr, Pittsburgh, PA 1978; **Fac Appt:** Prof Psychiatry, Univ Pittsburgh

Gorman, Jack Matthew MD (Psyc) - *Spec Exp:* Panic Disorder/Anxiety Disorders; Schizophrenia; **Hospital:** NY State Psychiatric Inst; **Address:** 1051 Riverside Drive, Unit 32, New York, NY 10032; **Phone:** (212) 543-5000; **Board Cert:** Psychiatry 1982; **Med School:** Columbia P&S 1977; **Resid:** Psychiatry, Columbia-Presby Med Ctr, New York, NY 1978-1980; **Fellow:** Psychopharmacology, Columbia-Presby Med Ctr, New York, NY 1980-1982; **Fac Appt:** Prof Psychiatry, Columbia P&S

Halmi, Katherine MD (Psyc) - *Spec Exp:* *Eating Disorders;* **Hospital:** NY Presby Hosp - Westchester Div; **Address:** 21 Bloomingdale Rd, White Plains, NY 10605; **Phone:** (914) 997-5875; **Board Cert:** Pediatrics 1970, Psychiatry 1977; **Med School:** Univ Iowa Coll Med 1965; **Resid:** Pediatrics, Univ Iowa Hosp, Iowa City, IA 1967-1968; Psychiatry, Univ Iowa Hosp, Iowa City, IA 1969-1972; **Fellow:** Child Development, Univ Iowa Hosp, Iowa City, IA 1969; **Fac Appt:** Prof Psychiatry, Cornell Univ-Weill Med Coll

Hendin, Herbert MD (Psyc) - *Spec Exp:* *Suicide; Post Traumatic Stress Disorder; Depression;* **Hospital:** Westchester Med Ctr (page 82); **Address:** 1045 Park Ave, Ste 3C, New York, NY 10028; **Phone:** (212) 348-4035; **Board Cert:** Psychiatry 1955; **Med School:** NYU Sch Med 1949; **Resid:** Psychiatry, Bellevue Hosp, New York, NY 1950-1952; Psychiatry, VA Med Ctr, New York, NY 1952-1953; **Fellow:** Psychiatry, Bellevue Hosp, New York, NY 1953-1956

Holland, Jimmie C B MD (Psyc) - *Spec Exp:* *Psychiatry of Cancer; Bereavement;* **Hospital:** Mem Sloan Kettering Cancer Ctr; **Address:** Dept Psyc & Behav Sci, 1242 Second Ave, Box 421, New York, NY 10021-6804; **Phone:** (212) 639-3904; **Board Cert:** Psychiatry 1967; **Med School:** Baylor Coll Med 1952; **Resid:** Psychiatry, Mass Genl Hosp, Boston, MA 1955; Psychiatry, EJ Meyer Meml Hosp, Buffalo, NY 1956-1957; **Fac Appt:** Prof Psychiatry, Cornell Univ-Weill Med Coll

Hollander, Eric MD (Psyc) - *Spec Exp:* *Obsessive-Compulsive Disorder; Anxiety Disorders;* **Hospital:** Mount Sinai Hosp (page 68); **Address:** 300 Central Park West, Ste 1C, New York, NY 10024-1513; **Phone:** (212) 873-4051; **Board Cert:** Psychiatry 1987; **Med School:** SUNY Hlth Sci Ctr 1982; **Resid:** Internal Medicine, Mount Sinai Hosp, New York, NY 1982-1983; Psychiatry, Mount Sinai Hosp, New York, NY 1983-1986; **Fellow:** Psychiatry, Columbia-Presby Med Ctr, New York, NY 1986-1988; **Fac Appt:** Prof Psychiatry, Mount Sinai Sch Med

Kavey, Neil B MD (Psyc) - *Spec Exp:* *Narcolepsy; Sleep Disorders;* **Hospital:** NY Presby Hosp - Columbia Presby Med Ctr (page 70); **Address:** Columbia Presby Med Ctr, Sleep Disorders Ctr, 161 Ft Washington Ave, New York, NY 10032; **Phone:** (212) 305-1860; **Board Cert:** Psychiatry 1976; **Med School:** Columbia P&S 1969; **Resid:** Psychiatry, Columbia Presby Med Ctr, New York, NY 1970-1973; **Fac Appt:** Clin Prof Psychiatry, Columbia P&S

Klagsbrun, Samuel C MD (Psyc) - *Spec Exp:* *Cancer; Terminal Illness;* **Hospital:** Four Winds Hosp; **Address:** Four Winds Hospital, 800 Cross River Rd, Katonah, NY 10536; **Phone:** (914) 763-8151; **Board Cert:** Psychiatry 1977; **Med School:** Univ Hlth Sci/Chicago Med Sch 1962; **Resid:** Psychiatry, Yale-New Haven Hosp, New Haven, CT 1963-1966; **Fac Appt:** Clin Prof Psychiatry, Albert Einstein Coll Med

Klein, Donald MD (Psyc) - *Spec Exp:* *Psychopharmacology; Depression; Anxiety Disorders;* **Hospital:** NY Presby Hosp - Columbia Presby Med Ctr (page 70); **Address:** 182 E 79th St, New York, NY 10021-0422; **Phone:** (212) 737-4166; **Board Cert:** Psychiatry 1959; **Med School:** SUNY Hlth Sci Ctr 1952; **Resid:** Psychiatry, Creedmoor State Hosp, Queens Village, NY 1953-1954; **Fac Appt:** Prof Psychiatry, Columbia P&S

Kupfer, David J. MD (Psyc) - *Spec Exp:* *Bipolar/Mood Disorders; Sleep Disorders/Apnea;* **Hospital:** Western Psy Inst & Clin; **Address:** Western Psychiatric Inst & Clin, 3811 O'Hara St, Pittsburgh, PA 15213; **Phone:** (412) 624-2353; **Board Cert:** Psychiatry 1978; **Med School:** Yale Univ 1965; **Resid:** Psychiatry, Yale-New Haven Hosp, New Haven, CT 1969-1970; Psychiatry, Natl Inst Mental Hlth, Bethesda, MD 1967-1969; **Fellow:** Psychiatry, Yale-New Haven Hosp, New Haven, CT 1966-1967; **Fac Appt:** Prof Psychiatry, Univ Pittsburgh

Lederberg, Marguerite MD (Psyc) - *Spec Exp:* Psychiatry of Cancer; **Hospital:** Mem Sloan Kettering Cancer Ctr; **Address:** 1242 2nd Ave, New York, NY 10021; **Phone:** (212) 639-3911; **Board Cert:** Pediatrics 1970, Psychiatry 1980; **Med School:** Yale Univ 1961; **Resid:** Pediatrics, Stanford Med Ctr, Stanford, CA 1962-1964; Psychiatry, Stanford Med Ctr, Stanford, CA 1972-1977; **Fellow:** Ambulatory Pediatrics, Stanford Med Ctr, Stanford, CA 1964-1968; **Fac Appt:** Clin Prof Psychiatry, Cornell Univ-Weill Med Coll

Liebowitz, Michael R MD (Psyc) - *Spec Exp:* Depression; Anxiety Disorders; **Hospital:** NY Presby Hosp - Columbia Presby Med Ctr (page 70); **Address:** 10 E 90th St, Ste 1A, New York, NY 10028; **Phone:** (212) 543-5366; **Board Cert:** Psychiatry 1978; **Med School:** Yale Univ 1969; **Resid:** Psychiatry, Med Ctr Hosp VT, Burlington, VT 1974-1975; Psychiatry, NY State Psyc Inst, New York, NY 1975-1977; **Fellow:** Psychiatry, NY State Psyc Inst, New York, NY 1977-1979; **Fac Appt:** Prof Psychiatry, Columbia P&S

Loewenstein, Richard MD (Psyc) - *Spec Exp:* Trauma Psychiatry; Dissociative Disorders; **Hospital:** Sheppard Pratt Hlth Sys; **Address:** 6501 N Charles St, Box 6815, Baltimore, MD 21204; **Phone:** (410) 938-5070; **Board Cert:** Psychiatry 1980; **Med School:** Yale Univ 1975; **Resid:** Psychiatry, Yale, New Haven, CT 1976-1979; **Fellow:** NIH,NIMH-Biol Psych Br, Bethesda, MD 1980-1982; **Fac Appt:** Assoc Clin Prof Psychiatry, Univ MD Sch Med

Manevitz, Alan MD (Psyc) - *Spec Exp:* Relationship Problems; Psychopharmacology; **Hospital:** NY Presby Hosp - NY Weill Cornell Med Ctr (page 70); **Address:** 60 Sutton Place South, Ste 1CN, New York, NY 10022; **Phone:** (212) 751-5072; **Board Cert:** Psychiatry 1987; **Med School:** Columbia P&S 1980; **Resid:** Psychiatry, NY Hosp, New York, NY 1980-1981; Psychiatry, NY Hosp, New York, NY 1981-1984; **Fellow:** Psychopharmacology, NY Hosp, New York, NY 1984-1985; **Fac Appt:** Assoc Clin Prof Psychiatry, Cornell Univ-Weill Med Coll

Marin, Deborah B MD (Psyc) - *Spec Exp:* Alzheimer's Disease; **Hospital:** Mount Sinai Hosp (page 68); **Address:** 1 Gustave Levy Pl, Box 1230, New York, NY 10029; **Phone:** (212) 659-8840; **Board Cert:** Psychiatry 1990; **Med School:** Mount Sinai Sch Med 1984; **Resid:** Psychiatry, Mount Sinai Hosp, New York, NY 1984-1988; **Fellow:** Psychiatry, NY Hosp-Cornell Med Ctr, New York, NY 1988-1991; **Fac Appt:** Assoc Prof Psychiatry, Mount Sinai Sch Med

McCann, Merle Clements MD (Psyc) - *Spec Exp:* Psychiatry - General; **Hospital:** Sheppard Pratt Hlth Sys; **Address:** Sheppard & Enoch Pratt Hosp, 6501 N Charles St, Baltimore, MD 21285; **Phone:** (410) 938-3000; **Board Cert:** Psychiatry 1986; **Med School:** Med Coll VA 1981; **Resid:** Psychiatry, Geo Wash Univ Hosp, Washington, DC 1982-1985; **Fac Appt:** Asst Clin Prof Psychiatry, Univ MD Sch Med

McHugh, Paul MD (Psyc) - *Spec Exp:* Neuro-Psychiatry; Huntington's Disease; **Hospital:** Johns Hopkins Hosp - Baltimore; **Address:** Johns Hopkins Hosp, 600 N Wolfe St, Meyer Bldg, rm 4-113, Baltimore, MD 21287-7413; **Phone:** (410) 955-3130; **Board Cert:** Neurology 1967, Psychiatry 1968; **Med School:** Harvard Med Sch 1956; **Resid:** Neurology, Mass Genl Hosp, Boston, MA 1957-1960; Psychiatry, Maudsley Hosp, London, England 1960-1961; **Fac Appt:** Prof Psychiatry, Johns Hopkins Univ

Pearlson, Godfrey D MD (Psyc) - *Spec Exp:* Schizophrenia; Psychiatric Neuro-Imaging; **Hospital:** Johns Hopkins Hosp - Baltimore; **Address:** Johns Hopkins Hospital, 600 N Wolfe St, Meyer Bldg, rm 3-166, Baltimore, MD 21287-7362; **Phone:** (410) 955-5135; **Board Cert:** Psychiatry 1980; **Med School:** England 1974; **Resid:** Psychiatry, Johns Hopkins Hosp, Baltimore, MD 1975-1978; **Fac Appt:** Prof Psychiatry, Johns Hopkins Univ

Rosse, Richard B MD (Psyc) - *Spec Exp:* Psychiatry - General; **Hospital:** VA Medical Center - Washington; **Address:** 50 Irving St NW, Ste 3A154, Washington, DC 20422-0001; **Phone:** (202) 745-8156; **Board Cert:** Psychiatry 1986; **Med School:** Univ MD Sch Med 1980; **Resid:** Psychiatry, Georgetown Univ Med Ctr, Washington, DC 1981-1984; **Fac Appt:** Assoc Prof Psychiatry, Georgetown Univ

Sadock, Benjamin MD (Psyc) - *Spec Exp:* Anxiety Disorders; Depression; Sexual Dysfunction; **Hospital:** NYU Med Ctr (page 71); **Address:** 4 E 89th St, rm 1E, New York, NY 10128-0656; **Phone:** (212) 263-6210; **Board Cert:** Psychiatry 1966; **Med School:** NY Med Coll 1959; **Resid:** Psychiatry, Bellevue Psyc Hosp, New York, NY 1960-1963; **Fac Appt:** Prof Psychiatry, NYU Sch Med

Sadock, Virginia MD (Psyc) - *Spec Exp:* Psychotherapy; Sexual Dysfunction; **Hospital:** NYU Med Ctr (page 71); **Address:** 4 E 89th St, New York, NY 10128; **Phone:** (212) 427-0885; **Board Cert:** Psychiatry 1975; **Med School:** NY Med Coll 1970; **Resid:** Psychiatry, NY Metropolitan Hosp, New York, NY 1970-1973; **Fac Appt:** Clin Prof Psychiatry, NYU Sch Med

Samberg, Eslee MD (Psyc) - *Spec Exp:* Psychoanalysis; **Hospital:** NY Presby Hosp - NY Weill Cornell Med Ctr (page 70); **Address:** 2211 Broadway, Ste 1DS, New York, NY 10024-6263; **Phone:** (212) 874-7725; **Board Cert:** Psychiatry 1983; **Med School:** Cornell Univ-Weill Med Coll 1978; **Resid:** Psychiatry, NY Hosp-Cornell Med Ctr, New York, NY 1979-1982; **Fac Appt:** Asst Clin Prof Psychiatry, Cornell Univ-Weill Med Coll

Shear, Mary Katherine MD (Psyc) - *Spec Exp:* Panic Disorder & Agoraphobia; Anxiety Disorders; Bereavement/Traumatic Grief; **Hospital:** UPMC - Presbyterian Univ Hosp; **Address:** 772 Bellfield Towers, 3811 O'Hara St, Pittsburgh, PA 15213; **Phone:** (412) 624-1340; **Board Cert:** Psychiatry 1981, Internal Medicine 1975; **Med School:** Tufts Univ 1972; **Resid:** Internal Medicine, Mt Sinai Hosp, New York, NY 1972-1976; Psychiatry, Payne Whitney Clin, New York, NY 1976-1979; **Fellow:** Psychosomatic Medicine, Montefiore Hosp, Bronx, NY 1979-1980; **Fac Appt:** Prof Psychiatry, Univ Pittsburgh

Simon, Robert Isaac MD (Psyc) - *Spec Exp:* Forensic Psychiatry; **Hospital:** Suburban Hosp - Bethesda; **Address:** 7921-D Glenbrook Rd, Bethesda, MD 20814; **Phone:** (301) 652-0010; **Board Cert:** Forensic Psychiatry 1994, Psychiatry 1969; **Med School:** Tufts Univ 1960; **Resid:** Psychiatry, Jackson Mem Hosp, Miami, FL 1963-1966; **Fac Appt:** Prof Psychiatry, Georgetown Univ

Stinnett, James MD (Psyc) - *Spec Exp:* Psychiatry - General; **Hospital:** Hosp Univ Penn (page 78); **Address:** Bldg Founders Fl 10 - rm 10.017, 3400 Spruce St, Philadelphia, PA 19104; **Phone:** (215) 662-2815; **Board Cert:** Psychiatry 1972; **Med School:** Univ Penn 1965; **Resid:** Psychiatry, Hosp Univ Penn, Philadelphia, PA 1965-1970; **Fac Appt:** Prof Psychiatry, Univ Penn

Stone, Michael H MD (Psyc) - *Spec Exp:* Personality Disorders; Psychoanalysis; Forensic Psychiatry; **Hospital:** NY Presby Hosp - Columbia Presby Med Ctr (page 70); **Address:** 225 Central Park West, Ste 114, New York, NY 10024; **Phone:** (212) 758-2000; **Board Cert:** Psychiatry 1971; **Med School:** Cornell Univ-Weill Med Coll 1958; **Resid:** Internal Medicine, Bellevue Hosp, New York, NY 1959-1961; Psychiatry, NYS Psych Inst, New York, NY 1963-1966; **Fellow:** Hematology, Meml Sloan Kettering Cancer Ctr, New York, NY 1961-1962; Medical Oncology, Meml Sloan Kettering Cancer Ctr, New York, NY 1962-1963; **Fac Appt:** Clin Prof Psychiatry, Columbia P&S

Sussman, Norman MD (Psyc) - *Spec Exp:* Psychopharmacology; Anxiety & Mood Disorders; **Hospital:** NYU Med Ctr (page 71); **Address:** 150 E 58th, Fl 27, New York, NY 10155; **Phone:** (212) 588-9722; **Board Cert:** Psychiatry 1980; **Med School:** NY Med Coll 1975; **Resid:** Psychiatry, Metropolitan Hosp Ctr, New York, NY 1975-1977; Psychiatry, Westchester Co Med Ctr, Westchester, NY 1977-1978; **Fac Appt:** Clin Prof Psychiatry, NYU Sch Med

Thase, Michael E MD (Psyc) - *Spec Exp:* Anxiety & Mood Disorders; Psychopharmocology; **Hospital:** UPMC - Presbyterian Univ Hosp; **Address:** 3811 O'Hara St, Pittsburgh, PA 15213; **Phone:** (412) 624-5070; **Board Cert:** Psychiatry 1984; **Med School:** Ohio State Univ 1979; **Resid:** Psychiatry, Western Psych Inst Clin, Pittsburgh, PA 1980-1983; **Fellow:** Research, Univ Pitts Sch Med, Pittsburgh, PA 1982-1984; **Fac Appt:** Prof Psychiatry, Univ Pittsburgh

Wait, Susan Braynard MD (Psyc) - *Spec Exp:* Post Traumatic Stress Disorder; Dissociative Disorders; **Hospital:** Sheppard Pratt Hlth Sys; **Address:** Sheppard Pratt Hlth System, 6501 N Charles St, Baltimore, MD 21285-6815; **Phone:** (410) 938-5076; **Board Cert:** Psychiatry 1993; **Med School:** Med Coll PA Hahnemann 1987; **Resid:** Psychiatry, Sheppard Pratt Hosp, Baltimore, MD 1987-1991; **Fac Appt:** Prof Psychiatry, Univ MD Sch Med

Walsh, B Timothy MD (Psyc) - *Spec Exp:* Eating Disorders; **Hospital:** NY State Psychiatric Inst; **Address:** NYS Psyc Inst-Unit 98, 1051 Riverside Dr, New York, NY 10032; **Phone:** (212) 543-5752; **Board Cert:** Psychiatry 1978; **Med School:** Harvard Med Sch 1972; **Resid:** Psychiatry, Bronx Muni Hosp Ctr, Bronx, NY 1974-1977; **Fac Appt:** Prof Psychiatry, Columbia P&S

Southeast

Ballenger, James MD (Psyc) - *Spec Exp:* Anxiety & Mood Disorders; Forensic Psychiatry; **Hospital:** Med Univ Hosp Authority; **Address:** Med Univ SC, Dept Psyc, 67 President St, Box 250861, Charleston, SC 29425; **Phone:** (843) 792-7693; **Board Cert:** Psychiatry 1977, Forensic Psychiatry 1999; **Med School:** Duke Univ 1970; **Resid:** Psychiatry, Mass Genl Hosp-Harvard, Boston, MA 1971-1974; **Fac Appt:** Prof Psychiatry, Med Univ SC

Blazer II, Dan G MD/PhD (Psyc) - *Spec Exp:* Psychiatry-Geriatric; Mood Disorders; **Hospital:** Duke Univ Med Ctr (page 60); **Address:** Duke Med Ctr, Dept Psyc, 3521 Hospital S, Box 3003, Durham, NC 27710-3003; **Phone:** (919) 684-4128; **Board Cert:** Psychiatry 1977, Geriatric Psychiatry 1991; **Med School:** Univ Tenn Coll Med, Memphis 1969; **Resid:** Psychiatry, Duke Univ Med Ctr, Durham, NC 1973-1975; **Fellow:** Liason Psychiatry, Montefiore Hosp, Bronx, NY 1975-1976; **Fac Appt:** Prof Psychiatry, Duke Univ

Davidson, Jonathan MD (Psyc) - *Spec Exp:* Anxiety & Mood Disorders; **Hospital:** Duke Univ Med Ctr (page 60); **Address:** Duke Univ Med Ctr, Box 3812, Durham, NC 27710; **Phone:** (919) 684-2880; **Board Cert:** Psychiatry 1979; **Med School:** England 1967; **Resid:** Psychiatry, Royal Edinburgh Hosp, Edinburgh, Scotland 1969-1972; **Fac Appt:** Prof Psychiatry, Duke Univ

Eisdorfer, Carl MD/PhD (Psyc) - *Spec Exp:* Aging and Dementitia; Alzheimer's Disease; **Hospital:** Univ of Miami - Jackson Meml Hosp; **Address:** 1695 NW Ninth Ave, Ste 3100, Miami, FL 33136-1024; **Phone:** (305) 355-9105; **Board Cert:** Psychiatry 1974; **Med School:** Duke Univ 1964; **Resid:** Psychiatry, Duke Univ Med Ctr, Durham, NC 1965-1967; **Fac Appt:** Prof Psychiatry, Univ Miami Sch Med

Kendler, Kenneth S MD (Psyc) - *Spec Exp:* Schizophrenia; Mood Disorders; **Hospital:** Med Coll of VA Hosp; **Address:** Dept Psychiatry, PO Box 980126, Richmond, VA 23298; **Phone:** (804) 828-8590; **Board Cert:** Psychiatry 1981; **Med School:** Stanford Univ 1976; **Resid:** Psychiatry, Yale-New Haven Hosp, New Haven, CT 1977-1980; **Fac Appt:** Prof Psychiatry, Med Coll VA

Mellman, Thomas MD (Psyc) - *Spec Exp:* Post-Traumatic Stress Disorder; Anxiety Disorders; Psychopharmacology; **Hospital:** Univ of Miami - Jackson Meml Hosp; **Address:** Univ Miami Dept Psy, 1400 NW 10th Ave, Ste 304A, Miami, FL 33136-1020; **Phone:** (603) 650-8558; **Board Cert:** Psychiatry 1989; **Med School:** Case West Res Univ 1982; **Resid:** Psychiatry, Univ Hospitals, Cleveland, OH 1982-1985; **Fellow:** Psychiatric Research, Ntl Inst Mental Hlth, Bethesda, MD 1985-1988

Powers, Pauline MD (Psyc) - *Spec Exp:* *Eating Disorders;* **Hospital:** Tampa Genl Hosp; **Address:** Univ S Fla, Dept Psych, 3515 E Fletcher Ave, Tampa, FL 33613-4706; **Phone:** (813) 974-2926; **Board Cert:** Psychiatry 1977; **Med School:** Univ Iowa Coll Med 1971; **Resid:** Psychiatry, Univ Iowa, Iowa City, IA 1972-1974; Psychiatry, Univ Calif-Davis, Santa Barbara, CA 1974-1975; **Fac Appt:** Prof Psychiatry, Univ S Fla Coll Med

Midwest

Andersen, Arnold MD (Psyc) - *Spec Exp:* *Eating Disorders;* **Hospital:** Univ of IA Hosp and Clinics; **Address:** Dept Psychiatry, 200 Hawkins Drive, rm 2880-JPP, Iowa City, IA 52242; **Phone:** (319) 356-1354; **Board Cert:** Psychiatry 1980; **Med School:** Cornell Univ-Weill Med Coll 1968; **Resid:** Psychiatry, NY Hosp, New York, NY 1969-1970; Psychiatry, Johns Hopkins Hosp, Baltimore, MD 1975-1976; **Fellow:** Psychiatry, Natl Inst Mental Hlth, Bethesda, MD 1974-1975; **Fac Appt:** Prof Psychiatry, Univ Iowa Coll Med

Astrachan, Boris MD (Psyc) - *Spec Exp:* *Community Psychiatry;* **Hospital:** Univ of IL at Chicago Med Ctr; **Address:** 912 S Wood St, Ste 709G, Chicago, IL 60612-7325; **Phone:** (312) 996-3580; **Board Cert:** Psychiatry 1966; **Med School:** Albany Med Coll 1956; **Resid:** Psychiatry, US Naval H, Philadelphia, PA 1957-1958; Psychiatry, Yale-New Haven Hosp, New Haven, CT 1961-1963; **Fac Appt:** Prof Psychiatry, Univ IL Coll Med

Cloninger, C Robert MD (Psyc) - *Spec Exp:* *Personality Disorders;* **Hospital:** Barnes-Jewish Hosp (page 55); **Address:** Wash Univ Sch Med, 660 S Euclid Ave, Box 8134, St Louis, MO 63110; **Phone:** (314) 362-7005; **Board Cert:** Psychiatry 1975; **Med School:** Washington Univ, St Louis 1970; **Resid:** Psychiatry, Barnes Hosp, St Louis, MO 1970-1973; Psychiatry, Renard Hosp, St Louis, MO 1970-1973; **Fac Appt:** Prof Psychiatry, Washington Univ, St Louis

Fawcett, Jan A MD (Psyc) - *Spec Exp:* *Depression;* **Hospital:** Rush-Presby - St Luke's Med Ctr (page 72); **Address:** 1725 W Harrison St, Ste 955, Chicago, IL 60612; **Phone:** (312) 942-5372; **Board Cert:** Psychiatry 1967; **Med School:** Yale Univ 1960; **Resid:** Psychiatry, Langley Porter Inst, San Francisco, CA 1961-1963; Psychiatry, Rochester Med Ctr, Rochester, NY 1963-1964

Greden, John MD (Psyc) - *Spec Exp:* *Anxiety & Mood Disorders; Depression;* **Hospital:** Univ of MI Hlth Ctr; **Address:** U Mich Med Ctr, Dept of Psyc, 1500 E Med Ctr Dr, Ann Arbor, MI 48109-0704; **Phone:** (734) 763-9629; **Board Cert:** Psychiatry 1975; **Med School:** Univ Minn 1967; **Resid:** Psychiatry, Univ Minn Med Ctr, Minneapolis, MN 1968-1969; Psychiatry, Walter Reed AMC, Washington, DC 1970-1972; **Fac Appt:** Prof Psychiatry, Univ Mich Med Sch

Greist, John MD (Psyc) - *Spec Exp:* *Anxiety & Mood Disorders; Behavioral Problems; Psychopharmacology;* **Hospital:** Univ WI Hosp & Clins; **Address:** 7617 Mineral Point Rd, Ste 300, Madison, WI 53717; **Phone:** (608) 827-2440; **Board Cert:** Psychiatry 1974; **Med School:** Indiana Univ 1965; **Resid:** Internal Medicine, Univ Wisc Hosp & Clin, Madison, WI 1966-1967; Psychiatry, Univ Wisc Hosp & Clin, Madison, WI 1967-1970; **Fellow:** Child & Adolescent Psychiatry, Univ Wisc Hosp & Clin, Madison, WI 1970-1971; **Fac Appt:** Clin Prof Psychiatry, Univ Wisc

Janicak, Philip G. MD (Psyc) - *Spec Exp:* *Psychopharmacology; Mood Disorders;* **Hospital:** Univ of IL at Chicago Med Ctr; **Address:** Univ IL at Chicago, Dept Psyc, 1601 W Taylor St, Chicago, IL 60612-4321; **Phone:** (312) 413-4507; **Board Cert:** Psychiatry 1978; **Med School:** Loyola Univ-Stritch Sch Med 1973; **Resid:** Psychiatry, McGaw Hosp/Loyola Med Ctr, Maywood, IL 1973-1976; **Fac Appt:** Prof Psychiatry, Univ IL Coll Med

Levine, Stephen B MD (Psyc) - *Spec Exp:* Sexual Dysfunction; Relationship Problems; **Hospital:** Univ Hosp of Cleveland; **Address:** 23230 Chagrin Blvd Bldg 3 - Ste 350, Beachwood, OH 44122-5402; **Phone:** (216) 831-2900; **Board Cert:** Psychiatry 1976; **Med School:** Case West Res Univ 1967; **Resid:** Psychiatry, Univ Hosps Cleveland, Cleveland, OH 1970-1973; **Fac Appt:** Clin Prof Psychiatry, Case West Res Univ

Uhde, Thomas W MD (Psyc) - *Spec Exp:* Anxiety & Mood Disorders; Depression; **Hospital:** Harper Hosp (page 59); **Address:** 4201 St. Antoine St, Ste 9B, Detroit, MI 48201; **Phone:** (313) 577-9553; **Board Cert:** Psychiatry 1984; **Med School:** Univ Louisville Sch Med 1975; **Resid:** Psychiatry, Yale-New Haven Hosp, New Haven, CT 1976-1979; **Fellow:** Psychiatry, Natl Inst Mental Hlth, Bethesda, MD 1979-1981; **Fac Appt:** Prof Psychiatry, Wayne State Univ

Zorumski, Charles F MD (Psyc) - *Spec Exp:* Neuro-Psychiatry; Psychopharmacology; **Hospital:** Barnes-Jewish Hosp (page 55); **Address:** 660 S Euclid Ave, Box CB8134, St Louis, MO 63110; **Phone:** (314) 747-2680; **Board Cert:** Psychiatry 1984; **Med School:** St Louis Univ 1978; **Resid:** Psychiatry, Barnes-Jewish Hosp, St Louis, MO 1978-1982; **Fac Appt:** Prof Psychiatry, Washington Univ, St Louis

Great Plains and Mountains

Davidson, Joyce Eileen MD (Psyc) - *Spec Exp:* Obsessive-Compulsive Disorder; Bipolar/Mood Disorders; Schizophrenia; **Hospital:** Menninger Clinic; **Address:** Menninger Clinic, Box 829, Topeka, KS 66601-0829; **Phone:** (785) 350-5442; **Board Cert:** Psychiatry 1988; **Med School:** Univ MO-Kansas City 1979; **Resid:** Psychiatry, Karl Menninger Sch Psyc, Topeka, KS 1980-1982; **Fellow:** Child & Adolescent Psychiatry, Karl Menninger Sch Psyc, Topeka, KS 1982-1984; **Fac Appt:** Prof Psychiatry, Karl Menninger Sch Psych

Menninger, W Walter MD (Psyc) - *Spec Exp:* Post Traumatic Stress Disorder; Forensic Psychiatry; **Hospital:** Menninger Clinic; **Address:** 5800 SW 6th St, Topeka, KS 66606; **Phone:** (785) 350-5830; **Board Cert:** Psychiatry 1963; **Med School:** Cornell Univ-Weill Med Coll 1957; **Resid:** Psychiatry, Topeka State Hosp, Topeka, KS 1958-1960; **Fellow:** Psychiatry, Menninger Fdn, Topeka, KS 1960-1961; **Fac Appt:** Prof Psychiatry, Karl Menninger Sch Psych

Mitchell, James E MD (Psyc) - *Spec Exp:* Eating Disorders; **Hospital:** MeritCare Hosp; **Address:** NeuroPsychological Research Inst, 700 1st Ave S, Box 1415, Fargo, ND 58107-1415; **Phone:** (701) 293-1335; **Board Cert:** Psychiatry 1979; **Med School:** Northwestern Univ 1972; **Resid:** Psychiatry, Fairview-Univ Med Ctr, Minneapolis, MN 1973-1976; **Fac Appt:** Prof Psychiatry, Univ ND Sch Med

Munich, Richard MD (Psyc) - *Spec Exp:* Psychotic Disorders; Psychoanalysis; Hospice Care; **Hospital:** Menninger Clinic; **Address:** Menninger Clinic, Box 829, Topeka, KS 66601; **Phone:** (785) 350-5530; **Board Cert:** Psychiatry 1982; **Med School:** Univ KY Coll Med 1965; **Resid:** Psychiatry, Yale New Haven Hosp, New Haven, CT 1966-1967; Psychiatry, Yale Psych Inst, New Haven, CT 1968-1970

Southwest

Altshuler, Kenneth Z. MD (Psyc) - *Spec Exp:* Psychotherapy; Psychoanalysis; **Hospital:** Zale Lipshy Univ Hosp; **Address:** 5323 Harry Hines Blvd, Dallas, TX 75390-9070; **Phone:** (214) 648-5588; **Board Cert:** Psychiatry 1961; **Med School:** SUNY Buffalo 1952; **Resid:** Psychiatry, VA Hosp, Bronx, NY 1955-1956; Psychiatry, NY Psychiatric Inst, New York, NY 1956-1958; **Fac Appt:** Prof Psychiatry, Univ Tex SW, Dallas

Bowden, Charles MD (Psyc) - *Spec Exp:* Bipolar/Mood Disorders; **Hospital:** Univ Hosp-San Antonio; **Address:** Univ Tex Hlth Sci Ctr, 7703 Floyd Curl Dr, San Antonio, TX 78230-3900; **Phone:** (210) 567-5391; **Board Cert:** Psychiatry 1970; **Med School:** Baylor Coll Med 1964; **Resid:** Psychiatry, NY State Psyc Inst/Columbia-Presby Med Ctr, New York, NY 1965-1968; **Fac Appt:** Prof Psychiatry, Univ Tex, San Antonio

Gabbard, Glen O. MD (Psyc) - *Spec Exp:* Personality Disorders-Borderline; Cognitive Psychiatry; **Hospital:** Baylor Univ Medical Ctr; **Address:** One Baylor Plaza, Houston, TX 77030; **Phone:** (713) 798-6397; **Board Cert:** Psychiatry 1979; **Med School:** Rush Med Coll 1975; **Resid:** Psychiatry, Menninger Sch Psyc, Topeka, KS 1975-1978; **Fellow:** Psychoanalysis, Topeka Inst Psychoan, Topeka, KS 1977-1984; **Fac Appt:** Clin Prof Psychiatry, Univ Kans

Hirschfeld, Robert, M A MD (Psyc) - *Spec Exp:* Mood Disorders; **Hospital:** Univ of Texas Hlth & Sci Ctr; **Address:** 301 University Blvd, Galveston, TX 77555-0429; **Phone:** (409) 772-4956; **Board Cert:** Psychiatry 1975; **Med School:** Univ Mich Med Sch 1968; **Resid:** Psychiatry, Stanford Med Ctr, Stanford, CA 1969-1972; **Fac Appt:** Prof Psychiatry, Univ Tex Med Br, Galveston

Mohl, Paul C. MD (Psyc) - *Spec Exp:* Psychopharmacology; Psychotherapy; **Hospital:** Zale Lipshy Univ Hosp; **Address:** 5323 Harry Hines Blvd, Dallas, TX 75390-9070; **Phone:** (214) 648-7365; **Board Cert:** Psychiatry 1977; **Med School:** Duke Univ 1971; **Resid:** Psychiatry, Duke Hospital, Durham, NC 1971-1974; **Fac Appt:** Prof Psychiatry, Univ Tex SW, Dallas

Moore, Constance A. MD (Psyc) - *Spec Exp:* Sleep Disorders/Apnea; **Hospital:** Baylor Univ Medical Ctr; **Address:** VA Affairs Med Ctr, 2002 Holcomb Blvd, MS 6C344, Houston, TX 77030; **Phone:** (713) 961-5055; **Board Cert:** Psychiatry 1991; **Med School:** Baylor Coll Med 1980; **Resid:** Psychiatry, Baylor Medical College, Houston, TX 1984; **Fac Appt:** Assoc Prof Psychiatry, Baylor Coll Med

Rush Jr, Augustus John MD (Psyc) - *Spec Exp:* Mood Disorders; **Hospital:** Zale Lipshy Univ Hosp; **Address:** Univ Tex-SW Med Ctr, Dept Psychiatry, 5323 Harry Hines Blvd, Dallas, TX 75390-9086; **Phone:** (214) 648-4600; **Board Cert:** Psychiatry 1976; **Med School:** Columbia P&S 1968; **Resid:** Psychiatry, Univ Penn, Philadelphia, PA 1972-1975; **Fac Appt:** Prof Psychiatry, Univ Tex SW, Dallas

Weiner, Myron MD (Psyc) - *Spec Exp:* Psychiatry-Geriatric; Alzheimer's Disease; **Hospital:** Zale Lipshy Univ Hosp; **Address:** Univ Texas SW Med Ctr, 5323 Harry Hines Blvd, Bldg NC6.102, Dallas, TX 75390-9070; **Phone:** (214) 648-5591; **Board Cert:** Psychiatry 1966, Geriatric Psychiatry 2001; **Med School:** Tulane Univ 1957; **Resid:** Psychiatry, Parkland Hosp, Dallas, TX 1960-1963; **Fellow:** Geriatric Psychiatry, Mt Sinai Med Ctr, New York, NY 1984-1985; **Fac Appt:** Prof Psychiatry, Univ Tex SW, Dallas

Yager, Joel MD (Psyc) - *Spec Exp:* Eating Disorders; **Hospital:** Univ NM Hosp; **Address:** Univ NM Sch Med, Dept Psyc, 2400 Tucker NE, Albuquerque, NM 87131-5326; **Phone:** (505) 272-5416; **Board Cert:** Psychiatry 1971; **Med School:** Albert Einstein Coll Med 1965; **Resid:** Psychiatry, Bronx Muni Hosp Ctr, New York, NY 1966-1969; **Fac Appt:** Prof Psychiatry, Univ New Mexico

West Coast and Pacific

Burt, Vivien Kleinman MD/PhD (Psyc) - *Spec Exp:* Women's Health-Mental Health; Impulse-Control Disorders; **Hospital:** UCLA Neuropsychiatric Hosp; **Address:** UCLA Neuropsyc Inst, 300 UCLA Med Plaza, Ste 2337, Los Angeles, CA 90095; **Phone:** (310) 206-5135; **Board Cert:** Psychiatry 1990; **Med School:** McGill Univ 1984; **Resid:** Psychiatry, UCLA-Neurpsyc Inst, Los Angeles, CA 1985-1988; **Fac Appt:** Assoc Prof Psychiatry, UCLA

Bystritsky, Alexander MD (Psyc) - *Spec Exp:* Obsessive-Compulsive Disorder; Anxiety Disorders; **Hospital:** UCLA Neuropsychiatric Hosp; **Address:** 300 UCLA Med Plaza, Ste 2200, Los Angeles, CA 90095-8346; **Phone:** (310) 206-5133; **Board Cert:** Psychiatry 1988; **Med School:** Russia 1977; **Resid:** Psychiatry, NYU Med Ctr, New York, NY 1981-1985; **Fellow:** RW Johnson/UCLA Sch Med, Los Angeles, CA 1985-1987; **Fac Appt:** Assoc Clin Prof Psychiatry, UCLA

Dunner, David Louis MD (Psyc) - *Spec Exp:* Anxiety & Mood Disorders; Bipolar/Mood Disorders; **Hospital:** Univ WA Med Ctr; **Address:** Ctr for Anxiety & Depression, 4225 Roosevelt Way, Ste 306C, Seattle, WA 98105-6099; **Phone:** (206) 221-3925; **Board Cert:** Psychiatry 1971; **Med School:** Washington Univ, St Louis 1965; **Resid:** Psychiatry, Barnes Hosp- Washington, Seattle, WA 1966-1969; **Fac Appt:** Prof Psychiatry, Univ Wash

Eisendrath, Stuart James MD (Psyc) - *Spec Exp:* Depression; Munchausen Syndrome; **Hospital:** UCSF Med Ctr; **Address:** UCSF Med Ctr, 401 Parnassus Ave, MC-0984, San Francisco, CA 94143-9911; **Phone:** (415) 476-7868; **Board Cert:** Psychiatry 1980; **Med School:** Med Coll Wisc 1974; **Resid:** Psychiatry, Langley Porter NPI, San Francisco, CA 1975-1978; **Fellow:** Liason Psychiatry, Langley Porter NPI, San Francisco, CA 1978-1979; **Fac Appt:** Prof Psychiatry, UCSF

Gitlin, Michael Jay MD (Psyc) - *Spec Exp:* Mood Disorders; **Hospital:** UCLA Neuropsychiatric Hosp; **Address:** 300 UCLA Med Plaza, Box 2200, Los Angeles, CA 90095; **Phone:** (310) 206-6546; **Board Cert:** Psychiatry 1981; **Med School:** Univ Penn 1975; **Resid:** Psychiatry, UCLA Med Ctr, Los Angeles, CA 1976-1979; **Fac Appt:** Prof Psychiatry, UCLA

Goin, Marcia Kraft MD (Psyc) - *Spec Exp:* Psychotherapy; Post-Traumatic Stress Disorder; **Address:** Dept of Psy & Behav Sciences, Bldg IRD 211, Los Angeles, CA 90089-9520; **Phone:** (213) 977-1129; **Board Cert:** Psychiatry 1965; **Med School:** Yale Univ 1958; **Resid:** Psychiatry, LA County-USC Sch Med Ctr, Los Angeles, CA 1959-1962; **Fellow:** Psychoanalysis, California Psychoanalytic Inst, Los Angeles, CA 1977-1977; **Fac Appt:** Clin Prof Psychiatry, Univ SC Sch Med

Guilleminault, Christian MD (Psyc) - *Spec Exp:* Sleep Disorders; Sleep Apnea; **Hospital:** Stanford Med Ctr; **Address:** 401 Quarry Rd, Ste 3301A, Stanford, CA 94305; **Phone:** (650) 723-6601; **Med School:** France 1968; **Fac Appt:** Prof Psychiatry, Stanford Univ

Liberman, Robert Paul MD (Psyc) - *Spec Exp:* Schizophrenia; Psychotic Disorders; Psychiatric Rehabilitation; **Hospital:** UCLA Neuropsychiatric Hosp; **Address:** UCLA, 300 Med Plaza, Ste 2263, Los Angeles, CA 90095; **Phone:** (310) 478-3711; **Board Cert:** Psychiatry 1969; **Med School:** Johns Hopkins Univ 1963; **Resid:** Psychiatry, Mass Mental Health Ctr, Boston, MA 1964-1967; **Fellow:** Psychiatry, Harvard Med Sch, Boston, MA 1966-1968; Psychiatry, UCSF, San Francisco, CA 1960-1961; **Fac Appt:** Prof Emeritus Psychiatry, UCLA

Marder, Stephen Robert MD (Psyc) - *Spec Exp:* Schizophrenia; Psychopharmacology; **Hospital:** VA Med Ctr - W Los Angeles; **Address:** West Los Angeles VA - Gr LA Hlth Svcs, 11301 Wilshire Blvd, Bldg MIRECC 210A, Los Angeles, CA 90073; **Phone:** (310) 268-3647; **Board Cert:** Psychiatry 1977; **Med School:** SUNY Buffalo 1971; **Resid:** Psychiatry, LAC-USC Med Ctr, Los Angeles, CA 1972-1975; **Fac Appt:** Prof Psychiatry, UCLA

Marmar, Charles MD (Psyc) - *Spec Exp:* Depression-Postpartum; Post-traumatic Stress Disorder; **Hospital:** VA Med Ctr - San Francisco; **Address:** 4150 Clement St, Bldg 8 - rm 3201, Box 116A, San Francisco, CA 94121; **Phone:** (415) 221-4810; **Board Cert:** Psychiatry 1982; **Med School:** Univ Manitoba 1970; **Resid:** Psychiatry, Univ Toronto Hosp, Toronto, Canada 1972-1976; **Fellow:** Anxiety Disorder, Langley Porter Inst-UCSF, San Francisco, CA 1977-1978; **Fac Appt:** Prof Psychiatry, UCSF

Neppe, Vernon Michael MD (Psyc) - *Spec Exp:* Forensic Psychiatry; Neuro-Psychiatry; **Hospital:** NW Hosp; **Address:** 10330 Meridian Ave N, Ste 380, Seattle, WA 98133-9463; **Phone:** (206) 527-6289; **Board Cert:** Geriatric Psychiatry 1991, Forensic Psychiatry 1994; **Med School:** South Africa 1973; **Resid:** Psychiatry, Johannesburgh, South Africa 1976-1980; **Fellow:** Psychopharmacology, NY Cornell Med Ctr, New York, NY 1982-1983; **Fac Appt:** Adjct Prof Psychiatry, St Louis Univ

Norman, Kim Peter MD (Psyc) - *Spec Exp:* Eating Disorders-Obesity; Schizophrenia; Personality Disorders; **Hospital:** UCSF Med Ctr; **Address:** UCSF-Langely Porter Psyc Inst, 505 Parnassus Avenue, San Francisco, CA 94143-6401; **Phone:** (415) 476-7402; **Board Cert:** Psychiatry 1983; **Med School:** Albert Einstein Coll Med 1977; **Resid:** Psychiatry, Langley Porter Psyc Inst, San Francisco, CA 1978-1981; **Fac Appt:** Asst Prof Psychiatry, UCSF

Pi, Edmond Hsin-Tung MD (Psyc) - *Spec Exp:* Psychopharmacology; Cross-Cultural Psychiatry; **Hospital:** LAC - King/Drew Med Ctr; **Address:** Charles R Drew Univ Med & Sci, 1731 E 120 St, Los Angeles, CA 90059-3051; **Phone:** (310) 668-4803; **Board Cert:** Psychiatry 1980; **Med School:** South Korea 1972; **Resid:** Psychiatry, SUNY-Stony Brook/Long Island Consortium, Stony Brook, NY 1975-1977; Psychiatry, Univ Kentucky Hosp-Chandler Med Ctr, Lexington, KY 1977-1978; **Fac Appt:** Prof Psychiatry, Charles Drew Univ Med & Sci

Pomer, Sydney Lawrence MD (Psyc) - *Spec Exp:* Psychoanalysis; **Hospital:** Cedars-Sinai Med Ctr; **Address:** 430 S Bundy Dr, Los Angeles, CA 90049; **Phone:** (310) 472-1580; **Board Cert:** Psychiatry 1953; **Med School:** Univ Toronto 1941; **Resid:** Psychiatry, VA Hosp, Palo Alto, CA 1946-1947; **Fellow:** Psychiatry, Mt Zion Hosp, San Francisco, CA 1947-1948; **Fac Appt:** Assoc Clin Prof Psychiatry, Univ SC Sch Med

Pynoos, Robert Sidney MD (Psyc) - *Spec Exp:* Post-Traumatic Stress Disorder; **Hospital:** UCLA Neuropsychiatric Hosp; **Address:** 300 UCLA Med Plaza, Los Angeles, CA 90095; **Phone:** (310) 206-8973; **Board Cert:** Psychiatry 1980; **Med School:** Columbia P&S **Fac Appt:** Prof Psychiatry, UCLA

Raskind, Murray MD (Psyc) - *Spec Exp:* Geriatric Psychiatry; Alzheimer's Disease; Post Traumatic Stress Disorder; **Hospital:** VA Puget Sound Hlth Care Sys; **Address:** VA Puget Sound Health Care System, Mental Hlth Svc 116, 1660 S Columbia Way, Seattle, WA 98108; **Phone:** (206) 768-5375; **Board Cert:** Psychiatry 1976, Geriatric Psychiatry 1991; **Med School:** Columbia P&S 1968; **Resid:** Psychiatry, Univ of Wash, Seattle, WA 1970-1973; Internal Medicine, Colum-Harlem Hosp Ctr, New York, NY 1969-1970; **Fac Appt:** Prof Psychiatry, Univ Wash

Reus, Victor Ivar MD (Psyc) - *Spec Exp:* Alzheimer's Disease; Bipolar/Mood Disorders; **Hospital:** UCSF Med Ctr; **Address:** 401 Parnassus Ave, San Francisco, CA 94143-0984; **Phone:** (415) 476-7478; **Board Cert:** Psychiatry 1977, Geriatric Psychiatry 1991; **Med School:** Univ MD Sch Med 1973; **Resid:** Psychiatry, Univ of WI, Madison, WI 1973-1976; **Fellow:** Psychiatry, NIMH, Bethesda, MD 1976-1978; **Fac Appt:** Prof Psychiatry, UCSF

Roy-Byrne, Peter MD (Psyc) - *Spec Exp:* Anxiety & Mood Disorders; Panic Disorder; **Hospital:** Univ WA Med Ctr; **Address:** 325 9th Ave, Box 359911, Seattle, WA 98104; **Phone:** (206) 341-4200; **Board Cert:** Psychiatry 1983; **Med School:** Tufts Univ 1978; **Resid:** Psychiatry, UCLA NPI, Los Angeles, CA 1979-1982; **Fellow:** Biological Psychiatry, Natl Inst Hlth, Bethesda, MD 1982-1984; **Fac Appt:** Prof Psychiatry, Univ Wash

Schatzberg, Alan F MD (Psyc) - *Spec Exp:* Anxiety & Mood Disorders; Psychopharmacology; **Hospital:** Stanford Med Ctr; **Address:** 401 Quarry Rd, Bldg PBSC305, MC 5717, Stanford, CA 94305-5717; **Phone:** (650) 723-6811; **Board Cert:** Psychiatry 1975; **Med School:** NYU Sch Med 1968; **Resid:** Psychiatry, Mass Mental Hlth Ctr, Boston, MA 1969-1972; **Fellow:** Psychiatry, Mass Mental Hlth Ctr/Harvard, Boston, MA 1969-1972; **Fac Appt:** Prof Psychiatry, Stanford Univ

739

Simpson, George M MD (Psyc) - *Spec Exp:* Schizophrenia; Depression; **Hospital:** LAC & USC Med Ctr; **Address:** LAC + USC Med Ctr, Psychiatric Outpatient Clinic, 1937 Hospital Pl, Bldg Grad Hall - rm 240, Los Angeles, CA 90033; **Phone:** (323) 226-5363; **Board Cert:** Psychiatry 1962; **Med School:** England 1955; **Resid:** Psychiatry, Royal Victoria Hosp-McGill Univ, Montreal, Canada 1956-1957; Psychiatry, Rockland State Hosp, Orangeburg, NY 1957-1959; **Fac Appt:** Prof Psychiatry, USC Sch Med

Spiegel, David MD (Psyc) - *Spec Exp:* Hypnosis; Psychiatry for Cancer; **Hospital:** Stanford Med Ctr; **Address:** Stanford Univ Sch Med, Dept Psyc-Behav Scis, PBS C231, MC-5718, Stanford, CA 94305-5718; **Phone:** (650) 723-6421; **Board Cert:** Psychiatry 1976; **Med School:** Harvard Med Sch 1971; **Resid:** Psychiatry, Mass Mntl Hlth Ctr-Harvard Med Sch, Boston, MA 1971-1974; Psychiatry, Cambridge Hosp-Harvard Med Sch, Boston, MA 1972-1974; **Fellow:** Community Psychiatry, Harvard Med Sch, Boston, MA 1973-1974; **Fac Appt:** Prof Psychiatry, Stanford Univ

Stein, Murray Brent MD (Psyc) - *Spec Exp:* Anxiety Disorders; Panic Disorder; Post Traumatic Stress Disorder; **Hospital:** VA San Diego Hlthcre Sys; **Address:** UCSD Sch Med, 9500 Gilman Dr, MC-0985, La Jolla, CA 92093-0985; **Phone:** (858) 622-6112; **Board Cert:** Psychiatry 1989; **Med School:** Univ Manitoba 1983; **Resid:** Psychiatry, Univ Toronto Hosp, Toronto, Canada 1985-1986; Psychiatry, Natl Inst Mental Hlth-NIH, Bethesda, MD 1986-1987; **Fellow:** Anxiety Disorder, Natl Inst Mental Hlth-NIH, Bethesda, MD 1987-1989; **Fac Appt:** Prof Psychiatry, UCSD

Zerbe, Kathryn J MD (Psyc) - *Spec Exp:* Eating Disorders; Women's Health-Mental Health; Psychoanalysis; **Hospital:** OR Hlth Sci Univ Hosp and Clinics; **Address:** 3181 SW Sam Jackson Park Rd, MC OP02, Oregon Hlth Sci Ctr, Portland, OR 97201; **Phone:** (503) 494-6572; **Board Cert:** Psychiatry 1984; **Med School:** Temple Univ 1978; **Resid:** Psychiatry, Menninger Clin, Topeka, KS 1978-1982; **Fac Appt:** Prof Psychiatry, Karl Menninger Sch Psych

Zisook, Sidney MD (Psyc) - *Spec Exp:* Bereavement/Traumatic Grief; Depression; **Hospital:** VA San Diego Hlthcre Sys; **Address:** Dept Psychiatry, 9500 Gilman Dr, MS 0603-R, La Jolla, CA 92093; **Phone:** (858) 534-4040; **Board Cert:** Psychiatry 1975; **Med School:** Loyola Univ-Stritch Sch Med 1969; **Resid:** Psychiatry, Mass Genl Hosp, Boston, MA 1970-1973; **Fellow:** Psychiatry, Harvard Med Sch, Boston, MA 1970-1973; **Fac Appt:** Prof Psychiatry, UCSD

PULMONOLOGY

(a subspecialty of INTERNAL MEDICINE)

An internist who treats diseases of the lungs and airways. The pulmonologist diagnoses and treats cancer, pneumonia, pleurisy, asthma, occupational diseases, bronchitis, sleep disorders, emphysema and other complex disorders of the lungs.

INTERNAL MEDICINE

An internist is a personal physician who provides long-term, comprehensive care in the office and the hospital, managing both common and complex illness of adolescents, adults and the elderly. Internists are trained in the diagnosis and treatment of cancer, infections and diseases affecting the heart, blood, kidneys, joints and digestive, respiratory and vascular systems. They are also trained in the essentials of primary care internal medicine which incorporates an understanding of disease prevention, wellness, substance abuse, mental health and effective treatment of common problems of the eyes, ears, skin, nervous system and reproductive organs.

Training required: Three years in internal medicine *plus* additional training and examination for certification in pulmonary disease

741

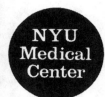

NYU Medical Center

550 First Avenue (at 31st Street)
New York, NY 10016
Physician Referral: (888) 7-NYU-MED
(888-769-8633) www.nyumedicalcenter.org

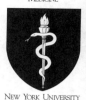

SCHOOL OF
MEDICINE

NEW YORK UNIVERSITY

PULMONOLOGY

Pulmonology at NYU Medical Center is characterized by its decisive commitment to diagnostic testing, excellence in patient care and rehabilitation, and research.

THE NYU MEDICAL CENTER PULMONARY FUNCTION LABORATORY
The newly renovated NYU Medical Center Pulmonary Function Laboratory is part of the **Department of Medicine/Division of Pulmonary and Critical Care** at **NYU School of Medicine**. Located in the **Rusk Institute of Rehabilitation Medicine**, the laboratory's technical capabilities for testing are state-of-the-art, offering exercise testing, nutritional assessments, and PFTs for indications such as the evaluation and follow-up of pulmonary symptoms and disorders, preoperative risk assessment, screening for smokers, and chemotherapy toxicity. Diagnostic testing and interpretation are performed by licensed pulmonary function technicians and technologists.

In addition to diagnostic testing, the laboratory is actively involved in research on obstructive airway dysfunction, regulation of breathing in neuromuscular disorders, pulmonary rehabilitation, and exercise physiology.

LUNG SURGERY AT NYU MEDICAL CENTER
We provide complete adult and pediatric general surgical and thoracic services, including surgery for congenital and acquired problems, tumor surgery, surgery on the lungs, esophageal surgery, and repair of chest wall deformities. We have over a decade of experience in using minimally invasive techniques to treat these problems. By using state-of-the-art instruments and techniques, often we can perform these procedures with minimal discomfort, little scarring and limited hospitalization.

PULMONARY REHABILITATION
Housed in the **Joan and Joel Smilow Cardiac Rehabilitation and Prevention Center** of the **Rusk Institute of Rehabilitation Medicine**, the cardiopulmonary rehabilitation unit is fully staff and equipped to handle both the inpatient and outpatient needs of the respiratory patient. The unit has dedicated inpatient beds for the hospitalized patients staffed by a Pulmonary Rehabilitation Team, comprised of pulmonologists, cardiologists, nurses, physical therapists, occupational therapists, psychologists, nutritionists, and social workers. Our exercise gym is equipped with exercise, monitoring, and resuscitation equipment for the safe and comprehensive delivery of services.

The program serves the rehabilitation needs of all patients with respiratory problems, including those suffering from obstructive pulmonary diseases such as asthma, emphysema, chronic bronchitis, and bronchiectasis—as well as those with musculoskeletal, neurological, and parenchymal restrictive diseases such as polio, spinal cord injury, muscular dystrophy, kyphoscoliosis, lung resection, sarcoidosis, and pulmonary fibrosis.

Treatment often involves a combination of physical therapy, including breathing exercises, relaxation, tracheobronchial drainage and aerobic exercises, and occupational therapy, including energy conservation techniques, and evaluation and prescription of self-help devices to facilitate daily living. Oxygen therapy is given to patients with hypoxemia (low blood oxygen level). Mechanical assistive devices are prescribed for patients with inadequate ventilation.

NYU MEDICAL CENTER

The Pulmonary Function Laboratory at NYU Medical Center offers several standard and specialized pulmonary tests, including:

- Spirometry (timed vital capacity, FEV1/FVC)
- Bronchodilator responsiveness (spirometry before and after bronchodilator administration)
- Flow volume loop
- Lung volumes (helium dilution and/or plethysmography)
- Maximum voluntary ventilation
- Diffusing capacity (single-breath carbon monoxide)
- Arterial and capillary blood gas analysis
- Pulse oximetry
- Airway resistance
- Maximal inspiratory and expiratory pressures
- Airway hyperactivity evaluation
- Pulmonary and Cardiopulmonary Exercise Tests
- Disability evaluations
- Nutritional assessment
- Oxygen dosage determinations

PHYSICIAN LISTINGS

Pulmonary Disease

New England

Braman, Sidney MD (Pul) - *Spec Exp:* *Asthma;* **Hospital:** Rhode Island Hosp; **Address:** Rhode Island Hosp, Div Pulm, 593 Eddy St, Providence, RI 02903; **Phone:** (401) 444-8410; **Board Cert:** Internal Medicine 1971, Pulmonary Disease 1972; **Med School:** Temple Univ 1967; **Resid:** Internal Medicine, Philadelphia Genl Hosp, Philadelphia, PA 1968-1969; **Fellow:** Pulmonary Disease, Univ Penn Med Ctr, Philadelphia, PA 1969-1970; **Fac Appt:** Assoc Prof Medicine, Brown Univ

Celli, Bartolome MD (Pul) - *Spec Exp:* *Chronic Obstructive Lung Disease (COPD); Mechanical Ventilation; Respiratory Failure;* **Hospital:** St Elizabeth's Med Ctr; **Address:** Dept Pulmonary Disease, 736 Cambridge St, Boston, MA 02135; **Phone:** (617) 789-2545; **Board Cert:** Critical Care Medicine 1987, Pulmonary Disease 1978; **Med School:** Venezuela 1971; **Resid:** Internal Medicine, St Vincent Hosp, Worcester, MA 1972-1973; Internal Medicine, Boston City Hosp, Boston, MA 1973-1976; **Fellow:** Pulmonary Disease, Boston Univ Med Ctr, Boston, MA 1974-1977; **Fac Appt:** Prof Medicine, Tufts Univ

Christiani, David MD (Pul) - *Spec Exp:* *Occupational Lung Disease;* **Hospital:** MA Genl Hosp; **Address:** 55 Fruit St, BUL-148, Boston, MA 02114; **Phone:** (617) 726-1721; **Board Cert:** Pulmonary Disease 1988, Occupational Medicine 1984; **Med School:** Tufts Univ 1976; **Resid:** Internal Medicine, Boston City Hosp, Boston, MA 1976-1979; Occupational Medicine, Harvard Sch Pub Health, Boston, MA 1979-1981; **Fellow:** Pulmonary Disease, Mass Genl Hosp, Boston, MA 1985-1987; **Fac Appt:** Prof Medicine, Harvard Med Sch

Fanta, Christopher MD (Pul) - *Spec Exp:* *Asthma;* **Hospital:** Brigham & Women's Hosp; **Address:** 75 Francis St, Tower4B, Boston, MA 02115; **Phone:** (617) 732-7420; **Board Cert:** Pulmonary Disease 1980, Critical Care Medicine 1991; **Med School:** Harvard Med Sch 1975; **Resid:** Internal Medicine, Peter Bent Brigham Hosp, Boston, MA 1976-1978; **Fellow:** Pulmonary Disease, Peter Bent Brigham Hosp, Boston, MA 1978-1980; **Fac Appt:** Assoc Prof Medicine, Harvard Med Sch

Friedman, Lloyd Neal MD (Pul) - *Spec Exp:* *Tuberculosis; Critical Care;* **Hospital:** Milford Hosp; **Address:** 300 Seaside Ave, Milford, CT 06460; **Phone:** (203) 876-4288; **Board Cert:** Critical Care Medicine 1999, Pulmonary Disease 1988; **Med School:** Yale Univ 1979; **Resid:** Internal Medicine, Beth Israel Med Ctr, New York, NY 1979-1980; Internal Medicine, Oregon Hlth Scis Univ, Portland, OR 1981-1983; **Fellow:** Pulmonary Intensive Care, Yale-New Haven Hosp, New Haven, CT 1985-1988; **Fac Appt:** Assoc Clin Prof Medicine, Yale Univ

Irwin, Richard Stephen MD (Pul) - *Spec Exp:* *Chronic Cough; Cardiac Respiratory Problems;* **Hospital:** U Mass Meml Hlth Care - Worcester; **Address:** 55 Lake Ave N, Worcester, MA -00008-9451; **Phone:** (508) 856-3121; **Board Cert:** Internal Medicine 1972, Pulmonary Disease 1974, Critical Care Medicine 1997; **Med School:** Tufts Univ 1968; **Resid:** Internal Medicine, Tufts-New England Med Ctr, Boston, MA 1969-1970; **Fellow:** Cardiac Respiratory Physiology, Columbia-Presby Hosp, New York, NY 1970-1972; **Fac Appt:** Prof Medicine, Univ Mass Sch Med

Mahler, Donald A MD (Pul) - *Spec Exp:* *Chronic Obstructive Lung Disease (COPD);* **Hospital:** Dartmouth - Hitchcock Med Ctr; **Address:** Dartmouth-Hitchcock Med Ctr, 1 Med Ctr Drive, Lebanon, NH 00067-7892; **Phone:** (603) 650-5533; **Board Cert:** Internal Medicine 1978, Pulmonary Disease 1980; **Med School:** Loyola Univ-Stritch Sch Med 1972; **Resid:** Internal Medicine, Dartmouth-Hitchcock Med Ctr, Lebanon, NH 1975-1977; **Fellow:** Pulmonary Disease, Yale-New Haven Hosp, New Haven, CT 1977-1980

Matthay, Richard MD (Pul) - *Spec Exp:* Lung Cancer; **Hospital:** Yale - New Haven Hosp; **Address:** 333 Cedar St, rm 105-LCI, Box 208057, New Haven, CT 06520-8057; **Phone:** (203) 785-4196; **Board Cert:** Pulmonary Disease 1976, Internal Medicine 1973; **Med School:** Tufts Univ 1970; **Resid:** Internal Medicine, Univ Colo Med Ctr, Denver, CO 1971-1973; **Fellow:** Pulmonary Disease, Univ Colo Med Ctr, Denver, CO 1973-1975; **Fac Appt:** Prof Medicine, Yale Univ

Metersky, Mark Lewis MD (Pul) - *Spec Exp:* Pulmonary Infections; Asthma; **Hospital:** Univ of Conn Hlth Ctr, John Dempsey Hosp; **Address:** Univ Conn Hlth Ctr, 263 Farmington Ave, Farmington, CT 06030; **Phone:** (860) 679-3343; **Board Cert:** Pulmonary Disease 1992, Critical Care Medicine 1993; **Med School:** NYU Sch Med 1985; **Resid:** Internal Medicine, Boston City Hosp, Boston, MA 1985-1988; **Fellow:** Pulmonary Critical Care Medicine, UCSD Med Ctr, San Diego, CA 1989-1992; **Fac Appt:** Assoc Prof Medicine, Univ Conn

Millman, Richard P MD (Pul) - *Spec Exp:* Sleep Disorders/Apnea; **Hospital:** Rhode Island Hosp; **Address:** Rhode Island Hosp, Pulmonology Div, 593 Eddy St, Providence, RI 02903-4923; **Phone:** (401) 444-3566; **Board Cert:** Internal Medicine 1979, Pulmonary Disease 1982, Critical Care Medicine 1999; **Med School:** Univ Penn 1976; **Resid:** Internal Medicine, Univ Mich Hosp, Ann Arbor, MI 1977-1979; **Fellow:** Pulmonary Disease, U Penn Med Ctr, Philadelphia, PA 1979-1981; **Fac Appt:** Prof Medicine, Brown Univ

Nardell, Edward MD (Pul) - *Spec Exp:* Tuberculosis; **Hospital:** Cambridge Hospital; **Address:** Cambridge Hosp., 1493 Cambridge Street, Cambridge, MA 02139; **Phone:** (617) 665-1029; **Board Cert:** Internal Medicine 1975, Pulmonary Disease 1982; **Med School:** Hahnemann Univ 1972; **Resid:** Internal Medicine, Hahnemann U Hosp., Philadelphia, PA 1973-1975; **Fellow:** Pulmonary Disease, Mass Genl Hosp., Boston, MA 1975-1977; **Fac Appt:** Assoc Prof Medicine, Harvard Med Sch

Parsons, Polly E. MD (Pul) - *Spec Exp:* Critical Care; **Hospital:** Fletcher Allen Hlthcare - UHC Campus; **Address:** Fletcher Allen Health Care / Patrick 310, 1111 Colchester Ave, Burlington, VT 05495; **Phone:** (802) 847-6177; **Board Cert:** Pulmonary Disease 1986, Critical Care Medicine 1989; **Med School:** Univ Ariz Coll Med 1978; **Resid:** Internal Medicine, Univ Colo Hosp, Denver, CO 1978-1981; **Fellow:** Pulmonary Disease, Univ Colo Hosp, Denver, CO 1982-1983; **Fac Appt:** Prof Pulmonary Disease, Univ VT Coll Med

Redlich, Carrie MD (Pul) - *Spec Exp:* Occupational Lung Disease; **Hospital:** Yale - New Haven Hosp; **Address:** 135 College St Fl 3, New Haven, CT 06510; **Phone:** (203) 737-2817; **Board Cert:** Internal Medicine 1986, Pulmonary Disease 1990, Occupational Medicine 1990; **Med School:** Yale Univ 1982; **Resid:** Internal Medicine, Yale-New Haven Hosp, New Haven, CT 1984-1986; Occupational Medicine, Yale-New Haven Hosp, New Haven, CT 1986-1987; **Fellow:** Pulmonary Disease, Univ Seattle, Seattle, WA 1987-1989; **Fac Appt:** Asst Prof Medicine, Yale Univ

Reilly Jr, John Joseph MD (Pul) - *Spec Exp:* Transplant Medicine-Lung; Emphysema; **Hospital:** Brigham & Women's Hosp; **Address:** 75 Francis St, Ste TW4B, Boston, MA 02115; **Phone:** (617) 732-7420; **Board Cert:** Pulmonary Disease 1986, Critical Care Medicine 1987; **Med School:** Harvard Med Sch 1981; **Resid:** Internal Medicine, Brigham & Women's Hosp, Boston, MA 1982-1984; **Fellow:** Pulmonary Disease, Brigham & Women's Hosp, Boston, MA 1984-1987; **Fac Appt:** Assoc Prof Medicine, Harvard Med Sch

Rochester, Carolyn MD (Pul) - *Spec Exp:* *Chronic Obstructive Lung Disease (COPD);* **Hospital:** Yale - New Haven Hosp; **Address:** Pulmonary & Critical Care Section, 333 Cedar St Bldg LCI - rm 105, Box 208057, New Haven, CT 06520-8057; **Phone:** (203) 785-3207; **Board Cert:** Critical Care Medicine 1991, Pulmonary Disease 1990; **Med School:** Columbia P&S 1983; **Resid:** Internal Medicine, Columbia Presby Med Ctr, New York, NY 1984-1986; **Fellow:** Pulmonary Disease, Colombia Presby Med Ctr, New York, NY 1986-1988; **Fac Appt:** Asst Prof Pulmonary Disease, Yale Univ

White, David P MD (Pul) - *Spec Exp:* *Sleep Disorders/Apnea;* **Hospital:** Brigham & Women's Hosp; **Address:** Brigham & Women's Hosp-Sleep Disorders Prog, 221 Longwood Ave, Boston, MA 02115; **Phone:** (617) 732-5778; **Board Cert:** Pulmonary Disease 1982, Critical Care Medicine 1997; **Med School:** Emory Univ 1975; **Resid:** Internal Medicine, Univ Colo Med Ctr, Denver, CO 1976-1978; **Fellow:** Pulmonary Disease, Univ Colo Med Ctr, Denver, CO 1979-1982; **Fac Appt:** Assoc Prof Medicine, Harvard Med Sch

Mid Atlantic

Arcasoy, Selim M MD (Pul) - *Spec Exp:* *Transplant-Lung; Pulmonary Critical Care;* **Hospital:** NY Presby Hosp - Columbia Presby Med Ctr (page 70); **Address:** 622 W 168th St, Ste PH 14 East - rm 104, New York, NY 10032; **Phone:** (212) 305-6589; **Board Cert:** Internal Medicine 1993, Critical Care Medicine 1997, Pulmonary Disease 1996; **Med School:** Turkey 1990; **Resid:** Internal Medicine, SUNY Downstate Med Ctr, Brooklyn, NY 1991-1993; **Fellow:** Pulmonary Critical Care Medicine, U Pittsburgh Med Ctr, Pittsburgh, PA 1994; **Fac Appt:** Assoc Prof Surgery, Columbia P&S

Greenberg, Harly MD (Pul) - *Spec Exp:* *Sleep Disorders/Apnea; Critical Care;* **Hospital:** Long Island Jewish Med Ctr; **Address:** Long Island Jewish Med Ctr, 270-05 76th Ave, New Hyde Park, NY 11040; **Phone:** (718) 470-6400; **Board Cert:** Internal Medicine 1985, Pulmonary Disease 1988, Critical Care Medicine 1989; **Med School:** NYU Sch Med 1982; **Resid:** Internal Medicine, North Shore Univ Hosp, Manhasset, NY 1982-1985; **Fellow:** Pulmonary Disease, NYU-Bellevue Hosp Ctr, New York, NY 1985-1987; **Fac Appt:** Asst Prof Medicine, Albert Einstein Coll Med

Hansen-Flaschen, John MD (Pul) - *Spec Exp:* *Interstitial Lung Disease; Diagnostic Problems; Chronic Obstructive Lung Disease (COPD);* **Hospital:** Hosp Univ Penn (page 78); **Address:** Hosp Univ PA, Dept Pulm and CCM, 3400 Spruce St, Bldg 3 Radvin - Ste F, Philadelphia, PA 19104; **Phone:** (215) 662-6003; **Board Cert:** Pulmonary Disease 1982, Critical Care Medicine 1988, Internal Medicine 1979; **Med School:** NYU Sch Med 1976; **Resid:** Internal Medicine, Hosp Univ PA, Philadelphia, PA 1977-1979; **Fellow:** Pulmonary Disease, Hosp Univ PA, Philadelphia, PA 1980-1981; Critical Care Medicine, Hosp Univ PA, Philadelphia, PA 1981-1982; **Fac Appt:** Prof Medicine, Univ Penn

Haponik, Edward Francis MD (Pul) - *Spec Exp:* *Sleep Disorders/Apnea; Critical Care;* **Hospital:** Johns Hopkins Bayview Med Ctr; **Address:** 600 N Wolfe St Bldg Blalock - rm 910, Baltimore, MD 21287; **Phone:** (410) 550-5864; **Board Cert:** Internal Medicine 1977, Pulmonary Disease 1980; **Med School:** Wake Forest Univ Sch Med 1974; **Resid:** Internal Medicine, N Carolina Bapt Hosp-Bowman Gray, Winston Salem, NC 1975; **Fellow:** Pulmonary Disease, Johns Hopkins Sch Med, Baltimore, MD 1978-1980; **Fac Appt:** Prof Medicine, Johns Hopkins Univ

Kamholz, Stephan MD (Pul) - *Spec Exp:* *AIDS/HIV;* **Hospital:** N Shore Univ Hosp at Manhasset; **Address:** 300 Community Drive, Manhasset, NY 11030; **Phone:** (516) 562-1310; **Board Cert:** Pulmonary Disease 1975, Critical Care Medicine 1997; **Med School:** NY Med Coll 1972; **Resid:** Internal Medicine, Montefiore Hosp Med Ctr, Bronx, NY 1972-1975; **Fellow:** Pulmonary Disease, Montefiore Hosp Med Ctr, Bronx, NY 1975-1977

Libby, Daniel MD (Pul) - *Spec Exp:* Asthma; Lung Cancer; Interstitial Lung Disease; **Hospital:** NY Presby Hosp - NY Weill Cornell Med Ctr (page 70); **Address:** 407 E 70th St, New York, NY 10021-5302; **Phone:** (212) 628-6611; **Board Cert:** Internal Medicine 1977, Pulmonary Disease 1987; **Med School:** Baylor Coll Med 1974; **Resid:** Internal Medicine, NY Hosp-Cornell Med Ctr, New York, NY 1974-1977; **Fellow:** Pulmonary Disease, NY Hosp-Cornell Med Ctr, New York, NY 1977-1979; **Fac Appt:** Clin Prof Medicine, Cornell Univ-Weill Med Coll

Nash, Thomas MD (Pul) - *Spec Exp:* Asthma; **Hospital:** NY Presby Hosp - NY Weill Cornell Med Ctr (page 70); **Address:** 310 E 72nd St, New York, NY 10021-4726; **Phone:** (212) 734-6612; **Board Cert:** Internal Medicine 1981, Infectious Disease 1984, Pulmonary Disease 1988; **Med School:** NYU Sch Med 1978; **Resid:** Internal Medicine, NY Hosp-Cornell Med Ctr, New York, NY 1978-1981; **Fellow:** Infectious Disease, NY Hosp-Cornell Med Ctr, New York, NY 1981-1985; Pulmonary Disease, Meml Sloan Kettering Cancer Ctr, New York, NY 1981-1985; **Fac Appt:** Assoc Clin Prof Medicine, NYU Sch Med

Niederman, Michael MD (Pul) - *Spec Exp:* Infectious Disease-Lung; Emphysema; Respiratory Failure & Pneumonia; **Hospital:** Winthrop - Univ Hosp; **Address:** 222 Station Plaza N, Ste 400, Mineola, NY 11501-3893; **Phone:** (516) 663-2834; **Board Cert:** Pulmonary Disease 1983, Critical Care Medicine 1997; **Med School:** Boston Univ 1977; **Resid:** Internal Medicine, Northwestern Univ Med Ctr, Chicago, IL 1977-1980; **Fellow:** Pulmonary Disease, Yale-New Haven Hosp, New Haven, CT 1980-1983; **Fac Appt:** Prof Medicine, SUNY Stony Brook

Pack, Allan I MD/PhD (Pul) - *Spec Exp:* Sleep Disorders & Aging; Sleep Disorders/Apnea; **Hospital:** Hosp Univ Penn (page 78); **Address:** Hosp Univ Penn, Dept Sleep & Respiratory Neurobiology, 991 Maloney Bldg/ 3600 Spruce Street, Philadelphia, PA 19104-4283; **Phone:** (215) 615-3669; **Med School:** Scotland 1967; **Resid:** Internal Medicine, Univ Glasgow, Scotland; **Fellow:** Pulmonary Disease, Univ Glasgow, Scotland; **Fac Appt:** Prof Medicine, Univ Penn

Reichman, Lee Brodersohn MD (Pul) - *Spec Exp:* Tuberculosis; Mycobacterial Infections; **Hospital:** UMDNJ-Univ Hosp-Newark; **Address:** NJ Med Sch, Nat Tuberculosis Ctr, 65 Bergen St, Ste GB1, Newark, NJ 07107-3001; **Phone:** (973) 972-3270; **Board Cert:** Internal Medicine 1972, Pulmonary Disease 1972; **Med School:** NYU Sch Med 1964; **Resid:** Internal Medicine, Bellevue Hosp, New York, NY 1964-1965; Internal Medicine, Harlem Hosp, New York, NY 1967-1969; **Fellow:** Pulmonary Disease, Harlem Hosp-Columbia P & S, New York, NY 1969-1970; **Fac Appt:** Prof Medicine, UMDNJ-NJ Med Sch, Newark

Rogers, Robert M MD (Pul) - *Spec Exp:* Pulmonary Alveolar Proteinosis; **Hospital:** UPMC - Presbyterian Univ Hosp; **Address:** UPMC, Dept Pulm Dis, Allergy, & Crit Care, 3459 5th Ave, rm NW628, Box MUH, Pittsburgh, PA 15203; **Phone:** (412) 692-2210; **Board Cert:** Pulmonary Disease 1969, Critical Care Medicine 1999; **Med School:** Univ Penn 1960; **Resid:** Internal Medicine, Univ Hosps Cleveland, Cleveland, OH 1961-1963; Pulmonary Disease, Case West Res, Cleveland, OH 1963-1964; **Fellow:** Pulmonary Disease, Univ Penn, Philadephia, PA 1964-1965; Physiology, Univ Penn, Philadelphia, PA 1966-1968; **Fac Appt:** Prof Medicine, Univ Pittsburgh

Rosen, Mark J MD (Pul) - *Spec Exp:* AIDS/HIV; Chronic Obstructive Lung Disease (COPD); Asthma; **Hospital:** Beth Israel Med Ctr - Petrie Division (page 58); **Address:** Beth Israel Med Ctr, Pul and CC Med, 1st Ave & 16th St, New York, NY 10003; **Phone:** (212) 420-2697; **Board Cert:** Pulmonary Disease 1998, Critical Care Medicine 1997; **Med School:** Brown Univ 1975; **Resid:** Internal Medicine, Mount Sinai Hosp, New York, NY 1975-1978; **Fellow:** Pulmonary Disease, Mount Sinai Hosp, New York, NY 1978-1980; Critical Care Medicine, St Vincent's Hosp & Med Ctr, New York, NY 1980; **Fac Appt:** Prof Medicine, Albert Einstein Coll Med

Schluger, Neil MD (Pul) - *Spec Exp:* Tuberculosis; Pulmonary Infections; **Hospital:** NY Presby Hosp - Columbia Presby Med Ctr (page 70); **Address:** 630 W 168th St Fl VC, Box 1206A, New York, NY 10032; **Phone:** (212) 305-9817; **Board Cert:** Pulmonary Disease 1992, Critical Care Medicine 1993; **Med School:** Univ Penn 1985; **Resid:** Internal Medicine, St Luke's Roosevelt Hosp Ctr, New York, NY 1985-1989; **Fellow:** Pulmonary Critical Care Medicine, NY Hosp-Cornell Med Ctr, New York, NY 1989-1992; **Fac Appt:** Assoc Prof Medicine, Columbia P&S

Schwab, Richard MD (Pul) - *Spec Exp:* Sleep Apnea; Sleep Disorders; **Hospital:** Hosp Univ Penn (page 78); **Address:** Univ of Penn Med Ctr, Dept Pulmonary and CCM, 3400 Spruce St, Bldg Ravdin 3 - Ste F, Philadelphia, PA 19104; **Phone:** (215) 662-3202; **Board Cert:** Critical Care Medicine 1991, Pulmonary Disease 1990; **Med School:** Univ Penn 1983; **Resid:** Internal Medicine, Jefferson Univ Hosp, Philadelphia, PA 1984-1986; **Fellow:** Pulmonary Critical Care Medicine, Jefferson Univ Hosp, Philadelphia, PA 1988-1991; **Fac Appt:** Asst Prof Medicine, Univ Penn

Smith, James P MD (Pul) - *Spec Exp:* Emphysema; Lung Cancer; Asthma; **Hospital:** NY Presby Hosp - NY Weill Cornell Med Ctr (page 70); **Address:** 170 E 77th St, New York, NY 10021-1912; **Phone:** (212) 879-2180; **Board Cert:** Internal Medicine 1967, Pulmonary Disease 1968; **Med School:** Georgetown Univ 1960; **Resid:** Internal Medicine, NY Hosp-Cornell Med Ctr, New York, NY 1960-1962; Internal Medicine, NY Hosp-Cornell Med Ctr, New York, NY 1964-1965; **Fellow:** Pulmonary Disease, NY Hosp-Cornell Med Ctr, New York, NY 1964-1966; **Fac Appt:** Clin Prof Medicine, Cornell Univ-Weill Med Coll

Steiger, David MD (Pul) - *Spec Exp:* Critical Care; **Hospital:** Hosp For Joint Diseases (page 61); **Address:** 305 2nd Ave, Ste 16, New York, NY 10003; **Phone:** (212) 598-6091; **Board Cert:** Pulmonary Disease 1992, Critical Care Medicine 1995; **Med School:** England 1981; **Resid:** Internal Medicine, St Luke's Roosevelt Hosp Ctr, New York, NY 1984-1989; **Fellow:** Pulmonary Disease, UCSF Med Ctr, San Francisco, CA 1989-1994; **Fac Appt:** Asst Prof Medicine, NYU Sch Med

Steinberg, Harry MD (Pul) - *Spec Exp:* Emphysema; Lung Cancer; **Hospital:** Long Island Jewish Med Ctr; **Address:** Long Island Jewish Med Ctr, Dept Med, 270-05 76th Ave, New Hyde Park, NY 11040-1496; **Phone:** (718) 470-7231; **Med School:** Temple Univ 1966; **Resid:** Internal Medicine, Long Island Jewish Med Ctr, New Hyde Park, NY 1967-1969; **Fellow:** Internal Medicine, Hosp Univ Penn, Philadelphia, PA 1972-1974; **Fac Appt:** Prof Medicine, Albert Einstein Coll Med

Stover-Pepe, Diane E MD (Pul) - *Spec Exp:* Lung Cancer; AIDS/HIV; Infectious Disease-Lung; **Hospital:** Mem Sloan Kettering Cancer Ctr; **Address:** 1275 York Ave Fl C - rm 678, New York, NY 10021; **Phone:** (212) 639-8380; **Board Cert:** Internal Medicine 1975, Pulmonary Disease 1978; **Med School:** Albert Einstein Coll Med 1970; **Resid:** Internal Medicine, Harlem Hosp Ctr, New York, NY 1971-1972; Internal Medicine, NY Hosp-Cornell Med Ctr, New York, NY 1974-1975; **Fellow:** Pulmonary Disease, Albert Einstein Med Ctr, Bronx, NY 1975; **Fac Appt:** Prof Medicine, Cornell Univ-Weill Med Coll

Teirstein, Alvin MD (Pul) - *Spec Exp:* Sarcoidosis; Interstitial Lung Disease; Lung Cancer; **Hospital:** Mount Sinai Hosp (page 68); **Address:** 1 Gustave Levy Pl, Box 1232, Mount Sinai Med Ctr, Pulmonary Associates, New York, NY 10029; **Phone:** (212) 241-5656; **Board Cert:** Internal Medicine 1961, Pulmonary Disease 1969; **Med School:** SUNY Downstate 1953; **Resid:** Internal Medicine, Mt Sinai Med Ctr, New York, NY 1955-1957; **Fellow:** Pulmonary Disease, Mt Sinai Med Ctr, New York, NY 1953-1954; Pulmonary Disease, VA Med Ctr, Bronx, NY 1954-1956; **Fac Appt:** Prof Medicine, Mount Sinai Sch Med

Terry, Peter Browne MD (Pul) - *Spec Exp:* Pulmonary Disease - General; **Hospital:** Johns Hopkins Hosp - Baltimore; **Address:** 600 N Wolfe St Bldg Blalock - rm 910, Baltimore, MD 21287; **Phone:** (410) 955-3467; **Board Cert:** Pulmonary Disease 1976, Internal Medicine 1973; **Med School:** St Louis Univ 1968; **Resid:** Internal Medicine, Univ Conn Hlth Ctr, Farmington, CT 1969-1970; Internal Medicine, Johns Hopkins Hosp, Baltimore, MD 1972-1973; **Fellow:** Pulmonary Disease, Johns Hopkins Hosp, Baltimore, MD 1973-1974; Pulmonary Disease, Mayo Clinic, Rochester, MN 1974-1975; **Fac Appt:** Prof Medicine, Johns Hopkins Univ

Thomashow, Byron MD (Pul) - *Spec Exp:* Emphysema; Asthma; **Hospital:** NY Presby Hosp - Columbia Presby Med Ctr (page 70); **Address:** 161 Fort Washington Ave, rm 311, New York, NY 10032; **Phone:** (212) 305-5261; **Board Cert:** Internal Medicine 1977, Pulmonary Disease 1980; **Med School:** Columbia P&S 1974; **Resid:** Internal Medicine, St Luke's-Roosevelt Hosp Ctr, New York, NY 1974-1977; Pulmonary Disease, St Luke's-Roosevelt Hosp Ctr, New York, NY 1977-1978; **Fellow:** Pulmonary Disease, Harlem Hosp Ctr, New York, NY 1978-1979; **Fac Appt:** Assoc Clin Prof Medicine, Columbia P&S

Tino, Gregory MD (Pul) - *Spec Exp:* Lung Volume Reduction; Chronic Obstructive Lung Disease (COPD); Interstitial Lung Disease; **Hospital:** Hosp Univ Penn (page 78); **Address:** Univ Penn Med Ctr, Pulmonary & Critical Care Div, 831 West Gates Bldg, Philadelphia, PA 19104; **Phone:** (215) 349-5303; **Board Cert:** Critical Care Medicine 1995, Pulmonary Disease 1992; **Med School:** Mount Sinai Sch Med 1986; **Resid:** Internal Medicine, Hosp Univ Penn, Philadelphia, PA 1986-1989; **Fellow:** Pulmonary Critical Care Medicine, Hosp Univ Penn, Philadelphia, PA 1989-1992; **Fac Appt:** Asst Prof Medicine, Univ Penn

White, Dorothy MD (Pul) - *Spec Exp:* Lung Cancer; AIDS/HIV; **Hospital:** Mem Sloan Kettering Cancer Ctr; **Address:** 1275 York Ave, rm C671, New York, NY 10021; **Phone:** (212) 639-8022; **Board Cert:** Pulmonary Disease 1984, Critical Care Medicine 1987; **Med School:** SUNY Hlth Sci Ctr 1977; **Resid:** Pulmonary Disease, NY Hosp-Cornell Med Ctr, New York, NY 1977-1981; **Fellow:** Pulmonary Disease, Yale-New Haven Hosp, New Haven, CT 1982-1984; **Fac Appt:** Assoc Prof Medicine, Cornell Univ-Weill Med Coll

Southeast

Bayly, Timothy C MD (Pul) - *Spec Exp:* Pulmonary Disease - General; **Hospital:** Inova Fairfax Hosp; **Address:** 5510 Alma Ln, Ste 300, Springfield, VA 22151; **Phone:** (703) 642-5990; **Board Cert:** Pulmonary Disease 1976, Internal Medicine 1975; **Med School:** Georgetown Univ 1972; **Resid:** Internal Medicine, Cornell Univ Med Coll, New York, NY 1974-1975; **Fellow:** Pulmonary Disease, Georgetown Univ Hosp, Washington, DC 1975-1976; **Fac Appt:** Asst Clin Prof Medicine, Georgetown Univ

Brooks, Stuart M MD (Pul) - *Spec Exp:* Occupational Lung Disease; **Hospital:** Tampa Genl Hosp; **Address:** USF Coll Pub Hlth, 13201 Bruce B Downs Blvd, Box 56 MDC, Tampa, FL 33612-3805; **Phone:** (813) 974-6626; **Board Cert:** Internal Medicine 1977, Pulmonary Disease 1969; **Med School:** Univ Cincinnati 1962; **Resid:** Internal Medicine, Boston City Hosp, Boston, MA 1963-1967; **Fellow:** Pulmonary Disease, Boston City Hosp, Boston, MA 1967-1969; **Fac Appt:** Prof Occupational Medicine, Univ S Fla Coll Med

Christman, Brian Wallace MD (Pul)* - *Spec Exp:* Pulmonary Hypertension; Lung Injury/ARDS; **Hospital:** Vanderbilt Univ Med Ctr (page 80); **Address:** Vanderbilt Univ Med Ctr, Div Pulm Med, 1161 21st Ave S, rm T1217, Nashville, TN 37232-2650; **Phone:** (615) 322-2386; **Board Cert:** Internal Medicine 1984, Critical Care Medicine 1999, Pulmonary Disease 1986; **Med School:** Univ Okla Coll Med 1981; **Resid:** Internal Medicine, Vanderbilt Univ Med Ctr, Nashville, TN 1982-1984; **Fellow:** Pulmonary Disease, Vanderbilt Univ Med Ctr, Nashville, TN 1984-1987; **Fac Appt:** Assoc Prof Medicine, Vanderbilt Univ

Cicale, Michael Jon MD (Pul) - *Spec Exp:* Pulmonary Disease - General; **Hospital:** Shands Hlthcre at Univ of FL (page 73); **Address:** Shands Healthcare at Univ FL, 1600 SW Archer Rd, Box 100255, Gainesville, FL 32610-0225; **Phone:** (352) 392-2666; **Board Cert:** Internal Medicine 1982, Pulmonary Disease 1984; **Med School:** Georgetown Univ 1979; **Resid:** Internal Medicine, Univ FL Med Ctr, Gainesville, FL 1979-1982; **Fellow:** Pulmonary Disease, Univ FL Med Ctr, Gainesville, FL 1982-1984; **Fac Appt:** Assoc Prof Medicine, Univ Fla Coll Med

Cooper, John Allen D MD (Pul) - *Spec Exp:* Drug Induced Lung Disease; Chronic Lung Disease-COPD; **Hospital:** Univ of Ala Hosp at Birmingham; **Address:** 215 Tinsley Harrison Tower, 1900 University Blvd, Birmingham, AL 35294; **Phone:** (205) 934-7941; **Board Cert:** Pulmonary Disease 1984, Critical Care Medicine 1989; **Med School:** Duke Univ 1978; **Resid:** Internal Medicine, University of Washington, Seattle, WA 1978-1987; Internal Medicine, University of Virginia, Charlottesville, VA 1979-1981; **Fellow:** Pulmonary Disease, Yale University, New Haven, CT 1981-1985; **Fac Appt:** Prof Medicine, Duke Univ

Cooper, William R MD (Pul) - *Spec Exp:* Critical Care; Asthma; Chronic Obstructive Lung Disease (COPD); **Hospital:** Virginia Beach Gen Hosp; **Address:** 1008 First Colonial Rd, Ste 103, Virginia Beach, VA 23454-3071; **Phone:** (757) 481-2515; **Board Cert:** Internal Medicine 1972, Pulmonary Disease 1974, Critical Care Medicine 1999; **Med School:** Univ VA Sch Med 1969; **Resid:** Internal Medicine, Cleveland Metro Genl Hosp, Cleveland, OH 1970-; Pulmonary Disease, Univ Virginia Hosp, Richmond, VA 1971-1973; **Fellow:** Pulmonary Disease, Mount Sinai Med Ctr, Miami Beach, FL 1973-1974

Donohue, James MD (Pul) - *Spec Exp:* Asthma; Chronic Obstructive Lung Disease (COPD); Sarcoidosis; **Hospital:** Univ of NC Hosp (page 77); **Address:** UNC Sch Med, Div Pulm Dis & CCM, 420 Burnett-Wolmack Bldg , MC CB#7020, Chapel Hill, NC 27599-7020; **Phone:** (919) 966-2531; **Board Cert:** Internal Medicine 1975, Pulmonary Disease 1976; **Med School:** UMDNJ-NJ Med Sch, Newark 1969; **Resid:** Internal Medicine, UMDNJ-Newark, Newark, NJ 1970-1971; Internal Medicine, NC Meml Hosp, Chapel Hill, NC 1973-1974; **Fellow:** Pulmonary Disease, Univ North Carolina, Chapel Hill, NC 1974-1976; **Fac Appt:** Prof Medicine, Univ NC Sch Med

Dunlap, Nancy Elizabeth MD/PhD (Pul) - *Spec Exp:* Tuberculosis; Critical Care; **Hospital:** Univ of Ala Hosp at Birmingham; **Address:** 2000 6th Ave S Fl 3/Admin, Birmingham, AL 35233; **Phone:** (205) 801-7900; **Board Cert:** Internal Medicine 1984, Pulmonary Disease 1988, Critical Care Medicine 1999; **Med School:** Duke Univ 1981; **Resid:** Internal Medicine, Univ Ala, Birmingham, AL 1982-1984; **Fellow:** Pulmonary Disease, Univ Ala, Birmingham, AL 1984-1987; **Fac Appt:** Prof Medicine, Univ Ala

Enelow, Richard Ian MD (Pul) - *Spec Exp:* Interstitial Lung Disease; Lung Disease; **Hospital:** Univ of VA Hlth Sys (page 79); **Address:** Div Pulmonary & Critical Care, Hosp Drive Fl 6 - rm 6590, Charlottesville, VA 22908; **Phone:** (804) 924-5270; **Board Cert:** Pulmonary Disease 1992, Internal Medicine 1986; **Med School:** Boston Univ 1983; **Resid:** Internal Medicine, New Eng-Deaconess Med Ctr, Boston, MA 1984-1986; **Fellow:** Pulmonary Disease, Univ VA Hlth Scis Ctr, Charlottesville, VA 1989-1992; **Fac Appt:** Assoc Prof Pulmonary Disease, Univ VA Sch Med

Fletcher, Eugene MD (Pul) - *Spec Exp:* Chronic Obstructive Lung Disease (COPD); **Hospital:** Univ Louisville Hosp; **Address:** 530 S Jackson St, rm A-3-L-01, Louisville, KY 40292; **Phone:** (502) 852-5841; **Board Cert:** Critical Care Medicine 1987, Pulmonary Disease 1980; **Med School:** Temple Univ 1971; **Resid:** Internal Medicine, Univ Colo Affil Hosp, Denver, CO 1972-1973; Internal Medicine, Fitzsimons Army Med Ctr, Denver, CO 1973-1974; **Fellow:** Pulmonary Disease, Univ Okla Hlth Scis Ctr, Oklahoma City, OK; **Fac Appt:** Prof Medicine, Univ Louisville Sch Med

Fulkerson Jr, William J MD (Pul) - *Spec Exp:* Respiratory Failure-Acute; Thromboembolic Disorders; **Hospital:** Duke Univ Med Ctr (page 60); **Address:** Duke Univ Med Ctr, Trent Drive, Box 3121, Durham, NC 27710; **Phone:** (919) 684-8076; **Board Cert:** Pulmonary Disease 1984, Critical Care Medicine 1996; **Med School:** Univ NC Sch Med 1977; **Resid:** Internal Medicine, Vanderbilt Univ Hosp, Nashville, TN 1977-1980; **Fellow:** Pulmonary Disease, Vanderbilt Univ Hosp, Nashville, TN 1981-1983; **Fac Appt:** Prof Medicine, Duke Univ

Goldman, Allan Larry MD (Pul) - *Spec Exp:* Occupational Lung Disease; Airway Disorders; **Hospital:** Tampa Genl Hosp; **Address:** USF Coll Med, Internal Med, 12901 Bruce B Downs Blvd, Box MDC19, Tampa, FL 33612-4799; **Phone:** (813) 974-2271; **Board Cert:** Pulmonary Disease 1972, Internal Medicine 1972; **Med School:** Univ Minn 1968; **Resid:** Internal Medicine, Brooke Army Hosp, San Antonio, TX 1969-1970; **Fellow:** Pulmonary Disease, Walter Reed Army Hosp, Washington, DC 1970-1972; **Fac Appt:** Prof Medicine, Univ S Fla Coll Med

Harman, Eloise M MD (Pul) - *Spec Exp:* Pulmonary Disease - General; **Hospital:** Shands Hlthcre at Univ of FL (page 73); **Address:** Shands at U F, 1600 SW Archer Rd, Box 100225, Gainesville, FL 32610-0225; **Phone:** (352) 392-2666; **Board Cert:** Pulmonary Disease 1976, Critical Care Medicine 1997; **Med School:** Johns Hopkins Univ 1970; **Resid:** Internal Medicine, Johns Hopkins Hosp, Baltimore, MD 1970-1972; **Fellow:** Pulmonary Disease, NY Hosp-Cornell Med Ctr, New York, NY 1972-1974; **Fac Appt:** Prof Medicine, Univ Fla Coll Med

Haynes, Johnson MD (Pul) - *Spec Exp:* Pulmonary Disease - General; **Hospital:** Univ of S Ala Med Ctr; **Address:** Univ S AL Med Ctr, 2451 Fillingim St, Ste 10G, Mobile, AL 36617; **Phone:** (251) 471-7888; **Board Cert:** Internal Medicine 1983, Pulmonary Disease 1986; **Med School:** Univ S Ala Coll Med 1980; **Resid:** Internal Medicine, Univ S AL Med Ctr, Mobile, AL 1981-1983; **Fellow:** Pulmonary Disease, Univ S AL Med Ctr, Mobile, AL 1984-1986; **Fac Appt:** Prof Medicine, Univ S Ala Coll Med

Heffner, John E MD (Pul) - *Spec Exp:* Critical Care; **Hospital:** Med Univ Hosp Authority; **Address:** Med Univ SC, Dept Pulm Med, 96 Jonathan Lucas St, Box 250623, Charleston, SC 29425; **Phone:** (843) 792-2153; **Board Cert:** Internal Medicine 1977, Pulmonary Disease 1982, Critical Care Medicine 1987; **Med School:** UCLA 1974; **Resid:** Internal Medicine, Univ Colo Med Ctr, Denver, CO 1973-1978; **Fac Appt:** Prof Medicine, Med Univ SC

Henke, David Carroll MD (Pul) - *Spec Exp:* Asthma; **Hospital:** Univ of NC Hosp (page 77); **Address:** Univ NC Med Sch-Chapel Hill, Dept Pulm Dis, rm 420, Box 7020, Chapel Hill, NC 27599-7020; **Phone:** (919) 966-2531; **Board Cert:** Pulmonary Disease 1988, Critical Care Medicine 1991; **Med School:** Univ NC Sch Med 1977; **Resid:** Internal Medicine, NC Memorial Hosp, Chapel Hill, NC 1978-1980; Dermatology, NC Meml NIEHS, Chapel Hill, NC 1982-1984; **Fellow:** Pulmonary Disease, NC Memorial Hosp, Chapel Hill, NC 1984-1987; **Fac Appt:** Assoc Prof Medicine, Univ NC Sch Med

Johnson, Bruce Ellsworth MD (Pul) - *Spec Exp:* Sleep Disorders/Apnea; **Hospital:** Virginia Beach Gen Hosp; **Address:** 1008 First Colonial Rd, Ste 103, Virginia Beach, VA 23454; **Phone:** (757) 481-2515; **Board Cert:** Critical Care Medicine 1991, Pulmonary Disease 1986; **Med School:** Med Coll GA 1978; **Fellow:** Pulmonary Disease, UVA Med Ctr, Charlottesville, VA 1981-1983

Koenig, Steven Michael MD (Pul) - *Spec Exp:* Sleep Disorders/Apnea; Occupational Lung Disease; Asthma; **Hospital:** Univ of VA Hlth Sys (page 79); **Address:** Univ Va Hlth System, Dept Med, Pulmonary Div, 100 Lee St W, Fl 6 - rm 6594, Box 800546, Charlottesville, VA 22908-0546; **Phone:** (804) 924-2228; **Board Cert:** Internal Medicine 1987, Pulmonary Disease 2000, Critical Care Medicine 2001; **Med School:** Univ Penn 1984; **Resid:** Internal Medicine, Univ Chicago, Chicago, IL 1984-1987; **Fellow:** Pulmonary Critical Care Medicine, Univ Chicago, Chicago, IL 1987-1990; **Fac Appt:** Assoc Prof Pulmonary Disease, Univ VA Sch Med

Light, Richard Wayne MD (Pul) - *Spec Exp:* *Pleural Disease;* **Hospital:** St Thomas Hosp - Nashville; **Address:** St Thomas Hosp, Pulm Dept, 4220 Harding Rd, Nashville, TN 37205; **Phone:** (615) 222-4445; **Board Cert:** Internal Medicine 1972, Pulmonary Disease 1974; **Med School:** Johns Hopkins Univ 1968; **Resid:** Internal Medicine, Johns Hopkins Hosp, Baltimore, MD 1969-1970; **Fellow:** Pulmonary Disease, Johns Hopkins Hosp, Baltimore, MD 1970-1972; **Fac Appt:** Prof Medicine, Vanderbilt Univ

Lorusso, Thomas MD (Pul) - *Spec Exp:* *Critical Care;* **Hospital:** Inova Fairfax Hosp; **Address:** 1800 Town Ctr Drive, Ste 419, Reston, VA 20190; **Phone:** (703) 620-3926; **Board Cert:** Critical Care Medicine 1993, Pulmonary Disease 1992; **Med School:** SUNY Syracuse 1987; **Resid:** Internal Medicine, Univ Hosp - SUNY, Stony Brook, NY 1988-1990; **Fellow:** Pulmonary Disease, Cedars Sinai Med Ctr, Los Angeles, CA 1990-1993

Loyd, James Emory MD (Pul) - *Spec Exp:* *Transplant Medicine-Lung; Interstitial Lung Disease; Pulmonary Fibrosis;* **Hospital:** Vanderbilt Univ Med Ctr (page 80); **Address:** Vanderbilt Univ Med Ctr, Div Pulm Med, Med Ctr North, rm T-1217, Nashville, TN 37232; **Phone:** (615) 322-2386; **Board Cert:** Internal Medicine 1978, Pulmonary Disease 1984, Critical Care Medicine 1997; **Med School:** W VA Univ 1973; **Resid:** Internal Medicine, Vanderbilt Univ Hosp, Nashville, TN 1974-1976; **Fellow:** Pulmonary Disease, Vanderbilt Univ Hosp, Nashville, TN 1976-1978; **Fac Appt:** Prof Medicine, Vanderbilt Univ

MacIntyre, Neil Ross MD (Pul) - *Spec Exp:* *Pulmonary Rehabilitation; Pulmonary Function Testing;* **Hospital:** Duke Univ Med Ctr (page 60); **Address:** 7951 Hospital North, Box 3911, Durham, NC 27710-0001; **Phone:** (919) 681-2720; **Board Cert:** Internal Medicine 1975, Pulmonary Disease 1980; **Med School:** Cornell Univ-Weill Med Coll 1972; **Resid:** Internal Medicine, NY Hosp-Cornell, New York, NY 1973-1975; **Fellow:** Pulmonary Disease, UCSF Med Ctr, San Francisco, CA 1978-1981; **Fac Appt:** Prof Medicine, Duke Univ

O'Brien, Richard MD (Pul) - *Spec Exp:* *Tuberculosis;* **Hospital:** Grady Hlth Sys; **Address:** CDC, Div TB Elimination, 1600 Clifton Rd NE, MS E-10, Atlanta, GA 30333; **Phone:** (404) 639-8123; **Board Cert:** Public Health & General Preventive Medicine 1980, Pulmonary Disease 1978; **Med School:** Univ VA Sch Med 1969; **Resid:** Internal Medicine, Emory Univ-Grady Meml Hosp., Atlanta, GA 1972-1974; **Fellow:** Pulmonary Disease, Emory Univ-Grady Meml Hosp., Atlanta, GA 1977-1978; **Fac Appt:** Asst Clin Prof Medicine, Emory Univ

Sahn, Steven A. MD (Pul) - *Spec Exp:* *Pleural Disease; Asthma;* **Hospital:** Med Univ Hosp Authority; **Address:** MUSC, Dept Pulmonary Med, 96 Jonathan Lucas St, Box 250623, Charleston, SC 29425; **Phone:** (843) 792-3167; **Board Cert:** Internal Medicine 1974, Pulmonary Disease 1974, Critical Care Medicine 1987; **Med School:** Univ Louisville Sch Med 1968; **Resid:** Internal Medicine, Univ Iowa Hosp, Iowa City, IA 1968-1971; **Fellow:** Pulmonary Disease, Univ Colorado Hlth Sci Ctr, Denver, CO 1971-1973; **Fac Appt:** Prof Medicine, Univ SC Sch Med

Schwartz, David A MD (Pul) - *Spec Exp:* *Occupational Lung Disease; Pulmonary Fibrosis; Asthma;* **Hospital:** Duke Univ Med Ctr (page 60); **Address:** Duke Univ Med Ctr, Box 2629, Durham, NC 27710; **Phone:** (919) 668-0380; **Board Cert:** Occupational Medicine 1987, Pulmonary Disease 1988; **Med School:** UCSD 1979; **Resid:** Internal Medicine, Boston City Hosp, Boston, MA 1981-1984; **Fellow:** Occupational Medicine, Harvard Sch Pub Hlth, Boston, MA 1984-1986; Pulmonary Disease, Univ of Seattle, Seattle, WA 1985-1988; **Fac Appt:** Asst Prof Medicine, Univ Iowa Coll Med

Shure, Deborah MD (Pul) - *Spec Exp:* Pulmonary Hypertension; Sarcoidosis; **Hospital:** Univ Hosps & Clins - Mississippi; **Address:** Dept Pulmonary Diseases, 2500 N State St, rm N-602, Jackson, MS 39216; **Phone:** (601) 984-5650; **Board Cert:** Pulmonary Disease 1980, Internal Medicine 1976; **Med School:** Albert Einstein Coll Med 1973; **Resid:** Internal Medicine, Bellevue Hosp, New York, NY 1973-1976; Internal Medicine, Bellevue Hosp, New York, NY 1976-1977; **Fellow:** Pulmonary Disease, UCSD Med Ctr, San Diego, CA 1977-1980; **Fac Appt:** Prof Medicine, Univ Miss

Sweet, Michael MD (Pul) - *Spec Exp:* Pulmonary Disease - General; **Hospital:** Martin Meml Hlth Sys; **Address:** 1100 E Ocean Blvd, Stuart, FL 34996-2590; **Phone:** (561) 283-4428; **Board Cert:** Internal Medicine 1977, Pulmonary Disease 1980; **Med School:** Univ Miami Sch Med 1974; **Resid:** Internal Medicine, U South FL Hosp, Tampa, FL 1975-1977; **Fellow:** Pulmonary Disease, U South Fl Hosp, Tampa, FL 1977-1979

Tapson, Victor MD/PhD (Pul) - *Spec Exp:* Pulmonary Hypertension; Transplant Medicine-Lung; Emphysema; **Hospital:** Duke Univ Med Ctr (page 60); **Address:** Duke Univ Med Ctr, Dept Pulmonary Critical Care Med, Box 31175, Durham, NC 27710; **Phone:** (919) 684-6237; **Board Cert:** Internal Medicine 1986, Pulmonary Disease 1990; **Med School:** Hahnemann Univ 1982; **Resid:** Internal Medicine, Duke Univ Med Ctr, Durham, NC 1983-1986; **Fellow:** Pulmonary Disease, Boston Univ, Boston, MA 1986-1989; **Fac Appt:** Assoc Prof Medicine, Duke Univ

Vaughey, Ellen MD (Pul) - *Spec Exp:* Critical Care; **Hospital:** Inova Fairfax Hosp; **Address:** 3289 Woodburn Rd, Ste 350, Annandale, VA 22003; **Phone:** (703) 641-8616; **Board Cert:** Pulmonary Disease 1992, Internal Medicine 1990; **Med School:** Georgetown Univ 1987; **Resid:** Internal Medicine, Thomas Jefferson Univ, Philadelphia, PA 1990; **Fellow:** Pulmonary Disease, Roger Williams Hosp-Brown Univ, Prividence, RI 1993

Wanner, Adam MD (Pul) - *Spec Exp:* Asthma; **Hospital:** Univ of Miami - Jackson Meml Hosp; **Address:** Univ Miami Sch Med, Div Pulm & Crit Care, Box 016960 (R-47), Miami, FL 33101; **Phone:** (305) 243-6387; **Board Cert:** Internal Medicine 1973, Pulmonary Disease 1974; **Med School:** Switzerland 1966; **Resid:** Internal Medicine, Kantonsspital Aarau, Switzerland 1968-1970; **Fellow:** Pulmonary Disease, Mt Sinai Med Ctr, Miami Beach, FL 1970-1972; **Fac Appt:** Prof Medicine, Univ Miami Sch Med

Wunderink, Richard MD (Pul) - *Spec Exp:* Infectious Disease-Lung; **Hospital:** Meth Hlth Care N - Memphis; **Address:** Univ Tenn Med Grp Heart Lung Ctr, 930 Madison, Ste 850, Memphis, TN 38104; **Phone:** (901) 726-8160; **Board Cert:** Internal Medicine 1983, Pulmonary Disease 1986, Critical Care Medicine 1997; **Med School:** Indiana Univ 1980; **Resid:** Internal Medicine, Butterworth Hosp, Grand Rapids, MI 1981-1983; **Fellow:** Pulmonary Disease, Henry Ford Hosp, Detroit, MI 1983-1985; **Fac Appt:** Assoc Prof Pulmonary Disease, Univ Tenn Coll Med, Memphis

Young, Keith Randall MD (Pul) - *Spec Exp:* Transplant Medicine-Lung; **Hospital:** Univ of Ala Hosp at Birmingham; **Address:** Univ AL Sch Med, 215 Tinsley Harrison Tower, 1900 University Blvd, Birmingham, AL 35294; **Phone:** (205) 934-5400; **Board Cert:** Internal Medicine 1982, Pulmonary Disease 1986, Allergy & Immunology 1987, Colon & Rectal Surgery 1989; **Med School:** Jefferson Med Coll 1978; **Resid:** Internal Medicine, Yale-New Haven Hosp, New Haven, CT 1979-1982; Pulmonary Disease, Yale-New Haven Hosp, New Haven, CT 1982-1985; **Fellow:** Allergy & Immunology, Nat Inst Hlth, Bethesda, MD 1985-1988; **Fac Appt:** Prof Medicine, Univ Ala

Midwest

Antony, Veena B. MD (Pul) - *Spec Exp:* Pleural Disease; **Hospital:** IN Univ Hosp (page 63); **Address:** VAMC 1481 W 10th St (111P), Indianapolis, IN 46202; **Phone:** (317) 554-0036; **Board Cert:** Internal Medicine 1979, Pulmonary Disease 1982; **Med School:** India 1974; **Resid:** Pulmonary Disease, Univ Co Hlth Sci Ctr; Pulmonary Disease, Natl Jewish Hosp-Asthma Ctr; **Fellow:** Internal Medicine, Kingsbrook Jewish Med Ctr

Arroliga, Alejandro C MD (Pul) - *Spec Exp:* Pulmonary Hypertension; **Hospital:** Cleveland Clin Fdn (page 57); **Address:** 9500 Euclid Ave, Ste 662, Cleveland, OH 44195; **Phone:** (216) 445-5765; **Board Cert:** Pulmonary Disease 1992, Critical Care Medicine 1993; **Med School:** Mexico 1984; **Resid:** Internal Medicine, Coney Island Hosp, Brooklyn, NY 1988-1990; **Fellow:** Pulmonary Disease, Yale-New Haven Hosp, New Haven, CT 1990-1993

Balk, Robert MD (Pul) - *Spec Exp:* Asthma; Emphysema; Respiratory Failure; **Hospital:** Rush-Presby - St Luke's Med Ctr (page 72); **Address:** 1725 W Harrison St, Bldg 3 - rm 054, Chicago, IL 60612; **Phone:** (312) 942-6744; **Board Cert:** Internal Medicine 1981, Pulmonary Disease 1986, Critical Care Medicine 1997; **Med School:** Univ MO-Kansas City 1978; **Resid:** Internal Medicine, Univ Missouri-Kansas City Affil Hosps, Kansas City, MO 1978-1981; **Fellow:** Pulmonary Critical Care Medicine, Univ Arkansas, Little Rock, AR 1981-1983; **Fac Appt:** Prof Medicine, Rush Med Coll

Cromydas, George MD (Pul) - *Spec Exp:* Emphysema; Lung Disease; **Hospital:** Advocate Lutheran Gen Hosp; **Address:** 1614 W Central Rd, Ste 205, Arlington Heights, IL 60005; **Phone:** (847) 818-1184; **Board Cert:** Pulmonary Disease 1984, Critical Care Medicine 1989; **Med School:** Univ IL Coll Med 1977; **Resid:** Internal Medicine, Univ IL Hosp & Clin, Chicago, IL 1977-1980; **Fellow:** Pulmonary Critical Care Medicine, Univ IL Hosp & Clin, Chicago, IL 1980-1982

Fahey, Patrick J MD (Pul) - *Spec Exp:* Lung Disease; **Hospital:** Loyola Univ Med Ctr; **Address:** 2160 1st Ave Bldg 102 - rm 7606, Maywood, IL 60153; **Phone:** (708) 216-3300; **Board Cert:** Pulmonary Disease 1978, Critical Care Medicine 1990; **Med School:** Univ Wisc 1973; **Resid:** Internal Medicine, St Elizabeth's Hosp, Boston, MA 1973-1976; **Fellow:** Pulmonary Disease, Strong Meml, Rochester, NY 1977-1980; **Fac Appt:** Prof Medicine, Loyola Univ-Stritch Sch Med

Geppert, Eugene MD (Pul) - *Spec Exp:* Cystic Fibrosis; Asthma; **Hospital:** Univ of Chicago Hosps (page 76); **Address:** 5758 S Maryland Ave Fl 5D, MC 9015, Chicago, IL 60637; **Phone:** (773) 702-9660; **Board Cert:** Pulmonary Disease 1978, Critical Care Medicine 1987; **Med School:** Yale Univ 1974; **Resid:** Internal Medicine, Univ Chicago Hosps, Chicago, IL 1975-1976; **Fellow:** Pulmonary Disease, UCSF Med Ctr, San Francisco, CA 1976-1979; **Fac Appt:** Asst Prof Medicine, Univ Chicago-Pritzker Sch Med

Glassroth, Jeffrey MD (Pul) - *Spec Exp:* Pulmonary Fibrosis; AIDS/HIV & Tuberculosis; Infectious Disease-Lung; **Hospital:** Univ WI Hosp & Clins; **Address:** Univ Wisc Med Sch- J5 219 CSC (2454), 600 Highland Ave, Madison, WI 53792; **Phone:** (608) 631-1792; **Board Cert:** Pulmonary Disease 1980, Critical Care Medicine 1989, Internal Medicine 1978; **Med School:** Univ Cincinnati 1973; **Resid:** Internal Medicine, Univ Cincinnati Med Ctr, Cincinnati, OH 1974-1978; **Fellow:** Pulmonary Disease, Boston Univ Med Ctr, Boston, MA 1978-1981; **Fac Appt:** Prof Pulmonary Disease, Univ Wisc

Gracey, Douglas Robert MD (Pul) - *Spec Exp:* Respiratory Failure; Chronic Obstructive Lung Disease (COPD); **Hospital:** Mayo Med Ctr & Clin - Rochester, MN; **Address:** Mayo Clinic, 200 1st St SW, Rochester, MN 55905-0002; **Phone:** (507) 284-2495; **Board Cert:** Internal Medicine 1969, Pulmonary Disease 1970; **Med School:** Northwestern Univ 1962; **Resid:** Internal Medicine, Mayo Grad Sch Med, Rochester, MN 1963-1966; **Fellow:** Pulmonary Disease, Mayo Grad Sch Med, Rochester, MN 1968-1969; **Fac Appt:** Prof Medicine, Mayo Med Sch

Grum, Cyril M MD (Pul) - *Spec Exp:* Asthma; Cystic Fibrosis; **Hospital:** Univ of MI Hlth Ctr; **Address:** Univ Michigan Med Ctr - Taubman Hlth Care Ctr, 1500 E Medical Center Dr, rm 3110-TC, Box 0368, Ann Arbor, MI 48109; **Phone:** (734) 936-5549; **Board Cert:** Pulmonary Disease 1982, Internal Medicine 1980; **Med School:** Med Coll Wisc 1977; **Resid:** Internal Medicine, Cleveland Clinic, Cleveland, OH; **Fellow:** Pulmonary Disease, Univ Michigan Hosps, Ann Arbor, MI; **Fac Appt:** Prof Medicine, Univ Mich Med Sch

Hall, Jesse MD (Pul) - *Spec Exp:* Respiratory Failure; Critical Care; Sleep Apnea; **Hospital:** Univ of Chicago Hosps (page 76); **Address:** 5841 S Maryland Ave, MC 6076, Chicago, IL 60637; **Phone:** (773) 702-1454; **Med School:** Univ Chicago-Pritzker Sch Med 1977; **Resid:** Internal Medicine, Univ Chicago Hosps, Chicago, IL 1978-1982; **Fac Appt:** Prof Pulmonary Disease, Univ Chicago-Pritzker Sch Med

Hunninghake, Gary MD (Pul) - *Spec Exp:* Sarcoidosis; Interstitial Lung Disease; **Hospital:** Univ of IA Hosp and Clinics; **Address:** Dept Pulmonary Disease, 200 Hawkins Drive, MC C-33-GH, Iowa City, IA 52242-1081; **Phone:** (319) 356-4187; **Board Cert:** Critical Care Medicine 1989, Pulmonary Disease 1980; **Med School:** Univ Kans 1972; **Resid:** Internal Medicine, Univ of KS Med Sch, Kansas City, KS 1972-1974; Pulmonary Disease, Natl Inst Hlth, Bethesda, MD 1974-1976; **Fac Appt:** Prof Medicine, Univ Iowa Coll Med

Hyers, Thomas Morgan MD (Pul) - *Spec Exp:* Thromboembolic Disorders; **Hospital:** St Joseph Hosp of Kirkwood; **Address:** 533 Couch Ave, Ste 140, St Louis, MO 63122; **Phone:** (314) 909-9779; **Board Cert:** Pulmonary Disease 1980, Critical Care Medicine 1999; **Med School:** Duke Univ 1968; **Resid:** Internal Medicine, Univ Wash Med Ctr, Seattle, WA 1972-1975; Pulmonary Disease, Univ Hosp, Denver, CO 1975-1977; **Fellow:** Pulmonary Disease, Natl Inst Hlth, Bethesda, MD 1969-1972; **Fac Appt:** Prof Medicine, St Louis Univ

Kaye, Mitchell MD (Pul) - *Spec Exp:* Chronic Obstructive Lung Disease (COPD); Asthma; Sleep Disorders/Apnea; **Hospital:** Fairview-Univ Med Ctr - Univ Campus; **Address:** Fairview Physicians Associates, 3400 W 66th St, Edina, MN 55435; **Phone:** (952) 928-1250; **Board Cert:** Pulmonary Disease 1990, Critical Care Medicine 1991; **Med School:** Univ Minn 1984; **Resid:** Internal Medicine, Univ Illinois Hosps & Clins, Chicago, IL 1984-1987; **Fellow:** Pulmonary Disease, Northwestern Univ Med Sch, Chicago, IL 1987-1989

Kollef, Marin Hristo MD (Pul) - *Spec Exp:* Critical Care; Infectious Disease-Lung; **Hospital:** Barnes-Jewish Hosp (page 55); **Address:** 660 S Euclid Ave, Box 80520, St Louis, MO 63110; **Phone:** (314) 454-8764; **Board Cert:** Pulmonary Disease 1988, Critical Care Medicine 1991; **Med School:** Univ Rochester 1983; **Resid:** Internal Medicine, Madigan Army Med Ctr, Tacoma, WA 1984-1986; **Fellow:** Pulmonary Disease, Madigan Army Med Ctr, Tacoma, WA 1986

Krowka, Michael Joseph MD (Pul) - *Spec Exp:* Hepatopulmonary Syndrome; **Hospital:** Mayo Med Ctr & Clin - Rochester, MN; **Address:** Div Pulmonary & Crit Care Med, 200 1st St SW, Rochester, MN 55905; **Phone:** (507) 284-2921; **Board Cert:** Internal Medicine 1983, Pulmonary Disease 1986; **Med School:** Univ Nevada 1980; **Resid:** Internal Medicine, Evanston Hosp, Chicago, IL 1981-1983; **Fellow:** Pulmonary Disease, Mayo Clinic, Rochester, MN 1983-1986; **Fac Appt:** Prof Pulmonary Disease, Mayo Med Sch

Lefrak, Stephen MD (Pul) - *Spec Exp:* Lung Volume Reduction; **Hospital:** Barnes-Jewish Hosp (page 55); **Address:** 4960 Children's Pl, Ste 4, St Louis, MO 63110; **Phone:** (314) 362-6044; **Board Cert:** Pulmonary Disease 1972, Critical Care Medicine 1987; **Med School:** SUNY Downstate 1965; **Resid:** Internal Medicine, Boston Univ Hosp, Boston, MA 1967-1968; Pulmonary Disease, Kings Co Hosp Ctr, Brooklyn, NY 1968-1969; **Fellow:** Cardiopulmonary Disease, Columbia-Presby Hosp, New York, NY 1969-1970

Lynch, Joseph P MD (Pul) - *Spec Exp:* Lung Transplant Care; Interstitial Lung Disease; Pulmonary Fibrosis; **Hospital:** Univ of MI Hlth Ctr; **Address:** 1500 E Med Ctr Drive, rm TC3915, Box 0360, Ann Arbor, MI 48109-0360; **Phone:** (734) 647-9342; **Board Cert:** Internal Medicine 1976, Pulmonary Disease 1980; **Med School:** Harvard Med Sch 1973; **Resid:** Internal Medicine, Univ Mich Med Ctr, Ann Arbor, MI 1974-1976; **Fellow:** Pulmonary Disease, Univ Mich Med Ctr, Ann Arbor, MI 1976-1978; **Fac Appt:** Prof Pulmonary Disease, Univ Mich Med Sch

Marini, John Joseph MD (Pul) - *Spec Exp:* Critical Care; **Hospital:** Regions Hosp - St Paul; **Address:** HealthPartners Ramsey Clin, Dept Pulm Crit Care, Jackson St Ctr for Intntl Health, 640 Jackson St, St Paul, MN 55101; **Phone:** (651) 254-4803; **Board Cert:** Pulmonary Disease 1978, Critical Care Medicine 1987; **Med School:** Johns Hopkins Univ 1973; **Resid:** Internal Medicine, Univ Washington Med Ctr, Seattle, WA 1974-1976; **Fellow:** Pulmonary Disease, Univ Washington Med Ctr, Seattle, WA 1976-1978; **Fac Appt:** Prof Medicine, Univ Minn

Martinez, Fernando J MD (Pul) - *Spec Exp:* Pulmonary Disease; Critical Care; **Hospital:** Univ of MI Hlth Ctr; **Address:** 1500 E Med Ctr Dr, 3916 Taubman Center, Ann Arbor, MI 48109; **Phone:** (734) 936-5201; **Board Cert:** Internal Medicine 1986, Critical Care Medicine 1999; **Med School:** Univ Fla Coll Med 1983; **Resid:** Internal Medicine, Beth Israel Hosp, Boston, MA 1984-1986; **Fellow:** Pulmonary Disease, Boston Univ, Boston, MA 1986-1989; **Fac Appt:** Prof Medicine, Univ Mich Med Sch

Mehta, Atul Chandrakant MD (Pul) - *Spec Exp:* Transplant Medicine-Lung; Lung Volume Reduction; Bronchoscopy; **Hospital:** Cleveland Clin Fdn (page 57); **Address:** Cleveland Clinic Foundation, 9500 Euclid Ave, Ste A-90, Cleveland, OH 44195-0002; **Phone:** (216) 444-2911; **Board Cert:** Internal Medicine 1981, Pulmonary Disease 1984, Critical Care Medicine 1991; **Med School:** India 1976; **Resid:** Internal Medicine, St Francis Med Ctr, Trenton, NJ 1978-1980; Internal Medicine, Easton Hosp, Easton, PA 1980-1981; **Fellow:** Pulmonary Disease, Cleveland Clin, Cleveland, OH 1981-1983; **Fac Appt:** Prof Medicine, Ohio State Univ

Popovich Jr, John MD (Pul) - *Spec Exp:* Lung Disease; Critical Care; **Hospital:** Henry Ford Hosp; **Address:** 2799 W Grand Blvd, Detroit, MI 48202; **Phone:** (313) 916-1828; **Board Cert:** Critical Care Medicine 1996, Pulmonary Disease 1980; **Med School:** Univ Mich Med Sch 1975; **Resid:** Internal Medicine, Henry Ford Hosp, Detroit, MI 1975-1978; **Fellow:** Pulmonary Disease, Henry Ford Hosp, Detroit, MI 1978-1980; **Fac Appt:** Asst Clin Prof Medicine, Univ Mich Med Sch

Prakash, Udaya MD (Pul) - *Spec Exp:* Bronchoscopy; **Hospital:** Mayo Med Ctr & Clin - Rochester, MN; **Address:** Div Pulmonary & Crit Care Med, 200 First St SW, Rochester, MN 55905; **Phone:** (507) 284-4162; **Board Cert:** Internal Medicine 1987, Pulmonary Disease 1976; **Med School:** India 1969; **Resid:** Internal Medicine, Mayo Clin, Rochester, MN 1972-1973; **Fellow:** Pulmonary Disease, Mayo Clin, Rochester, MN 1974-1976; **Fac Appt:** Prof Medicine, Mayo Med Sch

Silver, Michael MD (Pul) - *Spec Exp:* Chronic Obstructive Lung Disease (COPD); **Hospital:** Rush-Presby - St Luke's Med Ctr (page 72); **Address:** Professional Bldg 3, Rm 054, 1725 W Harrison St, Chicago, IL 60612; **Phone:** (312) 942-6744; **Board Cert:** Critical Care Medicine 1999, Pulmonary Disease 1988; **Med School:** Albany Med Coll 1981; **Resid:** Internal Medicine, Rush-Presby-St Luke's Med Ctr, Chicago, IL 1981-1985; **Fellow:** Pulmonary Critical Care Medicine, Rush-Presby-St Luke's Med Ctr, Chicago, IL 1985-1987; **Fac Appt:** Assoc Prof Medicine, Rush Med Coll

Stoller, James MD (Pul) - *Spec Exp:* Emphysema/Alpha-1 Antitrypsin Deficiency; **Hospital:** Cleveland Clin Fdn (page 57); **Address:** 9500 Euclid Ave, Desk A90, Cleveland, OH 44195; **Phone:** (216) 444-1960; **Board Cert:** Pulmonary Disease 1984, Internal Medicine 1982; **Med School:** Yale Univ 1979; **Resid:** Internal Medicine, Peter Bent Brigham Hosp, Boston, MA 1980-1982; **Fellow:** Pulmonary Disease, Brigham & Women's Hosp, Boston, MA 1982-1983

Tobin, Martin MD (Pul) - *Spec Exp:* Mechanical Ventilation; Chronic Obstructive Lung Disease (COPD); **Hospital:** Loyola Univ Med Ctr; **Address:** Dept Pulmonary & Critical Care, 2160 S First Ave Bldg 54 - rm 131, Maywood, IL 60153; **Phone:** (708) 202-2705; **Board Cert:** Critical Care Medicine 1987, Pulmonary Disease 1984; **Med School:** Ireland 1975; **Resid:** Internal Medicine, Trinity Coll Hosps, Dublin, Ireland 1976-1979; Pulmonary Disease, Kings Coll Hosp, London, England 1979-1980; **Fellow:** Pulmonary Critical Care Medicine, Mount Sinai Hosp, New York, NY 1980-1982; Pulmonary Critical Care Medicine, Univ Pittsburgh, Pittsburgh, PA 1982-1983; **Fac Appt:** Prof Medicine, Loyola Univ-Stritch Sch Med

Trulock, Elbert MD (Pul) - *Spec Exp:* Transplant Medicine-Lung; Emphysema & COPD; Pulmonary Hypertension; **Hospital:** Barnes-Jewish Hosp (page 55); **Address:** Wash Univ Sch Med, Dept Pulm, 660 S Euclid Ave, Box 8052, St Louis, MO 63110; **Phone:** (314) 454-8766; **Board Cert:** Internal Medicine 1981, Pulmonary Disease 1984; **Med School:** Emory Univ 1978; **Resid:** Internal Medicine, Barnes Hosp, St Louis, MO 1978-1981; **Fellow:** Pulmonary Disease, Wash Univ Med Ctr, St Louis, MO 1981-1983; **Fac Appt:** Prof Medicine, Washington Univ, St Louis

Wiedemann, Herbert P MD (Pul) - *Spec Exp:* Interstitial Lung Disease; Critical Care; **Hospital:** Cleveland Clin Fdn (page 57); **Address:** 9500 Euclid Ave, Desk A90, Cleveland, OH 44195; **Phone:** (216) 444-8335; **Board Cert:** Pulmonary Disease 1984, Critical Care Medicine 1987; **Med School:** Cornell Univ-Weill Med Coll 1977; **Resid:** Internal Medicine, Univ Wash Hosps, Seattle, WA 1977-1980; Internal Medicine, Harborview Hosp, Seattle, WA 1980-1981; **Fellow:** Pulmonary Disease, Yale Univ Sch Med, New Haven, CT 1981-1984

Great Plains and Mountains

Brown, Kevin K MD (Pul) - *Spec Exp:* Interstitial Lung Disease; Autoimmune Lung Disease; **Hospital:** Natl Jewish Med & Rsrch Ctr; **Address:** Natl Jewish Med & Research Ctr, 1400 Jackson St, rm F108, Denver, CO 80206; **Phone:** (303) 398-1621; **Board Cert:** Internal Medicine 1989, Pulmonary Disease 1992, Critical Care Medicine 1993; **Med School:** Univ Minn 1984; **Resid:** Internal Medicine, Providence Med Ctr, Portland, OR 1986-1989; **Fellow:** Pulmonary Disease, Maine Med Ctr, Portland, ME 1990-1992; Pulmonary Disease, Univ Colo Hlth Scis Ctr, Denver, CO 1992-1994; **Fac Appt:** Asst Prof Medicine, Univ Colo

Elliott, C Gregory MD (Pul) - *Spec Exp:* Pulmonary Hypertension; Thromboembolic Disorders; **Hospital:** LDS Hosp; **Address:** LDS Hosp, Dept Pulm, 325 8th Ave, Salt Lake City, UT 84143; **Phone:** (801) 408-1875; **Board Cert:** Internal Medicine 1976, Pulmonary Disease 1978; **Med School:** Univ MD Sch Med 1973; **Resid:** Internal Medicine, Univ Utah, Salt Lake City, UT 1976-1978; **Fellow:** Pulmonary Disease, Univ MD Hosp, Baltimore, MD 1974-1976; **Fac Appt:** Prof Medicine, Univ Utah

Harmon, Gary MD (Pul) - *Spec Exp:* Pulmonary Disease - General; **Hospital:** Overland Park Reg Med Ctr; **Address:** 10550 Quivira, Ste 480, Overland Park, KS 66215; **Phone:** (913) 599-3800; **Board Cert:** Pulmonary Disease 1986, Critical Care Medicine 1989; **Med School:** Univ Kans 1981; **Resid:** Pulmonary Disease, Univ Kansas Med Ctr, Kansas City, KS; Internal Medicine, Univ Kansas Med Ctr, Kansas City, KS

Iseman, Michael MD (Pul) - *Spec Exp:* Tuberculosis; Mycobacterial Infections; **Hospital:** Natl Jewish Med & Rsrch Ctr; **Address:** Natl Jewish Med & Rsch Ctr, 1400 Jackson St, rm B113, Denver, CO 80206; **Phone:** (303) 398-1667; **Board Cert:** Internal Medicine 1972, Pulmonary Disease 1976; **Med School:** Columbia P&S 1965; **Resid:** Internal Medicine, Bellevue Hosp, New York, NY 1965-1967; Internal Medicine, Harlem Hosp, New York, NY 1968-1970; **Fellow:** Pulmonary Disease, Harlem Hosp, New York, NY 1970-1972; **Fac Appt:** Prof Medicine, Univ Colo

Kaplan, James MD (Pul) - *Spec Exp:* Pulmonary Disease - General; **Hospital:** Overland Park Reg Med Ctr; **Address:** 10550 Quivira , Ste 480, Overland Park, KS 66215; **Phone:** (913) 599-3800; **Board Cert:** Pulmonary Disease 1990, Critical Care Medicine 1991; **Med School:** Univ MO-Kansas City 1984; **Resid:** Internal Medicine, Barnes Hosp, St Louis, MO 1984-1987; **Fellow:** Pulmonary Disease, Barnes Hosp-Wash Univ, St Louis, MO 1987-1989

Make, Barry J MD (Pul) - *Spec Exp:* Chronic Obstructive Lung Disease (COPD); Emphysema; **Hospital:** Natl Jewish Med & Rsrch Ctr; **Address:** Natl Jewish Med & Research Ctr, 1400 Jackson St, rm B107, Denver, CO 80206; **Phone:** (303) 398-1703; **Board Cert:** Internal Medicine 1973, Critical Care Medicine 1997; **Med School:** Jefferson Med Coll 1970; **Resid:** Internal Medicine, Univ Michigan, Ann Arbor, MI 1971-1973; **Fellow:** Pulmonary Disease, West Virginia Med Ctr, Morgantown, WV 1973-1974; Pulmonary Disease, Boston Univ Med Ctr, Boston, MA 1975-1976; **Fac Appt:** Prof Medicine, Univ Colo

Martin, Richard Jay MD (Pul) - *Spec Exp:* Asthma (Adult); Vocal Cord Disorders; **Hospital:** Natl Jewish Med & Rsrch Ctr; **Address:** Natl Jewish Med & Research Ctr, 1400 Jackson St, rm B-116, Denver, CO 80206-2761; **Phone:** (303) 398-1545; **Board Cert:** Internal Medicine 1976, Pulmonary Disease 1978; **Med School:** Univ Mich Med Sch 1971; **Resid:** Internal Medicine, Tulane, New Orleans, LA 1974-1976; **Fellow:** Pulmonary Disease, University of Okla, Oklahoma City, OK 1976-1978; **Fac Appt:** Prof Pulmonary Disease, Univ Colo

Newman, Lee MD (Pul) - *Spec Exp:* Occupational Lung Disease; **Hospital:** Natl Jewish Med & Rsrch Ctr; **Address:** 1400 Jackson Street, Denver, CO 80206; **Phone:** (303) 398-1725; **Board Cert:** Internal Medicine 1983, Pulmonary Disease 1986; **Med School:** Vanderbilt Univ 1980; **Resid:** Internal Medicine, Emory U Affil Prgm, Atlanta, GA 1982-1984; **Fellow:** Pulmonary Disease, Univ of Colo, Denver, CO 1984-1987; **Fac Appt:** Asst Prof Medicine, Univ Colo

Petty, Thomas L MD (Pul) - *Spec Exp:* Chronic Obstructive Lung Disease (COPD); Asthma; Respiratory Distress Syndrome(ARDS); **Hospital:** Presby - St Luke's Med Ctr; **Address:** 1850 High St, Denver, CO 80218-1235; **Phone:** (303) 839-6755; **Board Cert:** Internal Medicine 1965, Pulmonary Disease 1966; **Med School:** Univ Conn 1958; **Resid:** Univ Mich Hosp, Ann Arbor, MI 1959-1960; Univ Colo Med Ctr, Denver, CO 1960-1962; **Fellow:** Pulmonary Disease, Univ Colo Med Ctr, Denver, CO 1962-1963; **Fac Appt:** Prof Medicine, Univ Colo

Pingleton, Susan MD (Pul) - *Spec Exp:* Critical Care; **Hospital:** Univ Kansas Med Ctr; **Address:** 3901 Rainbow Blvd, Ste 4030 S, Kansas City, KS 66160; **Phone:** (913) 588-6044; **Board Cert:** Pulmonary Disease 1978, Critical Care Medicine 1991; **Med School:** Univ Kans 1972; **Resid:** Internal Medicine, Univ of Kansas Med Ctr, Kansas City, KS; **Fac Appt:** Prof Medicine, Univ Kans

Rodman, David MD (Pul) - *Spec Exp:* Cystic Fibrosis; Emphysema (Genetic); Bronchiectasis; **Hospital:** Univ Colo HSC - Denver; **Address:** Pulmonary Division, 4200 E Ninth Ave, MS C272, Denver, CO 80220-3706; **Phone:** (303) 315-7047; **Board Cert:** Pulmonary Disease 1988, Critical Care Medicine 1991; **Med School:** Univ Penn 1980; **Resid:** Internal Medicine, Univ Colorado Hosp, Denver, CO 1980-1983; Pulmonary Disease, Univ Colorado Hosp, Denver, CO 1983-1984; **Fellow:** Pulmonary Disease, Univ Colorado Hosp, Denver, CO 1985-1988; **Fac Appt:** Prof Medicine, Univ Colo

Rose, Cecile MD (Pul) - *Spec Exp:* Occupational Lung Disease; Sarcoidosis; Hypersensitivity Pneumonitis; **Hospital:** Natl Jewish Med & Rsrch Ctr; **Address:** 1400 Jackson Street, Denver, CO 80206-2761; **Phone:** (303) 398-1520; **Board Cert:** Occupational Medicine 1987, Pulmonary Disease 1986; **Med School:** Univ IL Coll Med 1980; **Resid:** Internal Medicine, Med Coll of VA Hosp, Richmond, VA 1981-1983; **Fellow:** Pulmonary Disease, Med Coll of VA Hosp, Richmond, VA 1983-1985; **Fac Appt:** Assoc Prof Medicine, Univ Colo

Schwarz, Marvin Ira MD (Pul) - *Spec Exp:* Interstitial Lung Disease; Pulmonary Vascular Disease; Lung Hemorrhage; **Hospital:** Univ Colo HSC - Denver; **Address:** Division of Pulmonary Science & Critical Care, 4200 Ninth Ave, Denver, CO 80262-0001; **Phone:** (303) 315-7047; **Board Cert:** Internal Medicine 1970, Pulmonary Disease 1971; **Med School:** Tulane Univ 1964; **Resid:** Internal Medicine, Charity Hosp, New Orleans, LA 1965-1967; **Fellow:** Pulmonary Disease, Charity Hosp, New Orleans, LA 1967-1969; **Fac Appt:** Prof Medicine, Univ Colo

Voelkel, Norbert F MD (Pul) - *Spec Exp:* Pulmonary Hypertension; Asthma; Emphysema; **Hospital:** Univ Colo HSC - Denver; **Address:** Univ Colorado Hlth Sci Ctr, 4200 E 9th Ave, rm 5525, Denver, CO 80262-0001; **Phone:** (303) 315-4211; **Med School:** Germany 1972; **Resid:** Internal Medicine, Univ Hamburg, Hamburg, Germany 1973-1977; **Fellow:** Research, Univ Colorado, Denver, CO 1977-1978; Pulmonary Disease, Univ Colorado, Denver, CO 1978-1981; **Fac Appt:** Prof Medicine, Univ Colo

Wenzel, Sally E MD (Pul) - *Spec Exp:* Asthma; **Hospital:** Natl Jewish Med & Rsrch Ctr; **Address:** Dept Medicine, Pulmonary Div, 1400 Jackson St, rm j114, Denver, CO 80206; **Phone:** (303) 398-1521; **Board Cert:** Pulmonary Disease 1986, Internal Medicine 1984; **Med School:** Univ Fla Coll Med 1981; **Resid:** Internal Medicine, NC Baptist Hosp, Winston Salem, NC 1981-1984; **Fellow:** Pulmonary Disease, Med Coll VA Hosp, Richmond, VA 1984-1986; **Fac Appt:** Asst Prof Medicine, Univ Colo

Southwest

Campbell, G. Douglas MD (Pul) - *Spec Exp:* Infectious Disease-Lung; **Hospital:** Louisiana State Univ Hosp; **Address:** LSUMC-Shrvprt, Div Pulm & CritCare, 1501 Kings Hwy, Shreveport, LA 71103; **Phone:** (318) 675-5920; **Board Cert:** Internal Medicine 1979, Pulmonary Disease 1986; **Med School:** Univ Miss 1976; **Resid:** Internal Medicine, Univ Miss Hosp, Jackson, MS 1977-1979; **Fellow:** Pulmonary Disease, Univ Tex Hlth Sci Ctr, San Antonio, TX 1981-1983; Infectious Disease, Univ Calgary HSC, Alberta, Canada 1983-1985; **Fac Appt:** Prof Medicine, Louisiana State Univ

Guidry, George Gary MD (Pul) - *Spec Exp:* Chronic Obstructive Lung Disease (COPD); **Hospital:** Our Lady of Lordes Reg Med Ctr - Lafayette; **Address:** 155 Hosp Dr, Ste 206, Lafayette, LA 70503-2852; **Phone:** (337) 234-3204; **Board Cert:** Internal Medicine 1988, Pulmonary Disease 1999; **Med School:** Louisiana State Univ 1985; **Resid:** Internal Medicine, LSU Med Ctr, Shreveport, LA 1985-1988; **Fellow:** Pulmonary Disease, LSU Med Ctr, Shreveport, LA 1988

Jenkinson, Stephen George MD (Pul) - *Spec Exp:* Lung Cancer; Chronic Obstructive Lung Disease (COPD); Asthma; **Hospital:** Audie L Murphy Meml Vets Hosp; **Address:** Audie Murphy VA Hosp, Dept Pulm, 7400 Merton Minter Blvd, San Antonio, TX 78229; **Phone:** (210) 617-5256; **Board Cert:** Pulmonary Disease 1978, Critical Care Medicine 1987; **Med School:** Louisiana State Univ 1973; **Resid:** Internal Medicine, LSU Med Ctr, Shreveport, LA 1973-1976; **Fellow:** Pulmonary Disease, LSU Med Ctr, Shreveport, LA 1976-1978; **Fac Appt:** Prof Medicine, Univ Tex, San Antonio

Levin, David C MD (Pul) - *Spec Exp:* Critical Care; **Hospital:** Univ OK Hlth Sci Ctr; **Address:** VA Hospital Med Ctr, 921 NE 13th St, Ste 111E, Oklahoma City, OK 73104; **Phone:** (405) 270-1573; **Board Cert:** Internal Medicine 1973, Pulmonary Disease 1976, Critical Care Medicine 1987; **Med School:** Case West Res Univ 1970; **Resid:** Internal Medicine, Univ Colorado Hlth Sci Ctr, Denver, CO 1971-1974; **Fellow:** Pulmonary Disease, Univ Colorado Hlth Sci Ctr, Denver, CO 1974-1975; **Fac Appt:** Prof Medicine, Univ Okla Coll Med

Perret, Phillip Samuel MD (Pul) - *Spec Exp:* Chronic Obstructive Lung Disease (COPD); **Hospital:** Our Lady of Lordes Reg Med Ctr - Lafayette; **Address:** 614 W St Mary Blvd, Lafayette, LA 70506; **Phone:** (337) 232-6435; **Board Cert:** Internal Medicine 1978, Pulmonary Disease 1980, Critical Care Medicine 1997; **Med School:** Emory Univ 1974; **Resid:** Internal Medicine, Emory Univ Hosp, Atlanta, GA 1974-1977; **Fellow:** Pulmonary Disease, Emory Univ Hosp, Atlanta, GA 1977-1979

Shellito, Judd Ernest MD (Pul) - *Spec Exp:* Pulmonary Infections; **Hospital:** Louisiana State Univ Hosp; **Address:** Louisiana State Univ Med Ctr, 1901 Perdido, Ste 3205, New Orleans, LA 70112-2865; **Phone:** (504) 568-4634; **Board Cert:** Internal Medicine 1977, Pulmonary Disease 1980, Critical Care Medicine 1989; **Med School:** Tulane Univ 1974; **Resid:** Internal Medicine, Evanston Hosp, Evanston, IL 1974-1978; **Fellow:** Pulmonary Critical Care Medicine, Univ New Mexico Hosp, Albuquerque, NM 1978-1980; **Fac Appt:** Prof Medicine, Louisiana State Univ

Weissler, Jonathan C MD (Pul) - *Spec Exp:* Interstitial Lung Disease; **Hospital:** Zale Lipshy Univ Hosp; **Address:** 5323 Harry Hines Blvd, Dallas, TX 75390-9034; **Phone:** (214) 648-5013; **Board Cert:** Pulmonary Disease 1984, Critical Care Medicine 1997; **Med School:** NYU Sch Med 1979; **Resid:** Internal Medicine, Univ Texas Hlth Sci Ctr, Dallas, TX 1979-1982; **Fellow:** Pulmonary Disease, Univ Texas HlthSci Ctr, Dallas, TX 1982-1985; **Fac Appt:** Prof Medicine, Univ Tex SW, Dallas

West Coast and Pacific

Albertson, Timothy MD/PhD (Pul) - *Spec Exp:* Critical Care; Transplant Medicine-Lung; **Hospital:** Univ CA - Davis Med Ctr; **Address:** UC Davis, Div Pulm Crit Care, 4150 V St, Ste 3400, Sacramento, CA 95817-9002; **Phone:** (916) 734-2111; **Board Cert:** Pulmonary Disease 1984, Critical Care Medicine 1996, Emergency Medicine 1997, Medical Toxicology 1995; **Med School:** UC Davis 1977; **Resid:** Internal Medicine, Univ Arizona, Tuscon, AZ 1979-1980; Internal Medicine, UC Davis Med Ctr, Sacramento, CA 1980-1981; **Fellow:** Pulmonary Critical Care Medicine, UC Davis Med Ctr, Sacramento, CA 1981-1983; **Fac Appt:** Prof Medicine, UC Davis

Balmes, John Randolph MD (Pul) - *Spec Exp:* Occupational Lung Disease; **Hospital:** San Francisco Gen Hosp; **Address:** 1001 Potrero Ave, Bldg 30 - Fl 5, San Francisco, CA 94110; **Phone:** (415) 206-4320; **Board Cert:** Internal Medicine 1979, Pulmonary Disease 1984; **Med School:** Mount Sinai Sch Med 1976; **Resid:** Internal Medicine, Mount Sinai Hosp, New York, NY 1977-1979; **Fellow:** Pulmonary Disease, Yale-New Haven Hosp, New Haven, CT 1979-1981; **Fac Appt:** Prof Medicine, UCSF

Bellamy, Paul Eric MD (Pul) - *Spec Exp:* Critical Care; **Hospital:** UCLA Med Ctr; **Address:** 200 UCLA Med Plaza, Ste 365B, Los Angeles, CA 90095; **Phone:** (310) 825-8061; **Board Cert:** Pulmonary Disease 1980, Critical Care Medicine 1987; **Med School:** SUNY Buffalo 1975; **Resid:** Internal Medicine, Univ Hosps Cleveland, Cleveland, OH 1976-1978; **Fellow:** Pulmonary Disease, UCLA Med Ctr, Los Angeles, CA 1978-1980; **Fac Appt:** Clin Prof Medicine, UCLA

Boushey Jr, Homer A MD (Pul) - *Spec Exp:* Asthma; Bronchitis; **Hospital:** UCSF Med Ctr; **Address:** UCSF Med Ctr, Dept Med, 505 Parnassus Ave, rm 1292-M, Box 0130, San Francisco, CA 94143-0130; **Phone:** (415) 476-8019; **Board Cert:** Internal Medicine 1972, Pulmonary Disease 1974; **Med School:** UCSF 1968; **Resid:** Internal Medicine, UCSF Med Ctr, San Francisco, CA 1969-1970; Internal Medicine, Beth Israel Hosp, Boston, MA 1970-1971; **Fellow:** Pulmonary Disease, Oxford Univ, Oxford, England 1971-1972; Pulmonary Disease, UCSF Hosp, San Francisco, CA 1972-1973; **Fac Appt:** Prof Medicine, UCSF

Catanzaro, Antonino MD (Pul) - *Spec Exp:* Tuberculosis; **Hospital:** UCSD Healthcare; **Address:** 200 W Arbor Dr, #8374, San Diego, CA 92103-8374; **Phone:** (619) 543-5550; **Board Cert:** Internal Medicine 1972, Pulmonary Disease 1976; **Med School:** SUNY Buffalo 1965; **Resid:** Internal Medicine, Georgetown Univ Hosp, Washington, DC 1968-1970; **Fellow:** Pulmonary Critical Care Medicine, Univ California San Diego Med Ctr, San Diego, CA 1970-1972; Research, Scripps Clin Rsch Fdn, La Jolla, CA 1970-1972; **Fac Appt:** Prof Medicine, UCSD

Gong Jr, Henry MD (Pul) - *Spec Exp:* Lung Disease; Environmental Diseases; **Hospital:** Rancho Los Amigos Natl Rehab Ctr; **Address:** Bldg Harriman - rm 145, 7601 E Imperial Hwy, Downey, CA 90242; **Phone:** (562) 401-7611; **Board Cert:** Pulmonary Disease 1980, Internal Medicine 1977; **Med School:** UC Davis 1973; **Resid:** Internal Medicine, Boston Hosp, Boston, MA 1974-1975; **Fellow:** Pulmonary Disease, UCLA Med Ctr, Los Angeles, CA 1975-1977; **Fac Appt:** Prof Preventive Medicine, USC Sch Med

Hopewell, Philip MD (Pul) - *Spec Exp:* AIDS/HIV; Tuberculosis; Infectious Disease-Lung; **Hospital:** San Francisco Gen Hosp; **Address:** 1001 Potrero Ave, Ste 5K1, Box 0841, San Francisco, CA 94110-1001; **Phone:** (415) 206-8313; **Board Cert:** Internal Medicine 1973, Pulmonary Disease 1974; **Med School:** W VA Univ 1965; **Resid:** Internal Medicine, UCSF Hosps, San Francisco, CA 1968-1971; **Fellow:** Pulmonary Disease, UCSF Hosp, San Francisco, CA 1971-1973; **Fac Appt:** Prof Medicine, UCSF

Huang, Laurence MD (Pul) - *Spec Exp:* AIDS/HIV; **Hospital:** San Francisco Gen Hosp; **Address:** 995 Potrero Ave, Bldg 80-Ward 84, San Francisco, CA 94110; **Phone:** (415) 476-4082; **Board Cert:** Pulmonary Disease 1996, Critical Care Medicine 1997; **Med School:** Columbia P&S 1989; **Resid:** Internal Medicine, Columbia-Presby Hosp, New York, NY 1990-1992; Pulmonary Critical Care Medicine, UCSF Med Ctr, San Francisco, CA 1992-1995; **Fac Appt:** Asst Clin Prof Medicine, UCSF

Hudson, Leonard MD (Pul) - *Spec Exp:* Critical Care; Lung Injury/ARDS; Respiratory Failure; **Hospital:** Univ WA Med Ctr; **Address:** 325 9th Ave, Box 359762, Seattle, WA 98104; **Phone:** (206) 731-3533; **Board Cert:** Internal Medicine 1973, Pulmonary Disease 1974; **Med School:** Univ Wash 1964; **Resid:** Internal Medicine, NY Hosp-Cornell Med Ctr, New York, NY 1965-1966; Internal Medicine, Univ Wash Hosps, Seattle, WA 1968-1969; **Fellow:** Pulmonary Disease, Univ Colo Med Ctr, Denver, CO 1970-1971; **Fac Appt:** Prof Medicine, Univ Wash

King Jr, Talmadge Everett MD (Pul) - *Spec Exp:* Interstitial Lung Disease; Bronchitis; Asthma; **Hospital:** San Francisco Gen Hosp; **Address:** 1001 Potrero Ave, Ste 5H22, San Francisco, CA 94110; **Phone:** (415) 206-6233; **Board Cert:** Internal Medicine 1977, Pulmonary Disease 1982; **Med School:** Harvard Med Sch 1974; **Resid:** Internal Medicine, Grady-Emory Univ Affil Hosp, Atlanta, GA 1975-1977; **Fellow:** Pulmonary Critical Care Medicine, Univ Colorado Hlth Sci Ctr, Denver, CO 1977-1979; **Fac Appt:** Prof Medicine, UCSF

Matthay, Michael Anthony MD (Pul) - *Spec Exp:* *Critical Care; ARDS/ALI;* **Hospital:** UCSF Med Ctr; **Address:** UCSF Med Ctr, 505 Parnasas Ave, rm M-917, Box 0624, San Francisco, CA 94143-0624; **Phone:** (415) 353-1206; **Board Cert:** Pulmonary Disease 1980, Critical Care Medicine 1987; **Med School:** Univ Penn 1973; **Resid:** Internal Medicine, Univ Colo Med Ctr, Denver, CO 1974-1976; **Fellow:** Surgery, UCLA Med Ctr, Los Angeles, CA 1977-1979; **Fac Appt:** Prof Medicine, UCSF

Mohsenifar, Zab MD (Pul) - *Spec Exp:* *Pulmonary Disease - General;* **Hospital:** Cedars-Sinai Med Ctr; **Address:** Cedars-Sinai Med Ctr, Dept Pulmonology, 8700 Beverly Blvd, rm 6732, Los Angeles, CA 90048-1804; **Phone:** (310) 423-4685; **Board Cert:** Internal Medicine 1978, Pulmonary Disease 1980; **Med School:** Iran 1973; **Resid:** Internal Medicine, Thomas Jefferson Univ Hosp, Philadelphia, PA; Internal Medicine, UCLA Med Ctr, Los Angeles, CA; **Fellow:** Pulmonary Disease, UCLA Med Ctr, Los Angeles, CA; **Fac Appt:** Prof Medicine, UCLA

Patterson, James R MD (Pul) - *Spec Exp:* *Pulmonary Disease - General;* **Hospital:** Providence Portland Med Ctr; **Address:** 507 NE 47th Ave, Ste 103, Portland, OR 97213; **Phone:** (503) 215-2300; **Board Cert:** Pulmonary Disease 1974, Internal Medicine 1972; **Med School:** Columbia P&S 1968; **Resid:** Internal Medicine, Columbia-Presby Med Ctr, New York, NY 1969-1970; **Fellow:** Pulmonary Disease, Fitzsimons Army Med Ctr, Denver, CO 1971-1973; **Fac Appt:** Clin Prof Medicine, Oregon Hlth Scis Univ

Raffin, Thomas Alfred MD (Pul) - *Spec Exp:* *LAM;* **Hospital:** Stanford Med Ctr; **Address:** 300 Pasteur Drive, Stanford, CA 94305-5236; **Phone:** (650) 723-6381; **Board Cert:** Internal Medicine 1976, Pulmonary Disease 1978, Critical Care Medicine 1987; **Med School:** Stanford Univ 1973; **Resid:** Internal Medicine, Peter Bent Brigham Hosp, Boston, MA 1973-1975; **Fellow:** Pulmonary Disease, Stanford Univ Med Ctr, Stanford, CA 1975-1978; **Fac Appt:** Prof Medicine, Stanford Univ

Raghu, Ganesh MD (Pul) - *Spec Exp:* *Interstitial Lung Disease; Pulmonary Fibrosis; Sarcoidosis;* **Hospital:** Univ WA Med Ctr; **Address:** 1959 NE Pacific St, Box 356166, Seattle, WA 98195; **Phone:** (206) 598-4615; **Board Cert:** Pulmonary Disease 1990, Critical Care Medicine 1991; **Med School:** India 1974; **Resid:** Internal Medicine, SUNY Buffalo, Buffalo, NY 1978-1981; Internal Medicine, U Rochester 1977-1978; **Fellow:** Critical Care Medicine, U Washington, Seattle, WA 1981-1984; **Fac Appt:** Prof Medicine, Univ Wash

Ries, Andrew MD (Pul) - *Spec Exp:* *Chronic Obstructive Lung Disease (COPD);* **Hospital:** UCSD Healthcare; **Address:** UCSD Med Ctr, 200 W Arbor Dr, San Diego, CA 92103-8377; **Phone:** (619) 543-7350; **Board Cert:** Pulmonary Disease 1980, Critical Care Medicine 1987; **Med School:** Yale Univ 1974; **Resid:** Internal Medicine, Bellevue Hosp Ctr, New York, NY 1975-1977; **Fellow:** Pulmonary Disease, UCSD Med Ctr, San Diego, CA 1977-1981; **Fac Appt:** Prof Medicine, UCSD

Rizk, Norman Wade MD (Pul) - *Spec Exp:* *Pulmonary & Critical Care; Asthma;* **Hospital:** Stanford Med Ctr; **Address:** 300 Pasteur Drive, Ste H3142, Stanford, CA 94305-5236; **Phone:** (650) 498-7746; **Board Cert:** Internal Medicine 1979, Pulmonary Disease 1984; **Med School:** Yale Univ 1976; **Resid:** Internal Medicine, San Fran Genl Hosp, San Francisco, CA 1977-1980; **Fellow:** Pulmonary Disease, Moffitt Hosp-UCSF, San Francisco, CA 1981-1983; **Fac Appt:** Prof Medicine, Stanford Univ

Rubin, Lewis MD (Pul) - *Spec Exp:* *Pulmonary Hypertension; Pulmonary Vascular Disease;* **Hospital:** UCSD Healthcare; **Address:** UCSD Med Ctr, 9300 Campus Pt Dr, Ste 7372, La Jolla, CA 92037; **Phone:** (858) 657-7105; **Board Cert:** Pulmonary Disease 1980, Critical Care Medicine 1989; **Med School:** Albert Einstein Coll Med 1975; **Resid:** Internal Medicine, Duke Univ Med Ctr, Durham, NC 1977-1978; **Fellow:** Pulmonary Disease, Duke Univ Med Ctr, Durham, NC 1978-1979; **Fac Appt:** Prof Medicine, UCSD

PULMONARY DISEASE

Sharma, Om Prakash MD (Pul) - *Spec Exp:* Sarcoidosis; **Hospital:** LAC & USC Med Ctr; **Address:** 1200 N State St, Bldg GNH 11900, Los Angeles, CA 90033; **Phone:** (323) 226-7923; **Board Cert:** Internal Medicine 1972; **Med School:** India 1959; **Resid:** Internal Medicine, Norwalk Hosp, Norwalk, CT 1962-1963; Internal Medicine, Einstein Med Coll Hosp, Bronx, NY 1963-1965; **Fellow:** Pulmonary Disease, Einstein Med Coll Hosp, Bronx, NY 1965-1966; Research, Royal Coll of Phys, London, England 1966-1969; **Fac Appt:** Prof Medicine, USC Sch Med

Stansell, John Dee MD (Pul) - *Spec Exp:* AIDS/HIV; **Hospital:** UCSF Med Ctr; **Address:** 995 Protrero Ave Bldg 80 Ward 84, San Francisco, CA 94110; **Phone:** (415) 502-4165; **Board Cert:** Internal Medicine 1989, Pulmonary Disease 1990; **Med School:** Geo Wash Univ 1985; **Resid:** Internal Medicine, Stanford Univ Hosp, Stanford, CA 1985-1988; **Fac Appt:** Assoc Clin Prof Medicine, UCSF

Tashkin, Donald P MD (Pul) - *Spec Exp:* Asthma; Chronic Obstructive Lung Disease (COPD); **Hospital:** UCLA Med Ctr; **Address:** UCLA Med Ctr, Dept Med, 200 UCLA Med Plaza, Ste 365B, Los Angeles, CA 90095; **Phone:** (310) 825-8061; **Board Cert:** Internal Medicine 1968, Pulmonary Disease 1972; **Med School:** Univ Penn 1961; **Resid:** Internal Medicine, VA Hosp, Philadelphia, PA 1962-1965; **Fellow:** Pulmonary Disease, UCLA Med Ctr, Los Angeles, CA 1967-1969; **Fac Appt:** Prof Medicine, UCLA

Tharratt, Robert Steven MD/PhD (Pul) - *Spec Exp:* Pulmonary Disease - General; **Hospital:** Univ CA - Davis Med Ctr; **Address:** UC Davis Med Ctr, Div Pulm Crit Care, 4150 V St, Ste 3400, Sacramento, CA 95817-2214; **Phone:** (916) 734-3564; **Board Cert:** Pulmonary Disease 1988, Critical Care Medicine 1999, Medical Toxicology 1995, Emergency Medicine 1997; **Med School:** UCLA 1983; **Fac Appt:** Prof Medicine, UC Davis

Theodore, James MD (Pul) - *Spec Exp:* Transplant Medicine-Heart & Lung; Pulmonary Fibrosis; Interstitial Lung Disease; **Hospital:** Stanford Med Ctr; **Address:** Standford Univ Med Ctr, Dept Pulm Critical Care, 300 Pasteur Dr, rm H3147, Stanford, CA 94305-5236; **Phone:** (650) 723-5200; **Board Cert:** Internal Medicine 1971; **Med School:** Univ Pittsburgh 1962; **Resid:** Internal Medicine, Univ Pitts Med Ctr, Pittsburgh, PA 1966-1967; Internal Medicine, Barnes Hosp, St Louis, MO 1967-1968; **Fellow:** Pulmonary Disease, Univ Pitts Med Ctr, Pittsburgh, PA 1963-1966; **Fac Appt:** Prof Medicine, Stanford Univ

Wallace, Jeanne Marie MD (Pul) - *Spec Exp:* AIDS/HIV; Pulmonary Infections; Asthma; **Hospital:** Olive View Med Ctr; **Address:** Olive View UCLA Med Ctr, 14445 Olive View Dr, Sylmar, CA 91342-1437; **Phone:** (818) 364-3205; **Board Cert:** Pulmonary Disease 1980, Critical Care Medicine 1991; **Med School:** UCLA 1974; **Resid:** Internal Medicine, UCSF Med Ctr, San Francisco, CA 1975-1977; **Fellow:** Pulmonary Disease, Univ Hosp, San Diego, CA 1978; **Fac Appt:** Assoc Prof Medicine, UCLA

Wilson, Archie MD/PhD (Pul) - *Spec Exp:* Pulmonary Disease - General; **Hospital:** UCI Med Ctr; **Address:** UC-Irvine Med Ctr, Dept Pulm, 101 The City Drive S Bldg 53 - rm 119, Orange, CA 92868-3298; **Phone:** (714) 456-5150; **Board Cert:** Internal Medicine 1970, Pulmonary Disease 1971; **Med School:** UCSF 1957; **Resid:** Internal Medicine, San Fran VA Hosp, San Francisco, CA 1958-1959; Pulmonary Disease, UCSF Med Ctr, San Francisco, CA 1959-1960; **Fellow:** Pulmonary Disease, UCLA Med Ctr, Los Angeles, CA 1966-1967; **Fac Appt:** Prof Medicine, UC Irvine

RADIATION ONCOLOGY

(a subspecialty of RADIOLOGY)

A subspecialist in radiation oncology deals with the therapeutic applications of radiant energy and its modifiers and the study and management of disease, especially malignant tumors.

RADIOLOGY

A radiologist utilizes radiologic methodologies to diagnose and treat disease. Physicians practicing in the field of radiology most often specialize in radiology, diagnostic radiology, radiation oncology or radiological physics.

Training required: Four years in radiology *plus* additional training and examination

NYU Medical Center

550 First Avenue (at 31st Street)
New York, NY 10016
Physician Referral: (888) 7-NYU-MED
(888-769-8633)   www.nyumedicalcenter.org

SCHOOL OF
MEDICINE

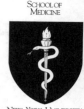

NEW YORK UNIVERSITY

RADIATION ONCOLOGY

High-quality radiation therapy requires both state-of-the-art equipment and expert personnel. Just as anybody who has a scalpel is not a world-class surgeon, the availability of modern equipment is necessary, but not sufficient, to ensure high-quality care.

The hallmark of Radiation Oncology at NYU Medical Center is our dedication to quality assurance. This begins with personalized care. Every patient's condition is discussed by the entire senior medical staff and every aspect of a patient's care is considered before a treatment plan is recommended.

As treatments have become more sophisticated, the ability of all Radiation Oncology facilities to cure tumors without harming patients has improved. Much of this success is attributable to the use of high power computers operated by highly trained, dedicated medical physicists. At NYU Medical Center, all our equipment is tested by our physics staff prior to use.

Radiation beams must be shaped to match their intended targets. In virtually all treatment machines, shortly after the beam is produced, it is "collimated" into a useful shape by blocking unwanted parts of the beam. Depending on the desired shape, additional blocking of the beam usually is required. We custom build most of the blocks that our patients require and have a dedicated block cutting room with a full time block cutting specialist.

Similarly, the calculations inherent in treatment planning are only as reliable as the attention to detail paid to them by the people performing them. All our calculations are independently double-checked by two medical physicists before a patient receives even one fraction of treatment. If a patient needs only one high dose fraction, the calculation is triple-checked prior to treatment.

Just as you would not expect to benefit from a meedicine the instant you swallow a pill, the full effects of radiation therapy typically occur after a course of treatment is complete. Consequently, we consider aftercare a critical component of our service. During each of these visits, your attending physician will review with you any changes in your condition, and will examine you to assess the status of your disease (hopefully, it will be gone) and the health of your normal tissues. If additional action is required, we will arrange it or prescribe needed medications.

NYU MEDICAL CENTER

For many patients, who have multiple medical problems, radiation therapy must be coordinated with other kinds of medical care. Often, radiation therapy must be combined with surgery and/or chemotherapy to produce the best result. Frequently, this raises questions about the condition of a patient's heart, lungs, kidneys, etc. One of the strengths of Cancer Care at NYU is the availability of specialist in any of these areas, who frequently work with us as a team.

Physician Referral
(888) 7-NYU-MED
(888-769-8633)
www.nyumedicalcenter.org

PHYSICIAN LISTINGS

New England

Choi, Noah C MD (RadRO) - *Spec Exp:* Lung Cancer; Esophageal Cancer; **Hospital:** MA Genl Hosp; **Address:** Mass Genl Hosp, Dept Rad Onc, 100 Blossom St, Bldg Cox - rm 307, Boston, MA 02114; **Phone:** (617) 726-8146; **Board Cert:** Therapeutic Radiology 1970; **Med School:** South Korea 1963; **Resid:** Radiation Oncology, Princess Margaret Hosp, Toronto, Canada 1970

D'Amico, Anthony V MD/PhD (RadRO) - *Spec Exp:* Prostate Cancer; Brachytherapy; **Hospital:** St Anne's Hosp; **Address:** 480 Hawthorne St, Ste 102, North Dartmouth, MA 02747; **Phone:** (508) 979-5858; **Board Cert:** Radiation Oncology 1999; **Med School:** Univ Penn 1990; **Resid:** Radiation Oncology, Penn U Hosp, Philadelphia, PA 1991-1994

Haffty, Bruce MD (RadRO) - *Spec Exp:* Breast Cancer; Lung Cancer; Head & Neck Cancer; **Hospital:** Yale - New Haven Hosp; **Address:** Dept Therapeutic Radiology, 20 York St, HRT-133, New Haven, CT 06504; **Phone:** (203) 785-2959; **Board Cert:** Radiation Oncology 1988; **Med School:** Yale Univ 1984; **Resid:** Radiation Oncology, Yale Univ, New Haven, CT 1985-1988; **Fac Appt:** Assoc Prof Radiology, Yale Univ

Harris, Jay R MD (RadRO) - *Spec Exp:* Breast Cancer; **Hospital:** Brigham & Women's Hosp; **Address:** 44 Binney St, Ste 1622, Boston, MA 02115; **Phone:** (617) 632-2291; **Board Cert:** Radiation Oncology 1999, Therapeutic Radiology 1976; **Med School:** Stanford Univ 1970; **Resid:** Radiation Oncology, Joint Ctr Rad Ther, Boston, MA 1973-1976; **Fellow:** Radium Therapy, Harvard Med Sch, Boston, MA 1976-1977; **Fac Appt:** Prof Radiation Oncology, Harvard Med Sch

Loeffler, Jay Steven MD (RadRO) - *Spec Exp:* Spinal Cord Tumors; Stereotactic Radiosurgery; Brain Tumors; **Hospital:** MA Genl Hosp; **Address:** Mass Gen Hosp, NE Proton Therapy Ctr, 100 Blossom St, Boston, MA 02114; **Phone:** (617) 724-1548; **Board Cert:** Therapeutic Radiology 1986; **Med School:** Brown Univ 1982; **Resid:** Radium Therapy, Harvard Joint Ctr, Boston, MA 1983-1986; Transplant Surgery, Harvard Joint Ctr, Boston, MA 1985-1986; **Fellow:** Cancer Biology, Harvard Sch Pub Hlth, Boston, MA 1984-1985; **Fac Appt:** Prof Radiation Oncology, Harvard Med Sch

Recht, Abram MD (RadRO) - *Spec Exp:* Breast Cancer; **Hospital:** Beth Israel Deaconess Med Ctr - Boston; **Address:** 330 Brookline Ave, Boston, MA 02215; **Phone:** (617) 667-2345; **Board Cert:** Therapeutic Radiology 1984; **Med School:** Johns Hopkins Univ 1980; **Resid:** Radiology, Joint Ctr Radium Therapy, Boston, MA 1981-1984; **Fac Appt:** Assoc Prof Radiology, Harvard Med Sch

Shipley, William MD (RadRO) - *Spec Exp:* Bladder Cancer; Prostate Cancer; **Hospital:** MA Genl Hosp; **Address:** 55 Fruit St Bldg Cox - Ste 302, Boston, MA 02114; **Phone:** (617) 726-8146; **Board Cert:** Therapeutic Radiology 1975; **Med School:** Harvard Med Sch 1966; **Resid:** Surgery, Mass Genl Hosp, Boston, MA 1967-1971; Radium Therapy, Mass Genl Hosp, Boston, MA 1971-1973; **Fellow:** Radium Therapy, Royal Marsden Hosp, Sutton, England 1973-1974; **Fac Appt:** Prof Radiology, Harvard Med Sch

Suit, Herman MD (RadRO) - *Spec Exp:* Sarcoma; **Hospital:** MA Genl Hosp; **Address:** 55 Fruit St, Boston, MA 02114; **Phone:** (617) 724-1155; **Board Cert:** Therapeutic Radiology 1958; **Med School:** Baylor Coll Med 1952; **Resid:** Radium Therapy, Jefferson Davis Hosp, Houston, TX 1953; Radium Therapy, Churchhill Hosp, Oxford, England 1954-1957; **Fac Appt:** Prof Radiation Oncology, Harvard Med Sch

Wazer, David E MD (RadRO) - *Spec Exp:* Breast Cancer; Melanoma; **Hospital:** New England Med Ctr - Boston; **Address:** 750 Washington St, Ste 359, Boston, MA 02111-1533; **Phone:** (617) 636-6161; **Board Cert:** Radiation Oncology 1988; **Med School:** NYU Sch Med 1982; **Resid:** Radiation Oncology, Tufts New England Med Ctr, Boston, MA 1985-1988; **Fellow:** Neurological Chemistry, NYU Med Ctr, New York, NY 1983-1984; **Fac Appt:** Prof Radiation Oncology, Tufts Univ

RADIATION ONCOLOGY
New England

Willett, Chris MD (RadRO) - *Spec Exp:* Gastrointestinal Cancer; **Hospital:** MA Genl Hosp; **Address:** 55 Fruit St, Boston, MA 02114; **Phone:** (617) 724-1548; **Board Cert:** Therapeutic Radiology 1986; **Med School:** Tufts Univ 1981; **Resid:** Radiation Oncology, Mass Genl Hosp, Boston, MA 1982-1986; **Fac Appt:** Prof Radiation Oncology, Harvard Med Sch

Mid Atlantic

Berg, Christine Dorothy MD (RadRO) - *Spec Exp:* Breast Cancer; **Hospital:** Suburban Hosp - Bethesda; **Address:** 6410 Rockledge Drive, Ste 640, Bethesda, MD 20817; **Phone:** (301) 896-3021; **Board Cert:** Therapeutic Radiology 1986, Radiation Oncology 1999; **Med School:** Northwestern Univ 1977; **Resid:** Internal Medicine, Northwestern Meml Hosp, Chicago, IL 1978-1981; Radiation Oncology, Georgetown Univ Hosp, Washington, DC 1984-1986; **Fellow:** Medical Oncology, Natl Cancer Inst-NIH, Bethesda, MD 1981-1984; **Fac Appt:** Assoc Prof Radiation Oncology, Georgetown Univ

Curran Jr, Walter J MD (RadRO) - *Spec Exp:* Lung Cancer; Brain Tumors; **Hospital:** Thomas Jefferson Univ Hosp; **Address:** Thomas Jefferson Univ Hosp, Dept Rad Onc, 111 S 11TH St, Philadelphia, PA 19107; **Phone:** (215) 955-6701; **Board Cert:** Therapeutic Radiology 1986; **Med School:** Med Coll GA 1982; **Resid:** Radiation Therapy, Hosp Univ Penn, Philadelphia, PA 1983-1986; **Fac Appt:** Prof Radiation Oncology, Jefferson Med Coll

Ennis, Ronald MD (RadRO) - *Spec Exp:* Brachytherapy; Prostate & Gynecologic Cancers; **Hospital:** NY Presby Hosp - Columbia Presby Med Ctr (page 70); **Address:** Columbia-Presby Med Ctr, Dept Rad Onc, 622 W 168th St, New York, NY 10032-3720; **Phone:** (212) 305-2991; **Board Cert:** Radiation Oncology 1995; **Med School:** Yale Univ 1990; **Resid:** Therapeutic Radiology, Yale-New Haven Hosp, New Haven, CT 1991-1994; **Fac Appt:** Assoc Prof Radiation Oncology, Columbia P&S

Fountain, Karen MD (RadRO) - *Spec Exp:* Radiation Therapy-Cancer; **Address:** 1129 Northern Blvd, Manhasset, NY 11030; **Phone:** (516) 365-6544; **Board Cert:** Therapeutic Radiology 1976, Radiation Oncology 2000; **Med School:** Univ MD Sch Med 1972; **Resid:** Radium Therapy, Univ Maryland Hosp, Baltimore, MD 1973-1974; Radium Therapy, Mayo Clinic, Rochester, MN 1974-1976; **Fac Appt:** Assoc Clin Prof Radiation Oncology, Columbia P&S

Glatstein, Eli MD (RadRO) - *Spec Exp:* Lymphoma; Lung Cancer; Photodynamic Therapy; **Hospital:** Hosp Univ Penn (page 78); **Address:** HUP Dept of Radiation Oncology, 3400 Spruce St Bldg Donner Fl 2, Philadelphia, PA 19104; **Phone:** (215) 662-3383; **Board Cert:** Therapeutic Radiology 1972; **Med School:** Stanford Univ 1964; **Resid:** Radium Therapy, Stanford Med Ctr, Stanford, CA 1967-1970; **Fellow:** Hammersmith Hosp, London, England 1970-1972; **Fac Appt:** Radiation Oncology, Univ Penn

Goodman, Robert L MD (RadRO) - *Spec Exp:* Breast Cancer; Lymphoma; **Hospital:** St Barnabas Med Ctr; **Address:** 94 Old Short Hills Rd, Livingston, NJ 07039; **Phone:** (973) 322-5637; **Board Cert:** Medical Oncology 1975, Therapeutic Radiology 1974; **Med School:** Columbia P&S 1966; **Resid:** Internal Medicine, Beth Israel Hosp, Boston, MA 1967-1970; Radium Therapy, Harvard Joint Ctr Rad Th, Boston, MA 1970-1972; **Fellow:** Hematology, Presby Hosp, New York, NY 1968-1969; Radiation Oncology, Harvard Medical Ctr, Boston, MA 1970-1974; **Fac Appt:** Adjct Prof Radiation Oncology

Harrison, Louis MD (RadRO) - *Spec Exp:* Brachytherapy; Head & Neck Cancer; **Hospital:** Beth Israel Med Ctr - Petrie Division (page 58); **Address:** Beth Israel Med Ctr, Dept Rad Onc, 10 Union Square East, New York, NY 10003-3314; **Phone:** (212) 844-8087; **Board Cert:** Therapeutic Radiology 1986; **Med School:** SUNY Hlth Sci Ctr 1982; **Resid:** Therapeutic Radiology, Yale-New Haven Hosp, New Haven, CT 1983-1986; **Fac Appt:** Prof Radiation Oncology, Albert Einstein Coll Med

Hilaris, Basil MD (RadRO) - *Spec Exp:* Prostate Cancer; Breast Cancer; Gynecologic Cancer; **Hospital:** Our Lady of Mercy Med Ctr; **Address:** 600 E 233rd St, Bronx, NY 10466-2604; **Phone:** (718) 920-9750; **Board Cert:** Radiation Oncology 1968; **Med School:** Greece 1955; **Resid:** Radiology, Meml Sloan Kettering Cancer Ctr, New York, NY 1957-1959; **Fellow:** Radiology, Mem-Sloan, New York, NY 1959-1964; **Fac Appt:** Prof Radiology, NY Med Coll

Isaacson, Steven MD (RadRO) - *Spec Exp:* Brain Tumors; **Hospital:** NY Presby Hosp - Columbia Presby Med Ctr (page 70); **Address:** Dept Radiation Oncolgy, 622 W 168th St, New York, NY 10032; **Phone:** (212) 305-2611; **Board Cert:** Radiation Oncology 1988, Otolaryngology 1978; **Med School:** Jefferson Med Coll 1973; **Resid:** Otolaryngology, Hosp Univ Penn, Philadelphia, PA 1975-1978; Radiation Oncology, SUNY Hlth Sci Ctr, Brooklyn, NY 1985-1988; **Fac Appt:** Asst Prof Radiation Oncology, Columbia P&S

Leibel, Steven A MD (RadRO) - *Spec Exp:* Prostate Cancer; **Hospital:** Mem Sloan Kettering Cancer Ctr; **Address:** 1275 York Ave, Dept Radiation Oncology, Box 22, New York, NY 10021-6007; **Phone:** (212) 639-6024; **Board Cert:** Therapeutic Radiology 1976, Radiation Oncology 1999; **Med School:** UCSF 1972; **Resid:** Radiation Oncology, UCSF Med Ctr, San Francisco, CA 1973-1976

Lepanto, Philip Bliss MD (RadRO) - *Spec Exp:* Radiation Oncology - General; **Hospital:** St Mary's Hosp - Huntington, WV; **Address:** Dept Radiation Therapy, 2900 First Ave, Huntington, WV 25702; **Phone:** (304) 526-1143; **Board Cert:** Therapeutic Radiology 1975; **Med School:** Univ Louisville Sch Med 1970; **Resid:** Radiology, U Penn Hosp, Philadelphia, PA 1971-1972; Radium Therapy, U Penn Hosp, Philadelphia, PA 1972-1975; **Fac Appt:** Clin Prof Radiology, Marshall Univ

McCormick, Beryl MD (RadRO) - *Spec Exp:* Breast Cancer; Eye Tumors/Cancer; **Hospital:** Mem Sloan Kettering Cancer Ctr; **Address:** 1275 York Ave, New York, NY 10021-6007; **Phone:** (212) 639-6828; **Board Cert:** Therapeutic Radiology 1977; **Med School:** UMDNJ-NJ Med Sch, Newark 1973; **Resid:** Therapeutic Radiology, Meml Sloan Kettering Canc Ctr, New York, NY 1974-1977; **Fac Appt:** Prof Radiation Oncology, Cornell Univ-Weill Med Coll

Minsky, Bruce MD (RadRO) - *Spec Exp:* Colon Cancer; **Hospital:** Mem Sloan Kettering Cancer Ctr; **Address:** Meml Sloan Kettering Cancer Ctr, Dept Rad Oncology, 1275 York Ave, New York, NY 10021; **Phone:** (212) 639-6817; **Board Cert:** Radiation Oncology 1987; **Med School:** Univ Mass Sch Med 1982; **Resid:** Radiation Oncology, Harvard Jt Ctr Rad Ther, Boston, MA 1983-1986

RADIATION ONCOLOGY

Nori, Dattatreyudu MD (RadRO) - *Spec Exp:* Breast Cancer; Prostate Cancer; Gynecologic Cancer; **Hospital:** NY Presby Hosp - NY Weill Cornell Med Ctr (page 70); **Address:** 525 E 68th St, New York, NY 10021-4870; **Phone:** (212) 746-3679; **Board Cert:** Radiation Oncology 1979; **Med School:** India 1970; **Resid:** Radiation Oncology, Meml Sloan Kettering, New York, NY 1973-1975; **Fellow:** Radiation Oncology, Meml Sloan Kettering, New York, NY 1976-1977; **Fac Appt:** Prof Radiation Oncology, Cornell Univ-Weill Med Coll

Pollack, Alan MD/PhD (RadRO) - *Spec Exp:* Prostate Cancer; **Hospital:** Fox Chase Cancer Ctr; **Address:** Fox Chase Cancer Ctr, Div Radiation Oncology, 7701 Burholme Ave, Philadelphia, PA 19111; **Phone:** (215) 728-2940; **Board Cert:** Radiation Oncology 1993; **Med School:** Univ Miami Sch Med 1987; **Resid:** Radium Therapy, MD Anderson Cancer Ctr, Houston, TX 1988-1992; **Fac Appt:** Prof Radiology, Univ Penn

Pollack, Jed MD (RadRO) - *Spec Exp:* Brain Tumors; Prostate Cancer; Head and Neck Cancer; **Hospital:** Long Island Jewish Med Ctr; **Address:** 270-05 76th Ave, Dept Rad Onc, New Hyde Park, NY 11040; **Phone:** (718) 470-7192; **Board Cert:** Therapeutic Radiology 1985; **Med School:** Univ New Mexico 1981; **Resid:** Therapeutic Radiology, Mem Sloan-Kett Cancer Ctr, New York, NY 1985; **Fac Appt:** Asst Clin Prof Radiation Oncology, Albert Einstein Coll Med

Schiff, Peter B MD/PhD (RadRO) - *Spec Exp:* Prostate Cancer; **Hospital:** NY Presby Hosp - Columbia Presby Med Ctr (page 70); **Address:** Columbia Presby Med Ctr, Dept Rad Onc, 622 W 168th St, New York, NY 10032-3720; **Phone:** (212) 305-2991; **Board Cert:** Radiation Oncology 1990; **Med School:** Albert Einstein Coll Med 1984; **Resid:** Internal Medicine, Meml Sloan Kettering Cancer Ctr, New York, NY 1984-1985; Radiation Oncology, Meml Sloan Kettering Cancer Ctr, New York, NY 1985-1988; **Fac Appt:** Prof Radiology, Columbia P&S

Solin, Lawrence MD (RadRO) - *Spec Exp:* Breast Cancer; **Hospital:** Hosp Univ Penn (page 78); **Address:** Univ Penn Med Ctr, Dept Rad Onc, 3400 Spruce St, 2 Donner Bldg, Philadelphia, PA 19104; **Phone:** (215) 662-7267; **Board Cert:** Therapeutic Radiology 1984, Radiation Oncology 1999; **Med School:** Brown Univ 1978; **Resid:** Surgery, Jefferson Univ Hosp, Philadelphia, PA 1979-1981; Radiation Oncology, Jefferson Univ Hosp/Hosp Univ Penn, Philadelphia, PA 1981-1984; **Fac Appt:** Prof Therapeutic Radiology, Univ Penn

Stock, Richard MD (RadRO) - *Spec Exp:* Prostate Cancer; **Hospital:** Mount Sinai Hosp (page 68); **Address:** 1184 5th Ave, Ste P-24, New York, NY 10029; **Phone:** (212) 241-7502; **Board Cert:** Radiation Oncology 1993; **Med School:** Mount Sinai Sch Med 1988; **Resid:** Radiation Oncology, Meml Sloan Kettering Canc Ctr, New York, NY 1989-1992; **Fac Appt:** Assoc Prof Radiation Oncology, Mount Sinai Sch Med

Southeast

Anscher, Mitchell MD (RadRO) - *Spec Exp:* Prostate Cancer; Brachytherapy; **Hospital:** Duke Univ Med Ctr (page 60); **Address:** Duke University Med Ctr, Dept Radiation Oncology, Box 3085, Durham, NC 27710; **Phone:** (919) 602-2113; **Board Cert:** Radiation Oncology 1987, Internal Medicine 1984; **Med School:** Med Coll VA 1981; **Resid:** Internal Medicine, St Marys Hosp, Waterbury, CT 1982-1984; Radiation Oncology, Duke Univ Med Ctr, Durham, NC 1984-1987; **Fac Appt:** Prof Radiation Oncology, Duke Univ

Brizel, David M MD (RadRO) - *Spec Exp:* Head & Neck Cancer; **Hospital:** Duke Univ Med Ctr (page 60); **Address:** Duke Univ Med Ctr,Dept Radiation Oncology, Box 3085, Durham, NC 27710; **Phone:** (919) 668-5637; **Board Cert:** Radiation Oncology 1987; **Med School:** Northwestern Univ 1983; **Resid:** Radiation Oncology, Mass Genl, Boston, MA 1984-1987; **Fac Appt:** Assoc Prof Radiology, Duke Univ

Ferree, Carolyn Ruth Black MD (RadRO) - *Spec Exp:* *Breast Cancer; Lymphoma; Radiation Oncology-Pediatric;* **Hospital:** Wake Forest Univ Baptist Med Ctr (page 81); **Address:** Wake Forest Univ Baptist Med Ctr, Medical Center Blvd, Winston Salem, NC 27157; **Phone:** (336) 716-4981; **Board Cert:** Therapeutic Radiology 1974; **Med School:** Wake Forest Univ Sch Med 1970; **Resid:** Therapeutic Radiology, NC Baptist Hosp, Winston Salem, NC 1971-1974; **Fac Appt:** Prof Radiation Oncology, Wake Forest Univ Sch Med

Halle, Jan MD (RadRO) - *Spec Exp:* *Breast & Lung Cancer;* **Hospital:** Univ of NC Hosp (page 77); **Address:** Univ North Carolina Sch Med, Dept Rad Onc, CB 7512, Chapel Hill, NC 27599; **Phone:** (919) 966-7700; **Board Cert:** Therapeutic Radiology 1982; **Med School:** Tufts Univ 1975; **Resid:** Radiation Oncology, North Carolina Meml-UNC, Chapel Hill, NC 1975-1981

Kelly, Maria MD (RadRO) - *Spec Exp:* *breast cancer; HDR; IMRT;* **Hospital:** Univ of VA Hlth Sys (page 79); **Address:** 2871 Ivy Rd, Charlottesville, VA; **Phone:** (434) 982-0777; **Board Cert:** Radiation Oncology 1992; **Med School:** Ireland 1983; **Resid:** Radiation Oncology, Univ. of VA Medical Center, Charlottesville, VA 1985-1990; **Fellow:** Radiation Oncology, University of VA Medical Center, Charlottesville, VA 1989-1990; **Fac Appt:** Assoc Prof Radiation Oncology, Univ VA Sch Med

Lewin, Alan MD (RadRO) - *Spec Exp:* *Radiation Oncology - General;* **Hospital:** Baptist Hosp - Miami; **Address:** 8900 N Kendall Dr, Miami, FL 33176-2118; **Phone:** (305) 596-6566; **Board Cert:** Therapeutic Radiology 1982, Medical Oncology 1981, Hematology 1978, Internal Medicine 1976; **Med School:** Geo Wash Univ 1973; **Resid:** Internal Medicine, Mt Sinai Hosp, New york, NY 1974-1976; **Fellow:** Radiation Oncology, Joint Ctr Rad Ther/ Harvard 1978-1980; Hematology and Oncology, Beth Israel Hosp/S. Far 1976-1978; **Fac Appt:** Prof Radiation Oncology, Univ Miami Sch Med

Marks, Lawrence MD (RadRO) - *Spec Exp:* *Breast Cancer; Lung Cancer;* **Hospital:** Duke Univ Med Ctr (page 60); **Address:** Duke University Medical Center, Box 3085, Durham, NC 27710; **Phone:** (919) 668-5640; **Board Cert:** Radiation Oncology 1989; **Med School:** Univ Rochester 1985; **Resid:** Radiation Oncology, Mass Genl Hosp, Boston, MA 1986-1989; **Fac Appt:** Prof Radiation Oncology, Duke Univ

Mendenhall, Nancy P MD (RadRO) - *Spec Exp:* *Breast Cancer; Lymphoma; Hodgkin's Disease;* **Hospital:** Shands Hlthcre at Univ of FL (page 73); **Address:** 2000 SW Archer Rd, Box 100385, Gainesville, FL 32610-0385; **Phone:** (352) 265-0287; **Board Cert:** Therapeutic Radiology 1985; **Med School:** Univ Fla Coll Med 1980; **Resid:** Radiology, Shands-Univ of Florida, Gainesville, FL 1981-1984; **Fac Appt:** Prof Radiation Oncology, Univ Fla Coll Med

Mendenhall, William M MD (RadRO) - *Spec Exp:* *Head & Neck Cancer; Stereotactic Radiosurgery; Colon Cancer;* **Hospital:** Shands Hlthcre at Univ of FL (page 73); **Address:** 1600 SW Archer Rd, Box 100385, Gainesville, FL 32610-0385; **Phone:** (352) 395-0287; **Board Cert:** Therapeutic Radiology 1983; **Med School:** Univ S Fla Coll Med 1978; **Resid:** Radiation Oncology, University of Florida, Gainesville, FL 1978-1983; **Fac Appt:** Prof Radiation Oncology, Univ Fla Coll Med

Prosnitz, Leonard MD (RadRO) - *Spec Exp:* *Lymphoma; Breast Cancer;* **Hospital:** Duke Univ Med Ctr (page 60); **Address:** Duke Univ Med Ctr, Box 3085, Durham, NC 27710; **Phone:** (919) 668-5640; **Board Cert:** Therapeutic Radiology 1970; **Med School:** SUNY Downstate 1961; **Resid:** Internal Medicine, Dartmouth Affil Hosps, New Haven, CT 1961-1963; Radiation Oncology, Yale-New Haven Hosp, New Haven, CT 1967-1969; **Fellow:** Hematology and Oncology, Yale-New Haven Hosp, New Haven, CT 1965-1967; **Fac Appt:** Prof Radiation Oncology, Duke Univ

RADIATION ONCOLOGY

Rich, Tyvin Andrew MD (RadRO) - *Spec Exp:* Colorectal Cancer; Chemoradiation (Comb. Modulated Therapy); Esophageal Cancer; **Hospital:** Univ of VA Hlth Sys (page 79); **Address:** Univ Va Hlth Sci Ctr, Dept Rad Onc, Box 800383, Charlottesville, VA 22908; **Phone:** (804) 924-5191; **Board Cert:** Radiation Oncology 1978; **Med School:** Univ VA Sch Med 1973; **Resid:** Radiation Oncology, Mass Genl Hosp, Boston, MA 1975-1978; **Fellow:** Radiation Oncology, Mt Vernon Hosp/Gray Lab, England 1978; **Fac Appt:** Prof Radiation Oncology, Univ VA Sch Med

Rosenman, Julian MD (RadRO) - *Spec Exp:* Lung Cancer; Breast Cancer; Prostate Cancer; **Hospital:** Univ of NC Hosp (page 77); **Address:** Univ NC-Dept Rad Onc, Box 7512, Chapel Hill, NC 27514-9722; **Phone:** (919) 966-1101; **Board Cert:** Therapeutic Radiology 1981; **Med School:** Univ Tex SW, Dallas 1977; **Resid:** Therapeutic Radiology, Mass Genl Hosp, Boston, MA 1978-1981; **Fac Appt:** Prof Radiation Oncology, Univ NC Sch Med

Sailer, Scott MD (RadRO) - *Spec Exp:* Head & Neck Cancer; Radiology-Pediatric; Genitourinary Cancer; **Hospital:** Univ of NC Hosp (page 77); **Address:** Univ North Carolina Schl Med, Dept Radiation Oncology CB 7512, Chapel Hill, NC 27599-7512; **Board Cert:** Radiation Oncology 1988; **Med School:** Harvard Med Sch 1984; **Resid:** Radiation Therapy, Mass Genl Hosp, Boston, MA 1985-1988; **Fac Appt:** Assoc Clin Prof Univ NC Sch Med

Shaw, Edward Gus MD (RadRO) - *Spec Exp:* Stereotactic Radiosurgery; Brain Tumors; **Hospital:** Wake Forest Univ Baptist Med Ctr (page 81); **Address:** Wake Forest Baptist Med Ctr, Med Center Blvd, Winston Salem, NC 27157-1029; **Phone:** (336) 716-4647; **Board Cert:** Radiation Oncology 1987; **Med School:** Rush Med Coll 1983; **Resid:** Radiation Oncology, Mayo Grad Sch Med, Rochester, MN 1984-1987; **Fac Appt:** Prof Radiation Oncology, Wake Forest Univ Sch Med

Tepper, Joel MD (RadRO) - *Spec Exp:* Gastrointestinal Cancer; Sarcoma; Colon Cancer; **Hospital:** Univ of NC Hosp (page 77); **Address:** North Carolina Clin Cancer Ctr, Dept Rad Onc - CB#7512, Chapel Hill, NC 27599-7512; **Phone:** (919) 966-0400; **Board Cert:** Therapeutic Radiology 1976; **Med School:** Washington Univ, St Louis 1972; **Resid:** Therapeutic Radiology, Mass Genl Hosp, Boston, MA 1973-1976; **Fellow:** Therapeutic Radiology, Mass Genl Hosp, Boston, MA 1976-1977; **Fac Appt:** Prof Radiation Oncology, Univ NC Sch Med

Turrisi III, Andrew Thomas MD (RadRO) - *Spec Exp:* Lung Cancer; Genitourinary Cancer-Male; Gastrointestinal Cancer; **Hospital:** Med Univ Hosp Authority; **Address:** Department of Radiation Oncology, 169 Ashley Ave, Box 250318, Charleston, SC 29425-5836; **Phone:** (843) 792-3273; **Board Cert:** Medical Oncology 1981, Therapeutic Radiology 2000; **Med School:** Georgetown Univ 1974; **Resid:** Internal Medicine, Georgetown Univ Hosp, Washington, DC 1975-1977; Radiation Oncology, Univ Penn Hosp, Philadelphia, PA 1980-1982; **Fellow:** Medical Oncology, Natl Cancer Inst-NIH, Bethesda, MD 1977-1980; **Fac Appt:** Prof Medicine, Med Univ SC

Midwest

Emami, Bahman MD (RadRO) - *Spec Exp:* Head & Neck Cancer; Lung Cancer; **Hospital:** Loyola Univ Med Ctr; **Address:** Loyola Univ Med Ctr, 2160 S First Ave, Ste 114B, Maywood, IL 60153-5590; **Phone:** (708) 216-2555; **Board Cert:** Therapeutic Radiology 1976; **Med School:** Iran 1968; **Resid:** Radium Therapy, Tufts Univ-New Eng Med Ctr, Boston, MA 1973-1976; **Fellow:** Radium Therapy, Tufts Univ-New England Med Ctr, Boston, MA 1976-1977; **Fac Appt:** Prof Radiation Oncology, Loyola Univ-Stritch Sch Med

Forman, Jeffrey D MD (RadRO) - *Spec Exp:* Prostate Cancer; Genitourinary Cancer; **Hospital:** Harper Hosp (page 59); **Address:** Harper Hosp, Dept Rad Onc, 3990 John R St, Detroit, MI 48021-2097; **Phone:** (313) 745-2593; **Board Cert:** Radiation Oncology 1986; **Med School:** NYU Sch Med 1982; **Resid:** Radiation Oncology, Johns Hopkins Hosp, Baltimore, MD 1983-1986; **Fellow:** Therapeutic Radiology, Johns Hopkins Hosp, Baltimore, MD 1986-1987; **Fac Appt:** Prof Radiation Oncology, Wayne State Univ

Kinsella, Timothy James MD (RadRO) - *Spec Exp:* Brain Tumors; Sarcoma; Gastrointestinal Cancer; **Hospital:** Univ Hosp of Cleveland; **Address:** U Hosp Cleveland- Dept Rad Onc, 11100 Euclid Ave, Bldg Bolwell B-200, Cleveland, OH 44106-6068; **Phone:** (216) 844-2530; **Board Cert:** Internal Medicine 1977, Medical Oncology 1979, Therapeutic Radiology 1980; **Med School:** Univ Rochester 1974; **Resid:** Internal Medicine, Mayo Clinic, Rochester, MN 1974-1976; Radiation Oncology, Joint Ctr for Rad Therapy, Boston, MA 1977-1980; **Fellow:** Medical Oncology, Dana Farber Cancer Ctr, Boston, MA 1976-1977; **Fac Appt:** Prof Radiation Oncology, Case West Res Univ

Lichter, Allen MD (RadRO) - *Spec Exp:* Lung Cancer; Breast Cancer; Prostate Cancer; **Hospital:** Univ of MI Hlth Ctr; **Address:** 1500 E Med Ctr Drive, UHB2 C490 Box0010, Ann Arbor, MI 48109-0010; **Phone:** (734) 936-8207; **Board Cert:** Therapeutic Radiology 1976; **Med School:** Univ Mich Med Sch 1972; **Resid:** Radiation Oncology, U Calif, San Francisco, CA 1973-1976; **Fac Appt:** Prof Radiation Oncology, Univ Mich Med Sch

Myerson, Robert J MD (RadRO) - *Spec Exp:* Colon Cancer; **Hospital:** Barnes-Jewish Hosp (page 55); **Address:** 4939 Children's Pl, Ste 5500CSRB, St. Louis, MO 63110; **Phone:** (314) 362-8510; **Board Cert:** Therapeutic Radiology 1985; **Med School:** Univ Miami Sch Med 1980; **Resid:** Radium Therapy, Univ Penn, Philadelphia, PA 1981-1984; **Fac Appt:** Prof Therapeutic Radiology, Washington Univ, St Louis

Pierce, Lori J MD (RadRO) - *Spec Exp:* Breast Cancer; **Hospital:** Univ of MI Hlth Ctr; **Address:** Univ Hosp, Dept Rad Onc, 1500 E Med Ctr Dr, rm B2C440, Box 0010, Ann Arbor, MI 48109-0010; **Phone:** (734) 936-4319; **Board Cert:** Radiation Oncology 1989; **Med School:** Duke Univ 1985; **Resid:** Radiation Oncology, Hosp Univ Penn, Philadelphia, PA 1986-1989; **Fac Appt:** Assoc Prof Radiation Oncology, Univ Mich Med Sch

Shina, Donald C MD (RadRO) - *Spec Exp:* Breast Cancer; **Hospital:** Univ Hosp - Cincinnati; **Address:** 11100 Euclid Ave, Cleveland, OH 44106; **Phone:** (216) 844-3103; **Board Cert:** Therapeutic Radiology 1981, Medical Oncology 1979, Internal Medicine 1977; **Med School:** Case West Res Univ 1974; **Resid:** Internal Medicine, Univ Hosps, Cleveland, OH 1975-1977; **Fellow:** Radiation Oncology, Univ Hosps, Cleveland, OH 1977-1980

Taylor, Marie E MD (RadRO) - *Spec Exp:* Breast Cancer; **Hospital:** Barnes-Jewish Hosp (page 55); **Address:** 660 S Euclid Ave, Box CB8224, St Louis, MO 63110; **Phone:** (314) 362-8587; **Board Cert:** Radiation Oncology 1987; **Med School:** Univ Wash 1982; **Resid:** Radiation Oncology, Univ Wash, Seattle, WA 1983-1986

Vicini, Frank A MD (RadRO) - *Spec Exp:* Breast Cancer; Prostate Cancer; Brachytherapy; **Hospital:** William Beaumont Hosp; **Address:** Dept Rad Onc, 3601 W 13 Mile Rd, Royal Oak, MI 48073; **Phone:** (248) 551-1219; **Board Cert:** Radiation Oncology 1999; **Med School:** Wayne State Univ 1985; **Resid:** Radiation Oncology, William Beaumont Hosp, Royal Oak, MI 1986-1989; **Fellow:** Radiation Oncology, Harvard Med Sch/Joint Ctr for Radiation Ther, Boston, MA 1989-1990; **Fac Appt:** Assoc Clin Prof Radiation Oncology, Univ Mich Med Sch

Weichselbaum, Ralph R MD (RadRO) - *Spec Exp:* Gene-Targeted Radiotherapy; Head & Neck Cancer; **Hospital:** Univ of Chicago Hosps (page 76); **Address:** Dept Radiation & Cellular Oncology, 5758 S Maryland Ave, MC-9006-DCAM, Chicago, IL 60637; **Phone:** (773) 702-0817; **Board Cert:** Therapeutic Radiology 1975; **Med School:** Univ IL Coll Med 1971; **Resid:** Therapeutic Radiology, Harvard Jt Ctr Rad Therapy, Cambridge, MA 1972-1975; **Fellow:** Radiology, Harvard Med Sch, Cambridge, MA 1974-1976

Wilson, J Frank MD (RadRO) - *Spec Exp:* Breast Cancer; Skin Cancer; **Hospital:** Froedtert Meml Lutheran Hosp; **Address:** Dept Radiation Oncology, 9200 W Wisconsin Ave, Milwaukee, WI 53226; **Phone:** (414) 805-4400; **Board Cert:** Therapeutic Radiology 1971; **Med School:** Univ MO-Columbia Sch Med 1965; **Resid:** Radiation Oncology, Penrose Cancer Hosp, Colorado Springs, CO 1966-1969; **Fellow:** Radium Therapy, NCI/NIH, Bethesda, MD 1969-1971; **Fac Appt:** Prof Radiation Oncology, Med Coll Wisc

Great Plains and Mountains

Smalley, Stephen R MD (RadRO) - *Spec Exp:* Colon Cancer; Gastrointestinal Cancer; **Hospital:** Olathe Med Ctr; **Address:** Olathe Med Ctr, 20375 W 151st St, Doctors Bldg, Ste 180, Olathe, KS 66061; **Phone:** (913) 768-7200; **Board Cert:** Internal Medicine 1982, Radiation Oncology 1987, Medical Oncology 1985; **Med School:** Univ MO-Kansas City 1979; **Resid:** Internal Medicine, Mayo Clinic, Rochester, MN 1979-1982; Radiation Oncology, Mayo Clinic, Rochester, MN 1984-1986; **Fellow:** Medical Oncology, Mayo Clinic, Rochester, MN 1982-1984; **Fac Appt:** Prof Radiation Oncology, Univ Kans

Tan, Donald Cheng-San MD (RadRO) - *Spec Exp:* Radiation Oncology - General; **Hospital:** Via Christi Reg Med Ctr - St Francis; **Address:** 929 N St. Francis Rd, Witchita, KS 67214; **Phone:** (316) 268-5908; **Board Cert:** Therapeutic Radiology 1971; **Med School:** Loma Linda Univ 1966; **Resid:** White Mem Med Ctr, Los Angeles, CA 1967-1970; **Fellow:** Therapeutic Radiology, M D Anderson Hosp, Houston, TX 1970-1971

Southwest

Ang, Kie-Kian MD/PhD (RadRO) - *Spec Exp:* Head & Neck Cancer; **Hospital:** Univ of TX MD Anderson Cancer Ctr, The; **Address:** UT MD Anderson Cancer Ctr, 1515 Holcombe Blvd, Box 97, Houston, TX 77030; **Phone:** (713) 792-3409; **Board Cert:** Radiation Oncology 1987; **Med School:** Belgium 1975; **Resid:** Radiation Oncology, Univ Hosp Louvian, Belgium 1976-1980; **Fac Appt:** Prof Radiology, Univ Tex, Houston

Cox, James D MD (RadRO) - *Spec Exp:* Lymphoma; Lung Cancer; **Hospital:** Univ of TX MD Anderson Cancer Ctr, The; **Address:** Univ Texas/MD Anderson Cancer Ctr, 1515 Holcombe Blvd, Box 97, Houston, TX 77030; **Phone:** (713) 792-3411; **Board Cert:** Radiation Oncology 1999, Therapeutic Radiology 1971; **Med School:** Univ Rochester 1965; **Resid:** Radiology, Penrose Cancer Hosp, Colorado Springs, CO 1966-1969; **Fellow:** Radiology, Inst Gustave-Roussy, Villejuif, France 1969-1970; **Fac Appt:** Prof Radiation Oncology, Univ Tex, Houston

Eifel, Patricia J MD (RadRO) - *Spec Exp:* Gynecologic Cancer; Cervical Cancer; **Hospital:** Univ of TX MD Anderson Cancer Ctr, The; **Address:** MD Anderson Cancer Ctr, Dept Radiation Oncology, 1515 Holcombe Blvd, rm B2.4859, Box 97, Houston, TX 77030-4009; **Phone:** (713) 792-3440; **Board Cert:** Therapeutic Radiology 1983; **Med School:** Stanford Univ 1977; **Resid:** Radiology, Stanford Univ Med Ctr, Stanford, CA 1978-1981; **Fellow:** Therapeutic Radiology, Stanford Univ Med Ctr, Stanford, CA 1981-1982; **Fac Appt:** Assoc Prof Radiology, Univ Tex, Houston

Gunderson, Leonard MD (RadRO) - *Spec Exp:* Gastrointestinal Cancer; Brachytherapy; **Hospital:** Mayo Clin Hosp - Scottsdale; **Address:** Div Radiation Oncology, 13400 E Shea Blvd, Scottsdale, AZ 85259; **Phone:** (480) 301-1735; **Board Cert:** Therapeutic Radiology 1975; **Med School:** Univ KY Coll Med 1969; **Resid:** Radiation Oncology, Latter Day Saints Hosp, Salt Lake City, UT 1970-1974

Herman, Terence Spencer MD (RadRO) - *Spec Exp:* Breast Cancer; Sarcoma; Brain Tumors; **Hospital:** Univ of Texas Hlth & Sci Ctr; **Address:** 7703 Floyd Curl Drive, MC 7889, San Antonio, TX 78229-3900; **Phone:** (210) 616-5648; **Board Cert:** Therapeutic Radiology 1985, Medical Oncology 1977; **Resid:** Internal Medicine, Univ Arizona, Tuscon, AZ 1973-1975; Radiation Oncology, Stanford Univ, Stanford, CA 1983-1985; **Fellow:** Medical Oncology, Univ Arizona, Tucson, AZ 1975-1977; **Fac Appt:** Prof Radiation Oncology, Univ Tex, San Antonio

Komaki, Ritsuko MD (RadRO) - *Spec Exp:* Lung Cancer; Thymoma; Esophageal Cancer; **Hospital:** Univ of TX MD Anderson Cancer Ctr, The; **Address:** 1515 Holcombe Blvd, Box 0097, Houston, TX 77030-4095; **Phone:** (713) 792-3420; **Board Cert:** Therapeutic Radiology 2001; **Med School:** Japan 1969; **Resid:** Radiation Oncology, Med Coll Wisc, Milwaukee, WI 1974-1978; **Fac Appt:** Prof Therapeutic Radiology, Univ Tex, Houston

McNeese, Marsha MD (RadRO) - *Spec Exp:* Breast Cancer; **Hospital:** Univ of TX MD Anderson Cancer Ctr, The; **Address:** Radiation Oncology, 1515 Holcombe Blvd, Box 97, Houston, TX 77030-4009; **Phone:** (713) 792-3400; **Board Cert:** Therapeutic Radiology 1978; **Med School:** Louisiana State Univ 1974; **Resid:** Radiation Oncology, Univ Texas/MD Anderson Cancer Ctr, Houston, TX 1975-1977; **Fac Appt:** Assoc Prof Radiation Oncology, Univ Tex, Houston

Medbery, Clinton A MD (RadRO) - *Spec Exp:* Breast Cancer; Gynecologic Cancer; **Hospital:** Presby Hosp - Oklahoma City; **Address:** Prebyterian Hospital, Dept Radiation Oncology, 700 NE 13th St, Oklahoma City, OK 73104-5004; **Phone:** (405) 271-6445; **Board Cert:** Internal Medicine 1980, Medical Oncology 1983, Radiation Oncology 1987; **Med School:** Med Univ SC 1976; **Resid:** Internal Medicine, Naval Hosp, Portsmouth, VA 1978-1980; Radiation Oncology, Natl Cancer Inst, Bethesda, MD 1984-1987; **Fellow:** Medical Oncology, Naval Hosp, Bethesda, MD 1980-1982

Pistenmaa, David A MD/PhD (RadRO) - *Spec Exp:* Stereotactic Radiosurgery; **Hospital:** St Paul Univ Hosp; **Address:** Univ Texas SW Med Sch, Dept Rad Onc, 5323 Harry Hines Blvd, Dallas, TX 75390-9183; **Phone:** (214) 648-6765; **Board Cert:** Therapeutic Radiology 1974; **Med School:** Stanford Univ 1970; **Fellow:** Radium Therapy, Stanford Univ, Stanford, CA 1970-1973; **Fac Appt:** Prof Radiation Oncology, Univ Tex SW, Dallas

Senzer, Neil Nathan MD (RadRO) - *Spec Exp:* Radiation Oncology - General; **Hospital:** Baylor Univ Medical Ctr; **Address:** 3535 Worth St, Dept Radiation Oncology, Dallas, TX 75246-2044; **Phone:** (214) 370-1400; **Board Cert:** Pediatrics 1976, Pediatric Hematology-Oncology 1978, Therapeutic Radiology 1985; **Med School:** SUNY Buffalo 1971; **Resid:** Pediatrics, Johns Hopkins Hosp, Baltimore, MD 1971-1974; Radiation Oncology, St Barnabas Med Ctr, Livingston, NJ 1982-1985; **Fellow:** Pediatric Hematology-Oncology, St Jude Chldns Rsch Hosp, Memphis, TN 1976-1978

Strom, Eric Alan MD (RadRO) - *Spec Exp:* Breast Cancer; Intensity Modulated Radiation Therapy; Multidisciplinary Care; **Hospital:** Univ of TX MD Anderson Cancer Ctr, The; **Address:** MD Anderson Cancer Ctr, Clin Rad Onc, 1515 Holcombe Blvd, Box 97, Houston, TX 77030; **Phone:** (713) 792-3400; **Board Cert:** Internal Medicine 1985, Radiation Oncology 1990; **Med School:** Northwestern Univ 1982; **Resid:** Internal Medicine, Univ Kentucky, Lexington, KY 1982-1985; Radiation Oncology, Univ Texas-MD Anderson Cancer Ctr, Houston, TX 1986-1990; **Fac Appt:** Assoc Prof Radiation Oncology, Univ Tex, Houston

West Coast and Pacific

Blasko, John Charles MD (RadRO) - *Spec Exp:* Radiation Therapy-Cancer; Prostate Cancer; **Hospital:** Swedish Med Ctr; **Address:** 1101 Madison, Ste 1101, Seattle, WA 98104; **Phone:** (206) 215-2480; **Board Cert:** Therapeutic Radiology 1976; **Med School:** Univ MD Sch Med 1969; **Resid:** Diagnostic Radiology, Maine Med Ctr, Portland, ME 1973-1974; Radium Therapy, Univ Wash, St Louis, MO 1974-1976; **Fac Appt:** Prof Radiation Oncology, Univ Wash

Donaldson, Sarah S MD (RadRO) - *Spec Exp:* Pediatric Cancers; Hodgkin's Disease; **Hospital:** Stanford Med Ctr; **Address:** 300 Pasteur Drive, rm A-083, Stanford, CA 94305; **Phone:** (650) 723-6195; **Board Cert:** Therapeutic Radiology 1974; **Med School:** Harvard Med Sch 1968; **Resid:** Radium Therapy, Stanford Univ Med Ctr, Stanford, CA 1969-1972; **Fellow:** Pediatric Hematology-Oncology, Inst Gustave-Roussy, France 1972-1973; Medical Oncology, MD Anderson Cancer Ctr, Houston, TX 1971; **Fac Appt:** Prof Radiation Oncology, Stanford Univ

Goffinet, Don R MD (RadRO) - *Spec Exp:* Breast Cancer; Melanoma; Sarcoma; **Hospital:** Stanford Med Ctr; **Address:** Dept Radiation Oncology, 300 Pasteur Drive, rm A-085-B, Stanford, CA 94305; **Phone:** (650) 723-6195; **Board Cert:** Therapeutic Radiology 1973; **Med School:** Stanford Univ 1964; **Resid:** Surgery, Stanford Univ, Stanford, CA 1965-1966; Surgery, Stanford Univ, Stanford, CA 1968-1972; **Fac Appt:** Prof Therapeutic Radiology, Stanford Univ

Halberg, Francine Erna MD (RadRO) - *Spec Exp:* Breast Cancer; **Hospital:** Marin Genl Hosp; **Address:** Marin Cancer Inst-Dept of Rad.Oncology, 1350 S Eliseo, Greenbrae, CA 94904-2011; **Phone:** (415) 925-7326; **Board Cert:** Internal Medicine 1981, Therapeutic Radiology 1984; **Med School:** Cornell Univ-Weill Med Coll 1978; **Resid:** Internal Medicine, USPHS Hosp, San Francisco, CA 1979-1981; **Fellow:** Radiation Oncology, Stanford Med Ctr, Palo Alto, CA 1981-1984; **Fac Appt:** Assoc Clin Prof Radiation Oncology, UCSF

Juillard, Guy Jean-Felix MD (RadRO) - *Spec Exp:* Head & Neck Cancer; Breast Cancer; Gynecologic Cancer; **Hospital:** UCLA Med Ctr; **Address:** 200 UCLA Med Plz, Ste B-265, Los Angeles, CA 90095; **Phone:** (310) 825-7145; **Board Cert:** Radiation Oncology 1991; **Med School:** France 1963; **Resid:** Radium Therapy, Inst Gustave Roussy, Villejuif, France 1961-1963; **Fac Appt:** Prof Radiation Oncology, UCLA

Petrovich, Zbigniew MD (RadRO) - *Spec Exp:* Eye Tumors/Cancer; Prostate Cancer; Macular Degeneration; **Hospital:** USC Norris Cancer Comp Ctr; **Address:** 1441 Eastlake Ave, Ste G356, Los Angeles, CA 90033; **Phone:** (323) 865-3072; **Board Cert:** Radiology 1971; **Med School:** Poland 1963; **Resid:** Radiology, St Boniface Genl Hosp, Winnipeg, Canada 1967-1968; **Fac Appt:** Prof Radiation Oncology, USC Sch Med

Phillips, Theodore Locke MD (RadRO) - *Spec Exp:* Radiation Therapy-Cancer; Head&Neck Cancer; Brain Tumors; **Hospital:** UCSF Med Ctr; **Address:** 505 Parnassus Ave, Ste L75, San Francisco, CA 94143-0226; **Phone:** (415) 353-8900; **Board Cert:** Therapeutic Radiology 1965; **Med School:** Univ Penn 1959; **Resid:** Radium Therapy, UCSF Med Ctr, San Francisco, CA 1960-1963; **Fac Appt:** Prof Radiation Oncology, UCSF

Quivey, Jeanne Marie MD (RadRO) - *Spec Exp:* Breast Cancer; **Hospital:** San Francisco Gen Hosp; **Address:** 505 Parnassus Ave, Ste L75, San Francisco, CA 94143; **Phone:** (415) 353-8900; **Board Cert:** Therapeutic Radiology 1974; **Med School:** UCSF 1970; **Resid:** Radium Therapy, UC - San Francisco Med Ctr, San Francisco, CA 1971-1974; **Fac Appt:** Prof Radiation Oncology, UCSF

Rose, Christopher Marshall MD (RadRO) - *Spec Exp:* Prostate Cancer; Breast Cancer; **Hospital:** Providence St Joseph Med Ctr; **Address:** St Joseph Med Ctr, Rad Ther, 501 S Buena Vista St, Burbank, CA 91505-4809; **Phone:** (818) 840-7925; **Board Cert:** Therapeutic Radiology 1979, Radiation Oncology 2000; **Med School:** Harvard Med Sch 1974; **Resid:** Internal Medicine, Beth Israel Deaconess, Boston, MA 1975-1976; Radium Therapy, Joint Ctr Rad Therapy, Boston, MA 1976-1979; **Fellow:** Research, British Inst Cancer Rsch, London, England 1978-1979; **Fac Appt:** Assoc Clin Prof Radiology, UCLA

Seagren, Stephen L MD (RadRO) - *Spec Exp:* Lung Cancer; Head & Neck Cancer; **Hospital:** UCSD Healthcare; **Address:** U California San Diego Med Ctr-Dept Rad Oncol, 200 W Arbor Dr, San Diego, CA 92103-8757; **Phone:** (619) 543-5303; **Board Cert:** Therapeutic Radiology 1977, Internal Medicine 1972, Medical Oncology 1977; **Med School:** Northwestern Univ 1967; **Resid:** Radiation Oncology, USCD, San Diego, CA 1976-1977; Internal Medicine, Univ Minn, Hennepin Co Genl Hosp, Minneapolis, MN 1968-1971; **Fellow:** Medical Oncology, LA Co-USC Med Ctr, Los Angeles, CA 1974-1975; Harob Genl Hosp, Los Angeles, CA 1975-1976; **Fac Appt:** Prof Radiology, UCSD

Selch, Michael T MD (RadRO) - *Spec Exp:* Brain Cancer; Lung Cancer; Pediatric Cancer; **Hospital:** UCLA Med Ctr; **Address:** 200 Med Plaza, Ste B265, Los Angeles, CA 90095-6591; **Phone:** (310) 825-4966; **Board Cert:** Therapeutic Radiology 1982; **Med School:** UCLA 1977; **Resid:** Radiation Oncology, UCLA Med Ctr, Los Angeles, CA 1979-1982; **Fac Appt:** Clin Prof Radiation Oncology, UCLA

Shank, Brenda MD/PhD (RadRO) - *Spec Exp:* Breast Cancer; Rectal Cancer; **Hospital:** Doctors Med Ctr; **Address:** 2000 Vale Rd, San Pablo, CA 94806; **Phone:** (510) 970-5239; **Board Cert:** Therapeutic Radiology 1980; **Med School:** UMDNJ-RW Johnson Med Sch 1976; **Resid:** Radium Therapy, Mem Sloan Kettering Cancer Ctr, New York, NY 1976-1979; **Fellow:** Mem Sloan Kettering Cancer Ctr, New York, NY 1979-1980

Streeter Jr, Oscar E MD (RadRO) - *Spec Exp:* Lung Cancer; Head & Neck Cancer; **Hospital:** USC Norris Cancer Comp Ctr; **Address:** 1441 Eastlake Ave, Ste G338, Los Angeles, CA 90033; **Phone:** (323) 865-3084; **Board Cert:** Radiation Oncology 1989; **Med School:** Howard Univ 1982; **Resid:** Radiation Oncology, Howard Univ, Washington, DC 1983-1986; **Fac Appt:** Assoc Prof Radiation Oncology, USC Sch Med

RADIOLOGY

A radiologist utilizes radiologic methodologies to diagnose and treat disease. Physicians practicing in the field of radiology most often specialize in radiology, diagnostic radiology, radiation oncology or radiological physics.

DIAGNOSTIC RADIOLOGY
A radiologist who utilizes X-ray, radionuclides, ultrasound and electromagnetic radiation to diagnose and treat disease.

RADIATION ONCOLOGY
A radiologist who deals with the therapeutic applications of radiant energy and its modifiers and the study and management of disease, especially malignant tumors.

NEURORADIOLOGY
A radiologist who diagnoses and treats diseases utilizing imaging procedures as they relate to the brain, spine and spinal cord, head, neck and organs of special sense in adults and children.

Training required: Four years

Certification in one of the following subspecialties requires additional training and examination.

Pediatric Radiology: A radiologist who is proficient in all forms of diagnostic imaging as it pertains to the treatment of diseases in the newborn, infant, child and adolescent. This specialist has knowledge of both imaging and interventional procedures related to the care and manegemtn of diseases of children. A pediatric radiologist must be highly knowledgeable of all organ systems as they relate to growth and development, congenital malformations, diseases peculiar to infants and children and diseases that begin in childhood but cause substantial residual impairment in adulthood.

Vascular and Interventional Radiology: A radiologist who diagnoses and treats diseases by various radiologic imaging modalities. These include fluoroscopy, digital radiography, computed tomography, sonography and magnetic resonance imaging.

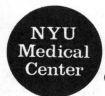

550 First Avenue (at 31st Street)
New York, NY 10016
Physician Referral: (888) 7-NYU-MED
(888-769-8633) www.nyumedicalcenter.org

SCHOOL OF
MEDICINE

NEW YORK UNIVERSITY

RADIOLOGY: The Diagnostic Core of Modern Medicine

In the past 10 years, radiology has undergone a technological revolution, intimately linked to dramatic developments in computer technology and physical engineering and their application to medical diagnostic imaging problems. Able to capture images of the body's structure and function with ever-greater precision, radiologists at NYU Medical Center use the new technologies to provide your doctor with an interpretation that integrates information gleaned from the imaging exam with the broader clinical picture.

EQUIPMENT

NYU Medical Center houses some of the most advanced radiology equipment in the world, including remote-controlled digital fluoroscopy and advanced digital subtraction angiography with three-dimensional capabilities. There are 6 high-field, large bore MRI units, an open MRI unit, ten CT units (seven of which are the latest high-speed spiral units), and one of the largest concentrations of SPECT cameras in the United States. More than 90 percent of the reports at NYU's Tisch Hospital are dictated directly into the radiology information system using computerized voice recognition technology.

FACULTY

The NYU Department of Radiology has a large and distinguished faculty with a significant national presence in their field. Among the faculty are 20 officers of national and regional scientific and professional societies, 11 members in selective societies, and numerous peer reviewers and editors of professional journals. They also are prolific authors of journal articles, books, and book chapters for academic texts.

At Faculty Practice Radiology, located on East 34th Street, patients are screened for colon cancer, lung cancer and coronary artery disease (CAD) via a low-dose, state-of-the-art, Subsecond Multisclice Siemens Plus 4 Volume Zoom CT scanner. Like breast cancer, early detection of lung cancer is widely considered crucial for improving survival rates. A CT lung screening will detect small, early-stage cancers that are not visible on conventional x-ray. Cardiac calcium scoring, also via high-speed CT scanning, measures calcification in the coronary arteries. Cardiac calcium scoring is a revolutionary tool in the diagnosis – and prevention – of coronary artery disease.

A DRIVER OF CROSS-DISCIPLINARY CLINICAL EXCELLENCE

Today, radiology is playing an increasingly pivotal role in medical research. With an explosion of imaging technologies, researchers at NYU are making rapid strides in the understanding of complex diseases, able to visualize anatomical and metabolic changes in the body at the molecular level. No longer a merely supportive discipline, radiology has been transformed into a dynamic driver of medical knowledge itself. For example, the new imaging technologies allow physicians to observe minute changes in tumor activity during cancer treatment, adjust the dosage accordingly, and monitor the disease process with a depth and precision that would have been unimaginable ten years ago.

Physician Referral
(888) 7-NYU-MED

(888-769-8633)

www.nyumedicalcenter.org

Physician Listings

New England

Kopans, Daniel B MD (DR) - *Spec Exp:* Breast Imaging; **Hospital:** MA Genl Hosp; **Address:** Mass Genl Hosp, 15 Parkman St Bldg WAC - rm 219, Boston, MA 02114-3117; **Phone:** (617) 726-3093; **Board Cert:** Diagnostic Radiology 1977; **Med School:** Harvard Med Sch 1973; **Resid:** Diagnostic Radiology, Mass Genl Hosp, Boston, MA 1974-1977; **Fac Appt:** Prof Radiology, Harvard Med Sch

McCarthy, Shirley MD/PhD (DR) - *Spec Exp:* Infertility; Gynecologic Cancer; **Hospital:** Yale - New Haven Hosp; **Address:** South Pavilion Fl 2 - rm 322, 20 York St, New Haven, CT 06520; **Phone:** (203) 785-5251; **Board Cert:** Diagnostic Radiology 1983; **Med School:** Yale Univ 1979; **Resid:** Radiology, Yale-New Haven Hosp, New Haven, CT 1980-1983; **Fellow:** Cross Sectional Imaging, UCSF Med Ctr, San Francisco, CA 1983-1984; **Fac Appt:** Prof Diagnostic Radiology, Yale Univ

Mid Atlantic

Austin, John MD (DR) - *Spec Exp:* Lung Cancer; **Hospital:** NY Presby Hosp - Columbia Presby Med Ctr (page 70); **Address:** 622 W 168th St, New York, NY 10032-3784; **Phone:** (212) 305-2986; **Board Cert:** Diagnostic Radiology 1970; **Med School:** Yale Univ 1965; **Resid:** Radiology, UCSF Med Ctr, San Francisco, CA 1966-1968; **Fellow:** Radiology, UCSF Med Ctr, San Francisco, CA 1968-1970; **Fac Appt:** Prof Radiology, Columbia P&S

Dalinka, Murray MD (DR) - *Spec Exp:* Bone Disorders; Musculoskeletal Disorders; **Hospital:** Hosp Univ Penn (page 78); **Address:** Hospital of Univ of Pa, Dept of Radiology, 3400 Spruce St, Philadelphia, PA 19104; **Phone:** (215) 662-3019; **Board Cert:** Radiology 1969; **Med School:** Univ Mich Med Sch 1964; **Resid:** Radiology, Montefiore Hosp, Bronx, NY 1965-1968; **Fac Appt:** Prof Radiology, Univ Penn

Dershaw, D David MD (DR) - *Spec Exp:* Breast Cancer; Radiology-Diagnostic; **Hospital:** Mem Sloan Kettering Cancer Ctr; **Address:** 1275 York Ave, New York, NY 10021-6007; **Phone:** (212) 639-7295; **Board Cert:** Diagnostic Radiology 1978; **Med School:** Jefferson Med Coll 1974; **Resid:** Diagnostic Radiology, New York Hosp, New York, NY 1975-1978; **Fellow:** Ultrasound, Thomas Jefferson Univ Hosp, Philadelphia, PA 1978-1979; **Fac Appt:** Prof Radiology, Cornell Univ-Weill Med Coll

Edelstein, Barbara A MD (DR) - *Spec Exp:* Breast Cancer; Women's Radiology; **Address:** 1045 Park Ave, New York, NY 10028; **Phone:** (212) 860-7700; **Board Cert:** Diagnostic Radiology 1983; **Med School:** NY Med Coll 1977; **Resid:** Diagnostic Radiology, Montefiore Hosp, New York, NY 1979-1982

Fishman, Elliot MD (DR) - *Spec Exp:* Thoracic Radiology; Abdominal Imaging; Cancer Imaging; **Hospital:** Johns Hopkins Hosp - Baltimore; **Address:** Johns Hopkins Hosp, Dept Radiology, 600 North Wolfe Street, Baltimore, MD 21287-0005; **Phone:** (410) 955-5173; **Board Cert:** Diagnostic Radiology 1981; **Med School:** Univ MD Sch Med 1977; **Resid:** Diagnostic Radiology, Sinai Hospital, Baltimore, MD 1977-1980; **Fellow:** Diagnostic Radiology, Johns Hopkins Hospital, Baltimore, MD 1980-1981; **Fac Appt:** Prof Radiology, Johns Hopkins Univ

Kurtz, Albert B MD (DR) - *Spec Exp:* Obstetrical Ultrasound; **Hospital:** Thomas Jefferson Univ Hosp; **Address:** Thomas Jefferson Univ Hosp, Dept Radiology, 111 S 11th St, rm 3350AB, Philadelphia, PA 19107; **Phone:** (215) 995-6343; **Board Cert:** Diagnostic Radiology 1977; **Med School:** St Louis Univ 1972; **Resid:** Internal Medicine, Montefiore Med Ctr, Bronx, NY 1973-1974; Diagnostic Radiology, Montefiore Med Ctr, Bronx, NY 1974-1977; **Fellow:** Ultrasound, Thomas Jefferson Univ Hosp, Philadelphia, PA 1977-1978; **Fac Appt:** Prof Radiology, Jefferson Med Coll

Mitnick, Julie MD (DR) - *Spec Exp:* Mammography; Breast Cancer; **Hospital:** NYU Med Ctr (page 71); **Address:** 650 1st Ave Fl 2, New York, NY 10016; **Phone:** (212) 686-4440; **Board Cert:** Diagnostic Radiology 1977; **Med School:** NYU Sch Med 1977; **Resid:** Diagnostic Radiology, NYU Med Ctr, New York, NY 1973-1977; **Fellow:** Pediatric Radiology, NYU Med Ctr, New York, NY 1977-1978; **Fac Appt:** Assoc Clin Prof Diagnostic Radiology, NYU Sch Med

Panicek, David MD (DR) - *Spec Exp:* Bone/Soft Tissue Disorders; Cross Sectional Imaging; **Hospital:** Mem Sloan Kettering Cancer Ctr; **Address:** 1275 York Ave, rm C278, New York, NY 10021; **Phone:** (212) 639-5825; **Board Cert:** Diagnostic Radiology 1984; **Med School:** Cornell Univ-Weill Med Coll 1980; **Resid:** Radiology, NY Hosp-Cornell, New York, NY 1981-1984; **Fac Appt:** Prof Radiology, Cornell Univ-Weill Med Coll

Sostman, H Dirk MD (DR) - *Spec Exp:* Diagnostic Radiology - General; **Hospital:** NY Presby Hosp - NY Weill Cornell Med Ctr (page 70); **Address:** 525 E 68th St, Starr Bldg, rm 8A37, New York, NY 10021-4870; **Phone:** (212) 746-2520; **Board Cert:** Diagnostic Radiology 1980, Nuclear Medicine 1996; **Med School:** Yale Univ 1976; **Resid:** Internal Medicine, Yale-New Haven Hosp, New Haven, CT 1976-1977; Diagnostic Radiology, Yale New Haven Hosp, New Haven, CT 1977-1979; **Fellow:** Nuclear Medicine, Yale-New Haven Hosp, New Haven, CT 1979-1980; Pulmonary Disease, Yale-New Haven Hosp, New Haven, CT 1980-1981; **Fac Appt:** Prof Radiology, Cornell Univ-Weill Med Coll

Teal, James S MD (DR) - *Spec Exp:* Interventional Radiology; **Hospital:** Howard Univ Hosp; **Address:** 2041 Georgia Ave NW, Washington, DC 20060-0001; **Phone:** (202) 865-1571; **Board Cert:** Diagnostic Radiology 1970; **Med School:** Univ Tex Med Br, Galveston 1965; **Resid:** Radiology, Mt Zion Hosp, San Francisco, CA 1965-1969; **Fellow:** Neurology, LAC Univ of SCA, Los Angeles, CA 1969-1970; **Fac Appt:** Prof Radiology, Howard Univ

White, Charles MD (DR) - *Spec Exp:* Thoracic Radiology; **Hospital:** University of MD Med Sys; **Address:** Dept Radiology, 22 S Greene St, Baltimore, MD 21201; **Phone:** (410) 328-8667; **Board Cert:** Radiology 1991, Internal Medicine 1987; **Med School:** SUNY Buffalo 1984; **Resid:** Internal Medicine, Columbia Presbyterian Hosp, New York, NY 1984-1987; Diagnostic Radiology, Columbia Presbyterian Hosp, New York, NY 1987-1991; **Fac Appt:** Assoc Prof Diagnostic Radiology, Univ MD Sch Med

Southeast

Hawkins Jr, Irvin MD (DR) - *Spec Exp:* Interventional Radiology; **Hospital:** Shands Hlthcre at Univ of FL (page 73); **Address:** Shands at U F, 1600 SW Archer Rd, Box 100374, Gainesville, FL 32610; **Phone:** (352) 395-0291; **Board Cert:** Diagnostic Radiology 1969; **Med School:** Univ MD Sch Med 1962; **Resid:** Radiology, Ohio State Univ, Columbus, OH 1965-1968; **Fellow:** Cardiology (Cardiovascular Disease), Shands Tchg Hosps, Gainesville, FL 1968-1970; **Fac Appt:** Prof Radiology, Univ Fla Coll Med

Mancuso, Anthony MD (DR) - *Spec Exp:* Head & Neck Diagnostic Imaging; Brain Neuroradiologic Diagnosis; Spine Neuroradiologic Diagnosis; **Hospital:** Shands Hlthcre at Univ of FL (page 73); **Address:** Shands HealthCare at Univ FLA, Dept Rad, 1600 SW Archer Rd, Gainesville, FL 32601; **Phone:** (352) 265-0296; **Board Cert:** Diagnostic Radiology 1978, Neuroradiology 1995; **Med School:** Univ Miami Sch Med 1973; **Resid:** Diagnostic Radiology, UCLA Med Ctr, Los Angeles, CA 1974-1977; **Fellow:** Neuroradiology, UCLA Med Ctr, Los Angeles, CA 1977-1978; **Fac Appt:** Prof Radiology, Univ Fla Coll Med

Pisano, Etta Driscoll MD (DR) - *Spec Exp:* *Breast Imaging;* **Hospital:** Univ of NC Hosp (page 77); **Address:** 101 Manning Dr, Box 7510, Chapel Hill, NC 27299-7510; **Phone:** (919) 966-6957; **Board Cert:** Diagnostic Radiology 1988; **Med School:** Duke Univ 1983; **Resid:** Diagnostic Radiology, Beth Israel Deaconess Hosp, Boston, MA 1984-1988

Midwest

Cavallino, Robert MD (DR) - *Spec Exp:* *Musculoskeletal Disorders;* **Hospital:** Advocate IL Masonic Med Ctr; **Address:** IL Masonic Med Ctr, Dept of Radiology, 836 W Wellington Ave, Chicago, IL 60657-4421; **Phone:** (773) 296-7820; **Board Cert:** Diagnostic Radiology 1968; **Med School:** Tufts Univ 1959; **Resid:** Radiology, New York Hosp, New York, NY 1964-1967; **Fac Appt:** Prof Radiology, Rush Med Coll

Monsees, Barbara MD (DR) - *Spec Exp:* *Mammography; Breast Cancer;* **Hospital:** Barnes-Jewish Hosp (page 55); **Address:** Mallinckrodt Inst of Radiology, 510 S Kingshighway Blvd, St Louis, MO 63110; **Phone:** (314) 454-7696; **Board Cert:** Diagnostic Radiology 1980; **Med School:** Washington Univ, St Louis 1975; **Resid:** Pediatrics, St Louis Chldns Hosp, St Louis, MO 1975-1977; Diagnostic Radiology, Mallinckrodt Inst Radiology, St Louis, MO 1977-1980; **Fac Appt:** Assoc Prof Radiology, Washington Univ, St Louis

Sagel, Stuart Steven MD (DR) - *Spec Exp:* *Lung Cancer; Occupational Lung Disease; Pulmonary Embolism;* **Hospital:** Barnes-Jewish Hosp (page 55); **Address:** Mallinckrodt Inst Rad-Barnes Hosp, 510 S Kingshighway Blvd, Box 8131, St Louis, MO 63110-1016; **Phone:** (314) 362-2927; **Board Cert:** Diagnostic Radiology 1970; **Med School:** Temple Univ 1965; **Resid:** Diagnostic Radiology, Yale New Haven Hosp, New Haven, CT 1966-1968; Diagnostic Radiology, UCSF, San Francisco, CA 1968-1970; **Fac Appt:** Prof Radiology, Washington Univ, St Louis

Southwest

Dodd III, Gerald Dewey MD (DR) - *Spec Exp:* *Ultrasound;* **Hospital:** Univ of Texas Hlth & Sci Ctr; **Address:** 7703 Floyd Curl Dr, MC-7800, San Antonio, TX 78229-3900; **Phone:** (210) 567-6470; **Board Cert:** Diagnostic Radiology 1987; **Med School:** Univ Tex, Houston 1983; **Resid:** Diagnostic Radiology, Univ Hosp, Cincinnati, OH 1984-1987; **Fellow:** Abdominal Imaging & Angio-Interventional, Univ Hosp, Cincinnati, OH 1987-1988; **Fac Appt:** Prof Radiology, Univ Tex, San Antonio

Huynh, Phan Tuong MD (DR) - *Spec Exp:* *Mammography;* **Hospital:** St Luke's Episcopal Hosp - Houston; **Address:** 6624 Fannin St Fl 10, Houston, TX 77030; **Phone:** (713) 791-8120; **Board Cert:** Diagnostic Radiology 1994; **Med School:** Univ VA Sch Med 1989; **Resid:** Radiology, Univ Virginia, Charlottesville, VA 1990-1994; **Fellow:** Mammography, Iniv Virginia, Charlottesville, VA 1994

Otto, Pamela MD (DR) - *Spec Exp:* *Mammography;* **Hospital:** Univ of Texas Hlth & Sci Ctr; **Address:** 7703 Floyd Curl Drive, MS 7800, San Antonio, TX 78229-3900; **Phone:** (210) 567-6488; **Board Cert:** Diagnostic Radiology 1993; **Med School:** Univ MO-Columbia Sch Med 1988; **Resid:** Radiology, U of Tx Hlth Sci Ctr., San Antonio, TX 1990-1993; **Fac Appt:** Assoc Prof Radiology, Univ Tex, San Antonio

Rivera, Frank James MD (DR) - *Spec Exp:* *Interventional Radiology;* **Hospital:** Parkland Mem Hosp; **Address:** UT Southwestern Medical Center, 5323 Harry Hines Blvd, Dallas, TX 75390-8896; **Phone:** (214) 648-8011; **Board Cert:** Diagnostic Radiology 1989, Vascular & Interventional Radiology 1998; **Med School:** Univ Tex, San Antonio 1982; **Resid:** Diagnostic Radiology, SUNY HSC, Syracuse, NY 1985-1989; **Fellow:** Vascular & Interventional Radiology, SUNY HSC, Syracuse, NY 1988-1989; **Fac Appt:** Asst Prof Radiology, Univ Tex SW, Dallas

West Coast and Pacific

Gomes, Antoinette Susan MD (DR) - *Spec Exp:* Cardiovascular Intervention Radiology; **Hospital:** UCLA Med Ctr; **Address:** MC 172115, 10833 Le Conte Ave, BL-141, CHS, Los Angeles, CA 90095; **Phone:** (310) 206-8909; **Board Cert:** Vascular & Interventional Radiology 1994, Diagnostic Radiology 1975; **Med School:** Med Coll PA Hahnemann 1969; **Resid:** Internal Medicine, LAC-USC MC, Los Angeles, CA 1970-1972; Diagnostic Radiology, Stanford Univ, CA 1972-1975; **Fellow:** Cardiovascular Radiology, UCLA Med Ctr, LA, CA 1975-1976; Cardiovascular Radiology, Univ Minn, MN 1976-1978; **Fac Appt:** Prof Radiology, UCLA

NEURORADIOLOGY

Mid Atlantic

Berenstein, Alejandro MD (NRad) - *Spec Exp:* Interventional Neuroradiology; Aneurysm-Cerebral; Endovascular Surgery; **Hospital:** Beth Israel Med Ctr - Singer Div (page 58); **Address:** Hyman Newman Inst Neurolgy & Neuro Surg, 170 E End Ave at 87th St, Fl 3, New York, NY 10128; **Phone:** (212) 870-9660; **Board Cert:** Diagnostic Radiology 1976, Neuroradiology 1995; **Med School:** Mexico 1970; **Resid:** Radiology, Mount Sinai Med Ctr, New York, NY 1973-1976; **Fellow:** Neuroradiology, NYU Med Ctr, New York, NY 1976-1978; **Fac Appt:** Prof Radiology, Albert Einstein Coll Med

Drayer, Burton P MD (NRad) - *Spec Exp:* Stroke; Parkinson's/Aging Brain; MRI & CT of Brain & Spine; **Hospital:** Mount Sinai Hosp (page 68); **Address:** 1 Gustave Levy Pl, Box 1234, New York, NY 10029; **Phone:** (212) 241-6403; **Board Cert:** Diagnostic Radiology 1978, Neuroradiology 1995, Neurology 1976; **Med School:** Univ Hlth Sci/Chicago Med Sch 1971; **Resid:** Neurology, Univ Vt Med Ctr, Burlington, VT 1972-1975; Radiology, Univ Pitt Hlth Ctr, Pittsburgh, PA 1975-1977; **Fellow:** Neuroradiology, Univ Pitt Hlth Ctr, Pittsburgh, PA 1977-1978; **Fac Appt:** Prof Radiology, Mount Sinai Sch Med

Grossman, Robert I MD (NRad) - *Spec Exp:* Neuroradiology - General; **Hospital:** Hosp Univ Penn (page 78); **Address:** Dept Radiology, 3400 Spruce St, Philadelphia, PA 19104; **Phone:** (215) 662-3064; **Board Cert:** Diagnostic Radiology 1979, Neuroradiology 1995; **Med School:** Univ Penn 1973; **Resid:** Neurological Surgery, Hosp Univ Penn, Philadelphia, PA 1974-1976; Radiology, Hosp Univ Penn, Philadelphia, PA 1976-1979; **Fellow:** Neuroradiology, Mass Genl Hosp, Boston, MA 1979-1981; **Fac Appt:** Prof Radiology, Univ Penn

Hurst, Robert W MD (NRad) - *Spec Exp:* Interventional Neuroradiology; **Hospital:** Hosp Univ Penn (page 78); **Address:** Dept Radiology/Neuroradiology, 3400 Spruce St, Philadelphia, PA 19104; **Phone:** (215) 662-3083; **Board Cert:** Diagnostic Radiology 1989, Neurology 1986, Neuroradiology 1995; **Med School:** Univ Tex, Houston 1981; **Resid:** Neurology, Univ Virginia, Charlottesville, VA 1982-1985; Radiology, Univ Virginia, Charlottesville, VA 1985-1989; **Fellow:** Neurological Radiology, Hosp Univ Penn, Philadelphia, PA 1989-1990; Interventional Radiology, NYU Med Ctr, New York, NY 1990-1991; **Fac Appt:** Assoc Prof Radiology, Univ Penn

Pile-Spellman, John MD (NRad) - *Spec Exp:* Interventional Neuroradiology; Intracranial Angioplasty & Stent; **Hospital:** NY Presby Hosp - Columbia Presby Med Ctr (page 70); **Address:** 177 Fort Washington Ave, Bldg MHB 8SK, New York, NY 10032-3713; **Phone:** (212) 305-6384; **Board Cert:** Diagnostic Radiology 1984; **Med School:** Tufts Univ 1978; **Resid:** Neurological Surgery, New England Med Ctr, Boston, MA 1979-1981; Neurological Radiology, Mass Genl Hosp, Boston, MA 1984-1986; **Fellow:** Interventional Neurological Radiology, NYU Med Ctr, New York, NY 1986; **Fac Appt:** Prof Radiology, Columbia P&S

Tenner, Michael MD (NRad) - *Spec Exp:* Neuroradiology - General; **Hospital:** Westchester Med Ctr (page 82); **Address:** NY Med Coll, Dept Radiology, Route 100, Valhalla, NY 10595; **Phone:** (914) 493-1927; **Board Cert:** Radiology 1967, Neuroradiology 1995; **Med School:** Univ MD Sch Med 1960; **Resid:** Radiology, Univ Maryland Hosp, Baltimore, MD 1961-1962; Radiology, Univ Maryland Hosp, Baltimore, MD 1964-1966; **Fellow:** Neuroradiology, Neurological Inst-Columbia Presby, New York, NY 1966-1968; **Fac Appt:** Prof Neuroradiology, NY Med Coll

NEURORADIOLOGY

Yousem, David Mark MD (NRad) - *Spec Exp:* Neuroradiology - General; **Hospital:** Johns Hopkins Hosp - Baltimore; **Address:** Johns Hopkins Hosp, 601 N Wolfe St, Bldg Houck - rm B-112, Baltimore, MD 21287; **Phone:** (410) 955-2353; **Board Cert:** Diagnostic Radiology 1987, Neuroradiology 1995; **Med School:** Univ Mich Med Sch 1983; **Resid:** Radiology, Johns Hopkins Hosp, Baltimore, MD 1984-1987; **Fellow:** Neuroradiology, Hosp Univ Penn, Philadelphia, PA 1988-1990; **Fac Appt:** Prof Radiology, Johns Hopkins Univ

Zimmerman, Robert A MD (NRad) - *Spec Exp:* Neuroradiology-Pediatric; **Hospital:** Chldn's Hosp of Philadelphia; **Address:** 34th & Civic Center Blvd, Philadelphia, PA 19104; **Phone:** (215) 590-2569; **Board Cert:** Radiology 1970, Neuroradiology 1995; **Med School:** Georgetown Univ 1964; **Resid:** Radiology, Hosp Univ Penn, Philadelphia, PA 1965-1969; **Fac Appt:** Prof Radiology, Univ Penn

Southeast

Dion, Jacques MD (NRad) - *Spec Exp:* Stroke; Intracranial Angioplasty & Stent; **Hospital:** Emory Univ Hosp; **Address:** Emory Univ Hosp, Dept Neuroradiology, 1364 Clifton Rd NE, rm A121, Atlanta, GA 30322; **Phone:** (404) 712-4991; **Board Cert:** Diagnostic Radiology 1982, Neuroradiology 1998; **Med School:** Canada 1978; **Resid:** Radiology, Harbor-UCLA Med Ctr, Torrance, CA 1979-1981; Radiology, Notre Dame Hosp, Montreal, Canada 1981-1983; **Fellow:** Neuroradiology, Univ Hospital, London, England 1983-1985; **Fac Appt:** Prof Radiology, Emory Univ

Joseph, Gregory J MD (NRad) - *Spec Exp:* Stroke; Aneurysm-Cerebral; Intracranial Angioplasty & Stent; **Hospital:** Presby Hosp - Charlotte; **Address:** Mecklenburg Radiology Assocs, 200 Hawthorne Ln, Charlotte, NC 28204; **Phone:** (704) 384-4057; **Board Cert:** Diagnostic Radiology 1989, Neuroradiology 1996; **Med School:** Georgetown Univ 1984; **Resid:** Diagnostic Radiology, Georgetown Univ Hosp, Washington, DC 1985-1989; Vascular & Interventional Radiology, Emory Univ Hosp, Atlanta, GA 1989-1991; **Fellow:** Neuroradiology, Emory Univ Hosp, Atlanta, GA 1991

Quencer, Robert MD (NRad) - *Spec Exp:* Spinal Cord Injury; **Hospital:** Univ of Miami - Jackson Meml Hosp; **Address:** Univ Miami, Dept Neuroradiology, 1150 NW 14th St, Ste 511, M828, Miami, FL 33136-2116; **Phone:** (305) 243-4701; **Board Cert:** Radiology 1972, Neuroradiology 1995; **Med School:** SUNY Syracuse 1967; **Resid:** Radiology, Columbia-Presbyterian Med Ctr, New York, NY 1968-1971; **Fellow:** Neuroradiology, Neurological Inst, New York, NY 1971-1972; **Fac Appt:** Prof Radiology, Univ Miami Sch Med

Midwest

Ball Jr, William S MD (NRad) - *Spec Exp:* Pediatric Neuroradiology; **Hospital:** Cincinnati Chldns Hosp Med Ctr; **Address:** Dept Neuroradiology, 3333 Burnet Ave, Cincinatti, OH 45229; **Phone:** (513) 636-8574; **Board Cert:** Diagnostic Radiology 1982, Pediatrics 1982, Neuroradiology 1999; **Med School:** Tulane Univ 1974; **Resid:** Pediatrics, Oschner Fdn Hosp, New Orleans, LA 1975-1977; Radiology, Univ New Mexico, Albuquerque, NM 1977-1978; **Fellow:** Pediatric Radiology, Chldns Hosp Med Ctr, Cincinnati, OH 1979-1981; Neuroradiology, Univ New Mexico Med Ctr, Albuquerque, NM 1978-1979; **Fac Appt:** Prof Radiology, Univ Cincinnati

Cross III, DeWitte T MD (NRad) - *Spec Exp:* Interventional Neuroradiology; **Hospital:** Barnes-Jewish Hosp (page 55); **Address:** Wash Univ, Dept Rad, 510 S Kingshighway Blvd, St Louis, MO 63110-1093; **Phone:** (314) 362-5580; **Board Cert:** Diagnostic Radiology 1985, Neuroradiology 1996; **Med School:** Univ Ala 1980; **Resid:** Diagnostic Radiology, Naval Hosp, Bethesda, MD 1982-1985; **Fellow:** Neuroradiology, NY Med Coll, Valhalla, NY 1987-1988; Neuroradiology, Columbia Univ, New York, NY 1988-1989; **Fac Appt:** Assoc Prof Radiology, Washington Univ, St Louis

Modic, Michael MD (NRad) - *Spec Exp:* MRI; **Hospital:** Cleveland Clin Fdn (page 57); **Address:** Cleveland Clinic, 9500 Euclid Ave, MC Hb-6, Cleveland, OH 44195; **Phone:** (216) 444-9308; **Board Cert:** Diagnostic Radiology 1979, Neuroradiology 1995; **Med School:** Case West Res Univ 1975; **Resid:** Radiology, Cleveland Clin Fdn, Cleveland, OH 1975-1978; **Fellow:** Neuroradiology, Cleveland Clin Fdn, Cleveland, OH 1978-1979; **Fac Appt:** Prof Radiology, Ohio State Univ

Great Plains and Mountains

Osborn, Anne G MD (NRad) - *Spec Exp:* Neuroradiology - General; **Hospital:** Univ Utah Hosp and Clin; **Address:** Dept Radiology, 50 N Medical Drive, rm 1A71-SOM, Salt Lake City, UT 84132; **Phone:** (801) 581-7553; **Board Cert:** Diagnostic Radiology 1974, Neuroradiology 1995; **Med School:** Stanford Univ 1970; **Resid:** Radiology, Stanford Univ Hosp, Stanford, CA 1971-1974; **Fellow:** Diagnostic Radiology, Univ Utah Hosp, Salt Lake City, UT 1974-1977; **Fac Appt:** Prof Radiology, Univ Utah

West Coast and Pacific

Atlas, Scott W MD (NRad) - *Spec Exp:* Stroke; MRI; **Hospital:** Stanford Med Ctr; **Address:** Stanford Univ Med Ctr, Dept Rad, 300 Pasteur Drive, rm S-047, Stanford, CA 94305-5105; **Phone:** (650) 723-7426; **Board Cert:** Diagnostic Radiology 1985, Neuroradiology 1995; **Med School:** Univ Chicago-Pritzker Sch Med 1981; **Resid:** Radiology, Northwestern Univ Med Ctr, Chicago, IL 1982-1985; **Fellow:** Neuroradiology, Hosp Univ Penn, Philadelphia, PA 1985-1987; **Fac Appt:** Prof Radiology, Stanford Univ

Barkovich, Anthony J MD (NRad) - *Spec Exp:* Pediatric Neuroradiology; **Hospital:** UCSF Med Ctr; **Address:** UCSF Med Ctr, Dept Neurorad, 505 Parnassus Ave, Box 0628, San Francisco, CA 94143; **Phone:** (415) 353-1655; **Board Cert:** Diagnostic Radiology 1984, Neuroradiology 2006; **Med School:** Geo Wash Univ 1980; **Resid:** Radiology, Letterman AMC, San Francisco, CA 1981-1984; **Fellow:** Neuroradiology, Walter Reed AMC, Washington, DC 1984-1986; **Fac Appt:** Prof Radiology, UCSF

Dillon, William P MD (NRad) - *Spec Exp:* Brain Tumors; **Hospital:** UCSF Med Ctr; **Address:** 505 Parnassus Ave, rm L 371, San Francisco, CA 94143; **Phone:** (415) 353-1668; **Board Cert:** Diagnostic Radiology 1982, Neuroradiology 1996; **Med School:** Loyola Univ-Stritch Sch Med 1978; **Resid:** Radiology, Univ Utah Hosp, Salt Lake City, UT 1979-1982; **Fellow:** Neuroradiology, UCSF Med Ctr, San Franciso, CA 1982-1983; **Fac Appt:** Prof Radiology, UCSF

Higashida, Randall T MD (NRad) - *Spec Exp:* Interventional Neuroradiology; Stroke; Intracranial Angioplasty & Stent; **Hospital:** UCSF Med Ctr; **Address:** UCSF Med Ctr, Dept Interven Neurorad, 505 Parnassus Ave, rm L352, San Francisco, CA 94143-0628; **Phone:** (415) 353-1863; **Board Cert:** Diagnostic Radiology 1984; **Med School:** Tulane Univ 1980; **Resid:** Radiology, UCLA Med Ctr, Los Angeles, CA 1981-1984; **Fellow:** Neuroradiology, UCLA Med Ctr, Los Angeles, CA 1984-1985; **Fac Appt:** Prof Radiology, UCSF

Teitelbaum, George P MD (NRad) - *Spec Exp:* Aneurysm-Brain; Stroke; Carotid Stenosis; **Hospital:** USC Univ Hosp - R K Eamer Med Plz; **Address:** USC Healthcare Consultation Center, 1510 San Pablo St, Ste 268, Los Angeles, CA 90033; **Phone:** (626) 351-3369; **Board Cert:** Diagnostic Radiology 1984, Vascular & Interventional Radiology 1995, Neuroradiology 1996; **Med School:** UCSD 1980; **Resid:** Radiology, UC Irvine Med Ctr, Orange, CA 1981-1984; Interventional Radiology, George Washington, Wash, DC 1984-1985; **Fellow:** Magnetic Resonance Imaging, Huntington Med Research Inst, Pasadena, CA 1987-1988; Interventional Neuroradiology, UCSF Med Ctr, San Francisco, CA 1992-1994; **Fac Appt:** Prof Neurological Surgery, USC Sch Med

Vinuela, Fernando MD (NRad) - *Spec Exp:* *Stroke; Intracranial Angioplasty & Stent; Aneurysm-Cerebral;* **Hospital:** UCLA Med Ctr; **Address:** UCLA Med Ctr, Dept Rad, 10833 Le Conte Ave, Box 951721, Los Angeles, CA 90095-1721; **Phone:** (310) 825-6576; **Board Cert:** Diagnostic Radiology 1979; **Med School:** Uruguay 1970; **Resid:** Radiology, Westminster Hosp, London, England 1974-1975; Radiology, Victoria Hosp, London, England 1975-1977; **Fellow:** Neuroradiology, Univ Hosp, London, England 1977-1979; **Fac Appt:** Prof Radiology, UCLA

RADIOLOGY

New England

Benson, Carol MD (Rad) - *Spec Exp:* Obstetrical Ultrasound; **Hospital:** Brigham & Women's Hosp; **Address:** Dept Radiology, 75 Francis St, Boston, MA 02115; **Phone:** (617) 732-6280; **Board Cert:** Diagnostic Radiology 1984; **Med School:** Univ Penn 1980; **Resid:** Radiology, NY Hosp-Cornell U, New York, NY 1981-1984; **Fellow:** Ultrasound, Brigham Womens, Boston, MA 1984-1985; **Fac Appt:** Assoc Prof Harvard Med Sch

Schepps, Barbara MD (Rad) - *Spec Exp:* Breast Imaging; **Hospital:** Rhode Island Hosp; **Address:** Director- Ann C Pappas Ctr for Breast Care, 593 Eddy St, Providence, RI 02903-4923; **Phone:** (401) 444-5184; **Board Cert:** Radiology 1973; **Med School:** Hahnemann Univ 1968; **Resid:** Radiology, Boston City Hosp, Boston, MA 1969-1972; **Fac Appt:** Clin Prof Radiology, Brown Univ

Mid Atlantic

Berdon, Walter MD (Rad) - *Spec Exp:* Radiology-Pediatric; **Hospital:** NY Presby Hosp - Columbia Presby Med Ctr (page 70); **Address:** Columbia Presby Med Ctr, Dept Radiology, 3959 Broadway, BHN 318, New York, NY 10032; **Phone:** (212) 305-9864; **Board Cert:** Radiology 1962, Pediatric Radiology 1995; **Med School:** SUNY Syracuse 1955; **Resid:** Internal Medicine, Montefiore Hosp, New York, NY 1956-1957; Radiology, Montefiore Hosp, New York, NY 1959-1962; **Fellow:** Pediatric Radiology, Coll P&S -Columbia Univ, New York, NY 1962-1964; **Fac Appt:** Prof Radiology, Columbia P&S

Haskal, Ziv MD (Rad) - *Spec Exp:* Uterine Fibroid Embolization; Angiography; Vascular & Interventional Radiology; **Hospital:** NY Presby Hosp - Columbia Presby Med Ctr (page 70); **Address:** Dept Interventional Radiology, 177 Fort Washington Ave, Ste 4-100, New York, NY 10032; **Phone:** (212) 305-8070; **Board Cert:** Vascular & Interventional Radiology 1999, Diagnostic Radiology 1991; **Med School:** Boston Univ 1986; **Resid:** Diagnostic Radiology, UCSF, San Francisco, CA 1987-1991; **Fellow:** Vascular & Interventional Radiology, UCSF, San Francisco, CA 1991-1992; **Fac Appt:** Prof Radiology, Columbia P&S

Kandarpa, Krishna MD (Rad) - *Spec Exp:* Vascular & Interventional Radiology; **Hospital:** NY Presby Hosp - NY Weill Cornell Med Ctr (page 70); **Address:** 525 E 68th St, L-515, New York, NY 10021-4870; **Phone:** (212) 746-2604; **Board Cert:** Diagnostic Radiology 1984, Vascular & Interventional Radiology 1996; **Med School:** Univ Miami Sch Med 1980; **Resid:** Radiology, Brigham & Women's-Harvard, Boston, MA 1981-1984; **Fellow:** Vascular & Interventional Radiology, Brigham & Women's-Harvard, Boston, MA 1984-1986; **Fac Appt:** Prof Radiology, Cornell Univ-Weill Med Coll

Kaye, Robin D MD (Rad) - *Spec Exp:* Interventional Radiology-Pediatric; **Hospital:** Chldn's Hosp of Philadelphia; **Address:** Children's Hosp Phila, Dept Radiology, 34th & Civic Ctr Blvd, Philadelphia, PA 19104; **Phone:** (215) 590-9940; **Board Cert:** Diagnostic Radiology 1991, Pediatric Radiology 1995; **Med School:** Univ Colo 1986; **Resid:** Internal Medicine, VA Med Ctr, Boise, ID 1987-1988; Diagnostic Radiology, Univ Colorado Hlth Sci Ctr, Denver, CO 1988-1990; **Fellow:** Pediatric Radiology, Chldns Hosp/Univ Colorado, Denver, CO 1990-1992; Pediatric Interventional Radiology, Childrens Hosp, Pittsburgh, PA 1992-1993

Leonidas, John MD (Rad) - *Spec Exp:* Radiology-Pediatric; **Hospital:** Long Island Jewish Med Ctr; **Address:** Dept Radiology, 270-05 76th Ave, New Hyde Park, NY 11040; **Phone:** (718) 470-3404; **Board Cert:** Pediatric Radiology 1995, Diagnostic Radiology 1969, Pediatrics 1964; **Med School:** Greece 1955; **Resid:** Pediatrics, Jewish Hosp, Brooklyn, NY 1961-1963; **Fellow:** Diagnostic Radiology, Columbia-Presby Med Ctr, New York, NY 1966-1969; **Fac Appt:** Prof Radiology, Albert Einstein Coll Med

Norton, Karen MD (Rad) - *Spec Exp:* Radiology-Pediatric; **Hospital:** Mount Sinai Hosp (page 68); **Address:** 1 Gustave Levy Pl, New York, NY 10029-6500; **Phone:** (212) 241-7418; **Board Cert:** Radiology 1984, Pediatric Radiology 1995; **Med School:** Mount Sinai Sch Med 1980; **Resid:** Pediatrics, NYU Med Ctr, New York, NY 1980-1981; Radiology, Mount Sinai Hosp, New York, NY 1981-1984; **Fellow:** Pediatric Pulmonology, Mount Sinai Hosp, New York, NY 1984-1985; **Fac Appt:** Asst Prof Pediatric Radiology, Mount Sinai Sch Med

Yoon, Sydney MD (Rad) - *Spec Exp:* Fibroid Embolization; Interventional Radiology Only; **Hospital:** St Francis Hosp - The Heart Ctr (page 74); **Address:** 100 Pt Washington Blvd, Dept Radiology, Roslyn, NY 11576-1348; **Phone:** (516) 562-6517; **Board Cert:** Vascular & Interventional Radiology 1998, Neuroradiology 1995, Diagnostic Radiology 1993, Internal Medicine 1989; **Med School:** Univ Chicago-Pritzker Sch Med 1986; **Resid:** Internal Medicine, Johns Hopkins Hosp, Baltimore, MD 1986-1989; Diagnostic Radiology, UCLA Med Ctr, Los Angeles, CA 1989-1993; **Fellow:** Neuroradiology, Columbia Presby Med Ctr, New York, NY 1993-1995; Vascular & Interventional Radiology, UCLA Med Ctr, Los Angeles, CA 1996-1997

Southeast

Becker, Gary J. MD (Rad) - *Spec Exp:* Vascular & Interventional Radiology; **Hospital:** Baptist Hosp - Miami; **Address:** 8900 N Kendall Drive, Miami, FL 33176; **Phone:** (305) 598-5990; **Board Cert:** Vascular & Interventional Radiology 1994, Diagnostic Radiology 1981; **Med School:** Indiana Univ 1977; **Resid:** Diagnostic Radiology, Ind U Med Ctr Hosp., Indianapolis, IN 1978-1981; **Fac Appt:** Clin Prof Radiology, Univ Miami Sch Med

Benenati, James Francis MD (Rad) - *Spec Exp:* Uterine Fibroid Embolization; Stent Grafts; Aneurysm-Abdominal Aortic; **Hospital:** Baptist Hosp - Miami; **Address:** 8900 N Kendall Dr, Miami, FL 33176; **Phone:** (305) 598-5990; **Board Cert:** Vascular & Interventional Radiology 1995, Diagnostic Radiology 1988; **Med School:** Univ S Fla Coll Med 1984; **Resid:** Radiation Oncology, Indiana Univ Hosp, Indianapolis, IN 1984-1988; **Fellow:** Cardiology (Cardiovascular Disease), Johns Hopkins Hosp, Baltimore, MD 1988-1989; **Fac Appt:** Prof Radiology, Univ Miami Sch Med

Coldwell, Douglas Michael MD (Rad) - *Spec Exp:* Vascular & Interventional Radiology; Chemoembolization; **Hospital:** Wake Forest Univ Baptist Med Ctr (page 81); **Address:** Medical Center Blvd, 2nd Fl, Winston-Salem, NC 27157-1088; **Phone:** (336) 716-4936; **Board Cert:** Diagnostic Radiology 1986, Vascular & Interventional Radiology 1995; **Med School:** Univ Tex Med Br, Galveston 1980; **Resid:** Diagnostic Radiology, Hershey Med Ctr-Penn St U, Hershey, PA 1980-1983; **Fellow:** Vascular & Interventional Radiology, MD Anderson Hosp-Tumor Inst, Houston, TX 1983-1984; **Fac Appt:** Prof Radiology, Univ MD Sch Med

Katzen, Barry MD (Rad) - *Spec Exp:* Radiology - General; **Hospital:** Baptist Hosp - Miami; **Address:** Miami Cardiac & Vasc Inst, 8900 N Kendall Dr, Miami, FL 33176-2118; **Phone:** (305) 598-5990; **Board Cert:** Diagnostic Radiology 1974, Vascular & Interventional Radiology 1994; **Med School:** Univ Miami Sch Med 1970; **Resid:** Radiology, NY Hosp Cornell Med Ctr, New York, NY 1971-1974

Midwest

Charboneau, J William MD (Rad) - *Spec Exp:* Ultrasound; Liver Cancer-Diagnosis & Ablation; Thyroid Cancer; **Hospital:** Mayo Med Ctr & Clin - Rochester, MN; **Address:** 200 First Street SW, Rochester, MN 55905-0002; **Phone:** (507) 284-2097; **Board Cert:** Diagnostic Radiology 1980; **Med School:** Univ Wisc 1976; **Resid:** Radiology, Mayo Clinic, Rochester, MN 1976-1980; **Fac Appt:** Prof Radiology, Mayo Med Sch

Goodman, Lawrence R MD (Rad) - *Spec Exp:* Thoracic Radiology; Radiology-Diagnostic; **Hospital:** Froedtert Meml Lutheran Hosp; **Address:** Froedtert Meml Lutheran Hosp, Dept Radiology, 9200 West Wisconsin Avenue, Milwaukee, WI 53226; **Phone:** (414) 805-3700; **Board Cert:** Diagnostic Radiology 1973; **Med School:** SUNY Downstate 1968; **Resid:** Radiology, Boston City Hosp, Boston, MA 1969-1972; **Fellow:** Thoracic Radiology, Univ California Hosp, CA 1972-1973

Martenson Jr, James A MD (Rad) - *Spec Exp:* Mucositis; Esophagitis; Therapeutic Radiology; **Hospital:** Mayo Med Ctr & Clin - Rochester, MN; **Address:** Dept Radiation Oncology, 200 First St SW, Rochester, MN 55905; **Phone:** (507) 284-4561; **Board Cert:** Therapeutic Radiology 1985; **Med School:** Univ Wash 1981; **Resid:** Radiation Oncology, Mayo Clinic, Rochester, MN 1981-1985; **Fac Appt:** Assoc Prof Radiology, Mayo Med Sch

McAlister, Bill MD (Rad) - *Spec Exp:* Radiology-Pediatric; **Hospital:** St Louis Children's Hospital; **Address:** 510 S Kingshighway Blvd, Saint Louis, MO 63110; **Phone:** (314) 454-6229; **Board Cert:** Pediatric Radiology 1994, Radiology 1961; **Med School:** Wayne State Univ 1954; **Resid:** Radiology, Cincinnati Genl Hosp, Cincinnati, OH 1957-1960; **Fac Appt:** Prof Radiology, Washington Univ, St Louis

Sivit, Carlos MD (Rad) - *Spec Exp:* Radiology-Pediatric; Abdominal Imaging; Emergency Radiology; **Hospital:** Rainbow Babies & Chldns Hosp; **Address:** Univ Hosps Cleveland, Dept Radiology, 11100 Euclid Ave, Cleveland, OH 44106; **Phone:** (216) 844-1172; **Board Cert:** Radiology 1987, Pediatric Radiology 1995; **Med School:** Univ VA Sch Med 1981; **Resid:** Pediatrics, Vanderbilt Univ Hosp, Nashville, TN 1981-1984; Radiology, George Washington Univ Hosp, Washington, DC 1984-1987; **Fellow:** Pediatric Radiology, Chldns Natl Med Ctr, Washington, DC 1987-1989; **Fac Appt:** Prof Radiology, Case West Res Univ

Great Plains and Mountains

Durham, Janette Denham MD (Rad) - *Spec Exp:* Vascular & Interventional Radiology; **Hospital:** Univ Colo HSC - Denver; **Address:** U Colo Hlth Sci Ctr, 4200 E Ninth Ave, Box A 030, Denver, CO 80262; **Phone:** (303) 372-6134; **Board Cert:** Diagnostic Radiology 1987, Vascular & Interventional Radiology 1996; **Med School:** Indiana Univ **Resid:** Ind Univ Hosp, Indianapolis, IN 1983-1987; **Fellow:** Mass Genl Hosp, Boston, MA 1987-1988; **Fac Appt:** Assoc Prof Radiology, Univ Colo

Kumpe, David A MD (Rad) - *Spec Exp:* Aneurysm-Brain; Stroke; Arterial Occlusions; **Hospital:** Univ Colo HSC - Denver; **Address:** Univ Hosp-Denver, Dept Radiology, 4200 E 9th Ave, Box A030, Denver, CO 80626; **Phone:** (303) 372-6141; **Board Cert:** Radiology 1972, Vascular & Interventional Radiology 1994; **Med School:** Harvard Med Sch 1967; **Resid:** Radiology, Mass Genl Hosp, Boston, MA 1968-1971; **Fellow:** Neurological Radiology, Zurich, Switzerland 1974-1975; Angiography, Zurich, Switzerland 1975-1976; **Fac Appt:** Prof Radiology, Univ Colo

Miller, Franklin MD (Rad) - *Spec Exp:* Interventional Radiology; **Hospital:** Univ Utah Hosp and Clin; **Address:** U of Utah School of Medicine, 50 N Medical Drive, Ste 1A71, Salt Lake City, UT 84132-0002; **Phone:** (801) 581-8188; **Board Cert:** Diagnostic Radiology 1973, Vascular & Interventional Radiology 1995; **Med School:** Temple Univ 1966; **Resid:** Diagnostic Radiology, Johns Hopkins Hosp, Baltimore, MD 1969-1972; **Fellow:** Vascular & Interventional Radiology, Johns Hopkins Hosp, Baltimore, MD 1972-1973; **Fac Appt:** Prof Radiology, Univ Utah

Southwest

Palmaz, Julio C. MD (Rad) - *Spec Exp:* Interventional Radiology; Endovascular Therapy; Intravascular Stents; **Hospital:** Univ of Texas Hlth & Sci Ctr; **Address:** 7703 Floyd Curl Drive, MS 7800, San Antonio, TX 78229-3900; **Phone:** (210) 567-5564; **Board Cert:** Diagnostic Radiology 1981, Vascular & Interventional Radiology 1994; **Med School:** Argentina 1971; **Resid:** Radiology, Rawson Hosp Bueno Aires, Argentina 1971-1974; **Fellow:** Vascular & Interventional Radiology, UC Davis VA Med Ctr, Martinez, CA 1977-1980; **Fac Appt:** Prof Radiology, Univ Tex, San Antonio

Seibert, Joanna J MD (Rad) - *Spec Exp:* Sickle Cell Screening; Radiology-Pediatric; **Hospital:** Arkansas Chldns Hosp; **Address:** Arkansas Children's Hospital-Dept Rad, 800 Marshall St, MS 105, Little Rock, AR 72202; **Phone:** (501) 320-1175; **Board Cert:** Diagnostic Radiology 1974, Pediatric Radiology 1994; **Med School:** Univ Tenn Coll Med, Memphis 1968; **Resid:** Radiology, Univ Tenn Coll Med, Memphis, TN 1970-1972; Radiology, Univ Iowa Hosp & Clinics, Iowa City, IA 1972-1973; **Fac Appt:** Prof Radiology, Univ Ark

West Coast and Pacific

Dake, Michael David MD (Rad) - *Spec Exp:* Interventional Radiology; **Hospital:** Stanford Med Ctr; **Address:** 300 Pasteur Drive, rm H-3647, MC 5642, Stanford, CA 94305; **Phone:** (650) 725-5204; **Board Cert:** Vascular & Interventional Radiology 1994, Pulmonary Disease 1986; **Med School:** Baylor Coll Med 1978; **Resid:** Internal Medicine, Baylor Hosp, Houston, TX 1978-1982; Radiology, UCSF Med Ctr, San Francisco, CA 1983-1986; **Fellow:** Pulmonary Disease, UCSF Med Ctr, San Francisco, CA 1982-1983; Interventional Radiology, UCSF Med Ctr, San Francisco, CA 1986-1987; **Fac Appt:** Assoc Prof Radiology, Stanford Univ

Keller, Frederick MD (Rad) - *Spec Exp:* Interventional Radiology; **Hospital:** OR Hlth Sci Univ Hosp and Clinics; **Address:** Dotter Interventional Inst, L-605, 3181 SW Sam Jackson Park Rd, Portland, OR 97201; **Phone:** (503) 494-7660; **Board Cert:** Vascular & Interventional Radiology 1994, Diagnostic Radiology 1977; **Med School:** Univ Penn 1968; **Resid:** Diagnostic Radiology, Univ Oreg Hlth Scis Ctr, Portland, OR 1974-1977; **Fac Appt:** Prof Diagnostic Radiology, Oregon Hlth Scis Univ

Valji, Karim MD (Rad) - *Spec Exp:* Interventional Radiology; **Hospital:** UCSD Healthcare; **Address:** UCSD Med Ctr, 200 W Arbor Dr, San Diego, CA 92103-8756; **Phone:** (619) 543-6607; **Board Cert:** Diagnostic Radiology 1989, Vascular & Interventional Radiology 1998; **Med School:** Harvard Med Sch 1982; **Resid:** Internal Medicine, UCSF, San Francisco, CA 1982-1984; Diagnostic Radiology, UCSD, San Diego, CA 1985-1988; **Fellow:** Angiography, UCSD, San Diego, CA 1988-1989; **Fac Appt:** Assoc Prof Radiology, Univ SD Sch Med

Wood, Beverly MD (Rad) - *Spec Exp:* Radiology-Pediatric; **Hospital:** LAC & USC Med Ctr; **Address:** 4650 Sunset Blvd, Los Angeles, CA 90033; **Phone:** (323) 442-2377; **Board Cert:** Diagnostic Radiology 1972, Pediatric Radiology 1994; **Med School:** Univ Rochester 1965; **Resid:** Radiology, Strong Meml Hosp, Rochester, NY 1968-1971; **Fellow:** Pediatric Radiology, Strong Meml Hosp, Rochester, NY 1971-1972; **Fac Appt:** Prof Radiology, USC Sch Med

REPRODUCTIVE ENDOCRINOLOGY

(a subspecialty of OBSTETRICS AND GYNECOLOGY)

An obstetrician/gynecologist who is capable of managing complex problems relating to reproductive endocrinology and infertility.

OBSTETRICS AND GYNECOLOGY

An obstetrician/gynecologist possesses special knowledge, skills and professional capability in the medical and surgical care of the female reproductive system and associated disorders. This physician serves as a consultant to other physicians and as a primary physician for women.

Training required: Four years plus two years in clinical practice before certification in obstetrics and gynecology is complete *plus* additional training and examination in reproductive endocrinology

NYU
Medical
Center

550 First Avenue (at 31st Street)
New York, NY 10016
Physician Referral: (888) 7-NYU-MED
(888-769-8633)   www.med.nyu.edu

SCHOOL OF
MEDICINE

NEW YORK UNIVERSITY

PROGRAM FOR IVF, REPRODUCTIVE SURGERY AND INFERTILITY

Today, thanks to promising new options in the treatment of infertility, specialists at NYU Medical Center can help more patients realize their dreams of parenthood. With unique expertise in all aspects of reproductive endocrinology, including the diagnosis and treatment of endometriosis, fibroids, problems with ovulation or sperm function, and recurrent pregnancy loss, NYU Medical Center uses the most advanced technology to assist infertile women and men who wish to conceive children.

From the initial diagnosis through all stages of treatment, couples receive state-of-the-art compassionate care based on their specific needs. After a comprehensive evaluation to determine the cause of infertility, couples are counseled on whether assisted reproduction is necessary. (Often, surgery can correct disorders that lead to infertility, like fibroids or endometriosis. Similarly, stimulation of a woman's ovaries with medication often results in pregnancy.) When the physician and couple agree that assisted reproduction is appropriate, the program offers:

- In Vitro Fertilization
- Donor Oocyte (Egg) and Sperm Services
- Intracytoplasmic Sperm Injection (injection of a single sperm directly into an egg)
- Assisted Hatching (creating an entry point in oocytes surrounded by tough tissue to assist sperm penetration)
- Preimplantation Genetic Diagnosis (for couples with a high risk of bearing children with specific genetic disorders)
- Cyropreservation (freezing embryos in liquid nitrogen to preserve them for future use)

and several male infertility treatments:

- Comprehensive evaluation of sperm health and fertility
- Testicular Biopsy
- Vasectomy Reversal
- Epididymal Repair (surgery to clear sperm pathways within penis)
- Microsurgical Sperm Aspiration (retrieval of sperm from inside the testes, when it is not present in the semen)
- Varicocele Repair (surgical reduction of enlarged veins around penis to reduce high temperature in groin area, which adversely impacts on fertility)

NYU MEDICAL CENTER

The Reproductive Endocrinologists at NYU Medical Center are dedicated not only to treating infertility, but also to researching its causes. Because of this first-hand knowledge of the latest breakthroughs in fertility treatment, our programs are among the most successful in the country. Among our achievements are:

- the first ICSI (Intracytoplasmic Sperm Injection) pregnancy

- the first Assisted Hatching pregnancy

- the first epididymal sperm retrieval

and

- the first embryo biopsy

in the world.

Physician Referral
(888) 7-NYU-MED
(888-769-8633)
www.med.nyu.edu

PHYSICIAN LISTINGS

Reproductive Endocrinology

New England

Barbieri, Robert MD (RE) - *Spec Exp:* Fibroids; Infertility-Female; Endometriosis; **Hospital:** Brigham & Women's Hosp; **Address:** Brigham & Womens Hosp, Dept Ob/Gyn, 75 Francis St, Boston, MA 02482; **Phone:** (617) 732-4265; **Board Cert:** Obstetrics & Gynecology 1997, Reproductive Endocrinology 1997; **Med School:** Harvard Med Sch 1977; **Resid:** Obstetrics & Gynecology, Peter Bent Brigham, Boston, MA 1980-1984; Internal Medicine, Peter Bent Brigham, Boston, MA 1977-1980; **Fac Appt:** Prof Obstetrics & Gynecology, Harvard Med Sch

Crowley, William MD (RE) - *Spec Exp:* Gonadotropin Deficiency; Kallmann Syndrome; **Hospital:** MA Genl Hosp; **Address:** Mass Genl Hosp-Bartlett Hall, Exten Bldg 5, Boston, MA 02114; **Phone:** (617) 726-5390; **Board Cert:** Internal Medicine 1974, Endocrinology, Diabetes & Metabolism 1977; **Med School:** Tufts Univ 1969; **Resid:** Internal Medicine, Mass Genl Hosp, Boston, MA 1970-1971; Internal Medicine, Mass Genl Hosp, Boston, MA 1973-1974; **Fellow:** Endocrinology, Diabetes & Metabolism, Mass Genl Hosp, Boston, MA 1974-1976; **Fac Appt:** Prof Medicine, Harvard Med Sch

Hill III, Joseph Albert MD (RE) - *Spec Exp:* Miscarriage-Recurrent; Infertility-Female; **Hospital:** Brigham & Women's Hosp; **Address:** 75 Francis St, ASB1-3, Boston, MA 02118; **Phone:** (617) 732-4222; **Board Cert:** Obstetrics & Gynecology 1989, Reproductive Endocrinology 1991; **Med School:** Med Coll GA 1981; **Resid:** Obstetrics & Gynecology, Med Coll Ga, Augusta, GA 1982-1985; **Fellow:** Reproductive Endocrinology, Brigham-Womens Hosp/Harvard, Boston, MA; **Fac Appt:** Prof Obstetrics & Gynecology, Harvard Med Sch

Isaacson, Keith B MD (RE) - *Spec Exp:* Infertility; Endometriosis; **Hospital:** MA Genl Hosp; **Address:** 214 Washington St, Newton, MA 02462; **Phone:** (617) 243-5205; **Board Cert:** Reproductive Endocrinology 1991, Obstetrics & Gynecology 1990; **Med School:** Med Coll GA 1983; **Resid:** Obstetrics & Gynecology, Ochsner Foundation Hosp., Houma, LA 1987; **Fellow:** Reproductive Endocrinology, Univ Penn, Philadelphia, PA 1989; **Fac Appt:** Assoc Prof Obstetrics & Gynecology, Harvard Med Sch

Keefe, David Lawrence MD (RE) - *Spec Exp:* Infertility-IVF; Reproductive Aging; **Hospital:** Women & Infants Hosp - Rhode Island; **Address:** Women & Infants Hosp, Dept OB/GYN, 101 Dudley St, Providence, RI 02905-2499; **Phone:** (401) 453-7500; **Board Cert:** Obstetrics & Gynecology 1993, Reproductive Endocrinology 1995; **Med School:** Georgetown Univ 1980; **Resid:** Psychiatry, Harvard Psych Srv/Camb Hosp, Boston, MA 1981-1983; Psychiatry, Univ Chicago Hosp & Clins, Chicago, IL 1983-1985; **Fellow:** Obstetrics & Gynecology, Yale New Haven Hosp, New Haven, CT 1985-1989; Reproductive Endocrinology, Yale New Haven Hosp, New Haven, CT 1989-1991; **Fac Appt:** Assoc Prof Obstetrics & Gynecology, Brown Univ

Luciano, Anthony Adolph MD (RE) - *Spec Exp:* Infertility; Endometriosis; **Hospital:** New Britain Gen Hosp; **Address:** 100 Grand St, Ste N3, New Britain, CT 06050; **Phone:** (860) 224-5467; **Board Cert:** Reproductive Endocrinology 1981, Obstetrics & Gynecology 1980; **Med School:** Univ Conn 1973; **Resid:** Obstetrics & Gynecology, Hartford Hosp, Hartford, CT 1974-1977; **Fellow:** Reproductive Endocrinology, Univ Conn Sch Med, Farmington, CT 1977-1979; **Fac Appt:** Prof Obstetrics & Gynecology, Univ Conn

Managaniello, Paul D. MD (RE) - *Spec Exp:* Infertility; Menopause; Operative Laparoscopy; **Hospital:** Dartmouth - Hitchcock Med Ctr; **Address:** One Medical Center Drive, Lebanon, NH 03756; **Phone:** (603) 650-8162; **Board Cert:** Obstetrics & Gynecology 1980, Reproductive Endocrinology 1984; **Resid:** Obstetrics & Gynecology, Thomas Jefferson Univ Hospital, Philadelphia, PA 1973-1977; **Fellow:** Gynecologic Endocrinology, Medical College of Georgia, Augusta, GA 1977-1979

REPRODUCTIVE ENDOCRINOLOGY

Schiff, Isaac MD (RE) - *Spec Exp:* Menopause Problems; Infertility-Female; **Hospital:** MA Genl Hosp; **Address:** Vincent Meml Hosp @ Mass Genl Hosp., 55 Fruit St., Bldg VBK - Ste 113, Boston, MA 02114; **Phone:** (617) 726-3001; **Board Cert:** Obstetrics & Gynecology 1998, Reproductive Endocrinology 1979; **Med School:** McGill Univ 1968; **Resid:** Surgery, New England Med. Ctr, Boston, MA 1974; Obstetrics & Gynecology, Boston Hosp. Women, Boston, MA 1971-1973; **Fellow:** Reproductive Endocrinology, Boston Hosp. Women, Boston, MA 1974-1976; **Fac Appt:** Prof Gynecologic Oncology, Harvard Med Sch

Mid Atlantic

Berga, Sarah Lee MD (RE) - *Spec Exp:* Infertility-IVF; Hormonal Replacement; Menstrual Disorders; **Hospital:** Magee Women's Hosp; **Address:** Magee-Women's Hosp, Dept ObGyn, 300 Halket St, Fl 4 - rm 4100, Pittsburgh, PA 15213-3180; **Phone:** (412) 641-1600; **Board Cert:** Obstetrics & Gynecology 1998, Reproductive Endocrinology 1998; **Med School:** Univ VA Sch Med 1980; **Resid:** Obstetrics & Gynecology, Harvard Med Sch/ Mass Genl Hosp, Boston, MA 1980-1984; **Fellow:** Reproductive Endocrinology, UCSD, San Diego, CA 1984-1986; **Fac Appt:** Prof Obstetrics & Gynecology, Univ Pittsburgh

Grifo, James MD/PhD (RE) - *Spec Exp:* Infertility; **Hospital:** NYU Med Ctr (page 71); **Address:** 660 1st Ave Fl 5, New York, NY 10016; **Phone:** (212) 263-7978; **Board Cert:** Reproductive Endocrinology 1994, Obstetrics & Gynecology 1991; **Med School:** Case West Res Univ 1984; **Resid:** Obstetrics & Gynecology, NY Hosp-Columbia, New York, NY 1985-1988; **Fellow:** Reproductive Endocrinology, Yale-New Haven Hosp, New Haven, CT 1988-1990; **Fac Appt:** Prof Reproductive Endocrinology, NYU Sch Med

Lobo, Rogerio MD (RE) - *Spec Exp:* Menopause Problems; **Hospital:** NY Presby Hosp - Columbia Presby Med Ctr (page 70); **Address:** 1790 Broadway Fl 2, New York, NY 10019; **Phone:** (212) 305-3696; **Board Cert:** Obstetrics & Gynecology 1981, Reproductive Endocrinology 1982; **Med School:** Georgetown Univ 1974; **Resid:** Obstetrics & Gynecology, Univ Chicago, Chicago, IL 1975-1978; **Fellow:** Reproductive Endocrinology, USC Med Ctr, Los Angeles, CA 1980; **Fac Appt:** Prof Obstetrics & Gynecology, Columbia P&S

McClamrock, Howard Dean MD (RE) - *Spec Exp:* Infertility; Blastocyst Transfer; Infertility-IVF; **Hospital:** University of MD Med Sys; **Address:** Univ Maryland, Dept OB/GYN, 419 W Redwood St, Ste 500, Baltimore, MD 21201; **Phone:** (800) 492-5538; **Board Cert:** Reproductive Endocrinology 1998, Obstetrics & Gynecology 1998; **Med School:** Univ NC Sch Med 1981; **Resid:** Obstetrics & Gynecology, Univ Maryland, Baltimore, MD 1982-1986; **Fellow:** Reproductive Endocrinology, Univ Maryland, Baltimore, MD 1986-1988; **Fac Appt:** Assoc Prof Obstetrics & Gynecology, Univ MD Sch Med

Oktay, Kutluk MD (RE) - *Spec Exp:* Transplant-Ovarian Tissue; Infertility-Female; **Hospital:** NY Presby Hosp - NY Weill Cornell Med Ctr (page 70); **Address:** Ctr for Reproductive Med & Infertility, 505 E 70th St, Fl 3, New York, NY 10021; **Phone:** (212) 746-1762; **Board Cert:** Obstetrics & Gynecology 1997, Reproductive Endocrinology 1999; **Med School:** Turkey 1986; **Resid:** Internal Medicine, Cook Co Hosp, Chicago, IL 1986-1989; Obstetrics & Gynecology, Univ Conn Hlt, Farmington, CT 1989-1993; **Fellow:** Reproductive Endocrinology, Univ Texas, San Antonio, TX 1993-1995; Reproductive Endocrinology, Univ Leeds, Leeds, England 1995-1996; **Fac Appt:** Asst Prof Obstetrics & Gynecology, Cornell Univ-Weill Med Coll

Rosenwaks, Zev MD (RE) - *Spec Exp:* Infertility-IVF; Genetic Disorders; **Hospital:** NY Presby Hosp - NY Weill Cornell Med Ctr (page 70); **Address:** 505 E 70th St, Ste 340, New York, NY 10021; **Phone:** (212) 746-1743; **Board Cert:** Obstetrics & Gynecology 1978, Reproductive Endocrinology 1981; **Med School:** SUNY Downstate 1972; **Resid:** Obstetrics & Gynecology, LIJ Med Ctr, New Hyde Park, NY 1972-1976; **Fellow:** Reproductive Endocrinology, Johns Hopkins Hosp, Baltimore, MD 1976-1978; **Fac Appt:** Prof Obstetrics & Gynecology, Cornell Univ-Weill Med Coll

Sauer, Mark MD (RE) - *Spec Exp:* Oocyte Donation; Infertility; **Hospital:** NY Presby Hosp - Columbia Presby Med Ctr (page 70); **Address:** 1790` Broadway Fl 2, New York, NY 10032; **Phone:** (212) 305-4665; **Board Cert:** Obstetrics & Gynecology 1987, Reproductive Endocrinology 1988; **Med School:** Univ Hlth Sci/Chicago Med Sch 1980; **Resid:** Obstetrics & Gynecology, Univ IL Med Ctr, Chicago, IL 1980-1984; **Fellow:** Reproductive Endocrinology, UCLA Med Ctr, Los Angeles, CA 1984-1986; **Fac Appt:** Prof Obstetrics & Gynecology, Columbia P&S

Wallach, Edward Eliot MD (RE) - *Spec Exp:* Fibroids; Infertility-IVF; Myomectomy; **Hospital:** Johns Hopkins Hosp - Baltimore; **Address:** Phipps Building, Rm 201, 600 N Wolfe St, Baltimore, MD 21287; **Phone:** (410) 955-7800; **Board Cert:** Obstetrics & Gynecology 1979, Reproductive Endocrinology 1975; **Med School:** Cornell Univ-Weill Med Coll 1958; **Resid:** Obstetrics & Gynecology, Kings Co Hosp, New York, NY 1959-1963; **Fellow:** Reproductive Endocrinology, Worcester Fdn Exptl Biol, Worcester, MA 1961-1962; **Fac Appt:** Prof Obstetrics & Gynecology, Johns Hopkins Univ

Zacur, Howard A. MD/PhD (RE) - *Spec Exp:* Prolactin Disorders; Uterine Fibroids; **Hospital:** Johns Hopkins Hosp - Baltimore; **Address:** 600 N Wolfe St Bldg Phipps - rm 247, Baltimore, MD 21205; **Phone:** (410) 583-2686; **Board Cert:** Obstetrics & Gynecology 1994, Reproductive Endocrinology 1984; **Med School:** Univ Miami Sch Med 1973; **Resid:** Obstetrics & Gynecology, Johns Hopkins Hosp, Baltimore, MD 1977-1980; **Fellow:** Reproductive Endocrinology, Johns Hopkins Hosp, Baltimore, MD 1981-1982; **Fac Appt:** Prof Reproductive Endocrinology, Johns Hopkins Univ

Southeast

Azziz, Ricardo MD (RE) - *Spec Exp:* Infertility-Surgical; Infertility-Female; Reproductive Endocrinology; **Hospital:** Univ of Ala Hosp at Birmingham; **Address:** Old Hillman Bldg, Ste 549, 618 S 20th St, Birmingham, AL 35294; **Phone:** (205) 934-5708; **Board Cert:** Obstetrics & Gynecology 1996, Reproductive Endocrinology 1996; **Med School:** Penn State Univ-Hershey Med Ctr 1981; **Fellow:** Reproductive Endocrinology, Johns Hopkins Hosp, Baltimore, MD 1985-1987; **Fac Appt:** Prof Obstetrics & Gynecology, Univ Ala

Blackwell, Richard MD/PhD (RE) - *Spec Exp:* Infertility-Female; Reproductive Medicine; Women's Medicine; **Hospital:** Univ of Ala Hosp at Birmingham; **Address:** 618 S 20th St, Birmingham, AL 35294; **Phone:** (205) 934-6090; **Board Cert:** Obstetrics & Gynecology 1982, Reproductive Endocrinology 1987; **Med School:** Baylor Coll Med 1975; **Resid:** Obstetrics & Gynecology, Univ Alabama Hosp, Birmingham, AL 1975-1979; **Fellow:** Reproductive Endocrinology, Univ Alabama Hosp, Birmingham, AL 1979-1981; Neurological Endocrinology, The Salk Institute, La Jolla, CA 1981-1982; **Fac Appt:** Prof Obstetrics & Gynecology, Univ Ala

DeVane, Gary Williams MD (RE) - *Spec Exp:* Infertility; Miscarriage-Recurrent; **Hospital:** Florida Hosp; **Address:** 3435 Pinehurst Ave, Orlando, FL 32804-4049; **Phone:** (407) 740-0909; **Board Cert:** Obstetrics & Gynecology 1977, Reproductive Endocrinology 1982; **Med School:** Baylor Coll Med 1971; **Resid:** Obstetrics & Gynecology, UCSD Hosp, San Diego, CA 1972-1975; **Fellow:** Reproductive Endocrinology, Univ Texas SW Hosp, Dallas, TX 1978-1980

Fritz, Marc Anthony MD (RE) - *Spec Exp:* Infertility; Menopause Problems; **Hospital:** Univ of NC Hosp (page 77); **Address:** Univ NC-CH, Dept Ob/Gyn, Campus Box 7570, Chapel Hill, NC 27599-7570; **Phone:** (919) 966-5283; **Board Cert:** Reproductive Endocrinology 1996, Obstetrics & Gynecology 1996; **Med School:** Tulane Univ 1977; **Resid:** Obstetrics & Gynecology, Wright State Univ, Dayton, OH 1978-1981; **Fellow:** Reproductive Endocrinology, Oregon Hlth Sci Univ, Portland, OR 1981-1983; **Fac Appt:** Prof Obstetrics & Gynecology, Univ NC Sch Med

Goodman, Neil MD (RE) - *Spec Exp:* Polycystic Ovarian Disease; Hormone Replacement Therap.; **Hospital:** Baptist Hosp - Miami; **Address:** 9150 SW 87th Ave, Ste 210, Miami, FL 33176-2313; **Phone:** (305) 595-6855; **Board Cert:** Internal Medicine 1973, Endocrinology, Diabetes & Metabolism 1975; **Med School:** Columbia P&S 1970; **Resid:** Internal Medicine, Beth Israel Hosp, Boston, MA 1971-1972; **Fellow:** Endocrinology, Mass Genl Hosp, Boston, MA 1972-1974; **Fac Appt:** Clin Prof Medicine, Univ Miami Sch Med

Hammond, Charles B MD (RE) - *Spec Exp:* Menopause Problems; **Hospital:** Duke Univ Med Ctr (page 60); **Address:** Duke Univ Med Ctr, Box 3853, Durham, NC 27710; **Phone:** (919) 684-3008; **Board Cert:** Obstetrics & Gynecology 1972, Reproductive Endocrinology 1974; **Med School:** Duke Univ 1961; **Resid:** Obstetrics & Gynecology, Duke Med Ctr, Durham, NC 1966-1968; Obstetrics & Gynecology, Duke Med Ctr, Durham, NC 1962-1963; **Fellow:** Gynecology, Duke Med Ctr, Durham, NC 1963-1964; **Fac Appt:** Prof Obstetrics & Gynecology, Duke Univ

Haney, Arthur F MD (RE) - *Spec Exp:* Infertility-Female; Reproductive Endocrinology; **Hospital:** Duke Univ Med Ctr (page 60); **Address:** Dept Obstetrics & Gynecology, Box 2971, Durham, NC 22710; **Phone:** (919) 684-2471; **Board Cert:** Obstetrics & Gynecology 1989, Reproductive Endocrinology 1981; **Med School:** Univ Ariz Coll Med 1972; **Resid:** Obstetrics & Gynecology, Duke Univ Med Ctr, Durham, NC 1972-1976; **Fellow:** Reproductive Endocrinology, Duke Univ Med Ctr, Durham, NC 1976-1978; **Fac Appt:** Prof Obstetrics & Gynecology, Duke Univ

Murphy, Ana Alvarez MD (RE) - *Spec Exp:* Infertility; Endometriosis; Pelvic Surgery; **Hospital:** Crawford Long Hosp of Emory Univ; **Address:** Reproductive Medicine & Fertility, 20 Linden Ave Fl 4, Atlanta, GA 30308; **Phone:** (404) 686-1843; **Board Cert:** Reproductive Endocrinology 1989, Obstetrics & Gynecology 1987; **Med School:** Univ Mich Med Sch 1980; **Resid:** Obstetrics & Gynecology, Johns Hopkins Univ, Baltimore, MD 1980-1984; **Fellow:** Reproductive Endocrinology, Johns Hopkins Univ, Baltimore, MD 1984-1986; **Fac Appt:** Prof Obstetrics & Gynecology, Emory Univ

Ory, Steven MD (RE) - *Spec Exp:* Infertility; **Hospital:** Northwest Med Ctr; **Address:** 2825 N State Road 7, Ste 302, Margate, FL 33063; **Phone:** (954) 247-6200; **Board Cert:** Reproductive Endocrinology 1984, Obstetrics & Gynecology 1983; **Med School:** Baylor Coll Med 1976; **Resid:** Obstetrics & Gynecology, Mayo Clinic, Rochester, MN 1976-1980; **Fellow:** Reproductive Endocrinology, Duke Univ, Durham, NC 1980-1982; **Fac Appt:** Assoc Clin Prof Obstetrics & Gynecology, Univ Miami Sch Med

Rock, John A MD (RE) - *Spec Exp:* Infertility-Female, Diagnostic; Endometriosis; Vaginal Abnormalities; **Hospital:** Emory Univ Hosp; **Address:** Emory Clinic, 1365 Clifton Rd, Bldg A - Fl 4, Atlanta, GA 30322; **Phone:** (404) 727-8704; **Board Cert:** Reproductive Endocrinology 1981, Obstetrics & Gynecology 2001; **Med School:** Louisiana State Univ 1972; **Resid:** Obstetrics & Gynecology, Duke Med Ctr, Durham, NC 1973-1976; **Fellow:** Reproductive Endocrinology, Johns Hopkins, Baltimore, MD 1976-1978; **Fac Appt:** Prof Obstetrics & Gynecology, Emory Univ

Steinkampf, Michael MD (RE) - *Spec Exp:* *Infertility;* **Hospital:** Univ of Ala Hosp at Birmingham; **Address:** 618 S 20th St, Birmingham, AL 35294-7333; **Phone:** (205) 934-1030; **Board Cert:** Obstetrics & Gynecology 1997, Reproductive Endocrinology 1997; **Med School:** Louisiana State Univ 1981; **Resid:** Obstetrics & Gynecology, Parkland Meml Hosp, Dallas, TX 1981-1985; **Fellow:** Reproductive Endocrinology, Univ Texas SW Med Sch, Dallas, TX 1985-1987; **Fac Appt:** Prof Obstetrics & Gynecology, Univ Ala

Younger, J Benjamin MD (RE) - *Spec Exp:* *Infertility-Female;* **Hospital:** Univ of Ala Hosp at Birmingham; **Address:** American Soc Reproductive Med, 1209 Montgomery Hwy, Birmingham, AL 35216-2809; **Phone:** (205) 978-5000; **Board Cert:** Obstetrics & Gynecology 1989; **Med School:** Tulane Univ 1962; **Resid:** Obstetrics & Gynecology, Duke Med Ctr, Durham, NC 1963-1965; **Fellow:** Reproductive Endocrinology, Duke Med Ctr, Durham, NC 1965-1966

Midwest

Barnes, Randall B MD (RE) - *Spec Exp:* *Endometriosis; Infertility; Polycystic Ovarian Disease;* **Hospital:** Northwestern Meml Hosp; **Address:** 675 NE St. Clair Fl 14 - Ste 200, Chicago, IL 60611; **Phone:** (312) 695-7269; **Board Cert:** Obstetrics & Gynecology 1986, Reproductive Endocrinology 1987; **Med School:** Johns Hopkins Univ 1979; **Resid:** Obstetrics & Gynecology, LAC-USC Med Ctr, Los Angeles, CA 1980-1983; **Fellow:** Reproductive Endocrinology, LAC-USC Med Ctr, Los Angeles, CA 1983-1985; **Fac Appt:** Assoc Prof Obstetrics & Gynecology, Univ Chicago-Pritzker Sch Med

Christman, Gregory MD (RE) - *Spec Exp:* *Infertility;* **Hospital:** Univ of MI Hlth Ctr; **Address:** Univ Mich, Med Sci Bldg I, 1301 Catherine St, rm 6428, Box 0617, Ann Arbor, MI 48109-0617; **Phone:** (734) 764-8142; **Board Cert:** Obstetrics & Gynecology 1994, Reproductive Endocrinology 1996; **Med School:** Univ Wisc 1983; **Resid:** Obstetrics & Gynecology, Univ Wisc Med Sch, Madison, WI 1983-1987; **Fellow:** Reproductive Endocrinology, Univ NC, Chapel Hill, NC 1990-1992; **Fac Appt:** Asst Prof Obstetrics & Gynecology, Univ Mich Med Sch

Diamond, Michael MD (RE) - *Spec Exp:* *Infertility-IVF; Infertility-Female; Polycystic Ovary Disease;* **Hospital:** Hutzel Hosp - Detroit (page 59); **Address:** Univ Ctr for Women's Med, 26400 W 12 Mile Rd, Southfield, MI 48034; **Phone:** (248) 352-6884; **Board Cert:** Obstetrics & Gynecology 1997, Reproductive Endocrinology 1997; **Med School:** Vanderbilt Univ 1981; **Resid:** Obstetrics & Gynecology, Vanderbilt Univ Med Ctr, Nashville, TN 1981-1985; Reproductive Endocrinology, Yale-New Haven Hosp, New Haven, CT 1985-1987; **Fac Appt:** Prof Obstetrics & Gynecology, Wayne State Univ

Dodds, William G MD (RE) - *Spec Exp:* *Infertility; Endometriosis; Infertility-IVF;* **Hospital:** Spectrum Health East; **Address:** 630 Kenmore Ave SE, Ste 100, Grand Rapids, MI 49546; **Phone:** (616) 988-2229; **Board Cert:** Obstetrics & Gynecology 1999, Reproductive Endocrinology 2000; **Med School:** Ohio State Univ 1982; **Resid:** Obstetrics & Gynecology, Ohio State Univ, Columbus, OH 1982-1986; **Fellow:** Reproductive Endocrinology, Ohio State Univ, Columbus, OH 1986-1988; **Fac Appt:** Assoc Prof Obstetrics & Gynecology, Univ Mich Med Sch

Dumesic, Daniel Anthony MD (RE) - *Spec Exp:* *Infertility-Female; Hormonal Disorders; Endometriosis/Pelvic Pain;* **Hospital:** Mayo Med Ctr & Clin - Rochester, MN; **Address:** Dept Ob/Gyn, Div Reproductive Endo, 200 1st St SW, Charlton Bldg, Rochester, MN 55905; **Phone:** (507) 284-9792; **Board Cert:** Obstetrics & Gynecology 1995, Reproductive Endocrinology 1999; **Med School:** Univ Wisc 1978; **Resid:** Obstetrics & Gynecology, Univ California San Fran Med Ctr, San Francisco, CA 1980-1982; **Fellow:** Reproductive Endocrinology, Univ California San Fran Med Ctr, San Francisco, CA 1985-1987; **Fac Appt:** Assoc Prof Obstetrics & Gynecology, Mayo Med Sch

Falcone, Tommaso MD (RE) - *Spec Exp:* Minimally Invasive Surgery; Infertility; Tubal Ligation Reversal-Microsurgery; **Hospital:** Cleveland Clin Fdn (page 57); **Address:** Cleveland Clin, Dept OB/Gyn, 9500 Euclid Ave, Box A81, Cleveland, OH 44195-0001; **Phone:** (216) 444-1758; **Board Cert:** Obstetrics & Gynecology 1998, Reproductive Endocrinology 1998; **Med School:** McGill Univ 1981; **Resid:** Obstetrics & Gynecology, McGill Univ, Montreal, CN 1983-1986; **Fellow:** Reproductive Endocrinology, McGill Univ, Montreal, CN 1987-1989

Jacobs, Laurence MD (RE) - *Spec Exp:* Infertility-IVF; Polycystic Ovary Disease; Endometriosis; **Hospital:** Advocate Lutheran Gen Hosp; **Address:** 3703 W Lake Ave, Ste 106, Glenview, IL 60025; **Phone:** (847) 215-8899; **Board Cert:** Obstetrics & Gynecology 1981; **Med School:** Northwestern Univ 1975; **Resid:** Obstetrics & Gynecology, Northwestern Meml Hosp, Chicago, IL 1975-1979; **Fellow:** Reproductive Endocrinology, Mayo Clinic, Rochester, MN 1986-1988; **Fac Appt:** Assoc Prof Obstetrics & Gynecology, Univ Chicago-Pritzker Sch Med

Kazer, Ralph MD (RE) - *Spec Exp:* Polycystic Ovary Disease; Infertility-IVF; **Hospital:** Northwestern Meml Hosp; **Address:** 675 N St Clair, Ste 14-200, Chicago, IL 60611; **Phone:** (312) 695-7269; **Board Cert:** Obstetrics & Gynecology 1996, Reproductive Endocrinology 1996; **Med School:** Tufts Univ 1979; **Resid:** Obstetrics & Gynecology, Tufts Univ, Boston, MA 1979-1983; **Fellow:** Reproductive Endocrinology, UC San Diego, San Diego, CA 1983-1986; **Fac Appt:** Assoc Prof Obstetrics & Gynecology, Northwestern Univ

Milad, Magdy P MD (RE) - *Spec Exp:* Reproductive Surgery; Infertility; Fibroids; **Hospital:** Northwestern Meml Hosp; **Address:** 675 N St Clair, Ste 14-200, Chicago, IL 60611; **Phone:** (312) 695-7269; **Board Cert:** Obstetrics & Gynecology 1994, Reproductive Endocrinology 1996; **Med School:** Wayne State Univ 1987; **Resid:** Obstetrics & Gynecology, William Beaumont Hosp, Royal Oaks, MI 1987-1991; **Fellow:** Reproductive Endocrinology, Mayo Clinic, Rochester, NY 1991-1993; **Fac Appt:** Assoc Prof Obstetrics & Gynecology, Northwestern Univ

Odem, Randall R MD (RE) - *Spec Exp:* Reproductive Surgery; **Hospital:** Barnes-Jewish Hosp (page 55); **Address:** 4444 Forest Park Ave, Ste 3100, St Louis, MO 63108; **Phone:** (314) 286-2400; **Board Cert:** Obstetrics & Gynecology 1998, Reproductive Endocrinology 1998; **Med School:** Univ Iowa Coll Med 1981; **Resid:** Obstetrics & Gynecology, U Ill Hosps, Chicago, IL 1981-1985; **Fellow:** Reproductive Endocrinology, Wash U Sch Med, St Louis, MO 1985-1987; **Fac Appt:** Assoc Prof Obstetrics & Gynecology, Washington Univ, St Louis

Ratts, Valerie Sue MD (RE) - *Spec Exp:* Polycystic Ovary Disease; Uterine Fibroids; **Hospital:** Barnes-Jewish Hosp (page 55); **Address:** 4444 Forest Park Ave, Ste 3100, St Louis, MO 63108; **Phone:** (314) 286-2400; **Board Cert:** Obstetrics & Gynecology 1995, Reproductive Endocrinology 1997; **Med School:** Johns Hopkins Univ 1987; **Resid:** Obstetrics & Gynecology, Johns Hopkins Hosp, Baltimore, MD 1987-1991; **Fellow:** Reproductive Endocrinology, Johns Hopkins Hosp, Baltimore, MD 1991-1993; **Fac Appt:** Asst Prof Obstetrics & Gynecology, Washington Univ, St Louis

Schreiber, James MD (RE) - *Spec Exp:* Menstrual Disorders; Infertility; **Hospital:** Barnes-Jewish Hosp (page 55); **Address:** 4911 Barnes Hospital Plaza, Box 8064, St Louis, MO 63110; **Phone:** (314) 362-7135; **Board Cert:** Obstetrics & Gynecology 1991, Reproductive Endocrinology 1982; **Med School:** Johns Hopkins Univ 1972; **Resid:** Obstetrics & Gynecology, USC-LA County, Los Angeles, CA 1972-1974; Obstetrics & Gynecology, USC-LA County, Los Angeles, CA 1976-1978; **Fellow:** Reproductive Endocrinology, Natl Inst of Hlth, Bethesda, MD 1974-1976; **Fac Appt:** Prof Obstetrics & Gynecology, Washington Univ, St Louis

Session, Donna Ruth MD (RE) - *Spec Exp:* Ultrasound Guided Surgery; Sonohysterography; Infertility-Female; **Hospital:** Mayo Med Ctr & Clin - Rochester, MN; **Address:** Dept Ob/Gyn, Div Reproductive Endo, 200 1st St SW, Bldg Charl - Fl 3A, Rochester, MN 55905; **Phone:** (507) 284-3176; **Board Cert:** Obstetrics & Gynecology 1994, Reproductive Endocrinology 1996; **Med School:** Eastern VA Med Sch 1986; **Resid:** Obstetrics & Gynecology, Winthrop Hosp, Mineola, NY 1986-1990; **Fellow:** Reproductive Endocrinology, Columbia Presby Med Ctr, New York, NY 1991-1993; **Fac Appt:** Asst Prof Obstetrics & Gynecology, Mayo Med Sch

Smith, Yolanda MD (RE) - *Spec Exp:* Infertility; **Hospital:** Univ of MI Hlth Ctr; **Address:** Women's Hosp, 1500 E Med Ctr Dr, Box 0276, Ann Arbor, MI 48109-0276; **Phone:** (734) 763-4323; **Board Cert:** Obstetrics & Gynecology 1997, Reproductive Endocrinology 1999; **Med School:** Wake Forest Univ Sch Med 1989; **Resid:** Obstetrics & Gynecology, Univ Mich Hosp, Ann Arbor, MI 1990-1993; **Fellow:** Reproductive Endocrinology, Johns Hopkins Hosp, Baltimore, MD 1993-1995; **Fac Appt:** Asst Prof Obstetrics & Gynecology, Univ Mich Med Sch

Wood Molo, Mary MD (RE) - *Spec Exp:* Infertility; Fibroids; **Hospital:** Rush-Presby - St Luke's Med Ctr (page 72); **Address:** 1725 W Harrison St, Ste 408 East, Chicago, IL 60612; **Phone:** (312) 997-2229; **Board Cert:** Reproductive Endocrinology 1994, Obstetrics & Gynecology 1991; **Med School:** Southern IL Univ 1982; **Resid:** Obstetrics & Gynecology, SIU Affil, Springfield, IL 1983-1984; Obstetrics & Gynecology, Rush Presby, Chicago, IL 1984-1987; **Fellow:** Reproductive Endocrinology, Rush Presby, Chicago, IL 1987-1989; **Fac Appt:** Asst Prof Obstetrics & Gynecology, Rush Med Coll

Zinaman, Michael MD (RE) - *Spec Exp:* Endometriosis; Infertility; Fibroids; **Hospital:** Loyola Univ Med Ctr; **Address:** Loyola Univ Med Ctr, Dept ObGyn, 2160 S First Ave, Maywood, IL 60153; **Phone:** (708) 327-1000; **Board Cert:** Obstetrics & Gynecology 1996, Reproductive Endocrinology 1996; **Med School:** SUNY Downstate 1981; **Resid:** Obstetrics & Gynecology, Univ Chicago Hosps, Chicago, IL 1981-1985; **Fellow:** Reproductive Endocrinology, Georgetown Univ, Washington, DC 1985-1987; **Fac Appt:** Prof Obstetrics & Gynecology, Loyola Univ-Stritch Sch Med

Great Plains and Mountains

Adashi, Eli Y MD (RE) - *Spec Exp:* Infertility-Female; **Hospital:** Univ Utah Hosp and Clin; **Address:** U Utah Sch Med, 30 N 1900 E, Ste 2 B 200, Salt Lake City, UT 84132; **Phone:** (801) 581-5490; **Board Cert:** Obstetrics & Gynecology 1991, Reproductive Endocrinology 1983; **Med School:** Israel 1972; **Resid:** Obstetrics & Gynecology, Tufts Univ Sch Med, Boston, MA 1974-1977; **Fellow:** Reproductive Endocrinology, Univ CA - San Diego, La Jolla, CA 1978-1981; Reproductive Endocrinology, Johns Hopkins Univ, Baltimore, MD 1977-1978; **Fac Appt:** Prof Obstetrics & Gynecology, Univ Utah

Richardson, Marilyn MD (RE) - *Spec Exp:* Reproductive Endocrinology - General; **Hospital:** Univ Kansas Med Ctr; **Address:** 21 N 12th St, Ste 400, Overland Park, KS 66204; **Phone:** (913) 588-6261; **Board Cert:** Reproductive Endocrinology 1987, Obstetrics & Gynecology 1985; **Med School:** Univ Kans 1979; **Resid:** Obstetrics & Gynecology, Univ of MO - Kansas School of Med, KS 1980-1983; **Fellow:** Reproductive Endocrinology, Univ of Texas Health Services, San Anonio, TX 1983-1985; **Fac Appt:** Asst Clin Prof Reproductive Endocrinology, Univ Kans

Schlaff, William D MD (RE) - *Spec Exp:* Infertility/Uterine Fibroids; Endometriosis; Vaginal Abnormalities; **Hospital:** Univ Colo HSC - Denver; **Address:** Univ Colo Hlth Scis Ctr, 1635 N Ursula St, Box F701, Aurora, CO 80010; **Phone:** (720) 848-1690; **Board Cert:** Obstetrics & Gynecology 1995, Reproductive Endocrinology 1997; **Med School:** Univ Mich Med Sch 1977; **Resid:** Obstetrics & Gynecology, Univ Mich Hosps, Ann Arbor, MI 1978-1981; **Fellow:** Reproductive Endocrinology, Johns Hopkins Med Ctr, Baltimore, MD 1983-1985; **Fac Appt:** Prof Obstetrics & Gynecology, Univ Colo

Surrey, Eric S MD (RE) - *Spec Exp:* Reproductive Endocrinology - General; **Hospital:** Univ Colo HSC - Denver; **Address:** 799 E Hamden Ave, Ste 300, Englewood, CO 80110; **Phone:** (303) 788-8300; **Board Cert:** Obstetrics & Gynecology 1998, Reproductive Endocrinology 1998; **Med School:** Univ Penn 1981; **Resid:** Obstetrics & Gynecology, UCLA Med. Ctr., Los Angeles, CA 1982-1986; **Fellow:** Reproductive Endocrinology, UCLA Med.Ctr., Los Angeles, CA 1986-1988

Southwest

Schenken, Robert S MD (RE) - *Spec Exp:* Infertility-Female; Endometriosis; **Hospital:** Univ of Texas Hlth & Sci Ctr; **Address:** Univ Texas Hlth Sci Ctr, Dept OB/GYN, 7703 Floyd Curl, MC-7836, San Antonio, TX 78229-3900; **Phone:** (210) 567-4930; **Board Cert:** Reproductive Endocrinology 1985, Obstetrics & Gynecology 1995; **Med School:** Baylor Coll Med 1977; **Resid:** Obstetrics & Gynecology, Bexar Co Hosp, San Antonio, TX 1978-1981; **Fellow:** Reproductive Endocrinology, Natl Inst Hlth, Bethesda, MD 1981-1982; Reproductive Endocrinology, Univ Texas Hlth Sci Ctr, San Antonio, TX 1982-1983; **Fac Appt:** Prof Obstetrics & Gynecology, Univ Tex, San Antonio

West Coast and Pacific

Burry, Kenneth Arnold MD (RE) - *Spec Exp:* Infertility-IVF; Menopause Problems; **Hospital:** OR Hlth Sci Univ Hosp and Clinics; **Address:** 1750 SW Harbor Way, Ste 100, Portland, OR 97201-5133; **Phone:** (503) 418-3744; **Board Cert:** Reproductive Endocrinology 1981, Obstetrics & Gynecology 1977; **Med School:** UC Irvine 1968; **Resid:** Obstetrics & Gynecology, Oreg Hlth Sci Univ and Clinics, Portland, OR 1971-1974; **Fellow:** Reproductive Endocrinology, Univ Wash Hosp, Seattle, WA 1974-1976; **Fac Appt:** Prof Obstetrics & Gynecology

Jaffe, Robert B MD (RE) - *Spec Exp:* Hormonal Disorders; Menopause Problems; **Hospital:** UCSF Med Ctr; **Address:** 505 Parnassus Ave, Ste HSW1656, San Francisco, CA 94143-0566; **Phone:** (415) 476-2269; **Board Cert:** Obstetrics & Gynecology 1967, Reproductive Endocrinology 1977; **Med School:** Univ Mich Med Sch 1957; **Resid:** Obstetrics & Gynecology, Univ Colo Med Ctr, Denver, CO 1959-1963; **Fellow:** Endocrinology, Univ Colo Med Ctr, Denver, CO 1958-1959; Reproductive Endocrinology, Karolinska Sjuktuset, Stockholm, Sweden 1963-1964; **Fac Appt:** Prof Obstetrics & Gynecology, UCSF

Marrs, Richard P MD (RE) - *Spec Exp:* Infertility-Female; Endometriosis; Fibroids; **Hospital:** Santa Monica - UCLA Med Ctr; **Address:** 1245 16th St, Ste 220, Santa Monica, CA 90404-1240; **Phone:** (310) 828-4008; **Board Cert:** Obstetrics & Gynecology 1980, Reproductive Endocrinology 1983; **Med School:** Univ Tex Med Br, Galveston 1974; **Resid:** Obstetrics & Gynecology, Univ Tex Hosps, Galveston, TX 1974-1977; **Fellow:** Reproductive Endocrinology, USC Med Ctr, Los Angeles, CA 1977-1979

Paulson, Richard John MD (RE) - *Spec Exp:* Infertility-IVF; Infertility-Egg Donation; Women of Advanced Reproductive Age; **Hospital:** LAC & USC Med Ctr; **Address:** USC Reproductive Endocrinology & Infertility, 1245 Wilshire Blvd, Ste 403, Los Angeles, CA 90017; **Phone:** (213) 975-9990; **Board Cert:** Obstetrics & Gynecology 1997, Reproductive Endocrinology 1997; **Med School:** UCLA 1980; **Resid:** Obstetrics & Gynecology, Harbor - UCLA Medical Center, Torrance, CA 1980-1984; **Fellow:** Reproductive Endocrinology, LAC - USC Med Ctr, Los Angeles, CA 1984-1986; **Fac Appt:** Prof Obstetrics & Gynecology, USC Sch Med

Polan, Mary Lake MD/PhD (RE) - *Spec Exp:* Menopause Problems; Infertility-IVF; **Hospital:** Stanford Med Ctr; **Address:** 300 Pasteur Drive, Ste HH333, Stanford, CA 94305-5317; **Phone:** (650) 723-5533; **Board Cert:** Obstetrics & Gynecology 1998, Reproductive Endocrinology 1999; **Med School:** Yale Univ 1975; **Resid:** Obstetrics & Gynecology, Yale-New Haven Hosp, New Haven, CT 1975-1978; **Fellow:** Reproductive Endocrinology, Yale New Haven Hosp, New Haven, CT 1979-1980; **Fac Appt:** Prof Obstetrics & Gynecology, Stanford Univ

Soules, Michael Roy MD (RE) - *Spec Exp: Reproductive Medicine; Infertility-Female;* **Hospital:** Univ WA Med Ctr; **Address:** 4225 Roosevelt Way NE, Ste 305, Seattle, WA 98105-6099; **Phone:** (206) 543-0670; **Board Cert:** Obstetrics & Gynecology 1993, Reproductive Endocrinology 1981; **Med School:** UCLA 1972; **Resid:** Obstetrics & Gynecology, Univ Colo Med Ctr, Denver, CO 1972-1976; **Fellow:** Reproductive Endocrinology, Duke Univ Hosp, Durham, NC 1976-1978; **Fac Appt:** Prof Obstetrics & Gynecology, Univ Wash

Taylor, Robert N MD (RE) - *Spec Exp: Endometriosis; Miscarriage-Recurrent;* **Hospital:** UCSF Med Ctr; **Address:** 350 Parnassus Ave, Ste 300, San Francisco, CA 94143-0310; **Phone:** (415) 476-2224; **Board Cert:** Obstetrics & Gynecology 1997, Reproductive Endocrinology 1997; **Med School:** Baylor Coll Med 1981; **Resid:** Obstetrics & Gynecology, UCSF Med Ctr, San Fransisco, CA 1981-1985; **Fellow:** Reproductive Endocrinology, UCSF Med Ctr, San Fransisco, CA 1984-1986; **Fac Appt:** Assoc Prof Obstetrics & Gynecology, UCSF

Winer, Sharon Ann MD (RE) - *Spec Exp: Hormonal Disorders; Infertility-Female;* **Hospital:** Cedars-Sinai Med Ctr; **Address:** 9400 Brighton Way, Ste 206, Beverly Hills, CA 90210-4709; **Phone:** (310) 274-9100; **Board Cert:** Obstetrics & Gynecology 1997, Reproductive Endocrinology 1997; **Med School:** USC Sch Med 1978; **Resid:** Obstetrics & Gynecology, LAC-USC Med Ctr, Los Angeles, CA 1978-1979; **Fellow:** Reproductive Endocrinology, USC Univ Hosp, Los Angeles, CA 1979-1982; Maternal & Fetal Medicine, Hammersmith, London, England 1982-1983; **Fac Appt:** Clin Prof Obstetrics & Gynecology, USC Sch Med

Yee, Billy MD (RE) - *Spec Exp: Infertility-IVF;* **Hospital:** Long Beach Meml Med Ctr; **Address:** 701 E 28th St, Ste 202, Long Beach, CA 90806-2773; **Phone:** (562) 427-2229; **Board Cert:** Obstetrics & Gynecology 1995, Reproductive Endocrinology 1995; **Med School:** UC Davis 1978; **Resid:** Obstetrics & Gynecology, LAC-USC Med Ctr, Los Angeles, CA 1979-1982; **Fellow:** Reproductive Endocrinology, LAC-USC Med Ctr, Los Angeles, CA 1983-1985; **Fac Appt:** Assoc Clin Prof Obstetrics & Gynecology, UC Irvine

RHEUMATOLOGY

An internist who treats diseases of joints, muscle, bones and tendons. This specialist diagnoses and treats arthritis, back pain, muscle strains, common athletic injuries and "collagen" diseases.

INTERNAL MEDICINE

An internist is a personal physician who provides long-term, comprehensive care in the office and the hospital, managing both common and complex illness of adolescents, adults and the elderly. Internists are trained in the diagnosis and treatment of cancer, infections and diseases affecting the heart, blood, kidneys, joints and digestive, respiratory and vascular systems. They are also trained in the essentials of primary care internal medicine which incorporates an understanding of disease prevention, wellness, substance abuse, mental health and effective treatment of common problems of the eyes, ears, skin, nervous system and reproductive organs.

Training required: Three years in internal medicine *plus* additional training and examination for certification in rheumatology

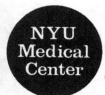

550 First Avenue (at 31st Street)
New York, NY 10016
Physician Referral: (888) 7-NYU-MED
(888-769-8633)   www.nyumedicalcenter.org

NYU Medical Center

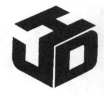

RHEUMATOLOGY

The Department of Rheumatology at the Hospital for Joint Diseases (HJD) is dedicated to the diagnosis and treatment of patients with rheumatic diseases – a group of conditions involving pain and inflammation of the joints, soft tissues, or other elements of the musculoskeletal system. In addition to rheumatoid arthritis, tendonitis, and osteoporosis, rheumatology also focuses on autoimmune diseases such as lupus and scleroderma. The department accomplishes its mission through a balanced combination of education, research, and clinical care.

Patients receive care at the Rheumatology Faculty Practice or at one of our two main rheumatology clinics.

FACULTY PRACTICE

Staffed by a select group of leading academic researchers and physicians, the practice provides comprehensive diagnosis and treatment of all rheumatologic conditions. Additionally, many of our physicians conduct clinical trials to evaluate the safety and efficacy of new medications.

GENERAL ARTHRITIS CLINIC

The General Arthritis Clinic serves two overlapping functions: the assessment of patients with musculoskeletal complaints, and the treatment of those with diagnosed inflammatory arthritis, degenerative arthritis, chronic musculoskeletal pain, or autoimmune diseases other than lupus. The clinic is staffed by a full complement of rheumatology attendings, including both full-time and voluntary faculty members. Orthopaedic attendings and residents are also on hand, as well as dentists specializing in TMJ disorders.

LUPUS CLINIC

In operation for 15 years, the Lupus Clinic is devoted solely to the treatment of patients with this multifaceted disease. Patients are seen regularly by rheumatologists, and have ready access to specialists in dermatology, nephrology, orthopaedics, and neurology, all of whom have expertise in systemic lupus erythematosus. The clinic also offers expertise in pregnancy and hormonal issues specific to patients with lupus.

AMBULATORY CLINICAL RESEARCH CENTER

Basic science and medicine converge at the Ambulatory Clinical Research Center, which focuses on developing improved treatments for rheumatic diseases. The center was established in 1992 to promote new initiatives in clinical investigation. Under its roof, researchers conduct protocols using a wide variety of new medications for the treatment of rheumatoid arthritis, osteoarthritis, systemic lupus erythematosus, and osteoporosis.

NYU MEDICAL CENTER

Founded in 1999, the NYU-HJD Center for Arthritis and Autoimmunity is a comprehensive program for the prevention, diagnosis, and treatment of musculoskeletal disorders. At the leading edge of research and clinical care, the center's uniqueness rests on its ability to integrate patient care across a variety of disciplines. Patients receive complete rheumatologic evaluations, orthopaedic and neurological consultative services, sophisticated diagnostic testing, physiotherapy, and complementary medicine, as well as opportunities to participate in clinical trials.

Physician Referral
(888) 7-NYU-MED
(888-769-8633)
www.nyumedicalcenter.org

PHYSICIAN LISTINGS

New England

Brenner, Michael B MD (Rhu) - *Spec Exp:* Gout/Pseudogout; Rheumatoid Arthritis; Lupus/SLE; **Hospital:** Brigham & Women's Hosp; **Address:** Arthritis Center, 75 Francis St, Boston, MA 02115; **Phone:** (617) 732-5325; **Board Cert:** Rheumatology 1982, Internal Medicine 1978; **Med School:** Vanderbilt Univ 1975; **Resid:** Internal Medicine, Vanderbilt Univ Hosp, Nashville, TN 1976-1979; **Fellow:** Rheumatology, UCLA Med Ctr, Los Angeles, CA 1979-1981; **Fac Appt:** Prof Medicine, Harvard Med Sch

Korn, Joseph H MD (Rhu) - *Spec Exp:* Scleroderma; Lupus; **Hospital:** Boston Med Ctr; **Address:** Boston Univ Sch Med, Div Rheumatology & Arthritis Ctr, 71 E Concord St, Boston, MA 02118; **Phone:** (617) 638-4486; **Board Cert:** Internal Medicine 1975, Rheumatology 1978; **Med School:** Columbia P&S 1972; **Resid:** Internal Medicine, North Carolina Meml Hosp, Chapel Hill, NC 1972-1975; **Fellow:** Rheumatology/Immunology, Med Ctr S Carolina, Charleston, SC 1975-1977; **Fac Appt:** Prof Medicine, Boston Univ

Polisson, Richard Paul MD (Rhu) - *Spec Exp:* Rheumatoid Arthritis; Lupus/SLE; **Hospital:** MA Genl Hosp; **Address:** The Arthritis Unit-Mass Genl Hosp, Bldg Bulfinch - rm 165, Boston, MA 02114; **Phone:** (617) 726-1581; **Board Cert:** Rheumatology 1984, Internal Medicine 1979; **Med School:** Duke Univ 1976; **Resid:** Natl Inst Hlth/NCI, Bethesda, MD 1978-1980; Internal Medicine, Duke U Med Ctr., Durham, NC 1977-1978; **Fellow:** Rheumatology, Mass Genl Hosp., Boston, MA 1980-1982; **Fac Appt:** Assoc Prof Rheumatology, Harvard Med Sch

Schoen, Robert Taylor MD (Rhu) - *Spec Exp:* Rheumatoid Arthritis; Lyme Disease; Osteoporosis; **Hospital:** Yale - New Haven Hosp; **Address:** 60 Temple St, Ste 6A, New Haven, CT 06510-2716; **Phone:** (203) 789-2255; **Board Cert:** Internal Medicine 1979, Rheumatology 1982; **Med School:** Columbia P&S 1976; **Resid:** Internal Medicine, Yale New haven Hosp, New Haven, CT 1977-1979; **Fellow:** Rheumatology, Brigham & Womens Hosp, Boston, MA 1979-1981; **Fac Appt:** Clin Prof Medicine, Yale Univ

Shadick, Nancy A MD (Rhu) - *Spec Exp:* Lupus/SLE; Rheumatoid Arthritis; Osteoarthritis; **Hospital:** Brigham & Women's Hosp; **Address:** Dept of Rheumatology, 45 Francis St, Boston, MA 02115-6105; **Phone:** (617) 732-5266; **Board Cert:** Internal Medicine 1989, Rheumatology 1992; **Med School:** NYU Sch Med 1986; **Resid:** Internal Medicine, Columbia-Presby Hosp, New York, NY 1986-1989; **Fellow:** Rheumatology, Brigham & Womens Hosp, Boston, MA 1989-1992; **Fac Appt:** Asst Prof Medicine, Harvard Med Sch

Weinblatt, Michael Eliot MD (Rhu) - *Spec Exp:* Rheumatoid Arthritis; **Hospital:** Brigham & Women's Hosp; **Address:** Brigham & Womens Hosp, 75 Francis St, Boston, MA 02115-6110; **Phone:** (617) 732-5331; **Board Cert:** Internal Medicine 1978, Rheumatology 1980; **Med School:** Univ MD Sch Med 1975; **Resid:** Internal Medicine, Univ Maryland Hosp, Baltimore, MD 1975-1978; **Fellow:** Rheumatology, Peter Bent Brigham Hosp, Boston, MA 1978-1980; **Fac Appt:** Prof Medicine, Harvard Med Sch

Mid Atlantic

Abramson, Steven B MD (Rhu) - *Spec Exp:* Arthritis; **Hospital:** Hosp For Joint Diseases (page 61); **Address:** 301 E 17th St, New York, NY 10003; **Phone:** (212) 598-6110; **Board Cert:** Internal Medicine 1977, Rheumatology 1980; **Med School:** Harvard Med Sch 1974; **Resid:** Internal Medicine, Bellevue Hosp/NYU, New York, NY 1974-1978; **Fellow:** Rheumatology, Bellevue Hosp/NYU, New York, NY 1978-1980; Rheumatology, NYU Med Ctr, New York, NY 1980-1983; **Fac Appt:** Prof Medicine, NYU Sch Med

Argyros, Thomas MD (Rhu) - *Spec Exp:* Lyme Disease; Lupus/SLE; **Hospital:** Lenox Hill Hosp (page 64); **Address:** 122 E 76th St, New York, NY 10021-2833; **Phone:** (212) 988-7680; **Board Cert:** Internal Medicine 1961; **Med School:** NYU Sch Med 1954; **Resid:** Internal Medicine, Lenox Hill Hosp, New York, NY 1957-1958; **Fellow:** Rheumatology, New York Univ Med Ctr, New York, NY 1964-1965; **Fac Appt:** Clin Prof Medicine, NYU Sch Med

Blume, Ralph MD (Rhu) - *Spec Exp:* Vasculitis; Lupus/SLE; Rheumatoid Arthritis; **Hospital:** NY Presby Hosp - Columbia Presby Med Ctr (page 70); **Address:** 161 Fort Washington Ave, Ste 537, New York, NY 10032-3713; **Phone:** (212) 305-5512; **Board Cert:** Internal Medicine 1972, Rheumatology 1974; **Med School:** Columbia P&S 1964; **Resid:** Internal Medicine, Columbia Presby Hosp, New York, NY 1964-1966; Internal Medicine, Columbia Presby Hosp, New York, NY 1968-1969; **Fellow:** Rheumatology, Columbia P&S, New York, NY 1968-1970; **Fac Appt:** Clin Prof Medicine, Columbia P&S

Bunning, Robert Daniel MD (Rhu) - *Spec Exp:* Exercise Therapy; Rheumatoid Arthritis; Musculoskeletal Disorders; **Hospital:** Natl Rehab Hosp; **Address:** Natl Rehab Hosp, 102 Irving St NW, Ste 2158, Washington, DC 20010-2921; **Phone:** (202) 877-1660; **Board Cert:** Internal Medicine 1984, Rheumatology 1986; **Med School:** Univ Cincinnati 1979; **Resid:** Internal Medicine, Wash Hosp Ctr, Washington, DC 1979-1981; Internal Medicine, Wash Hosp Ctr, Washington, DC 1981-1984; **Fellow:** Rheumatology, Wash Hosp Ctr, Washington, DC 1981-1983; **Fac Appt:** Asst Clin Prof Reproductive Endocrinology, Geo Wash Univ

Buyon, Jill P MD (Rhu) - *Spec Exp:* Lupus/SLE-Pregnancy; Lupus/SLE-Menopause; **Hospital:** Hosp For Joint Diseases (page 61); **Address:** Hosp Joint Dis, Rheum & Molecular Med, 305 E 2nd Ave, Fl 16, New York, NY 10003-2739; **Phone:** (212) 598-6516; **Board Cert:** Internal Medicine 1981, Rheumatology 1984; **Med School:** Albert Einstein Coll Med 1978; **Resid:** Internal Medicine, Albert Einstein, Bronx, NY 1979-1981; **Fellow:** Rheumatology, NYU Med Ctr, New York, NY 1981-1983; **Fac Appt:** Prof Medicine, NYU Sch Med

Clauw, Daniel J MD (Rhu) - *Spec Exp:* Fibromyalgia; Chronic Fatigue Syndrome; **Hospital:** Georgetown Univ Hosp; **Address:** GUMC - Lower Level, Gorman Bldg, 3800 Reservoir Rd NW, Washington, DC 20007; **Phone:** (202) 687-8233; **Board Cert:** Rheumatology 1990, Internal Medicine 1988; **Med School:** Univ Mich Med Sch 1985; **Resid:** Internal Medicine, Georgetown Univ Hosp, Washington, DC 1985-1988; Rheumatology, Georgetown Univ Hosp, Washington, DC 1988-1990; **Fac Appt:** Assoc Prof Medicine, Georgetown Univ

Cupps, Thomas R MD (Rhu) - *Spec Exp:* Vasculitis; Hepatitis B-Immune Response; **Hospital:** Georgetown Univ Hosp; **Address:** GUMC - Lower Level, Gorman Building, 3800 Reservoir Rd NW, Washington, DC 20007; **Phone:** (202) 687-8233; **Board Cert:** Allergy & Immunology 1981, Internal Medicine 1978; **Med School:** Stanford Univ 1975; **Resid:** Internal Medicine, Strong Meml Hosp, Rochester, NY 1975-1978; **Fellow:** Allergy & Immunology, Natl Inst of All & Inf Dis, Bethesda, MD

Farber, Martin Stuart MD/PhD (Rhu) - *Spec Exp:* Rheumatology - General; **Hospital:** Sunnyview Hosp; **Address:** Sunnyview Hosp, 1270 Belmont Ave, Schenectady, NY 12308; **Phone:** (518) 386-3644; **Board Cert:** Internal Medicine 1982, Rheumatology 1984; **Med School:** Albert Einstein Coll Med 1979; **Resid:** Internal Medicine, Boston City Hosp, Boston, MA 1980-1982; **Fellow:** Rheumatology, Boston Univ Sch Med, Boston, MA 1982-1984; **Fac Appt:** Asst Clin Prof Medicine, Albany Med Coll

Ginzler, Ellen MD (Rhu) - *Spec Exp:* *Lupus/SLE;* **Hospital:** Univ Hosp - Brklyn; **Address:** SUNY Hlth Sci Ctr, Dept Rheumatology, 450 Clarkson Ave, Box 42, Brooklyn, NY 11203-0042; **Phone:** (718) 270-1662; **Board Cert:** Internal Medicine 1972, Rheumatology 1974; **Med School:** Case West Res Univ 1969; **Resid:** Internal Medicine, Kings Co Hosp, Brooklyn, NY 1970-1971; Internal Medicine, Bellevue Hosp, New York, NY 1971-1972; **Fellow:** Rheumatology, Univ Hosp, Brooklyn, NY 1972-1974; **Fac Appt:** Prof Medicine, SUNY Hlth Sci Ctr

Gourley, Mark MD (Rhu) - *Spec Exp:* *Rheumatology - General;* **Hospital:** Washington Hosp Ctr; **Address:** Washington Hosp Ctr, Dept Rheumatology, 110 Irving St NW, Ste 2A66, Washington, DC 20010; **Phone:** (202) 877-6274; **Board Cert:** Rheumatology 1992, Internal Medicine 1988; **Med School:** Tulane Univ 1985; **Resid:** Internal Medicine, Univ Wisconsin Hosps & Clins, Madison, WI 1985-1988; **Fellow:** Rheumatology, Natl Inst Hlth, Bethesda, MD 1988-1996

Kagen, Lawrence MD (Rhu) - *Spec Exp:* *Musculoskeletal Disorders;* **Hospital:** Hosp For Special Surgery (page 62); **Address:** 535 E 70th St, Ste 714, New York, NY 10021; **Phone:** (212) 606-1449; **Board Cert:** Rheumatology 1974, Internal Medicine 1967; **Med School:** NYU Sch Med 1960; **Resid:** Internal Medicine, Presbyterian Hosp, New York, NY 1960-1965; **Fellow:** Rheumatology, Columbia P&S, New York, NY 1965-1966

Lahita, Robert MD (Rhu) - *Spec Exp:* *Lupus/SLE; Endocrinologic Joint Disorders; Vasculitis;* **Hospital:** St Vincent Cath Med Ctrs - Manhattan (page 75); **Address:** St Vincent's Hosp & Med Ctr, Dept Rheum, 115 E 61st St, Fl 11, New York, NY 10021; **Phone:** (212) 755-6550; **Board Cert:** Internal Medicine 1993, Rheumatology 1997; **Med School:** Jefferson Med Coll 1973; **Resid:** Internal Medicine, NY Hosp-Cornell, New York, NY 1974-1976; **Fellow:** Rheumatology, Rockefeller Hosp, New York, NY 1976-1978; **Fac Appt:** Prof Medicine, NY Med Coll

Lockshin, Michael Dan MD (Rhu) - *Spec Exp:* *Lupus/SLE;* **Hospital:** Hosp For Special Surgery (page 62); **Address:** 535 E 70th St, FL 6, New York, NY 10021; **Phone:** (212) 606-1461; **Board Cert:** Internal Medicine 1969, Rheumatology 1972; **Med School:** Harvard Med Sch 1963; **Resid:** Internal Medicine, Bellevue Hosp, New York, NY 1966-1968; **Fellow:** Rheumatology, Columbia-Presby Med Ctr, New York, NY 1968-1970; **Fac Appt:** Prof Rheumatology, Cornell Univ-Weill Med Coll

Medsger Jr, Thomas A MD (Rhu) - *Spec Exp:* *Scleroderma; Raynaud's Disease; Polymyositis & Dermatomyositis;* **Hospital:** UPMC - Presbyterian Univ Hosp; **Address:** Univ Arthritis Ctr - Liliane Kaufman Bldg, rm 900, 3471 Fifth Ave, Pittsburgh, PA 15213-3215; **Phone:** (412) 648-6970; **Board Cert:** Internal Medicine 1972, Rheumatology 1972; **Med School:** Univ Penn 1962; **Resid:** Internal Medicine, Univ Pittsburgh, Pittsburgh, PA 1966-1968; **Fellow:** Rheumatology, Univ Pittsburgh, Pittsburgh, PA 1965-1966; Rheumatology, Univ Tenn Coll Med, Memphis, TN 1968-1969; **Fac Appt:** Prof Medicine, Univ Pittsburgh

Mitnick, Hal J MD (Rhu) - *Spec Exp:* *Rheumatoid Arthritis; Psoriatic Arthritis; Osteoporosis;* **Hospital:** NYU Med Ctr (page 71); **Address:** 333 E 34th St, Ste 1C, New York, NY 10016-4956; **Phone:** (212) 889-7217; **Board Cert:** Internal Medicine 1976, Rheumatology 1978; **Med School:** NYU Sch Med 1972; **Resid:** Internal Medicine, Bellevue Hosp, New York, NY 1972-1976; **Fellow:** Rheumatology, New York Univ Med Ctr, New York, NY 1976-1978; **Fac Appt:** Clin Prof Medicine, NYU Sch Med

Oddis, Chester MD (Rhu) - *Spec Exp:* Polymyositis; Dermatomyositis; Connective Tissue Disease; **Hospital:** UPMC - Presbyterian Univ Hosp; **Address:** University Of Pittsburgh-Dept Med Rheum, 3500 Terrace St, S 703 BST, Pittsburgh, PA 15261; **Phone:** (412) 648-6970; **Board Cert:** Rheumatology 1986, Internal Medicine 1983; **Med School:** Penn State Univ-Hershey Med Ctr 1980; **Resid:** Internal Medicine, Hershey Med Ctr-Penn St Univ, Hershey, PA 1981-1984; **Fellow:** Rheumatology, Univ Pittsburgh, Pittsburgh, PA 1984-1986; **Fac Appt:** Prof Medicine, Univ Pittsburgh

Paget, Stephen MD (Rhu) - *Spec Exp:* Rheumatoid Arthritis; Lupus/SLE; **Hospital:** Hosp For Special Surgery (page 62); **Address:** 535 E 70th St, Fl 7, New York, NY 10021; **Phone:** (212) 606-1845; **Board Cert:** Internal Medicine 1974, Rheumatology 1976; **Med School:** SUNY Downstate 1971; **Resid:** Internal Medicine, Johns Hopkins Hosp, Baltimore, MD 1972-1973; **Fellow:** Rheumatology, Hosp Special Surg, New York, NY 1975; **Fac Appt:** Clin Prof Medicine, Cornell Univ-Weill Med Coll

Petri, Michelle Ann MD (Rhu) - *Spec Exp:* Lupus/SLE; Autoimmune Disease; **Hospital:** Johns Hopkins Hosp - Baltimore; **Address:** Div of Rheumatology, 1830 E Monument St, Ste 7500, Baltimore, MD 21205; **Phone:** (410) 955-3052; **Board Cert:** Internal Medicine 1983, Rheumatology 1986; **Med School:** Harvard Med Sch 1980; **Resid:** Internal Medicine, Mass Genl Hosp, Boston, MA 1980-1983; **Fellow:** Allergy & Immunology, Univ California San Fran Med Ctr, San Francisco, CA 1985; Rheumatology, Univ California San Fran Med Ctr, San Francisco, CA 1986; **Fac Appt:** Assoc Prof Medicine, Johns Hopkins Univ

Plotz, Paul MD (Rhu) - *Spec Exp:* Rheumatology - General; **Hospital:** Natl Inst of Hlth - Clin Ctr; **Address:** Building 10, Rm 9-N-244, 10 Center Drive, MC 1820, Bethseda, MD 20892-1820; **Phone:** (301) 496-1474; **Board Cert:** Internal Medicine 1970; **Med School:** Harvard Med Sch 1963; **Resid:** Internal Medicine, Beth Isrel Hosp, Boston, MA 1964-1965; **Fellow:** Rheumatology, Clin Ctr- NIH, Bethesda, MD 1965-1968

Sigal, Leonard H MD (Rhu) - *Spec Exp:* Lyme Disease; Lupus/SLE; Rheumatoid Arthritis; **Hospital:** Robert Wood Johnson Univ Hosp @ New Brunswick; **Address:** 125 Paterson St, New Brunswick, NJ 08901-1962; **Phone:** (732) 235-7210; **Board Cert:** Internal Medicine 1979, Rheumatology 1984; **Med School:** Stanford Univ 1976; **Resid:** Internal Medicine, Mount Sinai, New York, NY 1976-1979; Rheumatology, Yale Univ Sch Med, New Haven, CT 1981-1984; **Fac Appt:** Prof Medicine, Robert W Johnson Med Sch

Solomon, Gary MD (Rhu) - *Spec Exp:* Seronegative Arthritis; Rheumatoid Arthritis; Autoimmune Disease; **Hospital:** Hosp For Joint Diseases (page 61); **Address:** Hosp Joint Dis, Dept Rheumatology, 305 Second Ave, Ste 16, New York, NY 10003; **Phone:** (212) 598-6516; **Board Cert:** Internal Medicine 1980, Rheumatology 1982; **Med School:** Mount Sinai Sch Med 1977; **Resid:** Internal Medicine, Mount Sinai Med Ctr, New York, NY 1978-1980; **Fellow:** Rheumatology, Albert Einstein Coll Med, Bronx, NY 1980-1982; **Fac Appt:** Assoc Clin Prof Medicine, NYU Sch Med

Spiera, Harry MD (Rhu) - *Spec Exp:* Lupus/SLE; Scleroderma; Vasculitis; **Hospital:** Mount Sinai Hosp (page 68); **Address:** 1088 Park Ave, New York, NY 10128-1132; **Phone:** (212) 860-4000; **Board Cert:** Internal Medicine 1965, Rheumatology 1972; **Med School:** NYU Sch Med 1958; **Resid:** Internal Medicine, VA Med Ctr, Brooklyn, NY 1959-1960; Internal Medicine, Mount Sinai Hosp, New York, NY 1960-1961; **Fellow:** Rheumatology, Columbia-Presby Med Ctr, New York, NY 1961-1963; **Fac Appt:** Prof Medicine, Mount Sinai Sch Med

Weinstein, Arthur MD (Rhu) - *Spec Exp:* *Lyme Disease; Lupus/SLE; Complementary Medicine-Rheumatic Disease;* **Hospital:** Washington Hosp Ctr; **Address:** Washington Hospital, Director of Rheumatology, 110 Irving St NW, rm 2A-66, Washington, DC 20010; **Phone:** (202) 877-6274; **Board Cert:** Rheumatology 1976, Diagnostic Lab Immunology 1986; **Med School:** Univ Toronto 1967; **Resid:** Internal Medicine, Toronto Genl Hosp, Toronto, Canada 1967-1968; Internal Medicine, Toronto Welleley Hosp, Toronto, Canada 1968-1969; **Fellow:** Rheumatology, Hammersmith Hosp, London, England 1969-1971; Rheumatology, Toronto Wellesley Hosp, Toronto, Canada 1972-1973; **Fac Appt:** Prof Rheumatology, Geo Wash Univ

White, Barbara MD (Rhu) - *Spec Exp:* *Scleroderma;* **Hospital:** University of MD Med Sys; **Address:** 10 N Greene St, MS 1515, Baltimore, MD 21201; **Phone:** (410) 328-8667; **Board Cert:** Allergy & Immunology 1983, Rheumatology 1982; **Med School:** Univ Penn 1975; **Resid:** Internal Medicine, Univ Iowa, Iowa City, IA 1976-1978; **Fellow:** Allergy & Immunology, Univ Iowa, Iowa City, IA 1979-1981; Rheumatology, Univ Iowa, Iowa City, IA 1981-1982; **Fac Appt:** Prof Medicine, Univ MD Sch Med

Wigley, Frederick M MD (Rhu) - *Spec Exp:* *Scleroderma; Raynaud's Disease;* **Hospital:** Johns Hopkins Hosp - Baltimore; **Address:** 1830 E Monument Street, Ste 7500, Baltimore, MD 21205; **Phone:** (410) 955-3052; **Board Cert:** Internal Medicine 1975, Rheumatology 1980; **Med School:** Univ Fla Coll Med 1972; **Resid:** Internal Medicine, Johns Hopkins Hosp, Baltimore, MD 1972-1975; **Fellow:** Rheumatology, Johns Hopkins Hosp, Baltimore, MD 1977-1979; **Fac Appt:** Prof Medicine, Johns Hopkins Univ

Southeast

Allen, Nancy B MD (Rhu) - *Spec Exp:* *Vasculitis; Wegener's Granulomatosis; Lupus/SLE;* **Hospital:** Duke Univ Med Ctr (page 60); **Address:** Duke Univ Med Ctr, Box 3440, Durham, NC 27710; **Phone:** (919) 684-2965; **Board Cert:** Internal Medicine 1981, Rheumatology 1984; **Med School:** Tufts Univ 1978; **Resid:** Internal Medicine, Duke U Med Ctr, Durham, NC 1979-1981; **Fellow:** Rheumatology, Duke U Med Ctr, Durham, NC 1981-1983; **Fac Appt:** Prof Medicine, Duke Univ

Chatham, Walter W MD (Rhu) - *Spec Exp:* *Lupus/SLE; Fibromyalgia; Rheumatoid Arthritis;* **Hospital:** Univ of Ala Hosp at Birmingham; **Address:** Univ Alabama Birmingham Med Ctr, 1530 3rd Ave S, Ste THT 434, Birmingham, AL 35294-0006; **Phone:** (205) 934-4212; **Board Cert:** Internal Medicine 1983, Rheumatology 1988; **Med School:** Vanderbilt Univ 1980; **Resid:** Internal Medicine, North Carolina Meml Hosp-UNC, Chapel Hill, NC 1980-1982; Internal Medicine, North Carolina Meml Hosp-UNC, Chapel Hill, NC 1982-1983; **Fellow:** Rheumatology, Univ Alabama, Birmingham, AL 1986-1988; **Fac Appt:** Asst Prof Medicine, Univ Ala

Hadler, Nortin MD (Rhu) - *Spec Exp:* *Occupational Musculosketeal Disorders;* **Hospital:** Univ of NC Hosp (page 77); **Address:** University of NC, Dept Medicine, 3330 Thurston Building, Box 7280, Chapel Hill, NC 27599-7280; **Phone:** (919) 966-0566; **Board Cert:** Rheumatology 1974, Allergy & Immunology 1975, Internal Medicine 1973, Geriatric Medicine 1988; **Med School:** Harvard Med Sch 1968; **Resid:** Internal Medicine, Mass Genl Hosp, Boston, MA 1969-1973; **Fellow:** Rheumatology, Natl Inst Hlth, Bethesda, MD 1970-1972; Allergy & Immunology, Clin Res Ctr, London, England 1973-1974; **Fac Appt:** Prof Medicine, Univ NC Sch Med

Heck, Louis William MD (Rhu) - *Spec Exp:* *Lupus/SLE; Rheumatoid Arthritis;* **Hospital:** Univ of Ala Hosp at Birmingham; **Address:** 1717 6th Ave S, Birmingham, AL 35249; **Phone:** (205) 934-6485; **Board Cert:** Internal Medicine 1974, Rheumatology 1988; **Med School:** Indiana Univ 1970; **Resid:** Internal Medicine, Indiana Univ 1971-1972; **Fellow:** Allergy & Immunology, Natl Inst of Allergy & Inf Dis, Bethesda, MD 1972-1975; Rheumatology, Robert Bronton Hosp, Boston, MA 1975-1979; **Fac Appt:** Assoc Prof Medicine, Univ Ala

Kaplan, Stanley MD (Rhu) - *Spec Exp:* *Rheumatoid Arthritis;* **Hospital:** Baptist Memphis; **Address:** Univ Tenn Med Group, 7945 Wolf River Blvd, Ste 120, Germantown, TN 38138; **Phone:** (901) 448-7260; **Board Cert:** Internal Medicine 1965; **Med School:** Univ Tenn Coll Med, Memphis 1954; **Resid:** Internal Medicine, Univ Tenn Hosps, Memphis, TN 1958-1960; **Fellow:** Rheumatology, Univ Tenn Hosps, Memphis, TN 1960-1962; **Fac Appt:** Prof Medicine, Univ Tenn Coll Med, Memphis

Rahn, Daniel W MD (Rhu) - *Spec Exp:* *Rheumatoid Arthritis; Lyme Disease; Lupus/SLE;* **Hospital:** Med Coll of GA Hosp and Clin; **Address:** 1120 15th St, rm AA-311, Augusta, GA 30912; **Phone:** (706) 721-7346; **Board Cert:** Rheumatology 1982, Internal Medicine 1979; **Med School:** Yale Univ 1976; **Resid:** Internal Medicine, Yale New Haven Hosp, New Haven, CT 1972-1976; **Fellow:** Rheumatology, Yale Univ/Yale New Haven Hosp, New Haven, CT 1976-1978; **Fac Appt:** Prof Medicine, Med Coll GA

Sundy, John Sargent MD/PhD (Rhu) - *Spec Exp:* *Rheumatoid Arthritis; Gout; Lupus/SLE;* **Hospital:** Duke Univ Med Ctr (page 60); **Address:** Duke Univ Med Ctr, Box 3278, Durham, NC 27710; **Phone:** (919) 684-3956; **Board Cert:** Rheumatology 1998, Allergy & Immunology 1999; **Med School:** Hahnemann Univ 1991; **Resid:** Internal Medicine, Duke Univ Med Ctr, Durham, NC 1992-1993; **Fellow:** Rheumatology, Duke Univ Med Ctr, Durham, NC 1993-1996; Allergy & Immunology, Duke Univ Med Ctr, Durham, NC 1995-1998; **Fac Appt:** Assoc Prof Medicine, Duke Univ

Wise, Christopher Murray MD (Rhu) - *Spec Exp:* *Lupus/SLE; Sjogren's Syndrome; Rheumatoid Arthritis;* **Hospital:** Med Coll of VA Hosp; **Address:** Box 980647, Virginia Commonwealth Univ/MCV Campus, Richmond, VA 23298; **Phone:** (804) 828-9341; **Board Cert:** Internal Medicine 1980, Rheumatology 1982; **Med School:** Univ NC Sch Med 1977; **Resid:** Internal Medicine, Med Coll VA, Richmond, VA 1978-1980; **Fellow:** Rheumatology, Med Coll VA, Richmond, VA 1980; **Fac Appt:** Assoc Prof Medicine, Va Commonwealth Univ

Midwest

Adams, Elaine MD (Rhu) - *Spec Exp:* *Rheumatoid Arthritis; Lupus/SLE; Spondyloarthropathies;* **Hospital:** Loyola Univ Med Ctr; **Address:** Loyola Univ Med Ctr, Dept Rheumatology, 2160 S 1st Ave, Maywood, IL 60153-5590; **Phone:** (708) 216-3313; **Board Cert:** Internal Medicine 1981, Rheumatology 1984; **Med School:** Loyola Univ-Stritch Sch Med 1978; **Resid:** Internal Medicine, Loyola Univ Med Ctr, Maywood, IL 1979-1981; **Fellow:** Rheumatology, Univ Wisc Med Ctr, Madison, WI 1981-1983; **Fac Appt:** Assoc Prof Medicine, Loyola Univ-Stritch Sch Med

Barr, Walter Gerard MD (Rhu) - *Spec Exp:* *Scleroderma; Vasculitis; Stem Cell Transplant/Autoimmune Disease;* **Hospital:** Northwestern Meml Hosp; **Address:** 675 N Sinclair Ave, Ste 18-250, Chicago, IL 60611-5972; **Phone:** (312) 695-8628; **Board Cert:** Internal Medicine 1978, Rheumatology 1982; **Med School:** Loyola Univ-Stritch Sch Med 1975; **Resid:** Internal Medicine, Loyola Univ Med Ctr, Chicago, IL 1975-1978; **Fellow:** Rheumatology, Loyola Univ Med Ctr, Chicago, IL 1978-1979; Rheumatology, Mayo Clinic and Hosp, Rochester, MN 1979-1982; **Fac Appt:** Assoc Prof Medicine, Northwestern Univ

Brasington, Richard MD (Rhu) - *Spec Exp:* *Rheumatology - General;* **Hospital:** Barnes-Jewish Hosp (page 55); **Address:** Center For Advanced Medicine, Parkview Pl at Euclid Ave Fl 5 - Ste B & C, St Louis, MO 63108; **Phone:** (314) 286-2635; **Board Cert:** Internal Medicine 1985, Rheumatology 1986; **Med School:** Duke Univ 1980; **Resid:** Internal Medicine, Univ Iowa, Iowa City, IA 1981-1982; Internal Medicine, Univ Iowa, Iowa City, IA 1984-1985; **Fellow:** Rheumatology, Univ Iowa, Iowa City, IA 1982-1986; **Fac Appt:** Assoc Prof Medicine, Washington Univ, St Louis

Chang, Rowland Waton MD (Rhu) - *Spec Exp:* *Rheumatoid Arthritis; Arthritis Rehabilitation;* **Hospital:** Northwestern Meml Hosp; **Address:** 345 E Superior St, Fl 9, Chicago, IL 60611-2654; **Phone:** (312) 238-1156; **Board Cert:** Internal Medicine 1979, Rheumatology 1982; **Med School:** Tufts Univ 1976; **Resid:** Internal Medicine, Mt Auburn Hosp, Cambridge, MA 1977-1979; **Fellow:** Rheumatology, Hammersmith Hosp, London, England 1979-1980; Rheumatology, Brigham & Womens Hosp, Boston, MA 1980-1982; **Fac Appt:** Prof Medicine, Northwestern Univ

Chang-Miller, April MD (Rhu) - *Spec Exp:* *Connective Tissue Disorders;* *Spondyloarthropathies;* **Hospital:** Mayo Med Ctr & Clin - Rochester, MN; **Address:** Div of Rheumatology, 200 1st St SW, Rochester, MN 55905; **Phone:** (507) 284-2965; **Board Cert:** Rheumatology 1992, Internal Medicine 1986; **Med School:** Yale Univ 1983; **Resid:** Internal Medicine, Mayo Clinic, Rochester, MN 1983-1985; **Fellow:** Rheumatology, Mayo Clinic, Rochester, MN 1986-1989; Biochemical and Molecular Biology, Mayo Clinic, Rochester, MN 1989-1990; **Fac Appt:** Asst Prof Medicine, Mayo Med Sch

Crofford, Leslie MD (Rhu) - *Spec Exp:* *Fibromyalgia;* **Hospital:** Univ of MI Hlth Ctr; **Address:** 1500 E Med Center Dr, Bldg TC Reception D, Ann Arbor, MI 48109-0680; **Phone:** (734) 647-5900; **Board Cert:** Internal Medicine 1987, Rheumatology 1992; **Med School:** Univ Tenn Coll Med, Memphis 1984; **Resid:** Internal Medicine, Barnes/Wash Univ, St. Louis, MO 1984-1987; **Fellow:** Rheumatology, Natl Inst Hlth Clin Ctr, Bethesda, MD 1989-1992; **Fac Appt:** Assoc Prof Medicine, Univ Mich Med Sch

Curran, James Joseph MD (Rhu) - *Spec Exp:* *Rheumatoid Arthritis-Elderly; Lupus/SLE;* *Sjogren's Syndrome & Polymyositis;* **Hospital:** Univ of Chicago Hosps (page 76); **Address:** 5841 S Maryland Ave, MC-0930, Chicago, IL 60637-1463; **Phone:** (773) 702-1232; **Board Cert:** Internal Medicine 1980, Rheumatology 1982; **Med School:** Univ IL Coll Med 1976; **Resid:** Internal Medicine, Bethesda Naval Hosp, Bethesda, MD 1978-1980; **Fellow:** Rheumatology, Univ Chicago Hosp, Chicago, IL 1980-1982; **Fac Appt:** Clin Prof Medicine, Univ Chicago-Pritzker Sch Med

Duffy, Joseph MD (Rhu) - *Spec Exp:* *Eosinophilic Disorders; Spondyloarthropathies;* *Connective Tissue Disorders;* **Hospital:** Mayo Med Ctr & Clin - Rochester, MN; **Address:** Div Rheumatology, 200 1st St SW, Rochester, MN 55905; **Phone:** (507) 284-4550; **Board Cert:** Internal Medicine 1973, Rheumatology 1974; **Med School:** Univ Okla Coll Med **Resid:** Internal Medicine, Univ Cincinnati, Cincinnati, OH 1964-1965; **Fellow:** Rheumatology, Boston Univ Med Ctr, Boston, MA 1967-1968; Rheumatology, Baylor Coll of Med, Houston, TX 1971-1972

Ellman, Michael H MD (Rhu) - *Spec Exp:* *Scleroderma;* **Hospital:** Univ of Chicago Hosps (page 76); **Address:** Univ Chicago-Pritzker Sch Med, 5841 S Maryland Ave, MC-0930, Chicago, IL 60637-1463; **Phone:** (773) 702-1226; **Board Cert:** Internal Medicine 1969, Rheumatology 1972; **Med School:** Univ IL Coll Med 1964; **Resid:** Internal Medicine, Michael Reese Hosp, Chicago, IL 1968-1970; **Fellow:** Rheumatology, Univ Chicago Hosps, Chicago, IL 1970-1972; **Fac Appt:** Clin Prof Medicine, Univ Chicago-Pritzker Sch Med

Fischbein, Lewis Conrad MD (Rhu) - *Spec Exp:* *Rheumatoid Arthritis; Lupus/SLE;* **Hospital:** Barnes-Jewish Hosp (page 55); **Address:** One Barnes - Hospital Plz, East Pavilion , Ste 16422, St. Louis, MO 63110; **Phone:** (314) 367-9595; **Board Cert:** Internal Medicine 1977, Rheumatology 1980; **Med School:** Washington Univ, St Louis 1974; **Resid:** Internal Medicine, Barnes Jewish Hosp, St. Louis, MO 1975-1977; **Fellow:** Rheumatology, Barnes Jewish Hosp, St. Louis, MO 1977-1979; **Fac Appt:** Assoc Prof Medicine, Washington Univ, St Louis

RHEUMATOLOGY

Harrington, J Timothy MD (Rhu) - *Spec Exp:* *Arthritis;* **Hospital:** Univ WI Hosp & Clins; **Address:** Dept Rheumatology, One South Park St, Madison, WI 53715; **Phone:** (608) 287-2800; **Board Cert:** Internal Medicine 1972, Rheumatology 1972; **Med School:** Univ Wisc 1965; **Resid:** Internal Medicine, Mass Genl Hosp, Boston, MA 1966-1967; Internal Medicine, Parkland Meml Hosp, Dallas, TX 1969-1970; **Fellow:** Rheumatology, Univ Texas SW, Dallas, TX 1970-1971; **Fac Appt:** Prof Medicine, Univ Wisc

Hoffman, Gary Stuart MD (Rhu) - *Spec Exp:* *Vasculitis;* **Hospital:** Cleveland Clin Fdn (page 57); **Address:** 9500 Euclid Ave, MC-A50, Cleveland, OH 44195; **Phone:** (216) 445-6996; **Board Cert:** Internal Medicine 1976, Rheumatology 1978; **Med School:** Med Coll VA 1971; **Resid:** Internal Medicine, Dartmouth-Hitchcock Clin, Lebanon, NH 1972-1973; **Fellow:** Rheumatology, Dartmouth Univ, Lebanon, NH 1973-1974; **Fac Appt:** Prof Medicine, Ohio State Univ

Houk, John L MD (Rhu) - *Spec Exp:* *Rheumatology - General;* **Hospital:** Christ Hospital; **Address:** 2123 Auburn Ave, Ste 630, Cincinnati, OH 45219; **Phone:** (513) 585-1970; **Board Cert:** Internal Medicine 1972, Rheumatology 1994; **Med School:** Univ Cincinnati 1965; **Resid:** Internal Medicine, University Hospital, Cincinnati, OH 1969-1971; **Fellow:** Rheumatology, University Hospital, Cincinnati, OH 1971-1973; **Fac Appt:** Prof Medicine, Univ Cincinnati

Katz, Robert MD (Rhu) - *Spec Exp:* *Rheumatoid Arthritis; Lupus/SLE; Fibromyalgia;* **Hospital:** Rush-Presby - St Luke's Med Ctr (page 72); **Address:** 1725 W Harrison St, Ste 1039, Chicago, IL 60612; **Phone:** (312) 942-2159; **Board Cert:** Internal Medicine 1975, Rheumatology 1976; **Med School:** Univ MD Sch Med 1970; **Resid:** Internal Medicine, Washington Univ Med Ctr, St Louis, MO 1970-1972; **Fellow:** Rheumatology, Johns Hopkins, Baltimore, MD 1974-1976; **Fac Appt:** Assoc Prof Medicine, Rush Med Coll

Klearman, Micki MD (Rhu) - *Spec Exp:* *Arthritis; Lupus;* **Hospital:** Barnes-Jewish Hosp (page 55); **Address:** One Barnes-Jewish Hospital Plz, East Pavilion, Ste 16422, St. Louis, MO 63110; **Phone:** (314) 367-9595; **Board Cert:** Internal Medicine 1985, Rheumatology 1988; **Med School:** Washington Univ, St Louis 1981; **Resid:** Internal Medicine, Jewish Hosp, St Louis, MO 1982-1985; **Fellow:** Rheumatology, Wash University, St Louis, MO 1985-1987; **Fac Appt:** Assoc Prof Medicine, Washington Univ, St Louis

Luggen, Michael MD (Rhu) - *Spec Exp:* *Rheumatology;* **Hospital:** Univ Hosp - Cincinnati; **Address:** 2123 Auburn Ave, Ste 630, Cincinnati, OH 45219; **Phone:** (513) 585-1970; **Board Cert:** Rheumatology 1982, Internal Medicine 1978; **Med School:** Columbia P&S 1974; **Resid:** Internal Medicine, Cinn General Hosp, Cincinnati, OH 1975-1977; **Fellow:** Rheumatology, University Cinn, Cincinnati, OH 1980-1982; **Fac Appt:** Assoc Prof Medicine, Univ Cincinnati

Luthra, Harvinder Singh MD (Rhu) - *Spec Exp:* *Rheumatoid Arthritis; Ankylosing Spondilitis; Relapsing Polychondritis;* **Hospital:** St Mary's Hosp - Rochester, MN; **Address:** Mayo Clinic, 200 1st St SW, Rochester, MN 55905-0002; **Phone:** (507) 284-1227; **Board Cert:** Internal Medicine 1973, Rheumatology 1974; **Med School:** India 1967; **Resid:** Ophthalmology, Christian Med Coll, India 1968; Internal Medicine, Mount Sinai Hosp Med Ctr, Chicago, IL 1970-1972; **Fellow:** Rheumatology, Mayo Grad Sch, Rochester, MN 1972-1974; **Fac Appt:** Prof Medicine, Mayo Med Sch

McCune, W. Joseph MD (Rhu) - *Spec Exp:* *Lupus/SLE; Rheumatoid Arthritis;* **Hospital:** Univ of MI Hlth Ctr; **Address:** A Alfred Taubman Hlth Care Ctr, 1500 E Med Ctr, rm 3918, Box 0358, Ann Arbor, MI 48109-0358; **Phone:** (734) 936-5561; **Board Cert:** Rheumatology 1982, Internal Medicine 1978; **Med School:** Univ Cincinnati 1975; **Resid:** Rheumatology, Univ of Mich, Ann Arbor, MI 1975-1976; Internal Medicine, Brigham Womens Hosp, Boston, MA 1976-1978; **Fellow:** Rheumatology, Brigham Womens Hosp, Boston, MA 1978-1981; **Fac Appt:** Assoc Prof Medicine, Univ Mich Med Sch

Michalska, Margaret MD (Rhu) - *Spec Exp:* *Rheumatoid Arthritis; Connective Tissue Disorders;* **Hospital:** Rush-Presby - St Luke's Med Ctr (page 72); **Address:** 1725 W Harrison St, Ste 1017, Chicago, IL 60612; **Phone:** (312) 942-6641; **Board Cert:** Internal Medicine 1988, Rheumatology 1990; **Med School:** Poland 1979; **Resid:** Internal Medicine, Hines VA Hosp, Chicago, IL 1985-1988; **Fellow:** Biochemistry, Nortwestern Univ, Evanston, IL 1980-1985; Rheumatology, Rush - Presby St Lukes, Chicago, IL 1988-1990; **Fac Appt:** Asst Prof Medicine, Rush Med Coll

Moder, Kevin Gerard MD (Rhu) - *Spec Exp:* *Rheumatoid Arthritis; Lupus/SLE;* **Hospital:** Mayo Med Ctr & Clin - Rochester, MN; **Address:** Mayo Clinic, 200 1st St SW, Rochester, MN 55905-0002; **Phone:** (507) 284-4550; **Board Cert:** Internal Medicine 1990, Rheumatology 1994; **Med School:** Univ MO-Columbia Sch Med 1987; **Resid:** Internal Medicine, Mayo Med Clinic, Rochester, MN 1987-1990; **Fellow:** Rheumatology, Mayo Med Clinic, Rochester, MN 1990-1993; **Fac Appt:** Asst Prof Medicine, Mayo Med Sch

Moskowitz, Roland MD (Rhu) - *Spec Exp:* *Connective Tissue Disorders; Osteoarthritis;* **Hospital:** Univ Hosp - Cincinnati; **Address:** Division of Rheumatology, 11100 Euclid Avenue, Cleveland, OH 44106; **Phone:** (216) 844-8500; **Board Cert:** Internal Medicine 1961, Rheumatology 1974; **Med School:** Temple Univ 1953; **Resid:** Internal Medicine, Mayo Clinic, Rochester, MN 1954-1955; **Fellow:** Internal Medicine, Mayo Clin, Rochetser, MN 1957-1960; **Fac Appt:** Prof Medicine, Case West Res Univ

Nelson, Audrey May MD (Rhu) - *Spec Exp:* *Scleroderma; Rheumatoid Arthritis-Juvenile & Adult;* **Hospital:** St Mary's Hosp - Rochester, MN; **Address:** Mayo Medical Center, 200 1st St SW, Rochester, MN 55905-0001; **Phone:** (507) 284-4550; **Board Cert:** Internal Medicine 1971, Rheumatology 1972; **Med School:** Univ Minn 1965; **Resid:** Internal Medicine, Mayo Grad Sch, Rochester, MN 1966-1969; **Fellow:** Rheumatology, Mayo Grad Sch, Rochester, MN 1970-1971; **Fac Appt:** Prof Rheumatology, Mayo Med Sch

Pope, Richard M MD (Rhu) - *Spec Exp:* *Arthritis; Sjogren's Syndrome;* **Hospital:** Northwestern Meml Hosp; **Address:** 675 N St Claire, Ste 18-250, Chicago, IL 60611; **Phone:** (312) 695-8628; **Board Cert:** Rheumatology 1976, Internal Medicine 1973; **Med School:** Loyola Univ-Stritch Sch Med 1970; **Resid:** Internal Medicine, Michael Reese Hosp, Chicago, IL 1971-1972; **Fellow:** Rheumatology, Univ Wash Med Ctr, Seattle, WA 1972-1974; **Fac Appt:** Prof Rheumatology, Northwestern Univ

Great Plains and Mountains

Arend, Wiiliam Phelps MD (Rhu) - *Spec Exp:* *Arthritis; Rheumatoid Arthritis;* **Hospital:** Univ Colo HSC - Denver; **Address:** 4200 9th Ave, Denver, CO 80220-3700; **Phone:** (303) 315-6666; **Board Cert:** Internal Medicine 1971, Rheumatology 1980; **Med School:** Columbia P&S 1964; **Resid:** Internal Medicine, Univ Washington Hosp, Seattle, WA 1965-1966; Internal Medicine, Univ Washington Hosp, Seattle, WA 1968-1969; **Fellow:** Rheumatology, Univ Washington Hosp, Seattle, WA 1969-1971; **Fac Appt:** Prof Rheumatology, Univ Colo

Kotzin, Brian Leslie MD (Rhu) - *Spec Exp:* *Lupus/SLE;* **Hospital:** Univ Colo HSC - Denver; **Address:** U Colorado Hlth Sci Ctr, 4200 E 9th Ave, Denver, CO 80206; **Phone:** (303) 315-6977; **Board Cert:** Internal Medicine 1978, Rheumatology 1980; **Med School:** Stanford Univ 1975; **Resid:** Internal Medicine, Beth Israel Hosp, Boston, MA 1976-1977; **Fellow:** Rheumatology, Stanford Med Ctr, Palo Alto, CA 1978; **Fac Appt:** Prof Medicine, Univ Colo

West, Sterling MD (Rhu) - *Spec Exp:* Lupus/SLE; Vasculitis; Osteoporosis; **Hospital:** Univ Colo HSC - Denver; **Address:** Univ Colo Hlth Sci Ctr, 4200 E Ninth Ave, Box B 115, Denver, CO 80262; **Phone:** (303) 315-6665; **Board Cert:** Internal Medicine 1979, Rheumatology 1982; **Med School:** Emory Univ 1976; **Resid:** Internal Medicine, Fitzsimons Army Med Ctr, Aurora, CO 1976-1979; **Fellow:** Rheumatology, Fitzsimons Army Med Ctr, Aurora, CO 1979-1981; **Fac Appt:** Prof Medicine, Univ Colo

Williams, H James MD (Rhu) - *Spec Exp:* Arthritis; **Hospital:** Univ Utah Hosp and Clin; **Address:** Univ Utah Med Ctr, Med Div Rheum, 50 N Med Dr, 4B 200 SOM, Salt Lake City, UT 84132-0001; **Phone:** (801) 581-7724; **Board Cert:** Internal Medicine 1972, Rheumatology 1978; **Med School:** Univ Utah 1969; **Resid:** Internal Medicine, Duke Med Ctr, Durham, NC 1970-1972; Internal Medicine, Univ Utah Med Ctr, Salt Lake City, UT 1972-1973; **Fellow:** Rheumatology, Univ Utah Med Ctr, Salt Lake City, UT 1975-1977; **Fac Appt:** Prof Rheumatology, Univ Utah

Southwest

Arnett Jr, Frank Couchman MD (Rhu) - *Spec Exp:* Reiter's Syndrome; Spondylitis; Scleroderma; **Hospital:** Meml Hermann Hosp; **Address:** Hermann Prof Bldg, 6410 Fannin St, Ste 1100, Houston, TX 77030; **Phone:** (713) 704-6100; **Board Cert:** Rheumatology 1976, Clinical & Laboratory Immunology 1990; **Med School:** Univ Cincinnati 1968; **Resid:** Internal Medicine, Johns Hopkins Hosp, Baltimore, MD 1969-1970; **Fellow:** Rheumatology, Johns Hopkins Hosp, Baltimore, MD 1970-1972; **Fac Appt:** Prof Medicine, Univ Tex, Houston

Davis, William Eugene MD (Rhu) - *Spec Exp:* Lupus/SLE; Rheumatoid Arthritis; **Hospital:** Ochsner Found Hosp; **Address:** Ochsner Clinic, Rheum, 1514 Jefferson Hwy, #7N, New Orleans, LA 70121; **Phone:** (504) 842-3920; **Board Cert:** Internal Medicine 1987, Rheumatology 1988; **Med School:** Louisiana State Univ 1983; **Resid:** Internal Medicine, Ochsner Fdn Hosp, New Orleans, LA 1983-1986; **Fellow:** Rheumatology, Univ Michigan, Ann Arbor, MI 1986-1988

Hurd, Eric MD (Rhu) - *Spec Exp:* Rheumatoid Arthritis; **Hospital:** Baylor Univ Medical Ctr; **Address:** 712 N Washington St, Ste 200, Dallas, TX 75246; **Phone:** (214) 823-6503; **Board Cert:** Internal Medicine, Rheumatology; **Med School:** Univ Okla Coll Med 1962; **Resid:** Internal Medicine, Parkland Meml, Dallas, TX; Internal Medicine, St Johns Med Ctr

Lindsey, Stephen M MD (Rhu) - *Spec Exp:* Osteoporosis; Lupus/SLE; **Hospital:** Ochsner Found Hosp; **Address:** 9001 Summa Ave, Baton Rouge, LA 70809; **Phone:** (225) 761-5200; **Board Cert:** Internal Medicine 1975, Rheumatology 1980; **Med School:** Louisiana State Univ 1972; **Resid:** Internal Medicine, Letterman AMC, San Francisco, CA 1973-1975; **Fellow:** Rheumatology, Walter Reed AMC, Washington, DC 1977-1979

Lipstate, James Mitchell MD (Rhu) - *Spec Exp:* Arthritis; Osteoporosis; **Hospital:** Our Lady of Lordes Reg Med Ctr - Lafayette; **Address:** 401 Audubon Blvd, Ste 102B, Lafayette, LA 70503; **Phone:** (337) 237-7801; **Board Cert:** Internal Medicine 1983, Rheumatology 1986; **Med School:** Tulane Univ 1980; **Resid:** Internal Medicine, Univ Alabama Hosp, Birmingham, AL 1981-1983; **Fellow:** Rheumatology, Univ Alabama Hosp, Birmingham, AL 1983-1986; **Fac Appt:** Ass't Clin Prof Medicine, Louisiana State Univ

Malin, Jennifer MD (Rhu) - *Spec Exp:* Arthritis; **Hospital:** Our Lady of Lordes Reg Med Ctr - Lafayette; **Address:** 401 Audobon Blvd, Ste 102B, Lafayette, LA 70503-2676; **Phone:** (337) 237-7801; **Board Cert:** Internal Medicine 1991, Rheumatology 1996; **Med School:** Tulane Univ 1987; **Resid:** Obstetrics & Gynecology, Tulane Univ Sch Med, New Orleans, LA 1987-1988; Internal Medicine, Tulane Univ Sch Med, New Orleans, LA 1988-1991; **Fellow:** Rheumatology, Tulane Univ Sch Med, New Orleans, LA 1991-1993

Mayes, Maureen Davidica MD/PhD (Rhu) - *Spec Exp:* Scleroderma; **Hospital:** Univ of Texas Hlth & Sci Ctr; **Address:** U Tex Hlth Sci Ctr, 6341 Fannin, rm 5270, Houston, TX 77030; **Phone:** (713) 500-6900; **Board Cert:** Internal Medicine 1980, Rheumatology 1982; **Med School:** Eastern VA Med Sch 1976; **Resid:** Internal Medicine, Cleveland Clinic Fnd, Cleveland, OH 1978-1979; **Fellow:** Rheumatology, Cleveland Clinic Fnd, Cleveland, OH 1979-1981; **Fac Appt:** Prof Medicine, Univ Tex, Houston

Sessoms, Sandra Lee MD (Rhu) - *Spec Exp:* Arthritis; Lupus/SLE; **Hospital:** Methodist Hosp - Houston; **Address:** Methodist Hospital, 6550 Fannin St, Smith Tower, Ste 1057, Houston, TX 77030; **Phone:** (713) 986-8190; **Board Cert:** Internal Medicine 1981, Rheumatology 1984; **Med School:** Baylor Coll Med 1978; **Resid:** Internal Medicine, Baylor Coll Med, Houston, TX 1978-1979; **Fellow:** Rheumatology, Baylor Coll Med, Houston, TX 1981-1983; **Fac Appt:** Assoc Prof Medicine, Baylor Coll Med

West Coast and Pacific

Bobrove, Arthur M MD (Rhu) - *Spec Exp:* Inflammatory Muscle Disease; **Hospital:** Stanford Med Ctr; **Address:** 795 El Camino Real, Palo Alto, CA 94301; **Phone:** (650) 321-4121; **Board Cert:** Internal Medicine 1972, Rheumatology 1976; **Med School:** Temple Univ 1967; **Resid:** Internal Medicine, Univ Mich Hosp, Ann Arbor, MI 1968-1969; Internal Medicine, Univ Mich Hosp, Ann Arbor, MI 1971-1972; **Fellow:** Immunology, Stanford Univ Hosp, Stanford, CA 1972-1974; **Fac Appt:** Clin Prof Medicine, Stanford Univ

Clements, Philip Jordan MD (Rhu) - *Spec Exp:* Scleroderma; **Hospital:** UCLA Med Ctr; **Address:** UCLA Sch Med, Rehab 32-59, 1000 Veteran Ave, Los Angeles, CA 90095-1670; **Phone:** (310) 825-8414; **Board Cert:** Internal Medicine 1972, Rheumatology 1974; **Med School:** Indiana Univ 1965; **Resid:** Internal Medicine, Cedars-Sinai Med Ctr, Los Angeles, CA 1969-1971; **Fellow:** Rheumatology, UCLA Med Ctr, Los Angeles, CA 1971-1974; **Fac Appt:** Prof Medicine, UCLA

Ehresmann, Glenn Richard MD (Rhu) - *Spec Exp:* Rheumatology - General; **Hospital:** USC Univ Hosp - R K Eamer Med Plz; **Address:** USC Univ Hosp Rehabilitation Center, 1355 San Pablo St Bldg AHC Fl 1, Los Angeles, CA 90033; **Phone:** (323) 442-5100; **Board Cert:** Rheumatology 1978, Internal Medicine 1977; **Med School:** UC Irvine 1973; **Resid:** Internal Medicine, Los Angeles Co-USC Med Ctr, Los Angeles, CA 1976-1978; **Fellow:** Rheumatology, Los Angeles Co-USC Med Ctr, Los Angeles, CA 1976-1978

Gardner, Gregory MD (Rhu) - *Spec Exp:* Rheumatology - General; **Hospital:** Univ WA Med Ctr; **Address:** Arthritis Clinic, Medical Specialties, 1959 NE Pacific St, Box 356166, Seattle, WA 98195; **Phone:** (206) 598-7600; **Board Cert:** Rheumatology 1990, Internal Medicine 1987; **Med School:** Baylor Coll Med 1984; **Resid:** Internal Medicine, Univ of NC Hosp, Charleston, NC 1984-1987; **Fellow:** Rheumatology, Univ CA-San Diego Med Ctr, San Diego, CA 1987-1989

Gershwin, Merrill Eric MD (Rhu) - *Spec Exp:* Allergy; Rheumatoid Arthritis; **Hospital:** Univ CA - Davis Med Ctr; **Address:** UC Davis Sch of Med, Div Rheumatology, Box TB192, Davis, CA 95616; **Phone:** (530) 752-2884; **Board Cert:** Allergy & Immunology 1979, Rheumatology 1976; **Med School:** Stanford Univ 1971; **Resid:** Internal Medicine, New England Med Ctr, Boston, MA 1972-1973; **Fellow:** Rheumatology, Natl Inst Arth Med, Bethesda, MD 1973-1975; **Fac Appt:** Prof Medicine, UC Davis

Hahn, Bevra H MD (Rhu) - *Spec Exp:* Lupus/SLE; **Hospital:** UCLA Med Ctr; **Address:** 1000 Veteran Ave, Los Angeles, CA 90095; **Phone:** (310) 825-2448; **Board Cert:** Internal Medicine 1970, Rheumatology 1972; **Med School:** Johns Hopkins Univ 1964; **Resid:** Internal Medicine, Washington Univ - Barnes Hosp, St. Louis, MO 1965-1966; **Fellow:** Rheumatology, Johns Hopkins Hosp, Baltimore, MD 1966-1969; **Fac Appt:** Prof Medicine, UCLA

Harris Jr, Edward Day MD (Rhu) - *Spec Exp:* *Rheumatoid Arthritis; Osteoarthritis; Sclerodrma;* **Hospital:** Stanford Med Ctr; **Address:** Stanford Univ School of Med, 1000 Welch Rd, Ste 203, Palo Alto, CA 94304; **Phone:** (415) 723-5455; **Board Cert:** Internal Medicine 1968, Rheumatology 1976; **Med School:** Harvard Med Sch 1962; **Resid:** Internal Medicine, Mass Genl Hosp, Boston, MA 1963-1967; **Fellow:** Internal Medicine, Mass Genl Hosp, Boston, MA 1967-1969; **Fac Appt:** Prof Medicine, Stanford Univ

Kitridou, Rodanthi C MD (Rhu) - *Spec Exp:* *Lupus/SLE;* **Hospital:** USC Univ Hosp - R K Eamer Med Plz; **Address:** 1200 N State St, Box 386, Los Angeles, CA 90033-1029; **Phone:** (323) 442-5100; **Board Cert:** Internal Medicine 1972, Rheumatology 1972; **Med School:** Greece 1962; **Resid:** Internal Medicine, Hahnemann Hosp, Philadelphia, PA 1964-1966; **Fellow:** Rheumatology, Univ Penn Med Ctr, Philadelphia, PA 1967-1968; Rheumatology, VA Hosp, Philadephia, PA 1968-1969; **Fac Appt:** Prof Medicine, USC Sch Med

Quismorio Jr, Francisco P MD (Rhu) - *Spec Exp:* *Lupus/SLE; Connective Tissue Disorders;* **Hospital:** LAC & USC Med Ctr; **Address:** 2011 Zonal Ave, MC HMR711, Los Angeles, CA 90033-1034; **Phone:** (323) 442-1946; **Board Cert:** Internal Medicine 1975, Rheumatology 1976; **Med School:** Philippines 1964; **Resid:** Internal Medicine, Philippines General Hosp, Manila, Philippines 1964-1966; Internal Medicine, LAC USC Med Ctr, Los Angeles, CA 1970-1971; **Fellow:** Rheumatology, Univ Penn Hosp, Philadelphia, PA 1966-1968; Rheumatology, LAC USC Med Ctr, Los Angeles, CA 1968-1970; **Fac Appt:** Prof Medicine, USC Sch Med

Sack, Kenneth Edward MD (Rhu) - *Spec Exp:* *Rheumatology - General;* **Hospital:** UCSF Med Ctr; **Address:** 400 Parnassus Ave, Ste A555, San Francisco, CA 94143; **Phone:** (415) 353-2497; **Board Cert:** Internal Medicine 1973, Rheumatology 1978; **Med School:** Tufts Univ 1968; **Resid:** Internal Medicine, RI Hosp, Providence, RI 1969-1970; Internal Medicine, U Mich Hosp, Ann Arbor, MI 1972-1974; **Fellow:** Rheumatology, Univ Ala Hosp, Birmingham, AL 1977-1978; **Fac Appt:** Clin Prof Medicine, UCSF

Weiss, Arthur MD/PhD (Rhu) - *Spec Exp:* *Transduction; Signaling;* **Hospital:** UCSF Med Ctr; **Address:** Arthritis Clin, UCSF Ambulatory Care Bldg, 3rd and Parnassus Ave, Box 0795, San Francisco, CA 94143; **Phone:** (415) 476-1291; **Board Cert:** Internal Medicine 1983, Rheumatology 1986; **Med School:** Univ Chicago-Pritzker Sch Med 1979; **Resid:** Internal Medicine, UCSF, San Francisco, CA 1981-1983; **Fellow:** Rheumatology, UCSF, San Francisco, CA 1983-1985; **Fac Appt:** Prof Medicine, UCSF

Wener, Mark MD (Rhu) - *Spec Exp:* *Lupus/SLE; Vasculitis; Immune Disorders;* **Hospital:** Univ WA Med Ctr; **Address:** Univ Wash Med Ctr, Arthritis Clinic, 1959 NE Pacific St, Box 356166, Seattle, WA 98195-0001; **Phone:** (206) 598-4615; **Board Cert:** Internal Medicine 1978, Rheumatology 1980, Clinical & Laboratory Immunology 1986; **Med School:** Washington Univ, St Louis 1974; **Resid:** Internal Medicine, Univ Iowa Hosp, Iowa City, IA 1974-1978; **Fellow:** Rheumatology, Univ Iowa Hosp, Iowa City, IA 1978-1980; Immunology, Univ Wash, Seattle, WA 1980-1981; **Fac Appt:** Assoc Prof Laboratory Medicine, Univ Wash

Wofsy, David MD (Rhu) - *Spec Exp:* *Lupus/SLE;* **Hospital:** UCSF Med Ctr; **Address:** 533 Parnassus Ave, Box 0633, San Francisco, CA 94143; **Phone:** (415) 750-2104; **Board Cert:** Internal Medicine 1977, Rheumatology 1980; **Med School:** UCSD 1974; **Resid:** Internal Medicine, UCSF Hosps, San Francisco, CA 1975-1977; **Fellow:** Rheumatology, UCSF, San Francisco, CA 1977-1979; **Fac Appt:** Prof Medicine, UCSF

Sports Medicine

(a subspecialty of INTERNAL MEDICINE)

An internist trained to be responsible for continuous care in the field of sports medicine, not only for the enhancement of health and fitness, but also for the prevention of injury and illness. A sports medicine physician must have knowledge and experience in the promotion of wellness and the prevention of injury. Knowledge about special areas of medicine such as exercise physiology, biomechanics, nutrition, psychology, physical rehabilitation, epidemiology, physical evaluation, injuries (treatment and prevention and referral practice) and the role of exercise in promoting a healthy life style are essential to the practice of sports medicine. The sports medicine physician requires special education to provide the knowledge to improve the healthcare of the individual engaged in physical exercise (sports) whether as an individual or in team participation.

INTERNAL MEDICINE

An internist is a personal physician who provides long-term, comprehensive care in the office and the hospital, managing both common and complex illness of adolescents, adults and the elderly. Internists are trained in the diagnosis and treatment of cancer, infections and diseases affecting the heart, blood, kidneys, joints and digestive, respiratory and vascular systems. They are also trained in the essentials of primary care internal medicine which incorporates an understanding of disease prevention, wellness, substance abuse, mental health and effective treatment of common problems of the eyes, ears, skin, nervous system and reproductive organs.

Training required: Three years in internal medicine *plus* additional training and examination for certification in sports medicine

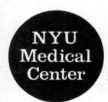

NYU Medical Center
550 First Avenue (at 31st St.), New York, NY 10016
Physician Referral: (888) 7-NYU-MED (888-769-8633)
www.nyumedicalcenter.org

Hospital for Joint Diseases
301 East 17th Street (at 2nd Ave.), New York, NY 10003
Physician Referral: (888) HJD-DOCS (888-453-3627)
www.jointdiseases.com

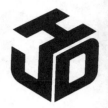

SPORTS MEDICINE

The NYU-Hospital for Joint Diseases (HJD) Sports Medicine Service, a joint program of NYU Medical Center and the Hospital for Joint Diseases, encompasses education, research, and clinical care that focuses on the treatment of athletic injuries. Its renowned specialists treat patients from high schools, colleges, and professional athletic teams, as well as recreational athletes of all ages.

Thousands of procedures are performed each year by the Service, including minimally invasive arthroscopic procedures for the knee, shoulder, elbow, and ankle. However, the majority of cases are treated nonoperatively. In fact, the proper treatment of athletic injuries starts with prevention. That's why the NYU-HJD Sports Medicine Service emphasizes education and rehabilitation to strengthen joints and prevent re-injury.

The Service's research focus is on chondrocyte (cartilage cell) transplantation. The earliest research in this area was performed at HJD, and the clinical studies conducted in Sweden and reported in the New England Journal of Medicine were a direct outgrowth of HJD's research. Continuing to pursue this exciting line of research, the Sports Medicine Service is pioneering the introduction of clinical articular chondrocyte transplantation in humans in the United States.

Hospital for Joint Diseases is the official hospital and team physicians of the New York Mets.

NYU MEDICAL CENTER

The Sports Medicine Service's expert staff covers numerous athletic events, including the U.S. Open Tennis Tournament, various Madison Square Garden activities, the Empire State Games, the New York Public School Athletic League, Catholic High Schools Athletic Association games, and the Maccabbi Games. Its physicians also serve in consultative and support capacities to a wide variety of New York City performing arts organizations.

Physician Referral
(888) 7-NYU-MED
(888-769-8633)
www.nyumedicalcenter.org

Physician Listings

Sports Medicine

Mid Atlantic

Altchek, David MD (SM) - *Spec Exp: Shoulder Surgery; Elbow Surgery; Knee Surgery;* **Hospital:** Hosp For Special Surgery (page 62); **Address:** 535 E 70st St, New York, NY 10021; **Phone:** (212) 606-1909; **Board Cert:** Orthopaedic Surgery 1990; **Med School:** Cornell Univ-Weill Med Coll 1982; **Resid:** Orthopaedic Surgery, Hosp For Special Surgery, New York, NY 1983-1987; **Fellow:** Sports Medicine, Hosp For Special Surgery, New York, NY 1987-1988; **Fac Appt:** Asst Prof Orthopaedic Surgery, Cornell Univ-Weill Med Coll

Kelly, Michael MD (SM) - *Spec Exp: Knee Surgery;* **Hospital:** Beth Israel Med Ctr - Singer Div (page 58); **Address:** 170 East End Ave Fl 4, New York, NY 10128; **Phone:** (212) 870-9747; **Board Cert:** Orthopaedic Surgery 1999; **Med School:** Georgetown Univ 1979; **Resid:** Surgery, St Vincent Hosp, New York, NY 1979-1981; Orthopaedic Surgery, Columbia-Presby Hosp, New York, NY 1981-1984; **Fellow:** Knee Surgery, Hosp For Special Surgery, New York, NY 1984-1985; **Fac Appt:** Asst Prof Orthopaedic Surgery, Columbia P&S

Levine, William MD (SM) - *Spec Exp: Arthroscopic Surgery; Sports Medicine; Shoulder & Knee Injuries;* **Hospital:** NY Presby Hosp - Columbia Presby Med Ctr (page 70); **Address:** 622 W 168th St Fl PH11 East Wing, New York, NY 10032; **Phone:** (212) 305-0762; **Board Cert:** Orthopaedic Surgery 1999; **Med School:** Case West Res Univ 1990; **Resid:** Surgery, Beth Israel Hosp, Boston, MA 1990-1991; Orthopaedic Surgery, New Eng Med Ctr Hosps, Boston, MA 1991-1995; **Fellow:** Shoulder Surgery, Columbia-Presby Med Ctr, New York, NY 1995-1996; Sports Medicine, Univ MD Med Ctr, Baltimore, MD 1997-1998; **Fac Appt:** Asst Prof Orthopaedic Surgery, Columbia P&S

Maharam, Lewis MD (SM) - *Spec Exp: Running Injuries; Primary Care Sports Med;* **Hospital:** Hosp For Joint Diseases (page 61); **Address:** 800A Fifth Ave, Ste 302, MC-10021, New York, NY 10021; **Phone:** (212) 308-2348; **Board Cert:** Sports Medicine 1990; **Med School:** Emory Univ 1985; **Resid:** Internal Medicine, Danbury Hosp, Danbury, CT 1986-1987; Internal Medicine, NY Infirm/Beekman Downtown, New York, NY 1987-1989; **Fellow:** Sports Medicine, Pascack Valley Hosp, Westwood, NJ 1989-1990

Nisonson, Barton MD (SM) - *Spec Exp: Knee Injuries; Shoulder & Knee Surgery;* **Hospital:** Lenox Hill Hosp (page 64); **Address:** 130 E 77th St, New York, NY 10021-1851; **Phone:** (212) 570-9120; **Board Cert:** Orthopaedic Surgery 1974; **Med School:** Columbia P&S 1966; **Resid:** Surgery, Columbia-Presby Med Ctr, New York, NY 1967-1968; **Fellow:** Orthopaedic Surgery, Columbia-Presby Med Ctr, New York, NY 1970-1973

Southeast

Andrews, James R MD (SM) - *Spec Exp: Shoulder, Elbow, Knee Surgery;* **Hospital:** Healthsouth Med Ctr - Birmingham; **Address:** 1201 11th Ave S, Ste 200, Birmingham, AL 35205-3410; **Phone:** (205) 930-0061; **Board Cert:** Orthopaedic Surgery 1974; **Med School:** Louisiana State Univ 1967; **Resid:** USPHS Hosp-Staten Island NY & USPHS Hosp, San Francisco, CA 1968; Orthopaedic Surgery, Touro Infirm-Tulane, New Orleans, LA 1969-1970; **Fellow:** Hand Surgery, VA Med Ctr, Charlottesville, VA 1972

Speer, Kevin MD (SM) - *Spec Exp: Irritated Cuff Repair;* **Hospital:** Duke Univ Med Ctr (page 60); **Address:** 3404 Wake Forest Rd, Ste 101, Raleigh, NC 27609; **Phone:** (919) 256-1511; **Board Cert:** Orthopaedic Surgery 1994; **Med School:** Johns Hopkins Univ 1985; **Resid:** Orthopaedic Surgery, Duke Univ Med Ctr, Durham, NC 1987-1991; **Fellow:** Sports Medicine, Hosp Special Surg, New York, NY 1991-1992; **Fac Appt:** Assoc Prof Orthopaedic Surgery, Duke Univ

Midwest

Noyes, Frank MD (SM) - *Spec Exp:* Knee Reconstruction; Meniscus & Ligament Transplants; Cartilage Regeneration & Transplant; **Hospital:** Deaconess Hosp - Indiana; **Address:** 621 E Mehring Way , rm 415, One Lytle Place, Cincinnati, OH 45202-3528; **Phone:** (513) 421-5100; **Board Cert:** Orthopaedic Surgery 1972; **Med School:** Geo Wash Univ 1966; **Resid:** Orthopaedic Surgery, University of Mich Med Ctr, Ann Arbor, MI 1967-1971; **Fellow:** Sports Medicine & Biomechanics, Aerospace Med Rsch Lab, US Airforce 1971-1975; **Fac Appt:** Clin Prof Orthopaedic Surgery, Univ Cincinnati

Paletta, George A MD (SM) - *Spec Exp:* Ankle Surgery; Knee Surgery; **Hospital:** Barnes-Jewish Hosp (page 55); **Address:** Dept Orthopaedic Surg, West Pavilion, Ste 11300, St Louis, MO 63110; **Phone:** (314) 747-2500; **Board Cert:** Orthopaedic Surgery 1998; **Med School:** Johns Hopkins Univ 1988; **Resid:** Orthopaedic Surgery, Cornell Univ Med Ctr, New York, NY 1990-1994; **Fellow:** Orthopaedic Surgery, Cleveland Clin Fnd, Cleveland, OH 1994-1995; **Fac Appt:** Asst Prof Orthopaedic Surgery, Washington Univ, St Louis

Schwenk, Thomas L MD (SM) - *Spec Exp:* Sports Medicine - General; **Hospital:** Univ of MI Hlth Ctr; **Address:** 1801 Briarwood Cir, Ann Arbor, MI 48108; **Phone:** (734) 998-7390; **Board Cert:** Family Practice 1996, Sports Medicine 1993; **Med School:** Univ Mich Med Sch 1975; **Resid:** Family Practice, Univ Utah Affil Hosps, Salt Lake City, UT 1975-1978; **Fellow:** Family Practice, Univ Utah Affil Hosps, Salt Lake City, UT 1980-1982; **Fac Appt:** Prof Family Practice, Univ Mich Med Sch

Shively, Robert A MD (SM) - *Spec Exp:* Ankle & Knee surgery; Knee Replacement; Shoulder Surgery; **Hospital:** Barnes-Jewish Hosp (page 55); **Address:** Washington Univ, 1 Barnes Plaza, Ste 11300, St Louis, MO 63110; **Phone:** (314) 362-4080; **Board Cert:** Orthopaedic Surgery 1981; **Med School:** Univ IL Coll Med 1969; **Resid:** Surgery, Carolinas Med Ctr Prgm, Charlotte, NC 1970-1971; Orthopaedic Surgery, St Louis Univ Sch Med, St Louis, MO 1975-1979; **Fellow:** Sports Medicine, Univ Okla Hlth Scis Ctr-Presby Hosp, Oklahoma City, OK 1979-1980; **Fac Appt:** Asst Prof Orthopaedic Surgery, Washington Univ, St Louis

West Coast and Pacific

Jobe, Frank Wilson MD (SM) - *Spec Exp:* Shoulder Surgery; Elbow Surgery; **Hospital:** Centinela Hosp Med Ctr; **Address:** 6801 Park Terr, Ste 400, Los Angeles, CA 90045; **Phone:** (310) 665-7200; **Board Cert:** Orthopaedic Surgery 1968; **Med School:** Loma Linda Univ 1956; **Resid:** Orthopaedic Surgery, Los Angeles Co Genl Hosp, Los Angeles, CA 1960-1964; **Fac Appt:** Clin Prof Orthopaedic Surgery, USC Sch Med

Schechter, David Louis MD (SM) - *Spec Exp:* Pain-Back; Sports Injuries; Muscle Pain-Stress Related; **Hospital:** Cedars-Sinai Med Ctr; **Address:** 50 N La Cienega Blvd , Ste 100, Beverly Hills, CA 90211; **Phone:** (310) 659-7414; **Board Cert:** Sports Medicine 1993, Family Practice 2001; **Med School:** NYU Sch Med 1984; **Resid:** Family Practice, UCLA/Santa Monica Hosp, Santa Monica, CA 1984-1987; **Fac Appt:** Assoc Clin Prof Family Practice, USC Sch Med

SURGERY

A surgeon manages a broad spectrum of surgical conditions affecting almost any area of the body. The surgeon establishes the diagnosis and provides the preoperative, operative and postoperative care to surgical patients and is usually responsible for the comprehensive management of the trauma victim and the critically ill surgical patient.

The surgeon uses a variety of diagnostic techniques, including endoscopy, for observing internal structures and may use specialized instruments during operative procedures. A general surgeon is expected to be familiar with the salient features of other surgical specialties in order to recognize problems in those areas and to know when to refer a patient to another specialist.

Training required: Five years

For a description of the subspecialty **Hand Surgery** *(see page 273)*, **Pediatric Surgery**, *(see page 666)* and **Vascular Surgery** *(see page 921)*

THE CENTER FOR MINIMALLY INVASIVE AND LAPAROSCOPIC SURGERY
MAIMONIDES MEDICAL CENTER

4802 Tenth Avenue • Brooklyn, NY 11219
Phone (718) 283-8860   Fax (718) 635-7102
www.maimonidesmed.org

Brooklyn's first center for minimally invasive surgery offers advanced laparoscopic procedures for a variety of conditions. The Medical Center's commitment to this form of surgery includes an investment in new surgical suites that will be dedicated to laparoscopic procedures. In addition, the center will establish training programs for both attending surgeons and residents.

Celia Divino, MD, heads the new center as Director of Minimally Invasive and Laparoscopic Surgery. Her associate, Brooke Gurland, MD, is a colorectal surgeon who also specializes in pelvic floor disease.

PIONEERING ROBOTIC SURGERY

Maimonides is also the first hospital in Brooklyn to perform robotic surgery with the da Vinci Surgical System. This revolutionary equipment makes minimally invasive operations easier, and also allows surgeons to pioneer procedures that have never or rarely been done laparoscopically. The purchase of this system is one of many innovations overseen by Chairman of Surgery Joseph Cunningham, MD.

Among the conditions that Maimonides can treat laparoscopically are appendicitis, gallstones, hernias, gastro-esophageal reflux disease, Crohn's disease, ulcerative colitis, inflammatory bowel disease, peptic ulcers, tumors and morbid obesity.

CENTER FOR MINIMALLY INVASIVE AND LAPAROSCOPIC SURGERY

One of the most exciting developments in surgery, **robotics** takes minimally invasive surgery to an even higher level of precision. Maimonides is proud to be the first hospital in Brooklyn to establish a center dedicated to this type of surgery. With benefits such as less pain, smaller scars and reduced chance of post-operative complications, minimally invasive surgery is expected to become the preferred method for many patients.

THE MOUNT SINAI HOSPITAL
MINIMALLY INVASIVE SURGERY

One Gustave L. Levy Place (Fifth Avenue and 98th Street)
New York, NY 10029-6574   Phone: (212) 241-6500
Physician Referral: 1-800-MD-SINAI (637-4624)
www.mountsinai.org

The expert surgeons at Mount Sinai continue to be at the forefront in the use of minimally invasive surgery techniques in highly advanced procedures, such as radical prostatectomies, radical nephrectomies, systectomies, and cryosurgery.

Using these advanced techniques, and with the advent of specialized state-of-the-art instruments, surgery to the gallbladder, prostate, stomach, heart, and intestines has become commonplace.

We also provide specialized and unique expertise in treating cancer of the kidney, bladder, and prostate, all with minimally invasive approaches.

Here are a few of the advanced procedures we perform:

Cardiac Surgeries
We perform many procedures using minimally invasive approaches, including **aortic valve replacement, mitral valve replacement, mitral valve repair,** and **off-pump coronary artery bypasses.**

Weight Loss Surgeries
Laparoscopic gastric bypass is the laparoscopic version of the "gold standard" weight-loss operation. The **Biliopancreatic diversion with Duodenal Switch** was first performed laparoscopically at Mount Sinai.

Urologic Surgery
We can perform most traditional open surgeries laparoscopically, including: **nephrectomy, nephroureterectomy, radical prostatectomy,** and **cystectomy.**

Transplant Surgeries
With **laparoscopic kidney donation,** we can remove kidneys from living donors using laparoscopic techniques.

Vascular Surgery
We can treat **abdominal aortic aneurysms** through insertion of a stent graft within the blood vessel itself.

Gynecologic Surgeries
We routinely treat **endometriosis, uterine fibroids, ovarian cysts,** and **urinary incontinence** by laparoscopy. **Uterine, cervical,** and **ovarian cancers** are also performed laparoscopically by our expert gynecologic oncologists.

THE MOUNT SINAI HOSPITAL

Our already excellent staff was recently joined by additional world-renowned physicians, including Dr. Scott J. Swanson, who is a pioneer in the field of minimally invasive lung and esophageal surgery, and Dr. Lishan Aklog, who is a leader in the development of minimally invasive cardiac surgery techniques.

In a recent *New York Magazine* ranking of the area's top minimally invasive surgeons in a variety of specialties, Mount Sinai's physicians were consistently at the top of the lists, including gynecologic oncology surgery, obstetrical surgery, colon and rectal surgery, liver and bilary surgery, thyroid surgery, hernia surgery, gastrointestinal surgery, thoracic surgery, and vascular surgery.

Compared with traditional open surgery, minimally invasive procedures result in less tissue trauma, less scarring, and faster postoperative recovery time. Although the techniques vary from procedure to procedure and among different surgical subspecialties, minimally invasive surgical procedures typically employ video cameras and lens systems to provide anatomic visualization within a region of the body.

THE MOUNT SINAI HOSPITAL
TRANSPLANTATION

One Gustave L. Levy Place (Fifth Avenue and 98th Street)
New York, NY 10029-6574   Phone: (212) 241-6500
Physician Referral: 1-800-MD-SINAI (637-4624)
www.mountsinai.org

Technological advances, along with improved medical therapies, continue to make hopes of a normal life after organ transplant a reality. Today, transplantation has become an accepted form of treatment for adults and children with a wide variety of diseases.

Intensely committed to clinical and basic science research, members of Mount Sinai's Transplant Institute investigate ways to improve organ preservation, reduce post-transplant complications, and the side effects of immunosuppression. They also focus on the prevention of disease after transplant, and overall quality of life after this relatively new medical miracle.

A History of Achievement
Mount Sinai surgeons were the first in New York State to perform liver transplantation, and also the first in the state to perform living donor liver transplantation. We perform more of these transplants than any other institution in the country.

Continuing The Tradition of Excellence
Mount Sinai is one of the few hospitals in the country with expertise in **small intestine/small bowel transplantation.** Working closely with each patient's referring physician, state-of-the-art procedures are performed that profoundly affect patients' lives. Treatment at the Hospital is not the end of the relationship, however: caregivers at Mount Sinai continue to work with the referring physician to help maintain the patient's optimum health level.

A Sampling Of Our Innovative Programs:
The Kidney/Pancreas Transplant Program began over 30 years ago, making Mount Sinai one of the first kidney transplant programs in the region. Today, the Hospital has performed over 1,000 kidney transplants and approximately 50 pancreas transplants or combination kidney/pancreas procedures, both for adults and children. Although pancreas transplantation has gained widespread acceptance in the United States, Mount Sinai is one of the few centers in the greater New York area that perform the operation, and is among the largest programs in the Northeast.

Our *Intestinal Transplant Program* is one of the most established and respected in the country. We offer a comprehensive approach to intestinal failure, and have developed a team approach that includes specialists from different fields working together to achieve the best possible result for the patient.

THE MOUNT SINAI HOSPITAL

U.S. News & World Report's "America's Best Hospitals" 2001 issue ranked Mount Sinai # 3 in intestine transplant and #1 in adult living-donor liver transplant and #2 in pediatric living-donor transplant.

The Recanati/Miller Transplantation Institute brings together clinical programs in adult and pediatric liver, kidney, pancreas, intestine and lung disease and includes a major research initiative.

We are one of the largest liver transplant centers in the United States, performing close to 200 procedures annually. Patients from around the world come to Mount Sinai for liver transplants, including living-donor and traditional surgeries.

The total volume of organ transplants at Mount Sinai places the hospital among the top three nationally.

NewYork-Presbyterian
The University Hospitals of Columbia and Cornell

Columbia Weill Cornell Transplantation Institute

Columbia Presbyterian Medical Center
622 West 168th Street
New York, NY 10032

NewYork Weill Cornell Medical Center
525 East 68th Street
New York, NY 10021

OVERVIEW:

The Columbia Weill Cornell Transplantation Institute is one of the leading centers of its kind in the United States. It brings together the outstanding transplantation programs of two major academic medical centers – Columbia Presbyterian and NewYork Weill Cornell – both recognized for their pioneering research and depth of clinical expertise in transplantation. The Institute's physicians and surgeons, who are leaders in their respective specialties, possess a level of unparalleled experience and skill that contributes to the strength of their individual transplantation programs, including:

- Heart – the world's largest and most experienced heart transplantation for adults and children. Offering surgical innovations and procedures not performed anywhere else.

- Kidney – one of the oldest kidney transplant programs in the country for treating adults and children with end-stage renal disease. A leader in transplanting kidneys from living related or unrelated donors using minimally invasive surgical procedure, laparoscopy.

- Pancreas – one of the largest whole organ pancreas transplant programs in the Northeast. Surgeons are among the most experienced in the country for transplanting the pancreas to treat Type I (juvenile) diabetes.

- Liver – dedicated to diagnosing and treating all forms of liver and biliary disease in adults and children. A leader in living donor transplantation in which a healthy person donates a portion of his or her liver, which can regenerate itself.

- Lung – a major single or double lung transplant program in the New York metropolitan area. Treats patients with severe end-stage pulmonary disease for which there is no alternative treatment other than transplantation.

Physician Referral: For a physician referral or to learn more about Columbia Weill Cornell Psychiatry call toll free **1-877-NYP-WELL** (1-877-697-9355) or visit our Web site at **www.nyp.org**.

INSTITUTE HIGHLIGHTS INCLUDE:

- The leading center for use of left ventricular assist devices (LVADs) as a bridge or an alternative to heart transplantation.

- In the forefront of developing and improving drugs to keep the body from rejecting a new organ.

- Actively involved in major research and clinical trials funded by NIH and the Juvenile Diabetes Research Foundation for islet cell transplantation, which shows promise for curing diabetes – the leading cause of kidney disease.

- Special state-of-the-art inpatient transplant units and comprehensive outpatient services.

NYU Medical Center

550 First Avenue (at 31st Street)
New York, NY 10016
Physician Referral: (888) 7-NYU-MED
(888-769-8633)
www.mininvasive.med.nyu.edu

SCHOOL OF MEDICINE

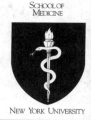

NEW YORK UNIVERSITY

MINIMALLY INVASIVE SURGERY AT NYU MEDICAL CENTER

NYU Medical Center has been at the forefront of minimally invasive surgery for two decades, treating conditions from heart disease, to prostate cancer, to obesity, to fetal anomalies in utero. Today, more patients are opting for minimally invasive procedures, a decision resulting in less pain, scarring, and surgical trauma. Post-operative recovery is also significantly reduced, allowing patients to resume their normal activities much sooner than with traditional surgery.

In 1996, surgeons at NYU Medical Center performed the world's first minimally invasive valve repair and replacement, as well as the world's first triple cardiac bypass surgery. NYU vascular surgeons and radiologists helped pioneer minimally invasive aneurysm repair. In 1997, the Center installed the city's first Gamma Knife, a neurosurgical tool that allows surgeons to remove brain tumors that were once inoperable.

The Department of Surgery at New York University School of Medicine is a highly regarded and nationally recognized academic department. The department comprises divisions of:

- Cardiothoracic Surgery
- Minimally Invasive Surgery
- Pediatric Surgery
- Plastic Surgery (reconstructive and cosmetic)
- Surgical Oncology
- Transplantation Surgery
- Vascular Surgery

Many faculty members receive national and international recognition for their work and hold leadership positions in both regional and national surgical societies. The department's goal is to develop leaders in clinical surgery and to provide the optimal academic surgical environment for patients, residents, and staff.

NYU MEDICAL CENTER

NYU is also taking the lead in noninvasive diagnostic procedures such as colonoscopy and bronchoscopy. MRI and CT scans have in many instances replaced the traditional angiogram to diagnose aortic aneurysm and vascular disease. For more information about these and other noninvasive tests, call 212-263-8904.

Physician Referral
(888) 7-NYU-MED

(888-769-8633)

www.mininvasive.med.nyu.edu

SHANDS TRANSPLANT CENTER AT THE UNIVERSITY OF FLORIDA

SHANDS AT THE UNIVERSITY OF FLORIDA

1600 SW Archer Road, Gainesville, FL 32610
Patient referral: 800.749.7424
Physician-to-physician referral: 800.633.2122
www.shands.org

WORLD-CLASS TRANSPLANT CARE

Since 1966, when University of Florida surgeons at Shands performed Florida's first successful kidney transplant, Shands Transplant Center at UF has expanded to offer the full range of transplant programs—kidney, kidney-pancreas, pancreas, liver, heart, lung and heart-lung. The center is one of only a handful of centers in the country that consistently performs more than 300 solid-organ transplants annually. Shands Transplant Center at UF is a leading referral center in the Southeast, and ranked 11th in the nation by volume of transplants performed in 2000.

The programs are truly multidisciplinary and draw on the combined skills and experience of experts in surgery, medicine, pediatrics, anesthesia, pathology, radiology, pharmacy, nursing, social work, physical therapy and psychology. Program members are recognized leaders in the field of transplantation. They are involved in research and clinical trials, and they are active on transplant policy-making committees.

SPECIALIZED SERVICES

The center offers both adult and pediatric transplant programs, each with dedicated physicians and support staff. The center provides transplant housing for patients and their immediate family, both on-site next to Shands at UF and off-site close to the medical center. Detailed patient education conferences, transplant support groups, and specialized clinics in areas such as compliance and lifestyle change also are available. Such experience and support results in patient and graft survival rates that are among the best in the country.

Services also include live-donor liver transplantation, a ventricular assist device program, and laparoscopic nephrectomy - hand-assisted, live-donor kidney removal using minimally invasive technology.

PHYSICIAN REFERRAL

The Shands Consultation Center is your link to UF physicians at the Shands Transplant Center at UF. For more information or to schedule an appointment, please call 800.749.7424 or visit our Web site at shands.org.

CLINICAL TRIALS AND RESEARCH

A variety of clinical trials and research efforts are fueled by collaboration among many specialists at UF's Health Science Center, including representatives from the Departments of Surgery, Physiology and Medicine at UF's College of Medicine; the Departments of Physical Therapy and Clinical and Health Psychology at UF's College of Health Professions; and the Department of Clinical Practice at UF's College of Pharmacy.

WESTCHESTER MEDICAL CENTER
WORLD-CLASS MEDICINE THAT'S NOT A WORLD AWAY.®

Valhalla Campus • *Valhalla, NY 10595* • *(914) 493-8251*

Website: www.worldclassmedicine.com

OVERVIEW

Several times a day STAT Flight, Westchester Medical Center's air and ground medical transport team, is called into action. STAT Flight responds around the clock to emergencies in the seven-county Hudson Valley region. Two highly trained helicopter teams, comprised of certified critical care flight nurses, veteran pilots and experienced paramedics, are based at the Medical Center and in Orange County, covering nearly 5,000 square miles at a moment's notice.

The STAT Flight team is trained to handle even the smallest of victims, with some transports involving babies weighing as little as two pounds. Our "mobile intensive care units" also include the STAT Flight ground team, dispatched when air transport is not an option. Whether by air or ground, the most severely ill or injured people from the region are ensured rapid transport to Westchester Medical Center's awaiting trauma team and Emergency Department. The Medical Center's on-site trauma team ensures that specialists, including cardiac surgeons, orthopaedic surgeons, burn specialists, neurosurgeons and obstetrical, neonatal and pediatric specialists, are available around the clock.

With the only Burn Center between New York City and the Canadian border, Westchester Medical Center offers hope for survival and a productive life to hundreds of burn victims each year. The Burn Center— named for a dedicated firefighter and burn center supporter, Hank Longo—has a team of 50 highly trained and dedicated burn specialists providing a full range of services from intensive care through rehabilitation. The unit is self-contained to minimize the risk of infection to the most susceptible of patients. It has private rooms and its own state-of-the-art operating rooms and treatment areas. Family rooms, day rooms and a kitchen make patients and families as comfortable as possible during what can be a long recovery period. The Burn Center is also home to the regional Advanced Wound Therapy and Hyperbaric Center, treating burn victims as well as people with a wide variety of injuries and wounds, including divers and victims of carbon monoxide poisoning. The Burn Center represents a commitment to a critical need in the region and the state. While other hospitals have closed similar units due to expense, Westchester Medical Center keeps its doors open to those devastated by burn injuries.

TRAUMA AND BURN CENTER

Known for our comprehensive emergency response system, including our award-winning STAT Flight team and Trauma and Burn teams, Westchester Medical Center has the distinction of being home to:

- The region's only Level 1 Trauma Center
- The only Adult Trauma Center, Pediatric Trauma Center and Burn Center in New York State accredited by the American College of Surgeons
- The only Burn Center between New York City and the Canadian border.
- The Regional Advanced Wound Therapy and Hyperbaric Center
- The region's only Pediatric Intensive Care facility
- The region's only hospital-based emergency air and ground transport program for critically ill and injured patients

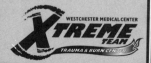

WESTCHESTER MEDICAL CENTER
WORLD-CLASS MEDICINE THAT'S NOT A WORLD AWAY.®

Valhalla Campus • Valhalla, NY 10595 • (914) 493-2504

Website: www.worldclassmedicine.com

OVERVIEW

The Transplant Center at Westchester Medical Center provides hundreds of people of all ages with a new lease on life every year. Our multidisciplinary team of physicians, nurse coordinators, social workers, nutritionists, psychiatrists and financial counselors work with patients and family members through each phase of the transplant experience. Our physicians, surgeons and transplant coordinators are able to provide the latest techniques in transplantation, and the team is committed to remaining at the forefront of this constantly evolving area of medicine.

In 1996, Westchester Medical Center performed the first-ever liver transplant in the Hudson Valley and, since then, has exceed all expectations. Since 1996, the Liver Transplant Program has performed 88 transplants, including four in children who received a segment of their parent's liver—a procedure that has been very successful at Westchester Medical Center. As an academic medical center, many patients benefit from drug studies currently underway prior to even considering liver transplantation.

The Kidney Transplant Program at Westchester Medical Center, now in its 13th year, has performed over 1,000 kidney transplants, making it the largest and busiest kidney program in New York State. Living-related kidney transplants are now performed regularly, providing improved graft survival rates, a decrease in immunosuppressive therapy and the ability to plan the time of transplantation.

Westchester Medical Center offers pancreas transplant, an accepted treatment for patients with end-stage renal disease and Type I diabetes. Successful pancreas transplantation can render the diabetic patient insulin free with an improved quality of life. Additionally, the Transplant Center performs hundreds of corneal transplants a year (most for children) and all types of bone marrow transplant.

The recently established Heart Transplant Program completes the Medical Center's Transplant program. Westchester Medical Center is now home to the only comprehensive heart failure, heart assist device and heart transplant program between New York City and Albany.

Westchester Medical Center is dedicated to all aspects of transplant and organ and tissue donation. For several years, we have been honored by the New York Organ Donor Network for our efforts.

TRANSPLANT CENTER

At the Transplant Center at Westchester Medical Center, we pride ourselves on providing transplant services that rival any major medical center. Our renowned physicians and surgeons work closely with a team of nurse coordinators, social workers, nutri-tionists, psychiatrists and financial counselors to guide patients and families through each phase of the transplant experience. We are committed to providing the latest techniques in transplantation and to staying at the forefront of this dynamic medical field.

Services at the Transplant Center include:

• Liver Transplant

• Kidney Transplant

• Pancreas Transplant

• Heart Transplant

• Corneal Transplant

• Bone Marrow Transplant

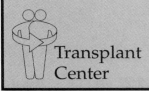

Transplant Center

PHYSICIAN LISTINGS

Surgery

New England

Auchincloss Jr, Hugh MD (S) - *Spec Exp:* Transplant-Kidney & Pancreas; Vascular Access; **Hospital:** Brigham & Women's Hosp; **Address:** Dept Transplant Surgery, 15 Francis St, rm PBB-215, Boston, MA 02115; **Phone:** (617) 732-6866; **Board Cert:** Surgery 1985; **Med School:** Harvard Med Sch 1976; **Resid:** Surgery, Mass General Hosp, Boston, MA 1977-1985; **Fellow:** Transplant Surgery, Mass General Hosp, Boston, MA 1985; **Fac Appt:** Assoc Prof Surgery, Harvard Med Sch

Becker, James MD (S) - *Spec Exp:* Inflammatory Bowel Disease; Colon Cancer; Gastrointestinal Disorders; **Hospital:** Boston Med Ctr; **Address:** Boston Med Ctr-Dept Surgery, 88 E Newton St, rm C500, Boston, MA 02118-2393; **Phone:** (617) 638-8600; **Board Cert:** Surgery 1999; **Med School:** Case West Res Univ 1975; **Resid:** Surgery, Univ Utah Med Ctr, Salt Lake City, UT 1975-1980; **Fellow:** Research, Mayo Clinic, Rochester, MN 1980-1982; **Fac Appt:** Prof Surgery, Boston Univ

Blackburn, George L MD/PhD (S) - *Spec Exp:* Obesity/Bariatric Surgery; Eating Disorders; **Hospital:** Beth Israel Deaconess Med Ctr - Boston; **Address:** 1 Autum St, Ste 1B, Boston, MA 02215; **Phone:** (617) 632-8543; **Board Cert:** Surgery 1972; **Med School:** Univ Kans 1965; **Resid:** Surgery, Boston City Hosp, Boston, MA 1965-1970; **Fac Appt:** Assoc Prof Surgery, Harvard Med Sch

Cady, Blake MD (S) - *Spec Exp:* Breast Cancer; Thyroid Cancer; **Hospital:** Women & Infants Hosp - Rhode Island; **Address:** Women & Infants Hosp - Breast Hlth Ctr, 101 Dudley St, Providence, RI 02905; **Phone:** (401) 453-7540; **Board Cert:** Surgery 1966; **Med School:** Cornell Univ-Weill Med Coll 1957; **Resid:** Surgery, Boston City Hosp, Boston, MA 1961-1965; Surgery, NY Meml Cancer Hosp, New York, NY 1965-1967; **Fac Appt:** Prof Surgery, Brown Univ

Cioffi, William MD (S) - *Spec Exp:* Trauma; **Hospital:** Rhode Island Hosp; **Address:** Rhode Island Hosp, Dept Surg, 2 Dudley St, Ste 470, Providence, RI 02905; **Phone:** (401) 553-8348; **Board Cert:** Surgery 1987, Surgical Critical Care 1988; **Med School:** Univ VT Coll Med 1981; **Resid:** Surgery, Med Ctr Hosp VT, Burlington, VT 1981-1986; **Fac Appt:** Assoc Prof Surgery, Brown Univ

Dudrick, Stanley MD (S) - *Spec Exp:* Critical Care; Laparoscopic Surgery; Total Parenteral Nutrition; **Hospital:** Bridgeport Hosp; **Address:** Dept Surgery, 8th Fl, 267 Grant St, Bridgeport, CT 06610; **Phone:** (203) 384-3273; **Board Cert:** Surgery 1968; **Med School:** Univ Penn 1961; **Resid:** Surgery, Hosp Univ Penn, Philadelphia, PA 1962-1967; **Fellow:** Research, Hosp Univ Penn, Philadelphia, PA 1962-1967; **Fac Appt:** Prof Surgery, Yale Univ

Hebert, James C MD (S) - *Spec Exp:* Biliary Surgery; **Hospital:** Fletcher Allen Hlth Care Med Ctr - Campus; **Address:** Fletcher Allen Hlth Care, 100 Colchester Ave, Fletcher 301, Burlington, VT 05401; **Phone:** (802) 656-5354; **Board Cert:** Surgery 2000; **Med School:** Univ VT Coll Med 1977; **Resid:** Surgery, Med Ctr Hosp, Burlington, VT 1978-1982; **Fac Appt:** Prof Surgery, Univ VT Coll Med

Iglehart, J Dirk MD (S) - *Spec Exp:* Breast Cancer; **Hospital:** Brigham & Women's Hosp; **Address:** Brigham & Women's Hosp, Sept Surgery, 75 Francis St, Boston, MA 02115; **Phone:** (617) 732-6437; **Board Cert:** Surgery 1995; **Med School:** Harvard Med Sch 1975; **Resid:** Surgery, Duke Univ Med Ctr, Durham, NC 1976-1981; Thoracic Surgery, Duke Univ Med Ctr, Durgam, NC 1981-1984; **Fac Appt:** Prof Surgery, Harvard Med Sch

Jenkins, Roger L MD (S) - *Spec Exp:* Transplant-Liver; **Hospital:** Lahey Cli.; **Address:** 41 Mall Rd, Ste 4W, Burlington, MA 01805; **Phone:** (781) 744-2500; **Board Cert:** Surgery 1993; **Med School:** Univ VT Coll Med 1977; **Resid:** Surgery, New Eng Deaconess Hosp, Boston, MA 1977-1982; **Fellow:** Transplant Surgery, Univ Pittsburgh Hosp, Pittsburgh, PA 1983; **Fac Appt:** Assoc Prof Surgery, Harvard Med Sch

Krag, David MD (S) - *Spec Exp:* Sentinel Lymph Node Mapping for BC; **Hospital:** Vermont Univ Coll of Med; **Address:** Surgery Given Bldg. E309C, Burlington, VT 05405; **Phone:** (802) 656-5830; **Board Cert:** Surgery 1996; **Med School:** Loyola Univ-Stritch Sch Med 1980; **Resid:** Surgery, UC Davis Medical Center, Davis, CA 1980-1983; **Fellow:** Surgical Oncology, UCLA Medical Center, Los Angeles, CA 1983-1984; **Fac Appt:** Assoc Prof Surgery, Univ VT Coll Med

Lipkowitz, George S. MD (S) - *Spec Exp:* Transplant-Kidney; **Hospital:** Baystate Med Ctr; **Address:** 208 Ashley Ave, West Springfield, MA 01089; **Phone:** (413) 750-3440; **Board Cert:** Surgery 1986; **Med School:** SUNY Downstate 1980; **Resid:** Surgery, SUNY Kings Co Hosp, Brooklyn, NY 1981-1985; **Fellow:** Transplant Surgery, SUNY Hlth Scis Ctr, Brooklyn, NY 1985-1986; **Fac Appt:** Assoc Prof Surgery, Tufts Univ

Monaco, Anthony MD (S) - *Spec Exp:* Transplant-Kidney; Transplant-Pancreas; **Hospital:** Beth Israel Deaconess Med Ctr - Boston; **Address:** Beth Israel Deaconess Med Ctr-The Transplant Center, 110 Francis St Fl 7, Boston, MA 02215; **Phone:** (617) 632-9822; **Board Cert:** Surgery 1963, Thoracic Surgery 1965; **Med School:** Harvard Med Sch 1956; **Resid:** Surgery, Mass Genl Hosp, Boston, MA 1957-1963; **Fellow:** Immunopathology, Mass Genl Hosp, Boston, MA 1960; **Fac Appt:** Prof Surgery, Harvard Med Sch

Osteen, Robert T MD (S) - *Spec Exp:* Breast Cancer; **Hospital:** Brigham & Women's Hosp; **Address:** Brigham & Women's Hosp- Dept Surgical Oncology, 75 Francis St, Boston, MA 02115-6110; **Phone:** (617) 732-6718; **Board Cert:** Surgery 1995; **Med School:** Duke Univ 1966; **Resid:** Surgery, Duke University Med Ctr, Durham 1967-1968; Surgery, PB Brigham, Boston, MA 1970-1975; **Fac Appt:** Assoc Prof Surgery, Harvard Med Sch

Salem, Ronald R MD (S) - *Spec Exp:* Cancer Surgery; Transplant-Liver; **Hospital:** Yale - New Haven Hosp; **Address:** Dept Surgery, 333 Cedar St, Box 208062, New Haven, CT 06520; **Phone:** (203) 785-3577; **Board Cert:** Surgery 1991; **Med School:** Zimbabwe 1978; **Resid:** Surgery, Hammersmith Hosp, London, England 1981-1985; Surgery, New Eng-Deaconess Hosp, Boston, MA 1987-1989; **Fac Appt:** Asst Prof Surgery, Yale Univ

Singer, Samuel MD (S) - *Spec Exp:* Soft Tissue Sarcoma; Melanoma; **Hospital:** Brigham & Women's Hosp; **Address:** Brigham & Women's Hosp, Div Surg Onc, 75 Francis St, Boston, MA 02115-6195; **Phone:** (617) 732-6980; **Board Cert:** Surgery 1998; **Med School:** Harvard Med Sch 1982; **Resid:** Surgery, Brigham & Women's Hosp, Boston, MA 1983-1988; **Fellow:** Surgical Oncology, Dana Farber Cancer Inst, Boston, MA 1988-1990; **Fac Appt:** Asst Prof Surgery, Harvard Med Sch

Smego, Douglas MD (S) - *Spec Exp:* Tumor Surgery; Laparoscopic Abdominal Surgery; **Hospital:** Stamford Hosp; **Address:** 1250 Summer St, Ste 303, Stamford, CT 06905-5318; **Phone:** (203) 327-6755; **Board Cert:** Surgery 1993; **Med School:** UMDNJ-NJ Med Sch, Newark 1977; **Resid:** Surgery, New York Hosp-Cornell Med Ctr, New York, NY 1978-1982; **Fellow:** Trauma, Univ Louisville, Louisville, KY 1982-1983

Smith, Barbara Lynn MD (S) - *Spec Exp:* Breast Cancer; **Hospital:** MA Genl Hosp; **Address:** Mass General Hosp-Gillette Ctr, 100 Blossom St Bldg Cox - Ste 1, Boston, MA 02114; **Phone:** (617) 724-4800; **Board Cert:** Surgery 1990; **Med School:** Harvard Med Sch 1983; **Resid:** Surgery, Brigham & Women's Hosp, Boston, MA 1983-1989; **Fac Appt:** Asst Prof Surgery, Harvard Med Sch

utton, John E. MD (S) - *Spec Exp:* Breast Cancer; **Hospital:** Dartmouth - Hitchcock Med Ctr; **address:** One Medical Center Drive, Lebanon, NH 03756; **Phone:** (603) 650-8022; **Board Cert:** urgery 1990, Surgical Critical Care 1995; **Med School:** Georgetown Univ 1974; **Resid:** Surgery, Dartmouth-Hitchcock Med Ctr, Lebanon, NH 1975-1981; **Fellow:** Critical Care Medicine, Dartmouth-Hitchcock Med Ctr, Lebanon, NH 1982-1983; **Fac Appt:** Prof Surgery, Dartmouth Med ch

anabe, Kenneth K MD (S) - *Spec Exp:* Liver Cancer; Colon & Rectal Cancer; Melanoma; **Hospital:** MA Genl Hosp; **Address:** Mass General Hosp.-Div. Surg. Onc., 100 Blossom St, Bldg Cox rm 626, Boston, MA 02114; **Phone:** (617) 726-8555; **Board Cert:** Surgery 1991; **Med School:** UCSD 985; **Resid:** Surgery, NY Cornell Hosp., New York, NY 1986-1990; **Fellow:** Surgical Oncology, MD Anderson Cancer Ctr., Houston, TX 1990; **Fac Appt:** Assoc Prof Surgery, Harvard Med Sch

ilney, Nicholas MD (S) - *Spec Exp:* Transplant-Kidney; **Hospital:** Brigham & Women's Hosp; **address:** 75 Francis St, Boston, MA 02115; **Phone:** (617) 732-6817; **Board Cert:** Surgery 1972; **Med chool:** Cornell Univ-Weill Med Coll 1962; **Resid:** Surgery, Peter Bent Brigham Hosp, Boston, MA 969-1971; **Fellow:** Cellular Immunology, Sir William Dunn Sch Path, Oxford, England 1971-1972; Cellular Immunology, Western Infirm Univ, Glasgow, Scotland 1972-1973; **Fac Appt:** Prof Surgery, Harvard Med Sch

Jdelsman, Robert MD (S) - *Spec Exp:* Parathyroid Minimally Invasive Surgery; Adrenal Minimally Invasive Surgery; **Hospital:** Yale - New Haven Hosp; **Address:** Yale School of Medicine, MB102 Bldg, 330 Cedar St, Box 208062, New Haven, CT 06520-8062; **Phone:** (203) 785-2697; **Board Cert:** Surgery 1990; **Med School:** Geo Wash Univ 1981; **Resid:** Surgery, Natl Inst Hlth, Bethesda, MD 1983-1986; Surgery, Johns Hopkins Univ Hosp, Baltimore, MD 1986-1989; **Fac Appt:** Prof Surgery, Yale Univ

Ward, Barbara MD (S) - *Spec Exp:* Breast Cancer; Tumor Surgery; **Hospital:** Greenwich Hosp; **address:** 77 Lafayette Pl, Greeenwich, CT 06830; **Phone:** (203) 863-4300; **Board Cert:** Surgery 991; **Med School:** Temple Univ 1983; **Resid:** Surgery, Yale-New Haven Hosp, New Haven, CT 984-1985; Surgery, Yale-New Haven Hosp, New Haven, CT 1987-1990; **Fellow:** Surgical Oncology, Natl Cancer Inst, Bethesda, MD 1985-1987; **Fac Appt:** Assoc Prof Surgery

Warshaw, Andrew L MD (S) - *Spec Exp:* Pancreatic Cancer; Pancreatic Surgery; **Hospital:** MA Genl Hosp; **Address:** 55 Fruit St, Bldg WHT 506, Boston, MA 02114-2696; **Phone:** (617) 726-8254; **Board Cert:** Surgery 1971, Surgical Critical Care 1986; **Med School:** Harvard Med Sch 1963; **Resid:** Surgery, Mass Genl Hosp, Boston, MA 1967-1971; Surgery, Mass Genl Hosp, Boston, MA 964-1965; **Fac Appt:** Prof Surgery, Harvard Med Sch

inner, Michael MD (S) - *Spec Exp:* Gastrointestinal Surgery; **Hospital:** Brigham & Women's Hosp; **Address:** 75 Francis St, Boston, MA 02115; **Phone:** (617) 732-8181; **Board Cert:** Surgery 1988; **Med School:** Univ Fla Coll Med 1971; **Resid:** Surgery, Johns Hopkins Hosp, Baltimore, MD 1973-974; Surgery, Johns Hoskins Hosp, Baltimore, MD 1976-1979; **Fac Appt:** Prof Surgery, Harvard Med Sch

Mid Atlantic

Alfonso, Antonio MD (S) - *Spec Exp:* Breast Cancer; Head & Neck Surgery; **Hospital:** Long Island Coll Hosp (page 58); **Address:** 100 Amity St, FL 1, Brooklyn, NY 11201-6005; **Phone:** (718) 375-3244; **Board Cert:** Surgery 1973; **Med School:** Philippines 1968; **Resid:** Surgery, Temple Univ Hosp, Philadelphia, PA 1968-1972; **Fellow:** Surgical Oncology, Meml Sloan Kettering Cancer Ctr, New York, NY 1972-1974; **Fac Appt:** Prof Surgery, SUNY Hlth Sci Ctr

Ashikari, Roy MD (S) - *Spec Exp:* Breast Cancer; **Hospital:** Saint Agnes Hosp; **Address:** 305 North St, White Plains, NY 10605-2299; **Phone:** (914) 681-9478; **Board Cert:** Surgery 1967; **Med School:** Japan 1958; **Resid:** Surgery, Mount Sinai Hosp, New York, NY 1961-1964; Surgery, Mem Sloan-Kettering Cancer Ctr, New York, NY 1966-1968; **Fellow:** Surgery, Mount Sinai Hosp, New York, NY 1964-1965; **Fac Appt:** Prof Surgery, NY Med Coll

Axelrod, Deborah MD (S) - *Spec Exp:* Breast Cancer; **Hospital:** St Vincent Cath Med Ctrs - Manhattan (page 75); **Address:** 325 W 15th St, New York, NY 10011; **Phone:** (212) 604-6004; **Board Cert:** Surgery 1989; **Med School:** Israel 1982; **Resid:** Surgery, Beth Israel Med Ctr, New York, NY 1983-1988; **Fellow:** Surgical Oncology, Meml Sloan Kettering Cancer Ctr, New York, NY 1985-1986; **Fac Appt:** Asst Prof Surgery, Albert Einstein Coll Med

Ballantyne, Garth MD (S) - *Spec Exp:* Laparoscopic Abdominal Surgery; Gastroesophageal Reflux; Colon Cancer; **Hospital:** Hackensack Univ Med Ctr; **Address:** 20 Prospect Ave, Ste 901, Hackensack, NJ 07601-1974; **Phone:** (201) 996-2959; **Board Cert:** Surgery 1984, Colon & Rectal Surgery 1985; **Med School:** Columbia P&S 1977; **Resid:** Surgery, Columbia, Bergen, NJ 1977-1978; Surgery, Columbia, Bergen, NJ 1978-1979; **Fellow:** Colon & Rectal Surgery, Mayo Clinic, Bergen, NJ 1983-1984; **Fac Appt:** Prof Surgery, UMDNJ-NJ Med Sch, Newark

Bartlett, Stephen Thomas MD (S) - *Spec Exp:* Transplant-Pancreas; Transplant-Kidney; **Hospital:** University of MD Med Sys; **Address:** 29 S Greene St, Ste 200, Baltimore, MD 21201; **Phone:** (410) 328-5408; **Board Cert:** Surgery 1995, Vascular Surgery (General) 1996; **Med School:** Univ Chicago-Pritzker Sch Med 1979; **Resid:** Surgery, Hosp Univ Penn, Philadelphia, PA 1980-1985; **Fellow:** Vascular Surgery (General), Northwestern Univ, Chicago, IL 1985-1986; **Fac Appt:** Prof Surgery, Univ MD Sch Med

Bass, Barbara MD (S) - *Spec Exp:* Surgery - General; **Hospital:** University of MD Med Sys; **Address:** 22 S Greene St, Ste S4B04, Baltimore, MD 21201; **Phone:** (410) 328-8346; **Board Cert:** Surgery 1996; **Med School:** Univ VA Sch Med 1979; **Resid:** Surgery, Geo Wash Univ, Washington, DC 1979-1982; Surgery, Geo Wash Univ, Washington, DC 1984-1986; **Fellow:** Surgery, Walter Reed Inst, Washington, DC 1982-1984; **Fac Appt:** Prof Surgery, Univ MD Sch Med

Bauer, Joel MD (S) - *Spec Exp:* Colon & Rectal Surgery; Inflammatory Bowel Disease; Laparoscopic Surgery; **Hospital:** Mount Sinai Hosp (page 68); **Address:** 25 E 69th St, New York, NY 10021-4925; **Phone:** (212) 517-8600; **Board Cert:** Surgery 1974; **Med School:** NYU Sch Med 1967; **Resid:** Surgery, Mount Sinai Hosp, New York, NY 1967-1973; **Fac Appt:** Prof Surgery, Mount Sinai Sch Med

Borgen, Patrick Ivan MD (S) - *Spec Exp:* Breast Cancer; **Hospital:** Mem Sloan Kettering Cancer Ctr; **Address:** 205 E 64th St, New York, NY 10021; **Phone:** (212) 639-5248; **Board Cert:** Surgery 1991; **Med School:** Louisiana State Univ 1984; **Resid:** Surgery, Ochsner Fdn Hosp, New Orleans, LA 1985-1989; **Fellow:** Surgical Oncology, Meml Sloan Kettering Canc Ctr, New York, NY 1989-1990; **Fac Appt:** Prof Surgery, Cornell Univ-Weill Med Coll

Brennan, Murray MD (S) - *Spec Exp:* Sarcoma; Tumor Surgery; **Hospital:** Mem Sloan Kettering Cancer Ctr; **Address:** 1275 York Ave, rm C1265, New York, NY 10021-6007; **Phone:** (212) 639-6586; **Board Cert:** Surgery 1975; **Med School:** New Zealand 1964; **Resid:** Surgery, Univ Otago Med Sch, Dunedin, New Zealand 1966-1969; **Fellow:** Surgery, Harvard Med Sch, Boston, MA 1970-1972; Surgery, Peter Bent Brigham Hosp, Cambridge, MA 1973-1975; **Fac Appt:** Prof Surgery, Cornell Univ-Weill Med Coll

Burdick, James Frederick MD (S) - *Spec Exp:* Transplant-Kidney; Vascular Surgery; **Hospital:** Johns Hopkins Hosp - Baltimore; **Address:** 600 N Wolfe St, Baltimore, MD 21287-8611; **Phone:** (410) 955-6875; **Board Cert:** Surgery 1997; **Med School:** Harvard Med Sch 1968; **Resid:** Surgery, Mass Genl Hosp, Boston, MA 1969-1970; Surgery, Mass Genl Hosp, Boston, MA 1973-1975; **Fellow:** Research, Mass Genl Hosp, Boston, MA 1976-1977; **Fac Appt:** Prof Surgery, Johns Hopkins Univ

Cameron, John MD (S) - *Spec Exp:* Pancreatic Cancer; **Hospital:** Johns Hopkins Hosp - Baltimore; **Address:** 720 Rutland Ave, Ross Bldg, Ste 759, Baltimore, MD 21205; **Phone:** (410) 955-0166; **Board Cert:** Surgery 1970, Thoracic Surgery 1971; **Med School:** Johns Hopkins Univ 1962; **Resid:** Surgery, Johns Hopkins Hosp, Baltimore, MD 1965-1970; **Fellow:** Thoracic Surgery, Johns Hopkins Hosp, Baltimore, MD 1970-1971; **Fac Appt:** Prof Surgery, Johns Hopkins Univ

Coit, Daniel G MD (S) - *Spec Exp:* Melanoma; Pancreatic & Stomach Cancer; **Hospital:** Meml Sloan Kettering Cancer Ctr; **Address:** 1275 York Ave, New York, NY 10021; **Phone:** (212) 639-8411; **Board Cert:** Surgery 1994; **Med School:** Univ Cincinnati 1976; **Resid:** Internal Medicine, New England Deaconess Hosp, Boston, MA 1977-1978; Surgery, New England Deaconess Hosp, Boston, MA 1978-1983; **Fellow:** Surgery, Meml Sloan Kettering Canc Ctr, New York, NY 1983-1985; **Fac Appt:** Assoc Prof Surgery, Cornell Univ-Weill Med Coll

Conti, David James MD (S) - *Spec Exp:* Transplant-Kidney; **Hospital:** Albany Medical Center; **Address:** Albany Med Ctr, 47 New Scotland Ave, MC 61GE, Albany, NY 12208; **Phone:** (518) 262-5614; **Board Cert:** Surgery 1998; **Med School:** Northwestern Univ 1981; **Resid:** Surgery, McGaw Med Ctr, Chicago, IL 1982-1987; **Fellow:** Surgery, Mass Genl Hosp, Boston, MA 1987-1989; **Fac Appt:** Prof Surgery, Albany Med Coll

Deitch, Edwin MD (S) - *Spec Exp:* Trauma; **Hospital:** UMDNJ-Univ Hosp-Newark; **Address:** Bldg MSB Fl G - rm 506, 185 S Orange Ave, Newark, NJ 07103; **Phone:** (973) 972-5045; **Board Cert:** Surgery 1997, Surgical Critical Care 1995; **Med School:** Univ MD Sch Med 1973; **Resid:** Surgery, US Public Hlth Svc Hosp, Baltimore, MD 1974-1976; Surgery, US Public Hlth Svc Hosp, New Orleans, LA 1976-1978; **Fac Appt:** Prof Surgery, UMDNJ-NJ Med Sch, Newark

Edge, Stephen B MD (S) - *Spec Exp:* Breast Cancer; **Hospital:** Roswell Park Cancer Inst; **Address:** Roswell Park Cancer Inst, Elm & Carlton Streets, Buffalo, NY 14263; **Phone:** (716) 845-8789; **Board Cert:** Surgery 1996; **Med School:** Case West Res Univ 1979; **Resid:** Surgery, Univ Hosp Cleveland, Cleveland, OH 1979-1986; **Fellow:** Surgical Oncology, Natl Cancer Inst, Bethesda, MD 1981-1984; **Fac Appt:** Assoc Prof Surgery, SUNY Buffalo

Edye, Michael MD (S) - *Spec Exp:* Laparoscopic Abdominal Surgery; Transplant-Living Kidney Donor; Gastroesophageal Reflux; **Hospital:** NYU Med Ctr (page 71); **Address:** NYU Med Ctr, Dept Surgery, 530 First Ave, rm 6A, New York, NY 10016; **Phone:** (212) 263-2350; **Med School:** Australia 1977; **Resid:** Surgery, St Vincents Hosp, Sidney, Australia 1978-1980; Surgery, Royal N Shore Hosp, Sidney, Australia 1981-1984; **Fac Appt:** Assoc Prof Surgery, NYU Sch Med

Emond, Jean Crawford MD (S) - *Spec Exp:* Transplant-Liver; Liver Cancer; **Hospital:** NY Presby Hosp - Columbia Presby Med Ctr (page 70); **Address:** 622 W 168th St, Ste PH14, New York, NY 10032; **Phone:** (212) 305-0914; **Board Cert:** Surgery 1985; **Med School:** Univ Chicago-Pritzker Sch Med 1979; **Resid:** Surgery, Cook Cty Hosp/Univ Ill, Chicago, IL 1980-1984; **Fellow:** Surgery, Hopital P Brousse/Univ de Paris Sud, Paris,France 1984-1985; Transplant Surgery, Univ Chicago Hosp, Chicago, IL 1985-1987; **Fac Appt:** Prof Surgery, Columbia P&S

Enker, Warren MD (S) - *Spec Exp:* Tumor Surgery; **Hospital:** Beth Israel Med Ctr - Petrie Division (page 58); **Address:** 350 E 17th St, Ste 1622, New York, NY 10003; **Phone:** (212) 420-3960; **Board Cert:** Surgery 1973; **Med School:** SUNY Hlth Sci Ctr 1967; **Resid:** Surgery, Univ Chicago Hosps-Clinics, Chicago, IL 1968-1972; **Fellow:** Immunopathology, Univ Chicago Hosps-Clinics, Chicago, IL 1972-1973; Immunopathology, Univ Minnesota, Minneapolis, MN 1973-1974; **Fac Appt:** Prof Surgery, Albert Einstein Coll Med

Estabrook, Alison MD (S) - *Spec Exp:* Breast Cancer; **Hospital:** St Luke's - Roosevelt Hosp Ctr - Roosevelt Div (page 58); **Address:** 425 W 59th St, Ste 7A, New York, NY 10019-1104; **Phone:** (212) 523-7500; **Board Cert:** Surgery 1985; **Med School:** NYU Sch Med 1978; **Resid:** Surgery, Columbia Presby Med Ctr, New York, NY 1979-1984; **Fellow:** Surgical Oncology, Columbia Presby Med Ctr, New York, NY 1981-1982; **Fac Appt:** Prof Surgery, NYU Sch Med

Ferzli, George MD (S) - *Spec Exp:* Laparoscopic Surgery; Endocrine Surgery; Breast Surgery; **Hospital:** Staten Island Univ Hosp-North Site; **Address:** 78 Cromwell Ave, Staten Island, NY 10304-3933; **Phone:** (718) 667-8100; **Board Cert:** Surgery 1993, Surgical Critical Care 1994; **Med School:** France 1979; **Resid:** Surgery, Staten Is Univ Hosp, Staten Island, NY 1980-1984; **Fac Appt:** Assoc Clin Prof Surgery, SUNY Downstate

Fowler, Dennis MD (S) - *Spec Exp:* Minimally Invasive Surgery; **Hospital:** NY Presby Hosp - NY Weill Cornell Med Ctr (page 70); **Address:** 525 E 68th St, Ste F763, New York, NY 10021; **Phone:** (212) 746-5599; **Board Cert:** Surgery 1998; **Med School:** Univ Kans 1973; **Resid:** Surgery, St Lukes Hosp, Kansas City, KS 1975-1979; **Fellow:** Surgical Endoscopy, Mass Genl Hosp, Boston, MA 1979-1980; **Fac Appt:** Assoc Prof Surgery, Cornell Univ-Weill Med Coll

Fraker, Douglas Leon MD (S) - *Spec Exp:* Tumor Surgery; **Hospital:** Hosp Univ Penn (page 78); **Address:** Hosp Univ Penn, Dept Surgery, 3400 Spruce St, 4 Silverstein, Philadelphia, PA 19104; **Phone:** (215) 662-7866; **Board Cert:** Surgery 1992; **Med School:** Harvard Med Sch 1983; **Resid:** Surgery, UCSF Med Ctr, San Francisco, CA 1984-1986; Surgery, UCSF Med Ctr, San Francisco, CA 1989-1991; **Fellow:** Surgical Oncology, Nat Cancer Inst, Bethesda, MD 1986-1989; **Fac Appt:** Prof Surgery, Univ Penn

Fung, John J MD/PhD (S) - *Spec Exp:* Transplant-Liver; Transplant-Kidney; **Hospital:** UPMC - Presbyterian Univ Hosp; **Address:** Falk Med Bldg, 3601 Fifth Ave, Ste 4th, Pittsburgh, PA 15213; **Phone:** (412) 648-3200; **Board Cert:** Surgery 1997; **Med School:** Univ Chicago-Pritzker Sch Med 1982; **Resid:** Surgery, Strong Memorial Hosp, Rochester, NY 1983-1988; **Fellow:** Transplant Surgery, Univ Pittsburgh, Pittsburgh, PA 1984-1986; **Fac Appt:** Assoc Prof Surgery, Univ Pittsburgh

Gagner, Michel MD (S) - *Spec Exp:* Parathyroid Endoscopic Surgery; Liver & Biliary Surgery; Robotic Surgery; **Hospital:** Mount Sinai Hosp (page 68); **Address:** 19 E 98th St, Ste 5A, Box 1103, New York, NY 10029; **Phone:** (212) 241-5339; **Board Cert:** Surgery 1990; **Med School:** Canada 1982; **Resid:** Surgery, Royal Victoria Hosp/McGill, Montreal, Canada 1982-1988; **Fellow:** Hepatobiliary Surgery, Hosp Paul-Brousse, Paris, France 1988-1989; Hepatobiliary Surgery, Lahey Clinic, Burlington, MA 1989-1990; **Fac Appt:** Assoc Prof Surgery, Mount Sinai Sch Med

Gibbs, John F MD (S) - *Spec Exp:* Liver Cancer; Hepatobiliary Cancer; **Hospital:** Roswell Park Cancer Inst; **Address:** Roswell Park Cancer Inst, Dept Surgical Oncology, Elm & Carlton Sts, Buffalo, NY 14263; **Phone:** (716) 845-5807; **Board Cert:** Surgery 1991; **Med School:** Univ SD Sch Med 1985; **Resid:** Surgery, Rush Presby-St Luke's Med Ctr, Chicago, IL 1986-1990; **Fellow:** Surgical Oncology, Roswell Park Cancer Inst, Buffalo, NY 1992-1996; **Fac Appt:** Asst Prof Surgery, SUNY Buffalo

Hardy, Mark MD (S) - *Spec Exp:* *Transplant-Kidney; Parathyroid Surgery;* **Hospital:** NY Presby Hosp - Columbia Presby Med Ctr (page 70); **Address:** 161 Fort Washington Ave, New York, NY 10032; **Phone:** (212) 305-5502; **Board Cert:** Surgery 1972; **Med School:** Albert Einstein Coll Med 1962; **Resid:** Surgery, Strong Meml Hosp, Rochester, NY 1963-1964; Surgery, Albert Einstein Med Ctr, Bronx, NY 1966-1971; **Fellow:** Transplant Surgery, Harvard Med Sch, Cambridge, MA 1968-1969; **Fac Appt:** Prof Surgery, Columbia P&S

Hoffman, John P MD (S) - *Spec Exp:* *Pancreatic Cancer; Surgical Oncology;* **Hospital:** Fox Chase Cancer Ctr; **Address:** Fox Chase Cancer Ctr, 7701 Burholme Ave, rm C308, Philadelphia, PA 19111-2412; **Phone:** (215) 728-3518; **Board Cert:** Surgery 1998; **Med School:** Case West Res Univ 1970; **Resid:** Surgery, Virginia Mason Hosp, Seattle, WA 1973-1977; **Fellow:** Surgical Oncology, Meml Sloan Kettering Cancer Ctr, New York, NY 1977-1980; **Fac Appt:** Prof Surgery, Temple Univ

Hofstetter, Steven MD (S) - *Spec Exp:* *Laparoscopic Gallbladder Surgery; Laparoscopic Appendix Surgery;* **Hospital:** NYU Med Ctr (page 71); **Address:** 530 1st Ave, Ste 6C, New York, NY 10016-6402; **Phone:** (212) 263-7302; **Board Cert:** Surgery 2000; **Med School:** SUNY Hlth Sci Ctr 1971; **Resid:** Surgery, Bellevue Hosp, New York, NY 1971-1976; **Fac Appt:** Assoc Prof Surgery, NYU Sch Med

Klein, Andrew S MD (S) - *Spec Exp:* *Transplant-Liver; Liver Cancer; Cirrhosis;* **Hospital:** Johns Hopkins Hosp - Baltimore; **Address:** Johns Hopkins Hosp, 600 N Wolfe St, Harvey 611, Baltimore, MD 21287-8611; **Phone:** (410) 955-5662; **Board Cert:** Surgery 1996; **Med School:** Johns Hopkins Univ 1979; **Resid:** Surgery, Johns Hopkins Hosp, Baltimore, MD 1980-1982; Surgery, Johns Hopkins Hosp, Baltimore, MD 1984-1986; **Fellow:** Transplant Surgery, UCLA-CHS, Los Angeles, CA 1987-1988; **Fac Appt:** Prof Surgery, Johns Hopkins Univ

Kraybill Jr, William G MD (S) - *Spec Exp:* *Sarcoma-Soft Tissue; Melanoma;* **Hospital:** Roswell Park Cancer Inst; **Address:** Roswell Park Cancer Inst, Dept Surgical Oncology, Elm & Carlton St, Buffalo, NY 14263; **Phone:** (716) 845-5807; **Board Cert:** Surgery 1995; **Med School:** Univ Cincinnati 1969; **Resid:** Surgery, Univ Oregon Hlth Sci Ctr, Portland, OR 1972-1978; **Fellow:** Surgical Oncology, Meml Sloan Kettering Cancer Ctr, New York, NY 1978-1980; **Fac Appt:** Assoc Prof Surgery, SUNY Buffalo

Leffall Jr, LaSalle D MD (S) - *Spec Exp:* *Breast Cancer; Head & Neck Surgery;* **Hospital:** Howard Univ Hosp; **Address:** 2041 Georgia Ave NW, Washington, DC 20060; **Phone:** (202) 865-6237; **Board Cert:** Surgery 1958; **Med School:** Howard Univ 1952; **Resid:** Surgery, Freedmens Hosp, Washington, DC 1953-1956; Surgery, DC Genl Hosp, Washington, DC 1954-1955; **Fellow:** Surgery, New York Meml Ctr, New York, NY 1957-1959; **Fac Appt:** Prof Emeritus Surgery, Howard Univ

Lillemoe, Keith Douglas MD (S) - *Spec Exp:* *Pancreatic & Biliary Surgery; Colon Surgery;* **Hospital:** Johns Hopkins Hosp - Baltimore; **Address:** Johns Hopkins Hosp Surg, 600 N Wolfe St, Baltimore, MD 21287-7495; **Phone:** (410) 955-7495; **Board Cert:** Surgery 1986; **Med School:** Johns Hopkins Univ 1978; **Resid:** Surgery, Johns Hopkins Hosp, Baltimore, MD 1979-1985; **Fac Appt:** Prof Surgery, Johns Hopkins Univ

Miller, Charles M MD (S) - *Spec Exp:* *Transplant-Liver; Liver & Biliary Surgery;* **Hospital:** Mount Sinai Hosp (page 68); **Address:** 1 Gustave Levy Pl, Box 1104, New York, NY 10029; **Phone:** (212) 241-8035; **Board Cert:** Surgery 1994; **Med School:** Mount Sinai Sch Med 1978; **Resid:** Surgery, Mount Sinai Hosp, New York, NY 1978-1983; **Fellow:** Transplant Surgery, Mount Sinai Hosp, New York, NY 1980-1981; Vascular Surgery (General), Mount Sinai Hosp, New York, NY 1983-1984; **Fac Appt:** Prof Surgery, Mount Sinai Sch Med

Nava-Villarreal, Hector MD (S) - *Spec Exp:* Esophageal Cancer; Stomach Cancer; **Hospital:** Roswell Park Cancer Inst; **Address:** Roswell Park Cancer Inst, Div UGI Endoscopy, Elm & Carlton Sts, Buffalo, NY 14263; **Phone:** (716) 845-5915; **Board Cert:** Surgery 1990; **Med School:** Mexico 1967; **Resid:** Surgery, Buffalo Genl Hosp, Buffalo, NY 1970-1974; **Fellow:** Surgical Oncology, Roswell Park Cancer Inst, Buffalo, NY 1974-1976; **Fac Appt:** Assoc Prof Surgery, SUNY Buffalo

Numann, Patricia MD (S) - *Spec Exp:* Breast Cancer; Thyroid Surgery; **Hospital:** Univ. Hosp.-SUNY Upstate Med. Univ.; **Address:** SUNY Hlth Sci Ctr, Dept Surg, 750 E Adams Street, rm 8140, Syracuse, NY 13210; **Phone:** (315) 464-4603; **Board Cert:** Surgery 1994; **Med School:** SUNY Syracuse 1965; **Resid:** Surgery, SUNY Upstate Med Ctr, Albany, NY 1966-1970; **Fac Appt:** Prof Surgery, SUNY Syracuse

Pachter, H Leon MD (S) - *Spec Exp:* Laparoscopic Adrenal Surgery; Laparoscopic Abdominal Surgery; **Hospital:** NYU Med Ctr (page 71); **Address:** 530 1st Ave, Ste 6C, New York, NY 10016; **Phone:** (212) 263-7302; **Board Cert:** Surgery 1999; **Med School:** NYU Sch Med 1971; **Resid:** Surgery, NYU Med Ctr, New York, NY 1972-1976; **Fac Appt:** Prof Surgery, NYU Sch Med

Peitzman, Andrew MD (S) - *Spec Exp:* Trauma; **Hospital:** UPMC - Presbyterian Univ Hosp; **Address:** UPP-Trauma Surgery, 3601 Fifth Ave, Bldg Falk - Ste 6B, Pittsburgh, PA 15213; **Phone:** (412) 648-9863; **Board Cert:** Surgery 1994, Surgical Critical Care 1997; **Med School:** Univ Pittsburgh 1976; **Resid:** Surgery, Univ Pittsburgh, Pittsburgh, PA 1977-1979; Surgery, Univ Pittsburgh, Pittsburgh, PA 1981-1984; **Fellow:** Surgery, NY Hosp-Cornell Univ, New York, NY 1979-1981; **Fac Appt:** Prof Surgery, Univ Pittsburgh

Petrek, Jeanne MD (S) - *Spec Exp:* Breast Cancer; **Hospital:** Mem Sloan Kettering Cancer Ctr; **Address:** 205 E 64th St, New York, NY 10021-6635; **Phone:** (212) 639-5246; **Board Cert:** Surgery 1978; **Med School:** Case West Res Univ 1973; **Resid:** Surgery, Brigham & Women's Hosp, Boston, MA 1974-1978; **Fellow:** Surgery, Meml Sloan-Kettering Canc Ctr, New York, NY 1978-1980

Pressman, Peter MD (S) - *Spec Exp:* Breast Cancer; **Hospital:** Beth Israel Med Ctr - Singer Div (page 58); **Address:** 425 E 61st St, Fl 8th, New York, NY 10021-3513; **Phone:** (212) 249-8040; **Board Cert:** Surgery 1967; **Med School:** Columbia P&S 1959; **Resid:** Surgery, Columbia-Presby Med Ctr, New York, NY 1959-1961; Surgery, Columbia-Presby Med Ctr, New York, NY 1961-1963; **Fac Appt:** Clin Prof Surgery, Albert Einstein Coll Med

Reiner, Mark MD (S) - *Spec Exp:* Laparoscopic Surgery-Gastrointestinal; Breast Cancer; **Hospital:** Mount Sinai Hosp (page 68); **Address:** 1010 5th Ave, New York, NY 10028; **Phone:** (212) 879-6677; **Board Cert:** Surgery 1990; **Med School:** SUNY Downstate 1974; **Resid:** Surgery, Mount Sinai Hosp, New York, NY 1974-1979; **Fac Appt:** Clin Prof Surgery, Mount Sinai Sch Med

Roh, Mark S MD (S) - *Spec Exp:* Liver Cancer; **Hospital:** Allegheny General Hosp; **Address:** Allegheny General Hospital, Dept Surgery, 320 E North Ave, Pittsburgh, PA 15212; **Phone:** (412) 359-6738; **Board Cert:** Surgery 1996; **Med School:** Ohio State Univ 1979; **Resid:** Surgery, U Hlth Ctr., Pittsburgh, PA 1984-1986; **Fellow:** Surgical Oncology, Meml Sloan-Kettering Cancer Ctr, New York, NY 1986-1987; **Fac Appt:** Prof Surgery, Med Coll PA Hahnemann

Rombeau, John L MD (S) - *Spec Exp:* Cancer-Colon; Cancer-Gastrointestinal; **Hospital:** Hosp Univ Penn (page 78); **Address:** Hosp Univ Penn, Dept Surg, 3400 Spruce St, 4 Silverstein, Philadelphia, PA 19104; **Phone:** (215) 662-2078; **Board Cert:** Surgery 1992, Colon & Rectal Surgery 1977; **Med School:** Loma Linda Univ 1967; **Resid:** Surgery, Good Samaritan Hosp, Los Angeles, CA 1970-1971; Surgery, LAC-USC Med Ctr, Los Angeles, CA 1971-1975; **Fellow:** Colon & Rectal Surgery, Cleveland Clinic, Cleveland, OH 1975-1976; **Fac Appt:** Prof Sports Medicine, Univ Penn

Rosato, Ernest F MD (S) - *Spec Exp:* Gastrointestinal Surgery; **Hospital:** Hosp Univ Penn (page 78); **Address:** Hosp Univ Penn, Dept Surg, 3400 Spruce St, 4 Silverstein, Philadelphia, PA 19104; **Phone:** (215) 662-2033; **Board Cert:** Surgery 1969; **Med School:** Univ Penn 1962; **Resid:** Surgery, Hosp Univ Penn, Philadelphia, PA 1963-1968; **Fac Appt:** Prof Surgery, Univ Penn

Rosenberg, Steven MD (S) - *Spec Exp:* Tumor Surgery; Melanoma; Kidney Cancer; **Hospital:** Natl Inst of Hlth - Clin Ctr; **Address:** National Cancer Institute, 9000 Rockville Pike Bldg 10 - rm 2-B-42, Bethesda, MD 20892; **Phone:** (301) 496-4164; **Board Cert:** Surgery 1975; **Med School:** Jefferson Med Coll 1964; **Resid:** Surgery, Peter Bent Brigham Hosp, Boston, MA 1968-1974

Roses, Daniel F MD (S) - *Spec Exp:* Breast Cancer; Melanoma; Thyroid & Parathyroid; **Hospital:** NYU Med Ctr (page 71); **Address:** 530 First Ave, Ste 6E, New York, NY 10016-6402; **Phone:** (212) 263-7330; **Board Cert:** Surgery 1975; **Med School:** NYU Sch Med 1969; **Resid:** Surgery, NYU - Bellevue Hosp, New York, NY 1969-1974; **Fellow:** Surgical Oncology, NYU - Bellevue Hosp, New York, NY 1976-1978; **Fac Appt:** Prof Surgery, NYU Sch Med

Salky, Barry A MD (S) - *Spec Exp:* Laparoscopic Surgery-Gastrointestinal; **Hospital:** Mount Sinai Hosp (page 68); **Address:** 1010 5th Ave, New York, NY 10028-0130; **Phone:** (212) 987-0410; **Board Cert:** Surgery 1998; **Med School:** Univ Tenn Coll Med, Memphis 1970; **Resid:** Surgery, Mount Sinai Hosp, New York, NY 1972-1973; Surgery, Mount Sinai Hosp, New York, NY 1975-1978; **Fac Appt:** Prof Surgery, Mount Sinai Sch Med

Schnabel, Freya MD (S) - *Spec Exp:* Breast Cancer; **Hospital:** NY Presby Hosp - Columbia Presby Med Ctr (page 70); **Address:** 161 Fort Washington Ave, Ste 1011, New York, NY 10032; **Phone:** (212) 305-1534; **Board Cert:** Surgery 1988; **Med School:** NYU Sch Med 1982; **Resid:** Surgery, NYU Med Ctr, New York, NY 1982-1987; **Fellow:** Surgery, Univ Hosp, Brooklyn, NY 1987-1988; **Fac Appt:** Assoc Clin Prof Surgery, Columbia P&S

Schwartz, Gordon F MD (S) - *Spec Exp:* Breast Cancer; **Hospital:** Thomas Jefferson Univ Hosp; **Address:** 1015 Chesnut St, Ste 510, Philadelphia, PA 19107-4305; **Phone:** (215) 627-8487; **Board Cert:** Surgery 1970; **Med School:** Harvard Med Sch 1960; **Resid:** Surgery, Columbia-Presby Med Ctr, New York, NY 1963-1968; **Fellow:** Oncology, Univ Penn, Philadelphia, PA 1968-1969; **Fac Appt:** Prof Surgery, Jefferson Med Coll

Shah, Jatin P MD (S) - *Spec Exp:* Head & Neck Surgery; Thyroid Surgery; **Hospital:** Mem Sloan Kettering Cancer Ctr; **Address:** 1275 York Ave, Ste C979, New York, NY 10021-6007; **Phone:** (212) 639-7604; **Board Cert:** Surgery 1975; **Med School:** India 1964; **Resid:** Surgery, SSG Hosp, Baroda, India 1964-1967; Surgery, NY Infirm, New York, NY 1972-1974; **Fellow:** Surgical Oncology, Meml Sloan-Kettering, New York, NY 1968-1972; **Fac Appt:** Prof Surgery, Cornell Univ-Weill Med Coll

Shaha, Ashok MD (S) - *Spec Exp:* Head & Neck Cancer; Thyroid & Parathyroid Surgery; **Hospital:** Mem Sloan Kettering Cancer Ctr; **Address:** 1275 York Ave, New York, NY 10021-6007; **Phone:** (212) 639-7649; **Board Cert:** Surgery 1992; **Med School:** India 1970; **Resid:** Surgery, Downstate Med Ctr, Brooklyn, NY 1977-1981; **Fellow:** Head and Neck Surgery, Meml Sloan Kettering Cancer Ctr, New York, NY 1981-1982; Surgical Oncology, Meml Sloan Kettering Cancer Ctr, New York, NY 1975-1976; **Fac Appt:** Prof Surgery, Cornell Univ-Weill Med Coll

Shapiro, Ron MD (S) - *Spec Exp:* Transplant-Kidney; Transplant-Pancreas; **Hospital:** UPMC - Presbyterian Univ Hosp; **Address:** 3601 5th Ave, Fl 4, Pittsburgh, PA 15213; **Phone:** (412) 648-3921; **Board Cert:** Surgery 1996; **Med School:** Stanford Univ 1980; **Resid:** Surgery, Mt Sinai Hosp, New York, NY 1980-1986; **Fac Appt:** Prof Surgery, Univ Pittsburgh

Sugarbaker, Paul H MD (S) - *Spec Exp:* Colon Cancer; Pseudomyxoma Peritonei; Tumor Surgery; **Hospital:** Washington Hosp Ctr; **Address:** Washington Cancer Inst, 110 Irving St NW, rm CG 175, Washington, DC 20010; **Phone:** (202) 877-3908; **Board Cert:** Surgery 1973; **Med School:** Cornell Univ-Weill Med Coll 1967; **Resid:** Surgery, Peter Bent Brigham Hosp, Boston, MA 1968-1973; **Fellow:** Surgery, Mass Genl Hosp, Boston, MA 1973-1976

Tartter, Paul MD (S) - *Spec Exp:* Breast Cancer; Breast Cancer in Elderly; Sentinel Node Biopsy; **Hospital:** St Luke's - Roosevelt Hosp Ctr - Roosevelt Div (page 58); **Address:** 425 W 59th St, Ste 7A, The Comprehensive Breast Center, New York, NY 10019; **Phone:** (212) 523-7500; **Board Cert:** Surgery 1983; **Med School:** Brown Univ 1977; **Resid:** Surgery, Mount Sinai Hosp, New York, NY 1977-1982; **Fac Appt:** Assoc Prof Surgery, Columbia P&S

Teperman, Lewis William MD (S) - *Spec Exp:* Transplant-Liver; Transplant-Kidney; **Hospital:** NYU Med Ctr (page 71); **Address:** 403 E 34th St Fl 3, New York, NY 10016; **Phone:** (212) 263-8134; **Board Cert:** Surgery 1997; **Med School:** Mount Sinai Sch Med 1981; **Resid:** Surgery, Columbia Presby Med Ctr, New York, NY 1981-1984; Surgery, LI Jewish Med Ctr, New Hyde Park, NY 1984-1986; **Fellow:** Transplant Surgery, Univ Pittsburgh, Pittsburgh, PA 1986-1988; **Fac Appt:** Asst Prof Surgery, NYU Sch Med

Yurt, Roger MD (S) - *Spec Exp:* Burns; Wound Healing/Care; **Hospital:** NY Presby Hosp - NY Weill Cornell Med Ctr (page 70); **Address:** 525 E 68th St, rm L706, New York, NY 10021-4885; **Phone:** (212) 746-5410; **Board Cert:** Surgery 1980; **Med School:** Univ Miami Sch Med 1972; **Resid:** Surgery, Parkland Meml Hosp, Dallas, TX 1972-1974; Surgery, NY Hosp-Cornell Med Ctr, New York, NY 1978-1980; **Fellow:** Internal Medicine, Brigham Hosp-Harvard, Cambridge, MA 1974-1978; **Fac Appt:** Prof Surgery, Cornell Univ-Weill Med Coll

Southeast

Albertson, David Allen MD (S) - *Spec Exp:* Endocrine Surgery; **Hospital:** Wake Forest Univ Baptist Med Ctr (page 81); **Address:** Wake Forest Univ Baptist Med Cntr, Medical Center Blvd, Winston Salem, NC 27157-1095; **Phone:** (336) 716-4442; **Board Cert:** Surgery 1998; **Med School:** Univ VA Sch Med 1972; **Resid:** Surgery, NC Bapt Hosp, Winston Salem, NC 1973-1977; **Fellow:** Endocrine Surgery, Boston Univ, Boston, MA 1977-1978; **Fac Appt:** Assoc Prof Surgery, Wake Forest Univ Sch Med

Baker, Christopher MD (S) - *Spec Exp:* Trauma; Colorectal Surgery; Critical Care; **Hospital:** Univ of NC Hosp (page 77); **Address:** Univ NC, Bldg Burnett-Womack - rm 215, Box 7210, Chapel Hill, NC 27599; **Phone:** (919) 966-4389; **Board Cert:** Surgery 1991, Surgical Critical Care 1996; **Med School:** Harvard Med Sch 1970; **Resid:** Surgery, UCSF, San Francisco, CA 1974-1975; Surgery, UCSF, San Francisco, CA 1975-1981; **Fellow:** Surgery, Yale Univ, New Haven, CT 1982-1989; **Fac Appt:** Prof Surgery, Univ NC Sch Med

Balch, Charles MD (S) - *Spec Exp:* Sentinel Node Surgery; Tumor Surgery; **Hospital:** Johns Hopkins Hosp - Baltimore; **Address:** 1900 Duke St, Ste 200, Alexandria, VA 22314; **Phone:** (703) 299-1081; **Board Cert:** Surgery 1997; **Med School:** Columbia P&S 1967; **Resid:** Surgery, U Alabama Med Ctr, Birmingham, AL 1970-1971; Surgery, U Alabama Med Ctr, Birmingham, AL 1973-1975; **Fellow:** Immunology, Scripps Clin-Rsch Fdn, La Jolla, CA 1971-1973; **Fac Appt:** Prof Surgery, Johns Hopkins Univ

Beauchamp, Robert Daniel MD (S) - *Spec Exp:* Breast Cancer; Colon & Rectal Cancer; **Hospital:** Vanderbilt Univ Med Ctr (page 80); **Address:** Medical Center North, D4316, 1161 21St Ave S, Nashville, TN 37232-2736; **Phone:** (615) 322-2391; **Board Cert:** Surgery 1997, Surgical Critical Care 1993; **Med School:** Univ Tex Med Br, Galveston 1982; **Resid:** Surgery, Univ Tex Med Br, Galveston, TX 1982-1987; **Fellow:** Cellular Molecular Biology, Vanderbilt Univ, Nashville, TN 1987-1989; **Fac Appt:** Prof Surgery, Vanderbilt Univ

Bland, Kirby MD (S) - *Spec Exp:* Breast Cancer; Colon Cancer; **Hospital:** Univ of Ala Hosp at Birmingham; **Address:** UAB, Dept Surgery Bldg BDB - rm 502, 1530 3rd Ave S, Birmingham, AL 35294-0012; **Phone:** (205) 975-5000; **Board Cert:** Surgery 1991; **Resid:** Surgery, Univ Fla Hosp, Gainesville, FL 1969-1970; Surgery, Univ Fla Hosp, Gainesville, FL 1972-1976; **Fellow:** Surgical Oncology, Univ Tex/Anderson Hosp, Houston, TX 1976-1977; **Fac Appt:** Prof Surgery

Bollinger, R Randal MD/PhD (S) - *Spec Exp:* Transplant-Kidney; Transplant-Pancreas; **Hospital:** Duke Univ Med Ctr (page 60); **Address:** Duke Univ Med Ctr, Box 2910, Durham, NC 27715-2910; **Phone:** (919) 684-5209; **Board Cert:** Surgery 1990; **Med School:** Tulane Univ 1970; **Resid:** Surgery, Duke Univ Med Ctr, Durham, NC 1970-1972; Surgery, Duke Univ Med Ctr, Durham, NC 1977-1980; **Fellow:** Immunology, Duke Univ Med Ctr, Durham, NC 1974-1976; **Fac Appt:** Prof Surgery, Duke Univ

Britt, L D MD (S) - *Spec Exp:* Surgery - General; **Hospital:** Sentara Norfolk Gen Hosp; **Address:** Dept Surgery, 825 Fairfax Ave, Ste 610, Norfolk, VA 23507; **Phone:** (757) 446-8950; **Board Cert:** Surgical Critical Care 1997, Surgery 1993; **Med School:** Harvard Med Sch 1977; **Resid:** Surgery, Barnes Hosp-Wash Univ, St Louis, MO 1978-1979; Surgery, Univ IL, Chicago, IL 1981-1984; **Fellow:** Trauma, Md Inst Emer Med Serv Sys, Baltimore, MD 1985-1986; **Fac Appt:** Prof Surgery, Eastern VA Med Sch

Cance, William George MD (S) - *Spec Exp:* Tumor Surgery; **Hospital:** Univ of NC Hosp (page 77); **Address:** 3010 Old Clinic Bldg, CB 7210, Chapel Hill, NC 27599-7210; **Phone:** (919) 966-5221; **Board Cert:** Surgery 1998; **Med School:** Duke Univ 1982; **Resid:** Surgery, Barnes Hosp-Wash Univ, St Louis, MO 1986-1988; **Fellow:** Surgical Oncology, Meml Sloan Kettering Canc Ctr, New York, NY 1989-1990; **Fac Appt:** Assoc Prof Surgery, Univ NC Sch Med

Carey, Larry C MD (S) - *Spec Exp:* Pancreatic Cancer; Bile Duct Cancer; **Hospital:** Tampa Genl Hosp; **Address:** 4 Columbia Drive, Ste 650, Tampa, FL 33606; **Phone:** (813) 259-0935; **Board Cert:** Surgery 1965, Critical Care Medicine 1987; **Med School:** Ohio State Univ 1959; **Resid:** Surgery, Milwaukee Co Genl Hosp, Milwaukee, WI 1960-1965; **Fac Appt:** Prof Surgery, Univ S Fla Coll Med

Carlson, Grant W MD (S) - *Spec Exp:* Breast Cancer; Breast Reconstruction; Head & Neck Cancer; **Hospital:** Crawford Long Hosp of Emory Univ; **Address:** Emory Clinic, 1365B Clifton Rd NE, Ste 1200, Atlanta, GA 30322; **Phone:** (404) 778-5233; **Board Cert:** Surgery 1996, Plastic Surgery 1993; **Resid:** Surgery, Emory Univ Hosp, Atlanta, GA 1983-1987; Plastic Surgery, Emory Univ Hosp, Atlanta, GA 1987-1989; **Fellow:** Surgical Oncology, MD Anderson, Houston, TX 1989-1991; **Fac Appt:** Prof Surgery

Copeland III, Edward M MD (S) - *Spec Exp:* Breast Cancer; Colon Cancer; **Hospital:** Shands Hlthcre at Univ of FL (page 73); **Address:** Shands Hlthcare Univ FL, 1600 SW Archer Rd, Box 100286, Gainesville, FL 32610; **Phone:** (352) 265-0622; **Board Cert:** Surgery 1971; **Med School:** Cornell Univ-Weill Med Coll 1963; **Resid:** Surgery, Univ Penn, Philadelphia, PA 1964-1969; Surgical Oncology, Univ TX MD Anderson Cancer Ctr, Houston, TX 1971-1972; **Fellow:** Research, Univ Penn, Philadelphia, PA 1966-1967; **Fac Appt:** Prof Surgery, Univ Fla Coll Med

Gadacz, Thomas R MD (S) - *Spec Exp:* Laparoscopic Surgery; **Hospital:** Med Coll of GA Hosp and Clin; **Address:** Dept Surgery, 1120 15th St, rm BI-4076, Augusta, GA 30912; **Phone:** (706) 721-4651; **Board Cert:** Surgery 1975; **Med School:** St Louis Univ 1966; **Resid:** Surgery, Univ Chicago Hosp, Chicago, IL 1967-1968; Surgery, Moffitt Hosp-UCSF, San Francisco, CA 1971-1974; **Fellow:** Gastroenterology, Mayo Clinic, Rochester, MN 1974; **Fac Appt:** Prof Surgery, Med Coll GA

Hanks, John B MD (S) - *Spec Exp:* Endocrine Surgery; Breast Surgery; Thyroid & Parathyroid Surgery; **Hospital:** Univ of VA Hlth Sys (page 79); **Address:** Dept Surgery, PO Box 800709, Charlottesville, VA 22908; **Phone:** (804) 924-0376; **Board Cert:** Surgery 1991; **Med School:** Univ Rochester 1973; **Resid:** Surgery, Duke Univ Med Ctr, Durham, NC 1972-1975; Surgery, Duke Univ Med Ctr, Durham, NC 1977-1982; **Fac Appt:** Prof Surgery, Univ VA Sch Med

Hinder, Ronald A MD (S) - *Spec Exp:* Gastroesophageal Reflux; Endoscopic Surgery; Gastrointestinal Cancers; **Hospital:** St Luke's Hosp; **Address:** Mayo/St Luke's Hosp, Dept General Surgery, 4500 San Pablo Rd, Jacksonville, FL 32234; **Phone:** (904) 953-2523; **Med School:** South Africa 1965; **Fac Appt:** Prof Surgery, Mayo Med Sch

Howard, Richard J MD (S) - *Spec Exp:* Transplant-Liver; Transplant-Kidney; Gastrointestinal Surgery; **Hospital:** Shands Hlthcre at Univ of FL (page 73); **Address:** Dept Surgery, 1600 SW Archer Rd, Ste 6142, Gainesville, FL 32610; **Phone:** (352) 265-0606; **Board Cert:** Surgery 1976; **Med School:** Yale Univ 1966; **Resid:** Surgery, Univ Minn Hosp, Minneapolis, MN 1969-1975; **Fac Appt:** Prof Surgery, Univ Fla Coll Med

Koruda, Mark Joseph MD (S) - *Spec Exp:* Gastrointestinal Surgery; Minimally Invasive Surgery; Inflammatory Bowel Disease; **Hospital:** Univ of NC Hosp (page 77); **Address:** Univ NC Chapel Hill - Div of Gastrointestinal Surgery, 405 Burnett Womack Bldg - CB 7210, Chapel Hill, NC 27599-7210; **Phone:** (919) 966-8436; **Board Cert:** Surgery 1999; **Med School:** Yale Univ 1981; **Resid:** Surgery, Hospital University PA, Philadelphia, PA 1981-1988; **Fac Appt:** Prof Surgery, Univ NC Sch Med

Leight, George MD (S) - *Spec Exp:* Breast Cancer; **Hospital:** Duke Univ Med Ctr (page 60); **Address:** Duke Univ Med Ctr, Dept Surgery, Erwin Rd, Box 3513, Durham, NC 27710; **Phone:** (919) 684-6849; **Board Cert:** Surgery 1999; **Med School:** Duke Univ 1972; **Resid:** Surgery, Duke Univ Med Ctr, Durham, NC 1973-1978; **Fac Appt:** Prof Surgery, Duke Univ

Luterman, Arnold MD (S) - *Spec Exp:* Burns; **Hospital:** Univ of S Ala Med Ctr; **Address:** Univ S. Alabama Dept. of Surgery, 2451 Fillingim St, Mobile, AL 36617; **Phone:** (251) 471-7993; **Board Cert:** Surgery 1996, Surgical Critical Care 1996; **Med School:** McGill Univ 1970; **Resid:** Surgery, Sinai Hospital, Baltimore, MD 1972; Surgery, Jewish Gen Hosp. McGill U, Montreal, Canada 1973-1976; **Fellow:** Trauma, University Wash 1974-1976; **Fac Appt:** Prof Surgery, Univ Ala

Lyerly, Herbert Kim MD (S) - *Spec Exp:* Breast Cancer; **Hospital:** Duke Univ Med Ctr (page 60); **Address:** Duke Univ Med Ctr, Box 2606, Durham, NC 27710-0001; **Phone:** (919) 681-8350; **Board Cert:** Surgery 1992; **Med School:** UCLA 1983; **Resid:** Surgery, Duke Univ Med Ctr, Durham, NC 1984-1990; **Fac Appt:** Prof Surgery, Duke Univ

McGrath, Patrick C MD (S) - *Spec Exp:* Breast Cancer; **Hospital:** Univ Kentucky Med Ctr; **Address:** Univ Kentucky Med Ctr, Dept Surgery, 800 Rose St, Lexington, KY 40536-0002; **Phone:** (859) 323-6346; **Board Cert:** Surgery 1996; **Med School:** Univ IL Coll Med 1980; **Resid:** Surgery, Med Coll Va, Richmond, VA 1980-1986; **Fellow:** Surgical Oncology, Med Coll Va, Richmond, VA 1986-1988; **Fac Appt:** Prof Surgery, Univ KY Coll Med

Meyer, Anthony A MD (S) - *Spec Exp:* Critical Care; **Hospital:** Univ of NC Hosp (page 77); **Address:** Univ NC-Sch Med, Dept Surg, Burnett Womack Bldg, Ste 136, Box CB7050, Chapel Hill, NC 27599-7210; **Phone:** (919) 966-4321; **Board Cert:** Surgery 1990, Surgical Critical Care 1994; **Med School:** Univ Chicago-Pritzker Sch Med 1977; **Resid:** Surgery, UCSF Med Ctr, San Francisco, CA 1978-1982; **Fac Appt:** Prof Surgery, Univ NC Sch Med

Miller, Joshua MD (S) - *Spec Exp:* Transplant-Kidney; Transplant-Pancreas; **Hospital:** Univ of Miami - Jackson Meml Hosp; **Address:** 1801 NW 9th Ave, Ste 519, Miami, FL 33136; **Phone:** (305) 355-5100; **Board Cert:** Thoracic Surgery 1971, Surgery 1970; **Med School:** Albert Einstein Coll Med 1961; **Resid:** Surgery, Yale-New Haven Hosp, New Haven, CT 1963-1966; Surgery, Yale-New Haven Hosp, New Haven, CT 1967-1968; **Fellow:** Cardiothoracic Transplantation, Yale-US Public Hlth Svc, New Haven, CT 1964-1965; **Fac Appt:** Prof Surgery, Univ Miami Sch Med

Minervini, Donald MD (S) - *Spec Exp:* Hernia; Laparoscopic Cholecystectomy; Breast Surgery; **Hospital:** Mount Sinai Med Ctr; **Address:** 4302 Alton Rd, Ste 820, Miami Beach, FL 33140-2893; **Phone:** (305) 531-7409; **Board Cert:** Surgery 1970; **Med School:** NY Med Coll 1964; **Resid:** Surgery, St Lukes Hosp, New York, NY 1965-1969

Newell, Kenneth MD/PhD (S) - *Spec Exp:* Transplant-Small Bowel; Transplant-Kidney; Transplant-Pancreas/Liver; **Hospital:** Emory Univ Hosp; **Address:** Emory Transplant Ctr, 1639 Pierce Drive, rm 5105 WMB, Atlanta, GA 30322; **Phone:** (404) 727-2489; **Board Cert:** Surgery 1999; **Med School:** Univ Mich Med Sch 1984; **Resid:** Surgery, Loyola Univ Med Ctr, Maywood, IL 1984-1989; **Fellow:** Transplant Surgery, Univ Chicago, Chicago, IL 1989; **Fac Appt:** Asst Prof Surgery, Emory Univ

Pappas, Theodore N MD (S) - *Spec Exp:* Laparoscopic Surgery; **Hospital:** Duke Univ Med Ctr (page 60); **Address:** Duke Univ Med Ctr, Box 3479, Durham, NC 27710-0001; **Phone:** (919) 681-3442; **Board Cert:** Surgery 1989; **Med School:** Ohio State Univ 1981; **Resid:** Surgery, Brigham & Womens Hosp, Boston, MA 1981-1988; **Fellow:** Gastroenterology, Wadworth VA Med Ctr, Los Angeles, CA 1983-1985; **Fac Appt:** Prof Surgery, Duke Univ

Polk Jr, Hiram C MD (S) - *Spec Exp:* Melanoma; Colon Cancer; Hiatal Hernia; **Hospital:** Univ Louisville Hosp; **Address:** Univ Louisville, Dept Surgery, Louisville, KY 40292-0001; **Phone:** (502) 583-8303; **Board Cert:** Surgery 1966; **Med School:** Harvard Med Sch 1960; **Resid:** Surgery, Barnes Hosp, St. Louis, MO 1960-1965; **Fac Appt:** Prof Surgery, Univ Louisville Sch Med

Reintgen, Douglas Scott MD (S) - *Spec Exp:* Melanoma-Sentinel Node; Breast Cancer-Sentinel Node; **Hospital:** H Lee Moffitt Cancer Ctr & Research Inst; **Address:** 12902 Magnolia Dr, Ste 3057A, Tampa, FL 33612-9416; **Phone:** (813) 972-8482; **Board Cert:** Surgery 1997; **Med School:** Duke Univ 1979; **Resid:** Surgery, Duke Univ Med Ctr, Durham, NC 1980-1987; **Fac Appt:** Prof Surgery, Univ S Fla Coll Med

Richardson, James David MD (S) - *Spec Exp:* Surgery - General; **Hospital:** Norton Hospital; **Address:** Univ Louisville, Dept Surg, 530 S Jackson St, Louisville, KY 40202-1675; **Phone:** (502) 852-5453; **Board Cert:** Thoracic Surgery 1999, Surgery 1992; **Med School:** Univ KY Coll Med 1970; **Resid:** Surgery, Univ Kentucky Med Ctr, Lexington, KY 1971-1972; Surgery, Univ Hosp-SW Texas Med Ctr, San Antonio, TX 1972-1976; **Fac Appt:** Prof Surgery, Univ Louisville Sch Med

Schirmer, Bruce David MD (S) - *Spec Exp:* Laparoscopic Surgery; Gastrointestinal/Liver Surgery; Pancreatic Surgery; **Hospital:** Univ of VA Hlth Sys (page 79); **Address:** UVA Health Systems, Dept Surgery, PO Box 800709, Charlottesville, VA 22908; **Phone:** (434) 924-2104; **Board Cert:** Surgery 1996; **Med School:** Duke Univ 1978; **Resid:** Surgery, Duke Med Ctr, Durham, NC 1980-1985; **Fac Appt:** Prof Surgery, Univ VA Sch Med

Stratta, Robert MD (S) - Spec Exp: *Transplant-Pancreas;* **Hospital:** Wake Forest Univ Baptist Med Ctr (page 81); **Address:** Wake Forest Univ Baptist Med Ctr, Dept General Surg, Medical Center Blvd, Winston-Salem, NC 27157-1095; **Phone:** (336) 716-6371; **Board Cert:** Surgery 1996, Surgical Critical Care 1991; **Med School:** Univ Chicago-Pritzker Sch Med 1980; **Resid:** Surgery, Univ Utah Med Ctr, Salt Lake City, UT 1980-1986; **Fellow:** Transplant Surgery, Univ Wisc Hosps & Clins, Madison, WI 1986-1988; **Fac Appt:** Prof Surgery, Wake Forest Univ Sch Med

Tzakis, Andreas MD (S) - Spec Exp: *Transplant-Liver; Transplant-Intestine;* **Hospital:** Univ of Miami - Jackson Meml Hosp; **Address:** 1801 NW 9th Ave, Ste 511, Miami, FL 33136; **Phone:** (305) 355-5011; **Board Cert:** Surgery 1993; **Med School:** Greece 1974; **Resid:** Surgery, Mt Sinai Hosp, New York, NY 1977-1979; Surgery, SUNY Stony Brook, Stony Brook, NY 1979-1983; **Fellow:** Transplant Surgery, Univ Pittsburgh Med Ctr, Pittburgh, PA 1983-1985; **Fac Appt:** Prof Surgery, Univ Miami Sch Med

Urist, Marshall MD (S) - Spec Exp: *Cancer Surgery; Breast Cancer; Melanoma;* **Hospital:** Univ of Ala Hosp at Birmingham; **Address:** Univ Alabama Sch Med, Dept Surg, 1922 7th Ave S, Bldg Kracke - Ste 321, Birmingham, AL 35294; **Phone:** (205) 934-3028; **Board Cert:** Surgery 2000; **Med School:** Univ Chicago-Pritzker Sch Med 1971; **Resid:** Surgery, Johns Hopkins Hosp, Baltimore, MD 1971-1978; **Fellow:** Surgical Oncology, Johns Hopkins Hosp, Baltimore, MD 1975-1976

Vogel, Stephen Burton MD (S) - Spec Exp: *Esophageal Cancer; Liver Cancer;* **Hospital:** Shands at Vista; **Address:** PO Box 100286, Gainesville, FL 32610-0286; **Phone:** (352) 265-0604; **Board Cert:** Surgery 1976; **Med School:** Univ Fla Coll Med 1967; **Resid:** Surgery, Univ Minn Hosp, Minneapolis, MN 1970-1975; **Fac Appt:** Prof Surgery, Univ Fla Coll Med

Willis, Irvin MD (S) - Spec Exp: *Pancreatic Surgery; Cancer Surgery;* **Hospital:** Mount Sinai Med Ctr; **Address:** 4302 Alton Rd, Ste 630, Miami Beach, FL 33140-2876; **Phone:** (305) 534-6050; **Board Cert:** Surgery 1970; **Med School:** Univ Cincinnati 1964; **Resid:** Surgery, Univ Miami-Jackson Meml, Miami, FL 1965-1969

Midwest

Bouwman, David L MD (S) - Spec Exp: *Breast Cancer;* **Hospital:** Barbara Ann Karmanos Cancer Inst; **Address:** Harper Hospital, Dept Surgery, 3990 John R, Detroit, MI 48201; **Phone:** (313) 745-8770; **Board Cert:** Surgery 1999; **Med School:** Johns Hopkins Univ 1971; **Resid:** Surgery, Johns Hopkins Hosp, Baltimore, MD 1972-1973; Surgery, Wayne State Univ Hosp, Detroit, MI 1975-1978; **Fac Appt:** Prof Surgery

Brems, John MD (S) - Spec Exp: *Transplant-Liver; Pancreatic Surgery; Obesity/Bariatric Surgery;* **Hospital:** Loyola Univ Med Ctr; **Address:** 2160 S 1st Ave, MC-EMS-3268, Maywood, IL 60153-3304; **Phone:** (708) 327-2774; **Board Cert:** Surgery 1995, Surgical Critical Care 1991; **Med School:** St Louis Univ 1981; **Resid:** Surgery, St Louis Univ, St Louis, MO 1982-1986; **Fellow:** Transplant Surgery, UCLA Med Ctr, Los Angeles, CA 1986-1987; **Fac Appt:** Prof Surgery, Loyola Univ-Stritch Sch Med

Chang, Alfred Edward MD (S) - Spec Exp: *Breast Cancer; Gastrointestinal Cancer;* **Hospital:** Univ of MI Hlth Ctr; **Address:** 1500 E Medical Center Dr., rm 3303, Box 0932, U-M Comprehensive Cncr and Ger. Ctr, Ann Arbor, MI 48109-0932; **Phone:** (734) 936-4392; **Board Cert:** Surgery 1991; **Med School:** Harvard Med Sch 1974; **Resid:** Surgery, Hosp U Penn, Philadelphia, PA 1979-1982; Surgery, Duke U Med Ctr., Durham, NC 1975-1976; **Fellow:** Medical Oncology, Natl Cancer Inst., Bethesda, MD 1976-1979; **Fac Appt:** Prof Surgery, Univ Mich Med Sch

Crowe, Joseph MD (S) - *Spec Exp:* Breast Cancer; Tumor Surgery; **Hospital:** Cleveland Clin Fdn (page 57); **Address:** 9500 Euclid Ave, rm A80, Cleveland, OH 44195; **Phone:** (216) 444-3024; **Board Cert:** Surgery 1994; **Med School:** Case West Res Univ 1978; **Resid:** Surgery, Univ Hosp Case-West Res, Cleveland, OH 1979-1983; **Fellow:** Surgical Oncology, Sloan Kettering Ctr, New York, NY 1983-1985

Donegan, William L MD (S) - *Spec Exp:* Breast Cancer; **Hospital:** Sinai Samaritan Med Ctr - AHC; **Address:** 950 N 12th St, Milwaukee, WI 53233-1306; **Phone:** (414) 219-6809; **Board Cert:** Surgery 1965; **Med School:** Wright State Univ 1959; **Resid:** Surgery, Barnes Hosp, St Louis, MO 1960-1964; **Fac Appt:** Prof Surgery, Med Coll Wisc

Donohue, John H MD (S) - *Spec Exp:* Gastrointestinal Cancers; **Hospital:** Mayo Med Ctr & Clin - Rochester, MN; **Address:** Mayo Clinic, Dept Surgery, 200 1st St SW, Rochester, MN 55905; **Phone:** (507) 284-0362; **Board Cert:** Surgery 1995; **Med School:** Harvard Med Sch 1986; **Fac Appt:** Prof Surgery, Mayo Med Sch

Eberlein, Timothy J MD (S) - *Spec Exp:* Breast Cancer; Tumor Surgery; **Hospital:** Barnes-Jewish Hosp (page 55); **Address:** 660 S Euclid Ave, Box 8109, St Louis, MO 63110; **Phone:** (314) 362-8021; **Board Cert:** Surgery 2007; **Med School:** Univ Pittsburgh 1977; **Resid:** Surgery, Peter Bent Brigham Hosp, Boston, MA 1978-1979; Surgery, Brigham-Womens Hosp, Boston, MA 1982-1985; **Fellow:** Allergy & Immunology, Natl Inst Hlth, Bethesda, MD 1979-1982; **Fac Appt:** Prof Washington Univ, St Louis

Ellison, Edwin Christopher MD (S) - *Spec Exp:* Transplant-Liver; Biliary Surgery; Pancreatic Cancer; **Hospital:** Ohio St Univ Med Ctr; **Address:** N729 Doan Hall, 410 W 10th Ave, Columbus, OH 43210-1236; **Phone:** (614) 293-4732; **Board Cert:** Surgery 1991; **Med School:** Univ Wisc **Resid:** Surgery, Ohio State Univ, Columbus, OH; **Fac Appt:** Assoc Prof Surgery, Ohio State Univ

Ferguson, Ronald MD (S) - *Spec Exp:* Transplant-Kidney; **Hospital:** Ohio St Univ Med Ctr; **Address:** 1654 Upham Drive Bldg Means Hall Fl 3, Columbus, OH 43210-1250; **Phone:** (614) 293-6322; **Board Cert:** Surgery 1981; **Med School:** Washington Univ, St Louis 1971; **Resid:** Surgery, Univ Minn Hosp, Minneapolis, MN 1972-1979; **Fellow:** Immunology, Univ Minn Hosp, Minneapolis, MN 1979-1980; **Fac Appt:** Prof Surgery, Ohio State Univ

Gabram, Sheryl MD (S) - *Spec Exp:* Breast Cancer; **Hospital:** Loyola Univ Med Ctr; **Address:** 2160 S First Ave, Bldg 110 - rm 3232, Maywood, IL 60153; **Phone:** (708) 216-8563; **Board Cert:** Surgery 1996, Surgical Critical Care 1989; **Med School:** Georgetown Univ 1982; **Resid:** Surgery, Washington Hospital Ctr., Washington, DC 1983-1987; **Fellow:** Trauma, Hartford Hospital, Hartford, CT 1987-1988; **Fac Appt:** Assoc Prof Surgery, Loyola Univ-Stritch Sch Med

Gamelli, Richard Louis MD (S) - *Spec Exp:* Burns; Trauma/Critical Care; **Hospital:** Loyola Univ Med Ctr; **Address:** Loyola Univ, Stritch School of Medicine, 2160 S First Ave, Bldg 110 - rm 3244, Maywood, IL 60153; **Phone:** (708) 216-8563; **Board Cert:** Surgery 1980; **Med School:** Univ VT Coll Med 1974; **Resid:** Surgery, VT Med Ctr Hosp, Burlington, VT 1975-1979; **Fac Appt:** Prof Surgery, Loyola Univ-Stritch Sch Med

Goulet Jr, Robert J MD (S) - *Spec Exp:* Breast Cancer; **Hospital:** IN Univ Hosp (page 63); **Address:** Indiana University Hosp, Cancer Pavilion, 535 Barnhill Drive, rm 431, Indianapolis, IN 46202-5112; **Phone:** (317) 274-3616; **Board Cert:** Surgery 1995; **Med School:** SUNY Downstate 1979; **Resid:** Surgery, SUNY-Downstate Med Ctr, Brooklyn, NY 1980-1986; **Fac Appt:** Assoc Clin Prof Surgery

Harkema, James M MD (S) - *Spec Exp:* Breast Cancer; **Hospital:** Sparrow Hospital; **Address:** Sparrow Professional Bldg, Breast Hlth Clinic, 1200 E Michigan Ave, Ste 655, Lansing, MI 48912; **Phone:** (517) 267-2461; **Board Cert:** Surgery 1975; **Med School:** Univ Mich Med Sch 1968; **Resid:** Surgery, Univ Michigan Hosp, Ann Arbor, MI 1969-1974; **Fac Appt:** Prof Surgery, Mich State Univ

Jochimsen, Peter R MD (S) - *Spec Exp:* Breast Cancer; **Hospital:** Univ of IA Hosp and Clinics; **Address:** Univ Iowa Hosps and Clinics, Dept Surgery, 200 Hawkins Drive, Iowa City, IA 52242; **Phone:** (319) 356-3584; **Board Cert:** Surgery 1973; **Med School:** Med Coll Wisc 1965; **Resid:** Surgery, Univ Minn Hosps, Minneapolis, MN 1966-1972; **Fac Appt:** Prof Surgery, Univ Iowa Coll Med

Kirby, Thomas MD (S) - *Spec Exp:* Transplant-Lung; Thoracic Surgery; **Hospital:** Univ Hosp of Cleveland; **Address:** 11100 Euclid Ave, Cleveland, OH 44106-5001; **Phone:** (216) 844-7267; **Board Cert:** Surgery 1995, Surgical Critical Care 1991; **Med School:** Univ Western Ontario 1978; **Resid:** Surgery, Univ Toronto, Toronto, Canada 1979-1984; **Fac Appt:** Prof Surgery, Case West Res Univ

Lewis Jr., Frank R. MD (S) - *Spec Exp:* Trauma-Cardiac; Trauma-Pulmonary; Trauma-Complex; **Hospital:** Henry Ford Hosp; **Address:** Henry Ford Hosp.-Dept. Surgery, 2799 W Grand Blvd, Detroit, MI 48202; **Phone:** (313) 916-3037; **Board Cert:** Surgery 1973; **Med School:** Univ MD Sch Med 1965; **Resid:** Surgery, UC San Francisco Med Ctr., San Francisco, CA 1967-1972; **Fellow:** Surgery, Univ Calif Hosp., CA 1972-1973; **Fac Appt:** Prof Surgery, Case West Res Univ

Maker, Vijay MD (S) - *Spec Exp:* Surgery - General; **Hospital:** Advocate IL Masonic Med Ctr; **Address:** 836 W Wellington Ave, Ste 4813, Chicago, IL 60657; **Phone:** (773) 296-5346; **Board Cert:** Surgery 1995; **Med School:** India 1967; **Resid:** Surgical Pathology, Mt Sinai Med Ctr, Chicago, IL 1969; Surgery, Mt Sinai Med Ctr, Chicago, IL 1969-1973; **Fac Appt:** Prof Surgery, Rush Med Coll

Matas, Arthur J MD (S) - *Spec Exp:* Transplant-Kidney; **Hospital:** Fairview-Univ Med Ctr - Univ Campus; **Address:** Dept Surg, 420 Delaware St SE, Minneapolis, MN 55455; **Phone:** (651) 221-3456; **Board Cert:** Surgery 1989; **Med School:** Univ Manitoba 1972; **Resid:** Surgery, Univ Minnesota Hosps, Minneapolis, MN 1973-1979; **Fellow:** Transplant Surgery, Univ Minnesota Hosps, Minneapolis, MN 1979-1980; **Fac Appt:** Prof Surgery, Univ Minn

Melvin, W Scott MD (S) - *Spec Exp:* Liver & Biliary Surgery; Pancreatic & Laparoscopic Surgery; **Hospital:** Ohio St Univ Med Ctr; **Address:** N729 Doan Hall, 410 W 10th Ave, Columbus, OH 43210-4030; **Phone:** (614) 293-4499; **Board Cert:** Surgery 1993; **Med School:** Med Coll OH 1987; **Resid:** Surgery, Univ Maryland, Baltimore, MD 1988-1992; **Fellow:** Gastrointestinal Surgery, Grant Med Ctr, Columbus, OH 1992-1993; **Fac Appt:** Asst Prof Surgery, Ohio State Univ

Millis, J Michael MD (S) - *Spec Exp:* Transplant-Liver; Transplant-Pancreas; Liver Cancer; **Hospital:** Univ of Chicago Hosps (page 76); **Address:** Univ Chicago, Dept Surg, 5841 S Maryland Ave, MC-5027, Chiciago, IL 60521; **Phone:** (773) 702-6319; **Board Cert:** Surgery 1993, Surgical Critical Care 1993; **Med School:** Univ Tenn Coll Med, Memphis 1985; **Resid:** Surgery, UCLA Med Ctr, Los Angeles, CA 1986-1992; **Fellow:** Transplant Surgery, UCLA Med Ctr, Los Angeles, CA 1992-1994; **Fac Appt:** Assoc Prof Surgery, Univ Chicago-Pritzker Sch Med

Morrow, Monica MD (S) - *Spec Exp:* Breast Cancer; **Hospital:** Northwestern Meml Hosp; **Address:** 675 N St Clair St, Ste 13-174, Chicago, IL 60611; **Phone:** (312) 926-9039; **Board Cert:** Surgery 1992; **Med School:** Jefferson Med Coll 1976; **Resid:** Surgery, Med Ctr Hosp of Vermont, Burlington, VT 1976-1981; **Fellow:** Surgical Oncology, Meml Sloan Kettering Cancer Ctr, New York, NY 1981-1983; **Fac Appt:** Prof Surgery, Northwestern Univ

Najarian, John S. MD (S) - *Spec Exp:* Transplant-Liver; Pediatric Transplant Surgery; **Hospital:** Fairview-Univ Med Ctr - Univ Campus; **Address:** Univ Minn, Dept Surgery, 420 Delaware St SE, Minneapolis, MN 55455; **Phone:** (612) 625-8444; **Board Cert:** Surgery 1961; **Med School:** UCSF 1952; **Resid:** Surgery, UCSF Med Ctr, San Francisco, CA 1955-1960; **Fellow:** Pathology, U Pittsburgh, Pittsburgh, PA 1960-1961; **Fac Appt:** Prof Surgery, Univ Minn

Prinz, Richard MD (S) - *Spec Exp:* Endocrine Surgery; Thyroid & Parathyroid Surgery; Pancreatic Surgery; **Hospital:** Rush-Presby - St Luke's Med Ctr (page 72); **Address:** 1653 W Congress Pkwy, Ste 785 Jelke, Chicago, IL 60612; **Phone:** (312) 942-6379; **Board Cert:** Surgery 1995; **Med School:** Loyola Univ-Stritch Sch Med 1972; **Resid:** Surgery, Barnes Hosp, St Louis, MO 1972-1974; Surgery, Loyola Univ Hosp, Chicago, IL 1974-1977; **Fellow:** Endocrinology, Diabetes & Metabolism, Hammersmith Hosp, London, England 1979-1980; **Fac Appt:** Prof Surgery, Rush Med Coll

Rikkers, Layton F MD (S) - *Spec Exp:* Liver & Biliary Surgery; **Hospital:** Univ WI Hosp & Clins; **Address:** Univ Wisc, Dept Surg, 600 Highland Ave, Clinic Sci Ctr, rm H4 710, Madison, WI 53792; **Phone:** (608) 265-8854; **Board Cert:** Surgery 1996; **Med School:** Stanford Univ 1970; **Resid:** Surgery, Univ Utah Hosp, Salt Lake City, UT 1971-1973; Surgery, Univ Utah Hosp, Salt Lake City, UT 1974-1976; **Fellow:** Hepatology, Royal Free Hosp, LondonEngland 1973-1974; **Fac Appt:** Prof Surgery, Univ Wisc

Robinson, David S MD (S) - *Spec Exp:* Breast Cancer; **Hospital:** St Luke's Hosp; **Address:** 4321 Washington St, Ste 1000, Kansas City, MO 64111; **Phone:** (816) 932-5350; **Board Cert:** Surgery 1993; **Resid:** Surgery, Univ Virginia Med Ctr, Chalottesville, VA 1973-1974; Surgery, Univ Virginia Med Ctr, Charlottesville, VA 1977-1978; **Fellow:** Oncology Research, UCLA Med Ctr, Los Angeles, CA 1974-1977; Surgical Oncology, Meml Sloan-Kettering Cancer Ctr, New York, NY 1980-1982

Rosen, Charles Burke MD (S) - *Spec Exp:* Transplant-Liver; **Hospital:** Mayo Med Ctr & Clin - Rochester, MN; **Address:** Dept Surgery/Div Transplantation, 200 First St SW, Charlton 10A, Rochester, MN 55905; **Phone:** (507) 266-6640; **Board Cert:** Surgery 1990; **Med School:** Mayo Med Sch 1984; **Resid:** Surgery, Mayo Clinic, Rochester, MN 1984-1989; **Fellow:** Transplant Surgery, Mayo Clinic, Rochester, MN 1989-1991

Saha, Sukamal MD (S) - *Spec Exp:* Sentinel Node Surgery; Colon Cancer; **Hospital:** McLaren Reg Med Ctr; **Address:** 3500 Calkins Rd, Flint, MI 48532; **Phone:** (810) 230-9600; **Board Cert:** Surgery 1989; **Med School:** India 1977; **Resid:** Surgery, Hahnemann Univ Hosp, Philadelphia, PA 1984-1985; Surgery, Easton Hosp, Easton, PA 1985-1987; **Fellow:** Surgical Oncology, Tulane Univ Med Ctr, New Orleans, LA 1987-1989

Schreiber, Helmut MD (S) - *Spec Exp:* Obesity/Bariatric Surgery; **Hospital:** St Vincent Charity Hosp; **Address:** St Vincent Chsrity Hosp, Cleveland Ctr for Bariatric Surgery, 2351 E 22nd St, Ste 208, Cleveland, OH 44115; **Phone:** (216) 363-2588; **Board Cert:** Surgery 1997; **Med School:** Ohio State Univ 1970; **Resid:** Surgery, Case West Res Affil Hosps, OH 1971-1975; **Fac Appt:** Assoc Clin Prof Surgery, Case West Res Univ

Scott-Conner, Carol E.H. MD/PhD (S) - *Spec Exp:* Laparoscopic Surgery; **Hospital:** Univ of IA Hosp and Clinics; **Address:** 200 Hawkins Dr., rm 1516JCP, U of IA Coll Med-Dept. Surgery, Iowa City, IA 52242-1086; **Phone:** (319) 356-0330; **Board Cert:** Surgery 1990, Surgical Critical Care 1998; **Med School:** NYU Sch Med 1976; **Resid:** Surgery, NYU Med Ctr, New York, NY 1977-1981; **Fac Appt:** Prof Surgery, Univ Iowa Coll Med

Shuck, Jerry M MD (S) - *Spec Exp:* *Thyroid Surgery;* **Hospital:** Univ Hosp of Cleveland; **Address:** 11100 Euclid Ave, Cleveland, OH 44106-5047; **Phone:** (216) 844-3871; **Board Cert:** Surgery 1967, Thoracic Surgery 1967; **Med School:** Univ Cincinnati 1959; **Resid:** Surgery, Cincinnati Genl Hosp, Cincinnati, OH 1960-1966; **Fac Appt:** Prof Surgery, Case West Res Univ

Sollinger, Hans W MD (S) - *Spec Exp:* *Transplant-Kidney; Transplant-Pancreas;* **Hospital:** Univ WI Hosp & Clins; **Address:** 600 Highland Ave, rm H5/701, Madison, WI 53792; **Phone:** (608) 263-9903; **Board Cert:** Surgery 1996; **Med School:** Germany 1974; **Resid:** Surgery, Univ Wisc Hosp, Madison, WI 1976-1980; **Fellow:** Immunological Biology, Univ Wisc Hosp, Madison, WI 1975-1977; **Fac Appt:** Prof Surgery, Univ Wisc

Soper, Nathaniel MD (S) - *Spec Exp:* *Laparoscopic Surgery; Gastroesophageal Reflux (GERD);* **Hospital:** Barnes-Jewish Hosp (page 55); **Address:** Barnes Jewish Hosp, Dept Surg, One Barnes Hosp Plaza, Ste 6108, Box 8109, St Louis, MO 63110-1036; **Phone:** (314) 454-8877; **Board Cert:** Surgery 1996; **Med School:** Univ Iowa Coll Med 1980; **Resid:** Surgery, Univ Utah Hosps, Salt Lake City, UT 1980-1986; **Fellow:** Digestive Dis, Mayo Clinic, Rochester, MN 1986-1988; **Fac Appt:** Prof Surgery, Washington Univ, St Louis

Sutherland, David MD (S) - *Spec Exp:* *Transplant-Pancreas;* **Hospital:** Fairview-Univ Med Ctr - Univ Campus; **Address:** 420 Delaware St SE Bldg MMC 280, Minneapolis, MN 55455; **Phone:** (612) 625-7600; **Board Cert:** Surgery 1978; **Med School:** Univ Minn 1966; **Resid:** Surgery, West Virginia Univ Hosp, Morgantown, VA 1966-1968; **Fellow:** Transplant Surgery, Univ Minn Hosps, Minneapolis, MN 1970-1975; **Fac Appt:** Prof Surgery, Univ Minn

Thistlethwaite, J Richard MD (S) - *Spec Exp:* *Transplant-Kidney; Transplant-Pancreas/Liver; Transplant-Pediatric;* **Hospital:** Univ of Chicago Hosps (page 76); **Address:** 5841 S Maryland Ave, rm J-517, MC 5026, Chicago, IL 60637; **Phone:** (773) 702-6104; **Board Cert:** Surgery 1996; **Med School:** Duke Univ 1977; **Resid:** Surgery, Mass Genl Hosp, Boston, MA 1977-1983; **Fellow:** Surgical Oncology, Natl Inst Health, Bethesda, MD 1979-1981; Transplant Surgery, Mass Genl Hosp, Boston, MA 1983-1984; **Fac Appt:** Prof Transplant Surgery, Univ Chicago-Pritzker Sch Med

Van Heerden, Jon MD (S) - *Spec Exp:* *Endocrine Surgery; Pheochromocytoma;* **Hospital:** Mayo Med Ctr & Clin - Rochester, MN; **Address:** Mayo Clinic, Dept Surgery, 200 1st St SW, Rochester, MN 55905; **Phone:** (507) 284-3364; **Board Cert:** Surgery 1981; **Med School:** South Africa 1961; **Resid:** Surgery, Groote Schuur Hosp, Cape Town, South Africa 1962-1964; Surgery, Mayo Clinic, Rochester, MN 1964-1970; **Fac Appt:** Prof Surgery, Mayo Med Sch

Walker, Alonzo P MD (S) - *Spec Exp:* *Breast Cancer;* **Hospital:** Froedtert Meml Lutheran Hosp; **Address:** Dept Surgery, 9200 W Wisconsin Ave, Milwaukee, WI 53226-3522; **Phone:** (414) 454-5737; **Board Cert:** Surgery 1992; **Med School:** Univ Fla Coll Med 1976; **Resid:** Surgery, Univ Maryland Hosps, Baltimore, MD 1978-1983; **Fac Appt:** Assoc Prof Surgery, Med Coll Wisc

Great Plains and Mountains

Edney, James A MD (S) - *Spec Exp:* *Breast Cancer;* **Hospital:** Nebraska Hlth Sys; **Address:** Univ Nebraska Med Ctr, Dept Surgery, 983280 Nebraska Medical Ctr, Omaha, NE 68198-3280; **Phone:** (402) 559-7272; **Board Cert:** Surgery 1990; **Med School:** Univ Nebr Coll Med 1975; **Resid:** Surgery, Univ Nebraska Med Ctr, Omaha, NE 1976-1980; **Fellow:** Surgical Oncology, Univ Colorado Med Ctr, Denver, CO 1980-1981; **Fac Appt:** Assoc Prof Surgery, Univ Nebr Coll Med

Karrer, Frederick Merrill MD (S) - *Spec Exp:* Liver Surgery-Complex; Transplant-Liver; Critical Care; **Hospital:** Chldn's Hosp - Denver; **Address:** Children's Hospital, Dept Surgery, 1950 Ogden St, Denver, CO 80218-1022; **Phone:** (303) 861-6571; **Board Cert:** Surgery 1996, Pediatric Surgery 1997, Surgical Critical Care 1998; **Med School:** Univ Nebr Coll Med 1979; **Resid:** Surgery, Univ Ariz, Tucson, AZ 1979-1984; Pediatric Surgery, Children's Meml Hosp, Chicago, IL 1986-1988; **Fellow:** Transplant Surgery, Univ Pittsburgh, Pittsburgh, PA 1985-1986; **Fac Appt:** Assoc Prof Surgery, Univ Colo

Moore, Ernest E MD (S) - *Spec Exp:* Trauma; Liver Trauma; Gastrointestinal Trauma; **Hospital:** Denver Health Med Ctr; **Address:** Denver Hlth Med Ctr, 777 Bannock St, MC 0206, Denver, CO 80204-4507; **Phone:** (303) 436-6558; **Board Cert:** Surgery 1996, Surgical Critical Care 1996; **Med School:** Univ Pittsburgh 1972; **Resid:** Surgery, Univ Vt Med Ctr, VT 1972-1976; **Fac Appt:** Prof Surgery, Univ Colo

Mulvihill, Sean Jordan MD (S) - *Spec Exp:* Gastrointestinal Surgery; **Hospital:** Univ Utah Hosp and Clin; **Address:** Univ Utah, Dept Surg, 50 N Medical Dr, Salt Lake City, UT 84132; **Phone:** (801) 581-7304; **Board Cert:** Surgery 1999; **Med School:** USC Sch Med 1981; **Resid:** Surgery, UCLA Med Ctr, Los Angeles, CA 1981-1987; **Fac Appt:** Prof Surgery, Univ Utah

Saffle, Jeffrey MD (S) - *Spec Exp:* Burns; Wound Healing/Care; **Hospital:** Univ Utah Hosp and Clin; **Address:** Univ Utah Hlth Sci Ctr, Dept Surg, 50 N Medical Dr, Salt Lake City, UT 84132; **Phone:** (801) 581-3595; **Board Cert:** Surgery 1983, Surgical Critical Care 1998; **Med School:** Univ Chicago-Pritzker Sch Med 1976; **Resid:** Surgery, Univ Utah Med Ctr, Salt Lake City, UT 1977-1982; **Fellow:** Burn Surgery, Univ Utah Med Ctr, Salt Lake City, UT 1979-1980; **Fac Appt:** Prof Surgery, Univ Utah

Shaw Jr, Byers Wendell MD (S) - *Spec Exp:* Transplant-Liver; **Hospital:** Nebraska Hlth Sys; **Address:** Nebraska Med Ctr, Transplant Ctr, Box 983280, Omaha, NE 68198-3285; **Phone:** (402) 559-4076; **Board Cert:** Surgery 1992, Surgical Critical Care 1996; **Med School:** Case West Res Univ 1976; **Resid:** Surgery, Univ Utah, Salt Lake City, UT 1977-1981; **Fellow:** Transplant Surgery, Univ Pittsburgh, Piitsburgh, PA 1981-1983; **Fac Appt:** Prof Surgery, Univ Nebr Coll Med

Southwest

Curley, Steven Alan MD (S) - *Spec Exp:* Colon & Rectal Cancer; Liver Cancer; **Hospital:** Univ of TX MD Anderson Cancer Ctr, The; **Address:** MD Anderson Cancer Ctr, Dept Surg Onc, 1515 Holcombe Blvd, Box 444, Houston, TX 77030; **Phone:** (713) 794-4957; **Board Cert:** Surgery 1997; **Med School:** Univ Tex, Houston 1982; **Resid:** Surgery, Univ New Mexico, Albuquerque, NM 1982-1988; **Fellow:** Surgical Oncology, MD Anderson Cancer Ctr, Houston, TX 1988-1990; **Fac Appt:** Surgery, Univ Tex, Houston

Dooley, William Chesnut MD (S) - *Spec Exp:* Breast Cancer; Metastatic Disease Mgmt; Tumors-Rare & Multiple; **Hospital:** Univ OK Hlth Sci Ctr; **Address:** 825 NE 10th St, Ste 3500, Oklahoma City, OK 73104; **Phone:** (405) 271-7867; **Board Cert:** Surgery 1997; **Med School:** Vanderbilt Univ 1982; **Resid:** Surgery, Oxford Univ, Oxford, England 1986; Surgery, Johns Hopkins, Baltimore, MD 1982-1987; **Fellow:** Medical Oncology, Johns Hopkins, Baltimore, MD 1987-1988; **Fac Appt:** Prof Surgery, Univ Okla Coll Med

Evans, Douglas Brian MD (S) - *Spec Exp:* Pancreatic Cancer; Thyroid Cancer; Endocrine Cancers; **Hospital:** Univ of TX MD Anderson Cancer Ctr, The; **Address:** UT MD Anderson Cancer Ctr, 1515 Holcombe Blvd, Box 444, Houston, TX 77030-4095; **Phone:** (713) 794-4324; **Board Cert:** Surgery 1996; **Med School:** Boston Univ 1983; **Resid:** Surgery, Dartmouth, Hanover 1984-1988; **Fellow:** Surgical Oncology, MD Anderson Cancer Inst, Houston, TX 1988-1990; **Fac Appt:** Prof Surgical Oncology, Univ Tex, Houston

Griswold, John A MD (S) - *Spec Exp:* Burns; **Hospital:** Univ Med Ctr - Lubbock; **Address:** Texas Tech Univ Hlth Scis Ctr, Dept Surgery, 3601 4th St, MS 8312, Lubbock, TX 79430; **Phone:** (806) 743-1615; **Board Cert:** Surgery 1999, Surgical Critical Care 1991; **Med School:** Creighton Univ 1981; **Resid:** Surgery, Texas Tech Univ Hlth Scis Ctr, Lubbock, TX 1982-1986; **Fellow:** Burn Surgery, Univ Washington, Seattle, WA 1986-1988

Halff, Glenn Alexander MD (S) - *Spec Exp:* Transplant-Liver; Liver Surgery; **Hospital:** Univ Hlth Sys - San Antonio; **Address:** Univ TX Hlth Sci Ctr San Antonio, Organ Transplantation Unit, 7703 Floyd Curl Drive, MC 7858, San Antonio, TX 78229-3900; **Phone:** (210) 567-5777; **Board Cert:** Surgical Critical Care 1990, Surgery 1998; **Med School:** Univ Tex, Houston **Resid:** Surgery, NYU Med Ctr, New York, NY 1983-1987; **Fellow:** Transplant Surgery, Univ of Pittsburgh, Pittsburgh, PA 1988-1989; **Fac Appt:** Assoc Prof Surgery, Univ Tex, San Antonio

Jackson, Gilchrist MD (S) - *Spec Exp:* Laparoscopic Surgery-Gastrointestinal; Tumor Surgery; Head & Neck Surgery; **Hospital:** St Luke's Episcopal Hosp - Houston; **Address:** 6624 Fannin St, Ste 1700, Houston, TX 77030-2329; **Phone:** (713) 442-1132; **Board Cert:** Surgery 1980; **Med School:** Univ KY Coll Med 1974; **Resid:** Parkland SW Hosps, Dallas, TX 1975-1979; **Fellow:** Surgical Oncology, MD Anderson Hosp, Houston, TX 1979-1980; **Fac Appt:** Assoc Clin Prof Baylor Coll Med

Kahan, Barry MD (S) - *Spec Exp:* Transplant-Kidney; **Hospital:** Meml Hermann Hosp; **Address:** 6431 Fannin St, rm 6-240, Houston, TX 77030-1501; **Phone:** (713) 500-7400; **Board Cert:** Surgery 1973; **Med School:** Univ Chicago-Pritzker Sch Med 1965; **Resid:** Surgery, Mass Genl Hosp, Boston, MA 1968-1972; **Fac Appt:** Prof Surgery, Univ Tex, Houston

Kelly, Keith A MD (S) - *Spec Exp:* Colon Cancer; **Hospital:** Mayo Clin Hosp - Scottsdale; **Address:** Mayo Clinic, Dept Genl Surg, 13400 E Shea Blvd, Scottsdale, AZ 85259; **Phone:** (480) 301-7157; **Board Cert:** Surgery 1989, Thoracic Surgery 1967; **Med School:** Univ Chicago-Pritzker Sch Med 1956; **Resid:** Surgery, Univ Wash Med Ctr, Seattle, WA 1957-1958; Surgery, Univ Wash Med Ctr, Seattle, WA 1961-1966; **Fellow:** Thoracic Surgery, Mayo Grad Sch Med, Rochester, MN 1966-1968; **Fac Appt:** Prof Surgery, Mayo Med Sch

Klimberg, V Suzanne MD (S) - *Spec Exp:* Breast Cancer; **Hospital:** UAMS; **Address:** Univ Arkansas Medical Sciences, 4301 W Markham, MS 725, Little Rock, AR 72205; **Phone:** (501) 686-6504; **Board Cert:** Surgery 1991; **Med School:** Univ Fla Coll Med 1984; **Resid:** Surgery, Univ Fla, Gainesville, FL 1985-1990; **Fellow:** Clinical Oncology, Univ Fla, Gainnsville, FL 1990-1991; Clinical Oncology, Univ Arkansas, Little Rock, AR 1990-1991; **Fac Appt:** Assoc Prof Surgery, Univ Ark

Lee, Jeffrey Edwin MD (S) - *Spec Exp:* Melanoma; Pancreatic Cancer; Adrenal Tumors; **Hospital:** Univ of TX MD Anderson Cancer Ctr, The; **Address:** UT MD Anderson Cancer Ctr, 1515 Holcombe Blvd, Box 444, Houston, TX 77030; **Phone:** (713) 792-7218; **Board Cert:** Surgery 1999; **Med School:** Stanford Univ 1984; **Resid:** Surgery, Stanford Univ Hosp, Palo Alto, CA 1985-1987; Surgery, Stanford Univ Hosp, Palo Alto, CA 1989-1991; **Fellow:** Immunology, Stanford Univ Sch Med, Palo Alto, CA 1987-1989; Surgical Oncology, Univ Tex-MD Anderson Cancer Ctr, Houston, TX 1991-1993; **Fac Appt:** Assoc Prof Surgery, Univ Tex, Houston

MacFadyen, Bruce MD (S) - *Spec Exp:* Laparoscopic Surgery; Gastrointestinal Surgery; Endoscopy; **Hospital:** Meml Hermann Hosp; **Address:** 6410 Fannin Street , Ste 1400, Houston, TX 77030-1501; **Phone:** (713) 704-6025; **Board Cert:** Surgery 1975; **Med School:** Hahnemann Univ 1968; **Resid:** Surgery, Hosp Univ Penn, Philadelphia, PA 1969-1972; Surgery, Hermann Hosp, Houston, TX 1972-1974; **Fac Appt:** Prof Surgery, Univ Tex, Houston

Peters, George N MD (S) - *Spec Exp:* Breast Cancer; **Hospital:** Univ Med Ctr - Lubbock; **Address:** University of Texas Center for Breast Care, Inwood Rd Fl 3, Dallas, TX 75301; **Phone:** (214) 648-7087; **Board Cert:** Surgery 1993; **Resid:** Surgery, Baylor Univ Med Ctr, Dallas, TX 1975-1979; **Fellow:** Surgical Oncology, Columbia-Presby Med Ctr, New York, NY 1979-1980

Ross, Merrick I MD (S) - *Spec Exp:* Sentinel Node Surgery; Breast Cancer; Melanoma; **Hospital:** Univ of TX MD Anderson Cancer Ctr, The; **Address:** Univ Texas, MD Anderson Cancer Ctr, 1515 Holcombe Blvd, Box 444, Houston, TX 77030; **Phone:** (713) 792-7217; **Board Cert:** Surgery 1997; **Med School:** Univ IL Coll Med 1980; **Resid:** Surgery, Univ Illinois Hosp & Clin, Chicago, IL 1980-1982; Surgery, Univ Illinois Hosp & Clin, Chicago, IL 1984-1987; **Fellow:** Research, Scripps Clin & Rsch, La Jolla, CA 1982-1984; Surgical Oncology, Univ TX-MD Anderson Cancer Ctr, Houston, TX 1987-1989; **Fac Appt:** Prof Surgery, Univ Tex, Houston

Schlinkert, Richard T MD (S) - *Spec Exp:* Gastrointestinal Surgery; Laparoscopic Surgery; Endocrine Surgery; **Hospital:** Mayo Clin Hosp - Scottsdale; **Address:** Mayo Clinic, Dept Surgery, 13400 E Shea Blvd, Scottsdale, AZ 85259-5404; **Phone:** (480) 301-6551; **Board Cert:** Surgery 1996; **Med School:** Med Coll OH 1980; **Resid:** Surgery, Mayo Clinic, Rochester, MN 1981-1986; **Fellow:** Hepatobiliary Surgery, Royal Infirmary, Glasgow, Scoltland 1986-1987; **Fac Appt:** Prof Surgery, Mayo Med Sch

Singletary, S Eva MD (S) - *Spec Exp:* Breast Cancer; **Hospital:** Univ of TX MD Anderson Cancer Ctr, The; **Address:** Univ Tex MD Anderson Canc Ctr, 1515 Holcombe Blvd, Box 444, Houston, TX 77030-4009; **Phone:** (713) 792-6937; **Board Cert:** Surgery 1994; **Med School:** Med Univ SC 1977; **Resid:** Surgery, Shands Hosp-Univ Florida, Gainesville, FL 1977-1983; **Fellow:** Surgery, MD Anderson Hosp, Houston, TX 1983-1985; **Fac Appt:** Prof Surgery, Univ Tex, Houston

Snyder III, William Henry MD (S) - *Spec Exp:* Thyroid Surgery; Parathyroid Surgery; Adrenal Surgery; **Hospital:** Zale Lipshy Univ Hosp; **Address:** Univ Texas SW Med Ctr, Dept Surg, 5323 Harry Hines Blvd, MC-9156, Dallas, TX 75390-9156; **Phone:** (214) 648-3510; **Board Cert:** Surgery 1971, Thoracic Surgery 1972; **Med School:** Baylor Coll Med 1962; **Resid:** Thoracic Surgery, Univ Cincinnati Affil Hosps, Cincinnati, OH 1965-1971; **Fac Appt:** Prof Surgery, Univ Tex SW, Dallas

Stewart, Ronald Mack MD (S) - *Spec Exp:* Trauma; **Hospital:** Univ of Texas Hlth & Sci Ctr; **Address:** Univ Texas Hlth Sci Ctr, Dept Surgery, 7703 Floyd Curl Dr, MC-7740, San Antonio, TX 78229-3900; **Phone:** (210) 567-3623; **Board Cert:** Surgery 1992, Surgical Critical Care 1993; **Med School:** Univ Tex, San Antonio 1985; **Resid:** Surgery, Univ Tex Hlth Sci Ctr, San Antonio, TX 1985-1991; **Fellow:** Trauma, Univ Tenn Coll Med, Memphis, TN 1991-1993; **Fac Appt:** Assoc Prof Surgery, Univ Tex, San Antonio

Stolier, Alan J MD (S) - *Spec Exp:* Breast Cancer; **Hospital:** Ochsner Found Hosp; **Address:** Ochsner Clinic, Dept Surgery, 1514 Jefferson Hwy, New Orleans, LA 70121; **Phone:** (504) 842-6406; **Board Cert:** Surgery 1994; **Med School:** Louisiana State Univ 1970; **Resid:** Surgery, Charity Hosp, New Orleans, LA 1971-1974; **Fellow:** Surgical Oncology, MD Anderson Hosp, Houston, TX 1975-1976

Wood, R Patrick MD (S) - *Spec Exp:* Transplant-Liver; Liver Surgery; Liver Cancer; **Hospital:** St Luke's Episcopal Hosp - Houston; **Address:** 6624 Fannin St, Ste 1200, Houston, TX 77030; **Phone:** (832) 355-8406; **Board Cert:** Surgery 1995, Surgical Critical Care 1992; **Med School:** Univ Rochester 1979; **Resid:** Surgery, NYU Med-Bellevue, New York, NY 1980-1984; **Fellow:** Transplant Surgery, U Pittsburgh, Pittsburgh, PA 1984-1985

West Coast and Pacific

Ascher, Nancy L MD (S) - *Spec Exp:* Transplant-Liver; Transplant-Kidney; **Hospital:** UCSF Med Ctr; **Address:** 513 Parnassus Ave, rm S320, San Francisco, CA 94143-0104; **Phone:** (415) 476-1236; **Board Cert:** Surgery 1991; **Med School:** Univ Mich Med Sch 1974; **Resid:** Surgery, Univ Minn Hosp, Minneapolis, MN 1975-1981; **Fellow:** Transplant Surgery, Univ Minn Hosp, Minneapolis, MN 1981-1982; **Fac Appt:** Prof Surgery, UCSF

Bilchik, Anton Joel MD (S) - *Spec Exp:* Cancer Surgery; Laparoscopic Surgery; **Hospital:** St John's Hlth Ctr; **Address:** John Wayne Cancer Institute, 2200 Santa Monica Blvd, Santa Monica, CA 90404-2302; **Phone:** (310) 449-5206; **Board Cert:** Surgery 1997; **Med School:** South Africa 1985; **Resid:** Surgery, UCLA, Los Angeles, CA 1991-1996; **Fellow:** John Wayne Cancer Inst., Santa Monica, CA 1996-1998; **Fac Appt:** Asst Clin Prof Surgery, UCLA

Busuttil, Ronald Wilfred MD/PhD (S) - *Spec Exp:* Transplant-Liver; **Hospital:** UCLA Med Ctr; **Address:** 10833 Le Conte Ave, rm 77-120, Los Angeles, CA 90095-7054; **Phone:** (310) 825-5318; **Board Cert:** Surgery 1997; **Med School:** Tulane Univ 1971; **Resid:** Surgery, UCLA, Los Angeles, CA 1972-1976; **Fellow:** Surgery, UCLA, Los Angeles, CA 1973-1975; **Fac Appt:** Prof Surgery, UCLA

Byrd, David MD (S) - *Spec Exp:* Tumor Surgery; Breast Cancer; **Hospital:** Univ WA Med Ctr; **Address:** Dept Surgery, 1959 NE Pacific St, Box 356410, Seattle, WA 98195; **Phone:** (206) 598-4477; **Board Cert:** Surgery 1998; **Med School:** Tulane Univ 1982; **Resid:** Surgery, Univ Wash Med Ctr, Seattle, WA 1983-1987; **Fellow:** Surgery, Univ Tex-Anderson Canc Ctr, Houston, TX 1989-1992; **Fac Appt:** Assoc Prof Surgery, Univ Wash

Chang, Helena MD (S) - *Spec Exp:* Breast Cancer; **Hospital:** UCLA Med Ctr; **Address:** 200 UCLA Medical Plaza, Ste B265-1, Revlon Breast Clinic, Los Angeles, CA 90095; **Phone:** (310) 825-2144; **Board Cert:** Surgery 1997; **Med School:** Temple Univ 1981; **Resid:** Surgery, Epis Hosp, Philadelphia, PA 1981-1986; **Fellow:** Surgical Oncology, Meml Sloan-Kettering, New York, NY 1986-1988; **Fac Appt:** Prof Surgery, UCLA

Clark, Orlo H MD (S) - *Spec Exp:* Thyroid Cancer; Pancreatic Cancer; Hyperparathyroidism; **Hospital:** UCSF - Mount Zion Med Ctr; **Address:** 2330 Post St, Ste 420, San Francisco, CA 94115; **Phone:** (415) 346-3200; **Board Cert:** Surgery 1974; **Med School:** Cornell Univ-Weill Med Coll 1967; **Resid:** Surgery, UCSF Med Ctr, San Francisco, CA 1967-1970; Surgery, UCSF Med Ctr, San Francisco, CA 1971-1973; **Fellow:** Surgery, Royal Med Sch London, London, England 1970-1971; **Fac Appt:** Prof Surgery, UCSF

Eilber, Frederick Richard MD (S) - *Spec Exp:* Tumor Surgery; Sarcoma; **Hospital:** UCLA Med Ctr; **Address:** 10833 Le Conte Ave, rm 54-14, Los Angeles, CA 90095; **Phone:** (310) 825-7086; **Board Cert:** Surgery 1973; **Med School:** Univ Mich Med Sch 1965; **Resid:** Surgery, Univ MD Hosp, Baltimore, MD 1966-1972; **Fellow:** Surgery, Univ TX MD Anderson Hosp, Houston, TX 1972-1973; **Fac Appt:** Prof Surgery, UCLA

Esquivel, Carlos Orlando MD (S) - *Spec Exp:* Transplant-Liver; **Hospital:** Stanford Med Ctr; **Address:** 750 Welch Rd, Ste 319, Palo Alto, CA 94304; **Phone:** (650) 498-5689; **Board Cert:** Surgical Critical Care 1999, Surgery 1994; **Med School:** Costa Rica 1975; **Resid:** Surgery, UC-Davis Med Ctr, Sacramento, CA 1977-1984; **Fellow:** Surgical Critical Care, Univ Hlth Ctr Pittsburgh, Pittsburgh, PA 1984-1985; **Fac Appt:** Prof Surgery, Stanford Univ

Esserman, Laura J MD (S) - *Spec Exp:* Breast Cancer; **Hospital:** UCSF - Mount Zion Med Ctr; **Address:** UCSF-Mt Zion Hosp, Dept Surg, 1600 Divisadero St, San Francisco, CA 94115; **Phone:** (415) 353-7111; **Board Cert:** Surgery 1992; **Med School:** Stanford Univ 1983; **Resid:** Surgery, Stanford Univ Med Ctr, Stanford, CA 1984-1991; **Fellow:** Medical Oncology, Stanford Univ Med Ctr, Stanford, CA 1990-1991; **Fac Appt:** Assoc Prof Surgery, UCSF

Essner, Richard MD (S) - *Spec Exp:* Sentinel Node Surgery; Melanoma; **Hospital:** St John's Hlth Ctr; **Address:** 2200 Santa Monica Blvd, Santa Monica, CA 90404; **Phone:** (310) 998-3906; **Board Cert:** Surgery 1994; **Med School:** Emory Univ 1985; **Resid:** Surgery, Univ NC Sch Med, Chapel Hill, NC 1985-1992; **Fac Appt:** Asst Clin Prof Surgery, USC Sch Med

Giuliano, Armando E MD (S) - *Spec Exp:* Sentinel Node Surgery; Breast Cancer; **Hospital:** St John's Hlth Ctr; **Address:** 2200 Santa Monica Blvd, Ste 113, Santa Monica, CA 90404; **Phone:** (310) 829-8089; **Board Cert:** Surgery 1999; **Med School:** Univ Chicago-Pritzker Sch Med 1973; **Resid:** Surgery, UCSF Med Ctr, San Francisco, CA 1974-1980; **Fellow:** Surgical Oncology, UCLA Med Ctr, Los Angeles, CA 1976-1980; **Fac Appt:** Prof Surgery, UCLA

Gower, Roland E MD (S) - *Spec Exp:* Breast Surgery; Biliary Surgery; Thyroid Surgery; **Hospital:** Providence Alaska Med Ctr; **Address:** 2841 De Barr Rd, Ste 41, Anchorage, AK 99508-2973; **Phone:** (907) 279-3564; **Board Cert:** Surgery 1997; **Med School:** Vanderbilt Univ 1971; **Resid:** Surgery, Kansas Med Ctr, KS 1971-1976

Hansen, Nora Marie MD (S) - *Spec Exp:* Sentinel Node Surgery; Breast Cancer; **Hospital:** St John's Hlth Ctr; **Address:** 2200 Santa Monica Blvd, Ste 113, Santa Monica, CA 90404; **Phone:** (310) 829-8089; **Board Cert:** Surgery 1996; **Med School:** NY Med Coll 1988; **Resid:** Surgery, Univ Chicago, Chicago, IL 1989-1995; **Fellow:** Surgical Oncology, Univ Chicago, Chicago, IL 1995-1996

Hoyt, David MD (S) - *Spec Exp:* Trauma; Critical Care; **Hospital:** UCSD Healthcare; **Address:** UCSD Med Ctr, Dept Surg, 200 W Arbor Drive, San Diego, CA 92103-9000; **Phone:** (619) 543-7200; **Board Cert:** Surgery 1994, Surgical Critical Care 1997; **Med School:** Case West Res Univ 1976; **Resid:** Surgery, UCSD Med Ctr, San Diego, CA 1977-1979; Surgery, UCSD Med Ctr, San Diego, CA 1982-1984; **Fellow:** Research, UCSD Med Ctr, San Diego, CA 1979-1980; Immunopathology, Scripps Clin, La Jolla, CA 1980-1982; **Fac Appt:** Prof Surgery, UCSD

Hunter, John G MD (S) - *Spec Exp:* Gastrointestinal Surgery; Laparoscopic Abdominal Surgery; **Hospital:** OR Hlth Sci Univ Hosp and Clinics; **Address:** Oregon Hlth Sci Univ Hosp, Dept Surgery, 3181 SW Sam Jackson Park Rd, Portland, OR 97201-3098; **Phone:** (503) 494-7758; **Board Cert:** Surgery 1997; **Med School:** Univ Penn 1981; **Resid:** Surgery, Univ Utah Med Ctr, Salt Lake City, UT 1982-1987; **Fellow:** Gastrointestinal Surgery, Mass Genl Hosp, Boston, MA 1987-1988; Pancreatic Endoscopy, Univ West Ontario, Canada 1988-1989; **Fac Appt:** Assoc Prof Surgery, Oregon Hlth Scis Univ

Knudson, Mary Margaret MD (S) - *Spec Exp:* Breast Cancer; Trauma; **Hospital:** UCSF Med Ctr; **Address:** UCSF Med Ctr, 400 Parnassus Ave, rm 655, San Fransisco, CA 94143; **Phone:** (415) 353-2161; **Board Cert:** Surgery 1992, Surgical Critical Care 1998; **Med School:** Univ Mich Med Sch 1976; **Resid:** Surgery, Beth Israel Hosp, Boston, MA 1977-1979; Surgery, Univ Mich Med Ctr, Ann Arbor, MI 1979-1982; **Fellow:** Pediatric Surgery, Stanford Univ Hosps, Stanford, CA 1982; **Fac Appt:** Assoc Prof Surgery, UCSF

Pellegrini, Carlos MD (S) - *Spec Exp:* Esophageal Surgery; Barrett's Esophagus; Laparoscopic Surgery; **Hospital:** Univ WA Med Ctr; **Address:** Univ Washington Med Ctr, Dept Surg, 1959 NE Pacific St, Box 356410, Seattle, WA 98195; **Phone:** (206) 543-3106; **Board Cert:** Surgery 1998; **Med School:** Argentina 1971; **Resid:** Surgery, Granadero Hosp, Argentina 1971-1975; Surgery, Chicago Hosps, Chicago, IL 1975-1979; **Fac Appt:** Prof Surgery, Univ Wash

Peters, Jeffrey Harold MD (S) - *Spec Exp:* Esophageal Surgery; Gastroesophageal Reflux; **Hospital:** USC Univ Hosp - R K Eamer Med Plz; **Address:** 1510 San Pablo St, Ste 514, Los Angeles, CA 90033-4612; **Phone:** (323) 442-5926; **Board Cert:** Surgical Critical Care 1994, Surgery 1998; **Med School:** Ohio State Univ 1981; **Resid:** Surgery, Johns Hopkins Hosp, Baltimore, MD 1985-1988; **Fellow:** Allergy & Immunology, Johns Hopkins Hosp, Baltimore, MD 1983-1985; Esophagy, Creighton Univ, Omaha, OK 1990; **Fac Appt:** Prof Surgery, USC Sch Med

Rassman, William Richard MD (S) - *Spec Exp:* Hair Restoration/Transplant; **Address:** 9911 W Pico Blvd, Ste 301, Los Angeles, CA 90035; **Phone:** (310) 553-9113; **Board Cert:** Surgery 1975; **Med School:** Med Coll VA 1966; **Resid:** Surgery, Cornell Med Ctr, New York, NY 1967-1969; Surgery, Dartmouth Med Ctr, Lebanon, NH 1971-1973

Selby, Robert Rick MD (S) - *Spec Exp:* Transplant-Liver; Transplant-Kidney; Transfusion Free Surgery; **Hospital:** USC Univ Hosp - R K Eamer Med Plz; **Address:** USC Univ Hosp, Dept Organ Transplant, 1510 San Pablo St, Ste 430, Los Angeles, CA 90033-4612; **Phone:** (323) 442-5908; **Board Cert:** Surgery 1999, Surgical Critical Care 1991; **Med School:** Univ MO-Columbia Sch Med 1979; **Resid:** Internal Medicine, Good Samaritan Hosp, Phoenix, AZ 1979-1981; Surgery, Good Samaritan Hosp, Phoenix, AZ 1981-1986; **Fellow:** Transplant Surgery, Presby Univ Hosp, Pittsburgh, PA 1987-1988; **Fac Appt:** Prof Surgery, USC Sch Med

Silverstein, Melvin J MD (S) - *Spec Exp:* Breast Cancer; **Hospital:** USC Norris Cancer Comp Ctr; **Address:** USC Norris Cancer Center, 1441 Eastlake Ave, rm 7415, MC-74, Los Angeles, CA 90033; **Phone:** (323) 865-3535; **Board Cert:** Surgery 1971; **Med School:** Albany Med Coll 1965; **Resid:** Surgery, Boston City Hosp-Tufts Univ, Boston, MA 1966-1970; **Fellow:** Surgical Oncology, UCLA, Los Angeles, CA 1972-1975; **Fac Appt:** Prof Surgery, USC Sch Med

Warren, Robert Samuel MD (S) - *Spec Exp:* Liver Cancer; Tumor Surgery; **Hospital:** UCSF Med Ctr; **Address:** UCSF Med Ctr-Ambulatory Care Ctr, 400 Parnassus Ave Fl 6 - rm A-655, Box 0338, San Francisco, CA 94122; **Phone:** (415) 353-2161; **Board Cert:** Surgery 1998; **Med School:** Univ Minn 1980; **Resid:** Surgery, Univ Minn, Minneapolis, MN 1980-1988; **Fellow:** Surgical Oncology, Meml Sloan-Kettering Canc Ctr, New York, NY 1983-1986; **Fac Appt:** Assoc Prof Surgery, UCSF

THORACIC SURGERY

A thoracic surgeon provides the operative, perioperative care and critical care of patients with pathologic conditions within the chest. Included is the surgical care of coronary artery disease, cancers of the lung, esophagus and chest wall, abnormalities of the trachea, abnormalities of the great vessels and heart valves, congenital anomalies, tumors of the mediastinum and diseases of the diaphragm. The management of the airway and injuries of the chest is within the scope of the specialty.

Thoracic surgeons have the knowledge, experience and technical skills to accurately diagnose, operate upon safely and effectively manage patients with thoracic diseases of the chest. This requires substantial knowledge of cardiorespiratory physiology and oncology, as well as capability in the use of heart assist devices, management of abnormal heart rhythms and drainage of the chest cavity, respiratory support systems, endoscopy and invasive and noninvasive diagnostic techniques.

Training required: Seven to eight years

Barnes-Jewish Hospital

BJC HealthCare℠

the primary adult hospital for
Washington University School of Medicine

216 S. Kingshighway
St. Louis, MO 63110
314-TOP-DOCS
(314-867-3627)
or toll free 1-866-867-3627
www.barnesjewish.org

THORACIC SURGERY

comprehensive thoracic surgery program

As part of a pulmonary program ranked fourth in the country by *U.S. News & World Report,* Barnes-Jewish Hospital's Thoracic Surgery program offers a world-class team of medical specialists. Known for its compassionate, expert care, the Thoracic Surgery program includes:

- patient care directed by some of the top thoracic surgeons in the nation

- a cohesive, focused team of thoracic oncologists, anesthesiologists and critical care staff

- access to the latest treatment options available in the areas of lung cancer and esophageal disorders

- dedicated thoracic surgery suites with specially trained nurses and the latest equipment

- one of only a handful of programs in the country to offer a dedicated general thoracic surgery inpatient unit.

one of the most active lung transplant centers in the world

In 1988, Barnes-Jewish Hospital became one of the first hospitals in the U.S. with a program fully dedicated to lung transplants. Substantially higher survival rates for all single and double lung transplant recipients distinguish our program from others. Having recently completed their 600th lung transplant, Washington University lung transplant specialists at Barnes-Jewish Hospital are noted for their many pioneering surgical and medical innovations:

- single-lung transplantation for emphysema and pulmonary hypertension

- bilateral sequential approach to double-lung transplantation for emphysema and cystic fibrosis

- the use of nitric oxide to manage lung injury when restoring blood flow after tranplantation

- lung volume reduction surgery for emphysema, which may be used as a "bridge" to tranplantation or eliminate the need for transplantation.

Advancing Medicine. Touching Lives.

"Everything we do is focused on helping our patients have a better quality of life than when they walked through our doors."

— G. Alexander Patterson, MD
Chief, Thoracic Surgery

If you need a thoracic surgeon go straight to the top. Call **314-TOP-DOCS** (314-867-3627) or toll free 1-866-867-3627. **www.barnesjewish.org**

550 First Avenue (at 31st Street)
New York, NY 10016
Physician Referral: (888) 7-NYU-MED
(888-769-8633) www.nyumedicalcenter.org

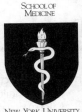

SCHOOL OF
MEDICINE

NEW YORK UNIVERSITY

NYU MEDICAL CENTER – A Leader in Minimally Invasive Thoracic Surgery

On the technological forefront of minimally invasive techniques, the Division of Thoracic Surgery at NYU Medical Center dedicates itself to the diagnosis and treatment of abdominal, lung, mediastinal, and chest wall problems. At NYU Hospitals Center, the majority of thoracic procedures are performed utilizing video-assisted equipment, which benefits surgeon and patient alike.

Use of video-assisted equipment means not only a more accurate and safe surgery, but it also means smaller incisions, an indispensable benefit to the patient, reducing discomfort, recovery time, and length of stay. Moving away from the traditional method of long incisions through the muscular abdominal wall, NYU's thoracic surgeons perform the same procedures through much smaller openings, with better results.

The Division of Thoracic Surgery at NYU Hospitals Center uses minimally invasive techniques to provide its patients maximum comfort and accuracy of diagnosis and treatment. Below are just some of the latest interventions performed by its doctors:

VIDEO-ASSISTED THORACOSCOPY

- Sympathectomy for Hyperhydrosis
- Pleural Biopsy
- Pleurectomy
- Pleurodesis
- Mediastinal Evaluation
- Lung Resection
- Lung Volume Reduction Procedures
- Esophageal Procedures

VIDEO-ASSISTED BRONCHOSCOPY

- Diagnostic Evaluation
- Laser Resection of Tumor
- Endobronchial Stent Insertion

VIDEO-ASSISTED MEDIASTINOSCOPY

- Staging Procedures
- Diagnostic Evaluations

NYU MEDICAL CENTER

The burgeoning field of minimally invasive thoracic surgery is constantly growing in leaps and bounds. In terms of its importance to the medical field, it has been compared to open-heart surgery, or even to anesthesia. Doctors at NYU Hospitals Center dedicate their time not only to unsurpassed clinical care, but also to contributions through research. For example, its surgeons have performed more minimally invasive port-access cardiac surgeries than any other hospital in the world, and their expertise in unparalleled.

Physician Referral
(888) 7-NYU-MED
(888-769-8633)
www.nyumedicalcenter.org

PHYSICIAN LISTINGS

Thoracic Surgery

New England

Akins, Cary W MD (TS) - *Spec Exp:* *Heart Valve Surgery; Coronary Artery Surgery; Aneurysm;* **Hospital:** MA Genl Hosp; **Address:** Mass Genl Hosp Dept Surgery, 55 Fruit St, WHT 503, Boston, MA 02114; **Phone:** (617) 726-8218; **Board Cert:** Thoracic Surgery 1997, Surgery 1976; **Med School:** Harvard Med Sch 1970; **Resid:** Surgery, Mass Genl Hosp, Boston, MA 1971-1975; **Fac Appt:** Clin Prof Surgery, Harvard Med Sch

Bredenberg, Carl Eric MD (TS) - *Spec Exp:* *Esophageal Surgery;* **Hospital:** Maine Med Ctr; **Address:** 887 Congress St, Ste 300, Portland, ME 04102; **Phone:** (207) 773-8161; **Board Cert:** Thoracic Surgery 1974, Vascular Surgery (General) 1993; **Med School:** Johns Hopkins Univ 1964; **Resid:** Surgery, Johns Hopkins Hosp, Baltimore, MD 1967-1972; **Fellow:** Research, Walter Reed Army Inst Rsch, Washington, DC 1965-1967; **Fac Appt:** Prof Surgery, Univ VT Coll Med

Cohn, Lawrence H MD (TS) - *Spec Exp:* *Heart Valve Surgery; Heart Disease-Congenital;* **Hospital:** Brigham & Women's Hosp; **Address:** 75 Francis St, Boston, MA 02115-6110; **Phone:** (617) 732-7678; **Board Cert:** Surgery 1970, Thoracic Surgery 1971; **Med School:** Stanford Univ 1962; **Resid:** Surgery, UCSF Med Ctr, San Francisco, CA 1966-1969; Cardiothoracic Surgery, Stanford Univ, Stanford, CA 1969-1971; **Fellow:** Surgery, Boston City Hosp, Boston, MA 1962-1964; **Fac Appt:** Prof Surgery, Harvard Med Sch

Elefteriades, John MD (TS) - *Spec Exp:* *Transplant-Heart; Aneurysm-Abdominal Aortic; Coronary Artery Surgery;* **Hospital:** Yale - New Haven Hosp; **Address:** 333 Cedar St, rm 121-FMB, New Haven, CT 06520; **Phone:** (203) 785-2705; **Board Cert:** Thoracic Surgery 1994; **Med School:** Yale Univ 1976; **Resid:** Surgery, Yale-New Haven Hosp, New Haven, CT 1977-1981; Thoracic Surgery, Yale-New Haven Hosp, New Haven, CT 1981-1983; **Fellow:** Thoracic Surgery, Yale-New Haven Hosp, New Haven, CT 1981-1983; **Fac Appt:** Prof Surgery, Yale Univ

Jonas, Richard A MD (TS) - *Spec Exp:* *Cardiac Surgery-Pediatric;* **Hospital:** Children's Hospital - Boston; **Address:** Children's Hospital- Cardiac Surgery, 300 Longwood Ave, Boston, MA 02115; **Phone:** (617) 355-7930; **Med School:** Australia 1974; **Resid:** Surgery, Royal Melbourne Hosp, Melbourne, Australia 1975-1979; Thoracic Surgery, Green Lane Hosp, Auckland, New Zealand 1980-1982; **Fellow:** Thoracic Surgery, Brigham & Women's Hosp, Boston, MA 1982-1984; **Fac Appt:** Prof Surgery, Harvard Med Sch

Kopf, Gary MD (TS) - *Spec Exp:* *Cardiac Surgery-Adult & Pediatric;* **Hospital:** Yale - New Haven Hosp; **Address:** 330 Orchard St, Ste 107, New Haven, CT 06511; **Phone:** (203) 785-2702; **Board Cert:** Thoracic Surgery 1982; **Med School:** Harvard Med Sch 1970; **Resid:** Surgery, Peter Bent Brigham Hosp, Boston, MA 1973-1977; Thoracic Surgery, Chldns Hosp Med Ctr, Boston, MA 1977-1980; **Fellow:** Surgery, Harvard/Brigham Hosp, Boston, MA 1973-1980; **Fac Appt:** Prof Surgery, Yale Univ

Mathisen, Douglas MD (TS) - *Spec Exp:* *Tracheal Surgery; Lung Cancer; Esophageal Cancer;* **Hospital:** MA Genl Hosp; **Address:** Mass Genl Hosp, 55 Fruit St, Bldg Blake 1570, Boston, MA 02114; **Phone:** (617) 726-6826; **Board Cert:** Surgery 1982, Thoracic Surgery 1984; **Med School:** Univ IL Coll Med 1974; **Resid:** Surgery, Mass Genl Hosp, Boston, MA 1974-1981; Thoracic Surgery, Mass Genl Hosp, Boston, MA 1981-1982; **Fellow:** Surgical Oncology, Natl Cancer Inst, Bethesda, MD 1977-1979; **Fac Appt:** Prof Surgery, Harvard Med Sch

Moncure, Ashby MD (TS) - *Spec Exp:* *Esophageal Cancer;* **Hospital:** MA Genl Hosp; **Address:** Mass Genl Hosp Bldg Wang ACC - Ste 335, 15 Parkman St, Boston, MA 02114; **Phone:** (617) 726-2819; **Board Cert:** Thoracic Surgery 1971, Vascular Surgery (General) 1989; **Med School:** Univ VA Sch Med 1960; **Resid:** Surgery, Mass Genl Hosp, Boston, MA 1961-1962; Thoracic Surgery, Frenchy Hosp, Bristol England 1967; **Fac Appt:** Assoc Prof Surgery, Harvard Med Sch

THORACIC SURGERY

Shahian, David MD (TS) - *Spec Exp:* Lung Cancer; **Hospital:** Lahey Cli.; **Address:** Lahey Clinic, Dept Thor and CV Surg, 41 Mall Rd, Burlington, MA 01805; **Phone:** (781) 744-8575; **Board Cert:** Thoracic Surgery 1990; **Med School:** Harvard Med Sch 1973; **Resid:** Surgery, Mass Genl Hosp, Boston, MA 1974-1978; **Fellow:** Thoracic Surgery, Rush Presby-St Lukes Hosp, Chicago, IL 1978-1980; **Fac Appt:** Assoc Clin Prof Surgery, Harvard Med Sch

Sugarbaker, David John MD (TS) - *Spec Exp:* Mesothelioma; **Hospital:** Brigham & Women's Hosp; **Address:** 75 Francis St, Boston, MA 02115-6110; **Phone:** (617) 732-5004; **Board Cert:** Surgery 1987, Thoracic Surgery 1999; **Med School:** Cornell Univ-Weill Med Coll 1979; **Resid:** Surgery, Brigham & Women's Hosp, Boston, MA 1980-1982; Surgery, Brigham & Women's Hosp, Boston, MA 1984-1986; **Fellow:** Thoracic Surgery, Toronto Genl Hosp, Toronto, CN 1986-1988; **Fac Appt:** Assoc Prof Surgery, Harvard Med Sch

Vander Salm, Thomas MD (TS) - *Spec Exp:* Heart Valve Surgery-Mitral; Cardiovascular Surgery; **Hospital:** U Mass Meml Hlth Care - Worcester; **Address:** 55 Lake Ave N, Worcester, MA 01655; **Phone:** (508) 856-2216; **Board Cert:** Surgery 1974, Thoracic Surgery 1994; **Med School:** Johns Hopkins Univ 1966; **Resid:** Surgery, Mass Genl Hosp, Boston, MA 1967-1968; Surgery, Johns Hopkins Hosp, Baltimore, MD 1968; **Fac Appt:** Prof Surgery, Univ Mass Sch Med

Wain, John MD (TS) - *Spec Exp:* Transplant-Lung; Emphysema; **Hospital:** MA Genl Hosp; **Address:** 55 Fruit St, Blake 1570, Boston, MA 02114; **Phone:** (617) 726-5200; **Board Cert:** Surgery 1986, Thoracic Surgery 1990; **Med School:** Jefferson Med Coll 1980; **Resid:** Surgery, Mass Genl Hosp, Boston, MA 1980-1985; Medical Oncology, City Hope Med Ctr, Duarte, CA 1985-1986; **Fellow:** Cardiothoracic Surgery, Mass Genl Hosp, Bostn, MA 1986-1988; **Fac Appt:** Asst Prof Thoracic Surgery, Harvard Med Sch

Wright, Cameron MD (TS) - *Spec Exp:* Lung Cancer; Esophageal Cancer; Tracheal Surgery; **Hospital:** MA Genl Hosp; **Address:** Division of Surgery, 55 Fruit St, Blake 1570, Boston, MA 02114-2696; **Phone:** (617) 726-5801; **Board Cert:** Surgery 1995, Thoracic Surgery 1997; **Med School:** Univ Mich Med Sch 1980; **Resid:** Surgery, Mass Genl Hosp, Boston, MA 1980-1986; Thoracic Surgery, Mass Genl Hosp, Boston, MA 1986-1988; **Fac Appt:** Assoc Prof Surgery, Harvard Med Sch

Mid Atlantic

Acinapura, Anthony MD (TS) - *Spec Exp:* Cardiothoracic Surgery; Vascular Surgery; **Hospital:** Maimonides Med Ctr (page 65); **Address:** Lutheran Med Ctr, 150 55th St, Ste 3524, Brooklyn, NY 11220; **Phone:** (718) 630-7351; **Board Cert:** Surgery 1971, Thoracic Surgery 1972; **Med School:** Georgetown Univ 1969; **Resid:** Surgery, Bellevue Hosp, New York, NY 1966-1969; Thoracic Surgery, Bellevue Hosp, New York, NY 1969-1971; **Fellow:** Surgery, Duke Univ Med Ctr, Durham, NC 1965-1966; **Fac Appt:** Prof Surgery, NY Med Coll

Acker, Michael A MD (TS) - *Spec Exp:* Transplant-Heart; Heart Assistance Devices; **Hospital:** Univ Penn - Presby Med Ctr; **Address:** 3400 Spruce St, 4 Silverstein Pavillion, Philadelphia, PA 19104-4227; **Phone:** (215) 349-8305; **Board Cert:** Thoracic Surgery 1992, Surgery 2000; **Med School:** Brown Univ 1981; **Resid:** Surgery, Hosp Univ Pennsylvania Hlth Sys, Philadelphia, PA 1982-1988; Thoracic Surgery, Johns Hopkins Hosp, Baltimore, MD 1988-1991; **Fac Appt:** Assoc Prof Surgery, Univ Penn

Adams, David H MD (TS) - *Spec Exp:* Minimally Invasive Cardiac Surgery; **Hospital:** Mount Sinai Hosp (page 68); **Address:** 1190 Fifth Ave Fl 2, New York, NY 10029; **Phone:** (212) 659-6800; **Board Cert:** Surgery 1992, Thoracic Surgery 1994; **Med School:** Duke Univ 1983; **Resid:** Surgery, Brigham & Women's Hosp, Boston, MA; Thoracic Surgery, Brigham & Women's Hosp, Boston, MA; **Fac Appt:** Prof Thoracic Surgery, Mount Sinai Sch Med

Aklog, Lishan MD (TS) - *Spec Exp:* Robotic Surgery-Cardiac; Minimally Invasive Surgery; Robotic Surgery-Mitral Valve; **Hospital:** Mount Sinai Hosp (page 68); **Address:** 1190 Fifth Ave Fl 2, New York, NY 10029; **Phone:** (212) 659-6800; **Board Cert:** Surgery 1997, Thoracic Surgery 2000; **Med School:** Harvard Med Sch 1989; **Resid:** Surgery, Brigham & Women's Hosp, Boston, MA 1990-1996; **Fellow:** Cardiothoracic Surgery, Brigham & Women's Hosp, Boston, MA 1996-1998

Alexander Jr., John C MD (TS) - *Spec Exp:* Minimally Invasive Cardiac Surgery; Robotic Surgery; **Hospital:** Hackensack Univ Med Ctr; **Address:** Hackensack Univ Med Ctr, Main Bldg, 30 Prospect Ave Fl 3, Hackensack, NJ 07601; **Phone:** (201) 996-2791; **Board Cert:** Thoracic Surgery 1992; **Med School:** Duke Univ 1972; **Resid:** Surgery, Duke Univ Med Ctr, Durham, NC 1972-1977; **Fellow:** Cardiothoracic Surgery, Duke Univ Med Ctr, Durham, NC 1979-1980; **Fac Appt:** Prof Surgery, UMDNJ-NJ Med Sch, Newark

Bains, Manjit MD (TS) - *Spec Exp:* Cardiothoracic Surgery; Esophageal Cancer; **Hospital:** Mem Sloan Kettering Cancer Ctr; **Address:** 1275 York Ave, New York, NY 10021; **Phone:** (212) 639-7450; **Board Cert:** Thoracic Surgery 1972; **Med School:** India 1963; **Resid:** Surgery, Rochester, Rochester, NY 1966-1970; **Fellow:** Thoracic Surgery, Sloan Kettering Cancer Ctr, New York, NY 1970-1972; **Fac Appt:** Clin Prof Surgery, Cornell Univ-Weill Med Coll

Baumgartner, William MD (TS) - *Spec Exp:* Thoracic Surgery - General; **Hospital:** Johns Hopkins Hosp - Baltimore; **Address:** 600 N Wolfe St, Blalock Bldg, Ste 618, Baltimore, MD 21287; **Phone:** (410) 955-5248; **Board Cert:** Surgery 1990, Thoracic Surgery 1991; **Med School:** Univ KY Coll Med 1973; **Resid:** Surgery, Stanford U Med Ctr, Stanford, CA 1974-1975; Thoracic Surgery, Stanford U Med Ctr, Stanford, CA 1975-1976; **Fac Appt:** Prof Surgery, Johns Hopkins Univ

Bavaria, Joseph MD (TS) - *Spec Exp:* Aortic Surgery-Thoracic; Transplant-Lung; Heart Valve Surgery; **Hospital:** Univ Penn - Presby Med Ctr; **Address:** Hosp of U Penn, 3400 Spruce St Fl 4, Philadelphia, PA 19104; **Phone:** (215) 662-2017; **Board Cert:** Surgery 1992, Thoracic Surgery 1993; **Med School:** Tulane Univ 1983; **Resid:** Surgery, U Penn, Philadelphia, PA 1983-1983; Surgery, U Penn, Philadelphia, PA 1984-1990; **Fellow:** Cardiothoracic Surgery, U Penn, Philadelphia, PA 1990-1992; **Fac Appt:** Assoc Prof Surgery, Univ Penn

Brodman, Richard Ferris MD (TS) - *Spec Exp:* Coronary Artery Surgery; **Hospital:** NY Presby Hosp - NY Weill Cornell Med Ctr (page 70); **Address:** NY Presby Hosp, Cardiothoracic Surgery, 525 E 68th St, MS F2103, New York, NY 10021-4870; **Phone:** (212) 746-1100; **Board Cert:** Thoracic Surgery 1997, Surgery 1977; **Med School:** Univ Fla Coll Med 1972; **Resid:** Surgery, Montefiore Hosp Med Ctr, Bronx, NY 1972-1976; Thoracic Surgery, Montefiore Hosp Med Ctr, Bronx, NY 1976-1978; **Fellow:** Univ Florida Sch Med, Gainesville, FL 1969-1970; **Fac Appt:** Prof Thoracic Surgery, Albert Einstein Coll Med

Colvin, Stephen MD (TS) - *Spec Exp:* Minimally Invasive Cardiac Surgery; Robotic Surgery; Heart Valve Repair; **Hospital:** NYU Med Ctr (page 71); **Address:** 530 1st Ave, Ste 9V, New York, NY 10016; **Phone:** (212) 263-6384; **Board Cert:** Thoracic Surgery 1984, Surgery 1979; **Med School:** Albert Einstein Coll Med 1969; **Resid:** Surgery, NYU/Bellevue Hosp, New York, NY 1969-1971; Thoracic Surgery, NYU/Bellevue Hosp, New York, NY 1976-1978; **Fellow:** Cardiothoracic Surgery, Natl Heart & Lung Inst, New York, NY 1971-1973; **Fac Appt:** Assoc Clin Prof Surgery, NYU Sch Med

Conte Jr, John V MD (TS) - *Spec Exp:* Transplant-Heart; Transplant-Lung; **Hospital:** Johns Hopkins Hosp - Baltimore; **Address:** 600 N Wolfe St Bldg Blalock - rm 618, Baltimore, MD 21287-4618; **Phone:** (410) 955-1753; **Board Cert:** Surgery 1993, Thoracic Surgery 1997; **Med School:** Georgetown Univ 1986; **Resid:** Thoracic Surgery, Standford Univ, Palo Alto, CA 1992-1995; Surgery, Georgetown Univ, Washington, DC 1987-1992

Cunningham Jr, Joseph N MD (TS) - *Spec Exp:* Coronary Artery Surgery; Minimally Invasive Cardiac Surgery; **Hospital:** Maimonides Med Ctr (page 65); **Address:** Cardiothoracic Dept, 4802 10th Ave, Brooklyn, NY 11219; **Phone:** (718) 283-8302; **Board Cert:** Surgery 1973, Thoracic Surgery 1975; **Med School:** Univ Ala 1966; **Resid:** Surgery, Parkland Meml Hosp, Dallas, TX 1967-1972; **Fellow:** Cardiology (Cardiovascular Disease), NYU Med Ctr, New York, NY 1972-1974; **Fac Appt:** Prof Surgery, SUNY Downstate

Furukawa, Satoshi MD (TS) - *Spec Exp:* Transplant-Heart & Lung; Cardiac Surgery-High Risk; Heart Valve Surgery; **Hospital:** Temple Univ Hosp; **Address:** 3401 N Broad St, Ste 300, Philadelphia, PA 19140-5189; **Phone:** (215) 707-3601; **Board Cert:** Surgery 1993, Thoracic Surgery 1996; **Med School:** Univ Penn 1984; **Resid:** Surgery, Univ Pennsylvania Hlth Sys, Philadelphia, PA 1984-1991; Thoracic Surgery, Univ Pennsylvania Hlth Sys, Philadelphia, PA 1991-1993; **Fac Appt:** Assoc Prof Thoracic Surgery, Temple Univ

Galloway, Aubrey MD (TS) - *Spec Exp:* Heart Disease-Congenital; Minimally Invasive Cardiac Surgery; Heart Valve Surgery; **Hospital:** NYU Med Ctr (page 71); **Address:** 530 1st Ave, Ste 9V, New York, NY 10016-6402; **Phone:** (212) 263-7185; **Board Cert:** Thoracic Surgery 1996; **Med School:** Tulane Univ 1978; **Resid:** Surgery, Univ CO Hosp, Denver, CO 1979-1983; Cardiothoracic Surgery, NYU Med Ctr, New York, NY 1983-1985; **Fellow:** Cardiothoracic Surgery, New York Univ Med Ctr, New York, NY 1983-1985; **Fac Appt:** Prof Surgery, NYU Sch Med

Gardner, Timothy Joseph MD (TS) - *Spec Exp:* Heart Failure; Coronary Artery Surgery; Heart Disease-Congenital; **Hospital:** Univ Penn - Presby Med Ctr; **Address:** Hosp Univ Penn, Dept Cardiothoracic Surgery, 3400 Spruce St , Bldg Silverstein - Fl 4, Philadelphia, PA 19104-4283; **Phone:** (215) 662-2022; **Board Cert:** Surgery 1975, Thoracic Surgery 1996; **Med School:** Georgetown Univ 1966; **Resid:** Surgery, Johns Hopkins Hosp, Baltimore, MD 1967-1968; Surgery, Johns Hopkins Hosp, Baltimore, MD 1971-1976; **Fellow:** Research, Johns Hopkins Hosp, Baltimore, MD 1970-1971; **Fac Appt:** Prof Surgery, Univ Penn

Graver, L Michael MD (TS) - *Spec Exp:* Heart Valve Surgery; Coronary Artery Surgery; Cardiac Surgery; **Hospital:** Long Island Jewish Med Ctr; **Address:** 270-05 76th Ave, New Hyde Park, NY 11040-1433; **Phone:** (718) 470-7460; **Board Cert:** Surgery 1993, Thoracic Surgery 1995; **Med School:** Albany Med Coll 1977; **Resid:** Surgery, St Luke's-Roosevelt Hosp Ctr, New York, NY 1977-1982; Cardiothoracic Surgery, Children's Hosp, Boston, MA 1982-1983; **Fellow:** Cardiothoracic Surgery, Deaconness Hosp, Boston, MA 1983-1985; **Fac Appt:** Assoc Prof Surgery, Albert Einstein Coll Med

Griepp, Randall MD (TS) - *Spec Exp:* Aneurysm-Abdominal Aortic; Endovascular Surgery; **Hospital:** Mount Sinai Hosp (page 68); **Address:** Mount Sinai Med Ctr, Dept Thoracic Surgery, Anneberg Bldg Fl 7 - rm 54, Box 1028, New York, NY 10029; **Phone:** (212) 241-8181; **Board Cert:** Thoracic Surgery 1997, Surgery 1977; **Med School:** Stanford Univ 1967; **Resid:** Thoracic Surgery, Stanford Univ Hosp, Stanford, CA 1968-1973; Internal Medicine, Bellevue Hosp Ctr, New York, NY 1967-1968; **Fellow:** Thoracic Surgery, Stanford Univ Hosp, Stanford, CA 1971-1972

Griffith, Bartley MD (TS) - *Spec Exp:* Transplant-Heart; **Hospital:** UPMC - Presbyterian Univ Hosp; **Address:** UPMC - Presbyterian Univ Hosp - CTS, 20 Lothrop St, Ste C700, Pittsburgh, PA 15213-2582; **Phone:** (412) 648-9254; **Board Cert:** Thoracic Surgery 1992, Surgery 1982; **Med School:** Jefferson Med Coll 1974; **Resid:** Surgery, Univ Hlth Ctr Hosp, Pittsburgh, PA 1978-1979; Thoracic Surgery, Univ Hlth Ctr Hosp, Pittsburgh, PA 1978-1979; **Fellow:** Research, Univ Hlth Ctr Hosp, Pittsburgh, PA 1977-1978; **Fac Appt:** Prof Surgery, Univ Pittsburgh

Grossi, Eugene A MD (TS) - *Spec Exp:* Coronary Artery Surgery; Mitral Valve- Minimally Invasive; Cardiac Tumors, Myxomas; **Hospital:** NYU Med Ctr (page 71); **Address:** NYU Med Ctr, 530 1st Ave, Ste 6D, New York, NY 10016-6402; **Phone:** (212) 263-7452; **Board Cert:** Thoracic Surgery 1993; **Med School:** Columbia P&S 1981; **Resid:** Surgery, NYU Med Ctr, New York, NY 1982-1987; Thoracic Surgery, NYU Med Ctr, New York, NY 1988-1991; **Fac Appt:** Assoc Prof Surgery, NYU Sch Med

Heitmiller, Richard F MD (TS) - *Spec Exp:* Esophageal Surgery; Esophageal Cancer; Lung Cancer; **Hospital:** Union Memorial Hosp - Baltimore; **Address:** 3333 N Calvert St, Ste 610, Baltimore, MD 21218; **Phone:** (410) 554-2063; **Board Cert:** Surgery 1997, Thoracic Surgery 1999; **Med School:** Johns Hopkins Univ 1979; **Resid:** Surgery, Mass Genl Hosp., Boston, MA 1980-1985; **Fellow:** Thoracic Surgery, Mass Genl Hosp., Boston, MA 1985-1987

Isom, O Wayne MD (TS) - *Spec Exp:* Cardiac Surgery; Coronary Artery Surgery; **Hospital:** NY Presby Hosp - NY Weill Cornell Med Ctr (page 70); **Address:** 525 E 68th St, rm M-404, New York, NY 10021; **Phone:** (212) 746-5151; **Board Cert:** Thoracic Surgery 1972, Surgery 1971; **Med School:** Univ Tex, Houston 1965; **Resid:** Surgery, Parkland Meml Hosp, Dallas, TX 1965-1970; **Fellow:** Thoracic Surgery, NYU Med Ctr, New York, NY 1970-1972

Kaiser, Larry Robert MD (TS) - *Spec Exp:* Lung Cancer; Esophageal Cancer; Mediastinal Tumors; **Hospital:** Hosp Univ Penn (page 78); **Address:** Silverstein Building, 4th FL, 3400 Spruce St, Philadelphia, PA 19104-4219; **Phone:** (215) 662-7538; **Board Cert:** Thoracic Surgery 1997, Surgery 1985; **Med School:** Tulane Univ 1977; **Resid:** Surgery, UCLA Med Ctr, Los Angeles, CA 1978-1983; Thoracic Surgery, Univ Toronto Hosps, Canada 1983-1985; **Fellow:** Surgical Oncology, UCLA Med Ctr, Los Angeles, CA 1979-1981; **Fac Appt:** Prof Surgery, Univ Penn

Kanda, Louis T MD (TS) - *Spec Exp:* Heart Valve Surgery; **Hospital:** Washington Hosp Ctr; **Address:** Cardio & Thor Surg Assocs, 106 Irving St NW, Bldg POB N. Tower - Fl 4300-N, Washington, DC 20010; **Phone:** (202) 829-5602; **Board Cert:** Thoracic Surgery 1991; **Med School:** Geo Wash Univ 1970; **Resid:** Surgery, Washington Hosp Ctr, Washington, DC 1971-1975; **Fellow:** Thoracic Surgery, Cleveland Clin Fdn, Cleveland, OH 1978-1980; **Fac Appt:** Asst Prof Surgery, Howard Univ

Katz, Nevin M MD (TS) - *Spec Exp:* Coronary Artery Surgery; Heart Valve Surgery; **Hospital:** G Washington Univ Hosp; **Address:** 2150 Pennsylvania Ave NW, Ste 6B, Washington, DC 20037; **Phone:** (202) 994-1928; **Board Cert:** Thoracic Surgery 2000; **Med School:** Case West Res Univ 1971; **Resid:** Cardiovascular Surgery, Boston Chldns Hosp, Birmingham, AL 1976; Cardiothoracic Surgery, Univ Alabama, Birmingham, AL 1978-1980; **Fellow:** Cardiovascular Surgery, Univ Alabama, Birmingham, AL 1977-1978; **Fac Appt:** Prof Surgery, Georgetown Univ

Keenan, Robert MD (TS) - *Spec Exp:* Transplant-Lung; Lung Surgery; **Hospital:** Allegheny General Hosp; **Address:** Allegheny Genl Hosp, O2 Level, 320 E North Ave, Pittsburgh, PA 15212; **Phone:** (412) 359-6137; **Board Cert:** Surgery 1990; **Med School:** Canada 1984; **Resid:** Surgery, Univ Toronto Med Ctr, Toronto, Canada 1985-1989; **Fellow:** Thoracic Surgery, Univ Pittsburgh Med Ctr, Pittsburgh, PA 1989-1990

Keller, Steven M MD (TS) - *Spec Exp:* Lung Cancer; Esophageal Cancer; Palmar Hyperhidrosis; **Hospital:** Montefiore Med Ctr (page 67); **Address:** Greene Medical Arts Pavilion, 3400 Bainbridge Ave, Ste 5B, Bronx, NY 10467-2404; **Phone:** (718) 920-7580; **Board Cert:** Surgery 1996, Thoracic Surgery 1998; **Med School:** Albany Med Coll 1977; **Resid:** Surgery, Mount Sinai Hosp, New York, NY 1979-1985; Thoracic Surgery, Mem Sloan Kettering Cancer Ctr, New York, NY 1985-1987; **Fellow:** Surgery, Natl Canc Ctr, Bethesda, MD 1981-1983; **Fac Appt:** Prof Thoracic Surgery, Albert Einstein Coll Med

Kormos, Robert MD (TS) - *Spec Exp:* Transplant-Heart; Heart-Artificial; **Hospital:** UPMC - Presbyterian Univ Hosp; **Address:** UPMC Presbyterian, 200 Lothrop St, Ste C700, Pittsburgh, PA 15213; **Phone:** (412) 648-8107; **Med School:** Canada 1976; **Resid:** Surgery, Toronto Western Hosp, Toronto, Canada; **Fellow:** Cardiothoracic Surgery, Toronto Genl Hosp, Toronto, Canada; Transplant Surgery, Univ Pitts Med Ctr, Pittsburgh, PA 1985-1987; **Fac Appt:** Assoc Prof Surgery, Univ Pittsburgh

Krellenstein, Daniel MD (TS) - *Spec Exp:* Thoracic Surgery - General; **Hospital:** Mount Sinai Hosp (page 68); **Address:** 16 E 98th St, Ste 1F, New York, NY 10029-6545; **Phone:** (212) 423-9311; **Board Cert:** Thoracic Surgery 1977, Surgery 1974; **Med School:** SUNY Buffalo 1964; **Resid:** Surgery, SUNY Downstate, Brooklyn, NY 1965-1972; **Fac Appt:** Assoc Clin Prof Thoracic Surgery, Mount Sinai Sch Med

Landreneau, Rodney MD (TS) - *Spec Exp:* Lung Cancer; Esophageal Cancer; Gastroesophageal Reflux; **Hospital:** Allegheny General Hosp; **Address:** Allegheny Genl Hosp, Dept Thor Surg, 320 E North Ave, Pittsburgh, PA 15212-4772; **Phone:** (412) 359-6412; **Board Cert:** Surgery 1984, Thoracic Surgery 1994; **Med School:** Louisiana State Univ 1965; **Resid:** Surgery, Parkland Meml Hosp, Dallas, TX 1978-1983; **Fellow:** Cardiothoracic Surgery, Univ Mich Med Ctr, Ann Arbor, MI 1983-1985; **Fac Appt:** Prof Surgery, Hahnemann Univ

Lang, Samuel MD (TS) - *Spec Exp:* Minimally Invasive Cardiac Surgery; **Hospital:** St Vincent Cath Med Ctrs - Manhattan (page 75); **Address:** 153 W 11th St, Spellman, 7th Fl, New York, NY 10011; **Phone:** (212) 604-2488; **Board Cert:** Thoracic Surgery 1996; **Med School:** Univ Ala 1978; **Resid:** Surgery, UCLA Med Ctr, Los Angeles, CA 1978-1982; Thoracic Surgery, NYU Med Ctr, New York, NY 1982-1983; **Fac Appt:** Prof Surgery, Cornell Univ-Weill Med Coll

Loulmet, Didier MD (TS) - *Spec Exp:* Heart Valve Surgery; Cardiac Robotic Surgery; Endoscopic Cardiac Surgery; **Hospital:** Lenox Hill Hosp (page 64); **Address:** Lenox Hill Hosp, William Black Hall, 130 E 77th St, Fl 4, New York, NY 10021; **Phone:** (212) 434-3000; **Med School:** France 1989; **Resid:** Cardiothoracic Surgery, Paris Univ Hosp, France 1989-1990; Cardiothoracic Surgery, Brigham & Women's Hosp, Boston, MA 1990-1991; **Fellow:** Pediatric Cardiac Surgery, Chldn's Hosp, Harvard Univ, Boston, MA 1991-1992

Mindich, Bruce MD (TS) - *Spec Exp:* Cardiac Surgery; **Hospital:** Valley Hosp, The; **Address:** 223 N Van Dien Ave, Ridgewood, NJ 07450-2736; **Phone:** (201) 447-8377; **Board Cert:** Thoracic Surgery 1998; **Med School:** SUNY Downstate 1972; **Resid:** Surgery, Jewish Hosp Med Ctr, Brooklyn, NY 1972-1975; Cardiothoracic Surgery, Mt Sinai Hosp, New York, NY 1975-1977; **Fellow:** Cardiothoracic Surgery, Cleveland Clinic, Cleveland, OH 1977-1978; Cardiology (Cardiovascular Disease), Univ Alabama Med Ctr, Birmingham, AL 1978

Oz, Mehmet Cengiz MD (TS) - *Spec Exp:* Transplant-Heart; Coronary Artery Surgery; Minimally Invasive Cardiac Surgery; **Hospital:** NY Presby Hosp - Columbia Presby Med Ctr (page 70); **Address:** New York Presbyterian Hospital, Dept of Surgery, 177 Ft Washington Ave Bldg MHB Fl 7 - Ste 435, New York, NY 10032; **Phone:** (212) 305-4434; **Board Cert:** Surgery 1992, Thoracic Surgery 1994; **Med School:** Univ Penn 1986; **Resid:** Surgery, Columbia Presby Med Ctr, New York, NY 1987-1991; **Fellow:** Thoracic Surgery, Columbia Presby Med Ctr, New York, NY 1991-1993; **Fac Appt:** Assoc Prof Surgery, Columbia P&S

Rose, Eric A MD (TS) - *Spec Exp:* Transplant-Heart; Cardiothoracic Surgery; **Hospital:** NY Presby Hosp - Columbia Presby Med Ctr (page 70); **Address:** 177 Fort Washington Ave, Ste 7-435, New York, NY 10032; **Phone:** (212) 305-6380; **Board Cert:** Thoracic Surgery 1992, Surgery 1975; **Med School:** Columbia P&S 1975; **Resid:** Surgery, Columbia Presby Med Ctr, New York, NY 1976-1979; Thoracic Surgery, Columbia Presby Med Ctr, New York, NY 1980-1981; **Fac Appt:** Prof Thoracic Surgery, Columbia P&S

Rusch, Valerie MD (TS) - *Spec Exp:* *Mesothelioma; Lung Cancer; Esophageal Cancer;* **Hospital:** Mem Sloan Kettering Cancer Ctr; **Address:** 1275 York Ave, Ste 867, New York, NY 10021-6094; **Phone:** (212) 639-5873; **Board Cert:** Surgery 2001, Thoracic Surgery 1992; **Med School:** Columbia P&S 1975; **Resid:** Surgery, Univ WA Med Ctr, Seattle, WA 1975-1980; Cardiothoracic Surgery, Univ WA Med Ctr, Seattle, WA 1980-1982; **Fac Appt:** Prof Surgery, Cornell Univ-Weill Med Coll

Samuels, Louis MD (TS) - *Spec Exp:* *Transplant-Heart; Artificial Heart;* **Hospital:** Hahnemann Univ Hosp; **Address:** Hahnemann Univ Hosp, Dept Cardiothor Surg, Broad & Vine St, Philadelphia, PA 19102; **Phone:** (215) 762-7802; **Board Cert:** Surgery 1994, Thoracic Surgery 1996; **Med School:** Hahnemann Univ 1987; **Resid:** Surgery, Hahnemann Hosp, Philadelphia, PA 1987-1992; Thoracic Surgery, Hahnemann Hosp, Philadelphia, PA 1992-1995; **Fac Appt:** Asst Prof Thoracic Surgery, Hahnemann Univ

Smith, Craig R MD (TS) - *Spec Exp:* *Robotic Surgery-Mitral Valve; Transplant-Heart; Endoscopic Coronary Artery Bypass;* **Hospital:** NY Presby Hosp - Columbia Presby Med Ctr (page 70); **Address:** 177 Fort Washington Ave, Fl 7th - rm 435, New York, NY 10032; **Phone:** (212) 305-8312; **Board Cert:** Thoracic Surgery 1986; **Med School:** Case West Res Univ 1977; **Resid:** Surgery, Strong Meml Hosp, Rochester, NY 1978-1982; **Fellow:** Cardiothoracic Surgery, Columbia Presby Med Ctr, New York, NY 1982-1984; **Fac Appt:** Prof Surgery, Columbia P&S

Sonett, Joshua R MD (TS) - *Spec Exp:* *Minimally Invasive Surgery-Lung; Transplant-Lung; Thoracic Oncology;* **Hospital:** NY Presby Hosp - Columbia Presby Med Ctr (page 70); **Address:** 622 W 168th St, Ste PH 14 East - rm 104, New York, NY 10032; **Phone:** (212) 305-8086; **Board Cert:** Thoracic Surgery 1997, Surgery 1994; **Med School:** E Carolina Univ 1988; **Resid:** Surgery, U Mass Med Ctr, Worcester, MA 1989-1993; **Fellow:** Thoracic Surgery, U Pittsburgh Med Ctr, Pittsburgh, PA 1993; Thoracic Surgery, Mem Sloane Kettering, New York, NY 1994

Strong III, Michael D MD (TS) - *Spec Exp:* *Coronary Artery Surgery; Heart Valve Surgery;* **Hospital:** Hahnemann Univ Hosp; **Address:** Dept Cardiothoracic Surgery, MS 111, Broad & Vine Sts, N Tower Bldg, Ste 744, Philadelphia, PA 19102; **Phone:** (215) 762-7802; **Board Cert:** Thoracic Surgery 1996, Surgery 1974; **Med School:** Jefferson Med Coll 1966; **Resid:** Surgery, Jefferson Hosp, Philadelphia, PA 1969-1973; Thoracic Surgery, Temple Univ Hosp, Philadelphia, PA 1973-1975; **Fac Appt:** Assoc Prof Thoracic Surgery, Hahnemann Univ

Subramanian, Valavanur MD (TS) - *Spec Exp:* *Minimally Invasive Cardiac Surgery; Coronary Artery Surgery;* **Hospital:** Lenox Hill Hosp (page 64); **Address:** 130 E 77th St, Fl 4, New York, NY 10021; **Phone:** (212) 737-9131; **Board Cert:** Surgery 1972, Thoracic Surgery 1974; **Med School:** India 1962; **Resid:** Surgery, NY Hosp-Cornell Hosp, New York, NY 1968-1972

Swanson, Scott James MD (TS) - *Spec Exp:* *Lung Cancer; Minimally Invasive Thoracic Surgery; Esophageal & Swallowing Disorders;* **Hospital:** Mount Sinai Hosp (page 68); **Address:** 1190 Fifth Ave Fl 2, New York, NY 10029; **Phone:** (212) 659-6800; **Board Cert:** Surgery 1991, Thoracic Surgery 1996; **Med School:** Harvard Med Sch 1985; **Resid:** Surgery, Brigham & Women's Hosp, Boston, MA 1986-1990; Thoracic Surgery, Brigham & Women's Hosp, Boston, MA 1992-1994

Tranbaugh, Robert MD (TS) - *Spec Exp:* *Coronary Artery Surgery; Heart Valve Disease;* **Hospital:** Beth Israel Med Ctr - Petrie Division (page 58); **Address:** 317 E 17th St Fl 11, New York, NY 10003; **Phone:** (212) 420-2584; **Board Cert:** Surgery 1984, Thoracic Surgery 1986; **Med School:** Univ Penn 1976; **Resid:** Surgery, UCSF Med Ctr, San Francisco, CA 1976-1983; Thoracic Surgery, UCSF Med Ctr, San Francisco, CA 1983-1985; **Fac Appt:** Asst Prof Thoracic Surgery, Albert Einstein Coll Med

Southeast

Alexander, James A MD (TS) - *Spec Exp: Transplant-Lung; Transplant-Heart; Cardiac Surgery-Adult & Pediatric;* **Hospital:** Shands Hlthcre at Univ of FL (page 73); **Address:** Univ of FL, Dept Surgery, Gainesville, FL 32610-0286; **Phone:** (352) 846-0364; **Board Cert:** Thoracic Surgery 1976, Surgical Critical Care 1993; **Med School:** Duke Univ 1966; **Resid:** Thoracic Surgery, Duke Univ, Durham, NC 1967-1974; **Fellow:** Thoracic Surgery, Duke Univ, Durham, NC; **Fac Appt:** Prof Thoracic Surgery, Univ Fla Coll Med

Craver, Joseph MD (TS) - *Spec Exp: Heart Bypass(off pump);* **Hospital:** Emory Univ Hosp; **Address:** Emory Clinic, 1365 Clifton Rd NE, Atlanta, GA 30322; **Phone:** (404) 778-3480; **Board Cert:** Surgery 1973, Thoracic Surgery 1975; **Med School:** Univ NC Sch Med 1967; **Resid:** Surgery, Mass Genl Hosp, Boston, MA 1968-1972; Thoracic Surgery, Univ Virginia Hosp, Charlottesvile, VA 1973-1974; **Fellow:** Cardiology (Cardiovascular Disease), Mass Genl Hosp, Boston, MA 1972; **Fac Appt:** Prof Surgery, Emory Univ

Daniel, Thomas M MD (TS) - *Spec Exp: Laparoscopic Esophageal Surgery; Thoracoscopic Lung Cancer Surgery; Thoracoscopic Sympathectomy;* **Hospital:** Univ of VA Hlth Sys (page 79); **Address:** Univ Virginia Hlth System, Dept of Surgery, Box 800679, Charlottesville, VA 22908-0679; **Phone:** (434) 924-5052; **Board Cert:** Surgery 1975, Thoracic Surgery 1994, Vascular Surgery (General) 1994; **Med School:** Univ VA Sch Med 1964; **Resid:** Internal Medicine, Grady Meml Hosp-Emory Univ, Atlanta, GA 1965-1966; Surgery, Duke Univ Med Ctr, Durham, NC 1968-1975; **Fac Appt:** Prof Surgery, Univ VA Sch Med

Dowling, Robert MD (TS) - *Spec Exp: Cardiac Surgery; Transplant-Heart;* **Hospital:** Jewish Hosp HlthCre Svcs Inc; **Address:** 201 Abraham Flexner Way, Ste 1200, Louisville, KY 40202; **Board Cert:** Surgery 1992, Thoracic Surgery 1995; **Med School:** Univ Pittsburgh 1985; **Resid:** Surgery, Presbyterian Hosp, Pittsburgh, PA; **Fellow:** Thoracic Surgery, Univ Pittsburgh Med Ctr, Pittsburgh, PA; **Fac Appt:** Surgery, Univ Louisville Sch Med

Drinkwater Jr, Davis C MD (TS) - *Spec Exp: Transplant-Heart; Cardiac Surgery;* **Hospital:** Vanderbilt Univ Med Ctr (page 80); **Address:** Vanderbilt Univ Med Ctr, Dept Cardiothoracic Surgery, 1301 22nd Ave, Ste 2986, Nashville, TN 37232-5734; **Phone:** (615) 343-9193; **Board Cert:** Surgery 1997, Thoracic Surgery 1995; **Med School:** Univ VT Coll Med 1976; **Resid:** Surgery, McGill Univ Med Ctr, Montreal, Canada 1976-1981; Cardiothoracic Surgery, McGill Univ Med Ctr, Montreal, Canada 1981-1983; **Fellow:** Cardiothoracic Surgery, Chldn's Hosp, Boston, MA 1983-1984; **Fac Appt:** Assoc Clin Prof Thoracic Surgery, Vanderbilt Univ

Egan, Thomas MD (TS) - *Spec Exp: Transplant-Lung; Thoracic Cancers;* **Hospital:** Univ of NC Hosp (page 77); **Address:** 108 Burnett Womack Bldg, CB7065, Chapel Hill, NC 27599; **Phone:** (919) 966-3381; **Board Cert:** Thoracic Surgery 1999; **Med School:** Univ Toronto 1984; **Resid:** Surgery, Univ Toronto, Toronto, Canada 1980-1982; Thoracic Surgery, Univ Toronto, Toronto, Canada 1984-1988; **Fellow:** Thoracic Surgery, Univ Toronto, Toronto, Canada 1982-1984; Thoracic Surgery, Washington Univ, St. Louis, MO 1988-1989; **Fac Appt:** Prof Surgery, Univ NC Sch Med

Glassford Jr, David M MD (TS) - *Spec Exp: Cardiac Surgery;* **Hospital:** St Thomas Hosp - Nashville; **Address:** Cardio Surg Assocs, 4230 Harding Rd, Ste 501W, Nashville, TN 37205; **Phone:** (615) 385-4781; **Board Cert:** Surgery 1998, Thoracic Surgery 1997; **Med School:** Univ Tex Med Br, Galveston 1970; **Resid:** Surgery, Univ Texas Med Br, Galveston, TX 1971-1975; Thoracic Surgery, Ochsner Clinic, New Orleans, LA 1975-1977; **Fac Appt:** Asst Clin Prof Thoracic Surgery, Vanderbilt Univ

Gray, Laman MD (TS) - *Spec Exp:* Cardiac Surgery; Transplant-Heart; **Hospital:** Jewish Hosp HlthCre Svcs Inc; **Address:** 201 Abraham Flexner Way, Ste 1200, Louisville, KY 40202-3841; **Phone:** (502) 583-8383; **Board Cert:** Thoracic Surgery 1975, Surgery 1973; **Med School:** Johns Hopkins Univ 1967; **Resid:** Surgery, Univ Hosp, Ann Arbor, MI 1968-1972; **Fac Appt:** Prof Surgery, Univ Louisville Sch Med

Guyton, Robert A MD (TS) - *Spec Exp:* Cardiac Surgery-Adult; **Hospital:** Crawford Long Hosp of Emory Univ; **Address:** Dept Cardiothoracic Surgery, 1365 Clifton Rd, Ste 2223, Atlanta, GA 30322; **Phone:** (404) 778-3836; **Board Cert:** Thoracic Surgery 1990, Surgery 1989; **Med School:** Harvard Med Sch 1971; **Resid:** Surgery, Mass Genl Hosp, Boston, MA 1973-1975; Mass Genl Hosp, Boston, MA 1979; **Fellow:** Natl Heart Lung Inst, Bethesda, MD 1973-1975

Hammon Jr, John W MD (TS) - *Spec Exp:* Cardiac Surgery; Thoracic Surgery; **Hospital:** Wake Forest Univ Baptist Med Ctr (page 81); **Address:** Wake Forest Univ Sch Med, Medical Center Blvd, Winston Salem, NC 27157-1096; **Phone:** (336) 716-6002; **Board Cert:** Thoracic Surgery 1997, Surgery 1978; **Med School:** Tulane Univ 1968; **Resid:** Thoracic Surgery, Duke Univ Med Ctr, Durham, NC 1969-1978; **Fac Appt:** Prof Thoracic Surgery, Wake Forest Univ Sch Med

Jones, Ellis MD (TS) - *Spec Exp:* Coronary Artery Surgery; **Hospital:** Emory Univ Hosp; **Address:** Dept Cardiothoracic Surgery, 1365 Clifton Rd, Atlanta, GA 30322; **Phone:** (404) 778-3484; **Board Cert:** Surgery 1972, Thoracic Surgery 1972; **Med School:** Emory Univ 1963; **Resid:** Surgery, Johns Hopkins Hosp, Baltimore, MD 1964-1965; **Fellow:** Thoracic Surgery, Johns Hopkins Hosp, Baltimore, MD 1967-1972; **Fac Appt:** Prof Thoracic Surgery, Emory Univ

Kiernan, Paul Chapman MD (TS) - *Spec Exp:* Vascular Surgery; **Hospital:** Inova Fairfax Hosp; **Address:** 3301 Woodburn Rd, Ste 301, Annandale, VA 22003; **Phone:** (703) 280-5858; **Board Cert:** Thoracic Surgery 1992; **Med School:** Georgetown Univ 1974; **Resid:** Surgery, Mayo Clin, Rochester 1975-1979; Thoracic Surgery, Mayo Clin, Rochester 1979-1981; **Fellow:** Vascular Surgery (General), Mayo Clin, Rochester 1981-1982; **Fac Appt:** Assoc Clin Prof Surgery, Georgetown Univ

Kirklin, James MD (TS) - *Spec Exp:* Transplant-Heart-Pediatric; Cardiac Surgery-Adult & Pediatric; **Hospital:** Univ of Ala Hosp at Birmingham; **Address:** Univ AL Med Ctr, Dept Thoracic Surg, 1530 3rd Ave S, Bldg Zeigler - rm 739, Birmingham, AL 35294-0007; **Phone:** (205) 934-3368; **Board Cert:** Surgery 1990, Thoracic Surgery 1981; **Med School:** Harvard Med Sch 1973; **Resid:** Surgery, Mass Genl Hosp, Boston, MA 1973-1974; Mass genl Hosp, Boston, MA 1978; **Fellow:** Cardiothoracic Surgery, Chldns Hosp Ctr, Boston, MA 1979; **Fac Appt:** Prof Surgery, Univ Ala

Kron, Irving L MD (TS) - *Spec Exp:* Coronary Artery Surgery; Transplant-Lung; **Hospital:** Univ of VA Hlth Sys (page 79); **Address:** Univ of Virginia Hlth Scis Ctr, Dept of Thoracic Surgery, Box 800679, Charlottesville, VA 22908; **Phone:** (804) 924-2158; **Board Cert:** Thoracic Surgery 2001, Surgical Critical Care 1996, Vascular Surgery (General) 1997, Surgery 2001; **Med School:** Med Coll Wisc 1975; **Resid:** Surgery, Maine Med Ctr, Portland, ME 1975-1980; Thoracic Surgery, Univ Virginia Med Ctr, Charlottesville, NC 1980-1982; **Fellow:** Thoracic Surgery, Univ Virginia Med Ctr, Charlottesville, NC 1980-1982; **Fac Appt:** Prof Thoracic Surgery, Univ VA Sch Med

Merrill, Walter H MD (TS) - *Spec Exp:* Cardiothoracic Surgery; Cardiac Surgery-Adult & Pediatric; Transplant-Heart; **Hospital:** Vanderbilt Univ Med Ctr (page 80); **Address:** Cardiac & Thoracic Surgery Department, 1301 S 22ND Ave, rm 2986T, Nashville, TN 37232-0001; **Phone:** (615) 322-0064; **Board Cert:** Thoracic Surgery 1991, Surgical Critical Care 1999; **Med School:** Johns Hopkins Univ 1974; **Resid:** Thoracic Surgery, Natl Inst Hlth, Bethesda, MD 1976-1978; Thoracic Surgery, Johns Hopkins Hosp, Baltimore, MD 1980-1982; **Fellow:** Pediatric Surgery, Hosp for Sick Children, London, England 1982-1983; **Fac Appt:** Prof Surgery, Vanderbilt Univ

Pacifico, Albert D MD (TS) - *Spec Exp:* Cardiac Surgery; Heart Disease-Congenital; **Hospital:** Univ of Ala Hosp at Birmingham; **Address:** Univ AL Hosp Birmingham, 1900 University Blvd Bldg THT - Ste 760, Birmingham, AL 35294; **Phone:** (205) 934-2344; **Board Cert:** Surgery 1971, Thoracic Surgery 1971; **Med School:** UMDNJ-NJ Med Sch, Newark 1964; **Resid:** Surgery, Mayo Grad Sch Med, Rochester, MN 1965-1966; Thoracic Surgery, Univ AL Hosp, Birmingham, AL 1970-1972; **Fellow:** Surgery, Univ AL Hosp, Birmingham, AL 1967-1968; **Fac Appt:** Prof Thoracic Surgery, Univ Ala

Perryman, Richard A MD (TS) - *Spec Exp:* Cardiothoracic Surgery-Pediatric; Cardiothoracic Surgery-Adult; **Hospital:** Joe Di Maggio Child. Hosp.; **Address:** Memorial Heart Ctr, 1150 N 35th Ave, Ste 440, Hollywood, FL 33021; **Phone:** (954) 962-5400; **Board Cert:** Thoracic Surgery 1994; **Med School:** England 1967; **Resid:** Thoracic Surgery, Duke Univ Med Ctr, Durham, NC 1969-1977; Thoracic Surgery, Univ Florida Med Coll, Gainesville, FL 1980-1981; **Fellow:** Cardiology (Cardiovascular Disease), Duke Univ Med Ctr, Durham, NC 1970-1971; **Fac Appt:** Prof Thoracic Surgery, Univ Miami Sch Med

Pierson III, Richard Norris MD (TS) - *Spec Exp:* Transplant-Lung; Lung Cancer; **Hospital:** Vanderbilt Univ Med Ctr (page 80); **Address:** Vanderbilt Univ Med Ctr, Dept Cardiothoracic Surgery, 1301 22nd Ave S, Ste 2986, Nashville, TN 37232-5734; **Phone:** (615) 322-0064; **Board Cert:** Surgery 1991, Thoracic Surgery 1994; **Med School:** Columbia P&S 1983; **Resid:** Surgery, Univ Mich, Ann Arbor, MI 1983-1990; **Fellow:** Cardiothoracic Surgery, Mass General Hosp, Boston, MA 1990-1992; **Fac Appt:** Asst Prof Thoracic Surgery, Vanderbilt Univ

Quintessenza, James MD (TS) - *Spec Exp:* Transplant Medicine-Heart; Coronary Artery Surgery; Cardiovascular Surgery; **Hospital:** All Children's Hosp; **Address:** 603 7th St S, Ste 450, St Petersburg, FL 33701-4734; **Phone:** (727) 822-6666; **Board Cert:** Thoracic Surgery 1989, Surgery 1987; **Med School:** Univ Fla Coll Med 1981; **Resid:** Surgery, Univ FL, Gainesville, FL 1982-1986; **Fellow:** Thoracic Surgery, UCSD, San Diego, CA 1986-1988

Smith, Peter Kent MD (TS) - *Spec Exp:* Coronary Artery Surgery; Heart Valve Surgery; **Hospital:** Duke Univ Med Ctr (page 60); **Address:** Duke Univ Med Ctr, Box 3442, Durham, NC 27710; **Phone:** (919) 684-2890; **Board Cert:** Surgery 1995, Thoracic Surgery 1998; **Med School:** Duke Univ 1977; **Resid:** Surgery, Duke Univ, Durham, NC 1977-1987; Thoracic Surgery, Duke Univ, Durham, NC 1984-1987; **Fac Appt:** Prof Surgery, Duke Univ

Staples, Edward D MD (TS) - *Spec Exp:* Transplant-Heart & Lung; Ventricular Assist Devices; **Hospital:** Shands Hlthcre at Univ of FL (page 73); **Address:** Shands Hlthcare at Univ FL, Dept CardioThoracic Surg, 1600 SW Archer Rd, Box 100286, Gainesville, FL 32610-0268; **Phone:** (352) 846-0362; **Board Cert:** Thoracic Surgery 1997, Surgical Critical Care 1993; **Med School:** Univ S Fla Coll Med 1977; **Resid:** Med Coll Virginia, Richmond, VA 1978-1979; Surgery, Univ Hosp, Jacksonville, FL 1979-1982; **Fellow:** Cardiothoracic Surgery, Univ Florida, Gainesville, FL 1982-1984; **Fac Appt:** Assoc Prof Surgery, Univ Fla Coll Med

Tedder, Mark MD (TS) - *Spec Exp:* Transplant Medicine-Heart; Cardiac Surgery; **Hospital:** St Thomas Hosp - Nashville; **Address:** Cardio Surg Assocs, 4230 Harding Rd, Ste 501, Nashville, TN 37205; **Phone:** (615) 385-4781; **Board Cert:** Surgery 1996, Thoracic Surgery 1998; **Med School:** Duke Univ 1988; **Resid:** Surgery, Duke Univ Med Ctr, Durham, NC 1988-1995; Cardiothoracic Surgery, Duke Univ Med Ctr, Durham, NC 1995-1997

Wilcox, Benson MD (TS) - *Spec Exp:* *Cardiothoracic Surgery;* **Hospital:** Univ of NC Hosp (page 77); **Address:** Univ North Carolina Sch of Med, 108 Burnett-Womack, Box 7065, Chapel Hill, NC 27599-7065; **Phone:** (919) 966-3381; **Board Cert:** Surgery 1965, Thoracic Surgery 1986; **Med School:** Univ NC Sch Med 1957; **Resid:** Surgery, Barnes Jewish Hosp, St Louis, MO 1958-1959; Surgery, NC Meml Hosp, Chapel Hill, NC 1959-1964; **Fellow:** Thoracic Surgery, Natl Inst Hlth, Bethesda, MD 1960-1962; **Fac Appt:** Prof Surgery, Univ NC Sch Med

Williams, Donald B MD (TS) - *Spec Exp:* *Cardiac Surgery;* **Hospital:** Mount Sinai Med Ctr; **Address:** 4300 Alton Rd, Ste 211, Miami Beach, FL 33140-2800; **Phone:** (305) 674-2780; **Board Cert:** Anatomic Pathology 1988, Thoracic Surgery 1990; **Med School:** Jefferson Med Coll 1974; **Resid:** Surgery, Dartmouth-Hitchcock Med Ctr, Lebanon, NH 1975-1979; **Fellow:** Thoracic Surgery, Mayo Clinic, Rochester, MN 1979-1981

Zorn, George L. MD (TS) - *Spec Exp:* *Transplant-Lung; Lung Cancer;* **Hospital:** Univ of Ala Hosp at Birmingham; **Address:** Univ Ala at Birm - Bldg 720THT, 1900 Univ Blvd, Birmingham, AL 35294; **Phone:** (205) 934-2536; **Board Cert:** Thoracic Surgery 1987, Surgery 1974; **Med School:** Emory Univ 1968; **Resid:** Surgery, Columbia - Presby Hosp, New York, NY 1969-1973; Thoracic Surgery, Univ Alabama, Birmingham, IL 1975-1977; **Fac Appt:** Assoc Prof Surgery, Univ Ala

Midwest

Bassett, Joseph MD (TS) - *Spec Exp:* *Heart Valve Surgery; Coronary Artery Surgery;* **Hospital:** William Beaumont Hosp; **Address:** 1663 W Big Beaver Rd, Troy, MI 48084; **Phone:** (248) 643-8633; **Board Cert:** Surgery 1967, Thoracic Surgery 1969; **Med School:** Wayne State Univ 1961; **Resid:** Surgery, Wayne State Univ Affil Hosp, Detroit, MI 1962-1966; Thoracic Surgery, Wayne State Univ Affil Hosp, Detroit, MI 1966-1968; **Fac Appt:** Assoc Clin Prof Surgery, Wayne State Univ

Behrendt, Douglas M. MD (TS) - *Spec Exp:* *Cardiothoracic Surgery;* **Hospital:** Univ of IA Hosp and Clinics; **Address:** Dept Surgery, 200 Hawkins Drive, Colloton Pavilion, Rm 1602-A, Iowa City, IA 52242; **Phone:** (319) 356-2761; **Board Cert:** Surgery 1972, Thoracic Surgery 1972; **Med School:** Harvard Med Sch 1963; **Resid:** Surgery, Mass Genl Hosp, Boston, MA 1964-1971; Cardiovascular Surgery, Natl Inst Hlth, Bethesda, MD 1967-1968; **Fellow:** Pediatric Cardiology, Hosp Sick Chldns, London, England 1969-1970; **Fac Appt:** Prof Thoracic Surgery, Univ Iowa Coll Med

Bolman III, Ralph Morton MD (TS) - *Spec Exp:* *Transplant-Heart; Cardiothoracic Surgery;* **Hospital:** Fairview-Univ Med Ctr - Univ Campus; **Address:** U Minnesota Physicians, Dept Cardio/Thoracic Surg, 516 Delaware St SE, Minneapolis, MN 55455; **Phone:** (612) 672-7422; **Board Cert:** Surgery 1991, Thoracic Surgery 1993; **Med School:** St Louis Univ 1973; **Resid:** Surgery, Duke Univ Med Ctr, Durham, NC 1974-1980; **Fellow:** Thoracic Surgery, Univ Minn Hosp, Minneapolis, MN 1980-1982

Brown, John W MD (TS) - *Spec Exp:* *Cardiac Surgery-Neonatal & Pediatric; Transplant-Heart; Heart Valve Surgery;* **Hospital:** Riley Chldrn's Hosp (page 588); **Address:** 545 Barnhill Dr, Emerson Hall 215, Indianapolis, IN 46202-5112; **Phone:** (317) 274-7150; **Board Cert:** Surgery 1977, Thoracic Surgery 1998; **Med School:** Indiana Univ 1970; **Resid:** Surgery, Univ Mich Med Ctr, Ann Arbor, MI 1974-1976; Cardiothoracic Surgery, Univ Mich Med Ctr, Ann Arbor, MI 1976-1978; **Fellow:** Natl Heart Lung-Blood Inst 1972-1974; **Fac Appt:** Assoc Prof Surgery, Indiana Univ

Cooper, Joel David MD (TS) - *Spec Exp:* *Transplant-Lung; Lung Volume Reduction;* **Hospital:** Barnes-Jewish Hosp (page 55); **Address:** Barnes-Jewish Hosp, Queeny Tower, 1 Barnes-Jewish Hosp Plaza, Ste 3108, St Louis, MO 63110-1013; **Phone:** (314) 362-6021; **Board Cert:** Surgery 1971, Thoracic Surgery 1972; **Med School:** Harvard Med Sch 1964; **Resid:** Surgery, Mass Genl Hosp, Boston, MA 1965-1968; Frenchay Hosp, Bristol England 1968; **Fellow:** Hammersmith Hosp, London England 1969; **Fac Appt:** Prof Surgery, Washington Univ, St Louis

Cosgrove III, Delos M MD (TS) - *Spec Exp:* Heart Valve Surgery; Minimally Invasive Surgery; **Hospital:** Cleveland Clin Fdn (page 57); **Address:** 9500 Euclid Ave, Cleveland, OH 44195; **Phone:** (216) 444-6733; **Board Cert:** Surgery 1975, Thoracic Surgery 1996; **Med School:** Univ VA Sch Med 1966; **Resid:** Surgery, Strong Meml Hosp, Rochester, NY 1967-1968; Surgery, Mass Genl Hosp, Boston, MA 1970-1972

Danielson, Gordon MD (TS) - *Spec Exp:* Heart Disease-Congenital; Ebstein's Anomaly; Heart Valve Disease; **Hospital:** Mayo Med Ctr & Clin - Rochester, MN; **Address:** Mayo Med Ctr, 200 1st St SW, Rochester, MN 55905-0001; **Phone:** (507) 255-7062; **Board Cert:** Surgery 1963, Thoracic Surgery 1963; **Med School:** Univ Penn 1956; **Resid:** Surgery, Univ Hosp - Univ MI, Ann Arbor, MI 1956-1957; Thoracic Surgery, Hosp Univ Penn, Philadelphia, PA 1957-1961; **Fellow:** Thoracic Surgery, Univ Hosp - Univ Penn, Philadelphia, PA 1962-1963; Cardiothoracic Surgery, Karolinska Sjukhuset, Stokholm, Sweden 1963-1964; **Fac Appt:** Prof Surgery, Mayo Med Sch

DeCamp Jr, Malcolm M MD (TS) - *Spec Exp:* Lung Surgery; Transplant-Lung; Esophageal Surgery; **Hospital:** Cleveland Clin Fdn (page 57); **Address:** Cleveland Clinic Foundation, 9500 Euclid Ave, Desk A-25, Cleveland, OH 44195; **Phone:** (216) 444-4053; **Board Cert:** Surgery 1991, Thoracic Surgery 1994; **Med School:** Univ Louisville Sch Med 1983; **Resid:** Surgery, Brighams & Womens Hosp, Boston, MA 1984-1986; Surgery, Brighams & Womens Hosp, Boston, MA 1988-1993; **Fac Appt:** Asst Prof Surgery, Harvard Med Sch

Deschamps, Claude MD (TS) - *Spec Exp:* Gastroesophageal Reflux; Achalasia; Esophageal/Lung Cancer; **Hospital:** St Mary's Hosp - Rochester, MN; **Address:** Mayo Clinic, Div Thoracic Surg, 200 First St SW, Rochester, MN 55905; **Phone:** (507) 284-8462; **Board Cert:** Surgery 1994; **Med School:** Univ Montreal 1979; **Resid:** Surgery, Univ Montreal Hosps, Canada 1980-1984; Thoracic Surgery, Univ Montreal Hosp, Montreal, Canada 1984-1985; **Fellow:** Thoracic Surgery, Mayo Clinic, Rochester, MN 1985-1987

Faber, L. Penfield MD (TS) - *Spec Exp:* Lung Cancer; Esophageal Cancer; Thoracic Cancers; **Hospital:** Rush-Presby - St Luke's Med Ctr (page 72); **Address:** 1725 W Harrison St, Ste 218, Chicago, IL 60612; **Phone:** (312) 738-3732; **Board Cert:** Surgery 1962, Thoracic Surgery 1963; **Med School:** Northwestern Univ 1956; **Resid:** Surgery, Rush Presby-St Luke's Med CtrHosp, Chicago, IL 1957-1961; Thoracic Surgery, Hines VA Hosp, Chicago, IL 1961-1963; **Fac Appt:** Prof Thoracic Surgery, Rush Med Coll

Ferguson, Mark MD (TS) - *Spec Exp:* Barrett's Esophagus; Esophageal Cancer; Lung Cancer; **Hospital:** Univ of Chicago Hosps (page 76); **Address:** 5841 S Maryland Ave, MC 5035, Chicago, IL 60637-1463; **Phone:** (773) 702-3551; **Board Cert:** Surgery 1993, Thoracic Surgery 1994; **Med School:** Univ Chicago-Pritzker Sch Med 1977; **Resid:** Surgery, Univ Chicago Hosps, Chicago, IL 1978-1982; **Fellow:** Cardiothoracic Surgery, Univ Chicago Hosps, Chicago, IL 1982-1984; **Fac Appt:** Prof Surgery, Univ Chicago-Pritzker Sch Med

Frederiksen, James W MD (TS) - *Spec Exp:* Cardiothoracic Surgery; **Hospital:** Northwestern Meml Hosp; **Address:** 201 E Huron St, Ste 10-105, Chicago, IL 60611; **Phone:** (312) 695-3121; **Board Cert:** Surgery 1980, Thoracic Surgery 1992; **Med School:** Harvard Med Sch 1972; **Resid:** Surgery, Peter Bent Brigham Hosp, Boston, MA 1973-1974; Cardiothoracic Surgery, Northwestern Meml Hosp, Chicago, IL 1976-1978; **Fellow:** Cardiothoracic Surgery, Johns Hopkins Hosp, Baltimore, MD 1974-1976; **Fac Appt:** Assoc Clin Prof Surgery, Northwestern Univ

Iannettoni, Mark D. MD (TS) - *Spec Exp:* Transplant-Lung; **Hospital:** Univ of MI Hlth Ctr; **Address:** Univ of Michigan Taubman Hlth Care Ctr, 1500 E Med Ctr Dr, rm TC2120, Box 0344, Ann Arbor, MI 48109-0344; **Phone:** (734) 763-7418; **Board Cert:** Thoracic Surgery 1994, Surgery 1993; **Med School:** SUNY Syracuse 1985; **Resid:** Thoracic Surgery, Univ Mich Med Sch, Ann Arbor, MI 1991-1993; Thoracic Surgery, SUNY Upstate, New York, NY 1986-1991; **Fellow:** Thoracic Surgery, Univ Mich Med Sch, Ann Arbor, MI 1993-1994; **Fac Appt:** Assoc Prof Thoracic Surgery, Univ Mich Med Sch

Jeevanandam, Valluvan MD (TS) - *Spec Exp:* Transplant-Heart; Heart Valve Surgery; Artificial Hearts; **Hospital:** Univ of Chicago Hosps (page 76); **Address:** 5841 S Maryland Ave, Ste E500, MC 5040, Chicago, IL 60637; **Phone:** (773) 702-2500; **Board Cert:** Surgery 1990, Thoracic Surgery 1993; **Med School:** Columbia P&S 1984; **Resid:** Surgery, Columbia-Presby Med Ctr, New York, NY 1985-1989; **Fellow:** Cardiothoracic Surgery, Columbia-Presby Med Ctr, New York, NY 1989-1991; **Fac Appt:** Assoc Prof Surgery, Univ Chicago-Pritzker Sch Med

Lytle, Bruce Whitney MD (TS) - *Spec Exp:* Heart Valve Surgery; Coronary Artery Surgery; Aortic Surgery; **Hospital:** Cleveland Clin Fdn (page 57); **Address:** Cleveland Clinic Fdn, 9500 Euclid Ave, MS F25, Cleveland, OH 44195; **Phone:** (216) 444-6962; **Board Cert:** Thoracic Surgery 1998; **Med School:** Harvard Med Sch 1971; **Resid:** Surgery, Mass Genl Hsop, Boston, MA 1971-1975; Shotley Bridge Hosp, England 1975-1976; **Fellow:** Thoracic Surgery, Mass Genl Hosp, Boston, MA 1977

McCarthy, Patrick McGuane MD (TS) - *Spec Exp:* Transplant-Heart; Maze Procedure; Left ventricular Assist Device (LVAD); **Hospital:** Cleveland Clin Fdn (page 57); **Address:** 9500 Euclid Ave, MS F25, Cleveland, OH 44195-0001; **Phone:** (216) 444-0648; **Board Cert:** Thoracic Surgery 1998; **Med School:** Loyola Univ-Stritch Sch Med 1980; **Resid:** Thoracic Surgery, Mayo Clinic, Rochester, MN 1985-1988; Surgery, Mayo Clinic, Rochester, MN 1980-1985; **Fellow:** Cardiothoracic Surgery, Stanford Univ, Palo Alto, CA 1988-1989

McGregor, Christopher MD (TS) - *Spec Exp:* Transplant-Heart & Lung; Cardiac Surgery; **Hospital:** Mayo Med Ctr & Clin - Rochester, MN; **Address:** Mayo Clinic - St Mary's Hospital, rm 6716, Rochester, MN 55905; **Phone:** (507) 255-6038; **Med School:** Scotland 1972; **Resid:** Surgery, Edinburgh Royal Infirm, Scotland 1973-1978; Surgery, Glasgow Royal Infirm, Scotland 1979-1981; **Fellow:** Cardiothoracic Transplantation, Stanford Univ Hosp, Stanford, CA 1983-1984; **Fac Appt:** Prof Surgery, Mayo Med Sch

Meyers, Bryan MD (TS) - *Spec Exp:* Lung Cancer; Esophageal Cancer; **Hospital:** Barnes-Jewish Hosp (page 55); **Address:** 3108 Queeny Tower, St Louis, MO 63110; **Phone:** (314) 362-8598; **Board Cert:** Surgery 1998, Thoracic Surgery 1999; **Med School:** Univ Chicago-Pritzker Sch Med 1986; **Resid:** Surgery, Mass Genl Hosp, Boston, MA 1990-1996; **Fellow:** Cardiothoracic Surgery, Barnes Hosp-Wash Univ, St Louis, MO 1996-1998; **Fac Appt:** Asst Prof Surgery, Washington Univ, St Louis

Michler, Robert MD (TS) - *Spec Exp:* Transplant-Heart; Robotic Heart Surgery; **Hospital:** Ohio St Univ Med Ctr; **Address:** 410 W 10th Ave Bldg Doan - rm N487, Columbus, OH 43210; **Phone:** (614) 293-5502; **Board Cert:** Surgery 1990, Thoracic Surgery 1988; **Med School:** Dartmouth Med Sch 1981; **Resid:** Surgery, Columbia Presby Med Ctr, New York, NY 1981-1987; Transplant Surgery, Columbia Presby Med Ctr, New York, NY 1984-1985; **Fellow:** Thoracic Surgery, Columbia Presby Med Ctr, New York, NY 1987-1989; Pediatric Surgery, Harvard Med Sch, Cambridge, MA 1989-1990; **Fac Appt:** Prof Surgery, Ohio State Univ

Orringer, Mark B MD (TS) - *Spec Exp:* Esophageal Cancer; Esophageal Disease, Benign; Cardiothoracic Surgery; **Hospital:** Univ of MI Hlth Ctr; **Address:** Sect of Genl Thoracic Surg, Taubman Hlth Care Ctr, Box 0344, 1500 E Medical Center Drive, rm 2120, Ann Arbor, MI 48109-0999; **Phone:** (734) 936-5800; **Board Cert:** Surgery 1973, Thoracic Surgery 1974; **Med School:** Univ Pittsburgh 1967; **Resid:** Thoracic Surgery, Johns Hopkins Hosp, Baltimore, MD 1968-1973; **Fac Appt:** Prof Thoracic Surgery, Univ Mich Med Sch

Pagani, Francis Domenic MD (TS) - *Spec Exp:* Transplant-Heart; **Hospital:** Univ of MI Hlth Ctr; **Address:** 2124G Taubman Ctr, 1500 E Med Ctr Drive, Ann Arbor, MI 48109-0348; **Phone:** (734) 647-2894; **Board Cert:** Surgery 1994, Thoracic Surgery 1996; **Med School:** Georgetown Univ 1986; **Resid:** Surgery, Georgetown Univ Med Ctr, Washinton, DC 1986-1993; Thoracic Surgery, Univ Michigan Hosp, Ann Arbor, MI 1993-1995; **Fac Appt:** Asst Prof Thoracic Surgery, Univ Mich Med Sch

Pairolero, Peter MD (TS) - *Spec Exp:* Chest Wall Tumors; **Hospital:** Mayo Med Ctr & Clin - Rochester, MN; **Address:** Div Thoracic Surgery, 200 1st St SW, Rochester, MN 55905-4317; **Phone:** (507) 284-2511; **Board Cert:** Thoracic Surgery 1974, Surgery 1972; **Med School:** Univ Mich Med Sch 1963; **Resid:** Surgery, Mayo Clinic, Rochester, MN 1966-1971; Thoracic Surgery, Mayo Clinic, Rochetser, MN 1971-1973; **Fellow:** Cerebrovascular Disease, Mayo Clinic, Rochester, MN 1968-1969

Pass, Harvey MD (TS) - *Spec Exp:* Lung Cancer; Mesothelioma; Clinical Trials for Cancer; **Hospital:** Harper Hosp (page 59); **Address:** Harper Hosp - Wayne State Univ, 3990 John R St, Ste 2102, Detroit, MI 48201; **Phone:** (313) 745-1413; **Board Cert:** Surgery 1981, Thoracic Surgery 1992; **Med School:** Duke Univ 1973; **Resid:** Surgery, Duke Univ Med Ctr, Durham, NC 1973-1975; Surgery, Univ Miss Med Ctr, Jackson, MI 1977-1980; **Fellow:** Cardiothoracic Surgery, MUSC Med Ctr, Charleston, SC 1980-1982; **Fac Appt:** Prof Surgery, Wayne State Univ

Patterson, George Alexander MD (TS) - *Spec Exp:* Transplant-Lung; **Hospital:** Barnes-Jewish Hosp (page 55); **Address:** One Barnes Jewish Hospital Plaza, Queeny Tower, Ste 3108, St Louis, MO 63110; **Phone:** (314) 362-6025; **Board Cert:** Surgery 1978, Thoracic Surgery 1981; **Med School:** Canada 1974; **Resid:** Surgery, Queens Univ, Kingston 1975-1978; Vascular Surgery (General), Unniv of Toronto 1978-1979; **Fellow:** Research, Toronto Genl Hosp, Toronto Canada 1980-1981; Research, Johns Hopkins Univ, Baltimore, MD 1981-1982; **Fac Appt:** Prof Surgery, Washington Univ, St Louis

Piccione, William MD (TS) - *Spec Exp:* Transplant-Heart; Heart Valve Surgery; **Hospital:** Rush-Presby - St Luke's Med Ctr (page 72); **Address:** 1725 W Harrison St, Ste 1156, Chicago, IL 60612; **Phone:** (312) 563-2762; **Board Cert:** Surgery 1997, Thoracic Surgery 1999; **Med School:** Univ Rochester 1980; **Resid:** Surgery, Harvard Surg Svc-New England Deaconess Hosp, Boston, MA 1981-1986; **Fellow:** Cardiothoracic Surgery, Rush Presbyterian-St Lukes Med Ctr, Chicago, IL 1986-1988; Thoracic Surgery, Meml Sloan Kettering, New York, NY 1988; **Fac Appt:** Assoc Prof Thoracic Surgery, Rush Med Coll

Schaff, Hartzell MD (TS) - *Spec Exp:* Heart Valve Surgery; Heart Disease-Congenital; Maze Procedure; **Hospital:** St Mary's Hosp - Rochester, MN; **Address:** Mayo Clin, Dept Cardiovasc Surg, 200 First St SW, Rochester, MN 55905-0001; **Phone:** (507) 255-7068; **Board Cert:** Thoracic Surgery 1992; **Med School:** Univ Okla Coll Med 1973; **Resid:** Surgery, Johns Hopkins Hosp, Baltimore, MD 1974-1978; Thoracic Surgery, Johns Hopkins Hosp, Baltimore, MD 1978-1980; **Fellow:** Surgery, Johns Hopkins Hosp, Baltimore, MD 1975-1976; **Fac Appt:** Prof Surgery, Mayo Med Sch

Silverman, Norman A MD (TS) - *Spec Exp:* Heart Valve Surgery; Aortic Surgery-Thoracic; Transplant-Heart; **Hospital:** Henry Ford Hosp; **Address:** Division of Cardiothoracic Surgery, 2799 W Grand Blvd, Detroit, MI 48202-2608; **Phone:** (313) 916-2695; **Board Cert:** Surgery 1989, Thoracic Surgery 2001; **Med School:** Boston Univ 1971; **Resid:** Surgery, Duke Univ Med Ctr, Durham, NC 1972-1973; Thoracic Surgery, Duke Univ Med Ctr, Durham, NC 1975-1980; **Fac Appt:** Prof Surgery, Case West Res Univ

Smedira, Nicholas MD (TS) - *Spec Exp:* Transplant-Heart; Transplant-Lung; **Hospital:** Cleveland Clin Fdn (page 57); **Address:** 9500 Euclid Ave, Ste F25, Cleveland, OH 44195; **Phone:** (216) 445-7052; **Board Cert:** Surgery 1992, Thoracic Surgery 1995; **Med School:** Univ Rochester 1995; **Resid:** Surgery, UCSF Med Ctr, San Francisco, CA 1984-1991; Thoracic Surgery, UCSF Med Ctr, San Francisco, CA 1992-1994

Stuart, Richard Scott MD (TS) - *Spec Exp:* Cardiac Surgery; **Hospital:** St Luke's Hosp; **Address:** 4320 Wornall Rd, Ste 50, Kansas City, MO 64111; **Phone:** (816) 931-3312; **Board Cert:** Surgical Critical Care 1993, Thoracic Surgery 1990; **Med School:** Johns Hopkins Univ 1981; **Resid:** Surgery, Johns Hopkins Hosp, Baltimore, MD 1982-1986; **Fellow:** Thoracic Surgery, Johns Hopkins Hosp, Baltimore, MD 1988-1989; **Fac Appt:** Assoc Prof Surgery, Johns Hopkins Univ

Sundt III, Thoralf Mauritz MD (TS) - *Spec Exp:* Heart Valve Surgery; Aneurysm-Aortic; Pulmonary Embolism; **Hospital:** Mayo Med Ctr & Clin - Rochester, MN; **Address:** Mayo Clinic, 200 First St SW, Rochester, MN 55905; **Phone:** (507) 255-7064; **Board Cert:** Surgery 2000, Thoracic Surgery 1993; **Med School:** Johns Hopkins Univ 1984; **Resid:** Surgery, Mass Genl Hosp, Boston, MA 1985-1991; Cardiothoracic Surgery, Wash Univ Sch Med, St Louis, MO 1991-1993; **Fellow:** Cardiothoracic Surgery, Harefield Hosp, London, England 1993-1994; **Fac Appt:** Assoc Prof Surgery, Mayo Med Sch

Turrentine, Mark W MD (TS) - *Spec Exp:* Cardiac Surgery-Pediatric; Transplant-Heart & Lung; **Hospital:** Riley Chldrn's Hosp (page 588); **Address:** 545 Barnhill Dr, Emerson Hall, Ste 215, Indianapolis, IN 46202; **Phone:** (317) 274-1121; **Board Cert:** Surgery 1989, Thoracic Surgery 1992; **Med School:** Univ Kans 1983; **Resid:** Surgery, Univ Kansas, Wichita, KS 1984-1988; Cardiothoracic Surgery, Indiana Univ Med Ctr, Indianapolis, IN 1989-1991; **Fellow:** Cardiothoracic Surgery, Texas Heart Inst, Houston, TX 1986; Transplant Surgery, Indiana Univ Med Ctr, Indianapolis, IN 1988-1989; **Fac Appt:** Assoc Prof Surgery, Indiana Univ

Great Plains and Mountains

Doty, Donald B MD (TS) - *Spec Exp:* Cardiac Surgery-Adult; **Hospital:** LDS Hosp; **Address:** 324 10th Ave, Ste 160, Salt Lake City, UT 84103; **Phone:** (801) 322-0563; **Board Cert:** Thoracic Surgery 1971, Surgery 1968; **Med School:** Stanford Univ 1962; **Resid:** Los Angeles Co Hosp, Los Angeles, CA 1963-1967; **Fellow:** Thoracic Surgery, Univ Ala Med Ctr, Birmingham, AL 1969-1971; **Fac Appt:** Clin Prof Thoracic Surgery, Univ Utah

Karwande, Shreekanth V MD (TS) - *Spec Exp:* Thoracic Surgery - General; **Hospital:** Univ Utah Hosp and Clin; **Address:** Univ Utah Med Ctr, Cardio Thors, 50 N Med Dr, Salt Lake City, UT 84132-0001; **Phone:** (801) 581-5311; **Board Cert:** Surgical Critical Care 1989, Thoracic Surgery 1993; **Med School:** India 1973; **Resid:** Surgery, Erie Co Med Ctr, Buffalo, NY 1976-1981; Surgery, NY Hosp-Cornell Med Ctr, New York, NY 1982-1985; **Fac Appt:** Assoc Prof Surgery, Univ Utah

Pomerantz, Marvin MD (TS) - *Spec Exp:* Tuberculosis; **Hospital:** Univ Colo HSC - Denver; **Address:** 4200 E Ninth Ave, Box C 310, Denver, CO 80262; **Phone:** (303) 315-8527; **Board Cert:** Surgery 1968, Thoracic Surgery 1968; **Med School:** Univ Rochester 1959; **Resid:** Surgery, Duke Univ Med Ctr, Durham, NC 1959-1963; Thoracic Surgery, Duke Univ Med Ctr, Durham, NC 1963-1967; **Fac Appt:** Prof Surgery, Univ Colo

Southwest

Antakli, Tamim MD (TS) - *Spec Exp:* Thoracic Surgery - General; **Hospital:** UAMS; **Address:** Dept Thoracic Surgery, 4301 W Markham St, Slot 713, Little Rock, AR 72205; **Phone:** (501) 686-7884; **Board Cert:** Thoracic Surgery 1997, Surgery 1994; **Med School:** Syria 1983; **Resid:** Surgery, Meth Hosp, Brooklyn, NY 1988-1993; Thoracic Surgery, Univ Arkansas Med Ctr, Little Rock, AR 1993-1996; **Fac Appt:** Asst Prof Surgery, Univ Ark

Cooley, Denton A MD (TS) - *Spec Exp:* Heart Valve Surgery; Aneurysm-Abdominal Aortic; **Hospital:** St Luke's Episcopal Hosp - Houston; **Address:** Tex Heart Inst, 1101 Bates Ave, Ste P-154, Houston, TX 77030; **Phone:** (713) 791-4900; **Board Cert:** Surgery 1951, Thoracic Surgery 1952; **Med School:** Johns Hopkins Univ 1944; **Resid:** Surgery, Johns Hopkins Hosp, Baltimore, MD 1945-1950; **Fellow:** Thoracic Surgery, Brompton Hosp Chest Dis, London England 1950-1951; **Fac Appt:** Clin Prof Surgery, Univ Tex, Houston

Copeland III, Jack G MD (TS) - *Spec Exp:* Transplant-Heart; Transplant-Heart & Lung; Artificial Heart; **Hospital:** Univ Med Ctr; **Address:** Univ Ariz Hlth Sci Ctr, 1501 N Campbell Rd, rm 4402, Box 245071, Tucson, AZ 85724-5071; **Phone:** (520) 626-6339; **Board Cert:** Thoracic Surgery 1997; **Med School:** Stanford Univ 1969; **Resid:** Surgery, UC-San Diego, San Diego, CA 1970-1971; Cardiovascular Surgery, Natl Inst Hlth, Bethesda, MD 1971-1973; **Fellow:** Cardiothoracic Surgery, Stanford Univ, Stanford, CA 1973-1977; **Fac Appt:** Prof Thoracic Surgery, Univ Ariz Coll Med

Coselli, Joseph S MD (TS) - *Spec Exp:* Aneurysm-Abdominal Aortic; Marfan's Syndrome; Vascular Surgery; **Hospital:** Methodist Hosp - Houston; **Address:** 6560 Fannin St, Ste 1100, Houston, TX 77030; **Phone:** (713) 790-4313; **Board Cert:** Surgery 1992, Thoracic Surgery 1993; **Med School:** Univ Tex Med Br, Galveston 1977; **Resid:** Surgery, Baylor Coll Med, Houston, TX 1977-1982; Thoracic Surgery, Baylor Coll Med, Houston, TX 1982-1984; **Fac Appt:** Assoc Prof Surgery, Baylor Coll Med

Frazier, Oscar Howard MD (TS) - *Spec Exp:* Transplant-Heart; Lung Surgery; **Hospital:** St Luke's Episcopal Hosp - Houston; **Address:** Texas Heart Inst, 1101 Bates, Ste P357, MC 3-147, Houston, TX 77030; **Phone:** (713) 791-4900; **Board Cert:** Surgery 1975, Thoracic Surgery 1997; **Med School:** Baylor Coll Med 1967; **Resid:** Surgery, Baylor Affil Hosp, Houston, TX 1970-1974; Thoracic Surgery, Texas Heart Inst, Houston, TX 1974-1976; **Fac Appt:** Prof Surgery, Univ Tex, Houston

Harrell Jr, James E MD (TS) - *Spec Exp:* Transplant-Heart; Cardiac Surgery-Pediatric; **Hospital:** Covenant Health Sys; **Address:** 3606 21st St, Ste 103, Lubbock, TX 79410; **Phone:** (806) 725-4425; **Board Cert:** Surgery 1995, Thoracic Surgery 1996; **Med School:** Baylor Coll Med 1978; **Resid:** Surgery, Univ Texas Hlth Science Ctr, Houston, TX 1980-1984; Thoracic Surgery, Baylor Coll Med, Houston, TX 1984-1986; **Fellow:** Cardiovascular Surgery, Hosp Sick Chldrn, London England 1986-1987

Harrison, Lynn MD (TS) - *Spec Exp:* Coronary Revascularization; **Hospital:** West Jefferson Med Ctr; **Address:** Louisiana St Univ Med Ctr Clins, 1111 Medical Center Blvd, Ste N504, Marrero, LA 70072; **Phone:** (504) 349-6606; **Board Cert:** Thoracic Surgery 1989; **Med School:** Univ Okla Coll Med 1970; **Resid:** Surgery, Duke Univ Hosp, Durham, NC 1971-1972; Thoracic Surgery, Duke Univ Hosp, Durham, NC 1974-1979; **Fellow:** Cardiothoracic Surgery, Duke Univ, Durham, NC 1978-1979; **Fac Appt:** Prof Surgery, Louisiana State Univ

Livesay, James J MD (TS) - *Spec Exp:* Coronary Artery Surgery; Heart Valve Surgery; **Hospital:** St Luke's Episcopal Hosp - Houston; **Address:** Surg Assocs of Texas, Box 20345, MC 1-194, Houston, TX 77225-0345; **Phone:** (832) 355-4976; **Board Cert:** Thoracic Surgery 1993, Surgery 1999; **Med School:** Baylor Coll Med 1973; **Resid:** Surgery, UCLA, Los Angeles, CA 1973-1979; Thoracic Surgery, Tex Heart Inst, Houston, TX 1979-1981; **Fellow:** Research, UCLA, Los Angeles, CA 1975-1976; **Fac Appt:** Assoc Prof Surgery, Univ Tex, Houston

Noon, George P MD (TS) - *Spec Exp:* Transplant-Heart; Transplant-Lung; Thoracic Vascular Surgery; **Hospital:** Methodist Hosp - Houston; **Address:** 6760 Fannin St, Ste 1860, Houston, TX 77030; **Phone:** (713) 790-3155; **Board Cert:** Thoracic Surgery 1966, Surgery 1966; **Med School:** Baylor Coll Med 1960; **Resid:** Surgery, Baylor Coll Med, Houston, TX 1961-1966; Surgery, Ben Taub Genl Hosp, Houston, TX 1965-1966; **Fac Appt:** Prof Surgery, Baylor Coll Med

Ott, David A MD (TS) - *Spec Exp:* Thoracic Surgery - General; **Hospital:** St Luke's Episcopal Hosp - Houston; **Address:** 1101 Bates St, Ste P-514, Houston, TX 77030-2607; **Phone:** (713) 791-4900; **Board Cert:** Thoracic Surgery 1997; **Med School:** Baylor Coll Med 1972; **Resid:** Surgery, Baylor Coll Med, Houston, TX 1972-1976; Vascular Surgery (General), Tex Heart Inst, Houston, TX 1976-1978; **Fac Appt:** Clin Prof Surgery, Baylor Coll Med

Putnam Jr, Joe B MD (TS) - *Spec Exp:* Lung Cancer; Esophageal Cancer; Sarcoma-Soft Tissue; **Hospital:** Univ of TX MD Anderson Cancer Ctr, The; **Address:** UT MD Anderson Cancer Ctr, 1515 Holcombe Blvd, Box 445, Houston, TX 77030-4009; **Phone:** (713) 792-6934; **Board Cert:** Thoracic Surgery 1997; **Med School:** Univ NC Sch Med 1979; **Resid:** Surgery, Univ Rochester, Rochester, NY 1984-1986; Thoracic Surgery, Univ Michigan, Ann Arbor, MI 1986-1988; **Fellow:** Surgical Oncology, NCI/NIH-Surg. Branch, Bethesda, MD 1981-1984; **Fac Appt:** Prof Surgery, Univ Tex, Houston

Reul, George J MD (TS) - *Spec Exp:* Coronary Artery Surgery; Aneurysm; Heart Valve Surgery; **Hospital:** St Luke's Episcopal Hosp - Houston; **Address:** Surg Assocs-Tex Heart Inst, 1101 Bates Ave, Ste P514, Houston, TX 77030-2607; **Phone:** (713) 791-4900; **Board Cert:** Surgery 1971, Thoracic Surgery 1971; **Med School:** Med Coll Wisc 1962; **Resid:** Surgery, Marquette Sch Med, Milwaukee, WI 1964-1969; Thoracic Surgery, Baylor Coll Med, Houston, TX 1969-1971; **Fac Appt:** Clin Prof Surgery, Univ Tex, Houston

Safi, Hazim Jawad MD (TS) - *Spec Exp:* Aneurysm-Abdominal Aortic; **Hospital:** Meml Hermann Hosp; **Address:** 6410 Fannin St, Ste 450, Houston, TX 77030; **Phone:** (713) 500-5304; **Board Cert:** Surgery 1994, Thoracic Surgery 1997; **Med School:** Iraq 1970; **Resid:** Surgery, Baylor Coll Of Med, Houston, TX 1977-1980; Radiation Oncology, Baylor Coll Of Med, Houston, TX 1980-1981; **Fellow:** Thoracic Surgery, Baylor Coll Of Med, Houston, TX 1981-1983; **Fac Appt:** Assoc Prof Surgery, Univ Tex, Houston

Trastek, Victor MD (TS) - *Spec Exp:* Lung Cancer; Esophageal Cancer; **Hospital:** Mayo Clin Hosp - Scottsdale; **Address:** Mayo Clinic, Dept Surg, 13400 E Shea Blvd, Scottsdale, AZ 85259; **Phone:** (480) 301-4608; **Board Cert:** Thoracic Surgery 1994; **Med School:** Univ Wisc 1976; **Resid:** Surgery, Mayo Clinic, Rochester, MN 1977-1981; Cardiothoracic Surgery, Mayo Clinic, Rochester, MN 1981-1984; **Fellow:** Thoracic Surgery, Toronto Genl Hosp, Toronto, Canada 1985

Turner, William F MD (TS) - *Spec Exp:* Coronary Artery Surgery; Cardiac Surgery; **Hospital:** E TX Med Ctr; **Address:** PO Box 150, Tyler, TX 75710-0150; **Phone:** (903) 595-6680; **Board Cert:** Surgery 1997, Thoracic Surgery 1998; **Med School:** Baylor Coll Med 1981; **Resid:** Surgery, Baylor Coll Med, Houston, TX 1983-1987; Thoracic Surgery, Baylor Coll Med, Houston, TX 1987-1989

Urschel Jr, Harold C MD (TS) - *Spec Exp:* *Thoracic Outlet Syndrome;* **Hospital:** Baylor Univ Medical Ctr; **Address:** 3600 Gaston Ave, Ste 1201, Dallas, TX 75246-1812; **Phone:** (214) 824-2503; **Board Cert:** Thoracic Surgery 1963, Surgery 1963; **Med School:** Harvard Med Sch 1955; **Resid:** Thoracic Surgery, Mass Genl Hosp, Boston, MA 1959-1961; Vascular Surgery (General), Mass Genl Hosp, Boston, MA 1956-1957; **Fac Appt:** Prof Thoracic Surgery, Univ Tex SW, Dallas

West Coast and Pacific

Bailey, Leonard Lee MD (TS) - *Spec Exp:* *Cardiac Surgery-Pediatric; Congenital Heart Surgery; Transplant-Heart-Pediatric;* **Hospital:** Loma Linda Children's Hosp; **Address:** Dept Surgery, 11175 Campus St, Ste 21120, Loma Linda, CA 92354; **Phone:** (909) 824-4200; **Board Cert:** Thoracic Surgery 1998, Surgery 1975; **Med School:** Loma Linda Univ 1969; **Resid:** Surgery, Loma Linda Univ Med Ctr, Loma Linda, CA 1970-1973; Thoracic Surgery, Loma Linda Univ Med Ctr, Loma Linda, CA 1973-1974; **Fellow:** Cardiovascular Surgery, Hosp Sick Chldn, Toronto, Canada 1974-1975; **Fac Appt:** Prof Surgery, Loma Linda Univ

Cohen, Robbin G MD (TS) - *Spec Exp:* *Minimally Invasive Surgery; Heart Valve Surgery;* **Hospital:** USC Univ Hosp - R K Eamer Med Plz; **Address:** 1510 San Pueblo St, Ste 415, USC Cardiothoracic, Los Angeles, CA 90033; **Phone:** (323) 442-5850; **Board Cert:** Thoracic Surgery 1999; **Med School:** Univ Colo 1980; **Resid:** Surgery, Stanford Univ Med Ctr, Stanford, CA 1981-1986; **Fellow:** Cardiothoracic Surgery, Stanford Univ Med Ctr, Stanford, CA 1986-1989; **Fac Appt:** Asst Prof Thoracic Surgery, USC Sch Med

De Meester, Tom R MD (TS) - *Spec Exp:* *Gastric Diseases; Esophageal Surgery;* **Hospital:** USC Univ Hosp - R K Eamer Med Plz; **Address:** 1510 San Pablo St, Ste 514, Los Angeles, CA 90033; **Phone:** (323) 442-5925; **Board Cert:** Surgery 1971, Thoracic Surgery 1971; **Med School:** Univ Mich Med Sch 1963; **Resid:** Surgery, Univ Mich Hosp, Ann Arbor, MI 1964-1965; Surgery, Johns Hopkins Hosp, Baltimore, MD 1965-1966; **Fellow:** Surgery, Johns Hopkins Hosp, Baltimore, MD 1967-1968; **Fac Appt:** Prof Surgery, USC Sch Med

Flachsbart, Keith D MD (TS) - *Spec Exp:* *Cardiac Surgery;* **Hospital:** Kaiser Permanente Med Ctr - SF; **Address:** 2350 Geary Blvd, San Francisco, CA 94115; **Phone:** (415) 202-3800; **Board Cert:** Thoracic Surgery 1990; **Med School:** Univ Nebr Coll Med 1971; **Resid:** Surgery, Rush-Presby St Lukes, Chicago, IL 1974-1978; Thoracic Surgery, Hosp Good Samaritan, Los Angeles, CA 1978-1980

Fontana, Gregory MD (TS) - *Spec Exp:* *Minimally Invasive Surgery; Cardiac Surgery-Pediatric;* **Hospital:** Cedars-Sinai Med Ctr; **Address:** 8700 Beverly Blvd, Ste 6215, Los Angeles, CA 90048; **Phone:** (310) 423-3851; **Board Cert:** Thoracic Surgery 1994, Surgery 1993; **Med School:** UCLA 1984; **Resid:** Surgery, Duke Univ Med Ctr, Durham, NC 1985-1990; **Fellow:** Thoracic Surgery, UCLA Med Ctr, Los Angeles, CA 1990-1993; Pediatric Cardiac Surgery, Chldns Hosp, Boston, MA 1993-1994; **Fac Appt:** Asst Clin Prof Surgery, UCLA

Gundry, Steven MD (TS) - *Spec Exp:* *Cardiac Surgery-Adult & Pediatric;* **Hospital:** Desert Regional Med Ctr; **Address:** 1180 N Indian Canyon Drive, Ste E318, Palm Springs, CA 92262; **Phone:** (760) 416-1376; **Board Cert:** Surgery 1993, Thoracic Surgery 1995; **Med School:** Med Coll GA 1977; **Resid:** Surgery, Univ Michigan Hosps, Ann Arbor, MI 1980-1983; Thoracic Surgery, Univ Michigan Hosps, Ann Arbor, MI 1983-1985; **Fellow:** Pediatric Cardiac Surgery, Hosp-Sick Chldn, London, England 1985-1986; **Fac Appt:** Prof Surgery, Loma Linda Univ

Hanley, Frank Louis MD (TS) - *Spec Exp:* Thoracic Surgery-Pediatric; **Hospital:** Stanford Med Ctr; **Address:** 300 Pasteur Drive, Stanford, CA 94305-5407; **Phone:** (650) 724-2925; **Board Cert:** Thoracic Surgery 1990, Surgery 1987; **Med School:** Tufts Univ 1978; **Resid:** Surgery, UCSF Med Ctr, San Francisco, CA 1978-1981; Cardiothoracic Surgery, UCSF Med Ctr, San Francisco, CA 1986-1988; **Fellow:** Research, UCSF Sch Med, San Francisco, CA 1981-1984; **Fac Appt:** Prof Surgery, UCSF

Holmes, E Carmack MD (TS) - *Spec Exp:* Lung Cancer; **Hospital:** UCLA Med Ctr; **Address:** UCLA Med Ctr, Dept of Surgery, 10833 Le Conte Ave, Los Angeles, CA 90095-1749; **Phone:** (310) 825-7017; **Board Cert:** Thoracic Surgery 1974, Surgery 1973; **Med School:** Univ NC Sch Med 1964; **Resid:** Surgery, Johns Hopkins Hosp, Baltimore, MD 1965-1973; Surgery, Natl Cancer Inst 1966-1969; **Fac Appt:** Prof Surgery, UCLA

Kay, Jerome Harold MD (TS) - *Spec Exp:* Cardiac Surgery; Lung Surgery; **Hospital:** Good Samaritan Hosp - Los Angeles; **Address:** 1127 Wilshire Blvd, Ste 600, Los Angeles, CA 90017-3907; **Phone:** (213) 250-5711; **Board Cert:** Surgery 1955, Thoracic Surgery 1957; **Med School:** UCSF **Resid:** Surgery, McKinney VA Hosp 1946-1950; Surgery, Johns Hopkins Hosp, Baltimore, MD 1950-1954; **Fellow:** Thoracic Surgery, Johns Hopkins Hosp, BAltimore, MD 1950-1952

Laks, Hillel MD (TS) - *Spec Exp:* Heart Disease-Congenital; Transplant-Heart; **Hospital:** UCLA Med Ctr; **Address:** UCLA Med Ctr, Div Cardiothoracic Surg, 10833 Le Conte Ave, rm 62-182 A, Los Angeles, CA 90095-1741; **Phone:** (310) 206-8232; **Board Cert:** Surgery 1975, Thoracic Surgery 1996; **Med School:** Africa 1965; **Resid:** Surgery, Peter Bent Brigham Hosp, Boston, MA 1967-1969; Thoracic Surgery, Peter Bent Brigham Hosp, Boston, MA 1969-1973; **Fac Appt:** Prof Surgery, UCLA

Little, Alex G MD (TS) - *Spec Exp:* Thoracic Surgery - General; **Hospital:** Univ Med Ctr-Las Vegas; **Address:** 2040 W Charleston Blvd, Ste 601, Las Vegas, NV 89102; **Phone:** (702) 671-2339; **Board Cert:** Surgery 1998, Thoracic Surgery 1990; **Med School:** Johns Hopkins Univ 1974; **Resid:** Thoracic Surgery, Univ Chicago Hosp, Chicago, IL 1979-1981; Surgery, Univ Chicago Hosp, Chicago, IL 1977-1979; **Fac Appt:** Prof Thoracic Surgery, Univ Nevada

McKenna Jr, Robert J MD (TS) - *Spec Exp:* Lung Cancer; Gastroesophageal Reflux; Minimally Invasive Surgery; **Hospital:** Cedars-Sinai Med Ctr; **Address:** 8635 W 3rd St, Ste 975W, Los Angeles, CA 90048-6101; **Phone:** (310) 652-0530; **Board Cert:** Thoracic Surgery 1997, Surgery 1983; **Med School:** USC Sch Med 1977; **Resid:** Surgery, Stanford University Hosp, Stanford, CA 1978-1982; Surgery, Good Samaritan Hosp, Los Angeles, CA 1985-1987; **Fellow:** Thoracic Surgery, MD Anderson Tumor Inst, Houston, TX 1982-1983; **Fac Appt:** Clin Prof Thoracic Surgery, UCLA

Miller, David Craig MD (TS) - *Spec Exp:* Endovascular Stent-Grafting; Thoracic Aortic Surgery; **Hospital:** Stanford Med Ctr; **Address:** Stanford Univ Sch Med, Falk Research Bldg, 300 Pasteur, MC 5407, Stanford, CA 94305-5247; **Phone:** (650) 725-3826; **Board Cert:** Thoracic Surgery 1988, Vascular Surgery (General) 1993; **Med School:** Stanford Univ 1972; **Resid:** Thoracic Surgery, Standford Univ Med Ctr, Standford, CA 1973-1978; **Fac Appt:** Prof Thoracic Surgery, Stanford Univ

Morton, Donald Lee MD (TS) - *Spec Exp:* Melanoma; Sentinel Node Surgery; Breast Cancer; **Hospital:** St John's Hlth Ctr; **Address:** John Wayne Cancer Inst, 2200 Santa Monica Blvd, Santa Monica, CA 90404; **Phone:** (310) 829-8363; **Board Cert:** Thoracic Surgery 1969, Surgery 1967; **Med School:** UCSF 1958; **Resid:** Surgery, Natnl Cancer Inst-NIH, Bethesda, MD 1960-1962; Thoracic Surgery, UC- San Francisco, San Francisco, CA 1962-1966; **Fellow:** Surgery, Cancer Rsch Inst-UCSF, San Francisco, CA 1962-1966; **Fac Appt:** Prof Emeritus Surgery, UCLA

Reitz, Bruce Arnold MD (TS) - *Spec Exp:* *Transplant-Heart; Heart Valve Surgery;* **Hospital:** Stanford Med Ctr; **Address:** 300 Pasteur Drive, Stanford, CA 94305-5407; **Phone:** (650) 725-4497; **Board Cert:** Thoracic Surgery 1991, Surgery 1980; **Med School:** Yale Univ 1970; **Resid:** Thoracic Surgery, Stanford Univ Hosp, Palo Alto, CA 1971-1972; Thoracic Surgery, Natl Heart Inst-NIH, Bethesda, MD 1972-1974; **Fac Appt:** Prof Thoracic Surgery, Stanford Univ

Robbins, Robert Clayton MD (TS) - *Spec Exp:* *Thoracic Surgery - General;* **Hospital:** Stanford Med Ctr; **Address:** 300 Pasteur Drive, Ste A265, Stanford, CA 94305; **Phone:** (650) 723-5044; **Board Cert:** Thoracic Surgery 1994, Surgery 1990; **Med School:** Univ Miss 1983; **Resid:** Surgery, Univ Miss Med Ctr, Jackson, MS 1984-1988; **Fellow:** Thoracic Surgery, Stanford Univ, Stanford, CA 1989-1991; **Fac Appt:** Asst Prof Thoracic Surgery, Stanford Univ

Starnes, Vaughn A MD (TS) - *Spec Exp:* *Transplant-Heart & Lung -Pediatric; Heart Valve Surgery; Ross Procedure;* **Hospital:** USC Univ Hosp - R K Eamer Med Plz; **Address:** USC Cardiothoracic Surg, 1510 San Pablo St, Ste 415, Los Angeles, CA 90033; **Phone:** (323) 442-5849; **Board Cert:** Surgery 1985, Thoracic Surgery 1998; **Med School:** Univ NC Sch Med 1977; **Resid:** Surgery, Vanderbilt Univ Hosp, Nashville, TN 1977-1984; Cardiovascular Surgery, Stanford Unv Hosp, Stanford, CA 1984-1986; **Fellow:** Cardiothoracic Transplantation, Stanford Unv Hosp, Stanford, CA 1986-1987; Pediatric Cardiac Surgery, Univ NC Hosp, Chapel Hill, NC 1987; **Fac Appt:** Prof Surgery, USC Sch Med

Trento, Alfredo MD (TS) - *Spec Exp:* *Transplant-Heart; Cardiac Surgery-Adult & Pediatric;* **Hospital:** Cedars-Sinai Med Ctr; **Address:** Cedars-Sinai Med Ctr, Dept Cardiothor Surg, 8700 Beverly Blvd, North Tower - rm 6215, Los Angeles, CA 90048; **Phone:** (310) 423-3851; **Board Cert:** Surgery 1984, Thoracic Surgery 1995; **Med School:** Italy 1975; **Resid:** Surgery, Univ Mass Med Ctr, Worcester, MA 1977-1982; Thoracic Surgery, Univ Pittsburgh, Pittsburgh, PA 1983-1985; **Fellow:** Cardiothoracic Surgery, Univ Mass-Coord Surg Prog, Worcester, MA 1982; **Fac Appt:** Prof Surgery, UCLA

Ungerleider, Ross M MD (TS) - *Spec Exp:* *Heart Disease-Congenital; Cardiac Surgery-Adult & Pediatric;* **Hospital:** Doernbecher Chldns Hosp; **Address:** 3181 SW Sam Jackson Park Rd, L353, Portland, OR 97201; **Phone:** (503) 418-5443; **Board Cert:** Thoracic Surgery 1997; **Med School:** Rush Med Coll 1977; **Resid:** Surgery, Duke Univ Med Ctr, Durham, NC 1978-1979; Thoracic Surgery, Duke Univ Med Ctr, Durham, NC 1981-1987; **Fellow:** Thoracic Surgery, Duke Univ Med Ctr, Durham, NC 1979-1981; **Fac Appt:** Prof Surgery, Duke Univ

Verrier, Edward MD (TS) - *Spec Exp:* *Coronary Artery Surgery; Heart Valve Surgery;* **Hospital:** Univ WA Med Ctr; **Address:** UWMC, Ste AA-115, Box 356310, 1959 NE Pacific St, Seattle, WA 98195-6310; **Phone:** (206) 543-3093; **Board Cert:** Surgery 1992, Thoracic Surgery 1993; **Med School:** Tufts Univ 1974; **Resid:** Surgery, UCSF Med Ctr, San Francisco, CA 1980-1982; Thoracic Surgery, UCSF Med Ctr, San Francisco, CA 1982-1984; **Fellow:** Thoracic Surgery, UCSF Med Ctr, San Francisco, CA 1977-1980; **Fac Appt:** Prof Thoracic Surgery, Univ Wash

Wells, Winfield J MD (TS) - *Spec Exp:* *Tracheal Surgery-Pediatric; Congenital Heart Surgery;* **Hospital:** Chldns Hosp - Los Angeles; **Address:** Children's Hosp, Div Cardiothoracic Surgery, 4650 Sunset Blvd, MS 66, Los Angeles, CA 90027; **Phone:** (323) 669-4148; **Board Cert:** Thoracic Surgery 1987; **Med School:** USC Sch Med 1970; **Resid:** Surgery, Columbia-Presby Med Ctr, New York, NY 1971-; **Fac Appt:** Assoc Prof Surgery, USC Sch Med

Whyte, Richard MD (TS) - *Spec Exp:* Lung Cancer; Esophageal Cancer; **Hospital:** Stanford Med Ctr; **Address:** Stanford Univ Sch Med, Div Thor Surg, 300 Pasteur Dr, Bldg CVRB - rm 205, Stanford, CA 94305; **Phone:** (650) 723-6649; **Board Cert:** Surgery 1991, Thoracic Surgery 1993; **Med School:** Univ Pittsburgh 1983; **Resid:** Surgery, Mass Genl Hosp, Boston, MA 1983-1990; Thoracic Surgery, Univ Michigan Hosp, Ann Arbor, MI 1991-1992; **Fac Appt:** Assoc Prof Thoracic Surgery, Stanford Univ

Wood, Douglas MD (TS) - *Spec Exp:* Lung & Esophageal Cancer; Tracheal Tumors/Tracheal stenosis; **Hospital:** Univ WA Med Ctr; **Address:** Division of Cardiothoracic Surgery, 1959 Pacific NE, Bldg AA - rm 115, Box 356310, MC-356310, Seattle, WA 98195-6310; **Phone:** (206) 685-3228; **Board Cert:** Thoracic Surgery 1993, Surgery 1999; **Med School:** Harvard Med Sch 1983; **Resid:** Surgery, Mass Genl Hosp, Boston, MA 1983-1989; Thoracic Surgery, Massachusetts General Hospital, Boston, MA 1989-1991; **Fellow:** Surgical Critical Care, Massachusetts General Hospital, Boston, MA 1989-1991; **Fac Appt:** Assoc Prof Surgery, Univ Wash

UROLOGY

A urologist manages benign and malignant medical and surgical disorders of the genitourinary system and the adrenal gland. This specialist has comprehensive knowledge of, and skills in, endoscopic, percutaneous and open surgery of congenital and acquired conditions of the urinary and reproductive systems and their contiguous structures.

Training required: Five years

CLEVELAND CLINIC UROLOGICAL INSTITUTE
THE CLEVELAND CLINIC

9500 Euclid Avenue, Cleveland, OH 44195
Phone: 800/223-2273, Ext. 45600
www.clevelandclinic.org/urology

A NATIONAL LEADER IN UROLOGY

The Cleveland Clinic Urological Institute provides the highest quality of care for adult and pediatric patients with routine or complex urological disorders. Successful results in the practice and science of urology have won the Urological Institute international acclaim as one of the most progressive and accomplished urologic groups in the country.

INNOVATIVE CARE

In the treatment of kidney disease, the Institute has made numerous pioneering contributions including the development of "bench surgery," a technique designed to repair the kidney outside the body and then transplant it back into the patient.

The Institute is also a recognized leader in partial nephrectomies, or kidney-sparing surgery, for the treatment of kidney cancer. In 2001, the 1000th kidney-sparing procedure was performed, representing the largest experience in the world with this type of reconstructive procedure. Another treatment option performed here for kidney cancer is cryoablation, a minimally invasive treatment that uses a freezing probe to destroy the cancerous portion of the kidney. The Institute is one of the world's most experienced with this procedure.

In prostate cancer, the Institute has the largest experience in the United States with laparoscopic prostatectomy. Laparoscopic patients enjoy a shortened hospital stay, quicker recovery, less pain and the same result as any conventional surgical techniques done in the United States.

DEFINING THE STATE OF THE ART

The Cleveland Clinic Urological Institute has been instrumental in perfecting and refining many laparoscopic techniques that offer patients improved outcomes. These techniques are now routinely used for many urological diseases and conditions including prostate cancer, kidney and bladder cancer, urinary incontinence and in removing and transplanting kidneys in live-donor transplants.

As one of only a handful of centers in the world skilled in using the latest versions of robotic surgery systems, the Cleveland Clinic Urological Institute is leading the way in developing the surgery of the future.

ONE OF THE BEST

With 46 full-time urologists, the Cleveland Clinic Urological Institute is the largest and most comprehensive urological group in the world. Many procedures have been developed or perfected here and adopted around the world. These include laparoscopic urological surgery, female incontinence procedures, kidney-sparing surgery for kidney cancer, kidney-artery reconstruction and kidney transplantation. The Institute also offers innovative treatment for sexual dysfunction, male infertility and testicular and bladder cancer. The latest and most effective treatments are provided for virtually every urological disorder in adults and children.

Because of its clinical and academic achievements, the Urological Institute has consistently received national and international recognition. *U.S.News & World Report* ranks the Cleveland Clinic Urological Institute one of the top two urological groups in the United States.

THE MOUNT SINAI HOSPITAL
UROLOGY

One Gustave L. Levy Place (Fifth Avenue and 98th Street)
New York, NY 10029-6574   Phone: (212) 241-6500
Physician Referral: 1-800-MD-SINAI (637-4624)
www.mountsinai.org

The Mount Sinai prides itself on adapting the latest technologic advancements and results of translational and clinical research to the assessment and treatment of urologic problems.

Conditions treated include:

Prostate Cancer – Having pioneered the use of radioactive seeds, the Department offers a full range of surgical and radiation treatments in the management of localized prostate cancer. For more advanced disease, treatment may integrate the use of new vaccines, gene therapy, new agents in chemotherapy, and hormonal therapy.

Bladder Cancer – As recognized leaders in the assessment and treatment of all forms of bladder cancer, Mount Sinai's specialists employ knowledge of tumor markers and understanding of biologic aspects of bladder cancer to determine the most effective treatment approaches, such as the use of minimally invasive tools, which help preserve and maximize quality of life.

Kidney Cancer – When feasible, Mount Sinai employs minimally invasive surgical techniques, minimizing pain and recovery time. Such techniques may be applied to remove all or a portion of a kidney. Other modalities – such as freezing, high radio frequency, and sonic energy – may be recommended to treat small kidney cancers while preserving maximal function.

Prostatic Enlargement – The latest technologies and treatments are applied for their effect in relieving urinary problems, including frequency, pain, burning, and retention.

Urinary Dysfunction – For men and women, Mount Sinai provides comprehensive resources for the evaluation and treatment, both medical and surgical, of urinary incontinence, neuro-urologic problems, and pelvic pain syndrome.

Urologic Stone Disease – Mount Sinai's expertise in the minimally invasive treatment of kidney stone disease complements the use of various lasers, sonic energies, and extracorporeal shock wave lithotripsy. The program also emphasizes kidney stone prevention.

Pediatric Conditions – Mount Sinai has a strong reputation in the treatment of urologic problems in children, especially in reconstructive treatment, involving, when appropriate, minimally invasive procedures.

Male Infertility – State-of-the-art approaches using medications and in vitro fertilization techniques result in a high success rate.

Sexuality-related Health Concerns – For both men and women, sexuality-related issues are addressed through application of current medical and surgical approaches.

THE MOUNT SINAI HOSPITAL

Minimally Invasive Urologic Surgery – Mount Sinai has developed an extensive program in this rapidly growing area. Mount Sinai is currently the only facility in the greater New York area in which complex and extensive procedures are performed laparoscopically or endoscopically for treatment of various urologic cancers, reconstruction for various anatomic abnormalities, and management of stone disease. These approaches provide for a rapid and virtually painless recovery and rapid return to normal activity.

The Deane Prostate Health Center – The Center offers a new multidisciplinary facility for the assessment and treatment of all aspects of prostatic disease, including cancer, benign enlargement, and inflammation. Activities through the Center are designed to empower the patient and his family to understand the nature of prostatic condition and decide upon the optimum treatment that may create lasting benefit and enhance quality of life.

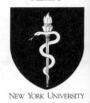

NYU Medical Center
550 First Avenue (at 31st Street)
New York, NY 10016
Physician Referral: (888) 7-NYU-MED
(888-769-8633) www.nyumedicalcenter.org

SCHOOL OF MEDICINE

NEW YORK UNIVERSITY

UROLOGY

NYU Medical Center's urologists are internationally renowned specialists who have pioneered numerous advances in the surgical and pharmacological treatment of urological disease. They are an interdisciplinary team of physicians, nurses, and allied health professionals dedicated to providing the highest-quality state-of-the-art care. All of our doctors are also faculty at NYU School of Medicine who specialize in all aspects of urological disease. Our programs include:

Urologic Oncology – aggressively treating and curing urologic cancers while maintaining the highest quality of life. Cancers of the prostate, kidney, bladder, and teste are the most common malignancies treated in this program. Since treating cancer often requires a multidisciplinary approach, urologists work closely with NYU's medical and radtiation oncologists to tailor treatment to each patient's priorities and objectives.

Minimally Invasive Surgery – committed to developing new technologies to treat even the most complex disorders more effectively and less invasively, so patients experience less pain and a quicker recovery.

Male Fertility and Sexual Health – collaborating closely with the world-renowned NYU *In Vitro* Fertilization Program, the fertility treatment program uses state-of-the-art technology and a multidisciplinary approach to diagnose and treat the underlying causes of both male and female sexual dysfunction.

Benign Prostatic Diseases – developing innovative medical and surgical therapies for benign prostatic diseases, such as benign prostatic hyperplasia (BPH, or enlarged prostate) and prostatitis (infection in the prostate).

Female Urology and Incontinence –expertise in the many urological problems unique to women, including recurrent urinary tract infections, pelvic pain, prolapse, and sexual dysfunction.

Pediatric Urology and Reconstructive Surgery – treating urologic diseases in children.

NYU MEDICAL CENTER

National Institutes for Health funding for NYU urological research is among the highest for a Urology department in thenation. To assure the continued cross-fertilization of research and patient care, basic scientists with primary academic appointments work closely with the NYU Medical Center urologists on research, leading to a superior understanding of clinical problems.

Physician Referral
(888) 7-NYU-MED

(888-769-8633)

www.nyumedicalcenter.org

Physician Listings

Urology

New England

Althausen, Alex F MD (U) - *Spec Exp:* *Urologic Cancer;* **Hospital:** MA Genl Hosp; **Address:** One Hawthorne Pl, Ste 109, Boston, MA 02114-2333; **Phone:** (617) 523-5250; **Board Cert:** Urology 1976; **Med School:** Tufts Univ 1966; **Resid:** Surgery, Albany Med Ctr, Albany, NY 1967-1968; Urology, Mass Genl Hosp, Boston, MA 1970-1974; **Fac Appt:** Assoc Prof Surgery, Harvard Med Sch

Dretler, Stephen P. MD (U) - *Spec Exp:* *Kidney Stones;* **Hospital:** MA Genl Hosp; **Address:** 15 Parkman St, Ste 486, Boston, MA 02114-3139; **Phone:** (617) 726-3512; **Board Cert:** Urology 1975; **Med School:** Tufts Univ 1964; **Resid:** Surgery, Mass Genl Hosp, Boston, MA 1965; Urology, Mass Genl Hosp, Boston, MA 1971; **Fellow:** Nephrology, Mass Genl Hosp, Boston, MA 1968; **Fac Appt:** Clin Prof Surgery, Harvard Med Sch

Goldstein, Irwin MD (U) - *Spec Exp:* *Erectile Dysfunction;* **Hospital:** Boston Med Ctr; **Address:** 720 Harrison Ave, Ste 606, Boston, MA 02118-2334; **Phone:** (617) 638-8485; **Board Cert:** Urology 1982; **Med School:** McGill Univ 1975; **Resid:** Urology, Boston Univ Med Ctr, Boston, MA 1977-1980; Surgery, Boston Univ Med Ctr, Boston, MA 1977; **Fellow:** Urology, Boston Univ Med Ctr, Boston, MA 1981; **Fac Appt:** Assoc Prof Urology, Boston Univ

Gomery, Pablo MD (U) - *Spec Exp:* *Neuro-Urology; Erectile Dysfunction;* **Hospital:** MA Genl Hosp; **Address:** Mass Genl Hosp-Dept Urology, Bldg ACC528, Boston, MA 02114; **Phone:** (617) 724-6208; **Board Cert:** Urology 2000; **Med School:** Albert Einstein Coll Med 1974; **Resid:** Urology, Mass Genl Hosp, Boston, MA 1977-1980; Surgery, New England Deaconess, Boston, MA 1975-1977

Heney, Niall M MD (U) - *Spec Exp:* *Urologic Cancer;* **Hospital:** MA Genl Hosp; **Address:** Mass General Hosp, Dept Urology, 15 Parkman St, Boston, MA 02114; **Phone:** (617) 726-3011; **Board Cert:** Urology 1977; **Med School:** Ireland 1965; **Resid:** Urology, Reg Hosp, Galway, Ireland 1968-1972; Urology, Mass Genl Hosp, Boston, MA; **Fac Appt:** Prof Medicine, Harvard Med Sch

Libertino, John A. MD (U) - *Spec Exp:* *Kidney Reconstruction; Prostate Cancer; Adrenal Disorders;* **Hospital:** Lahey Cli.; **Address:** 41 Mall Rd, Lahey Medical Clinic, Burlington, MA 01803; **Phone:** (781) 744-8420; **Board Cert:** Urology 1973; **Med School:** Georgetown Univ 1965; **Resid:** Urology, Yale-New Haven Hosp., New Haven, CT 1967-1970; Urology, U Rochester-Strong Meml Hosp., Rochester, NY 1967; **Fellow:** Surgery, Yale-New Haven Hosp., New Haven, CT 1968; **Fac Appt:** Assoc Clin Prof Surgery, Harvard Med Sch

McDougal, William Scott MD (U) - *Spec Exp:* *Urinary Reconstruction; Urologic Cancer; Prostate Cancer;* **Hospital:** MA Genl Hosp; **Address:** Mass Genl Hosp, 55 Fruit St, Bldg GRB - rm 1102, Boston, MA 02114; **Phone:** (617) 726-3010; **Board Cert:** Urology 1992, Surgery 1975; **Med School:** Cornell Univ-Weill Med Coll 1968; **Resid:** Surgery, Univ Hosps Cleveland, Cleveland, OH 1969-1975; **Fellow:** Physiology, Yale Med Sch, New Haven, CT 1971-1972; **Fac Appt:** Prof Urology, Harvard Med Sch

McGovern, Francis MD (U) - *Spec Exp:* *Prostate Cancer;* **Hospital:** MA Genl Hosp; **Address:** 1 Hawthorne Pl, Ste 109, Boston, MA 02114; **Phone:** (617) 523-5250; **Board Cert:** Urology 1999; **Med School:** Case West Res Univ 1983; **Resid:** Urology, Mass Genl Hosp., Boston, MA 1984-1989

Oates, Robert Davis MD (U) - *Spec Exp:* Infertility-Male; Vasectomy Reversal; **Hospital:** Boston Med Ctr; **Address:** Boston Univ Med Ctr, Dept Urology, 720 Harrison Ave, Ste 606, Boston, MA 02118-2334; **Phone:** (617) 638-8485; **Board Cert:** Urology 1990; **Med School:** Boston Univ 1982; **Resid:** Urology, Boston Univ Hosp, Boston, MA 1984-1987; Surgery, Boston Univ Hosp, Boston, MA 1983-1984; **Fellow:** Reproductive Medicine, Baylor Coll Med, Houston, TX 1987-1988; **Fac Appt:** Assoc Prof Urology, Boston Univ

Retik, Alan MD (U) - *Spec Exp:* Urinary Reconstruction-Pediatric; **Hospital:** Children's Hospital - Boston; **Address:** Chldn's Hosp, Dept Urology, 300 Longwood Ave Bldg Hunnewell - rm 390, Boston, MA 02115-5724; **Phone:** (617) 731-6220; **Board Cert:** Urology 1969; **Med School:** Cornell Univ-Weill Med Coll 1957; **Resid:** Surgery, Strong Meml Hosp, Rochester, MN 1958-1961; Urology, Peter Bent Brigham Hosp, Boston, MA 1962-1965; **Fellow:** Pediatric Urology, Hosp Sich Chldn, London, England 1966-1967; **Fac Appt:** Prof Urology, Harvard Med Sch

Richie, Jerome MD (U) - *Spec Exp:* Prostate Cancer; Testicular Cancer; Kidney Cancer; **Hospital:** Brigham & Women's Hosp; **Address:** Division of Urology, 75 Francis St, Boston, MA 02115-6106; **Phone:** (617) 732-6325; **Board Cert:** Urology 1977; **Med School:** Univ Tex Med Br, Galveston 1969; **Resid:** Surgery, UCLA Med Ctr, Los Angeles, CA 1969-1971; Urology, UCLA Med Ctr, Los Angeles, CA 1971-1975; **Fac Appt:** Prof Urology, Harvard Med Sch

Sigman, Mark MD (U) - *Spec Exp:* Infertility-Male; Vasectomy Reversal; **Hospital:** Rhode Island Hosp; **Address:** 2 Dudley St, Ste 175, Providence, RI 02905-3247; **Phone:** (401) 421-0710; **Board Cert:** Urology 2000; **Med School:** Univ Conn 1981; **Resid:** Urology, Univ VA, Charlottesville, VA 1983-1987; Surgery, Univ VA, Charlottesville, VA 1982-1983; **Fellow:** Male Reproduction, Baylor Coll Med, Houston, TX 1987-1989; **Fac Appt:** Assoc Prof Urology, Brown Univ

Weiss, Robert M MD (U) - *Spec Exp:* Urology-Pediatric; **Hospital:** Yale - New Haven Hosp; **Address:** Yale Univ Sch Med, Dept of Urol, 800 Howard Ave, New Haven, CT 06520; **Phone:** (203) 785-2815; **Board Cert:** Urology 1970; **Med School:** SUNY Downstate 1960; **Resid:** Surgery, Beth Israel Hosp, New York, NY 1963-1967; Urology, Columbia Presby, New York, NY 1963-1967; **Fellow:** Pharmacology, Columbia Presby, New York, NY 1964-1965; **Fac Appt:** Prof Urology, Yale Univ

Mid Atlantic

Alexander, Richard B MD (U) - *Spec Exp:* Prostate Disease; **Hospital:** University of MD Med Sys; **Address:** 419 W Redwood St, Ste 320, Baltimore, MD 21201; **Phone:** (410) 328-5544; **Board Cert:** Urology 1999; **Med School:** Johns Hopkins Univ 1981; **Resid:** Urology, Johns Hopkins, Baltimore, MD 1983-1988; Surgery, Vanderbilt Univ Affl Hosps, Nashville, TN 1981-1983; **Fac Appt:** Assoc Prof Urology, Univ MD Sch Med

Bander, Neil MD (U) - *Spec Exp:* Prostate Cancer; **Hospital:** NY Presby Hosp - NY Weill Cornell Med Ctr (page 70); **Address:** 525 E 68th St, rm F940, New York, NY 10021; **Phone:** (212) 746-5460; **Board Cert:** Urology 1983; **Med School:** Univ Conn 1974; **Resid:** Urology, Bellevue Hosp, New York, NY 1975-1977; Urology, U Conn, Farmington, CT 1977-1980; **Fellow:** Urologic Oncology, Meml Sloan Kettering Cancer Ctr, New York, NY 1980-1983; **Fac Appt:** Prof Urology, Cornell Univ-Weill Med Coll

Belman, A Barry MD (U) - *Spec Exp:* Urology-Pediatric; Hypospadias; **Hospital:** Chldns Natl Med Ctr - DC; **Address:** Chldns Natl Med Ctr, 111 Michigan Ave NW, Washington, DC 20010; **Phone:** (202) 884-5042; **Board Cert:** Urology 1973; **Med School:** Northwestern Univ 1964; **Resid:** Urology, Northwestern Univ Med Ctr, Chicago, IL 1964-1970; **Fac Appt:** Prof Urology, Geo Wash Univ

Benson, Mitchell C MD (U) - *Spec Exp:* *Prostate Cancer; Incontinence;* **Hospital:** NY Presby Hosp - Columbia Presby Med Ctr (page 70); **Address:** 161 Ft Washington Ave, Ste 1153, New York, NY 10032-3713; **Phone:** (212) 305-5201; **Board Cert:** Urology 1984; **Med School:** Columbia P&S 1977; **Resid:** Surgery, Mount Sinai Med Ctr, New York, NY 1977-1979; Urology, Columbia-Presby Hosp, New York, NY 1979-1982; **Fellow:** Medical Oncology, Johns Hopkins Hosp, Baltimore, MD 1982-1984; **Fac Appt:** Prof Urology, Columbia P&S

Blaivas, Jerry G MD (U) - *Spec Exp:* *Uro-Gynecology; Bladder/Prostate Problems; Urology-Female;* **Hospital:** NY Presby Hosp - NY Weill Cornell Med Ctr (page 70); **Address:** 400 E 56th St, New York, NY 10022; **Phone:** (212) 308-6565; **Board Cert:** Urology 1978; **Med School:** Tufts Univ 1964; **Resid:** Surgery, Boston Med Ctr, Boston, MA 1969-1971; Urology, New England Med Ctr, Boston, MA 1973-1976; **Fac Appt:** Clin Prof Urology, Cornell Univ-Weill Med Coll

Burnett II, Arthur L MD (U) - *Spec Exp:* *Prostate Cancer; Erectile Dysfunction;* **Hospital:** Johns Hopkins Hosp - Baltimore; **Address:** 600 N Wolfe St, Marburg Bldg, Ste 407, Baltimore, MD 21287; **Phone:** (410) 614-3986; **Board Cert:** Urology 1998; **Med School:** Johns Hopkins Univ 1988; **Resid:** Urology, Johns Hopkins Hosp, Baltimore, MD 1990-1994; Surgery, Johns Hopkins Hosp, Baltimore, MD 1989-1990; **Fac Appt:** Prof Urology, Johns Hopkins Univ

Droller, Michael J MD (U) - *Spec Exp:* *Urologic Cancer; Bladder/Prostate Cancer; Kidney Cancer;* **Hospital:** Mount Sinai Hosp (page 68); **Address:** 5 E 98th St Fl 6th, Box 1272, New York, NY 10029-6501; **Phone:** (212) 241-3868; **Board Cert:** Urology 1979; **Med School:** Harvard Med Sch 1968; **Resid:** Surgery, Peter Bent Brigham Hosp, Boston, MA 1969-1970; Urology, Stanford Univ Med Ctr, Palo Alto, CA 1972-1976; **Fellow:** Immunology, Univ Stockholm, Sweden 1976-1977; **Fac Appt:** Prof Urology, Mount Sinai Sch Med

Eid, Jean Francois MD (U) - *Spec Exp:* *Erectile Dysfunction; Urological Prosthesis; Incontinence;* **Hospital:** NY Presby Hosp - NY Weill Cornell Med Ctr (page 70); **Address:** 50 E 69th St, New York, NY 10021; **Phone:** (212) 536-6690; **Board Cert:** Urology 1999; **Med School:** Cornell Univ-Weill Med Coll 1982; **Resid:** Surgery, NY Hosp-Cornell Med Ctr, New York, NY 1983-1984; Urology, NY Hosp-Cornell Med Ctr, New York, NY 1984-1988; **Fac Appt:** Assoc Clin Prof Urology, Cornell Univ-Weill Med Coll

Fisch, Harry MD (U) - *Spec Exp:* *Infertility-Male;* **Hospital:** NY Presby Hosp - Columbia Presby Med Ctr (page 70); **Address:** 944 Park Ave, Ste 1C, New York, NY 10028; **Phone:** (212) 879-0800; **Board Cert:** Urology 1999; **Med School:** Mount Sinai Sch Med 1983; **Resid:** Surgery, Montefiore Hosp Med Ctr, Bronx, NY 1983-1985; Urology, Montefiore Hosp Med Ctr, Bronx, NY 1985-1989; **Fac Appt:** Asst Prof Urology, Columbia P&S

Goldstein, Marc MD (U) - *Spec Exp:* *Infertility-Male; Vasectomy Reversal; Vasectomy-Scalpelless;* **Hospital:** NY Presby Hosp - NY Weill Cornell Med Ctr (page 70); **Address:** 525 E 68th St, rm F900, Box 580, New York, NY 10021; **Phone:** (212) 746-5470; **Board Cert:** Urology 1982; **Med School:** SUNY Downstate 1972; **Resid:** Surgery, Columbia-Presby Med Ctr, New York, NY 1972-1974; Urology, SUNY Hlth Sci Ctr, Brooklyn, NY 1977-1980; **Fellow:** Reproductive Endocrinology, Rockefeller Univ, New York, NY 1980-1982; **Fac Appt:** Prof Urology, Cornell Univ-Weill Med Coll

Gribetz, Michael MD (U) - *Spec Exp:* *Prostate Disease; Sexual Dysfunction; Urology-Female;* **Hospital:** Mount Sinai Hosp (page 68); **Address:** 1155 Park Ave, New York, NY 10128-1209; **Phone:** (212) 831-1300; **Board Cert:** Urology 1980; **Med School:** Albert Einstein Coll Med 1973; **Resid:** Surgery, Montefiore Hosp Med Ctr, Bronx, NY 1973-1975; Urology, Mount Sinai, New York, NY 1975-1978; **Fac Appt:** Asst Prof Urology, Mount Sinai Sch Med

Hensle, Terry MD (U) - *Spec Exp:* Urology-Pediatric; **Hospital:** NY Presby Hosp - Columbia Presby Med Ctr (page 70); **Address:** 3959 Broadway, Ste 219N, New York, NY 10032-1551; **Phone:** (212) 305-8510; **Board Cert:** Urology 1978; **Med School:** Cornell Univ-Weill Med Coll 1968; **Resid:** Surgery, Boston City Hosp, Boston, MA 1969-1973; Urology, Mass Genl Hosp, Boston, MA 1973-1976; **Fellow:** Pediatric Urology, Mass Genl Hosp, Boston, MA 1976-1977; Pediatric Urology, Great Ormond St Hosp, London, UK 1977-1978; **Fac Appt:** Prof Urology, Columbia P&S

Herr, Harry Wallace MD (U) - *Spec Exp:* Bladder Cancer; Urologic Tumors; **Hospital:** Mem Sloan Kettering Cancer Ctr; **Address:** Meml Sloan Kettering Canc Ctr, Dept Urology, 1275 York Ave, New York, NY 10021; **Phone:** (646) 422-4411; **Board Cert:** Urology 1976; **Med School:** UCSF 1969; **Resid:** Urology, UC Irvine, Orange, CA 1970-1974; **Fellow:** Urology, Meml Sloan Kettering Canc Ctr, New York, NY 1974-1976; **Fac Appt:** Assoc Prof Surgery, Cornell Univ-Weill Med Coll

Huben, Robert P MD (U) - *Spec Exp:* Prostate Cancer; Urologic Cancer; **Hospital:** Roswell Park Cancer Inst; **Address:** Roswell Park Cancer Inst, Urology Clin, Elm & Carlton Sts, Buffalo, NY 14263-0001; **Phone:** (716) 845-3159; **Board Cert:** Urology 1983; **Med School:** Cornell Univ-Weill Med Coll 1976; **Resid:** Urology, East Virginia Med Ctr, Norfolk, VA 1977-1981; **Fellow:** Medical Oncology, Roswell Park Meml Inst, Buffalo, NY 1981-1982

Irwin, Robert J MD (U) - *Spec Exp:* Urology - General; **Hospital:** UMDNJ-Univ Hosp-Newark; **Address:** 185 S Orange Ave, Ste G536, Newark, NJ 07103; **Phone:** (973) 972-4488; **Board Cert:** Urology 1976; **Med School:** Harvard Med Sch 1967; **Resid:** Urology, Mass Genl Hosp, Boston, MA 1971-1974; **Fellow:** Chemical Pathology, Guys Hosp Med Sch, London England 1964-1965; **Fac Appt:** Prof Urology, UMDNJ-NJ Med Sch, Newark

Jacobs, Stephen C MD (U) - *Spec Exp:* Laparoscopic Nephrectomy; Prostate Cancer; Kidney Cancer; **Hospital:** University of MD Med Sys; **Address:** 22 S Greene St, rm S8D18, Baltimore, MD 21201; **Phone:** (410) 328-5544; **Board Cert:** Urology 1979; **Med School:** Case West Res Univ 1971; **Resid:** Urology, Peter Bent Brigham Hosp, Boston, MA 1975-1977; Surgery, UC San Diego, San Diego, CA 1972-1975; **Fac Appt:** Prof Urology, Univ MD Sch Med

Jarow, Jonathan MD (U) - *Spec Exp:* Infertility-Male; Prostate Cancer; Erectile Dysfunction; **Hospital:** Johns Hopkins Hosp - Baltimore; **Address:** Johns Hopkins Hosp, 601 N Caroline St Fl 4, Baltimore, MD 21287; **Phone:** (410) 955-3617; **Board Cert:** Urology 1999; **Med School:** Northwestern Univ 1980; **Resid:** Surgery, Johns Hopkins, Baltimore, MD 1981-1982; Urology, Johns Hopkins, Baltimore, MD 1982-1986; **Fellow:** Andrology, Baylor Univ, Houston, TX 1987; **Fac Appt:** Asst Prof Urology, Wake Forest Univ Sch Med

Kavoussi, Louis Rapheal MD (U) - *Spec Exp:* Laparoscopic Surgery; Endourology; Kidney Stones; **Hospital:** Johns Hopkins Hosp - Baltimore; **Address:** 601 N Wolfe St, Baltimore, MD 21287; **Phone:** (410) 955-6101; **Board Cert:** Urology 1999; **Med School:** SUNY Buffalo 1983; **Resid:** Surgery, Barnes Hosp/Wash Univ Sch Med, St Louis, MO 1983-1985; Urology, Barnes Hosp/Wash Univ Sch Med, St Louis, MO 1985-1989; **Fac Appt:** Prof Urology, Johns Hopkins Univ

Kirschenbaum, Alexander Michael MD (U) - *Spec Exp:* Prostate Cancer; Bladder Surgery; **Hospital:** Mount Sinai Hosp (page 68); **Address:** 5 E 98th St, New York, NY 10029; **Phone:** (646) 422-0926; **Board Cert:** Urology 1997; **Med School:** Mount Sinai Sch Med 1980; **Resid:** Surgery, Mount Sinai Hosp, New York, NY 1980-1982; Urology, Mount Sinai Hosp, New York, NY 1982-1985; **Fellow:** Urologic Oncology, Mount Sinai Hosp, New York, NY 1985-1987; **Fac Appt:** Assoc Prof Urology, Mount Sinai Sch Med

Lepor, Herbert MD (U) - *Spec Exp:* Prostate Cancer; Kidney Cancer; **Hospital:** NYU Med Ctr (page 71); **Address:** 150 E 32nd St, New York, NY 10016; **Phone:** (646) 825-6300; **Board Cert:** Urology 1987; **Med School:** Johns Hopkins Univ 1975; **Resid:** Urology, Johns Hopkins Hosp, Baltimore, MD 1981-1986; **Fac Appt:** Prof Urology, NYU Sch Med

Levitt, Selwyn MD (U) - *Spec Exp:* Urology-Pediatric; Voiding Dysfunction; **Hospital:** Long Island Jewish Med Ctr; **Address:** 833 Northern Blvd, Ste 270, Great Neck, NY 11021; **Phone:** (516) 466-6953; **Board Cert:** Urology 1972; **Med School:** South Africa 1961; **Resid:** Urology, Bronx Muni Hosp, Bronx, NY 1963-1967; **Fellow:** Pediatric Urology, Babies Hosp, New York, NY 1967-1968; Pediatric Urology, Hosp for Sick Chldrn, London, England 1968-1969; **Fac Appt:** Clin Prof Urology, NY Med Coll

Lowe, Franklin MD (U) - *Spec Exp:* Prostate Disease; Alternative Medicine; **Hospital:** St Luke's - Roosevelt Hosp Ctr - Roosevelt Div (page 58); **Address:** 425 W 59th St, Ste 3A, New York, NY 10019; **Phone:** (212) 523-7790; **Board Cert:** Urology 1995; **Med School:** Columbia P&S 1979; **Resid:** Surgery, Johns Hopkins Hosp, Baltimore, MD 1979-1981; Urology, Johns Hopkins Hosp, Baltimore, MD 1981-1984; **Fac Appt:** Assoc Clin Prof Urology, Columbia P&S

Macchia, Richard MD (U) - *Spec Exp:* Prostate Disease; Prostate Cancer; Voiding Dysfunction-Urinary; **Hospital:** Univ Hosp - Brklyn; **Address:** SUNY Downstate Medical School, Dept of Urology, 445 Lenox Rd, Box 79, Brooklyn, NY 11203-2098; **Phone:** (718) 270-2554; **Board Cert:** Urology 1977; **Med School:** NY Med Coll 1969; **Resid:** Surgery, St Vincent's Hosp & Med Ctr, Brooklyn, NY 1970; Urology, SUNY Downstate Medical School, Brooklyn, NY 1971-1974; **Fellow:** Urologic Oncology, Meml Sloan Kettering Cancer Ctr, New York, NY 1975-1976; **Fac Appt:** Prof Urology, SUNY Downstate

Malkowicz, Bruce MD (U) - *Spec Exp:* Urologic Cancer; **Hospital:** Hosp Univ Penn (page 78); **Address:** Univ Penn Hospital, 1st Floor Rhoades, 3400 Spruce St, Philadelphia, PA 19104; **Phone:** (215) 662-2893; **Board Cert:** Urology 2000; **Med School:** Univ Penn 1981; **Resid:** Surgery, Hosp Univ Penn, Philadelphia, PA 1982-1983; Urology, Hosp Univ Penn, Philadelphia, PA 1983-1987; **Fellow:** Urologic Oncology, USC Med Ctr, Los Angeles, CA 1987-1998; Urologic Oncology, Hosp Univ Penn/Wistar Inst, Philadelphia, PA 1988-1990; **Fac Appt:** Assoc Prof Urology, Univ Penn

Melman, Arnold MD (U) - *Spec Exp:* Erectile Dysfunction; Incontinence; **Hospital:** Montefiore Med Ctr (page 67); **Address:** 969 Park Ave, Ste 1G, New York, NY 10028; **Phone:** (212) 639-1561; **Board Cert:** Urology 1976; **Med School:** Univ Rochester 1966; **Resid:** Urology, Strong Meml Hosp, Rochester, NY 1966-1968; Urology, UCLA Med Ctr, Los Angeles, CA 1970-1974; **Fellow:** Nephrology, Cedars-Sinai Med Ctr, Los Angeles, CA 1971-1972; **Fac Appt:** Prof Urology, Albert Einstein Coll Med

Mostwin, Jacek Lech MD/PhD (U) - *Spec Exp:* Prostate Cancer; **Hospital:** Johns Hopkins Hosp - Baltimore; **Address:** 600 N Wolfe St, Bldg Marburg - Ste 401C, Baltimore, MD 21287; **Phone:** (410) 955-4461; **Board Cert:** Urology 1997; **Med School:** Univ MD Sch Med 1975; **Resid:** Urology, Johns Hopkins Hosp., Baltimore, MD 1979-1983; Surgery, U Mich., Ann Arbor, MI 1976-1978; **Fac Appt:** Prof Urology, Johns Hopkins Univ

Nagler, Harris M MD (U) - *Spec Exp:* Vasectomy Reversal; Infertility-Male; Erectile Dysfunction; **Hospital:** Beth Israel Med Ctr - Petrie Division (page 58); **Address:** 10 Union Square E, Ste 3A, New York, NY 10003; **Phone:** (212) 844-8900; **Board Cert:** Urology 1982; **Med School:** Temple Univ 1975; **Resid:** Urology, Columbia Presby Hosp, New York, NY 1976-1980; **Fellow:** Reproductive Medicine, Columbia Presby Hosp, New York, NY 1980-1981; **Fac Appt:** Prof Urology, Albert Einstein Coll Med

Naslund, Michael MD (U) - *Spec Exp:* Prostate Cancer; Prostate Disease; **Hospital:** University of MD Med Sys; **Address:** Maryland Prostate Ctr, 419 W Redwood St, Ste 320, Baltimore, MD 21201; **Phone:** (410) 328-0800; **Board Cert:** Urology 2000; **Med School:** Johns Hopkins Univ 1981; **Resid:** Urology, Johns Hopkins Hosp, Baltimore, MD 1983-1987; Surgery, Johns Hopkins Hosp, Baltimore, MD 1982-1983; **Fac Appt:** Assoc Prof Surgery, Univ MD Sch Med

Nelson, Joel Byron MD (U) - *Spec Exp:* Prostate Cancer; **Hospital:** UPMC - Presbyterian Univ Hosp; **Address:** UPMC Shadyside Med Ctr, 5200 Centre Ave, Ste 209, Pittsburgh, PA 15232; **Phone:** (412) 605-3013; **Board Cert:** Urology 1998; **Med School:** Northwestern Univ 1988; **Resid:** Urology, Northwestern Mem Hosp, Chicago, IL 1988-1994; **Fellow:** Urology, Johns Hopkins Hosp, Baltimore, MD; **Fac Appt:** Prof Urology, Univ Pittsburgh

Nitti, Victor MD (U) - *Spec Exp:* Voiding Dysfunction; Urology-Female; Incontinence-Female; **Hospital:** NYU Med Ctr (page 71); **Address:** NYU Med Ctr, Dept Urology, 540 First Ave, New York, NY 10016-6402; **Phone:** (212) 263-1086; **Board Cert:** Urology 1994; **Med School:** UMDNJ-NJ Med Sch, Newark 1985; **Resid:** Surgery, Univ Hosp- SUNY Hlth Sci Ctr, Brooklyn, NY 1985-1987; Urology, Univ Hosp-SUNY Hlth Sci Ctr, Brooklyn, NY 1987-1991; **Fellow:** Urology, UCLA Med Ctr, Los Angeles, CA 1991-1992; **Fac Appt:** Assoc Prof Urology, NYU Sch Med

Olsson, Carl MD (U) - *Spec Exp:* Prostate Cancer; Kidney Cancer; Bladder Cancer; **Hospital:** NY Presby Hosp - Columbia Presby Med Ctr (page 70); **Address:** Irving Pavilion Fl 11 - rm 1102, 161 Fort Washington Ave, New York, NY 10032-3713; **Phone:** (212) 305-0100; **Board Cert:** Urology 1995; **Med School:** Boston Univ 1963; **Resid:** Internal Medicine, Boston Univ Hosp, Boston, MA 1964-1966; Urology, Boston VA, Boston, MA 1966-1969; **Fellow:** Urology, Cleveland Clinic Fdn, Cleveland, OH 1966; **Fac Appt:** Prof Urology, Columbia P&S

Scardino, Peter MD (U) - *Spec Exp:* Bladder Cancer; Prostate Cancer; **Hospital:** Mem Sloan Kettering Cancer Ctr; **Address:** 1275 York Ave, New York, NY 10021; **Phone:** (646) 422-4329; **Board Cert:** Urology 1981; **Med School:** Duke Univ 1971; **Resid:** Internal Medicine, Mass Genl Hosp, Boston, MA 1972-1973; Urology, UCLA Med Ctr, Los Angeles, CA 1976-1979; **Fellow:** Urology, Natl Cancer Inst, Bethesda, MD 1973-1976

Schlegel, Peter MD (U) - *Spec Exp:* Prostate Cancer; Infertility-Male; **Hospital:** NY Presby Hosp - NY Weill Cornell Med Ctr (page 70); **Address:** 525 E 68th St Fl 907A, New York, NY 10021-4870; **Phone:** (212) 746-5491; **Board Cert:** Urology 2000; **Med School:** Univ Mass Sch Med 1983; **Resid:** Surgery, Johns Hopkins Hosp, Baltimore, MD 1983-1985; Urology, Johns Hopkins Hosp, Baltimore, MD 1985-1989; **Fellow:** Medical Oncology, Johns Hopkins Hosp, Baltimore, MD 1986-1987; Male Reproduction, NY Hosp-Cornell Med Ctr, New York, NY 1989-1991; **Fac Appt:** Assoc Prof Urology, Cornell Univ-Weill Med Coll

Smith, Arthur D MD (U) - *Spec Exp:* Kidney Stones; Laparoscopic Surgery; **Hospital:** Long Island Jewish Med Ctr; **Address:** Long Island Jewish Med Ctr, 270-05 76th Ave, Fl 4th, New Hyde Park, NY 11040; **Phone:** (718) 470-7221; **Board Cert:** Urology 1980; **Med School:** South Africa 1962; **Resid:** Surgery, Baragwanannath Hosp, Johannesburg, So Africa 1966; Genl Hosp, Johannesburg, So Africa; **Fellow:** Urology, Johannesburg Hosp, Johannesburg, So Africa; **Fac Appt:** Prof Urology, Albert Einstein Coll Med

Snyder III, Howard M MD (U) - *Spec Exp:* Urology-Pediatric; Genital Reconstruction; Reconstructive Urologic Surgery; **Hospital:** Chldn's Hosp of Philadelphia; **Address:** Chldrns Hosp, Dept Ped Urology, 34th St & Civic Ctr Blvd, Wood Bldg, Fl 3, Philadelphia, PA 19104; **Phone:** (215) 590-2754; **Board Cert:** Urology 1982, Pediatric Surgery 1995, Surgery 1996; **Med School:** Harvard Med Sch 1969; **Resid:** Surgery, Peter Bent Brigham Hosp, Boston, MA 1970-1973; Pediatric Surgery, Boston Chldns Hosp Med Ctr, Boston, MA 1973-1974; **Fac Appt:** Prof Urology, Univ Penn

Sosa, R Ernest MD (U) - *Spec Exp:* *Kidney Stones; Laparoscopic Surgery; Laser Surgery;* **Hospital:** NY Presby Hosp - NY Weill Cornell Med Ctr (page 70); **Address:** 525 E 68th St Fl 9 - rm F940, New York, NY 10021-4870; **Phone:** (212) 746-5362; **Board Cert:** Urology 1996; **Med School:** Cornell Univ-Weill Med Coll 1978; **Resid:** Surgery, NY Hosp-Cornell Med Ctr, New York, NY 1979-1980; Urology, NY Hosp-Cornell Med Ctr, New York, NY 1980-1984; **Fellow:** Renal Physiology, NY Hosp-Cornell Med Ctr, New York, NY 1984-1986; **Fac Appt:** Assoc Prof Urology, Cornell Univ-Weill Med Coll

Vapnek, Jonathan M MD (U) - *Spec Exp:* *Incontinence; Urology-Female; Neurogenic Bladder;* **Hospital:** Mount Sinai Hosp (page 68); **Address:** 5 E 98th St Fl 6, New York, NY 10029-6501; **Phone:** (212) 241-4812; **Board Cert:** Urology 1995; **Med School:** UCSD 1986; **Resid:** Surgery, UCSD Med Ctr, San Diego, CA 1987-1988; Urology, UCSF, San Francisco, CA 1988-1992; **Fellow:** Urology, UC Davis, Sacramento, CA 1992-1993; **Fac Appt:** Asst Prof Urology, Mount Sinai Sch Med

Vaughan, Edwin D MD (U) - *Spec Exp:* *Urologic Cancer; Adrenal Disorders; Prostate Disease;* **Hospital:** NY Presby Hosp - NY Weill Cornell Med Ctr (page 70); **Address:** New York Presby Hosp, Dept Urology, 525 E 68th St, Ste F901, Box 94, New York, NY 10021-4870; **Phone:** (212) 746-5480; **Board Cert:** Urology 1986; **Med School:** Univ VA Sch Med 1965; **Resid:** Surgery, Vanderbilt Univ, Nashville, TN 1966-1967; Urology, Univ VA Hlth Sci Ctr, Charlottesville, VA 1969-1971; **Fellow:** Internal Medicine, Columbia Univ, NY, NY 1971-1973; **Fac Appt:** Prof Urology, Cornell Univ-Weill Med Coll

Waldbaum, Robert MD (U) - *Spec Exp:* *Prostate Cancer; Prostate Disease; Urologic Cancer;* **Hospital:** N Shore Univ Hosp at Manhasset; **Address:** 535 Plandome Rd, Ste 3, Manhasset, NY 11030-1961; **Phone:** (516) 627-6188; **Board Cert:** Urology 1973; **Med School:** Columbia P&S 1962; **Resid:** Surgery, Columbia Presby Med Ctr, New York, NY 1965-1966; Urology, New York Hosp-Cornell, New York, NY 1966-1970; **Fac Appt:** Clin Prof Urology, Cornell Univ-Weill Med Coll

Walsh, Patrick MD (U) - *Spec Exp:* *Prostate Cancer; Urologic Cancer;* **Hospital:** Johns Hopkins Hosp - Baltimore; **Address:** Johns Hopkins Hosp-Brady Urological Inst, 600 N Wolfe St, Bldg Marbu - Fl rg - rm 134, Baltimore, MD 21287-2101; **Phone:** (410) 614-3377; **Board Cert:** Urology 1975; **Med School:** Case West Res Univ 1964; **Resid:** Urology, UCLA Med Ctr, Los Angeles, CA 1967-1971; Pediatric Surgery, Boston Chldn's Hosp, Boston, MA 1966-1967; **Fellow:** Endocrinology, Diabetes & Metabolism, Harbor Genl Hospital, Torrance, CA 1968-1970; **Fac Appt:** Prof Urology, Johns Hopkins Univ

Wein, Alan J MD (U) - *Spec Exp:* *Neuro-Urology; Prostate Cancer; Incontinence;* **Hospital:** Hosp Univ Penn (page 78); **Address:** Dept Urology, 1 Rhoads Pavilion, 3400 Spruce St, Philadelphia, PA 19104; **Phone:** (215) 662-2891; **Board Cert:** Urology 1995; **Med School:** Univ Penn 1966; **Resid:** Surgery, Hosp Univ Penn, Philadelphia, PA 1969-1972; Urology, Hosp Univ Penn, Philadelphia, PA 1967-1968; **Fellow:** Urology, Hosp Univ Penn, Philadelphia, PA 1968-1969; **Fac Appt:** Prof Urology, Univ Penn

Southeast

Abramson, Edward G MD (U) - *Spec Exp:* *Urology - General;* **Hospital:** Inova Alexandria Hosp; **Address:** 1707 Osage St, Ste 301, Alexandria, VA 22302; **Phone:** (703) 836-8010; **Board Cert:** Urology 1977; **Med School:** Univ VA Sch Med 1967; **Resid:** Surgery, George Washington Univ Hosp, Washington, DC 1968-1969; Urology, George Washington Univ Hosp, Washington, DC 1969-1972; **Fac Appt:** Asst Clin Prof Urology, Geo Wash Univ

Albala, David Mois MD (U) - *Spec Exp:* Laparoscopic Surgery; Kidney Stones; Prostate Surgery; **Hospital:** Duke Univ Med Ctr (page 60); **Address:** Duke Univ Med Ctr, Green Zone, Trent Drive Bldg DUMC #3457, Durham, NC 27710; **Phone:** (919) 684-5416; **Board Cert:** Urology 2001; **Med School:** Mich State Univ 1983; **Resid:** Surgery, Dartmouth-Hitchcock Med Ctr, Lebanon, NH 1984-1985; Urology, Dartmouth-Hitchcock Med Ctr, Lebanon, NH 1986-1990; **Fellow:** Endourology, Wash Univ Med Ctr, St Louis, MO 1990-1991; **Fac Appt:** Prof Urology, Duke Univ

Assimos, Dean George MD (U) - *Spec Exp:* Kidney & Ureteral Stones; Reconstructive Renal Surgery; **Hospital:** Wake Forest Univ Baptist Med Ctr (page 81); **Address:** Wake Forest Univ Baptist Med Ctr, Dept Urology, Medical Center Blvd, Winston-Salem, NC 27157; **Phone:** (336) 716-4131; **Board Cert:** Urology 1995; **Med School:** Loyola Univ-Stritch Sch Med 1977; **Resid:** Surgery, Northwestern Univ Hosp, Chicago, IL 1978-1979; Urology, Northwestern Univ Hosp, Chicago, IL 1979-1983; **Fellow:** Urology, Bowman Gray Sch Med, Winston-Salem, NC 1983-1984; **Fac Appt:** Prof Surgery, Wake Forest Univ Sch Med

Beall, Michael E MD (U) - *Spec Exp:* Urology - General; **Hospital:** Inova Fairfax Hosp; **Address:** 8503 Arlington Blvd, Ste 310, Fairfax, VA 22030; **Phone:** (703) 876-1791; **Board Cert:** Urology 1979; **Med School:** Geo Wash Univ 1972; **Resid:** Surgery, Geo Wash Univ Hosp, Washington, DC 1972-1974; Urology, Geo Wash Univ Hosp, Washington, DC 1974-1977; **Fac Appt:** Assoc Clin Prof Urology, Geo Wash Univ

Belker, Arnold MD (U) - *Spec Exp:* Infertility-Male; Vasectomy Reversal; Microsurgery; **Hospital:** Jewish Hosp HlthCre Svcs Inc; **Address:** 250 E Liberty St, Ste 602, Louisville, KY 40202; **Phone:** (502) 584-0651; **Board Cert:** Urology 1969; **Med School:** Univ Louisville Sch Med 1958; **Resid:** Urology, Univ Iowa Hosps, Iowa City, IA 1962-1965; Surgery, Louisville Genl Hosp, Louisville, KY 1961-1962; **Fellow:** Nephrology, Louisville Genl Hosp, Louisville, KY 1965-1966; **Fac Appt:** Clin Prof Surgery, Univ Louisville Sch Med

Broderick, Gregory MD (U) - *Spec Exp:* Erectile Dysfunction; Voiding Dysfunction; Urethral Strictures; **Hospital:** St Luke's Hosp; **Address:** Mayo Clinic, Dept Urol, 4500 San Pablo Rd, Jacksonville, FL 32224; **Phone:** (904) 953-7330; **Board Cert:** Urology 1992; **Med School:** UCSF 1983; **Resid:** Surgery, UCSF Med Ctr, San Francisco, CA 1983-1985; Urology, UCSF Med Ctr, San Francisco, CA 1985-1988; **Fellow:** Neurourology, UC Davis, Sacramento, CA 1989-1990; **Fac Appt:** Prof Urology, Mayo Med Sch

Carson, Culley MD (U) - *Spec Exp:* Erectile Dysfunction; Kidney Stones; Peyronie's Disease; **Hospital:** Univ of NC Hosp (page 77); **Address:** Univ North Carolina, Dept Urol, 427 Burnett-Womack Bldg, Chapel Hill, NC 27599-7235; **Phone:** (919) 966-2571; **Board Cert:** Urology 1980; **Med School:** Geo Wash Univ 1971; **Resid:** Surgery, Dartmouth Hitchcock Med Ctr, Hanover, NH 1972-1973; **Fellow:** Urology, Mayo Clinic, Rochester, MN 1975-1978; **Fac Appt:** Prof Urology, Univ NC Sch Med

Harty, James MD (U) - *Spec Exp:* Urologic Cancer; **Hospital:** Norton Hospital; **Address:** 210 E Gray St, Ste 1000, Louisville, KY 40202; **Phone:** (502) 629-5904; **Board Cert:** Urology 1979; **Med School:** Ireland 1969; **Resid:** Surgery, Johns Hopkins Hosp, Baltimore, MD 1972-1973; Urology, Johns Hopkins Hosp, Baltimore, MD 1973-1977; **Fac Appt:** Prof Surgery, Univ Louisville Sch Med

Howards, Stuart S MD (U) - *Spec Exp:* Infertility-Male; Urology-Pediatric; **Hospital:** Univ of VA Hlth Sys (page 79); **Address:** Dept Urology, PO Box 800422, Charlottesville, VA 22908; **Phone:** (804) 924-9559; **Board Cert:** Urology 1975; **Med School:** Columbia P&S 1963; **Resid:** Surgery, Peter Bent Brigham-Chldns Hosp, Boston, MA 1963-1965; Urology, Peter Bent Brigham Hosp, Boston, MA 1968-1971; **Fellow:** Renal Physiology, Natl Inst Hlth, Bethesda, MD 1965-1968; **Fac Appt:** Prof Urology, Univ VA Sch Med

Irby III, Pierce B MD (U) - *Spec Exp:* Kidney Stones; **Hospital:** Carolinas Med Ctr; **Address:** 1416 E Moorehead St, Ste 101, Charlotte, NC 28204; **Phone:** (704) 355-8686; **Board Cert:** Urology 1994; **Med School:** Uniformed Srvs Univ, Bethesda 1983; **Resid:** Urology, Letterman Army Med Ctr, San Francisco, CA 1986-1990; **Fellow:** Endourology, UCSF Med Ctr, San Francisco, CA 1991-1992

Jordan, Gerald MD (U) - *Spec Exp:* Incontinence; Urethral Reconstruction; **Hospital:** Sentara Norfolk Gen Hosp; **Address:** 400 W Brambleton Ave, Ste 100, Norfolk, VA 23510; **Phone:** (757) 457-5125; **Board Cert:** Urology 1984; **Med School:** Univ Tex, San Antonio 1977; **Resid:** Urology, Naval Reg Med Ctr, Portsmouth, VA 1977-1978; **Fellow:** Reconstructive Surgery, Eastern Va Med Sch, Norfolk, VA 1982-1984; **Fac Appt:** Prof Urology, Eastern VA Med Sch

Kennelly, Michael Joseph MD (U) - *Spec Exp:* Incontinence; Voiding Dysfunction; Pelvic Reconstruction; **Hospital:** Carolinas Med Ctr; **Address:** McKay Urology, 1416 E Morehead St, Ste 101, Charlotte, NC 28204; **Phone:** (704) 355-8686; **Board Cert:** Urology 1997; **Med School:** Univ Cincinnati 1989; **Resid:** Urology, Univ Mich Med Ctr, Ann Arbor, MI 1991-1994; **Fellow:** Neurology, Univ Tex Hlth Sci Ctr, Houston, TX 1994-1995; **Fac Appt:** Clin Prof Urology, Univ NC Sch Med

Lewis, Ronald W MD (U) - *Spec Exp:* Erectile Dysfunction; **Hospital:** Med Coll of GA Hosp and Clin; **Address:** Dept Urology, 1120 15th St, rm BA-8412, Augusta, GA 30912; **Phone:** (706) 721-2546; **Board Cert:** Urology 1976; **Med School:** Tulane Univ 1968; **Resid:** Urology, Naval Reg Med Ctr, Oakland, CA 1970-1974; **Fellow:** Research, Tulane Univ-Delta Reg, Covington, LA 1976-1977; **Fac Appt:** Prof Urology, Med Coll GA

Lloyd Jr, Lewis K MD (U) - *Spec Exp:* Interstitial Cystitis; **Hospital:** Univ of Ala Hosp at Birmingham; **Address:** Univ Ala Med Ctr, Div Urol, 1530 3rd Ave S Bldg MEB - rm 606, Birmingham, AL 35294-0001; **Phone:** (205) 975-0088; **Board Cert:** Urology 1976; **Med School:** Tulane Univ 1966; **Resid:** Urology, Tulane Univ Hosp, New Orleans, LA 1970-1974; **Fac Appt:** Prof Surgery, Univ Ala

Lockhart, Jorge L MD (U) - *Spec Exp:* Kidney Stones; **Hospital:** Tampa Genl Hosp; **Address:** 12902 Magnolia Drive, Tampa, FL 33612; **Phone:** (813) 979-3980; **Board Cert:** Urology 1980; **Med School:** Uruguay 1973; **Resid:** Urology, Duke Univ Med Ctr, Durham, NC 1974-1977; **Fellow:** Urodynamics, Duke Univ Med Ctr, Durham, NC 1977-1978; **Fac Appt:** Prof Surgery, Univ S Fla Coll Med

Marshall, Fray F MD (U) - *Spec Exp:* Urologic Cancer; Prostate Cancer; **Hospital:** Emory Univ Hosp; **Address:** Emory Clin, Dept Urology, 1365 Clifton Rd, Fl A3225, Atlanta, GA 30322; **Phone:** (404) 778-5951; **Board Cert:** Urology 1977; **Med School:** Univ VA Sch Med 1969; **Resid:** Urology, Mass Genl Hosp, Boston, MA 1972-1975; Surgery, Univ Mich Hosp, Ann Arbor, MI 1970-1972; **Fac Appt:** Prof Urology, Emory Univ

McCullough, David L MD (U) - *Spec Exp:* Genitourinary Cancer; Kidney Stones; **Hospital:** Wake Forest Univ Baptist Med Ctr (page 81); **Address:** Dept Urology- Medical Center Blvd, Winston-Salem, NC 27157; **Phone:** (336) 716-4131; **Board Cert:** Urology 1995; **Med School:** Wake Forest Univ Sch Med 1964; **Resid:** Urology, Mass Genl Hosp, Boston, MA 1969-1972; Surgery, Univ Hosp-Case Western Res Univ, Cleveland, OH 1965-1966; **Fac Appt:** Prof Urology, Wake Forest Univ Sch Med

Milam, Douglas F MD (U) - *Spec Exp:* Urodynamics; Voiding Dysfunction; **Hospital:** Vanderbilt Univ Med Ctr (page 80); **Address:** Vanderbilt Univ Med Ctr North, Dept Urol, rm A-1302, Nashville, TN 37232-2765; **Phone:** (615) 322-2142; **Board Cert:** Urology 1994; **Med School:** W VA Univ 1986; **Resid:** Surgery, Univ Utah, Salt Lake City, UT 1987-1988; Urology, Univ Utah, Salt Lake City, UT 1988-1991; **Fac Appt:** Asst Prof Urology, Vanderbilt Univ

Noseworthy, John MD (U) - *Spec Exp:* Multiple Sclerosis (Incontinence); Urologic Surgery-Pediatric; **Hospital:** Baptist Health; **Address:** 807 Children's Way, Nemours Children's Clinic, Jacksonville, FL 32207; **Phone:** (904) 390-3740; **Board Cert:** Urology 1981, Pediatric Surgery 1991; **Med School:** Harvard Med Sch 1970; **Resid:** Surgery, Univ Hosps-Case West Res, Cleveland, OH 1971-1978; Urology, Univ Hosps-Case West Res, Cleveland, OH 1974-1978; **Fellow:** Pediatric Surgery, Chldns Hosp Med Ctr, Boston, MA 1978-1980; **Fac Appt:** Assoc Prof Surgery

Paulson, David F MD (U) - *Spec Exp:* Urologic Cancer; **Hospital:** Duke Univ Med Ctr (page 60); **Address:** Duke Univ Med Ctr, Box 2977, Durham, NC 27710-0001; **Phone:** (919) 684-5057; **Board Cert:** Urology 1974; **Med School:** Duke Univ 1964; **Resid:** Surgery, Duke Univ Med Ctr, Durham, NC 1965-1966; Urology, Duke Univ Med Ctr, Durham, NC 1969-1972; **Fellow:** Surgery, Natl Cancer Inst, Bethesda, MD 1966-1969; **Fac Appt:** Prof Urology, Duke Univ

Rowland, Randall MD (U) - *Spec Exp:* Urologic Cancer; **Hospital:** Univ Kentucky Med Ctr; **Address:** University of Kentucky Med Ctr, Div Urology, 800 Rose St, rm MS269, Lexington, KY 40536-0298; **Phone:** (859) 323-6677; **Board Cert:** Urology 1980; **Med School:** Northwestern Univ 1972; **Resid:** Urology, Northwestern Meml Hosp, Chicago, IL 1973-1978; **Fac Appt:** Prof Urology, Univ KY Coll Med

Sanders, William Holt MD (U) - *Spec Exp:* Prostate Cancer; Kidney Stones; Bladder Cancer; **Hospital:** St Joseph's Hosp - Atlanta; **Address:** 5669 Peachtree Dunwoody Rd, Ste 350, Atlanta, GA 30342-1721; **Phone:** (404) 255-3822; **Board Cert:** Urology 1996; **Med School:** Emory Univ 1988; **Resid:** Urology, Yale Sch of Med, New Haven, CT 1991-1993

Schellhammer, Paul MD (U) - *Spec Exp:* Urology - General; **Hospital:** Sentara Norfolk Gen Hosp; **Address:** 600 Gresham Dr, Norfolk, VA 23507; **Phone:** (757) 668-3000; **Board Cert:** Urology 1999; **Med School:** Cornell Univ-Weill Med Coll 1966; **Resid:** Surgery, U Hosps, Cleveland, OH 1967-1968; Urology, Med Coll Va, Richmond, VA 1970-1973; **Fellow:** Urology, Meml Hosp-Am Canc Soc, New York, NY 1973-1974; **Fac Appt:** Prof Urology, Eastern VA Med Sch

Shaban, Stephen F MD (U) - *Spec Exp:* Infertility-Male; **Hospital:** Univ of NC Hosp (page 77); **Address:** 427 Burnett-Womack Bldg, Box CB7235, Chapel Hill, NC 27599-7235; **Phone:** (919) 966-8217; **Board Cert:** Urology 1993; **Med School:** Mount Sinai Sch Med 1982; **Resid:** Urology, Univ S Fla, Tampa, FL 1983-1987; **Fellow:** Male Reproduction, Baylor Coll Med, Houston, TX 1987-1988; **Fac Appt:** Assoc Prof Surgery, Univ NC Sch Med

Smith, Joseph A MD (U) - *Spec Exp:* Urologic Cancer; Prostate Cancer; Bladder Cancer; **Hospital:** Vanderbilt Univ Med Ctr (page 80); **Address:** Vanderbilt Univ Med Ctr, Dept Urol Surgery, A-1302 MCN, Nashville, TN 37232-2765; **Phone:** (615) 343-0234; **Board Cert:** Urology 2000; **Med School:** Univ Tenn Coll Med, Memphis 1974; **Resid:** Surgery, Parkland Meml Hosp, Dallas, TX 1975-1976; Urology, Univ Utah, Salt Lake City, UT 1976-1979; **Fellow:** Urologic Oncology, Meml Sloan Kettering Cancer Ctr, New York, NY 1979-1980; **Fac Appt:** Prof Urology, Vanderbilt Univ

Soloway, Mark MD (U) - *Spec Exp:* Urologic Cancer; Kidney Cancer; Bladder Cancer; **Hospital:** Univ of Miami - Jackson Meml Hosp; **Address:** Univ Miami, Dept Urol, PO Box 016960, MA14, Miami, FL 33101; **Phone:** (305) 243-6596; **Board Cert:** Urology 1977; **Med School:** Case West Res Univ 1968; **Resid:** Surgery, Univ Hosps Cleveland, Cleveland, OH 1969-1970; Urology, Univ Hosps Cleveland, Cleveland, OH 1972-1975; **Fellow:** Surgery, Natl Cancer Inst, Bethesda, MD 1970-1972; **Fac Appt:** Prof Urology, Univ Miami Sch Med

Steers, William D MD (U) - *Spec Exp:* Incontinence; Impotence; **Hospital:** Univ of VA Hlth Sys (page 79); **Address:** UVA Health System, Dept Urology, PO Box 800422, Charlotteville, VA 22908; **Phone:** (804) 924-9107; **Board Cert:** Urology 1999; **Med School:** Ohio Univ, Coll Osteo Med 1980; **Resid:** Urology, Univ Tex Hlth Sci Ctr, Houston, TX 1981-1986; **Fellow:** Neurology, Univ Pitts Med Ctr, Pittsburgh, PA 1986-1988; **Fac Appt:** Prof Urology, Univ VA Sch Med

Teigland, Chris Michael MD (U) - *Spec Exp:* Urologic Cancer; **Hospital:** Carolinas Med Ctr; **Address:** Mckay Urology, 1461 E Morehead St, Ste 101, Charlotte, NC 28204; **Phone:** (704) 355-3686; **Board Cert:** Urology 1999; **Med School:** Duke Univ 1980; **Resid:** Surgery, Univ Utah Affil Hosps, UT 1981-1982; Urology, Univ Texas SW Med Ctr, TX 1983-1987; **Fac Appt:** Assoc Clin Prof Surgery, Univ NC Sch Med

Wajsman, Zew Lew MD (U) - *Spec Exp:* Urologic Cancer; **Hospital:** Shands Hlthcre at Univ of FL (page 73); **Address:** Shands Hlthcare at Univ Florida, Dept Surgery, 1600 SW Archer Rd, Box 100286, Gainesville, FL 32610-0247; **Phone:** (352) 392-2501; **Board Cert:** Urology 1979; **Med School:** Israel 1965; **Resid:** Surgery, Central Emek Hosp, Afula, Israel 1969-1970; Urology, Central Emek Hosp, Afula, Israel 1970-1973; **Fellow:** Urology, Rosewell Park Meml Inst, Buffalo, NY 1973-1975; **Fac Appt:** Prof Urology, Univ Fla Coll Med

Walker III, R Dixon MD (U) - *Spec Exp:* Urology-Pediatric; Genitourinary Congenital Abnormality; **Hospital:** Shands Hlthcare at Univ of FL (page 73); **Address:** Shands Hlthcare at Univ FL, 1600 SW Archer Rd, Box 100286, Gainesville, FL 32610-0247; **Phone:** (352) 392-2501; **Board Cert:** Urology 1972; **Med School:** Univ Miami Sch Med 1963; **Resid:** Surgery, Shands Hosp-Univ Fla, Gainesville, FL 1964-1968; **Fac Appt:** Prof Surgery, Univ Fla Coll Med

Webster, George David MD (U) - *Spec Exp:* Reconstructive Urology; Urology-Female; Urodynamics; **Hospital:** Duke Univ Med Ctr (page 60); **Address:** Duke Univ Med Ctr -Dept Urol, Box 3146, Durham, NC 27710-3146; **Phone:** (919) 684-2516; **Board Cert:** Urology 1981; **Med School:** England 1968; **Resid:** Urology, Inst Urol, London UK 1973-1974; Harare Hosp, Salisbury, UK 1970-1972; **Fellow:** Urology, Duke Univ Med Ctr, Durham, NC 1975-1978; **Fac Appt:** Prof Urology, Duke Univ

Midwest

Bahnson, Robert MD (U) - *Spec Exp:* Laparoscopic Surgery; Urethral Reconstruction; **Hospital:** Ohio St Univ Med Ctr; **Address:** 456 West 10th Avenue, Div of Urology 4960 UHC, Columbus, OH 43210-1228; **Phone:** (614) 293-8155; **Board Cert:** Urology 1995; **Med School:** Tufts Univ 1979; **Resid:** Surgery, Northwestern U, Chicago, IL 1980-1981; Urology, Northwestern U, Chicago, IL 1981-1983; **Fellow:** Urology, Northwestern U, Chicago, IL 1983-1984; Research, U of Pittsburgh, Pittsburgh, PA 1989-1991; **Fac Appt:** Prof Urology, Ohio State Univ

Bloom, David A MD (U) - *Spec Exp:* Urology-Pediatric; Voiding Dysfunction; Genitourinary Reconstruction; **Hospital:** Univ of MI Hlth Ctr; **Address:** Taubman Health Care Center- Urology Dept, 1500 E Medical Ctr Dr, Ann Arbor, MI 48109-0330; **Phone:** (734) 936-7030; **Board Cert:** Urology 1982, Surgery 1977; **Med School:** SUNY Buffalo 1971; **Resid:** Urology, UCLA Med Ctr, Los Angeles, CA 1976-1980; Surgery, UCLA Med Ctr, Los Angeles, CA 1971-1976; **Fellow:** Pediatrics, Inst Urol-St Peters Hosp, London, England 1977-1978; **Fac Appt:** Prof Urology, Univ Mich Med Sch

Brendler, Charles B MD (U) - *Spec Exp:* Prostate Cancer; **Hospital:** Univ of Chicago Hosps (page 76); **Address:** 5758 S Maryland Ave, Ste 2D, MC 9010, Chicago, IL 60637; **Phone:** (773) 702-1860; **Board Cert:** Urology 1981; **Med School:** Univ VA Sch Med 1974; **Resid:** Surgery, Duke Univ Med Ctr, Durham, NC 1974-1976; Urology, Duke Univ Med Ctr, Durham, NC 1976-1979; **Fellow:** Prostate Cancer, Johns Hopkins Hosp, Baltimore, MD 1980-1981; **Fac Appt:** Prof Urology, Univ Chicago-Pritzker Sch Med

Bruskewitz, Reginald C MD (U) - *Spec Exp:* Urologic Cancer; Prostate Disease; **Hospital:** Univ WI Hosp & Clins; **Address:** 600 Highland Avenue, rm G-5329, Madison, WI 53792; **Phone:** (608) 263-4757; **Board Cert:** Urology 1981; **Med School:** Univ Wisc 1973; **Resid:** Urology, Univ Wisc, Madsion, WI 1974-1978; **Fellow:** Urology, UCLA, Los Angeles, CA 1978-1979; **Fac Appt:** Assoc Prof Surgery, Univ Wisc

Bushman, Wade MD (U) - *Spec Exp:* Neurourology; Urodynamics; Female Urology; **Hospital:** Northwestern Meml Hosp; **Address:** Northwestern Univ Med Sch, Dept Urol, 303 E Chicago Ave, Bldg Tarry 11-715, Chicago, IL 60611-3008; **Phone:** (312) 695-8146; **Board Cert:** Urology 1997; **Med School:** Univ Chicago-Pritzker Sch Med 1986; **Resid:** Urology, Univ VA Med Ctr, Charlottesville, VA 1988-1992; **Fac Appt:** Asst Prof Urology, Northwestern Univ

Catalona, William J MD (U) - *Spec Exp:* Urologic Cancer; Prostate Cancer; **Hospital:** Barnes-Jewish Hosp (page 55); **Address:** Washington Univ Med Ctr, Dept Urology, 4960 Chldns Pl, St Louis, MO 63110-1002; **Phone:** (314) 362-8200; **Board Cert:** Urology 1978; **Med School:** Yale Univ 1968; **Resid:** Surgery, UC San Francisco, San Francisco, CA 1969-1970; Urology, Johns Hopkins Hosp, Baltimore, MD 1972-1976; **Fellow:** Surgical Oncology, Natl Cancer Inst, Bethesda, MD 1970-1972; **Fac Appt:** Prof Urology, Washington Univ, St Louis

Chodak, Gerald MD (U) - *Spec Exp:* Prostate Cancer; Prostate Disease; **Hospital:** Louis A Weiss Mem Hosp; **Address:** 4646 N Marine Dr, Suite A5500, Chicago, IL 60640; **Phone:** (773) 564-5006; **Board Cert:** Urology 1984; **Med School:** SUNY Buffalo 1975; **Resid:** Surgery, UCLA Med Ctr, California, CA 1976-1977; Urology, Brigham & Womens Hosp, Boston, MA 1977-1979; **Fellow:** Research, Harvard Chldns Hosp, Boston, MA 1981-1982; **Fac Appt:** Prof Surgery, Univ Chicago-Pritzker Sch Med

Flanigan, Robert C MD (U) - *Spec Exp:* Prostate Cancer; Bladder Cancer; Transplant-Kidney; **Hospital:** Loyola Univ Med Ctr; **Address:** Loyola Univ Med-Fahey Bldg 54, 2160 S First Ave, rm 245, Maywood, IL 60153; **Phone:** (708) 216-5100; **Board Cert:** Surgery 1998, Urology 1980; **Med School:** Case West Res Univ 1972; **Resid:** Surgery, Case West Univ Med Ctr, Cleveland, OH 1973-1978; Urology, Case West Univ Med Ctr, Cleveland, OH 1973-1978; **Fac Appt:** Prof Urology, Loyola Univ-Stritch Sch Med

Gluckman, Gordon MD (U) - *Spec Exp:* Urinary Tract Infections; Erectile Dysfunction; **Hospital:** Advocate Lutheran Gen Hosp; **Address:** Parkside Center, 1875 Dempster St, Ste 506, Park Ridge, IL 60068; **Phone:** (847) 823-4700; **Board Cert:** Urology 1997; **Med School:** Northwestern Univ 1989; **Resid:** Surgery, UCSF, San Francisco, CA 1990-1991; Urology, UCSF, San Francisco, CA 1991-1995

Gujral, Saroj K MD (U) - *Spec Exp:* Urologic Cancer; Urology-Female; **Hospital:** Albert Lea Med Ctr-Mayo Hlth Sys; **Address:** 404 W Fountain St, Albert Lea, MN 56007; **Phone:** (507) 373-2384; **Board Cert:** Urology 1979; **Med School:** India 1970; **Resid:** Urology, Suburban Hosp, Bethesda, MD 1973-1978; Urology, Dalhousie U Med Ctrs, Halifax, Canada 1979

Klein, Eric A MD (U) - *Spec Exp:* Prostate Cancer; Bladder Cancer; Urologic Cancer; **Hospital:** Cleveland Clin Fdn (page 57); **Address:** Cleveland Clinic Fdn, Dept Urol, Sect Urol-Onc, 9500 Euclid Ave, Fl A100, Cleveland, OH 44195-0001; **Phone:** (216) 444-5591; **Board Cert:** Urology 1999; **Med School:** Univ Pittsburgh 1981; **Resid:** Urology, Cleveland Clinic Fdn, Cleveland, OH 1981-1986; **Fellow:** Urologic Oncology, Meml Sloan Kettering Canc Ctr, New York, NY 1986-1989; **Fac Appt:** Assoc Prof Surgery, Ohio State Univ

Kozlowski, James Michael MD (U) - *Spec Exp:* Prostate Cancer; Continent Urinary Diversions; Laparoscopic Surgery; **Hospital:** Northwestern Meml Hosp; **Address:** 675 N St Clair, Bldg Galter - Ste 150, Chicago, IL 60611; **Phone:** (312) 695-8146; **Board Cert:** Surgery 1993, Urology 1983; **Med School:** Northwestern Univ 1975; **Resid:** Surgery, Northwestern Univ-McGraw, Chicago, IL 1975-1979; Urology, Northwestern Univ-McGraw, Chicago, IL 1977-1981; **Fellow:** Research, Natl Cancer Inst-Frederick Canc Rsch, Chicago, IL 1982-1984; **Fac Appt:** Assoc Prof Urology, Northwestern Univ

Levine, Laurence Adan MD (U) - *Spec Exp:* Erectile Dysfunction; Infertility-Male; Impotence-Peyronies Disease; **Hospital:** Rush-Presby - St Luke's Med Ctr (page 72); **Address:** 1725 W Harrison St, Ste 917, Chicago, IL 60612; **Phone:** (312) 829-1820; **Board Cert:** Urology 1999; **Med School:** Univ Colo 1980; **Resid:** Surgery, Tufts-New England Med Ctr, Boston, MA 1980-1982; Urology, Brigham & Women's Hosp/Harvard, Boston, MA 1983-1987; **Fac Appt:** Prof Urology, Rush Med Coll

Mc Vary, Kevin MD (U) - *Spec Exp:* Prostate Cancer; Erectile Dysfunction; **Hospital:** Northwestern Meml Hosp; **Address:** 675 N St Clair, Ste 20-150, Chicago, IL 60611-4813; **Phone:** (312) 695-8146; **Board Cert:** Urology 1991; **Med School:** Northwestern Univ 1983; **Resid:** Surgery, Northwestern Meml Hosp, Chicago, IL 1984-1985; Urology, Northwestern Meml Hosp, Chicago, IL 1985-1988; **Fellow:** Urology, Northwestern Meml Hosp, Chicago, IL; **Fac Appt:** Assoc Prof Urology, Northwestern Univ

Menon, Mani MD (U) - *Spec Exp:* Prostate Cancer; Transplant-Kidney; **Hospital:** Henry Ford Hosp; **Address:** Henry Ford Hlth Sys, Dept Urol, 1 Ford Pl, Ste 2F, Detroit, MI 48202-2689; **Phone:** (313) 874-4754; **Board Cert:** Urology 1982; **Med School:** India 1969; **Resid:** Urology, Bryn Mawr Hosp, Bryn Mawr, PA 1973-1974; Urology, Johns Hopkins Hosp, Baltimore, MD 1974-1980; **Fellow:** Transplant Surgery, Johns Hopkins Univ, Baltimore, MD 1976-1977; **Fac Appt:** Prof Surgery, Univ Mass Sch Med

Montague, Drogo K. MD (U) - *Spec Exp:* Erectile Dysfunction; Incontinence; **Hospital:** Cleveland Clin Fdn (page 57); **Address:** Cleveland Clinic Foundation-Urological Inst, 9500 Euclid Ave, Cleveland, OH 44195-5041; **Phone:** (216) 444-5590; **Board Cert:** Urology 1975; **Med School:** Univ Mich Med Sch 1968; **Resid:** Surgery, Cleveland Clinic, Cleveland, OH 1969-1970; Urology, Cleveland Clinic, Cleveland, OH 1970-1973; **Fac Appt:** Prof Urology, Ohio State Univ

Montie, James MD (U) - *Spec Exp:* Bladder Cancer; Prostate Cancer; **Hospital:** Univ of MI Hlth Ctr; **Address:** 1500 E Medical Ctr Dr, A. Alfred Taubman Hlth Care Ctr-Sec Urol, rm 2918, Box 0330, Ann Arbor, MI 48109; **Phone:** (734) 647-8903; **Board Cert:** Urology 1978; **Med School:** Univ Mich Med Sch 1971; **Resid:** Urology, Cleveland Clinic Foundation 1973-1976; **Fellow:** Urology, Memorial Sloan-Kettering, New York, NY 1978-1979; **Fac Appt:** Prof Urology, Univ Mich Med Sch

Mulcahy, John J. MD (U) - *Spec Exp:* Erectile Dysfunction; Incontinence; Penile Prostheses; **Hospital:** IN Univ Hosp (page 63); **Address:** 535 Barnhill, Ste 420, Indianapolis, IN 46202-2859; **Phone:** (317) 278-7560; **Board Cert:** Urology 1976; **Med School:** Georgetown Univ 1966; **Resid:** Urology, Mayo Clinic, Rochester, MN 1972-1974; Urology, Mayo Clinic, Rochester, MN 1967-1969; **Fellow:** Physiology, Univ Mich, Ann Arbor, MI 1969-1972; **Fac Appt:** Prof Urology, Indiana Univ

Novick, Andrew MD (U) - *Spec Exp:* Transplant-Kidney; Adrenal Disorders; Urologic Cancer; **Hospital:** Cleveland Clin Fdn (page 57); **Address:** 9500 Euclid Ave, rm A100, Cleveland, OH 44195; **Phone:** (216) 444-5584; **Board Cert:** Urology 1979; **Med School:** McGill Univ 1972; **Resid:** Cleveland Clinic, Cleveland, OH 1974-1977; Royal Victoria Hosp, Montreal, CN 1973-1974

Ohl, Dana Alan MD (U) - *Spec Exp:* Infertility-Male; Erectile Dysfunction; **Hospital:** Univ of MI Hlth Ctr; **Address:** Univ Mich Med Ctr, Dept Urology, 1500 E Med Ctr, Ann Arbor, MI 48109-0330; **Phone:** (734) 936-7030; **Board Cert:** Urology 1999; **Med School:** Univ Mich Med Sch 1982; **Resid:** Urology, Univ Mich Hosps, Ann Arbor, MI 1983-1987; **Fac Appt:** Assoc Prof Urology, Univ Mich Med Sch

Pryor, Jon L MD (U) - *Spec Exp:* Infertility-Male; Erectile Dysfunction; Vasectomy and Vasectomy Reversal; **Hospital:** Fairview-Univ Med Ctr - Univ Campus; **Address:** Dept Urology, 420 Delaware St SE, Box MMC394, Minneapolis, MN 55455-0374; **Phone:** (612) 625-0662; **Board Cert:** Urology 1994; **Med School:** Univ Minn 1983; **Resid:** Urology, Univ Va, Charlottesville, VA 1985-1989; **Fellow:** Infertility, Univ Minn, Minneapolis, MN 1989-1991

Resnick, Martin MD (U) - *Spec Exp:* Prostate Cancer; **Hospital:** Univ Hosp of Cleveland; **Address:** 11100 Euclid Ave, 11100 Euclid Ave, Cleveland, OH 44106-5046; **Phone:** (216) 844-3011; **Board Cert:** Urology 1977; **Med School:** Wake Forest Univ Sch Med 1969; **Resid:** Surgery, Univ Hosps Cleveland, Cleveland, OH 1970-1971; Urology, Northwestern Med Ctr, Cleveland, OH 1971-1975; **Fac Appt:** Prof Urology, Case West Res Univ

Rink, Richard C MD (U) - *Spec Exp:* Urology-Pediatric; Reconstructive Urology; Genital Reconstruction; **Hospital:** Riley Chldrn's Hosp (page 588); **Address:** Indiana Univ Med Ctr, 702 Barhill Ave, Ste 1739, Indianapolis, IN 46202; **Phone:** (317) 274-7472; **Board Cert:** Urology 1996; **Med School:** Indiana Univ 1978; **Resid:** Surgery, Emory Univ Med Ctr, Atlanta, GA 1979-1980; Urology, Indiana Univ Med Ctr, Indianapolis, IN 1980-1984; **Fellow:** Pediatrics, Chldns Hosp-Harvard, Boston, MA 1984-1985; **Fac Appt:** Prof Pediatrics, Indiana Univ

Ross, Lawrence S MD (U) - *Spec Exp:* Infertility-Male; Impotence; Prostate Disease; **Hospital:** Univ of IL at Chicago Med Ctr; **Address:** 900 N Michigan Ave, Ste 1420, Chicago, IL 60611; **Phone:** (312) 440-5127; **Board Cert:** Urology 1974; **Med School:** Univ Chicago-Pritzker Sch Med 1965; **Resid:** Urology, Michael Reese Hosp, Chicago, IL 1966-1970; **Fac Appt:** Prof Urology, Univ IL Coll Med

Sandlow, Jay Ira MD (U) - *Spec Exp:* Infertility-Male; Varicoceles; Vasectomy & Vasectomy Reversal; **Hospital:** Univ of IA Hosp and Clinics; **Address:** Univ Iowa Hosp & Clinics, Dept Urology, 200 Hawkins Dr, 3241 RCP, Iowa City, IA 52242; **Phone:** (319) 356-2421; **Board Cert:** Urology 1997; **Med School:** Rush Med Coll 1987; **Resid:** Surgery, Univ Iowa Hosps & Clinics, Iowa City, IA 1987-1989; Urology, Univ Iowa Hosps & Clinics, Iowa City, IA 1989-1993; **Fellow:** Infertility, Univ Iowa Hosps & Clinics, Iowa City, IA 1993-1995; **Fac Appt:** Assoc Prof Urology, Univ Iowa Coll Med

Schaeffer, Anthony MD (U) - *Spec Exp:* Interstitial Cystitis; Incontinence; **Hospital:** Northwestern Meml Hosp; **Address:** 675 N St Clair St Bldg Galter Fl 20 - Ste 150, Chicago, IL 60611; **Phone:** (312) 695-8146; **Board Cert:** Urology 1978; **Med School:** Northwestern Univ 1968; **Resid:** Surgery, Northwestern Meml Hosp, Chicago, IL 1969-1970; Urology, Stanford Med Ctr, Stanford, CA 1972-1976; **Fac Appt:** Prof Urology, Northwestern Univ

Seftel, Allen D MD (U) - *Spec Exp:* Sexual Dysfunction; Infertility-Male; Prostate Disease; **Hospital:** Univ Hosp of Cleveland; **Address:** Univ Hosp-Cleveland, 11100 Euclid Ave, MS 5046, Cleveland, OH 44106-5046; **Phone:** (216) 844-7632; **Board Cert:** Urology 1995; **Med School:** SUNY Downstate 1984; **Resid:** Urology, SUNY Downstate Med Ctr, Brooklyn, NY 1986-1987; Urology, Univ Hosps-Case West Res, Cleveland, OH 1987-1990; **Fellow:** Reproductive Medicine, Boston Univ Med Ctr, Boston, MA 1990-1992; **Fac Appt:** Assoc Prof Urology, Case West Res Univ

Thomas, Anthony J. MD (U) - *Spec Exp:* *Infertility-Male; Vasectomy Reversal; Microsurgery;* **Hospital:** Cleveland Clin Fdn (page 57); **Address:** Dept Urology, 9500 Euclid Ave, rm A-100, Cleveland, OH 44195-0002; **Phone:** (216) 444-5600; **Board Cert:** Urology 1978; **Med School:** Univ Cincinnati 1969; **Resid:** Urology, Wayne State Univ Affil Hosp, Detroit, MI 1973-1976

Totonchi, Emil MD (U) - *Spec Exp:* *Urology - General;* **Hospital:** Advocate IL Masonic Med Ctr; **Address:** 860 N Clark St, Chicago, IL 60610-3218; **Phone:** (312) 944-2848; **Board Cert:** Urology 1984; **Med School:** Iraq 1968; **Resid:** Surgery, United Kingdom 1972-1977; Urology, Cook County Hosp, Chicago, IL 1978-1982; **Fellow:** Surgery, Univ Illinois, Chicago, IL 1977-1978

Uehling, David T MD (U) - *Spec Exp:* *Urology-Pediatric;* **Hospital:** Univ WI Hosp & Clins; **Address:** 600 Highland Ave, rm G5/333, Madison, WI 53792; **Phone:** (608) 263-4757; **Board Cert:** Urology 1967; **Med School:** Northwestern Univ 1959; **Resid:** Urology, Northwestern Univ, Chicago, IL 1960-1964; **Fellow:** Pediatric Urology, Chldns Meml Hosp, Chicago, IL 1964; **Fac Appt:** Prof Surgery, Univ Wisc

Williams, Richard D MD (U) - *Spec Exp:* *Kidney Cancer; Bladder Cancer; Prostate Cancer;* **Hospital:** Univ of IA Hosp and Clinics; **Address:** Univ Iowa, Dept Urol, 200 Hawkins Dr, Iowa City, IA 52242-1089; **Phone:** (319) 356-0760; **Board Cert:** Urology 1979; **Med School:** Univ Kans 1970; **Resid:** Surgery, Univ Minn Hosps & Clins, Minneapolis, MN 1971-1972; Urology, Univ Minn Hosps & Clins, Minneapolis, MN 1972-1976; **Fellow:** Urologic Oncology, Univ Minn Hosps & Clins, Minneapolis, MN 1976-1979; **Fac Appt:** Prof Urology, Univ Iowa Coll Med

Great Plains and Mountains

Cartwright, Patrick MD (U) - *Spec Exp:* *Urology-Pediatric;* **Hospital:** Primary Children's Med Ctr; **Address:** Primary Chldns Hosp, 100 N Medical Dr, Ste 2200, Salt Lake City, UT 84113-1100; **Phone:** (801) 588-3300; **Board Cert:** Urology 1992; **Med School:** Univ Tex SW, Dallas 1984; **Resid:** Urology, Univ Utah Affil Hosp, Salt Lake City, UT 1984-1989; **Fellow:** Pediatric Urology, Chldns Hosp, Philadelphia, PA 1989-1990; **Fac Appt:** Assoc Prof Surgery, Univ Utah

Koyle, Martin Allan MD (U) - *Spec Exp:* *Genitourinary Reconstruction-Complex; Transplant-Kidney-Pediatric; Urologic Surgery-Pediatric;* **Hospital:** Chldn's Hosp - Denver; **Address:** Chldrn's Hosp, 1056 E 19th Ave, rm B-463, Denver, CO 80218-1007; **Phone:** (303) 837-2680; **Board Cert:** Urology 1986; **Med School:** Canada 1976; **Resid:** Surgery, Hlth Scis Ctr, Winnipeg, Canada 1977-1978; Urology, Brigham-Womens Hosp, Boston, MA 1980-1984; **Fellow:** Transplant Surgery, Pacific Med Ctr, San Francisco, CA 1981-1982; **Fac Appt:** Prof Surgery, Univ Colo

Middleton, Richard MD (U) - *Spec Exp:* *Urology - General;* **Hospital:** Univ Utah Hosp and Clin; **Address:** University of Utah Med Ctr, 50 N Med Dr., Salt Lake City, UT 84132-1001; **Phone:** (801) 581-4703; **Board Cert:** Urology 1970; **Med School:** Cornell Univ-Weill Med Coll 1958; **Resid:** Surgery, NY Hosp-Cornell Med Ctr, New York, NY 1959-1961; Urology, NY Hosp-Cornell Med Ctr, New York, NY 1963-1967; **Fac Appt:** Prof Urology, Univ Utah

Southwest

Bardot, Stephen F MD (U) - *Spec Exp:* *Urologic Cancer; Prostate Cancer;* **Hospital:** Ochsner Found Hosp; **Address:** Ochsner Clinic, 1514 Jefferson Hwy, New Orleans, LA 70121; **Phone:** (504) 842-4083; **Board Cert:** Urology 1993; **Med School:** Univ Kans 1985; **Resid:** Surgery, St Luke's Hosp, Kansas City, MO 1985-1987; Urology, Kansas City Univ Med Ctr, Kansas City, KS 1987-1990; **Fellow:** Urologic Oncology, Cleveland Clinic, Cleveland, OH 1990-1991

Basler, Joseph W MD (U) - *Spec Exp:* Prostate Cancer; Urologic Cancer; **Hospital:** Audie L Murphy Meml Vets Hosp; **Address:** 7703 Floyd Curl Dr, MC-7845, San Antonio, TX 78229-3900; **Phone:** (210) 567-5640; **Board Cert:** Urology 1992; **Med School:** Univ MO-Columbia Sch Med 1984; **Resid:** Surgery, Univ Missouri, Columbia, MO 1984-1986; Urology, Barnes Hosp/Wash Univ, St Louis, MO 1986-1990; **Fac Appt:** Assoc Prof Surgery, Univ Tex, San Antonio

Boone, Timothy Bolton MD/PhD (U) - *Spec Exp:* Neuro-Urology; Urinary Reconstruction; Incontinence; **Hospital:** Methodist Hosp - Houston; **Address:** Scurlock Tower, 6560 Fannin, Ste 2100, Houston, TX 77030-2769; **Phone:** (713) 798-4001; **Board Cert:** Urology 1995; **Med School:** Univ Tex, Houston 1985; **Resid:** Surgery, Univ Tex SW, Dallas, TX 1986-1987; Urology, Univ Tex SW, Dallas, TX 1987-1991; **Fac Appt:** Prof Urology, Baylor Coll Med

Buch, Jeffrey Phillip MD (U) - *Spec Exp:* Infertility-Male; **Hospital:** Baylor-Richardson Med Ctr; **Address:** 1600 Coit Rd, Ste 304A, Plano, TX 75075; **Phone:** (972) 612-8037; **Board Cert:** Urology 1997; **Med School:** Univ Mich Med Sch 1980; **Resid:** Surgery, Albany Med Ctr, Albany, NY 1981-1982; Urology, Albany Med Ctr, Albany, NY 1982-1985; **Fellow:** Urology, Baylor Coll Med, Houston, TX 1985-1987

Culkin, Daniel J MD (U) - *Spec Exp:* Urology-Pediatric; **Hospital:** VA Med Ctr; **Address:** Oklahoma Univ HSC, Div Urol, 920 S L Young Blvd, WP 3150, Oklahoma City, OK 73104-5020; **Phone:** (405) 271-6900; **Board Cert:** Urology 1987; **Med School:** Creighton Univ 1979; **Resid:** Surgery, Loyola Univ Med Ctr, Maywood, IL 1980-1981; Urology, Loyola Univ Med Ctr, Maywood, IL 1981-1983; **Fellow:** Endourology, Loyola Univ Med Ctr, Maywood, IL 1983-1984; **Fac Appt:** Prof Urology, Univ Okla Coll Med

Fuselier Jr, Harold A MD (U) - *Spec Exp:* Kidney Stones; Prostate Disease; Erectile Dysfunction; **Hospital:** Ochsner Found Hosp; **Address:** Ochsner Clinic, 1514 Jefferson Hwy, Fl 10N, New Orleans, LA 70121-2483; **Phone:** (504) 842-4083; **Board Cert:** Urology 1974; **Med School:** Louisiana State Univ 1967; **Resid:** Urology, Alton Ochsner Med Fdn, New Orleans, LA 1970-1973; Urology, Mobile Genl Hosp, Mobile, AL 1973-1974; **Fac Appt:** Prof Urology, Louisiana State Univ

Greene, Graham MD (U) - *Spec Exp:* Urologic Cancer; **Hospital:** UAMS; **Address:** 4301 W Markham, Slot 774, Little Rock, AR 72205; **Phone:** (501) 296-1545; **Board Cert:** Urology 1999; **Med School:** Dalhousie Univ 1994; **Resid:** Urology, Victoria Genl, Halifax, Canada 1990-1994; **Fellow:** Medical Oncology, M.D. Anderson Cancer Ctr, Houston, TX 1994-1997; **Fac Appt:** Asst Prof Urology, Univ Ark

Lipshultz, Larry MD (U) - *Spec Exp:* Infertility-Male; Microsurgery; Erectile Dysfunction; **Hospital:** St Luke's Episcopal Hosp - Houston; **Address:** 6560 Fannin St, Ste 2100, Houston, TX 77030-2706; **Phone:** (713) 798-4001; **Board Cert:** Urology 1977; **Med School:** Univ Penn 1968; **Resid:** U Penn Hosp., Philadelphia, PA 1969-1971; **Fellow:** Reproductive Medicine, U Tex., Houston, TX; **Fac Appt:** Prof Urology, Baylor Coll Med

McConnell, John Dowling MD (U) - *Spec Exp:* Prostate Cancer; **Hospital:** Zale Lipshy Univ Hosp; **Address:** Dept Urology, 5323 Harry Hines Blvd, Dallas, TX 75235; **Phone:** (214) 648-5630; **Board Cert:** Urology 1996; **Med School:** Loyola Univ-Stritch Sch Med 1978; **Resid:** Urology, Univ Texas Hlth Sci Ctr-Parkland, Dallas, TX 1980-1984; Surgery, Univ Texas Hlth Sci Ctr-Parkland, Dallas, TX 1979-1980; **Fac Appt:** Prof Urology, Univ Tex SW, Dallas

Miles, Brian J MD (U) - *Spec Exp:* Prostate Cancer; Kidney Cancer; Bladder Cancer; **Hospital:** Methodist Hosp - Houston; **Address:** Scurlock Tower, 6560 Fannin St, Ste 2100, Houston, TX 77030; **Phone:** (713) 798-4001; **Board Cert:** Urology 1984; **Med School:** Univ Mich Med Sch 1974; **Resid:** Urology, Walter Reed Army Med Ctr, Washington, DC 1978-1982; **Fac Appt:** Prof Urology, Baylor Coll Med

Sagalowsky, Arthur I MD (U) - *Spec Exp:* Urologic Cancer; Transplant-Kidney; **Hospital:** Zale Lipshy Univ Hosp; **Address:** Univ Tex SW Med Ctr, Dept Urol, 5323 Harry Hines Blvd, Dallas, TX 75390-9110; **Phone:** (214) 648-3976; **Board Cert:** Urology 1980; **Med School:** Indiana Univ 1973; **Resid:** Surgery, Indiana Univ Hosps, Indianapolis, IN 1973-1975; Urology, Indiana Univ Hosps, Indianapolis, IN 1975-1978; **Fellow:** Clinical Pharmacology, Univ Tex SW Med Ctr, Dallas, TX 1978-1980; **Fac Appt:** Prof Urology, Univ Tex SW, Dallas

Strand, William MD (U) - *Spec Exp:* Urology-Pediatric; Laparoscopic Nephrectomy; **Hospital:** Chldns Med Ctr of Dallas; **Address:** Children's Med Ctr, Dept Urol, 6300 Harry Hines Blvd, Ste 1401, Dallas, TX 75235; **Phone:** (214) 456-2444; **Board Cert:** Urology 1991; **Med School:** Mayo Med Sch 1983; **Resid:** Surgery, Naval Med Ctr, San Diego, CA 1983-1984; Urology, National Naval Med Ctr, Bethesda, MD 1984-1988; **Fac Appt:** Assoc Prof Urology, Univ Tex SW, Dallas

Swanson, David A MD (U) - *Spec Exp:* Genitourinary Cancer; Organ-Conserving Surgery; **Hospital:** Univ of TX MD Anderson Cancer Ctr, The; **Address:** Univ Tex MD Anderson Cancer Ctr, Dept Urol, 1515 Holcombe Blvd, Box 110, Houston, TX 77030-4095; **Phone:** (713) 792-3250; **Board Cert:** Urology 1977; **Med School:** Univ Penn 1967; **Resid:** Surgery, Harbor Genl Hosp, Torrance, CA 1967-1969; Urology, UC Davis, Sacramento, CA 1972-1975; **Fellow:** Urologic Oncology, Univ Tex-MD Anderson Hosp, Houston, TX 1976-1978; **Fac Appt:** Prof Urology, Univ Tex, Houston

Thompson Jr, Ian M MD (U) - *Spec Exp:* Prostate Cancer; Prostate Surgery; **Hospital:** Univ of Texas Hlth & Sci Ctr; **Address:** Univ Tex Hlth Scis Ctr, Dept Urology, 7703 Floyd Curl, MC 78229, San Antonio, TX 78229-3900; **Phone:** (210) 567-5643; **Board Cert:** Urology 1997; **Med School:** Tulane Univ 1980; **Resid:** Urology, Brooke Army Med Ctr, San Antonio, TX 1981-1985; **Fellow:** Medical Oncology, Meml Sloan-Kettering Canc Ctr, New York, NY 1987-1988; **Fac Appt:** Prof Surgery, Univ Tex, San Antonio

von Eschenbach, Andrew C MD (U) - *Spec Exp:* Prostate Cancer; **Hospital:** Univ of TX MD Anderson Cancer Ctr, The; **Address:** Univ Tex - MD Anderson Cancer Ctr, 1515 Holcombe Blvd, Box 405, Houston, TX 77030-4009; **Phone:** (713) 792-2570; **Board Cert:** Urology 1978; **Med School:** Georgetown Univ 1967; **Resid:** Surgery, Penn Hosp, Philadelphia, PA 1971-1972; Transplant Surgery, Penn Hosp, Philadelphia, PA 1972-1975; **Fellow:** Urologic Oncology, Univ Texas-MD Anderson Hosp, Houston, TX 1976-1977; **Fac Appt:** Prof Urology, Univ Tex, Houston

Winters, Jack Christian MD (U) - *Spec Exp:* Voiding Dysfunction; Urology-Female; Urinary Reconstruction; **Hospital:** Ochsner Found Hosp; **Address:** Ochsner Clinic, 1514 Jefferson Hwy, Fl 10N, New Orleans, LA 70121; **Phone:** (504) 842-4083; **Board Cert:** Urology 1997; **Med School:** Louisiana State Univ 1988; **Resid:** Surgery, Ochner Fdn Hosp, New Orleans, LA 1988-1990; Urology, Ochner Fdn Hosp, New Orleans, LA 1990-1994; **Fellow:** Female Urology, Cleveland Clinic Fdn, Cleveland, OH 1994-1995

West Coast and Pacific

Berger, Richard E MD (U) - *Spec Exp:* Infertility-Male; Infectious Disease; Urologic Surgery; **Hospital:** Univ WA Med Ctr; **Address:** 1959 NE Pacific St, Box 356510, Seattle, WA 98105; **Phone:** (206) 598-4203; **Board Cert:** Urology 1981; **Med School:** Univ Chicago-Pritzker Sch Med 1973; **Resid:** Surgery, Univ Colo Hlth Sci Ctr, Denver, CO 1974-1975; Urology, Univ Wash Med Ctr, Seattle, WA 1975-1979; **Fellow:** Infectious Disease, Univ Wash Med Ctr, Seattle, WA 1976-1977; **Fac Appt:** Prof Urology, Univ Wash

Boyd, Stuart D MD (U) - *Spec Exp:* Incontinence; Impotence; Urologic Cancer; **Hospital:** USC Norris Cancer Comp Ctr; **Address:** 1441 Eastlake Ave, Ste 7416, Los Angeles, CA 90033-4525; **Phone:** (323) 865-3704; **Board Cert:** Urology 1984; **Med School:** UCLA 1975; **Resid:** Urology, UCLA, Los Angeles, CA 1978-1982; **Fac Appt:** Prof Urology, USC Sch Med

Carroll, Peter Robert MD (U) - *Spec Exp:* Urology - General; **Hospital:** UCSF Med Ctr; **Address:** 400 Parnassus Ave, Ste 610, San Francisco, CA 94143-0330; **Phone:** (415) 476-1611; **Board Cert:** Urology 1998; **Med School:** Georgetown Univ 1979; **Resid:** Surgery, UC San Francisco Med Ctr, San Francisco, CA 1980-1984; **Fellow:** Urology, Mem Sloan Kettering Cancer Ctr, New York, NY 1984-1986; **Fac Appt:** Prof Urology, UCSF

Clayman, Ralph V MD (U) - *Spec Exp:* Kidney Stones; Endourology; **Hospital:** UCI Med Ctr; **Address:** 101 The City Drive Bldg 26, MC 81, UCI Med Ctr, Dept of Urology, Orange, CA 92868; **Phone:** (714) 456-6068; **Board Cert:** Urology 1981; **Med School:** UCSD 1973; **Resid:** Urology, Univ Minn, Minneapolis, MN 1974-1979; **Fac Appt:** Prof Urology, Washington Univ, St Louis

Danoff, Dudley S MD (U) - *Spec Exp:* Prostate Cancer; Bladder Cancer; Kidney Cancer; **Hospital:** Cedars-Sinai Med Ctr; **Address:** 8631 W 3rd St, Ste 915-E, Los Angeles, CA 90048; **Phone:** (310) 854-9898; **Board Cert:** Urology 1974; **Med School:** Yale Univ 1963; **Resid:** Urology, Yale Med Ctr, New Haven, CT 1964-1965; Urology, Columbia P&S, New York, NY 1965-1969

de Kernion, Jean Bayhi MD (U) - *Spec Exp:* Urologic Cancer; Kidney Cancer; **Hospital:** UCLA Med Ctr; **Address:** UCLA Med Ctr, Dept Urol, 10833 Le Conte Ave, Box 951738, Los Angeles, CA 90095; **Phone:** (310) 206-6453; **Board Cert:** Urology 1975, Surgery 1973; **Med School:** Louisiana State Univ 1965; **Resid:** Surgery, Univ Hosps-Case West Res, Cleveland, OH 1966-1967; Urology, Univ Hosps-Case West Res, Cleveland, OH 1969-1973; **Fellow:** Urologic Oncology, Natl Cancer Inst, Bethesda, MD 1967-1969; **Fac Appt:** Prof Urology, UCLA

Fuchs, Eugene F MD (U) - *Spec Exp:* Infertility-Male; Kidney Stones; Vasectomy Reversal; **Hospital:** OR Hlth Sci Univ Hosp and Clinics; **Address:** 1750 SW Harbor Way, Ste 230, Portland, OR 97201; **Phone:** (503) 525-0071; **Board Cert:** Urology 1977; **Med School:** Univ VT Coll Med 1970; **Resid:** Urology, U Oregon, Portland, OR 1971-1975; **Fac Appt:** Prof Urology, Oregon Hlth Scis Univ

Gill, Harcharan Singh MD (U) - *Spec Exp:* Urologic Cancer; **Hospital:** Stanford Med Ctr; **Address:** 300 Pasteur Drive, Stanford, CA 94305; **Phone:** (650) 723-6024; **Board Cert:** Urology 1995; **Med School:** Kenya 1977; **Resid:** Urology, Inst of Urol, London, England; Urology, Univ Penn, Philidelphia, PA 1986-1991; **Fellow:** Urology, Univ Penn, Philidelphia, PA 1985-1986; **Fac Appt:** Prof Urology, Stanford Univ

Holden, Stuart MD (U) - *Spec Exp:* Kidney Cancer; **Hospital:** Cedars-Sinai Med Ctr; **Address:** 8631 W 3rd St, Ste 915E, Los Angeles, CA 90048; **Phone:** (310) 854-9898; **Board Cert:** Urology 1977; **Med School:** Cornell Univ-Weill Med Coll 1968; **Resid:** Surgery, NY Hosp-Cornell, New York, NY 1969-1970; Urology, Emory Univ Hosp, Atlanta, GA 1972-1975; **Fellow:** Urology, Sloan Kettering Cancer Ctr, New York, NY 1976-1978

Huffman, Jeffry Lee MD (U) - *Spec Exp:* Kidney Stones; Kidney Cancer; Bladder/Prostate Cancer; **Hospital:** USC Univ Hosp - R K Eamer Med Plz; **Address:** USC Care Med Grp, 1510 San Pablo St, Ste 649, Los Angeles, CA 90033; **Phone:** (323) 442-5955; **Board Cert:** Urology 1995; **Med School:** Loyola Univ-Stritch Sch Med 1978; **Resid:** Urology, Univ Chicago/Pritzker, New York, NY 1980-1983; **Fellow:** Urologic Oncology, Memorial Sloan Kettering Cancer Ctr, New York, NY 1983-1985; **Fac Appt:** Prof Urology, USC Sch Med

Lieskovsky, Gary MD (U) - *Spec Exp:* Prostate Cancer; **Hospital:** USC Norris Cancer Comp Ctr; **Address:** 1441 Eastlake Ave, Ste 7416, Los Angeles, CA 90089; **Phone:** (323) 865-3702; **Board Cert:** Urology 1980; **Med School:** Canada 1973; **Resid:** Urology, Univ Alberta Hosp, Edmonton, Canada 1974-1978; **Fellow:** Urology, UCLA Med Ctr, Los Angeles, CA 1979-1980; **Fac Appt:** Prof Urology, USC Sch Med

Lue, Tom F MD (U) - *Spec Exp: Impotence; Peyronie's disease;* **Hospital:** UCSF Med Ctr; **Address:** 2330 Post St, Ste 600, San Francisco, CA 94115; **Phone:** (415) 353-7344; **Board Cert:** Urology 1983; **Med School:** Taiwan 1972; **Resid:** Surgery, Brookdale Hosp, Brooklyn, NY 1976-1978; Urology, SUNY Downstate Med Ctr, Brooklyn, NY 1978-1981; **Fellow:** Urology, UCSF, San Francisco, CA 1981-1982; **Fac Appt:** Prof Urology, UCSF

McAninch, Jack MD (U) - *Spec Exp: Trauma;* **Hospital:** San Francisco Gen Hosp; **Address:** San Francisco Genl Hosp, Dept Urology, 1001 Potrero Ave, Ste 3A20, San Francisco, CA 94110-3518; **Phone:** (415) 476-3372; **Board Cert:** Urology 1972; **Med School:** Univ Tex Med Br, Galveston 1964; **Resid:** Darnall Army Hosp, Fort Hood, TX; Letterman AMC, San Francisco, CA 1966-1969; **Fac Appt:** Prof Urology, UCSF

McClure, Robert Dale MD (U) - *Spec Exp: Infertility-Male;* **Hospital:** Virginia Mason Med Ctr; **Address:** Virginia Mason Med Ctr, 1100 9th Ave, Box 900, Seattle, WA 98101-2756; **Phone:** (206) 223-6179; **Board Cert:** Urology 1979; **Med School:** Canada 1968; **Resid:** Urology, McGill Univ Hosp, Montreal, Canada 1970-1975; **Fellow:** Endocrinology, Univ Washington Med Ctr, Seattle, WA 1975-1977

Padma-Nathan, Harin MD (U) - *Spec Exp: Erectile Dysfunction;* **Hospital:** USC Norris Cancer Comp Ctr; **Address:** 9100 Wilshire Blvd, East Tower, Ste 360, Beverly Hills, CA 90212; **Phone:** (310) 858-4455; **Med School:** Dalhousie Univ 1980; **Resid:** Urology, Dalhoise Univ, Halifax, Canada 1981-1985; **Fellow:** Urology, Boston Univ Med Ctr, Boston, MA 1985-1988; **Fac Appt:** Clin Prof Urology, USC Sch Med

Payne, Christopher K MD (U) - *Spec Exp: Interstitial Cystitis; Pelvic Prolapse & Reconstruction; Incontinence-Female;* **Hospital:** Stanford Med Ctr; **Address:** Stanford Med Ctr MC-5314, 300 Pasteur Dr, Ste 287, Stanford, CA 94305-5118; **Phone:** (650) 723-6024; **Board Cert:** Urology 1995; **Med School:** Vanderbilt Univ 1986; **Resid:** Urology, Univ Penn, Philadelphia, PA 1987-1992; **Fellow:** Urology, UCLA, Los Angeles, CA 1992-1993; **Fac Appt:** Assoc Prof Urology, Stanford Univ

Rajfer, Jacob MD (U) - *Spec Exp: Erectile Dysfunction;* **Hospital:** LAC - Harbor - UCLA Med Ctr; **Address:** 1000 W Carson St, Box 5, Torrance, CA 90509; **Phone:** (310) 222-2727; **Board Cert:** Urology 1980; **Med School:** Northwestern Univ 1972; **Resid:** Surgery, St Josephs Hosp, Denver, CO 1973-1974; Urology, Johns Hopkins Hosp, Baltimore, MD 1976-1978; **Fellow:** Research, Johns Hopkins Hosp, Baltimore, MD 1975-1976; **Fac Appt:** Prof Urology, UCLA

Raz, Shlomo MD (U) - *Spec Exp: Incontinence-Female; Urology-Female;* **Hospital:** UCLA Med Ctr; **Address:** 924 Westwood Blvd, Ste 520, Los Angeles, CA 90024-2926; **Phone:** (310) 794-0206; **Board Cert:** Urology 1979; **Med School:** Uruguay 1938; **Resid:** Surgery, Hadassah Univ Hosp, Jerusalem, Israel 1967-1973; **Fellow:** Urology, UCLA Med Ctr, Los Angeles, CA 1974-1975; **Fac Appt:** Assoc Prof Urology, UCLA

Salvatierra, Oscar MD (U) - *Spec Exp: Transplant-Kidney;* **Hospital:** Stanford Med Ctr; **Address:** 703 Welch Rd, Ste H2, Palo Alto, CA 94304; **Phone:** (650) 498-5481; **Board Cert:** Urology 1970; **Med School:** USC Sch Med 1961; **Resid:** Urology, LAC-USC Med Ctr, Los Angeles, CA 1962-1966; **Fellow:** Transplant Surgery, UCSF, San Francisco, CA 1972-1973; **Fac Appt:** Prof Urology, Stanford Univ

Schmidt, Joseph MD (U) - *Spec Exp: Prostate Cancer;* **Hospital:** UCSD Healthcare; **Address:** 200 W Arbor Drive, San Diego, CA 92103-8897; **Phone:** (619) 543-5904; **Board Cert:** Urology 1971; **Med School:** Univ IL Coll Med 1961; **Resid:** Surgery, Rush-Presby-St Lukes Hosp, Chicago, IL 1962-1963; Urology, Johns Hopkins Hosp, Baltimore, MD 1963-1967; **Fac Appt:** Prof Urology, UCSD

Sharlip, Ira Dorian MD (U) - *Spec Exp:* *Erectile Dysfunction; Infertility-Male; Vasectomy Reversal;* **Hospital:** CA Pacific Med Ctr - Pacific Campus; **Address:** 2100 Webster St, Ste 222, San Francisco, CA 94115-2376; **Phone:** (415) 202-0250; **Board Cert:** Internal Medicine 1972, Urology 1977; **Med School:** Univ Penn 1965; **Resid:** Internal Medicine, Hosp Univ Penn, Philadelphia, PA 1966-1967; Urology, UCSF Medical Center, San Francisco, CA 1972-1975; **Fellow:** Urology, Middlesex Hosp, Waltham, MA 1975-1976; **Fac Appt:** Asst Clin Prof Urology, UCSF

Shortliffe, Linda MD (U) - *Spec Exp:* *Urology-Pediatric;* **Hospital:** Stanford Med Ctr; **Address:** Stanford U Med Ctr, Dept Ped Urol, rm S-287, 300 Pasteur Dr, Stanford, CA 94305-5118; **Phone:** (650) 725-5530; **Board Cert:** Urology 1983; **Med School:** Stanford Univ 1975; **Resid:** Surgery, Tufts Med Ctr, Boston, MA 1976-1977; Urology, Stanford U Med Ctr, Stanford, CA 1977-1981; **Fac Appt:** Prof Urology, Stanford Univ

Skinner, Donald George MD (U) - *Spec Exp:* *Bladder Cancer; Urologic Cancer;* **Hospital:** USC Univ Hosp - R K Eamer Med Plz; **Address:** 2025 Zonal Ave, rm 5900, Los Angeles, CA 90033; **Phone:** (323) 865-3707; **Board Cert:** Urology 1974; **Med School:** Yale Univ 1964; **Resid:** Urology, Mass Genl Hosp, Boston, MA 1964-1966; Surgery, Mass Genl Hosp, Boston, MA 1968-1971; **Fac Appt:** Prof Urology, USC Sch Med

Skinner, Eila C MD (U) - *Spec Exp:* *Urologic Cancer; Urinary Reconstruction; Urology-Female;* **Hospital:** LAC & USC Med Ctr; **Address:** USC-Keck Sch Med, Dept Urol, NOR 7416 Bldg, MC-9178, Los Angeles, CA 90033-1034; **Phone:** (323) 865-3705; **Board Cert:** Urology 1992; **Med School:** USC Sch Med 1983; **Resid:** Urology, LAC-USC Med Ctr, Los Angeles, CA 1984-1988; **Fellow:** Urologic Oncology, LAC-USC Med Ctr, Los Angeles, CA 1988-1990; **Fac Appt:** Assoc Clin Prof Urology, USC Sch Med

Smith, Robert B MD (U) - *Spec Exp:* *Urologic Cancer;* **Hospital:** UCLA Med Ctr; **Address:** UCLA Sch Med, Div Urology, 760 Westwood Plaza, Los Angeles, CA 90024; **Phone:** (310) 825-9273; **Board Cert:** Urology 1972; **Med School:** UCLA 1963; **Resid:** Surgery, UCLA Med Ctr, Los Angeles, CA 1964-1965; Urology, UCLA Med Ctr, Los Angeles, CA 1965-1969; **Fac Appt:** Prof Surgery, UCLA

Stoller, Marshall Leedy MD (U) - *Spec Exp:* *Kidney Stones; Laparoscopic Surgery;* **Hospital:** UCSF Med Ctr; **Address:** 400 Panassus Ave Fl 6, San Francisco, CA 94143; **Phone:** (415) 353-2200; **Board Cert:** Urology 1999; **Med School:** Baylor Coll Med 1981; **Resid:** Urology, UCSF, San Francisco, CA 1983-1987; Surgery, UCSF, San Francisco, CA 1981-1983; **Fellow:** Urology, Prince Henry Hosptial, Sydney, Australia 1985-1986; **Fac Appt:** Prof Urology, UCSF

Stone, Anthony MD (U) - *Spec Exp:* *Urology-Female; Voiding Dysfunction;* **Hospital:** Univ CA - Davis Med Ctr; **Address:** 4860 1st St, Ste 3500, Sacramento, CA 95817-2214; **Phone:** (916) 734-2823; **Board Cert:** Urology 1997; **Med School:** Scotland 1972; **Resid:** Urological Renal Transplant, Western Genl Hosp, Glasgow, Scotland 1978-1980; Urology, Cardiff Royal Infirm, Cardiff, Wales 1980-1983; **Fellow:** Urodynamics, Duke Univ Med Ctr, Durham, NC 1983-1986; **Fac Appt:** Prof Urology, UC Davis

Tomera, Kevin M MD (U) - *Spec Exp:* *Urologic Cancer; Voiding Dysfunction;* **Hospital:** Alaska Regional Med Ctr; **Address:** 1200 Airport Heights Drive, Ste 101, Anchorage, AK 99508-2944; **Phone:** (907) 276-2803; **Board Cert:** Urology 1995; **Med School:** Northwestern Univ 1978; **Resid:** Urology, Mayo Clinic, Rochester, MN 1980-1983

Winfield, Howard Neil MD (U) - *Spec Exp:* Kidney Stones; Laparaoscopic Surgery; **Hospital:** Stanford Med Ctr; **Address:** Stanford Hlth Svcs, Dept Urol-S287, 300 Pasteur, Stanford, CA 94305; **Phone:** (650) 858-3916; **Board Cert:** Urology 1999; **Med School:** McGill Univ 1978; **Resid:** Urology, McGill Univ Tchg Hosp, Montreal, Canada 1981-1984; **Fellow:** Urology, UCLA, Los Angeles, CA 1985-1986; Urology, Washington University, St. Louis, MO 1984-1985; **Fac Appt:** Assoc Prof Urology, Stanford Univ

VASCULAR SURGERY (GENERAL)

(a subspecialty of SURGERY)

A surgeon with expertise in the management of surgical disorders of the blood vessels, excluding the intercranial vessels or the heart.

SURGERY

A surgeon manages a broad spectrum of surgical conditions affecting almost any area of the body. The surgeon establishes the diagnosis and provides the preoperative, operative and postoperative care to surgical patients and is usually responsible for the comprehensive management of the trauma victim and the critically ill surgical patient.

The surgeon uses a variety of diagnostic techniques, including endoscopy, for observing internal structures and may use specialized instruments during operative procedures. A general surgeon is expected to be familiar with the salient features of other surgical specialties in order to recognize problems in those areas and to know when to refer a patient to another specialist.

Training required: Five years in surgery *plus* additional training and examination

THE VASCULAR INSTITUTE
MAIMONIDES MEDICAL CENTER

4802 Tenth Avenue • Brooklyn, NY 11219
Phone (718) 283-7957   Fax (718) 283-8599
www.maimonidesmed.org

The Vascular Institute at Maimonides Medical Center has helped thousands of patients prevent the most serious circulatory complications of hypertension, diabetes, arteriosclerosis and other diseases. A nationally recognized Center of Excellence established in 1992 by Enrico Ascher, MD, the Institute sets the standard for medical quality in stroke prevention, chronic wound treatment, limb salvage surgery, varicose vein treatment, balloon angioplasties and stents, and diagnosis and treatment of circulatory blockages.

The Vascular Institute consists of the following divisions and services:

THE DIVISION OF VASCULAR SURGERY

Stroke prevention: Through balloon angioplasty and stents as well as a simplified technique for carotid endarterectomy, Dr. Ascher and his colleagues have pioneered innovative and less invasive approaches to stroke prevention.
The Vein Center: Several effective and safe procedures are used to remove unwanted varicose veins.
The Endovascular Center: One of the busiest of its kind, the center uses minimally invasive techniques to repair aneurysms and blocked arteries.

THE VASCULAR DIAGNOSTIC LABORATORY

This is the largest noninvasive lab in New York State and employs the most advanced technology to assess patients. Thanks to dedicated physicians and a multimillion-dollar investment in sophisticated equipment, patients receive full and speedy evaluations—and most can do so without undergoing invasive angiograms.

THE WOUND TREATMENT CENTER

The first in Brooklyn and Staten Island to focus on the needs of patients with chronic non-healing wounds of the extremities, the center has had a remarkable number of patients reporting dramatic improvements in their condition.

THE VASCULAR INSTITUTE

Enrico Ascher, MD, founder of The Vascular Institute, is known as the best option to save a dying limb. He views amputation as a rare last resort, focusing instead on following an aggressive treatment program. As a result, The Vascular Institute saves almost two-thirds of limbs that had been deemed unreconstructable.

NewYork-Presbyterian
The University Hospitals of Columbia and Cornell
Columbia Weill Cornell Vascular Center

Columbia Presbyterian Medical Center
622 West 168th Street
New York, NY 10032

NewYork Weill Cornell Medical Center
525 East 68th Street
New York, NY 10021

OVERVIEW:

Vascular disease can affect people of all ages and requires a wide range of expertise for appropriate and effective therapies. The Columbia Weill Cornell Vascular Care Center offers a comprehensive and integrated program for the prevention, diagnosis and treatment of diverse problems relating to arteries and veins throughout the body, including the heart, abdomen, kidneys, legs, neck and brain.

The Center brings together medical and surgical experts of two internationally renowned academic medical centers – Columbia Presbyterian and NewYork Weill Cornell – who bring a depth of experience to treating even the most unusual vascular conditions. Patients benefit from the Vascular Care Center's proven cutting edge technologies, innovative programs and groundbreaking research.

The Columbia Weill Cornell Vascular Care Center meets the needs of its patients through:
- Programs that emphasize prevention measures;
- Rigorous screenings and integrated care for patients at risk for life-threatening vascular diseases, such as strokes and abdominal aortic aneurysms;
- Innovative applications of non-invasive diagnostic technologies, including CT scans, ultrasound, MRI and MRA;
- Advances in the latest drug therapies;
- State-of-the-art surgical and minimally invasive treatments;
- New approaches in the treatment of blood clots;
- Basic and clinical research to develop more effective procedures for diagnosis and treatment.

Physician Referral: For a physician referral or to learn more about the Columbia Weill Cornell Vascular Center call toll free **1-877-NYP-WELL** (1-877-697-9355) or visit our website at **www.nyp.org**.

COMPREHENSIVE SERVICES INCLUDE:

- Lipid Control Centers, where adults and children at risk for inherited or acquired cholesterol and lipid are evaluated and treated.

- Comprehensive Stroke Centers with an interdisciplinary Acute Stroke Team on call round the clock.

- Comprehensive Abdominal Aortic Aneurysm Program to detect and treat one of the leading causes of death, particularly in men.

- Hypertension Center for treating blocked kidney arteries, which can cause high blood pressure and kidney failure.

- Amputation Prevention Program for treating vascular blockages leading to difficulty walking or the loss of a leg.

- Gene Therapy Center includes a program to treat blocked arteries in legs.

- Wound Healing Program offers a hyperbaric oxygen chamber, growth factors and gene therapy to treat poorly healing wounds.

NYU Medical Center

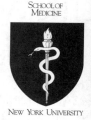

NEW YORK UNIVERSITY

550 First Avenue (at 31st Street)
New York, NY 10016
Physician Referral: (888) 7-NYU-MED
(888-769-8633)
www.mininvasive.med.nyu.edu

VASCULAR SURGERY
A KINDER, GENTLER APPROACH TO ANEURYSM REPAIR

When a patient has heart disease, aneurysms, or bulges in the aorta are often an unfortunate, potentially deadly symptom. Most aortic aneurysms occur in areas damaged by artherosclerosis, a condition in which the arteries become hardened from the buildup of cholesterol and other material over many years. It is estimated that one to five percent of people over the age of 65 have an aneurysm. There are usually few symptoms, although some people may feel deep back pain. Severe, excruciating pain is usually the first symptom of a rupture.

Ten years ago, a patient with an aortic aneurysm would have undergone an extensive operation to repair it. Today, NYU Medical Center is among a select group of institutions worldwide that offer minimally invasive surgical solutions to complex aortic problems.

The new, minimally invasive procedure involves making small incisions in the groin and inserting a stent graft, which the surgeon guides to the exact position in the artery needed to ease pressure and prevent rupture. Usually, patients require no blood transfusion and are able to leave the hospital just one or two days after surgery.

As the site of early FDA testing of one of the newest devices used in endovascular surgery, NYU Medical Center is leading the way in both clinical and scientific research in the burgeoning field of vascular surgery. It also is a major training center, where vascular surgeons learn and perfect the latest minimally invasive techniques. NYU's outstanding specialists continue to achieve high rates of success with the new stent graft procedure, even in patients over 75 years of age. Judging from the pace of research at NYU, it is extremely likely that the new techniques will be used to treat other types of conditions in the very near future.

NYU MEDICAL CENTER

At NYU Medical Center, we pride ourselves on delivering the highest quality care. Our emphasis on the newest surgical technologies is not an end in itself, but a way to ease pain and decrease recovery time, as well as achieve the best possible outcomes. In conventional aneurysm repair, the surgeon performs an open-chest procedure, involving blood transfusions, intensive care, and lengthy hospital stays. With the new devices and minimally invasive techniques, out patients not only get well – they return to normal activity and improved quality of life as soon as one week after surgery.

Physician Referral
(888) 7-NYU-MED
(888-769-8633)
www.mininvasive.med.nyu.edu

924
Sponsored Page

Physician Listings

Vascular Surgery (General)

New England

Abbott, William Martin MD (GVS) - *Spec Exp:* Vascular Surgery (General) - General; **Hospital:** MA Genl Hosp; **Address:** Dept Surgery, 15 Parkman St, WAC-458, Boston, MA 02114; **Phone:** (617) 726-8250; **Board Cert:** Vascular Surgery (General) 1992, Surgery 1971; **Med School:** Stanford Univ 1961; **Resid:** Surgery, Mass Genl Hosp, Boston, MA 1962-1965; Surgery, Mass Genl Hosp, Boston, MA 1969-1971; **Fellow:** Surgery, Mass Genl Hosp, Boston, MA 1965-1966; **Fac Appt:** Prof Surgery, Harvard Med Sch

Belkin, Michael MD (GVS) - *Spec Exp:* Aneurysm; Arterial Bypass Surgery; Carotid Artery Surgery; **Hospital:** Brigham & Women's Hosp; **Address:** Brigham & Women's Hosp, 75 Francis St, Boston, MA 02115; **Phone:** (617) 732-6816; **Board Cert:** Vascular Surgery (General) 2010, Surgical Critical Care 2003; **Med School:** Univ Conn 1982; **Resid:** Surgery, Hartford Hosp, Hartford, CT 1982-1987; **Fellow:** Vascular Surgery (General), Boston Univ/Brigham-Womens Hosp, Boston, MA 1987-1989; **Fac Appt:** Assoc Prof Surgery, Harvard Med Sch

Brewster, David C MD (GVS) - *Spec Exp:* Aneurysm-Abdominal Aortic; Endovascular Surgery; **Hospital:** MA Genl Hosp; **Address:** One Hawthorne Pl, Ste 111, Boston, MA 02114; **Phone:** (617) 523-4293; **Board Cert:** Vascular Surgery (General) 1991, Surgery 1975; **Med School:** Columbia P&S 1967; **Resid:** Surgery, Mass Genl Hosp, Boston, MA 1968-1975; **Fellow:** Vascular Surgery (General), Mass Genl Hosp, Boston, MA 1975-1976; **Fac Appt:** Clin Prof Surgery, Harvard Med Sch

Cambria, Richard P MD (GVS) - *Spec Exp:* Aneurysm-Abdominal Aortic; Cerebrovascular Disease; Renovascular Disease; **Hospital:** MA Genl Hosp; **Address:** Mass Genl Hosp, Surgery, 15 Parkman St, MS WAC 458, Boston, MA 02114-3117; **Phone:** (617) 726-8278; **Board Cert:** Surgery 1994, Vascular Surgery (General) 1994; **Med School:** Columbia P&S 1977; **Resid:** Surgery, Mass Genl Hosp, Boston, MA 1977-1978; **Fellow:** Vascular Surgery (General), Mass Genl Hosp, Boston, MA 1983-1984; **Fac Appt:** Prof Surgery, Harvard Med Sch

Cronenwett, Jack MD (GVS) - *Spec Exp:* Peripheral Vascular Surgery; Aneurysm-Abdominal Aortic; **Hospital:** Dartmouth - Hitchcock Med Ctr; **Address:** Dartmouth Hitchcock Med Ctr, Sect Vasc Surg, 1 Med Ctr Drive, Lebanon, NH 03756; **Phone:** (603) 650-8670; **Board Cert:** Vascular Surgery (General) 1991, Surgery 1989; **Med School:** Stanford Univ 1973; **Resid:** Surgery, Univ Mich Hosp, Ann Arbor, MI 1974-1979; **Fellow:** Vascular Surgery (General), Univ Tenn Hosp, Memphis, TN 1979-1980; **Fac Appt:** Prof Surgery, Dartmouth Med Sch

Gibbons, Gary William MD (GVS) - *Spec Exp:* Diabetic Leg/Foot Surgery; **Hospital:** Boston Med Ctr; **Address:** 732 Harrison Ave, Preston Bldg, Fl 2, Boston, MA 02118; **Phone:** (617) 414-6843; **Board Cert:** Vascular Surgery (General) 1992; **Med School:** Univ Cincinnati 1971; **Resid:** Surgery, New England Deaconess Hosp, Boston, MA 1972-1976; **Fellow:** Nutrition, New England Deaconess Hosp, Boston, MA 1974; **Fac Appt:** Prof Surgery, Boston Univ

Hallett Jr, John MD (GVS) - *Spec Exp:* Aneurysm-Abdominal Aortic; **Hospital:** Eastern Maine Med Ctr; **Address:** Eastern Maine Med Ctr, 489 State St, Bangor, ME 04401; **Phone:** (207) 973-4295; **Board Cert:** Vascular Surgery (General) 1993, Surgery 1999; **Med School:** Duke Univ 1973; **Resid:** Surgery, Wilford Hall USAF Med Ctr, San Antonio, TX 1974-1978; **Fellow:** Vascular Surgery (General), Mass Genl Hosp-Harvard Med Sch, Boston, MA 1979

Lo Gerfo, Frank W MD (GVS) - *Spec Exp:* Arterial Bypass Surgery-Leg; Diabetic Leg/Foot; **Hospital:** Beth Israel Deaconess Med Ctr - Boston; **Address:** BIDMC - Div Vascular Surgery, 110 Francis St, Ste 5B, Boston, MA 02215; **Phone:** (617) 632-9955; **Board Cert:** Surgery 1972, Vascular Surgery (General) 2004; **Med School:** Univ Rochester 1966; **Resid:** Surgery, Boston Univ Hosp, Boston, MA 1967-1971; **Fac Appt:** Prof Surgery, Harvard Med Sch

Mackey, William C. MD (GVS) - *Spec Exp:* Carotid Artery Surgery; Aneurysm-Abdominal Aortic; **Hospital:** New England Med Ctr - Boston; **Address:** 750 Washington St, Ste 1035, Boston, MA 02111-1526; **Phone:** (617) 636-5927; **Board Cert:** Vascular Surgery (General) 1995, Surgical Critical Care 1997; **Med School:** Duke Univ 1977; **Resid:** Surgery, NY Hosp-Cornell Med Ctr, New York, NY 1978-1982; **Fellow:** Vascular Surgery (General), Tufts Univ-New Eng Med Ctr, Boston, MA 1982-1984; **Fac Appt:** Prof Surgery, Tufts Univ

Whittemore, Anthony D MD (GVS) - *Spec Exp:* Carotid Artery Surgery; Aortic Surgery; Aneurysm-Abdominal Aortic; **Hospital:** Brigham & Women's Hosp; **Address:** 75 Francis St, Boston, MA 02115-6195; **Phone:** (617) 732-8515; **Board Cert:** Surgery 1987, Vascular Surgery (General) 1992; **Med School:** Columbia P&S 1970; **Resid:** Surgery, Columbia-Presby Med Ctr, New York, NY 1970-1976; **Fellow:** Vascular Surgery (General), Peter Bent Brigham Hosp, Boston, MA 1976-1977; **Fac Appt:** Prof Surgery, Harvard Med Sch

Mid Atlantic

Adelman, Mark MD (GVS) - *Spec Exp:* Carotid Artery Surgery; Aneurysm-Abdominal Aortic; Minimally Invasive Surgery; **Hospital:** NYU Med Ctr (page 71); **Address:** 530 1st Ave, Ste 6F, New York, NY 10016-6402; **Phone:** (212) 263-7311; **Board Cert:** Vascular Surgery (General) 1993, Surgery 1999; **Med School:** NYU Sch Med 1985; **Resid:** Surgery, New York Univ, New York, NY 1986-1990; **Fellow:** Vascular Surgery (General), New York Univ, New York, NY 1990-1991; **Fac Appt:** Assoc Prof Vascular Surgery (General), NYU Sch Med

Ascher, Enrico MD (GVS) - *Spec Exp:* Carotid Artery Surgery; Aneurysm; Limb Salvage; **Hospital:** Maimonides Med Ctr (page 65); **Address:** 4802 10th Ave Fl 4 - rm 0, Brooklyn, NY 11219-2844; **Phone:** (718) 283-7957; **Board Cert:** Surgery 1984, Vascular Surgery (General) 1995; **Med School:** Brazil 1974; **Resid:** Surgery, NY Med Coll, Valhalla, NY 1976-1981; **Fellow:** Vascular Surgery (General), Montefiore Hosp Med Ctr, Bronx, NY 1981-1982; **Fac Appt:** Prof Surgery, SUNY Downstate

Atnip, Robert G MD (GVS) - *Spec Exp:* Aneurysm-Abdominal Aortic; Aneurysm-Peripheral; **Hospital:** Penn State Univ Hosp - Milton S Hershey Med Ctr; **Address:** Penn State Milton S Hershey Med Ctr, 500 University Drive, rm C 4628, Box 850, Hershey, PA 17033; **Phone:** (717) 531-8866; **Board Cert:** Surgery 1985, Surgical Critical Care 1990; **Med School:** Univ Ala 1978; **Resid:** Surgery, Mass Genl Hospital, Boston, MA 1979-1984; **Fellow:** Vascular Surgery (General), Mass Genl Hospital, Boston, MA 1984-1985; **Fac Appt:** Assoc Prof Surgery, Penn State Univ-Hershey Med Ctr

Benvenisty, Alan I MD (GVS) - *Spec Exp:* Cardiovascular Surgery; Peripheral Vascular Surgery; **Hospital:** NY Presby Hosp - Columbia Presby Med Ctr (page 70); **Address:** 161 Fort Washington Ave, rm 638, New York, NY 10032; **Phone:** (212) 305-8055; **Board Cert:** Surgery 1994, Vascular Surgery (General) 1999; **Med School:** Columbia P&S 1978; **Resid:** Surgery, Columbia-Presby Med Ctr, New York, NY 1979-1983; **Fellow:** Vascular Surgery (General), Columbia-Presby Med Ctr, New York, NY 1983-1984; **Fac Appt:** Assoc Clin Prof Surgery, Columbia P&S

Brener, Bruce MD (GVS) - *Spec Exp:* Endovascular Stent Grafts; Minimally Invasive Surgery; **Hospital:** Newark Beth Israel Med Ctr; **Address:** Millburn Surgical Assoc, 225 Millburn Ave, Ste 104B, Millburn, NJ 07041; **Phone:** (973) 379-5888; **Board Cert:** Surgery 1972, Vascular Surgery (General) 1993; **Med School:** Harvard Med Sch 1966; **Resid:** Surgery, Chldns Hosp, Boston, MA 1967-1968; Surgery, Peter Bent Hosp, Boston, MA 1968-1972; **Fellow:** Surgery, Mass Genl Hosp, Boston, MA 1972-1973; **Fac Appt:** Clin Prof Surgery, UMDNJ-NJ Med Sch, Newark

Calligaro, Keith D MD (GVS) - *Spec Exp:* *Aneurysm-Abdominal Aortic;* **Hospital:** Pennsylvania Hosp (page 78); **Address:** 700 Spruce St, Ste 101, Philadelphia, PA 19106; **Phone:** (215) 829-5000; **Board Cert:** Surgery 1997, Vascular Surgery (General) 1990; **Med School:** Rutgers Univ 1982; **Resid:** Surgery, U Hlth Scis/Chicago Med. Sch, Chicago, IL 1984-1987; Surgery, St. Barnabas Med. Ctr., Livingston, NJ 1982-1984; **Fac Appt:** Assoc Clin Prof Surgery, Univ Penn

Cohen, Jon MD (GVS) - *Spec Exp:* *Aneurysm-Abdominal Aortic; Carotid Artery Surgery;* **Hospital:** Long Island Jewish Med Ctr; **Address:** LIJ Med Ctr, Vascular Surgery, 270-05 76th Ave, New Hyde Park, NY 11040; **Phone:** (718) 470-7377; **Board Cert:** Vascular Surgery (General) 1996, Surgery 1994; **Med School:** Univ Miami Sch Med 1979; **Resid:** Surgery, Cornell Med Ctr, New York, NY 1980-1984; Vascular Surgery (General), Brigham & Women's, Boston, MA 1984-1985; **Fellow:** Vascular Surgery (General), Brigham & Women's, Boston, MA 1984-1985; **Fac Appt:** Prof Surgery, Albert Einstein Coll Med

Comerota, Anthony J MD (GVS) - *Spec Exp:* *Endovascular Surgery;* **Hospital:** Temple Univ Hosp; **Address:** Temple Univ Hosp, Dept Surg, Broad & Ontario Sts, Parkinsons Pavilion- FL 14, Philadelphia, PA 19140; **Phone:** (215) 707-3622; **Board Cert:** Surgery 1987, Vascular Surgery (General) 1994; **Med School:** Temple Univ 1974; **Resid:** Surgery, Temple Univ Hosp, Philadelphia, PA 1974-1978; **Fellow:** Vascular Surgery (General), Good Samaritan Hosp, Cincinnati, OH 1979-1981; **Fac Appt:** Prof Surgery, Temple Univ

Dardik, Herbert MD (GVS) - *Spec Exp:* *Limb Salvage; Carotid Artery Surgery; Stroke;* **Hospital:** Englewood Hosp & Med Ctr; **Address:** 350 Engle St, Englewood, NJ 07631-1823; **Phone:** (201) 894-3698; **Board Cert:** Surgery 1966, Vascular Surgery (General) 1983; **Med School:** NYU Sch Med 1960; **Resid:** Surgery, Montefiore Hosp Med Ctr, Bronx, NY 1960-1965; **Fac Appt:** Clin Prof Surgery, Mount Sinai Sch Med

Darling, Ralph Clement MD (GVS) - *Spec Exp:* *Aneurysm-Abdominal Aortic; Carotid Artery Surgery;* **Hospital:** Albany Medical Center; **Address:** Albany Med Ctr, Vascular Inst, 47 New Scotland Ave, MC 157, Albany, NY 12208; **Phone:** (518) 262-5640; **Board Cert:** Surgery 1999, Vascular Surgery (General) 1995, Surgical Critical Care 1995; **Med School:** Univ Cincinnati 1984; **Resid:** Vascular Surgery (General), Havard-Deaconess Hosp, Boston, MA 1984-1989; **Fellow:** Vascular Surgery (General), Albany Med Ctr Hosp, Albany, NY 1990-1991; **Fac Appt:** Prof Surgery, Albany Med Coll

Fantini, Gary A MD (GVS) - *Spec Exp:* *Vein Disease; Wound Healing/Care; Thoracic Outlet Syndrome;* **Hospital:** NY Presby Hosp - NY Weill Cornell Med Ctr (page 70); **Address:** 635 Madison Ave Fl 7, New York, NY 10022; **Phone:** (212) 317-4550; **Board Cert:** Surgery 1999, Vascular Surgery (General) 1992; **Med School:** Albert Einstein Coll Med 1983; **Resid:** Surgery, NY Hosp-Cornell Med Ctr, New York, NY 1983-1989; **Fellow:** Vascular Surgery (General), UCSF Med Ctr, San Francisco, CA 1989-1990; **Fac Appt:** Assoc Prof Surgery, Cornell Univ-Weill Med Coll

Giangola, Gary MD (GVS) - *Spec Exp:* *Carotid Artery Surgery; Aneurysm-Aortic; Diabetic Leg/Foot;* **Hospital:** St Luke's - Roosevelt Hosp Ctr - Roosevelt Div (page 58); **Address:** 425 W 59th St, Ste 7B, New York, NY 10019-1104; **Phone:** (212) 523-8700; **Board Cert:** Surgery 1986, Vascular Surgery (General) 1988; **Med School:** NYU Sch Med 1980; **Resid:** Surgery, New York Univ Med Ctr, New York, NY 1981-1985; **Fellow:** Vascular Surgery (General), New York Univ Med Ctr, New York, NY 1985-1986; **Fac Appt:** Assoc Clin Prof Surgery, NYU Sch Med

Green, Richard M MD (GVS) - *Spec Exp:* *Aneurysm-Abdominal Aortic; Carotid Artery Surgery;* **Hospital:** Strong Memorial Hosp - URMC; **Address:** Univ Rochester, Dept Surg, 601 Elmwood Ave, Box 652, Rochester, NY 14642; **Phone:** (716) 275-6772; **Board Cert:** Surgery 1993, Vascular Surgery (General) 1993; **Med School:** Univ Rochester 1970; **Resid:** Surgery, Strong Meml Hosp, Rochester, NY 1971-1976; **Fac Appt:** Prof Surgery, Univ Rochester

VASCULAR SURGERY (GENERAL)

Harrington, Elizabeth MD (GVS) - ***Spec Exp:*** *Carotid Artery Surgery; Aneurysm-Aortic; Arterial Bypass Surgery-Leg;* **Hospital:** Mount Sinai Hosp (page 68); **Address:** 1225 Park Ave, Ste 1D, New York, NY 10128-1758; **Phone:** (212) 876-7400; **Board Cert:** Surgery 1999, Vascular Surgery (General) 1997; **Med School:** NY Med Coll 1975; **Resid:** Surgery, Mount Sinai Hosp, New York, NY 1975-1980; **Fellow:** Vascular Surgery (General), Mount Sinai Hosp, New York, NY 1980-1981; **Fac Appt:** Assoc Prof Vascular Surgery (General), Mount Sinai Sch Med

Hobson II, Robert Wayne MD (GVS) - ***Spec Exp:*** *Vascular Surgery (General) - General;* **Hospital:** Saint Michael's Med Ctr; **Address:** UMDNJ-New Jersey Med Sch, Bldg 6, 30 Bergen St, rm 620, Newark, NJ 07107; **Phone:** (973) 972-6633; **Board Cert:** Surgery 1972, Vascular Surgery (General) 1992; **Med School:** Geo Wash Univ 1963; **Resid:** Surgery, Walter Reed AMC, Washington, DC 1967-1971; **Fellow:** Vascular Surgery (General), Walter Reed AMC, Washington, DC 1972-1973; **Fac Appt:** Prof Surgery, UMDNJ-NJ Med Sch, Newark

Hollier, Larry Harold MD (GVS) - ***Spec Exp:*** *Aortic Surgery; Carotid Artery Surgery; Endovascular Surgery;* **Hospital:** Mount Sinai Hosp (page 68); **Address:** 5 E 98th St, Fl 14th, Box 1263, New York, NY 10029; **Phone:** (212) 241-7646; **Board Cert:** Surgery 1976, Vascular Surgery (General) 1983; **Med School:** Louisiana State Univ 1968; **Resid:** Surgery, Charity Hosp, New Orleans, LA 1968-1973; **Fellow:** Vascular Surgery (General), Baylor Med Ctr, Dallas, TX 1973-1974; **Fac Appt:** Prof Surgery, Mount Sinai Sch Med

Kent, K Craig MD (GVS) - ***Spec Exp:*** *Carotid Artery Disease; Endovascular Surgery-Abdominal Aneurys; Lower Limb Arterial Disease;* **Hospital:** NY Presby Hosp - NY Weill Cornell Med Ctr (page 70); **Address:** 530 E 70th St, rm M014, New York, NY 10021-9800; **Phone:** (212) 746-5192; **Board Cert:** Surgery 1997, Vascular Surgery (General) 1998; **Med School:** UCSF 1981; **Resid:** Surgery, UCSF Med Ctr, San Francisco, CA 1981-1986; **Fellow:** Vascular Surgery (General), Brigham & Women's Hosp, Boston, MA 1986-1988; **Fac Appt:** Prof Vascular Surgery (General), Cornell Univ-Weill Med Coll

Makaroun, Michel MD (GVS) - ***Spec Exp:*** *Endovascular Surgery; Aneurysm; Carotid Artery Disease;* **Hospital:** UPMC - Presbyterian Univ Hosp; **Address:** Presby-Univ Hosp. A-1011, Pittsburgh, PA 15213; **Phone:** (412) 648-4000; **Board Cert:** Surgery 1993, Vascular Surgery (General) 1998; **Med School:** Lebanon 1978; **Resid:** Surgery, Anerican U Hosp., Lebanon 1978-1980; Surgery, U Pittsburgh, Pittsburgh, PA 1980-1985; **Fac Appt:** Prof Surgery, Univ Pittsburgh

Perler, Bruce Alan MD (GVS) - ***Spec Exp:*** *Carotid Artery Surgery; Aneurysm; Stroke;* **Hospital:** Johns Hopkins Hosp - Baltimore; **Address:** Johns Hopkins Hosp-Surg, 600 N Wolfe St, Bldg Harvey - Ste 611, Baltimore, MD 21287-8611; **Phone:** (410) 955-2618; **Board Cert:** Vascular Surgery (General) 1997, Surgery 1982; **Med School:** Duke Univ 1976; **Resid:** Surgery, Mass Genl Hosp, Boston, MA 1976-1981; **Fellow:** Vascular Surgery (General), Mass Genl Hosp, Boston, MA 1981-1982; **Fac Appt:** Prof Surgery, Johns Hopkins Univ

Ricotta, John MD (GVS) - ***Spec Exp:*** *Aneurysm; Carotid Artery Surgery;* **Hospital:** Stony Brook Univ Hosp; **Address:** SUNY Dept Surgery, HSC, Fl 19 - rm 020, Stony Brook, NY 11794-8191; **Phone:** (631) 444-7875; **Board Cert:** Surgery 2000, Vascular Surgery (General) 1995; **Med School:** Johns Hopkins Univ 1973; **Resid:** Surgery, Johns Hopkins Hosp, Baltimore, MD 1973-1977; **Fellow:** Surgery, Johns Hopkins Hosp, Baltimore, MD 1977-1979; **Fac Appt:** Prof Surgery, SUNY Stony Brook

Riles, Thomas MD (GVS) - ***Spec Exp:*** *Aneurysm-Abdominal Aortic; Carotid Artery Surgery;* **Hospital:** NYU Med Ctr (page 71); **Address:** NYU Med Ctr, Univ Vascular Assoc, 530 1st Ave, Fl 6F, New York, NY 10016; **Phone:** (212) 263-7311; **Board Cert:** Vascular Surgery (General) 1992, Surgery 1990; **Med School:** Baylor Coll Med 1969; **Resid:** Surgery, NYU Med Ctr, New York, NY 1970-1976; **Fellow:** Vascular Surgery (General), NYU Med Ctr, New York, NY 1976-1977; **Fac Appt:** Prof Surgery, NYU Sch Med

Shah, Dhiraj MD (GVS) - *Spec Exp:* Carotid Artery Surgery; **Hospital:** Albany Medical Center; **Address:** Albany Med Coll-Dept Surg, 47 New Scotland Ave MC 157, Albany, NY 12208-3412; **Phone:** (518) 262-5640; **Board Cert:** Vascular Surgery (General) 1983, Surgery 1977; **Med School:** Bangladesh 1965; **Resid:** Surgery, St Peters Hosp, Albany, NY 1971-1975; **Fellow:** Research, Albany Med Ctr, Albany, NY 1975-1976; **Fac Appt:** Prof Surgery, Albany Med Coll

Steed, David Luther MD (GVS) - *Spec Exp:* Wound Healing/Care; **Hospital:** UPMC - Presbyterian Univ Hosp; **Address:** 200 Lothrop St Bldg PUH - rm A-1011, Pittsburgh, PA 15213; **Phone:** (412) 648-4000; **Board Cert:** Vascular Surgery (General) 1997, Surgical Critical Care 1995; **Med School:** Univ Pittsburgh 1973; **Resid:** Surgery, Univ Pitts Med Ctr, Pittsburgh, PA 1974-1976; Surgery, Univ Pitts Med Ctr, Pittsburgh, PA 1977-1980; **Fellow:** Thoracic Surgery, UCLA Med Ctr, Los Angeles, CA 1976-1977; **Fac Appt:** Prof Surgery, Univ Pittsburgh

Todd, George MD (GVS) - *Spec Exp:* Minimally Invasive Vascular Surgery; Aneurysm-Abdominal Aortic; **Hospital:** St Luke's - Roosevelt Hosp Ctr - Roosevelt Div (page 58); **Address:** St Luke's-Roosevelt Hosp Ctr, Dept Surgery, 1000 10th Ave, Fl 5 - rm RG77, New York, NY 10019; **Phone:** (212) 523-7481; **Board Cert:** Surgery 1980, Vascular Surgery (General) 1986; **Med School:** Penn State Univ-Hershey Med Ctr 1974; **Resid:** Vascular Surgery (General), Columbia-Presby, New York, NY 1974-1979; **Fellow:** Vascular Surgery (General), Columbia-Presby, New York, NY 1979-1980; **Fac Appt:** Prof Surgery, Columbia P&S

Turner, James MD (GVS) - *Spec Exp:* Esophageal Varices; Laparoscopic Surgery; **Hospital:** NY Hosp Med Ctr of Queens; **Address:** 56-45 Main St, Flushing, NY 11355; **Phone:** (718) 445-0220; **Board Cert:** Surgery 1995, Surgical Critical Care 1995; **Med School:** Eastern VA Med Sch 1970; **Resid:** Surgery, NYU Med Ctr, New York, NY 1970-1975; **Fac Appt:** Assoc Clin Prof Surgery, Cornell Univ-Weill Med Coll

Veith, Frank James MD (GVS) - *Spec Exp:* Limb Salvage; Aneurysm-Aortic; Endovascular Surgery; **Hospital:** Montefiore Med Ctr (page 67); **Address:** Montefiore Med Ctr-Vascular, 111 E 210th St, Bronx, NY 10467-2490; **Phone:** (718) 920-4757; **Board Cert:** Surgery 1961, Vascular Surgery (General) 1991, Thoracic Surgery 1968; **Med School:** Cornell Univ-Weill Med Coll 1955; **Resid:** Surgery, Peter Bent Brigham Hosp, Boston, MA 1955-1960; **Fellow:** Vascular Surgery (General), Harvard Med, Cambridge, MA 1962-1963; **Fac Appt:** Prof Surgery, Albert Einstein Coll Med

Webster Jr., Marshall W. MD (GVS) - *Spec Exp:* Thoracic Vascular Surgery; **Hospital:** UPMC - Presbyterian Univ Hosp; **Address:** 200 Lothrop St, Ste A-1011, Pittsburgh, PA 15213; **Phone:** (412) 648-4000; **Board Cert:** Surgery 1971, Vascular Surgery (General) 1971; **Med School:** Johns Hopkins Univ 1964; **Resid:** Surgery, U Pittsburgh, Pittsburgh, PA 1965-1970; **Fac Appt:** Prof Surgery, Univ Pittsburgh

Williams, G. Melville MD (GVS) - *Spec Exp:* Peripheral Vascular Surgery; Aneurysm-Abdominal Aortic; **Hospital:** Johns Hopkins Hosp - Baltimore; **Address:** 600 N Wolfe St Bldg Harvey - Ste 611, Baltimore, MD 21287; **Phone:** (410) 955-5165; **Board Cert:** Vascular Surgery (General) 1994, Surgery 1966; **Med School:** Harvard Med Sch 1957; **Resid:** Surgery, Mass Genl Hosp, Boston, MA 1962-1964; Surgery, Mass Genl Hosp, Boston, MA 1958-1960; **Fac Appt:** Prof Surgery, Johns Hopkins Univ

Southeast

Bandyk, Dennis MD (GVS) - ***Spec Exp:*** *Vascular Graft Infection; Infrainguinal Bypass;* **Hospital:** Tampa Genl Hosp; **Address:** Harborside Med Tower, 4 Columbia Dr, Ste 650, Tampa, FL 33606; **Phone:** (813) 259-0921; **Board Cert:** Vascular Surgery (General) 1991, Surgery 1988; **Med School:** Univ Mich Med Sch 1975; **Resid:** Surgery, Univ Wash Hosp, Seattle, WA 1976-1980; **Fellow:** Vascular Surgery (General), Univ Wash Hosp, Seattle, WA 1980-1981; **Fac Appt:** Prof Surgery, Univ S Fla Coll Med

Dean, Richard H MD (GVS) - ***Spec Exp:*** *Hypertension-Renovascular;* **Hospital:** Wake Forest Univ Baptist Med Ctr (page 81); **Address:** Wake Forest Univ Sch Med, Med Center Blvd, Winston Salem, NC 27157-1003; **Phone:** (336) 716-4424; **Board Cert:** Surgery 1975, Vascular Surgery (General) 1983; **Med School:** Med Coll VA 1968; **Resid:** Surgery, Vanderbilt Univ Hosp, Nashville, TN 1969-1974; **Fellow:** Vascular Surgery (General), Northwestern Univ Hosp, Chicago, IL 1974-1975; **Fac Appt:** Prof Surgery, Wake Forest Univ Sch Med

Flynn, Timothy Carlyle MD (GVS) - ***Spec Exp:*** *Aneurysm; Carotid Artery Surgery;* **Hospital:** Shands Hlthcre at Univ of FL (page 73); **Address:** Shands Hlthcare Univ FL, Dept Surg, PO Box 100286, Gainesville, FL 32610-0286; **Phone:** (352) 374-6013; **Board Cert:** Vascular Surgery (General) 1994, Surgical Critical Care 1998; **Med School:** Baylor Coll Med 1974; **Resid:** Surgery, Univ Texas, Houston, TX 1977-1980; **Fac Appt:** Prof Surgery, Univ Fla Coll Med

Hansen, Kimberley J MD (GVS) - ***Spec Exp:*** *Aortic & Visceral Artery Reconstruction; Renovascular Disease; Carotid Artery Surgery;* **Hospital:** Wake Forest Univ Baptist Med Ctr (page 81); **Address:** Wake Forest Univ Sch Med, Dept Genl Surg, Medical Center Blvd, Winston-Salem, NC 27157-1095; **Phone:** (336) 716-4151; **Board Cert:** Vascular Surgery (General) 1998, Surgical Critical Care 1992; **Med School:** Univ Ala 1980

Keagy, Blair Allen MD (GVS) - ***Spec Exp:*** *Mesenteric Occlusive Disease;* **Hospital:** Univ of NC Hosp (page 77); **Address:** Univ North Carolina Hosp, Bldg Burnett-Womack - rm 210, Chapel Hill, NC 27599; **Phone:** (919) 966-3391; **Board Cert:** Vascular Surgery (General) 1998, Surgery 1989; **Med School:** Univ Pittsburgh 1970; **Resid:** Surgery, Univ North Carolina, Chapel Hill, NC 1971-1977; **Fellow:** Vascular Surgery (General), Univ North Carolina, Chapel Hill, NC 1978; **Fac Appt:** Prof Thoracic Surgery, Univ NC Sch Med

Lumsden, Alan Boyd MD (GVS) (relocated to Houston, TX) - ***Spec Exp:*** *Aortic Stent Grafts; Minimally Invasive Surgery;* **Hospital:** Methodist Hosp - Houston, St Luke's Episcopal Hosp - Houston; **Address:** 6550 Fannin St, Ste 1661, Houston, TX 77030; **Phone:** (713) 798-5700; **Board Cert:** Vascular Surgery (General) 1993, Surgery 1990; **Med School:** Scotland 1981; **Resid:** Surgery, Emory Univ Hosp, Atlanta, GA 1983-1989; **Fellow:** Vascular Surgery (General), Emory Univ Hosp, Atlanta, GA 1990; **Fac Appt:** Prof Vascular Surgery (General), Emory Univ

McCann, Richard L MD (GVS) - ***Spec Exp:*** *Vascular Surgery (General) - General;* **Hospital:** Duke Univ Med Ctr (page 60); **Address:** Duke Univ Med Ctr, Box 2990, Durham, NC 27710; **Phone:** (919) 684-2620; **Board Cert:** Surgery 1992, Vascular Surgery (General) 1996; **Med School:** Cornell Univ-Weill Med Coll 1974; **Resid:** Surgery, Duke Univ Med Ctr, Durham, NC 1975-1983; **Fac Appt:** Prof Surgery, Duke Univ

Rosenthal, David MD (GVS) - ***Spec Exp:*** *Stroke; Aneurysm;* **Hospital:** Atlanta Med Ctr; **Address:** 315 Blvd NE, Ste 412, Atlanta, GA 30312; **Phone:** (404) 524-0095; **Board Cert:** Vascular Surgery (General) 1991; **Med School:** SUNY Downstate 1973; **Resid:** Surgery, Tufts-New Eng Med Ctr, Boston, MA 1973-1977; **Fellow:** Vascular Surgery (General), Tufts-New Eng Med Ctr, Boston, MA 1977-1978; **Fac Appt:** Clin Prof Surgery, Med Coll GA

eeger, James M MD (GVS) - *Spec Exp:* *Lower Limb Arterial Disease; Aneurysm-Aortic;* **ospital:** Shands Hlthcre at Univ of FL (page 73); **Address:** Univ FL, Dept Vasc Surg, 1600 SW rcher Rd, Bldg JHMHC - rm 6165, Box 100286, Gainesville, FL 32610-0286; **Phone:** (352) 265-0605; **oard Cert:** Surgery 1990, Vascular Surgery (General) 1992; **Med School:** Med Coll GA 1973; **esid:** Surgery, Univ UT Med Ctr, Salt Lake City, UT; **Fellow:** Vascular Surgery (General), Eastern A Med Sch, Norfolk, VA; **Fac Appt:** Prof Surgery, Univ Fla Coll Med

ivina, Manuel MD (GVS) - *Spec Exp:* *Vascular Surgery (General) - General;* **Hospital:** Mount nai Med Ctr; **Address:** 4300 Alton Rd Bldg Greenspan - Ste 212A, Miami Beach, FL 33140-2800; **hone:** (305) 674-2760; **Board Cert:** Surgery 1987; **Med School:** Peru 1969; **Resid:** Surgery, Mt Sinai led Ctr, Miami Beach, FL 1970-1975; **Fellow:** Vascular Surgery (General), Mt Sinai Med Ctr, liami Beach, FL 1975-1976

Midwest

aker, William MD (GVS) - *Spec Exp:* *Carotid Artery Surgery; Aneurysm-Abdominal Aortic;* **ospital:** Loyola Univ Med Ctr; **Address:** Loyola Univ Med Ctr, 2160 S 1st Ave, Fl 3, Maywood, IL 0153-5590; **Phone:** (708) 327-2685; **Board Cert:** Surgery 1970, Vascular Surgery (General) 1991; **led School:** Univ Chicago-Pritzker Sch Med 1962; **Resid:** Surgery, Univ Iowa Hosp, Iowa City, IA 963-1964; Surgery, U Chicago Hosp-Clin, Chicago, IL 1966-1969; **Fellow:** Vascular Surgery General), U Calif, San Francisco, CA 1969-1970; **Fac Appt:** Prof Surgery, Loyola Univ-Stritch Sch led

eebe, Hugh Grenville MD (GVS) - *Spec Exp:* *Endovascular Surgery;* **Hospital:** Toledo Hosp; **ddress:** 2109 Hughes Drive, Ste 400, Toledo, OH 43606; **Phone:** (419) 471-2088; **Board Cert:** urgery 1971, Vascular Surgery (General) 1995; **Med School:** Univ Rochester 1964; **Resid:** Surgery, trong Meml Hosp, Rochester, NY 1965-1969; **Fac Appt:** Clin Prof Surgery, Univ Mich Med Sch

erguer, Ramon MD/PhD (GVS) - *Spec Exp:* *Cerebrovascular Disease; Aortic Branch Surgery;* *horacic Aortic Surgery;* **Hospital:** Harper Hosp (page 59); **Address:** DMC-WSU Harper Hosp. ept. Vascular Surgery, 3990 John R, Detroit, MI 48201; **Phone:** (313) 745-8637; **Board Cert:** ascular Surgery (General) 1983, Surgery 1970; **Med School:** Spain 1963; **Resid:** Surgery, Henry ord Hospital, Detroit, MI 1964-1969; **Fellow:** Vascular Surgery (General), Henry Ford Hosp, etroit, MI 1969-1970; **Fac Appt:** Prof Surgery, Wayne State Univ

herry Jr., Kenneth J. MD (GVS) - *Spec Exp:* *Vascular Reconstruction; Aortic Graft Infection;* **ospital:** St Mary's Hosp - Rochester, MN; **Address:** Mayo Clinic-Rochester, Div Vasc Surg, 200 irst St SW, Rochester, MN; **Phone:** (507) 284-2644; **Board Cert:** Surgery 1981, Vascular Surgery General) 1993; **Med School:** Univ VA Sch Med 1974; **Resid:** Surgery, Univ VA Hosp, harlottesville, VA 1975-1980; Vascular Surgery (General), Univ California San Fran Med Ctr, San rancisco, CA 1980-1981; **Fac Appt:** Prof Surgery, Mayo Med Sch

orson, John MD (GVS) - *Spec Exp:* *Carotid Artery Surgery; Vascular Disease in the Elderly;* *imb Salvage;* **Hospital:** Univ of IA Hosp and Clinics; **Address:** Univ Iowa Hosps, Div Vas Surg, 200 lawkins Drive Bldg JCP 1537, Iowa City, IA 52242-1009; **Phone:** (319) 356-1639; **Board Cert:** urgery 1991, Vascular Surgery (General) 1992; **Med School:** Scotland 1968; **Resid:** Surgery, Univ losp Wales, Cardiff, Wales, UK 1971-1975; Surgery, Boston Univ Med Ctr, Boston, MA 1977-1980; **ellow:** Vascular Research, Boston Univ Med Ctr, Boston, MA 1975-1977; Vascular Surgery General), Mass Genl Hosp/Harvard, Boston, MA 1980-1981; **Fac Appt:** Prof Surgery, Univ Iowa oll Med

Gewertz, Bruce MD (GVS) - *Spec Exp:* Carotid Artery Surgery; Peripheral Vascular Surgery; Aneurysm-Aortic; **Hospital:** Univ of Chicago Hosps (page 76); **Address:** Univ Chicago, Dept Vascular Surgery, 5841 S Maryland Ave, Bldg SBRI - rm J557, MC-5028, Chicago, IL 60637-1463; **Phone:** (773) 702-6128; **Board Cert:** Vascular Surgery (General) 1993; **Med School:** Jefferson Med Coll 1972; **Resid:** Surgery, Univ Mich Hosp, Ann Arbor, MI 1972-1977; **Fac Appt:** Prof Surgery, Univ Chicago-Pritzker Sch Med

Gloviczki, Peter MD (GVS) - *Spec Exp:* Aneurysm-Abdominal Aortic; Ischemia-Critical Limb; Vein Disorders; **Hospital:** Mayo Med Ctr & Clin - Rochester, MN; **Address:** Mayo Clin, Div Vasc Surg, West 6B, 200 First Street SW, Rochester, MN 55905-0001; **Phone:** (507) 284-4652; **Board Cert:** Surgery 1988, Vascular Surgery (General) 1989; **Med School:** Hungary 1972; **Resid:** Vascular Surgery (General), Semmelweis Med Sch, Budapest,Hungary 1977-1980; Surgery, Mayo Clin, Rochester, MN 1984-1987; **Fellow:** Vascular Surgery (General), Mayo Clin, Rochester, MN 1983; **Fac Appt:** Prof Surgery, Mayo Med Sch

Greenfield, Lazar MD (GVS) - *Spec Exp:* Pulmonary Embolism; Deep Venous Thrombosis; Carotid Artery Surgery; **Hospital:** Univ of MI Hlth Ctr; **Address:** 1500 E Medical Center Drive, Box TC2320, Ann Arbor, MI 48109-0346; **Phone:** (734) 936-5850; **Board Cert:** Thoracic Surgery 1967, Surgery 1980; **Med School:** Baylor Coll Med 1958; **Resid:** Johns Hopkins Hosp, Baltimore, MD 1961-1966; **Fellow:** Natl Heart Inst, Washington, DC 1959-1961; **Fac Appt:** Prof Surgery, Univ Mich Med Sch

Hertzer, Norman Ray MD (GVS) - *Spec Exp:* Carotid Artery Surgery; Aneurysm-Abdominal Aortic; **Hospital:** Cleveland Clin Fdn (page 57); **Address:** 9500 Euclid Ave, Ste S-61, Cleveland, OH 44195-0001; **Phone:** (216) 444-5705; **Board Cert:** Vascular Surgery (General) 1993, Surgery 1973; **Med School:** Indiana Univ 1967; **Resid:** Vascular Surgery (General), Cleveland Clin Hosp, Cleveland, OH 1974-1975; Surgery, Cleveland Clin Hosp, Cleveland, OH 1968-1972

Hodgson, Kim John MD (GVS) - *Spec Exp:* Aneurysm; Carotid Angioplasty; Endovascular Surgery; **Hospital:** St John's Hosp - Springfield; **Address:** 800 N Rutledge, Ste D346, Springfield, IL 62702; **Phone:** (217) 545-8856; **Board Cert:** Vascular Surgery (General) 1995, Surgery 1995; **Med School:** Univ Penn 1981; **Resid:** Surgery, Albany Med Ctr, Albany, NY 1982-1986; **Fellow:** Vascular Surgery (General), Southern Ill Univ, Springfield, IL 1986-1987; **Fac Appt:** Prof Vascular Surgery (General), Southern IL Univ

Merrick III, Hollis W. MD (GVS) - *Spec Exp:* Vascular Surgery (General) - General; **Hospital:** Med Coll of Ohio Hosps; **Address:** 3065 Arlington Ave, Toledo, OH 43614-2570; **Phone:** (419) 383-4421; **Board Cert:** Surgery 1988; **Med School:** McGill Univ 1964; **Resid:** Surgery, Royal Victoria Hospital, Montreal, CN 1967-1972; **Fac Appt:** Prof Surgery, Med Coll OH

Ouriel, Kenneth MD (GVS) - *Spec Exp:* Thrombolytic Therapy; **Hospital:** Cleveland Clin Fdn (page 57); **Address:** 9500 Euclid Ave/Desk S61, Cleveland, OH 44195; **Phone:** (216) 445-3464; **Board Cert:** Vascular Surgery (General) 1995, Surgery 1995; **Med School:** Univ Chicago-Pritzker Sch Med 1981; **Resid:** Vascular Surgery (General), Strong Meml Hosp-Univ Roch, Rochester, MN 1982-1986; **Fellow:** Vascular Surgery (General), Strong Meml Hosp-Univ Roch, Rochester, MN 1986-1987

Pearce, William MD (GVS) - *Spec Exp:* Aneurysm-Abdominal Aortic; Stroke; Claudication; **Hospital:** Northwestern Meml Hosp; **Address:** Northwestern Meml Hosp - Galter Pavilion, 675 N St Clair St, Ste 19-100, Chicago, IL 60611-2647; **Phone:** (312) 695-2714; **Board Cert:** Vascular Surgery (General) 1992, Surgical Critical Care 1999; **Med School:** Univ Colo 1975; **Resid:** Internal Medicine, Mayo Grad Sch Med/Mayo Fdn, Rochester, MN 1975-1976; Surgery, Univ Co Hlth Sci Ctr, Denver, CO 1976-1980; **Fellow:** Cardiology (Cardiovascular Disease), Northwestern Meml Hosp, Chicago, IL 1981-1982; **Fac Appt:** Prof Surgery, Northwestern Univ

eddy, Daniel MD (GVS) - *Spec Exp:* Aneurysm-Aortic; Carotid Artery Surgery; **Hospital:** Henry ord Hosp; **Address:** Henry Ford Hosp, Dept Vascular Surgery, 2799 W Grand Blvd, Detroit, MI 8202-2608; **Phone:** (313) 916-3156; **Board Cert:** Surgery 1998, Vascular Surgery (General) 1991; **Med School:** Univ Mich Med Sch 1973; **Resid:** Vascular Surgery (General), Wayne State Univ, etroit, MI 1974-1978; **Fellow:** Vascular Surgery (General), Wayne State Univ, Detroit, MI 1978-979

hepard, Alexander D MD (GVS) - *Spec Exp:* Arterial Bypass Surgery-Leg; **Hospital:** Henry ord Hosp; **Address:** 2799 W Grand Blvd, Detroit, MI 48202; **Phone:** (313) 916-3155; **Board Cert:** urgery 1992, Vascular Surgery (General) 1994; **Med School:** Johns Hopkins Univ 1976; **Resid:** urgery, Johns Hopkins Hosp, Baltimore, MD 1976-1982; **Fellow:** Vascular Surgery (General), New ngland Med Ctr, Boston, MA 1983-1985; **Fac Appt:** Asst Prof Surgery, Johns Hopkins Univ

icard, Gregorio Arquel MD (GVS) - *Spec Exp:* Aneurysm-Abdominal Aortic; **Hospital:** arnes-Jewish Hosp (page 55); **Address:** CB8109 660 S Euclid Ave, St Louis, MO 63110; **Phone:** 314) 362-7841; **Board Cert:** Vascular Surgery (General) 1992, Surgery 1996; **Med School:** Univ uerto Rico 1972; **Resid:** Surgery, Barnes Hosp, St Louis, MO 1973-1977; **Fellow:** Transplant urgery, Wash Univ Hosp, St Louis, MO 1977-1978; **Fac Appt:** Prof Surgery, Washington Univ, St ouis

tanley, James MD (GVS) - *Spec Exp:* Peripheral Vascular Surgery; Renovascular Disease; **lospital:** Univ of MI Hlth Ctr; **Address:** Univ Hosp, Dept Vasc Surg, 1500 E Med Ctr Drive Bldg TC - te 2210, Ann Arbor, MI 48109-0329; **Phone:** (734) 936-5786; **Board Cert:** Surgery 1973, Vascular urgery (General) 1991; **Med School:** Univ Mich Med Sch 1964; **Resid:** Surgery, Univ Mich Med :tr, Ann Arbor, MI 1967-1972; **Fac Appt:** Prof Surgery, Univ Mich Med Sch

owne, Jonathan MD (GVS) - *Spec Exp:* Peripheral Vascular Surgery; Thoracic Outlet yndrome; **Hospital:** Froedtert Meml Lutheran Hosp; **Address:** Med Coll Wisconsin, 9200 W Visconsin Ave, Milwaukee, WI 53226; **Phone:** (414) 456-6970; **Board Cert:** Surgery 1973, Vascular urgery (General) 1991; **Med School:** Univ Rochester 1967; **Resid:** Surgery, Univ Mich Med Ctr, Michigan, MI 1968-1969; Surgery, Univ Nebraska Coll Med, Nebraska, WI 1969-1972; **Fellow:** 'ascular Surgery (General), Baylor Coll Med, Houston, TX 1974-1975; **Fac Appt:** Prof Vascular urgery (General), Med Coll Wisc

'ao, James MD (GVS) - *Spec Exp:* Peripheral vascular disease; Sports injuries; **Hospital:** Jorthwestern Meml Hosp; **Address:** 675 N St Clair St, Ste 19-100, Chicago, IL 60611; **Phone:** (312) 95-2714; **Board Cert:** Vascular Surgery (General) 1983, Surgery 1967; **Med School:** Taiwan 1961; **esid:** Surgery, Cook Co Hosp, Chicago, IL 1962-1967; **Fellow:** Vascular Surgery (General), St Mary's Hosp, London, England 1967-1968; **Fac Appt:** Prof Surgery, Northwestern Univ

Southwest

Clagett, George Patrick MD (GVS) - *Spec Exp:* Aneurysm-Abdominal Aortic; **Hospital:** Parkland Mem Hosp; **Address:** Univ Tex SW Med Ctr, 5323 Harry Hines Blvd, Dallas, TX 75390-9157; **Phone:** (214) 648-3516; **Board Cert:** Surgery 1996, Vascular Surgery (General) 1991; **Med School:** Jniv VA Sch Med **Resid:** Surgery, Univ Mich, Ann Harbor, MI 1974-1976; **Fellow:** Vascular Surgery General), Walter Reed Army Med Ctr, Washington, DC 1978-1979; Research, Harvard Med Sch, 3oston, MA 1972-1974; **Fac Appt:** Prof Surgery, Univ Tex SW, Dallas

Eidt, John MD (GVS) - *Spec Exp:* Arterial Bypass Surgery; Critical Care; **Hospital:** UAMS; **Address:** 4301 W Markham St, Slot 520-2, Little Rock, AR 72205; **Phone:** (501) 686-6176; **Board :ert:** Vascular Surgery (General) 1996, Surgical Critical Care 1990; **Med School:** Univ Tex SW,)allas 1981; **Resid:** Surgery, Brigham-Womens Hosp, Boston, MA 1981-1986; **Fellow:** Vascular urgery (General), Univ Tex SW Med Ctr, Dallas, TX 1987; **Fac Appt:** Assoc Prof Surgery, Univ Ark

VASCULAR SURGERY (GENERAL)

Money, Samuel MD (GVS) - *Spec Exp:* Aneurysm-Abdominal Aortic; Arterial Bypass Surgery-Leg; Endovascular Surgery; **Hospital:** Ochsner Found Hosp; **Address:** Department of Surgery, 1514 Jefferson Hwy, New Orleans, LA 70121-2429; **Phone:** (504) 842-4070; **Board Cert:** Surgery 1991, Vascular Surgery (General) 1995; **Med School:** SUNY Downstate 1983; **Resid:** Surgery, Kings Co Med Ctr, Brooklyn, NY 1983-1990; **Fellow:** Vascular Surgery (General), Ochsner Clinic, New Orleans, LA 1991-1993; **Fac Appt:** Assoc Clin Prof Surgery, Tulane Univ

West Coast and Pacific

Ahn, Samuel S MD (GVS) - *Spec Exp:* Thoracic Outlet Syndrome; **Hospital:** UCLA Med Ctr; **Address:** UCLA Med Ctr, 200 UCLA Medical Plaza, Ste 526, Los Angeles, CA 90095; **Phone:** (310) 206-3885; **Board Cert:** Surgery 1994, Vascular Surgery (General) 1997; **Med School:** Univ Tex SW, Dallas 1978; **Resid:** Surgery, UCLA Med Ctr, Los Angeles, CA 1979-1984; **Fellow:** Vascular Surgery (General), UCLA Med Ctr, Los Angeles, CA 1984-1986; **Fac Appt:** Prof Surgery, UCLA

Andros, George MD (GVS) - *Spec Exp:* Aneurysm-Aortic; Carotid Artery Surgery; **Hospital:** Providence St Joseph Med Ctr; **Address:** 2701 W Alameda Ave, Ste 606, Encino, CA 91505-4402; **Phone:** (818) 845-7242; **Board Cert:** Surgery 1970, Vascular Surgery (General) 1983; **Med School:** Univ Chicago-Pritzker Sch Med 1960; **Resid:** Surgery, Mass Genl Hosp, Boston, MA 1965-1969

Bergan, John Jerome MD (GVS) - *Spec Exp:* Vein Disease; Vein Disease/Leg Ulcers; **Hospital:** Scripps Meml Hosp - La Jolla; **Address:** 9850 Genesee Ave, Ste 410, La Jolla, CA 92037-1229; **Phone:** (858) 550-0330; **Board Cert:** Vascular Surgery (General) 1991, Surgery 1960; **Med School:** Indiana Univ 1954; **Resid:** Surgery, Northwestern Meml Hosp, Chicago, IL 1955-1959; **Fac Appt:** Prof Surgery, UCSD

Flanigan, Preston D. MD (GVS) - *Spec Exp:* Aneurysm-Abdominal Aortic; **Hospital:** St Joseph's Hosp - Orange; **Address:** 1310 W Stewart Dr, Ste 407, Orange, CA 92868-3855; **Phone:** (714) 997-4961; **Board Cert:** Surgery 1978, Vascular Surgery (General) 1983; **Med School:** Jefferson Med Coll 1972; **Resid:** Surgery, St Joseph-Mercy Hosp, Ann Arbor, MI 1974-1977; **Fellow:** Vascular Surgery (General), Northwest Med Ctr 1977-1978; **Fac Appt:** Clin Prof Surgery, UC Irvine

Grey, Douglas P MD (GVS) - *Spec Exp:* Vascular Surgery (General) - General; **Hospital:** KFH San Francisco Med Ctr; **Address:** 2238 Geary Blvd, Fl 2, San Francisco, CA 94115; **Phone:** (415) 833-3383; **Board Cert:** Thoracic Surgery 1993, Vascular Surgery (General) 1993; **Med School:** UC Irvine 1975; **Resid:** Surgery, Peter Bent Brigham Hosp, Boston, MA 1976-1980; Thoracic Surgery, Texas Heart Inst, Houston, TX 1980-1982; **Fac Appt:** Clin Prof Surgery, UCSF

Johansen, Kaj MD/PhD (GVS) - *Spec Exp:* Portal Hypertension; Trauma; Vascular Access; **Hospital:** Swedish Med Ctr Providence Campus; **Address:** 1600 E Jefferson St, Ste 110, Seattle, WA 98122; **Phone:** (206) 860-5945; **Board Cert:** Surgery 1979, Vascular Surgery (General) 1983; **Med School:** Univ Wash 1970; **Resid:** Surgery, UCSD, San Diego, CA 1975-1978; Surgery, UCSD, San Diego, CA 1971-1972; **Fellow:** Vascular Surgery (General), UCSD, San Diego, CA 1972-1977; **Fac Appt:** Prof Surgery, Univ Wash

Moore, Wesley Sanford MD (GVS) - *Spec Exp:* Aneurysm-Abdominal Aortic; Carotid Artery Surgery; Arterial Reconstruction; **Hospital:** UCLA Med Ctr; **Address:** Dept Surgery, Box 956904, Los Angeles, CA 90095-6904; **Phone:** (310) 825-9641; **Board Cert:** Surgery 1966, Vascular & Interventional Radiology 1983; **Med School:** UCSF 1959; **Resid:** Surgery, Univ California San Fran Med Ctr, San Francisco, CA 1960-1964; **Fellow:** Research, VA Hosp-Natl Inst Hlth, San Francisco, CA 1966-1967; **Fac Appt:** Prof Surgery, UCLA

bel, Michael MD (GVS) - *Spec Exp:* Carotid Artery Surgery; Vein Disease; **Hospital:** Puget ound Hosp; **Address:** East Side Specialty Clinic, 1700 116th Ave NE, Bellevue, WA 98004; **Phone:** (25) 646-7777; **Board Cert:** Vascular Surgery (General) 1996, Surgery 1992; **Med School:** Albert nstein Coll Med 1975; **Resid:** Surgery, Beth Israel Hosp/Harvard, Boston, MA 1976-1982; **Fellow:** ascular Surgery (General), NYU Med Ctr, New York, NY 1982-1983; **Fac Appt:** Prof Surgery, Univ Vash

aylor, Lloyd M MD (GVS) - *Spec Exp:* Vascular Surgery (General) - General; **Hospital:** OR Hlth ci Univ Hosp and Clinics; **Address:** 3181 SW Sam Jackson Park Rd, MC OP-11, Portland, OR 7201; **Phone:** (503) 494-7593; **Board Cert:** Vascular Surgery (General) 1987, Surgery 1983; **Med chool:** Duke Univ 1973; **Resid:** Surgery, U Oreg Hlth Sci Ctr, Portland, OR 1977-1981; Surgery, U Oreg Hlth Sci Ctr, Portland, OR 1981-1982; **Fellow:** Vascular Surgery (General), Oreg Hlth Sci U, ortland, OR 1982-1983; **Fac Appt:** Prof Surgery, Oregon Hlth Scis Univ

Vhite, Rodney Allen MD (GVS) - *Spec Exp:* Vascular Surgery; Aneurysm; **Hospital:** LAC - larbor - UCLA Med Ctr; **Address:** Harbor-UCLA Med Ctr, 1000 W Carson St, Box 11, Torrance, CA 0502; **Phone:** (310) 222-2704; **Board Cert:** Surgery 1988, Vascular Surgery (General) 1994; **Med chool:** SUNY Syracuse 1974; **Resid:** Surgery, LA Co Harbor-UCLA, Torrance, CA 1975-1979; ellow: Vascular Surgery (General), LA Co Harbor-UCLA, Torrance, CA 1979-1980; **Fac Appt:** Prof urgery, UCLA

ellin, Albert E MD (GVS) - *Spec Exp:* Vascular Surgery (General) - General; **Hospital:** LAC & JSC Med Ctr; **Address:** 1200 N State St, rm 9610, Los Angeles, CA 90033; **Phone:** (323) 226-7737; **oard Cert:** Vascular Surgery (General) 1991, Surgery 1970; **Med School:** USC Sch Med 1962; **esid:** Surgery, LAC-USC Med Ctr, Los Angeles, CA 1965-1969; **Fellow:** Vascular Surgery (General), LAC-USC Med Ctr, Los Angeles, CA 1969-1970; **Fac Appt:** Prof Surgery, USC Sch Med

arins, Christopher Kristaps MD (GVS) - *Spec Exp:* Carotid Artery Surgery; Aneurysm-Abdominal Aortic; **Hospital:** Stanford Med Ctr; **Address:** Dept Vascular Surgery, 300 Pasteur Ave, te H-3630 - rm H-3600, Stanford, CA 94305; **Phone:** (650) 725-5227; **Board Cert:** Vascular Surgery (General) 1991, Surgery 1975; **Med School:** Johns Hopkins Univ 1968; **Resid:** Surgery, Univ Michigan Hosp, Ann Arbor, MI 1969-1974; **Fellow:** Surgery, Johns Hopkins Hosp, Baltimore, MD 1971-1972; **Fac Appt:** Prof Surgery, Stanford Univ

APPENDICES

Appendix A

AMERICAN BOARD OF MEDICAL SPECIALTIES

THE STATEMENT OF PURPOSE INCLUDED IN THE ARTICLES OF INCORPORATION IS:

- *To improve the standards of medical care.*

- *To act as spokesman for all approved specialty boards, as a group.*

- *To resolve problems encountered among and between specialty boards.*

- *To deal with the applications for approval of proposed new specialty boards, new types of certification, modification of existing types of certification, and related matters.*

- *To endeavor to avoid duplication of effort by specialty boards.*

- *To establish and maintain standards of organization and operation of specialty boards.*

Following is a list of the addresses of the various medical specialty boards approved by the ABMS. Note that there are 24 board organizations for 25 medical specialties. Psychiatry and Neurology share the same board.

To find out if a physician is certified, consumers can call the individual boards which will provide information for a fee, or they can contact the ABMS at (866) 275-2267 (no fee) or www.abms.org.

BOARD SPECIALTIES

■ **American Board of Allergy and Immunology**
510 Walnut Street, Suite 1701
Philadelphia, PA 19106-3699
(215) 592-9466
General Certification in Allergy and Immunology; with Added Qualification in Diagnostic Laboratory Immunology. Certifications awarded since 1989 are valid for 10 years. For those certified prior to 1989 there is no recertification requirement.

■ **American Board of Anesthesiology**
4101 Lake Boone Trail
Suite 510
Raleigh, NC 27607-7506
(919) 881-2570
General Certification in Anesthesiology; with Special and Added Qualifications in Critical Care Medicine and Pain Management. Certifications awarded since 2000 are valid for 10 years.

■ **American Board of Colon and Rectal Surgery**
20600 Eureka Road, Suite 600
Taylor, MI 48180
(734) 282-9400
General Certification is in Colon and Rectal Surgery. Certifications awarded since 1991 are valid for 8 years.

■ **American Board of Dermatology**
Henry Ford Hospital
One Ford Place
Detroit, MI 48202
(313) 874-1088
General Certification in Dermatology; with Special Qualifications in Dermatopathology, Dermatological Immunology/Diagnostic and Laboratory Immunology. Certifications awarded since 1991 are valid for 10 years. For those certified prior to 1991, there is no recertification requirement.

■ **American Board of Emergency Medicine**
3000 Coolidge Road
East Lansing, MI 48823
(517) 332-4800
General Certification in Emergency Medicine; with Special and Added Qualifications in Pediatric Emergency Medicine and Sports Medicine. Certifications are valid for a 10-year period.

942

■ **American Board of Family Practice**
2228 Young Drive
Lexington, KY 40505
(859) 269-5626
General Certification in Family Practice; with Added Qualifications in Geriatric Medicine and Sports Medicine. Certifications are valid for a 7-year period.

■ **American Board of Internal Medicine**
510 Walnut Street, Suite 1700
Philadelphia, PA 19106-3699
(215) 446-3500, (800) 441-ABIM
General Certification in Internal Medicine; with Special Qualifications in Cardiovascular Disease, Critical Care Medicine, Endocrinology, Diabetes and Metabolism, Gastroenterology, Hematology, Infectious Disease, Medical Oncology, Nephrology, Pulmonary Disease, and Rheumatology; and Added Qualifications in Adolescent Medicine, Cardiac Electrophysiology, Diagnostic Laboratory Immunology, Geriatric Medicine and Sports Medicine. Certifications awarded since 1990 are valid for 10 years. For those certified prior to 1990 there is no recertification requirement.

■ **American Board of Medical Genetics**
9650 Rockville Pike
Bethesda, MD 20814
(301) 571-1825
General Certification in Clinical Genetics, Medical Genetics, Clinical Biochemical Genetics, Clinical Cytogenetics, Clinical Biochemical/Molecular Genetics and Clinical Molecular Genetics. Certifications are valid for a 10-year period.

■ **American Board of Neurological Surgery**
6550 Fannin Street
Suite 2139
Houston, TX 77030-2701
(713) 790-6015
General Certification in Neurological Surgery. Certifications awarded since 1999 are valid for 10 years.

■ **American Board of Nuclear Medicine**
900 Veteran Avenue, Room 13-152
Los Angeles, CA 90024-1786
(310) 825-6787
General Certification in Nuclear Medicine. Certifications awarded since 1992 are valid for 10 years. For those certified prior to 1992, there is no recertification requirement.

APPENDIX A

■ **American Board of Obstetrics and Gynecology**
2915 Vine Street
Dallas, TX 75204
(214) 871-1619
General Certification in Obstetrics and Gynecology; with Special Qualifications in Gynecologic Oncology, Maternal and Fetal Medicine, Reproductive Endocrinology and Added Qualification in Critical Care. Certifications awarded since 1986 are valid for 10 years. For those certified prior to 1986, there is no recertification requirement.

■ **American Board of Ophthalmology**
111 Presidential Boulevard, Suite 241
Bala Cynwyd, PA 19004
(610) 664-1175
Certifications awarded since 1992 are valid for 10 years. For those certified prior to 1992, there is no recertification requirement.

■ **American Board of Orthopaedic Surgery**
400 Silver Cedar Court
Chapel Hill, NC 27514
(919) 929-7103
General Certification in Orthopaedic Surgery; with Added Qualification in Hand Surgery. Certifications awarded since 1986 are valid for 10 years. For those certified prior to 1986, there is no recertification requirement.

■ **American Board of Otolaryngology**
3050 Post Oak Boulevard, Suite 1700
Houston, TX 77056
(713) 850-0399
General Certification in Otolaryngology; with Added Qualification in Otology/Neurotology and Pediatric Otolaryngology. Presently, there is no recertification requirement.

■ **American Board of Pathology**
P.O. Box 25915
Tampa, FL 33622-5915
(813) 286-2444
General Certification in Anatomic and Clinical Pathology, Anatomic Pathology and Clinical Pathology; with Special Qualifications in Blood Banking/Transfusion Medicine, Chemical Pathology, Dermatopathology, Forensic Pathology, Hematology, Immunopathology, Medical Microbiology, Neuropathology and Pediatric Pathology and Added Qualification in Cytopathology. Certifications awarded since 1997 are valid for 10 years.

American Board of Pediatrics

111 Silver Cedar Court
Chapel Hill, NC 27514-1651
(919) 929-0461
General Certification in Pediatrics; with Special Qualifications in Adolescent Medicine, Allergy & Immunology, Pediatric Cardiology, Pediatric Critical Care Medicine, Pediatric Emergency Medicine, Pediatric Endocrinology, Pediatric Gastroenterology, Pediatric Hematology-Oncology, Pediatric Infectious Diseases, Pediatric Nephrology, Pediatric Pulmonology, Neonatal-Perinatal Medicine and Pediatric Rheumatology. Added Qualifications in Diagnostic Laboratory Immunology, Medical Toxicology and Sports Medicine. Certifications valid for 7 years.

American Board of Physical Medicine and Rehabilitation

21 First Street, S.W., Suite 674
Rochester, MN 55902
(507) 282-1776
General Certification in Physical Medicine and Rehabilitation; with Special Qualifications in Spinal Cord Injury Medicine. Certifications awarded since 1993 are valid for 10 years.

American Board of Plastic Surgery

Seven Penn Center, Suite 400
1635 Market Street
Philadelphia, PA 19103-2204
(215) 587-9322
General Certification in Plastic Surgery; with Added Qualification in Hand Surgery. Certifications are valid for a 10-year period.

American Board of Preventive Medicine

330 South Wells Street, Suite 1018
Chicago, IL 60606
(312) 939-2276
General Certification in Aerospace Medicine, Occupational Medicine and Public Health and General Preventive Medicine; with Added Qualification in Underseas Medicine and Medical Toxicology. In the subspecialty of Underseas Medicine and Medical Toxicology certifications are valid for a 10-year period.

American Board of Psychiatry & Neurology

500 Lake Cook Road, Suite 335
Deerfield, IL 60015
(847) 945-7900
General Certification in Psychiatry, Neurology and Neurology with Special Qualification in Child Neurology; with Special Qualification in Child and Adolescent Psychiatry and Added Qualification in Addiction Psychiatry, Clinical Neurophysiology, Forensic Psychiatry and Geriatric Psychiatry. Certifications are valid for a 10-year period.

APPENDIX A

■ **American Board of Radiology**
5441 E. Williams Boulevard
Tucson, AZ 85711
(520) 790-2900
General Certification in Diagnostic Radiology or Radiation Oncology; with Special Competency in Nuclear Radiology and Added Qualifications in Neuroradiology, Pediatric Radiology and Vascular and Interventional Radiology. Radiation Physics is a non-clinical certification. Certificates are valid for a 10-year period.

■ **American Board of Surgery**
1617 John F. Kennedy Boulevard, Suite 860
Philadelphia, PA 19103-1847
(215) 568-4000
General Certification in Surgery; with Special Qualifications in Pediatric Surgery and General Vascular Surgery and Added Qualifications in Surgery of the Hand, Surgical Critical Care and General Vascular Surgery. Certifications are valid for a 10-year period.

■ **American Board of Thoracic Surgery**
One Rotary Center, Suite 803
Evanston, IL 60201
(847) 475-1520
General Certification in Thoracic Surgery. Certifications awarded since 1976 are valid for 10 years. For those certified prior to 1976, there is no recertification requirement.

■ **American Board of Urology**
2216 Ivy Road, Suite 210
Charlottesville, VA 22903
(434) 979-0059
General Certification in Urology. Certifications awarded as of 1985 are valid for 10 years. For those certified prior to 1985, there is no recertification requirement.

Appendix B

OSTEOPATHIC BOARDS

American Osteopathic Association
142 E Ontario Street
Chicago, IL 60611
(800) 621-1773

GENERAL CERTIFICATION

- **American Osteopathic Board of Anesthesiology**
  Anesthesiology
  - No time-limited certificates

- **American Osteopathic Board of Dermatology**
  Dermatology
  - No time-limited certificates

- **American Osteopathic Board of Emergency Medicine**
  Emergency Medicine
  - Beginning 1/1/94, 10-year certificates

- **American Osteopathic Board of Family Physicians**
  Family Practice
  - Beginning 3/1/97, 8-year certificates

- **American Osteopathic Board of Internal Medicine**
  Internal Medicine
  - Beginning 1/1/93, 10-year certificates

- **American Osteopathic Board of Neurology and Psychiatry**
  Neurology
  Psychiatry
  - Beginning 1/1/96, 10-year certificates

- **American Osteopathic Board of Obstetrics and Gynecology**
  Obstetrics and Gynecology
  - No time-limited certificates

APPENDIX B

■ **American Osteopathic Board of Ophthalmology and Otorhinolaryngology**
Ophthalmology
  • Beginning 1/1/00, 10-year certificates
Otorhinolaryngology
Facial Plastic Surgery
Otorhinolaryngology and Facial Plastic Surgery
  • Beginning 1/1/02, 10-year certificates

■ **American Osteopathic Board of Orthopaedic Surgery**
Orthopaedic Surgery
  • Beginning 1/1/94, 10-year certificates

■ **American Osteopathic Board of Pathology**
Laboratory Medicine
Anatomic Pathology
Anatomic Pathology and Laboratory Medicine
  • Beginning 1/1/95, 10-year certificates

■ **American Osteopathic Board of Pediatrics**
Pediatrics
  • Beginning 1/1/95, 7-year certificates

■ **American Osteopathic Board of Preventive Medicine**
Preventive Medicine/Aerospace Medicine
Preventive Medicine/Occupational-Environmental Medicine
Preventive Medicine/Public Health
  • Beginning 1/1/94, 10-year certificates

■ **American Osteopathic Board of Proctology**
Proctology
  • No time-limited certificates

■ **American Osteopathic Board of Radiology**
Diagnostic Radiology
Radiation Oncology
  • No time-limited certificates

■ **American Osteopathic Board of Rehabilitation Medicine**
Rehabilitation Medicine
  • No time-limited certificates

■ **American Osteopathic Board of Special Proficiency in Osteopathic Manipulative Medicine**
Special Proficiency in Osteopathic Manipulative Medicine
• Beginning 1/1/95, 10-year certificates

■ **American Osteopathic Board of Surgery**
Surgery (general)
Plastic and Reconstructive Surgery
Thoracic Cardiovascular Surgery
Urological Surgery
General Vascular Surgery
• Beginning 1/1/97, 10-year certificates

Consumers may call the American Osteopathic Association at (800) 621-1773 for general certification information.

APPENDIX C

SELF-DESIGNATED MEDICAL SPECIALTIES

This list of self-designated medical specialty groups was obtained from the American Board of Medical Specialties. However, it is important to point out that these groups are not recognized by the ABMS, the governing board for the recognized twenty-four medical specialty boards (listed in Appendix A).

The organizations listed below range from highly organized groups that are attempting to formalize training and certification in their field to informal groups interested in a particular aspect of medicine.

If you wish to obtain information from any of these groups you will have to do some detective work. Because so many are informal, the location, phone and mailing addresses change frequently, depending upon the person who is functioning as secretary or administrator.

The best way to track down one of these groups is to consult the doctor listings to find a doctor who has expressed a special interest in that field, and call his or her office. You might also call a nearby academic health center in the area to see if they have a faculty or staff member known to be involved in that particular medical interest. If that fails, take the same approach with your community hospital.

APPENDIX C

A

Abdominal Surgeons
Acupuncture Medicine
Addiction Medicine
Addictionology
Adolescent Psychiatry
Aesthetic Plastic Surgery
Alcoholism and Other Drug
  Dependencies (AMSAODD)
Algology (Chronic Pain)
Alternative Medicine
Ambulatory Anesthesia
Ambulatory Foot Surgery
Anesthesia
Arthroscopic Surgery
Arthroscopy (Board of North America)

B

Bariatric Medicine
Bionic Psychology
Bloodless Medicine & Surgery

C

Chelation Therapy
Chemical Dependence
Clinical Chemistry
Clinical Ecology
Clinical Medicine and Surgery
Clinical Neurology
Clinical Neurophysiology
Clinical Neurosurgery
Clinical Nutrition
Clinical Orthopaedic Surgery
Clinical Pharmacology
Clinical Polysomnography
Clinical Psychiatry
Clinical Psychology
Clinical Toxicology
Cosmetic Plastic Surgery
Cosmetic Surgery
Council of Non-Board Certified Physicians
Critical Care in Medicine & Surgery

D

Dermalogy
Disability Analysis
Disability Evaluating Physicians

E

Electrodiagnostic Medicine
Electroencephalography
Electromyography & Electrodiagnosis
Environmental Medicine
Epidemiology (College)
Eye Surgery

F

Facial Cosmetic Surgery
Facial Plastic & Reconstructive Surgery
Family Practice, Certification
Forensic Examiners
Forensic Psychiatry
Forensic Toxicology

H

Hand Surgery
Head, Facial & Neck Pain & TMJ Orthopaedics
Health Physics
Homeopathic Physicians
Homeotherapeutics
Hypnotic Anesthesiology, National Board for

I

Independent Medical Examiners
Industrial Medicine & Surgery
Insurance Medicine
International Cosmetic & Plastic
  Facial Reconstructive Standards
Interventional Radiology

L

Laser Surgery
Law in Medicine
Longevity Medicine/Surgery

SELF-DESIGNATED MEDICAL SPECIALTIES

M

Malpractice Physicians
Maxillofacial Surgeons
Medical Accreditation (American Federation for)
Medical Hypnosis
Medical Laboratory Immunology
Medical-Legal Analysis of Medicine & Surgery
Medical Legal & Workers
  Comp. Medicine & Surgery
Medical-Legal Consultants
Medical Management
Medical Microbiology
Medical Preventics (Academy)
Medical Psychotherapists
Medical Toxicology
Microbiology (Medical Microbiology)
Military Medicine
Mohs Micrographic Surgery &
  Cutaneous Oncology

N

Neuroimaging
Neurologic & Orthopaedic Dental
  Medicine and Surgery
Neurological & Orthopaedic Medicine
Neurological & Orthopaedic Surgery
Neurological Microsurgery
Neurology
Neuromuscular Thermography
Neuro-Orthopaedic Dental Medicine & Surgery
Neuro-Orthopaedic Electrodiagnosis
Neuro-Orthopaedic Laser Surgery
Neuro-Orthopaedic Psychiatry
Neuro-Orthopaedic Thoracic Medicine/Surgery
Neurorehabilitation
Nutrition

O

Orthopaedic Medicine
Orthopaedic Microneurosurgery
Otorhinolaryngology

P

Pain Management (American Academy of)

Pain Management Specialties
Pain Medicine
Palliative Medicine
Percutaneous Diskectomy
Plastic Esthetic Surgeons
Prison Medicine
Professional Disability Consultants
Psychiatric Medicine
Psychiatry (American National Board of)
Psychoanalysis (American Examining
  Board in)
Psychological Medicine (International)

Q

Quality Assurance & Utilization Review

R

Radiology & Medical Imaging
Rheumatologic Surgery
Rheumatological & Reconstructive Medicine
Ringside Medicine & Surgery

S

Skin Specialists
Sleep Medicine (Polysomnography)
Spinal Cord Injury
Spinal Surgery
Sports Medicine
Sports Medicine/Surgery

T

Toxicology
Trauma Surgery
Traumatologic Medicine & Surgery
Tropical Medicine

U

Ultrasound Technology
Urologic Allied Health Professionals
Urological Surgery

W

Weight Reduction Medicine

APPENDIX D

PATIENT RIGHTS

YOUR RIGHTS IN THE HOSPITAL

The following Bill of Rights is one that has been adopted by the American Hospital Association (AHA) and is in use in many hospitals throughout the nation.

The patient has the right to:

- *Considerate and respectful care.*

- *Complete information about his/her treatment and condition in terms the patient can reasonably understand.*

- *Know the identity of physicians, nurses, and others involved in their care, as well as when those involved are students, residents, or other trainees.*

- *Information necessary to give informed consent prior to the start of any procedure or treatment.*

- *Refuse treatment and be informed of the consequences.*

- *Have an advance directive (such as a living will, health care proxy, or durable power of attorney) for health care.*

- *Privacy concerning his/her treatment.*

- *Have all records and communications regarding medical treatment kept confidential.*

- *Expect the hospital, within the limits of its capabilities, to respond to a request for services.*

- *Obtain information regarding the relationship of the hospital to any other health care institutions.*

- *Be advised if the hospital proposes human experimentation which affects his/her care.*

APPENDIX D

- *Reasonable continuity of care.*
- *An explanation of the bill, regardless of payment source.*
- *Know what hospital rules and regulations apply to patient contact.*

(Source: American Hospital Association, Chicago, IL)

According to the American Hospital Association, this version of the Patient's Bill of Rights is the most recent; it was last edited in 1992. However, the AHA now has a website: www.aha.org/resource/pbillofrights.asp which lists the bill of rights. Consumers can also obtain an up-to-date copy, free of charge, by calling the AHA's resource Department at (312) 422-2050.

APPENDIX E

HOSPITAL LISTINGS

Following is an alphabetical listing of hospitals noted in doctors' entries. The abbreviations as they appear in the listings are in italics below. Due to the many mergers taking place in the hospital industry these days, the names on this list may have changed subsequent to publication of this guide.

Abbott - Northwestern Hospital
Abbott - Northwestern Hosp
800 E 28th St
Minneapolis, MN 55407
Midwest
(612) 863-4000

Advocate Christ Medical Center
Advocate Christ Med Ctr
4440 W 95th St
Oak Lawn, IL 60453
Midwest
(708) 425-8000

Advocate Illinois Masonic Medical Center
Advocate IL Masonic Med Ctr
836 W Wellington Ave
Chicago, IL 60657-5147
Midwest
(773) 975-1600

Advocate Lutheran General Hospital
Advocate Lutheran Gen Hosp
1775 Dempster St
Park Ridge, IL 60068
Midwest
(847) 723-2210

Alaska Native Medical Center
Alaska Native Medical Ctr
4315 Diplomacy Dr
Anchorage, AK 99508
West Coast and Pacific
(907) 563-2662

Alaska Regional Medical Center
Alaska Regional Med Ctr
2801 DeBarr Rd
Anchorage, AK 99508
West Coast and Pacific
(907) 276-1131

Albany Medical Center
Albany Medical Center
43 New Scotland Ave
Albany, NY 12208
Mid Atlantic
(518) 262-3125

Albert Einstein Medical Center
Albert Einstein Med Ctr
5501 Old York Road
Philadelphia, PA 19141
Mid Atlantic
(215) 456-7890

Institutions in bold are profiled in this edition of the Castle Connolly Guide.

Albert Lea Medical Center-Mayo Health System
Albert Lea Med Ctr-Mayo Hlth Sys
404 W Fountain St
Albert Lea, MN 56007
Midwest
(507) 373-2384

Alfred I Dupont Hospital for Children
Alfred I Dupont Hosp for Children
1600 Rockland Rd
Wilmington, DE 19803
Mid Atlantic
(302) 651-4000

All Children's Hospital
All Children's Hosp
801 Sixth Street South
St. Petersburg, FL 33701
Southeast
(727) 898-7451

Allegheny General Hospital
Allegheny General Hosp
320 E. North Avenue
Pittsburgh, PA 15212
Mid Atlantic
(412) 359-3131

Alta Bates Summit Medical Center - Ashby Campus
Alta Bates Summit Med Ctr - Ashby Campus
2450 Ashby Avenue
Berkeley, CA 94705
West Coast and Pacific
(510) 204-4444

Anne Bates Leach Eye Hosp
Anne B Leach Eye Hosp
900 NW 17th St PO Box 16680
Miami, FL 33136
Southeast
(305) 326-6000

Arkansas Children's Hospital
Arkansas Chldns Hosp
800 Marshall St
Little Rock, AR 72202
Southwest
(501) 320-1100

Arlington Hospital
Arlington Hosp
1701 N George Mason Dr
Arlington, VA 22205-3698
Southeast
(703) 558-5000

Armed Forces Institute of Pathology
Armed Forces Inst of Path
6825 16th St NW, Bldg 54
Washington, DC 20306-6000
Mid Atlantic
(202) 782-2100

Arthur G. James Cancer Hospital & Research Institute
Arthur G James Cancer Hosp & Research Inst
300 West 10th Avenue
Columbus, OH 43210
Midwest
(614) 293-3300

Atlanta Medical Center
Atlanta Med Ctr
303 Parkway Dr. NE
Atlanta, GA 3031
Southeast
(404) 265-4000

Institutions in bold are profiled in this edition of the Castle Connolly Guide.

Atlantic Medical Center - Daytona
Atlantic Med Ctr - Daytona
400 N Clyde Morris Blvd
Daytona Beach, FL 32114
Southeast
(904) 239-5000

Audie L Murphy Memorial Veterans
Hospital
Audie L Murphy Meml Vets Hosp
7400 Merton Minter Blvd
San Antonio, TX 78229
Southwest
(210) 617-5300

Baptist Health
Baptist Health
800 Prudential Drive
Jacksonville, FL 32207
Southeast
(904) 202-2000

Baptist Hospital
Baptist Hosp
2000 Church St
Nashville, TN 37236
Southeast
(615) 284-5555

Baptist Hospital - Miami
Baptist Hosp - Miami
8900 N Kendall Dr
Miami, FL 33176
Southeast
(305) 596-1960

Baptist Medical Center - San Antonio
Baptist Med Ctr - San Antonio
111 Dallas St
San Antonio, TX 78205
Southwest
(210) 297-7000

Baptist Memphis
Baptist Memphis
6019 Walnut Grove Rd
Memphis, TN 38120
Southeast
(901) 226-5000

Barbara Ann Karmanos Cancer Institute
Barbara Ann Karmanos Cancer Inst
110 E Warren Ave
Detroit, MI 48201
Midwest
(800) 527-6266

Barnes-Jewish Hospital
Barnes-Jewish Hosp
One Barnes-Jewish Hospital Plaza
St. Louis, MO 63110
Midwest
(314) 362-5000

Baylor University Medical Center
Baylor Univ Medical Ctr
3500 Gaston Avenue
Dallas, TX 75246
Southwest
(214) 820-0111

Baylor-Richardson Medical Center
Baylor-Richardson Med Ctr
401 West Campbell Road
Richardson, TX 75080
Southwest
(972) 498-4000

Baystate Medical Center
Baystate Med Ctr
759 Chestnut Street
Springfield, MA 01199
New England
(413) 794-0000

Institutions in bold are profiled in this edition of the Castle Connolly Guide.

Ben Taub General Hospital
Ben Taub General Hosp
1504 Taub Loop
Houston, TX 77001
Southwest
(713) 793-2000

Beth Israel Deaconess Medical Center - Boston
Beth Israel Deaconess Med Ctr - Boston
330 Brookline Ave
Boston, MA 02215
New England
(617) 667-7000

Beth Israel Medical Center - Herbert & Nell Singer Division
Affiliate, Continuum Health Partners, Inc.
Beth Israel Med Ctr - Singer Div
170 East End Avenue @ 87th Street
New York, NY 10128
Mid Atlantic
(212) 870-9000

Beth Israel Medical Center - Milton & Caroll Petrie Division
Affiliate, Continuum Health Partners, Inc.
Beth Israel Med Ctr - Petrie Division
First Avenue @ 16th Street
New York, NY 10003
Mid Atlantic
(212) 420-2000

Boca Raton Community Hosp
Boca Raton Comm Hosp
800 Meadows Road
Boca Raton, FL 33486
Southeast
(561) 395-7100

Boston Medical Center
Boston Med Ctr
1 Boston Medical Center Pl
Boston, MA 02118
New England
(617) 638-8000

Bridgeport Hospital
Bridgeport Hosp
267 Grant St
Bridgeport, CT 06610
New England
(203) 384-3000

Brigham & Women's Hospital
Brigham & Women's Hosp
75 Francis St
Boston, MA 02115
New England
(617) 732-5500

Brooklyn Hospital Center-Downtown
Brooklyn Hosp Ctr-Downtown
121 DeKalb Avenue
Brooklyn, NY 11201
Mid Atlantic
(718) 250-8000

Broward General Medical Center
Broward General Med Ctr
1600 S Andrews Ave
Fort Lauderdale, FL 33316
Southeast
(954) 355-4400

Bryn Mawr Hospital
Bryn Mawr Hosp
130 Bryn Mawr Ave
Bryn Mawr, PA 19010-3143
Mid Atlantic
(610) 526-3000

Institutions in bold are profiled in this edition of the Castle Connolly Guide.

Buffalo General Hospital
Buffalo General Hosp
100 High Street
Buffalo, NY 14203
Mid Atlantic
(716) 859-5600

Burke Rehabilitation Hospital
Burke Rehab Hosp
785 Mamaroneck Avenue
White Plains, NY 10605
Mid Atlantic
(914) 597-2500

Butler Hospital
Butler Hosp
345 Blackstone Blvd
Providence, RI 02906
New England
(401) 455-6200

Cabrini Medical Center
Cabrini Med Ctr
227 East 19th Street
New York, NY 10003
Mid Atlantic
(212) 995-6000

California Pacific Medical Center - Davies
Campus
CA Pacific Med Ctr - Davies Campus
Castro & Duboce St
San Francisco, CA 94114
West Coast and Pacific
(415) 565-6000

California Pacific Medical Center - Pacific
Campus
CA Pacific Med Ctr - Pacific Campus
2333 Buchanan St
San Francisco, CA 94115
West Coast and Pacific
(415) 600-6000

Cambridge Hospital
Cambridge Hospital
1493 Cambridge Street
Cambridge, MA 02139
New England
(617) 665-1000

Campbell Clinic
Campbell Clin
1400 S Germantown Rd
Germantown, TN 38138
Southeast
(901) 759-3100

Cancer Institute of New Jersey, The
Cancer Inst of NJ, The
195 Little Albany St
New Brunswick, NJ 08901
Mid Atlantic
(732) 235-2465

Carolinas Medical Center
Carolinas Med Ctr
1000 Blythe Blvd
Charlotte, NC 28203-5871
Southeast
(704) 355-2000

Cedars Medical Center - Miami
Cedars Med Ctr - Miami
1400 NW 12 Ave
Miami, FL 33136
Southeast
(305) 325-5511

Cedars-Sinai Medical Center
Cedars-Sinai Med Ctr
8700 Beverly Boulevard
Los Angeles, CA 90048
West Coast and Pacific
(310) 423-3277

Institutions in bold are profiled in this edition of the Castle Connolly Guide.

Centennial Medical Center
Centennial Med Ctr
2300 Patterson Street
Nashville, TN 37203
Southeast
(615) 342-1000

Centinela Hospital Medical Center
Centinela Hosp Med Ctr
555 East Hardy Street
Inglewood, CA 90301
West Coast and Pacific
(310) 673-4660

Century City Hospital
Century City Hosp
2070 Century Park East
Los Angeles, CA 90067
West Coast and Pacific
(310) 553-6211

Children's Healthcare of Atlanta -
Eggleston
Chldns Hlthcare of Atlanta - Eggleston
1405 NE Clifton Rd
Atlanta, GA 30322
Southeast
(404) 325-6000

Children's Healthcare of Atlanta -
Scottish Rite
Chldn's Hlthcre of Atlanta - Scottish Rite
1001 Johnson Ferry Rd
Atlanta, GA 30342
Southeast
(404) 250-5437

Children's Hospital - Birmingham
Children's Hospital - Birmingham
1600 7th Ave South
Birmingham, AL 35233
Southeast
(205) 939-9100

Children's Hospital - Boston
Children's Hospital - Boston
300 Longwood Avenue
Boston, MA 02115
New England
(617) 355-8555

Children's Hospital - Columbus, OH
Chldn's Hosp - Columbus, OH
700 Children's Drive
Columbus, OH 43205
Midwest
(614) 722-2000

Children's Hospital - Los Angeles
Chldns Hosp - Los Angeles
4650 Sunset Blvd
Los Angeles, CA 90027
West Coast and Pacific
(323) 660-2450

Children's Hospital - New Orleans
Children's Hospital - New Orleans
200 Henry Clay Ave
New Orleans, LA 70118
Southwest
(504) 899-9511

Children's Hospital and Clinics -
Minneapolis
Chldns Hosp and Clinics - Minneapolis
2525 Chicago Ave S
Minneapolis, MN 55404
Midwest
(612) 813-6000

Children's Hospital and Health Center
Children's Hosp and Hlth Ctr - San Diego
3020 Childrens Way
San Diego, CA 92123
West Coast and Pacific
(858) 576-1700

Institutions in bold are profiled in this edition of the Castle Connolly Guide.

Children's Hospital and Regional Medical
Center - Seattle
Chldns Hosp and Regl Med Ctr - Seattle
4800 Sand Point Way NE
Seattle, WA 98105
West Coast and Pacific
(206) 526-2000

Children's Hospital at OU Medical Center,
The
Chldn's Hosp at OU Med Ctr
940 NE13th Street
Oklahoma City, OK 73104
Southwest
(405) 271-5437

Children's Hospital of Michigan
Affiliate, Detroit Medical Center
Chldns Hosp of Michigan
3901 Beaubian Blvd
Detroit, MI 48201
Midwest
(313) 745-5437

Children's Hospital of Pittsburgh
Chldn's Hosp of Pittsbrgh
3705 Fifth Avenue
Pittsburgh, PA 15213
Mid Atlantic
(412) 692-5325

Children's Hospital of Wisconsin
Chldrns Hosp - Wisconsin
9000 W Wisconsin Ave
Wauwatosa, WI 53226
Midwest
(414) 266-2000

Children's Medical Center of Dallas
Chldns Med Ctr of Dallas
1935 Motor St
Dallas, TX 75235
Southwest
(214) 456-7000

Children's Memorial Hospital
Children's Mem Hosp
2300 Children's Plaza
Chicago, IL 60614
Midwest
(773) 880-4000

Children's Memorial Hospital - Omaha
Children's Mem Hosp - Omaha
8301 Dodge St
Omaha, NE 68101
Great Plains and Mountains

Children's Mercy Hospitals & Clinics
Chldns Mercy Hosps & Clinics
2401 Gilham Rd
Kansas City, MO 64108
Midwest
(816) 234-3000

Children's National Medical Center - DC
Chldns Natl Med Ctr - DC
111 Michigan Ave NW
Washington, DC 20010
Mid Atlantic
(202) 884-5000

Chippenham Johnston-Willis Medical
Center
CJW Med Ctr
1401 Johnston-Willis Dr
Richmond, VA 23235
Southeast
(804) 320-3911

Institutions in bold are profiled in this edition of the Castle Connolly Guide.

Christ Hospital, The
Christ Hospital
2139 Auburn Ave
Cincinnati, OH 45219
Midwest
(513) 585-2000

Christus St Joseph's Hospital
Christus St Joseph's Hosp
1919 La Branch St
Houston, TX 77002
Southwest
(713) 757-1000

Cincinnati Children's Hospital Medical
Center
Cincinnati Chldns Hosp Med Ctr
3333 Burnet Ave
Cincinnati, OH 45229-3039
Midwest
(800) 344-2462

Citrus Memorial Hospital
Citrus Memorial Hosp
502 West Highland Boulevard
Iverness, FL 34452
Southeast
(352) 726-1551

City of Hope National Medical Center &
Beckman Research
City of Hope Natl Med Ctr & Beckman Rsch
1500 E Duarte Rd
Duarte, CA 91010
West Coast and Pacific
(626) 359-8111

Clarkson Bishop Memorial Hospital
Clarkson Bishop Mem Hosp
Dewey Ave @ 44th St
Omaha, NE 68101

Great Plains and Mountains
Cleveland Clinic Florida
Cleveland Clin FL
2950 Cleveland Blvd
Weston, FL 33331
Southeast
(954) 659-5000

Cleveland Clinic Foundation
Cleveland Clin Fdn
9500 Euclid Avenue
Cleveland, OH 44195
Midwest
(800) 223-2273

Columbus Hospital
Columbus Hosp
495 N 13th Street
Newark, NJ 07107
Mid Atlantic
(973) 268-1400

Community Memorial Hospital - San
Buena Ventura
Comm Mem Hosp - San Buena Ventura
147 N Brent St
Ventura, CA 93003
West Coast and Pacific
(805) 652-5011

Cook Children's Medical Center
Cook Children's Med Ctr
801 7th Ave
Fort Worth, TX 76104-2796
Southwest
(817) 885-4000

Cooper Medical Center
Cooper Med Ctr
One Cooper Plaza
Lebanon, NJ 03756
New England
(609) 342-2000

Institutions in bold are profiled in this edition of the Castle Connolly Guide.

Covenant Health System
Covenant Health Sys
3615 19th St
Lubbock, TX 79410
Southwest
(806) 792-1011

Craig Hospital
Craig Hospital
3425 S Clarkson
Englewood, CO 80110-2899
Great Plains and Mountains
(303) 789-8000

Crawford Long Hospital of Emory
University
Crawford Long Hosp of Emory Univ
550 Peachtree Street NorthEast
Atlanta, GA 30365
Southeast
(404) 686-4411

Crouse Hospital
Crouse Hosp
736 Irving Ave
Syracuse, NY 13210-1607
Mid Atlantic
(315) 470-7111

Dana Farber Cancer Institute
Dana Farber Cancer Inst
44 Binney St
Boston, MA 02115
New England
(617) 632-3000

Dartmouth - Hitchcock Medical Center
Dartmouth - Hitchcock Med Ctr
1 Medical Center Dr
Lebanon, NH 03756-0002
New England
(603) 650-5000

Deaconess Hospital - Indiana
Deaconess Hosp - Indiana
600 Mary St
Evansville, IN 47747-0002
Midwest
(812) 450-5000

Denver Health Medical Center
Denver Health Med Ctr
777 Bannock St
Denver, CO 80204
Great Plains and Mountains
(303) 436-6000

Desert Regional Medical Center
Desert Regional Med Ctr
1150 N Indian Canyon Dr
Palm Springs, CA 92262
West Coast and Pacific
(760) 323-6511

Doctors Medical Center
Doctors Med Ctr
2000 Vale Rd
San Pablo, CA 94806
West Coast and Pacific
(510) 970-5000

Doernbecher Children's Hospital/Oregon
Health Science University
Doernbecher Chldns Hosp
3181 SW Sam Jackson Park Rd
Portland, OR 97201-3098
West Coast and Pacific
(503) 494-8811

Institutions in bold are profiled in this edition of the Castle Connolly Guide.

Duke University Medical Center
Affiliate, Duke University Health
System
Duke Univ Med Ctr
Erwin Rd
Durham, NC 27710
Southeast
(919) 684-8111

East Jefferson General Hospital
E Jefferson Genl Hosp
4200 Houma Blvd
Metairie, LA 70006-2973
Southwest
(504) 454-4000

East Texas Medical Center
E TX Med Ctr
1000 South Beckham Ave.
Tyler, TX 75701
Southwest
(903) 597-0351

Eastern Maine Medical Center
Eastern Maine Med Ctr
489 State St
Bangor, ME 04401
New England
(207) 973-7000

Eastmoreland Hospital
Eastmoreland Hosp
2900 SE Steele St
Portland, OR 97202-4590
West Coast and Pacific
(503) 234-0411

Eden Medical Center
Eden Med Ctr
20103 Lake Chabot Rd
Castro Valley, CA 94546
West Coast and Pacific
(510) 537-1234

Edward W Sparrow Hospital
Sparrow Hospital
1215 E Michigan Ave
Lansing, MI 48912
Midwest
(517) 483-2505

Emory University Hospital
Emory Univ Hosp
1364 Clifton Rd NE
Atlanta, GA 30322
Southeast
(404) 712-7021

Englewood Hospital & Medical Center
Englewood Hosp & Med Ctr
350 Engle Street
Englewood, NJ 07631
Mid Atlantic
(201) 894-3000

Evanston Hospital
Evanston Hosp
2650 Ridge Ave
Evanston, IL 60201
Midwest
(847) 570-2000

Fairview Southdale Hospital
Fairview Southdale Hosp
6401 France Ave S
Edina, MN 55435-2199
Midwest
(952) 924-5000

Fairview-University Medical Center -
Riverside Campus
Fairview-Univ Med Ctr - Riverside Campus
2450 Riverside Ave S
Minneapolis, MN 55454
Midwest
(612) 672-6000

Institutions in bold are profiled in this edition of the Castle Connolly Guide.

Fairview-University Medical Center -
University Campus
Fairview-Univ Med Ctr - Univ Campus
420 Delaware St S
Minneapolis, MN 55455
Midwest
(612) 273-3000

Fletcher Allen Health Care Medical
Center - Campus
Fletcher Allen Hlth Care Med Ctr - Campus
111 Colchester Ave (Burgess 1)
Burlington, VT 05401
New England
(802) 847-0000

Fletcher Allen Healthcare - UHC Campus
Fletcher Allen Hlthcare - UHC Campus
1 S Prospect St
Burlington, VT 05401
New England
(802) 847-0000

Florida Hospital
Florida Hosp
400 Celebration Pl
Celebration, FL 34747
Southeast
(407) 303-4000

Florida Hospital Apopka
Florida Hospital Orlando Apopka
201 North Park Ave
Apopka, FL 32703
Southeast
(407) 889-1001

Forsyth Medical Center
Forsyth Med Ctr
3333 Silas Creek Pkwy
Winston-Salem, NC 27103
Southeast
(336) 718-5000

Four Winds Hospital
Four Winds Hosp
800 Cross River Road
Katonah, NY 10536
Mid Atlantic
(914) 763-8151

Fox Chase Cancer Center
Fox Chase Cancer Ctr
7701 Burholme Avenue
Philadelphia, PA 19111
Mid Atlantic
(215) 728-6900

Froedtert Memorial Lutheran Hospital
Froedtert Meml Lutheran Hosp
9200 W Wisconsin Ave
Milwaukee, WI 53226
Midwest
(414) 805-6644

Geisinger Health System
Geisinger Hlth Sys
100 N. Academy Avenue
Danville, PA 17822
Mid Atlantic
(570) 271-6000

George Washington University Hospital
G Washington Univ Hosp
901 23rd St NW
Washington, DC 20037
Mid Atlantic
(202) 715-4000

Georgetown University Hospital
Georgetown Univ Hosp
3800 Reservoir Rd NW
Washington, DC 20007
Mid Atlantic
(202) 784-3000

Institutions in bold are profiled in this edition of the Castle Connolly Guide.

Gillette Children's Specialty Healthcare
Gillette Chldn's Specialty Hlthcre
200 University Ave E
St Paul , MN 55101
Midwest
(651) 291-2848

Glenbrook Hospital
Glenbrook Hosp
2100 Pfingsten Rd
Glenview, IL 60025
Midwest
(847) 657-5800

Goleta Valley Cottage Hospital
Goleta Vly Cottage Hosp
351 S Patterson Ave
Goleta, CA 93111
West Coast and Pacific
(805) 967-3411

Good Samaritan Hosp - Cincinnati
Good Samaritan Hosp - Cincinnati
375 Dixmyth Ave
Cincinnati, OH 45220
Midwest
(513) 872-1400

Good Samaritan Hospital - Los Angeles
Good Samaritan Hosp - Los Angeles
1225 Wilshire Boulevard
Los Angeles, CA 90017
West Coast and Pacific
(213) 977-2121

Good Samaritan Regional Medical Center
- Phoenix
Good Samaritan Regl Med Ctr - Phoenix
1111 E McDowell Rd
Phoenix, AZ 85060
Southwest
(602) 239-2000

Good Samaritan Medical Center - W
Palm Beach
Good Samaritan Med Ctr - W Palm Beach
111309 North Flager Drive
West Palm Beach, FL 33401
Southeast
(561) 655-5511

Grady Health System
Grady Hlth Sys
80 Jesse Hill Jr Dr
Atlanta, GA 30303
Southeast
(404) 616-4307

Greater Baltimore Medical Center
Greater Baltimore Med Ctr
6701 N Charles St
Baltimore, MD 21204
Mid Atlantic
(443) 849-2000

Green Hospital - Scripps Clinic
Green Hosp - Scripps Clinic
10666 N. Torrey Pines Road
La Jolla, CA 92037
West Coast and Pacific
(858) 455-9100

Greenwich Hospital
Greenwich Hosp
Five Perryridge Road
Greenwich, CT 06830
New England
(203) 863-3000

H Lee Moffitt Cancer Center & Research
Institute
H Lee Moffitt Cancer Ctr & Research Inst
12902 Magnolia Drive
Tampa, FL 33612-9497
Southeast
(813) 972-4673

Institutions in bold are profiled in this edition of the Castle Connolly Guide.

Hackensack University Medical Center
Hackensack Univ Med Ctr
30 Prospect Avenue
Hackensack, NJ 07601
Mid Atlantic
(201) 996-2000

Hahnemann University Hospital
Hahnemann Univ Hosp
Broad & Vine St
Philadelphia, PA 19102
Mid Atlantic
(215) 762-7000

Hamot Medical Center
Hamot Med Ctr
201 State Street
Erie, PA 16550-0001
Mid Atlantic
(814) 877-6000

Harborview Medical Center
Harborview Med Ctr
325 9th Ave
Seattle, WA 98104-2499
West Coast and Pacific
(206) 223-3000

Harlem Hospital Center
Harlem Hosp Ctr
506 Lenox Avenue
New York, NY 10037
Mid Atlantic
(212) 939-1000

Harper Hospital
Affiliate, Detroit Medical Center
Harper Hosp
3990 John R St
Detroit, MI 48201-2097
Midwest
(313) 745-8040

Hartford Hospital
Hartford Hosp
80 Seymour St, Box 5037
Hartford, CT 06102-5037
New England
(860) 545-5000

Health Midwest - Overland Park Regional
Medical Center
Overland Park Reg Med Ctr
10500 Quivira Rd
Overland Park, KS 66215
Great Plains and Mountains
(913) 541-5000

Healthsouth Doctor's Hospital
Healthsouth Doctor's Hosp
5000 University Dr
Coral Gables, FL 33146
Southeast
(305) 666-2111

Healthsouth Medical Center -
Birmingham
Healthsouth Med Ctr - Birmingham
1201 11th Ave S
Birmingham, AL 35205-5299
Southeast
(205) 930-7000

Hebrew Rehabilitation Center for the
Aged
Hebrew Rehab Ctr for the Aged
1200 Centre St
Boston, MA 02131
New England
(617) 325-8000

Institutions in bold are profiled in this edition of the Castle Connolly Guide.

APPENDIX E

Helen Ellis Memorial Hospital
Helen Ellis Memorial Hosp
1395 S Pinellas Avenue
Tarpon Springs, FL 34689
Southeast
(727) 942-5000

Hennepin County Medical Center
Hennepin Cnty Med Ctr
701 Park Ave S
Minneapolis, MN 55415
Midwest
(612) 347-2121

Henry Ford Hospital
Henry Ford Hosp
2799 W Grand Blvd
Detroit, MI 48202
Midwest
(313) 916-2600

Hershey Medical Center - Universtiy
Hospital
Hershey Med Ctr - Univ Hosp
500 University Drive
Hershey, PA 17033
Mid Atlantic
(717) 531-8521

Highland Park Hospital
Highland Park Hosp
718 Glenview Ave
Highland Park, IL 60035
Midwest
(847) 432-8000

Hoag Memorial Hospital Presbyterian
Hoag Meml Hosp Presby
One Hoag Drive
Newport Beach, CA 92663
West Coast and Pacific
(949) 645-8600

Hospital for Joint Diseases
Affiliate, NYU Medical Center
Hosp For Joint Diseases
301 East 17th Street
New York, NY 10003
Mid Atlantic
(212) 598-6000

Hospital for Special Surgery
Hosp For Special Surgery
535 East 70th Street
New York, NY 10021
Mid Atlantic
(212) 606-1000

Hospital of St Raphael's
Hosp of St Raphael's
1450 Chapel Street
New Haven, CT 06511
New England
(203) 789-3000

Hospital of the University of
Pennsylvania
Affiliate, University of Pennsylvania
Health System
Hosp Univ Penn
3400 Spruce Street
Philadelphia, PA 19104
Mid Atlantic
(215) 662-4000

Howard University Hospital
Howard Univ Hosp
2041 Georgia Ave NW
Washington, DC 20060
Mid Atlantic
(202) 865-6100

Institutions in bold are profiled in this edition of the Castle Connolly Guide.

Hutzel Hospital - Detroit
Affiliate, Detroit Medical Center
Hutzel Hosp - Detroit
4707 St Antoine Blvd
Detroit, MI 48201-1498
Midwest
(313) 745-7555

Indian River Memorial Hosp
Indian River Mem Hosp
1000 36th St
Vero Beach, FL 32960
Southeast
(561) 567-4311

Indiana University Hospital
Affiliate, Clarian Health System
IN Univ Hosp
550 N University Blvd
Indianapolis, IN 46202
Midwest
(317) 962-2000

Inova Alexandria Hospital
Inova Alexandria Hosp
4320 Seminary Rd
Alexandria, VA 22304
Southeast
(703) 504-3000

Inova Fair Oaks Hospital
Inova Fair Oaks Hosp
3600 Joseph Siewick Dr
Fairfax, VA 22033
Southeast
(703) 391-3600

Inova Fairfax Hospital
Inova Fairfax Hosp
3300 Gallows Road
Falls Church, VA 22042
Southeast
(703) 698-1110

Intergris Baptist Medical Center -
Oklahoma
Intergris Baptist Med Ctr - OK
3300 NW Expressway
Oklahoma City, OK 73112-9028
Southwest
(405) 949-3011

Jewish Hospital HealthCare Services, Inc.
Jewish Hosp HlthCre Svcs Inc
217 E. Chestnut Street
Louisville, KY 40202
Southeast
(502) 587-4011

JFK Medical Center - Atlantis
JFK Med Ctr - Atlantis
5301 S Congress Ave
Atlantis, FL 33462
Southeast
(561) 642-3791

JFK Medical Center - Edison
JFK Med Ctr - Edison
65 James Street
Edison, NJ 08818
Mid Atlantic
(732) 321-7000

Joe Di Maggio Children's Hospital
Joe Di Maggio Child. Hosp.
3501 Johnson St, Ste 520
Hollywood, FL 33021
Southeast
(954) 987-2000

Johns Hopkins Bayview Medical Center
Johns Hopkins Bayview Med Ctr
4940 Eastern Avenue
Baltimore, MD 21224
Mid Atlantic
(410) 550-0100

Institutions in bold are profiled in this edition of the Castle Connolly Guide.

Johns Hopkins Hospital - Baltimore
Johns Hopkins Hosp - Baltimore
600 N Wolfe
Baltimore, MD 21287
Mid Atlantic
(410) 955-5000

Kaiser Foundation Hospital - Anaheim
Kaiser Foundation Hosp - Anaheim
441 North Lakeview Avenue
Anaheim, CA 92807
West Coast and Pacific
(714) 279-4000

Kaiser Permanente Medical Center - San
Francisco
Kaiser Permanente Med Ctr - SF
1200 El Camino Real
South San Francisco, CA 94080
West Coast and Pacific
(650) 742-2000

Kapiolani Medical Center for Women &
Children
Kapiolani Med Ctr for Women & Chldn
1319 Punahou St
Honolulu, HI 96826
West Coast and Pacific
(808) 983-6000

Kessler Institute for Rehabilitation - East
Orange
Kessler Inst for Rehab - East Orange
240 Central Ave
East Orange, NJ 07018
Mid Atlantic
(973) 414-4700

Kessler Institute for Rehabilitation - West
Orange
Kessler Inst for Rehab - W Orange
1199 Pleasant Valley Way
West Orange, NJ 07052-1499
Mid Atlantic
(973) 243-6800

KFH San Francisco Medical Center
KFH San Francisco Med Ctr
2425 Geary Blvd
San Francisco, CA 94115
West Coast and Pacific
(415) 202-2000

KPH Panorama City Medical Center
KPH Panorama City Med Ctr
13652 Cantara St
Panorama City, CA 91402
West Coast and Pacific
(818) 375-2000

La Rabida Children's Hospital
La Rabida Children's Hosp
E 65th at Lake Michigan
Chicago, IL 60649
Midwest
(773) 363-6700

LAC & USC Medical Center
LAC & USC Med Ctr
1200 N State St
Los Angeles, CA 90033-4525
West Coast and Pacific
(323) 226-2622

LAC - Harbor - UCLA Medical Center
LAC - Harbor - UCLA Med Ctr
1000 W Carson St
Torrance, CA 90509-2059
West Coast and Pacific
(310) 222-2345

Institutions in bold are profiled in this edition of the Castle Connolly Guide.

LAC - King/Drew Medical Center
LAC - King/Drew Med Ctr
12021 South Wilmington Avenue
Los Angeles, CA 90059
West Coast and Pacific
(310) 668-4321

LAC - Olive View - UCLA Medical Center
LAC - Olive View - UCLA Med Ctr
14445 Olive View Drive
Sylmar, CA 91342
West Coast and Pacific
(818) 364-1555

Lahey Clinic
Lahey Cli.
41 Mall Road
Burlington, MA 01805
New England
(781) 744-5100

Lake Forest Hospital
Lake Forest Hosp
660 N Westmoreland Road
Lake Forest, IL 60045
Midwest
(847) 234-5600

LDS Hospital
LDS Hosp
8th Ave & C St
Salt Lake City, UT 84143
Great Plains and Mountains
(801) 408-1100

Le Bonheur Children's Medical Center
Le Bonheur Chldns Med Ctr
50 N Dunlap
Memphis, TN 38103-2893
Southeast
(901) 572-3000

Legacy Good Samaritan Hospital and
Medical Center
Legacy Good Samaritan Hosp and Med Ctr
1015 NW 22nd Ave
Portland, OR 97210-3025
West Coast and Pacific
(503) 413-7711

Lenox Hill Hospital
Lenox Hill Hosp
100 East 77th Street
New York, NY 10021
Mid Atlantic
(212) 434-2000

Loma Linda Children's Hospital
Loma Linda Children's Hosp
11234 Anderson St
Loma Linda, CA 92354
West Coast and Pacific
(714) 824-4710

Loma Linda University Behavioral
Medical Center - Redlands
Loma Linda Univ Behav Med Ctr - Redlands
1710 Barton Road
Redlands, CA 92373
West Coast and Pacific
(909) 793-9333

Loma Linda University Medical Center
Loma Linda Univ Med Ctr
11234 Anderson St
Loma Linda, CA 92354
West Coast and Pacific
(909) 824-0800

Long Beach Memorial Medical Center
Long Beach Meml Med Ctr
2801 Atlantic Ave
Long Beach, CA 90806
West Coast and Pacific
(562) 933-2000

Institutions in bold are profiled in this edition of the Castle Connolly Guide.

**Long Island College Hospital
Affiliate, Continuum Health
Partners, Inc.**
Long Island Coll Hosp
**339 Hicks Street
Brooklyn, NY 11201
Mid Atlantic
(718) 780-1000**

Long Island Jewish Medical Center
Long Island Jewish Med Ctr
270-05 76th Avenue
New Hyde Park, NY 11040
Mid Atlantic
(516) 470-7000

Los Alamitos Medical Center
Los Alamitos Med Ctr
3751 Katella Ave
Los Alamitos, CA 90720
West Coast and Pacific
(562) 598-1311

Louis A Weiss Memorial Hospital
Louis A Weiss Mem Hosp
4646 N Marine Dr
Chicago, IL 60640
Midwest
(773) 878-8700

Louisiana State University Hospital
Louisiana State Univ Hosp
1501 Kings Highway P.O. Box 33932
Shreveport, LA 71130
Southwest
(318) 675-4239

Loyola University Medical Center
Loyola Univ Med Ctr
2160 S 1st Ave
Maywood, IL 60153
Midwest
(708) 216-9000

Magee Rehabilitation Hospital
Magee Rehab Hosp
1513 Race St
Philadelphia, PA 19102-1177
Mid Atlantic
(215) 587-3000

Magee Women's Hospital
Magee Women's Hosp
300 Halket Street
Pittsburgh, PA 15213
Mid Atlantic
(412) 641-1000

Maimonides Medical Center
Maimonides Med Ctr
**4802 Tenth Avenue
Brooklyn, NY 11219
Mid Atlantic
(718) 283-6000**

Maine Medical Center
Maine Med Ctr
22 Bramhall St
Portland, ME 04102
New England
(207) 871-0111

Manhattan Eye, Ear & Throat Hospital
Manhattan Eye, Ear & Throat Hosp
210 East 64th Street
New York, NY 10021
Mid Atlantic
(212) 838-9200

Marin General Hospital
Marin Genl Hosp
250 Bon Air Rd
Greenbrae, CA 94904
West Coast and Pacific
(415) 925-7000

Institutions in bold are profiled in this edition of the Castle Connolly Guide.

Martin Memorial Health System
Martin Meml Hlth Sys
300 Hospital Dr
Stuart, FL 34994
Southeast
(561) 287-5200

Mary Shiels Hospital
Mary Shiels Hosp
3515 Howell St
Dallas, TX 75204
Southwest
(214) 443-3000

Maryland General Hospital
Maryland Genl Hosp
827 Linden Ave
Baltimore, MD 21201
Mid Atlantic
(410) 225-8000

Maryland Psychiatric Research Center
Maryland Psyc Research Ctr
Maple & Locust, Box 21247
Baltimore, MD 21228
Mid Atlantic
(410) 402-7666

Massachusetts Eye & Ear Infirmary
Mass Eye & Ear Infirmary
243 Charles Street
Boston, MA 02114
New England
(617) 573-5520

Massachusetts General Hospital
MA Genl Hosp
55 Fruit St
Boston, MA 02114
New England
(617) 726-2000

Massachusetts Mental Health Center
MA Mental Hlth Ctr
74 Fenwood Rd
Boston, MA 02115
New England
(617) 626-9300

Mayo Clinical Hospital - Scottsdale
Mayo Clin Hosp - Scottsdale
13400 E Shea Blvd
Scottsdale, AZ 85259
Southwest
(480) 301-8000

Mayo Medical Center & Clinic -
Rochester, MN
Mayo Med Ctr & Clin - Rochester, MN
200 First St SW
Rochester, MN 55905
Midwest
(507) 284-2511

McLaren Regional Medical Center
McLaren Reg Med Ctr
401 S. Ballenger Highway
Flint, MI 48532
Midwest
(810) 342-2000

McLean Hospital
McLean Hosp
115 Mill St
Belmont, MA 02478
New England
(617) 855-2000

Medical Center of Central Georgia
Med Ctr of Central GA
777 Hemlock Street
Macon, GA 31201
Southeast
(478) 633-1000

Institutions in bold are profiled in this edition of the Castle Connolly Guide.

Medical College of Georgia Hospital and Clinic
Med Coll of GA Hosp and Clin
1120 15th Street
Augusta, GA 30912
Southeast
(706) 721-0211

Medical College of Ohio Hospitals
Med Coll of Ohio Hosps
3000 Arlington Ave
Toledo, OH 43614
Midwest
(419) 383-4000

Medical College of Virginia Hospitals
Med Coll of VA Hosp
401 N 12th St, Box 980510
Richmond, VA 23298-0570
Southeast
(804) 828-9000

Medical University Hospital Authority
Med Univ Hosp Authority
169 Ashley Ave
Charleston, SC 29425
Southeast
(843) 792-2300

Memorial Hermann Hospital
Meml Hermann Hosp
6411 Sannin St
Houston, TX 77030
Southwest
(713) 704-4000

Memorial Medical Center - Baptist Campus
Meml Med Ctr - Baptist Campus
2700 Napoleon Ave
New Orleans, LA 70115
Southwest
(504) 899-9311

Memorial Medical Center - Savannah
Meml Med Ctr - Savannah
4700 Waters Ave
Savannah, GA 31404
Southeast
(912) 350-8000

Memorial Regional Hospital- Hollywood
Mem Reg Hosp - Hollywood
3501 Johnson Street
Hollywood, FL 33021
Southeast
(954) 987-2000

Memorial Sloan Kettering Cancer Center
Mem Sloan Kettering Cancer Ctr
1275 York Avenue
New York, NY 10021
Mid Atlantic
(212) 639-2000

Menninger Clinic
Menninger Clinic
5800 SW 6th Ave or PO Box 829
Topeka, KS 66601-0829
Great Plains and Mountains
(785) 350-5000

Mercy Health Center - Oklahoma City
Mercy Hlth Ctr - Oklahoma City
4300 W Memorial Rd
Oklahoma City, OK 73120
Southwest
(405) 755-1515

Mercy Hospital & Medical Center - San Diego
Mercy Hosp & Med Ctr - San Diego
4077 5th Ave
San Diego, CA 92103
West Coast and Pacific
(619) 294-8111

Institutions in bold are profiled in this edition of the Castle Connolly Guide.

Mercy Hospital - Coon Rapids
Mercy Hosp - Coon Rapids
4050 Coon Rapids Blvd
Coon Rapids, MN 55433-2522
Midwest
(763) 421-8888

Mercy Hospital - Miami, FL
Mercy Hosp - Miami, FL
3663 S Miami Ave
Miami, FL 33133
Southeast
(305) 854-4400

MeritCare Hospital
MeritCare Hosp
720 Fourth Street North
Fargo, ND 58122
Great Plains and Mountains
(701) 234-6000

Methodist Health Care North - Memphis
Meth Hlth Care N - Memphis
3960 New Covington Pike
Memphis, TN 38128
Southeast
(901) 384-5200

Methodist Healthcare Central - Memphis
Hospital
Meth Healthcare Central - Memphis Hosp
1265 Union Ave
Memphis, TN 38104
Southeast
(901) 726-7000

Methodist Hospital - Houston
Methodist Hosp - Houston
6565 Fannin St, D200
Houston, TX 77030
Southwest
(713) 790-3311

Methodist Hospital - Indianapolis
Affiliate, Clarian Health System
Methodist Hosp - Indianapolis
1701 N Senate Blvd
Indianapolis, IN 46202
Midwest
(317) 962-2000

Methodist Hospital Healthsystem -
Minnesota
Methodist Hosp - Minnesota
6500 Excelsior Blvd
Minneapolis, MN 55426-4700
Midwest
(952) 993-5000

Miami Children's Hospital
Miami Children's Hosp
3100 SW 62nd Ave
Miami, FL 33155
Southeast
(305) 666-6511

Miami Heart Institute - North Campus
Miami Heart Inst - North Campus
4701 Meridian Ave
Miami Beach, FL 33140
Southeast
(305) 672-1111

Michael Reese Hospital & Medical Center
Michael Reese Hosp & Med Ctr
2929 S Ellis Ave
Chicago, IL 60616
Midwest
(312) 791-2000

Milford Hospital
Milford Hosp
300 Seaside Ave
Milford, CT 06460
New England
(203) 876-4000

Institutions in bold are profiled in this edition of the Castle Connolly Guide.

Millard Fillmore Hospitals
Millard Fillmore Hosp
3 Gates Cir
Buffalo, NY 14209
Mid Atlantic
(716) 887-4600

Mills - Peninsula Health Center Hospital
Mills - Peninsula Hlth Ctr Hosp
1783 El Camino Real
Burlingame, CA 94010
West Coast and Pacific
(650) 696-5400

Montclair - Baptist Medical Center
Montclair - Baptist Med Ctr
800 Montclair Rd
Birmingham, AL 35213-1984
Southeast
(205) 592-1000

Montefiore Medical Center
Affiliate, Montefiore Medical Center
Montefiore Med Ctr
111 East 210 Street
Bronx, NY 10467
Mid Atlantic
(718) 920-4321

Montefiore Medical Center - Weiler-
Einstein Division
Affiliate, Montefiore Medical Center
Montefiore Med Ctr - Weiler-Einstein
Div
1825 Eastchester Road
Bronx, NY 10461
Mid Atlantic
(718) 904-2000

Moss Rehab Hospital
Moss Rehab Hosp
1200 W Tabor Rd
Philadelphia, PA 19141
Mid Atlantic
(215) 456-9900

Motts Children's Hospital
Motts Chldns Hosp
1500 E Medical Center Drive
Ann Arbor, MI 48109
Midwest
(734) 936-4000

Mount Auburn Hospital
Mount Auburn Hosp
330 Mount Auburn Street
Cambridge, MA 02238
New England
(617) 492-3500

Mount Sinai Hospital
Affiliate, Mount Sinai Hospital
Mount Sinai Hosp
One Gustave L. Levy Pl
New York, NY 10029
Mid Atlantic
(212) 241-6500

Mount Sinai Medical Center
Mount Sinai Med Ctr
4300 Alton Rd
Miami Beach, FL 33140
Southeast
(305) 674-2121

Muhlenberg Regional Medical Center
Muhlenberg Regional Med Ctr
Park Avenue and Randolph Road
Plainfield, NJ 07061
Mid Atlantic
(908) 668-2000

Institutions in bold are profiled in this edition of the Castle Connolly Guide.

National Institutes of Health - Clinical
Center
Natl Inst of Hlth - Clin Ctr
9000 Rockville Pike, Building 10
Bethesda, MD 20892
Mid Atlantic
(301) 496-2563

National Jewish Medical & Research
Center
Natl Jewish Med & Rsrch Ctr
1400 Jackson Street
Denver, CO 80206-2762
Great Plains and Mountains
(303) 388-4461

National Rehabilitation Hospital
Natl Rehab Hosp
102 Irving Street NorthWest
Washington, DC 20010
Mid Atlantic
(202) 877-1000

Nebraska Health System
Nebraska Hlth Sys
987400 Nebraska Med Ctr.
Omaha, NE 68198-7400
Great Plains and Mountains
(402) 559-2000

Nebraska Health System - Clarkson
Nebraska Hlth Sys - Clarkson
4350 Dewey Ave
Omaha, NE 68105-1018
Great Plains and Mountains
(402) 552-2000

Nebraska Methodist Hospital
Nebraska Meth Hosp
8303 Dodge St
Omaha, NE 68114
Great Plains and Mountains
(402) 354-4000

New Britain General Hospital
New Britain Gen Hosp
100 Grand St
New Britain, CT 06050
New England
(860) 224-5666

New England Baptist Hospital
New England Baptist
125 Parker Hill Avenue
Boston, MA 02120
New England
(617) 754-5800

New England Medical Center
New England Med Ctr - Boston
750 Washington St
Boston, MA 02111
New England
(617) 636-5000

New Orleans Adolescent Hosp
New Orleans Adol Hosp
210 State St
New Orleans, LA 70118-5735
Southwest
(504) 897-3400

**New York Eye & Ear Infirmary
Affiliate, Continuum Health
Partners, Inc.**
New York Eye & Ear Infirm
310 East 14th Street
New York, NY 10003
Mid Atlantic
(212) 979-4000

Institutions in bold are profiled in this edition of the Castle Connolly Guide.

New York Hospital Medical Center of
Queens
NY Hosp Med Ctr of Queens
56-45 Main Street
Flushing, NY 11355
Mid Atlantic
(718) 670-1231

New York State Psychiatric Institute
NY State Psychiatric Inst
1051 Riverside Dr
New York, NY 10032
Mid Atlantic
(212) 543-5000

New York- Presbyterian Hospital
NY Presby Hosp
161 Fort Washington Avenue
New York, NY 10032
Mid Atlantic
(212) 305-3710

Newark Beth Israel Medical Center
Newark Beth Israel Med Ctr
201 Lyons Ave
Newark, NJ 07112
Mid Atlantic
(973) 926-7000

Newton - Wellesley Hospital
Newton - Wellesley Hosp
2014 Washington Street
Newton, MA 02462
New England
(617) 243-6000

**NewYork Presbyterian Hospital -
Columbia Presbyterian Medical
Center
Affiliate, NewYork-Presbyterian
Health System**
*NY Presby Hosp - Columbia Presby
Med Ctr*
**622 W 168th St
New York, NY 10032
Mid Atlantic
(212) 305-2500**

**NewYork Presbyterian Hospital -
NewYork Weill Cornell Medical
Center
Affiliate, NewYork-Presbyterian
Health System**
*NY Presby Hosp - NY Weill Cornell
Med Ctr*
**525 E 68th St
New York, NY 10021
Mid Atlantic
(212) 746-5454**

NewYork Presbyterian Hospital -
Westchester Division
NY Presby Hosp - Westchester Div
21 Bloomingdale Rd
White Plains, NY 10605
Mid Atlantic
(914) 682-9100

North Central Baptist Hospital
N Central Baptist Hosp
520 Madison Oak Dr.
San Antonio, TX 78258
Southwest
(210) 297-4000

Institutions in bold are profiled in this edition of the Castle Connolly Guide.

North Oaks Medical Center
North Oaks Med Ctr
15790 Paul Vega MD Dr
Hammond, LA 70403
Southwest
(985) 230-6601

North Shore University Hospital at
Manhasset
N Shore Univ Hosp at Manhasset
300 Community Dr
Manhasset, NY 11030
Mid Atlantic
(516) 562-0100

Northern Westchester Hospital Center
Northern Westchester Hosp Ctr
400 East Main Street
Mount Kisco, NY 10549
Mid Atlantic
(914) 666-1200

Northwest Hospital
NW Hosp
1550 N 115th St
Seattle, WA 98133-0806
West Coast and Pacific
(206) 364-0500

Northwest Medical Center
Northwest Med Ctr
2801 N State Rd 7
Margate, FL 33063
Southeast
(954) 974-0400

Northwestern Memorial Hospital
Northwestern Meml Hosp
251 E Huron St
Chicago, IL 60611
Midwest
(312) 926-2000

Norton Hospital
Norton Hospital
200 E Chestnut St
Louisville, KY 40202
Southeast
(502) 629-8000

NYU Downtown Hospital
Affiliate, NYU Medical Center
NYU Downtown Hosp
170 William Street
New York, NY 10038
Mid Atlantic
(212) 312-5000

NYU Medical Center
Affiliate, NYU Medical Center
NYU Med Ctr
540 First Avenue
New York, NY 10016
Mid Atlantic
(212) 263-7300

Ochsner Foundation Hospital
Ochsner Found Hosp
1516 Jefferson Hwy
New Orleans, LA 70121-2484
Southwest
(504) 842-3000

Ohio State University Medical Center
Ohio St Univ Med Ctr
410 W 10th Avenue
Columbus, OH 43210
Midwest
(614) 293-8000

Olathe Medical Center
Olathe Med Ctr
20333 W 151st St
Olathe, KS 66061-5352
Great Plains and Mountains
(913) 791-4200

Institutions in bold are profiled in this edition of the Castle Connolly Guide.

Olive View Medical Center
Olive View Med Ctr
14445 Olive View Dr
Sylmar, CA 91342
West Coast and Pacific
(818) 364-1555

Oregon Health Science University
Hospital and Clinics
OR Hlth Sci Univ Hosp and Clinics
3181 SW Sam Jackson Park Rd
Portland, OR 97201-3098
West Coast and Pacific
(503) 494-8311

Orlando Regional Medical Center
Orlando Reg Med Ctr
1414 Kuhl Avenue
Orlando, FL 32806
Southeast
(407) 841-5111

Orthopaedic Hospital
Orthopaedic Hosp
2400 South Flower Street
Los Angeles, CA 90007
West Coast and Pacific
(213) 742-1000

Orthopedic Specialty Hospital, The
TOSH - The Ortho Spec Hosp
5848 S 300 East
Salt Lake City, UT 84107
Great Plains and Mountains
(801) 269-4000

Our Lady of Lourdes Regional Medical
Center - Lafayette
Our Lady of Lordes Reg Med Ctr - Lafayette
611 ST Landry St
Lafayette, LA 70506-4697
Southwest
(337) 289-2000

Our Lady of Mercy Medical Center
Our Lady of Mercy Med Ctr
600 E 233rd St
Bronx, NY 10466
Mid Atlantic
(718) 920-9000

Overlake Hospital Medical Center
Ovelake Hosp Med Ctr
1035 116th Ave NE
Bellevue, WA 98004-4687
West Coast and Pacific
(425) 688-5000

Parkland Memorial Hospital
Parkland Mem Hosp
5201 Harry Hines Boulevard
Dallas, TX 75235
Southwest
(214) 590-8000

Penn State University Hospital - Milton
S.Hershey Medical Center
*Penn State Univ Hosp - Milton S Hershey
Med Ctr*
500 University Dr, Box 850
Hershey, PA 17033
Mid Atlantic
(717) 531-8803

**Pennsylvania Hospital
Affiliate, University of Pennsylvania
Health System**
Pennsylvania Hosp
**800 Spruce Street
Philadelphia, PA 19107
Mid Atlantic
(215) 829-3000**

Institutions in bold are profiled in this edition of the Castle Connolly Guide.

Phillips Eye Institute
Phillips Eye Inst
2215 Park Ave S
Minneapolis, MN 55404
Midwest
(612) 336-6000

Presbyterian - St Luke's Medical Center
Presby - St Luke's Med Ctr
1719 E 19th Ave
Denver, CO 80218
Great Plains and Mountains
(303) 839-6000

Presbyterian Hospital - Albuquerque
Presbyterian Hospital - Albuquerque
1100 Central Ave SE
Albuquerque, NM 87106
Southwest
(505) 841-1234

Presbyterian Hospital - Charlotte
Presby Hosp - Charlotte
200 Hawthorne Ln
Charlotte, NC 28204-2528
Southeast
(704) 384-4000

Presbyterian Hospital - Oklahoma City
Presby Hosp - Oklahoma City
700 NE 13th Street
Oklahoma City, OK 73104
Southwest

Presbyterian Hospital of Dallas
Presby Hosp - Dallas
8200 Walnut Hill Lane
Dallas, TX 75231
Southwest
(214) 345-8400

Primary Children's Medical Center
Primary Children's Med Ctr
100 N Medical Drive
Salt Lake City, UT 84113-1100
Great Plains and Mountains
(801) 588-2000

Providence Portland Medical Center
Providence Portland Med Ctr
4805 NE Glisan St
Portland, OR 97313-2967
West Coast and Pacific
(503) 215-1111

Promina Piedmont Hospital
Promina Piedmont Hosp
1968 Peachtree Road NorthWest
Atlanta, GA 30309
Southeast
(404) 605-5000

Providence Alaska Medical Center
Providence Alaska Med Ctr
3200 Providence Drive
Anchorage, AK 99508-4615
West Coast and Pacific
(907) 562-2211

Providence Hospital - Southfield
Providence Hosp - Southfield
16001 Nine Mile Road
Southfield, MI 48075
Midwest
(248) 424-3000

Providence Portland Medical Center
Providence Portland Med Ctr
4805 NE Glisan
Portland, OR 97213-2967
West Coast and Pacific
(503) 215-1111

Institutions in bold are profiled in this edition of the Castle Connolly Guide.

Providence Saint Joseph Medical Center
Providence St Joseph Med Ctr
501 South Buena Vista St.
Burbank, CA 91505
West Coast and Pacific
(818) 843-5111

Puget Sound Hospital
Puget Sound Hosp
215 S 36th St, Box 11412
Tacoma, WA 98411
West Coast and Pacific
(206) 474-0561

Queen's Medical Center - Honolulu
Queen's Med Ctr - Honolulu
1301 Punchbowl Street
Honolulu, HI 96813
West Coast and Pacific
(808) 538-9011

Rainbow Babies & Children's Hospital
Rainbow Babies & Chldns Hosp
11100 Euclid Ave
Cleveland, OH 44106
Midwest
(216) 844-1000

Rancho Los Amigos National
Rehabilitation Center
Rancho Los Amigos Natl Rehab Ctr
7601 East Imperial Highway
Downey, CA 90242
West Coast and Pacific
(562) 401-7111

Rapid City Regional Hospital
Rapid City Reg Hosp
353 Fairmount Blvd
Rapid City, SD 57701
Great Plains and Mountains
(605) 719-1000

Regions Hospital - St Paul
Regions Hosp - St Paul
640 Jackson Street
St Paul, MN 55101
Midwest
(651) 221-3456

Rehabilitation Institute - Chicago
Rehab Inst - Chicago
345 E. Superior Street
Chicago, IL 60611
Midwest
(312) 238-1000

Rhode Island Hospital
Rhode Island Hosp
593 Eddy Street
Providence, RI 02903
New England
(401) 444-4000

Riley Children's Hospital
Affiliate, Clarian Health System
Riley Chldrn's Hosp
702 Barnhill Drive
Indianapolis, IN 46202
Midwest
(317) 962-2000

Robert Wood Johnson University Hospital
@ New Brunswick
Robert Wood Johnson Univ Hosp @ New Brunswick
1 Robert Wood Johnson Pl
New Brunswick, NJ 08903
Mid Atlantic
(732) 828-3000

Institutions in bold are profiled in this edition of the Castle Connolly Guide.

Rochester General Hospital
Rochester Gen Hosp
1425 Portland Avenue
Rochester, NY 14621
Mid Atlantic
(585) 922-4000

Rochester Methodist Hospital
Rochester Meth Hosp
201 W Center St
Rochester, MN 55905-3003
Midwest
(507) 266-8596

Rockefeller University
Rockefeller Univ
1230 York Avenue
New York, NY 10021
Mid Atlantic
(212) 327-8000

Roswell Park Cancer Institute
Roswell Park Cancer Inst
Elm and Carlton Streets
Buffalo, NY 14263
Mid Atlantic
(716) 845-5770

**Rush-Presbyterian - St Luke's
Medical Center**
Rush-Presby - St Luke's Med Ctr
**1653 W Congress Parkway
Chicago, IL 60612-3833
Midwest
(312) 942-5000**

**Rusk Institute of Rehabilitation
Medicine
Affiliate, NYU Medical Center**
Rusk Inst of Rehab Med
**400 East 34th Street
New York, NY 10016
Mid Atlantic
(212) 263-7300**

Sacred Heart Medical Center
Sacred Heart Med Ctr
1255 Hilyard St
Eugene, OR 97440-3700
West Coast and Pacific
(541) 686-7300

Saint Agnes Hospital
Saint Agnes Hosp
305 North St
White Plains, NY 10605
Mid Atlantic
(914) 681-4500

Saint Joseph Hospital
Saint Joseph Hosp
2900 N Lake Shore Dr
Chicago, IL 60657
Midwest
(773) 665-3000

Saint Michael's Medical Center
Saint Michael's Med Ctr
268 Dr. Martin Luther King, Jr. Blvd
Newark, NJ 07102
Mid Atlantic
(973) 877-5000

Institutions in bold are profiled in this edition of the Castle Connolly Guide.

**Saint Vincent Catholic Medical
Centers - St Vincent's Manhattan
Affiliate, Saint Vincent Catholic
Medical Centers**
St Vincent Cath Med Ctrs - Manhattan
**170 West 12th Street
New York, NY 10011
Mid Atlantic
(212) 604-7000**

**Saint Vincent Catholic Medical
Centers - St Vincent's Staten Island
Affiliate, Saint Vincent Catholic
Medical Centers**
*St Vincent Cath Med Ctr - Staten
Island*
**355 Bard Ave
Staten Island, NY 10310-1699
Mid Atlantic
(718) 818-1234**

San Francisco General Hospital
San Francisco Gen Hosp
1001 Potrero Avenue
San Francisco, CA 94110
West Coast and Pacific
(415) 206-8000

Santa Clara Valley Medical Center
Santa Clara Valley Med Ctr
751 S Bascom Avenue
San Jose, CA 95128
West Coast and Pacific
(408) 885-5000

Santa Monica - UCLA Medical Center
Santa Monica - UCLA Med Ctr
1250 16th Street
Santa Monica, CA 90404
West Coast and Pacific
(310) 319-4000

Sarasota Memorial Hospital
Sarasota Mem Hosp
1700 S Tamiami Trail
Sarasota, FL 34239
Southeast
(941) 917-9000

Schneider's Children's Hospital
Schneider's Chldns Hosp
269-01 76th Ave
New Hyde Park, NY 11040
Mid Atlantic
(718) 470-3000

Schwab Rehabilitation Hospital
Schwab Rehab Hosp
1401 S. California Boulevard
Chicago, IL 60608
Midwest
(773) 522-2010

Scripps Memorial Hospital - La Jolla
Scripps Meml Hosp - La Jolla
9888 Genesee Ave
La Jolla, CA 92037
West Coast and Pacific
(858) 457-4123

Self Regional Healthcare
Self Regional Healthcare
1325 Spring St
Greenwood, SC 29646
Southeast
(864) 227-4111

Sentara Leigh Hospital
Sentara Leigh Hosp
830 Kempsville Rd
Norfolk, VA 23502-3981
Southeast
(757) 466-6000

Institutions in bold are profiled in this edition of the Castle Connolly Guide.

Sentara Norfolk General Hospital
Sentara Norfolk Gen Hosp
600 Gresham Drive
Norfolk, VA 23507
Southeast
(757) 668-3000

Sentara Virginia Beach General Hospital
Virginia Beach Gen Hosp
1060 First Colonial Rd
Virginia Beach, VA 23454
Southeast
(757) 395-8000

Shadyside Hospital - Pittsburgh
Shadyside Hosp - Pittsburgh
5230 Center Ave
Pittsburgh, PA 15232
Mid Atlantic
(412) 623-2121

Shands at Vista
Shands at Vista
8900 NW 39th Ave
Gainesville, FL 32606
Southeast
(352) 265-5497

Shands Healthcare at University of
Florida
Shands Hlthcre at Univ of FL
1600 SW Archer Road
Gainesville, FL 32610
Southeast
(352) 265-0111

Shands Jacksonville
Shands Jacksonville
655 W 8th St
Jacksonville, FL 32209
Southeast
(904) 244-0411

Sharp Memorial Hospital
Sharp Mem Hosp
7901 Frost Street
San Diego, CA 92103
West Coast and Pacific
(858) 541-3400

Sheppard Pratt Health System
Sheppard Pratt Hlth Sys
6501 N Charles St
Baltimore, MD 21285-6815
Mid Atlantic
(410) 938-3000

Silver Hill Hospital
Silver Hill Hosp
208 Valley Rd
New Canaan, CT 06840-3899
New England
(203) 966-3561

Sinai Hospital - Baltimore
Sinai Hosp - Baltimore
2401 West Belvedere Avenue
Baltimore, MD 21215
Mid Atlantic
(410) 601-5134

Sinai Samaritan Medical Center - Aurora
Health Care
Sinai Samaritan Med Ctr - AHC
945 N. 12th Street, PO Box 342
Milwaukee, WI 53201
Midwest
(414) 649-7500

Sinai-Grace Hospital - Detroit
Affiliate, Detroit Medical Center
Sinai-Grace Hosp - Detroit
6071 W. Outer Drive
Detroit, MI 48235
Midwest
(313) 966-3300

Institutions in bold are profiled in this edition of the Castle Connolly Guide.

South Shore Hospital - Miami Beach
South Shore Hosp - Miami Bch
630 Alton Rd
Miami Beach, FL 33139
Southeast
(305) 672-2100

Southwest Texas Methodist Hospital
SW Texas Methodist Hosp
7700 Floyd Curl Drive
San Antonio, TX 78201
Southwest

Sparrow Health System - St Lawrence
Sparrow Health System - St Lawrence
1210 W Saginaw St0
Lansing, MI 48915-1999
Midwest
(517) 372-8220

Spaulding Rehabilitation Hospital
Spauding Rehab Hosp
125 Nashua Street
Boston, MA 02114
New England
(617) 720-6400

Spectrum Health East
Spectrum Health East
1840 Wealthy St SE
Grand Rapids, MI 49506
Midwest
(616) 774-7444

SSM St Mary's Health Center - St Louis
SSM St Mary's Hlth Ctr - St Louis
6420 Clayton Rd
St. Louis, MO 63117
Midwest
(314) 768-8000

St Alexius Medical Center
St Alexius Med Ctr
1555 Barrington Rd
Hoffman Estates, IL 60194
Midwest
(847) 843-2000

St Alphonsus Regional Medical Center
St Alphonsus Reg Med Ctr
1055 N Curtis Rd
Boise, ID 83706-1370
Great Plains and Mountains
(208) 367-2121

St Anne's Hospital
St Anne's Hosp
795 Middle Street
Fall River, MA 02721
New England
(508) 674-5741

St Barnabas Medical Center
St Barnabas Med Ctr
94 Old Short Hills Rd
Livingston, NJ 07039-5672
Mid Atlantic
(973) 322-5000

St Christopher's Hospital for Children
St Christopher's Hosp for Children
Erie Avenue at Front Street
Philadelphia, PA 19134
Mid Atlantic
(215) 427-5337

St Elizabeth's Medical Center
St Elizabeth's Med Ctr
736 Cambridge Street
Brighton, MA 02135
New England
(617) 789-3000

Institutions in bold are profiled in this edition of the Castle Connolly Guide.

St Francis Hospital & Medical Center
St Francis Hosp & Med Ctr
114 Woodland Street
Hartford, CT 06105
New England
(860) 714-4000

St Francis Hospital - Evanston
St Francis Hosp - Evanston
355 Ridge Ave
Evanston, IL 60202
Midwest
(847) 316-4000

St Francis Hospital - The Heart Center
St Francis Hosp - The Heart Ctr
100 Port Washington Boulevard
Roslyn, NY 11576
Mid Atlantic
(516) 562-6000

St Francis Medical Center of Santa Barbara
St Francis Med Ctr of Santa Barbara
601 E. Micheltorena St
Santa Barbara, CA 93103
West Coast and Pacific
(805) 962-7661

St John Hospital and Medical Center
St John Hosp and Med Ctr
22101 Moross Road
Detroit, MI 48236-2172
Midwest
(313) 343-4000

St John's Health Center
St John's Hlth Ctr
1328 22nd St
Santa Monica, CA 90404
West Coast and Pacific
(310) 829-5511

St John's Hospital - Springfield
St John's Hosp - Springfield
800 E. Carpenter Street
Springfield, IL 62769
Midwest
(217) 544-6464

St John's Mercy Medical Center - St Louis
St John's Mercy Med Ctr - St Louis
615 S New Ballas Rd
St Louis, MO 63141
Midwest
(314) 569-6000

St Joseph Hospital
St Joseph Hosp
172 Kinsley St
Nashua, NH 03060
New England
(603) 882-3000

St Joseph Hospital of Kirkwood
St Joseph Hosp of Kirkwood
525 Couch Ave
St Louis, MO 63122
Midwest
(314) 966-1500

St Joseph Medical Center
St Joseph Med Ctr
7601 Osler Drive
Baltimore, MD 21208
Mid Atlantic

St Joseph Mercy Hospital - Ann Arbor
St Joseph Mercy Hosp - Ann Arbor
5301 E Huron River Dr, Box 992
Ann Arbor, MI 48106
Midwest
(734) 712-3456

Institutions in bold are profiled in this edition of the Castle Connolly Guide.

APPENDIX E

St Joseph Mercy Oakland
St Joseph Mercy - Oakland
44405 Woodward Ave
Pontiac, MI 48341
Midwest
(248) 858-3000

St Joseph's Hospital & Medical Center - Phoenix
St Joseph's Hosp & Med Ctr - Phoenix
350 West Thomas Road
Phoenix, AZ 85013-4496
Southwest
(602) 406-3000

St Joseph's Hospital - Atlanta
St Joseph's Hosp - Atlanta
5665 Peachtree Dunwoody Road
NorthEast
Atlanta, GA 30342
Southeast
(404) 851-7001

St Joseph's Hospital - Orange
St Joseph's Hosp - Orange
1100 West Stewart Drive
Orange, CA 92868
West Coast and Pacific
(714) 633-9111

St Joseph's Hospital - Tampa
St Joseph's Hosp - Tampa
3001 W Martin Luther King Jr Blvd
Tampa, FL 33607
Southeast
(813) 870-4000

St Jude Children's Research Hospital
St Jude Children's Research Hosp
332 N Lauderdale St
Memphis, TN 38105
Southeast
(901) 495-3300

St Louis Children's Hospital
St Louis Children's Hospital
One Children's Place
St Louis, MO 63110
Midwest
(314) 454-6000

St Louis University Hospital
St Louis Univ Hospital
3635 Vista at Grand Blvd
St. Louis, MO 63110
Midwest
(314) 577-8000

St Luke's - Roosevelt Hospital Center - Roosevelt Division
Affiliate, Continuum Health Partners, Inc.
St Luke's - Roosevelt Hosp Ctr - Roosevelt Div
1000 Tenth Avenue
New York, NY 10019
Mid Atlantic
(212) 523-4000

St Luke's Episcopal Hospital - Houston
St Luke's Episcopal Hosp - Houston
6720 Bertner Avenue
Houston, TX 77030
Southwest
(713) 785-8537

St Luke's Hospital
St Luke's Hosp
4401 Wornhall Road
Kansas City, MO 64111
Midwest
(816) 932-2000

Institutions in bold are profiled in this edition of the Castle Connolly Guide.

St Luke's Hospital
St Luke's Hosp
4201 Belfort Rd
Jacksonville, FL 32216
Southeast
(904) 296-3700

St Lukes Hospital
St Lukes Hosp
232 S Woods Mill Rd
Chesterfield, MO 63017
Midwest
(314) 434-1500

St Mary's Hospital - Huntington, WV
St Mary's Hosp - Huntington, WV
2900 1st Ave   .
Huntington, WV 25702-1272
Mid Atlantic
(304) 526-1234

St Mary's Hospital - Rochester, MN
St Mary's Hosp - Rochester, MN
1216 2nd St SW
Rochester, MN 55902
Midwest
(507) 255-5123

St Mary's Medical Center .
St Mary's Med Ctr
1050 Linden Avenue
Long Beach, CA 90813
West Coast and Pacific
(562) 491-9000

St Mary's Medical Center - Duluth
St Mary's Med Ctr - Duluth
407 E 3rd St
Duluth, MN 55805-1984
Midwest
(218) 726-4000

St Mary's Medical Center - San Francisco
St Mary's Med Ctr - San Fran
450 Stanyan Street
San Francisco, CA 94117
West Coast and Pacific
(415) 668-1000

St Mary's Medical Center - West Palm
Beach
St Mary's Med Ctr - W Palm Bch
901 45th St
West Palm Beach, FL 33407
Southeast
(561) 844-6300

St Mary's Mercy Medical Center
St. Mary's Mercy Med Ctr
200 Jefferson Ave SE
Grand Rapids, MI 49503
Midwest
(616) 752-6090

St Paul University Hospital
St Paul Univ Hosp
5909 Harry Hines Boulevard
Dallas, TX 75235
Southwest
(214) 879-1000

St Thomas Hospital - Nashville
St Thomas Hosp - Nashville
4220 Harding Road
Nashville, TN 37205
Southeast
(615) 222-2111

St Vincent Charity Hospital
St Vincent Charity Hosp
2351 E 22nd St
Cleveland, OH 44115-3197
Midwest
(216) 861-6200

Institutions in bold are profiled in this edition of the Castle Connolly Guide.

St Vincent's Hospital - Carmel
St Vincent's Hosp - Carmel
13500 N Meridian Street
Carmel, IN 46032-1496
Midwest
(317) 573-7000

St Vincent's Hospital and Health Center - Indianapolis
St Vincent's Hosp and Hlth Ctr - Indianapolis
2001 West 86th Street
Indianapolis, IN 46260-1991
Midwest
(317) 338-7000

St Vincent's Medical Center - Jacksonville
St Vincent's Med Ctr - Jacksonville
1800 Barrs Street
Jacksonville, FL 32214
Southeast
(904) 308-7300

St Vincent's Medical Center - Los Angeles
St Vincent's Med Ctr - Los Angeles
2131 W 3rd St
Los Angeles, CA 90057
West Coast and Pacific
(213) 484-7111

St. Alexius Medical Center
St. Alexius Med Ctr - Bismarck
900 E Broadway Ave
Bismarck, ND 58501
Great Plains and Mountains
(701) 530-7000

St. Luke's Regional Medical Center
St. Luke's Reg Med Ctr - Boise
190 E Bannock St
Boise, ID 83712
Great Plains and Mountains

Stamford Hospital
Stamford Hosp
Shelburne Rd @ W Broad St, Box 9317
Stamford, CT 06904
New England
(203) 325-7000

Stanford Medical Center
Stanford Med Ctr
300 Pasteur Dr
Stanford, CA 94305
West Coast and Pacific
(650) 723-4000

Staten Island University Hospital - North Site
Staten Island Univ Hosp-North Site
475 Seaview Avenue
Staten Island, NY 10305
Mid Atlantic
(718) 226-9000

Stony Brook University Hospital
Stony Brook Univ Hosp
Nicolls Rd
Stony Brook, NY 11794
Mid Atlantic
(631) 689-8333

Strong Memorial Hospital - Medical Center
Strong Memorial Hosp - URMC
601 Elmwood Avenue
Rochester, NY 14642
Mid Atlantic
(716) 275-7685

Suburban Hospital Healthcare Systems
Suburban Hosp - Bethesda
8600 Old Georgetown Road
Bethesda, MD 20814
Mid Atlantic
(301) 896-3100

Institutions in bold are profiled in this edition of the Castle Connolly Guide.

Sunnyview Hospital and Rehabilitation
Center
Sunnyview Hosp
1270 Belmont Ave
Schenectady, NY 12308-2198
Mid Atlantic
(518) 382-4500

Sunrise Hospital & Medical
Center/Sunrise Children's Hospital
*Sunrise Hosp & Med Ctr/Sunrise Chldn's
Hosp*
3186 Maryland Pkwy
Las Vegas, NV 89109-2306
West Coast and Pacific
(702) 731-8000

Swedish Covenant Hospital
Swedish Covenant Hosp
5145 N California Ave
Chicago, IL 60625
Midwest
(773) 878-8200

Swedish Medical Center
Swedish Med Ctr
747 Broadway
Seattle, WA 98122
West Coast and Pacific
(206) 386-6000

Swedish Medical Center - Englewood
Swedish Med Ctr - Englewood
501 E Hampden Ave
Englewood, CO 80110-2795
Great Plains and Mountains
(303) 788-5000

Swedish Medical Center Providence
Campus
Swedish Med Ctr Providence Campus
500 17th Ave
Seattle, WA 98122
West Coast and Pacific
(206) 320-2000

Tacoma General Hospital
Tacoma Gen Hosp
315 S Martin Luther King Jr Way
Tacoma, WA 98405
West Coast and Pacific
(206) 552-1000

Tampa General Hospital
Tampa Genl Hosp
PO BOX 1289
Tampa, FL 33601
Southeast
(844) 251-7000

Temple University Hospital
Temple Univ Hosp
3401 N Broad St
Philadelphia, PA 19140-5189
Mid Atlantic
(215) 707-2000

Texas Children's Hospital - Houston
TX Chldns Hosp - Houston
6621 Fannin
Houston, TX 77030
Southwest
(832) 824-1000

Institutions in bold are profiled in this edition of the Castle Connolly Guide.

Texas Scottish Rite Hospital for Children - Dallas
Texas Scottish Rite Hosp for Children - Dallas
2222 Welborn
Dallas, TX 75219
Southwest
(214) 521-3168

The Children's Hospital - Denver
Chldn's Hosp - Denver
1056 east 19th Ave
Denver, CO 80218
Great Plains and Mountains
(303) 861-8888

The Children's Hospital of Buffalo
Chldn's Hosp of Buffalo
219 Bryant St.
Buffalo, NY 14222
Mid Atlantic
(716) 878-7000

The Children's Hospital of Philadelphia
Chldn's Hosp of Philadelphia
34th and Civic Center Boulevard
Philadelphia, PA 19104
Mid Atlantic
(215) 590-1000

The Parkinson's Institute/Movement Disorders Treament Center
Parkinson's Inst/Movement Disorders Treatmt Ctr
1170 Morse Ave
Sunnyvale, CA 94089-1605
West Coast and Pacific
(408) 734-2800

The Woman's Hospital of Texas
Woman's Hosp TX
7600 Fannin St
Houston, TX 77054
Southwest
(713) 790-1234

Thomas Jefferson University Hospital
Thomas Jefferson Univ Hosp
111 S 11th St
Philadelphia, PA 19107
Mid Atlantic
(215) 955-6000

TIRR
TIRR
1333 Moursund
Houston, TX 77030
Southwest
(713) 799-5000

Toledo Hospital
Toledo Hosp
2142 N Cove Blvd
Toledo, OH 43606
Midwest
(419) 291-4000

Tulane University Medical Center Hospital & Clinic
Tulane Univ Med Ctr Hosp & Clinic
1415 Tulane Avenue
New Orleans, LA 70112
Southwest
(504) 588-5263

U Mass Memorial Health Care - Worcester
U Mass Meml Hlth Care - Worcester
55 Lake Avenue North
Worcester, MA 01655-0002
New England
(508) 856-0011

Institutions in bold are profiled in this edition of the Castle Connolly Guide.

UCLA Medical Center
UCLA Med Ctr
10833 Le Conte Avenue
Los Angeles, CA 90095
West Coast and Pacific
(310) 825-9111

UCLA Neuropsychiatric Hospital
UCLA Neuropsychiatric Hosp
760 Westwood Plaza
Los Angeles, CA 90024
West Coast and Pacific
(310) 825-9989

UCLA-Sepulveda VA Greater LA Health
Care System
UCLA-Sepulveda VA Grtr LA Hlth Care Sys
16111 Plummer St
North Hills, CA 91343
West Coast and Pacific
(818) 891-7711

UCSF - Mount Zion Medical Center
UCSF - Mount Zion Med Ctr
1600 Divisadero Street
San Francisco, CA 94115
West Coast and Pacific
(415) 567-6600

UMDNJ-University Hospital-Newark
UMDNJ-Univ Hosp-Newark
150 Bergen St
Newark, NJ 07103-2406
Mid Atlantic
(973) 972-4300

Union Memorial Hospital - Baltimore
Union Memorial Hosp - Baltimore
201 E University Pkwy
Baltimore, MD 21218
Mid Atlantic
(410) 554-2000

University Community Hospital
University Comm Hosp
3100 E Fletcher Avenue
Tampa, FL 33613
Southeast
(813) 971-6000

University Community Hospital of
Carrollwood
University Comm Hosp of Carrollwood
7171 N Dale Mabry
Tampa, FL 33614
Southeast
(813) 932-2222

University Health System
Univ Hlth Sys - San Antonio
4502 Medical Drive
San Antonio, TX 78229
Southwest
(210) 358-4000

University Hospital
Univ Hosp-San Antonio
4502 Medical Drive
San Antonio, TX 78229
Southwest
(210) 358-4000

University Hospital & Clinics- Mississippi
Univ Hosps & Clins - Mississippi
2500 North State Street
Jackson, MS 39216
Southeast
(601) 984-1000

University Hospital - Brooklyn
Univ Hosp - Brklyn
450 Clarkson Ave
Brooklyn, NY 11203
Mid Atlantic
(718) 270-1000

Institutions in bold are profiled in this edition of the Castle Connolly Guide.

University Hospital - Charlotte
Unv Hosp- Charlotte, NC
8800 N Tryon St
Charlotte, NC 28262-8415
Southeast
(704) 548-6000

University Hospital - Cincinnati
Univ Hosp - Cincinnati
234 Goodman Street
Cincinnati, OH 45219
Midwest
(513) 584-1000

University Hospital - SUNY Upstate
Medical University
Univ. Hosp.- SUNY Upstate Med. Univ.
750 E Adams Street
Syracuse, NY 13210
Mid Atlantic
(315) 464-5540

University Hospitals of Cleveland
Univ Hosp of Cleveland
11100 Euclid Ave
Cleveland, OH 44106
Midwest
(216) 844-1000

University Medical Center - Las Vegas
Univ Med Ctr-Las Vegas
1800 W Charleston Blvd
Las Vegas, NV 89102
West Coast and Pacific
(702) 383-2000

University Medical Center - Lubbock
Univ Med Ctr - Lubbock
602 Indiana Ave
Lubbock, TX 79415-3364
Southwest
(806) 743-3111

University Medical Center- Tucson
Univ Med Ctr
1501 N. Campbell Ave
Tucson, AZ 85724-5128
Southwest
(520) 694-0111

University of Alabama Hospital at
Birmingham
Univ of Ala Hosp at Birmingham
619 South 19th Street
Birmingham, AL 35249-6544
Southeast
(205) 934-4011

University of Arkansas for Medical
Sciences
UAMS
4301 W Markham St
Little Rock, AR 72205
Southwest
(501) 686-7000

University of California - Davis Medical
Center
Univ CA - Davis Med Ctr
2315 Stockton Boulevard
Sacramento, CA 95817
West Coast and Pacific
(916) 734-3096

University of California - Irvine Medical
Center
UCI Med Ctr
101 The City Drive
Orange, CA 92868
West Coast and Pacific
(714) 456-6011

Institutions in bold are profiled in this edition of the Castle Connolly Guide.

University of California - San Diego
Healthcare
UCSD Healthcare
200 West Arbor Drive
San Diego, CA 92103
West Coast and Pacific
(619) 543-6222

University of California - San Francisco
Medical Center
UCSF Med Ctr
500 Parnassus Avenue
San Francisco, CA 94143
West Coast and Pacific
(415) 476-1000

University of Chicago Hospitals
Univ of Chicago Hosps
5841 S Maryland Ave
Chicago, IL 60637
Midwest
(773) 702-1000

University of Colorado Health & Science
Center
Univ Colo HSC - Denver
4200 E. 9th Avenue
Denver, CO 80262
Great Plains and Mountains
(303) 372-0000

University of Connecticut Health Center,
John Dempsey Hospital
Univ of Conn Hlth Ctr, John Dempsey Hosp
263 Farmington Ave
Farmington, CT 06030
New England
(860) 679-2100

University of Illinois at Chicago Eye and
Ear Infirmary
Univ of IL at Chicago Eye and Ear Infi
1855 W Taylor St
Chicago, IL 60612
Midwest
(312) 996-6500

University of Illinois at Chicago Medical
Center
Univ of IL at Chicago Med Ctr
1740 W Taylor St.
Chicago, IL 60612
Midwest
(312) 996-7000

University of Iowa Hospitals and Clinics
Univ of IA Hosp and Clinics
200 Hawkins Drive
Iowa City , IA 52242
Midwest
(319) 356-3155

University of Kansas Medical Center
Univ Kansas Med Ctr
3901 Rainbow Boulevard
Kansas City, KS 66160
Great Plains and Mountains
(913) 588-5000

University of Kentucky Medical Center
Univ Kentucky Med Ctr
800 Rose Street
Lexington, KY 40536
Southeast
(859) 323-5000

University of Louisville Hospital
Univ Louisville Hosp
530 S. Jackson Street
Louisville, KY 40202
Southeast
(502) 562-3000

Institutions in bold are profiled in this edition of the Castle Connolly Guide.

University of Maryland Medical System
University of MD Med Sys
22 S Greene St
Baltimore, MD 21201
Mid Atlantic
(410) 328-8667

University of Miami - Jackson Memorial
Hospital
Univ of Miami - Jackson Meml Hosp
1611 NW 12th Ave
Miami, FL 33136
Southeast
(305) 585-1111

University of Miami Hosp &
Clinics/Sylvestor Comp Cancer Cntr
*Univ of Miami & Clinics/Sylvestor Comp
Cancer Ctr*
1475 NW 12th Ave
Miami, FL 33136
Southeast
(305) 243-6418

University of Michigan Health Center
Univ of MI Hlth Ctr
1500 E. Medical Center Drive
Ann Arbor, MI 48109
Midwest
(734) 936-4000

University of Missouri Hospitals & Clinics
Univ of Missouri Hosp & Clinics
One Hospital Drive
Columbia, MO 65212
Midwest
(573) 882-4141

University of New Mexico Hospital
Univ NM Hosp
2211 Lomas Boulevard, N.E.
Albuquerque, NM 87106
Southwest
(505) 272-2111

**University of North Carolina
Hospitals**
Univ of NC Hosp
101 Manning Drive, Box 7600
Chapel Hill, NC 27514-4335
Southeast
(919) 966-4131

University of Oklahoma Health Science
Center
Univ OK Hlth Sci Ctr
1100 N Lindsay
Oklahoma City, OK 73104
Southwest
(405) 271-4000

University of Pennsylvania - Presbyterian
Medical Center
Univ Penn - Presby Med Ctr
51 N 39th St
Philadelphia, PA 19104
Mid Atlantic
(215) 662-8000

University of South Alabama Medical
Center
Univ of S Ala Med Ctr
2451 Fillingim Street
Mobile, AL 36617
Southeast
(334) 471-7000

Institutions in bold are profiled in this edition of the Castle Connolly Guide.

University of Tennessee Bowld Hospital
Univ of Tenn Bowld Hosp
951 Court Ave
Memphis, TN 38103
Southeast
(901) 448-4000

University of Texas Health & Science
Center
Univ of Texas Hlth & Sci Ctr
7703 Floyd Curl Drive
San Antonio, TX 78229
Southwest
(210) 567-7000

University of Texas MD Anderson Cancer
Center, The
Univ of TX MD Anderson Cancer Ctr, The
1515 Holcombe Boulevard
Houston, TX 77030
Southwest
(713) 792-2121

University of Texas Medical Branch
Hospitals at Galveston
Univ of TX Med Brch Hosps at Galveston
301 University Boulevard
Galveston, TX 77555
Southwest
(409) 772-1011

University of Utah Hospital and Clinics
Univ Utah Hosp and Clin
50 N Medical Dr
Salt Lake City, UT 84132-0001
Great Plains and Mountains
(801) 581-2121

**University of Virginia Health
Systems**
Univ of VA Hlth Sys
Lee Street
Charlottesville, VA 22908-0001
Southeast
(434) 924-0211

University of Washington Medical Center
Univ WA Med Ctr
1959 NE Pacific Street, Box 35-356355
Seattle, WA 98195
West Coast and Pacific
(206) 598-3300

University of Wisconsin Hospital &
Clinics
Univ WI Hosp & Clins
600 Highland Avenue
Madison, WI 53792
Midwest
(608) 263-6400

UPMC - Presbyterian University Hospital
UPMC - Presbyterian Univ Hosp
200 Lothrop Street
Pittsburgh, PA 15213
Mid Atlantic
(412) 647-2345

Upstate University Medical Hospital
Upstate Univ Med Hosp
750 E Adams St
Syracuse, NY 13210-2306
Mid Atlantic
(315) 464-5540

Institutions in bold are profiled in this edition of the Castle Connolly Guide.

USC Norris Cancer Comprehensive
Center
USC Norris Cancer Comp Ctr
1441 Eastlake Avenue
Los Angeles, CA 90033
West Coast and Pacific
(323) 865-3000

USC University Hospital - Richard K.
Eamer Medical Plaza
USC Univ Hosp - R K Eamer Med Plz
1500 San Pablo St
Los Angeles, CA 90033
West Coast and Pacific
(323) 442-8444

VA Connecticut Healthcare System
VA Conn Hlthcre Sys
950 Campbell Ave
West Haven, CT 06516
New England
(203) 932-5711

VA Medical Center - Atlanta
VA Med Ctr - Atlanta
1670 Clairmont Rd
Decatur, GA 30003
Southeast
(404) 321-6111

VA Medical Center - San Francisco
VA Med Ctr - San Francisco
4150 Clement St
San Francisco, CA 94121
West Coast and Pacific
(415) 221-4810

VA Medical Center - West Los Angeles
VA Med Ctr - W Los Angeles
11301 Wilshire Blvd
Los Angeles, CA 90073
West Coast and Pacific
(310) 478-3711

VA Pittsburgh Health Care System
VA Pittsburgh Hlth Care Sys
University Drive
Pittsburgh, PA 15240
Mid Atlantic
(412) 688-6000

VA San Diego Healthcare System
VA San Diego Hlthcre Sys
3350 La Jolla Village Drive
San Diego, CA 92161
West Coast and Pacific
(858) 552-8585

Valley Children's Hospital
Valley Chldns Hosp
9300 Valley Children's Pl
Madera, CA 93638
West Coast and Pacific
(559) 353-5000

Valley Hospital, The
Valley Hosp, The
223 N Van Dien Ave
Ridgewood, NJ 07450
Mid Atlantic
(201) 447-8000

Vanderbilt University Medical Center
Vanderbilt Univ Med Ctr
University Hospital 1211 22nd Ave.
South
Nashville, TN 37232
Southeast
(615) 322-5000

Vermont University College of Medicine
Vermont Univ Coll of Med
80 University Heights
Burlington, VT 05405-0068
New England
(802) 656-4094

Institutions in bold are profiled in this edition of the Castle Connolly Guide.

Veterans Affairs Medical Center - Indianapolis
VA Med Ctr
1481 W 10th St
Indianapolis, IN 46202
Midwest
(317) 554-0000

Veterans Affairs Medical Center - Little Rock
VA Med Ctr
4300 W. 7th Street
Little Rock, AR 72205
Southwest
(501) 257-1000

Veterans Affairs Medical Center - Oklahoma City
VA Med Ctr
921 NE 13th St
Oklahoma City, OK 73104
Southwest
(405) 270-5133

Veterans Affairs Medical Center - Washington
VA Medical Center - Washington
50 Irving Street, N.W.
Washington, DC 20422
Mid Atlantic
(202) 745-8100

Veterans Affairs Puget Sound Health Care System
VA Puget Sound Hlth Care Sys
1660 South Columbian Way
Seattle, WA 98108
West Coast and Pacific
(206) 764-2299

Via Christi Regional Medical Center- St. Francis Campus
Via Christi Reg Med Ctr - St Francis
929 N St. Francis Rd
Witchita, KS 67214
Great Plains and Mountains
(316) 268-5000

Via Health System-Genesee Hospital
Via Hlth Sys-Genesee Hosp
224 Alexander Street
Rochester, NY 14607
Mid Atlantic
(716) 922-6000

Virginia Mason Medical Center
Virginia Mason Med Ctr
1100 Ninth Ave, Box 900
Seattle, WA 98111
West Coast and Pacific
(206) 223-6600

Wake Forest University Baptist Medical Center
Wake Forest Univ Baptist Med Ctr
Medical Center Blvd
Winston-Salem, NC 27157-1015
Southeast
(336) 716-2011

WakeMed New Bern Avenue Campus
WakeMed New Bern
3000 New Bern Ave
Raleigh, NC 27610
Southeast
(919) 350-8000

Washington Hospital Center
Washington Hosp Ctr
110 Irving St NW
Washington, DC 20010
Mid Atlantic
(202) 877-7000

Institutions in bold are profiled in this edition of the Castle Connolly Guide.

Washington University Medical Center
Washington Univ Med Ctr
4444 Forest Park Ave
St Louis, MO 63108
Midwest
(314) 935-5100

Wesley Woods Geriatric Hospital
Wesley Woods Ger Hosp
1821 Clifton Road
Atlanta, GA 30329
Southeast
(404) 728-6200

West Hills Medical Center
West Hills Med Ctr
7300 Medical Center drive
West Hills, CA 91307
West Coast and Pacific
(818) 676-4100

West Jefferson Medical Center
West Jefferson Med Ctr
1101 Medical Ctr Blvd
Marrero, LA 70072
Southwest
(504) 347-5511

West Virginia University Hospital - Ruby
Memorial
WV Univ Hosp - Ruby Memorial
1 Medical Center Drive
Morgantown, WV 26506
Mid Atlantic
(304) 598-4000

Westchester Medical Center
Westchester Med Ctr
95 Grasslands Road
Valhalla, NY 10595
Mid Atlantic
(914) 493-7000

Western Psychiatric Institute & Clinic
Western Psy Inst & Clin
3811 O'Hara St
Pittsburgh, PA 15213-2593
Mid Atlantic
(412) 624-2100

Western Wake Medical Center
Western Wake Med Ctr
1900 Kildaire Farm Rd
Cary , NC 27511-6616
Southeast
(919) 233-2300

William Beaumont Hospital
William Beaumont Hosp
3601 West 13 Mile Road
Royal Oak, MI 48073
Midwest
(248) 551-5000

William S Hall Psychiatric Institute
William S Hall Psyc Inst
1800 Colonial Drive, PO Box 202
Columbia, SC 29202-6827
Southeast
(803) 898-1693

Wills Eye Hospital
Wills Eye Hosp
900 Walnut Street
Philadelphia, PA 19107-5598
Mid Atlantic
(215) 928-3000

Winthrop - University Hospital
Winthrop - Univ Hosp
259 1st St
Mineola, NY 11501
Mid Atlantic
(516) 663-0333

Institutions in bold are profiled in this edition of the Castle Connolly Guide.

Wolfson Children's Hospital @ Baptist
Medical Center
*Wolfson Children's Hosp @ Baptist Med
Cen*
800 Prudential Drive
Jacksonville, FL 32207
Southeast
(904) 393-2000

Women & Infants Hospital - Rhode Island
Women & Infants Hosp - Rhode Island
101 Dudley Street
Providence, RI 02905
New England
(401) 274-1100

Yale - New Haven Hospital
Yale - New Haven Hosp
20 York St
New Haven, CT 06504
New England
(203) 688-4242

Zale Lipshy University Hospital
Zale Lipshy Univ Hosp
5151 Harry Hines Boulevard
Dallas, TX 75235
Southwest
(214) 590-3101

Institutions in bold are profiled in this edition of the Castle Connolly Guide.

APPENDIX F

MEDICAL SCHOOLS

The following is a list of U.S. and Canadian medical schools and the abbreviations used for each in the doctor listings. The abbreviations as they appear in the listings are in italics below.

ALABAMA

University of Alabama School of
Medicine University of Alabama at
Birmingham
U Ala Sch Med

University of South Alabama College of
Medicine
U South Ala Coll Med

ARIZONA

University of Arizona College of
Medicine
Arizona Health Sciences Center
U Ariz Coll Med

ARKANSAS

University of Arkansas College of
Medicine
U Ark Sch Med

CALIFORNIA

University of California Davis School of
Medicine
UC Davis

University of California Irvine
College of Medicine
UC Irvine

University of California San Diego School
of Medicine
UC San Diego

Loma Linda University School of
Medicine
Loma Linda U

University of California Los Angeles
UCLA School of Medicine
UCLA

University of Southern California School
of Medicine
USC Sch Med

College of Osteopathic Medicine
of the Pacific
Coll of Osteo Med-Pacific

University of California San Francisco
School of Medicine
UC San Francisco

Stanford University School of Medicine
Stanford U

COLORADO

University of Colorado School of Medicine
U Colo Sch Med

CONNECTICUT

University of Connecticut School of Medicine
U Conn Sch Med

Yale University School of Medicine
Yale U Sch Med

DISTRICT OF COLUMBIA

George Washington University School of Medicine and Health Science
Geo Wash U Sch Med

Georgetown University School of Medicine
Georgetown U

Howard University College of Medicine
Howard U

FLORIDA

University of Florida College of Medicine
U Fla Coll Med

University of Miami School of Medicine
U Miami Sch Med

Nova Southeastern University, College of Osteopathic Medicine
Nova SE Univ, Coll of Osteo Med

University of South Florida College of Medicine
U South Fla Coll Med

Florida College of Osteopathic Medicine
FL Coll of Osteo Med

GEORGIA

Emory University School of Medicine
Emory U Sch Med

Morehouse School of Medicine
Morehouse Sch Med

Medical College of Georgia School of Medicine
Med Coll Ga

Mercer University School of Medicine
Mercer U Sch Med, Macon, GA

HAWAII

University of Hawaii John A. Burns School of Medicine
U Hawaii JA Burns Sch Med

ILLINOIS

Arizona College of Osteopathic Medicine, Midwestern University
Ariz Coll of Osteo Med

Chicago College of Osteopathic Medicine, Midwestern University
Chicago Coll of Osteo Med

Northwestern University Medical School
Northwestern U

Rush Medical College of Rush University
Rush Med Coll

University of Chicago (Div Bio Sci) Pritzker School of Medicine
U Chicago-Pritzker Sch Med

University of Illinois College of Medicine
U Ill Coll Med

Loyola University of Chicago - Stritch School of Medicine
Loyola U-Stritch Sch Med, Maywood

University of Health Sciences Chicago Medical School
U Hlth Sci/Chicago Med Sch

Southern Illinois University School of Medicine
Southern Ill U

INDIANA

Indiana University School of Medicine
Ind U Sch Med

IOWA

University of Osteopathic Medicine
U of Osteo Med-IA

University of Iowa College of Medicine
U Iowa Coll Med

KANSAS

University of Kansas Medical Center School of Medicine
U Kans Sch Med

KENTUCKY

University of Kentucky College of Medicine
U Ky Coll Med

University of Louisville School of Medicine
KY Sch Med, Louisville

LOUISIANA

Louisiana State University School of Medicine New Orleans
LSU Sch Med, New Orleans

Tulane University School of Medicine
Tulane U

Louisiana State University School Of Medicine Shreveport
LSU Med Ctr, Shreveport

MARYLAND

Johns Hopkins University School of Medicine
Johns Hopkins U

University of Maryland School of Medicine
U Md Sch Med

F. Edward A. Hebert School of Medicine Uniformed Services University of Health Sciences
Uniformed Srvs U, Bethesda

MASSACHUSETTS

Boston University School of Medicine
Boston U

Harvard Medical School
Harvard Med Sch

Tufts University School of Medicine
Tufts U

University of Massachusetts Medical School
U Mass Sch Med

MICHIGAN

University of Michigan Medical School
U Mich Med Sch

Wayne State University School of Medicine
Wayne State U

Michigan State University College of Human Medicine
Mich St U

Michigan State University College of Osteopathic Medicine
Mich St Coll of Osteo Med

MINNESOTA

University of Minnesota Duluth School of Medicine
U Minn-Duluth Sch Med

University of Minnesota Medical School
U Minn

Mayo Medical School
Mayo Med Sch

MISSISSIPPI

University of Mississippi School of Medicine
U Miss Sch Med

MISSOURI

University of Missouri Columbia School of Medicine
U Mo-Columbia Sch Med

Kirksville College of Osteopathic Medicine
Kirksville Coll of Osteo Med

University of Health Sciences/College of Osteopathic Medicine
U of Hlth Sci, Coll of Osteo Med

University of Missouri Kansas City School of Medicine
U Mo-Kansas City Sch Med

Saint Louis University School of Medicine
St Louis U

Washington University School of Medicine
Wash U, St. Louis

NEBRASKA

Creighton University School of Medicine
Creighton U

University of Nebraska College of Medicine
U Nebr Coll Med

NEVADA

University of Nevada School of Medicine
U Nevada

NEW HAMPSHIRE

Dartmouth Medical School
Dartmouth Med Sch

NEW JERSEY

University of Medicine and Dentistry of New Jersey
UMDNJ-NJ Med Sch, Newark

University of Medicine and Dentistry of New Jersey
UMDNJ-RW Johnson Med Sch

University of Medicine and Dentistry
of New Jersey/School of Osteopathic
Medicine
UMD-NJ Sch of Osteo Med

NEW MEXICO

University of New Mexico
School of Medicine
U New Mexico

NEW YORK

Albany Medical College
Albany Med Coll

Albert Einstein College of
Medicine of Yeshiva University
Albert Einstein Coll Med

Columbia University College
of Physicians and Surgeons
Columbia P&S

Cornell University Medical College
Cornell U

Mt. Sinai School of Medicine of
the City University of New York
Mt Sinai Sch Med

New York College of Osteopathic
Medicine
NY Coll of Osteo Med

New York Medical College
NY Med Coll

New York University School
of Medicine
NYU Sch Med

State University of New York at Buffalo
School of Medicine & Biomedical
Sciences
SUNY Buffalo

State University of New York Health
Science Center at Brooklyn
SUNY Health Sci Ctr, Bklyn

State University of New York Health
Science Center at Syracuse
SUNY Hlth Sci Ctr, Syracuse

State University of New York at Stony
Brook Health Sciences Center
SUNY Hlth Sci Ctr, Stony Brook

University of Rochester
School of Medicine and Dentistry
U Rochester

NORTH CAROLINA

University of North Carolina at Chapel
Hill School of Medicine
U NC Sch Med

Duke University School of Medicine
Duke U

East Carolina University School
of Medicine
E Carolina U

Bowman Gray School of Medicine
Bowman Gray

NORTH DAKOTA

University of North Dakota
School of Medicine
U ND Sch Med

OHIO

University of Cincinnati
College of Medicine
U Cincinnati

Case Western Reserve University
School of Medicine
Case West Res U

Ohio University, College
of Osteopathic Medicine
OH Coll of Osteo Med

Ohio State University
College of Medicine
Ohio State U

Wright State University
School of Medicine
Wright State U Sch Med

Northeastern Ohio University
College of Medicine
NE Ohio U

Medical College of Ohio
MC Ohio, Toledo

OKLAHOMA

University of Oklahoma
College of Medicine
U Okla Coll Med

Oklahoma State University
College of Osteopathic Medicine
OSU Coll of Osteo Med

OREGON

Oregon Health Science
University School of Medicine
U Oreg/Hlth Sci U, Portland

PENNSYLVANIA

Lake Erie College
of Osteopathic Medicine
Lake Erie Coll of Osteo Med

Pennsylvania State University
College of Medicine
Penn St U-Hershey Med Ctr

Hahnemann University
School of Medicine
Hahnemann U

Jefferson Medical College
of Thomas Jefferson University
Jefferson Med Coll

Medical College of Pennsylvania
Med Coll Penn

Philadelphia College
of Osteopathic Medicine
Philadelphia Coll of Osteo Med

Temple University
School of Medicine
Temple U

University of Pennsylvania
School of Medicine
U Penn

University of Pittsburgh
School of Medicine
U Pittsbrgh

PUERTO RICO

Universidad Central del Caribe School of
Medicine
U del Caribe Escuela Med Cayey

Ponce School of Medicine
Ponce Med Sch

University of Puerto Rico School of
Medicine
U Puerto Rico

RHODE ISLAND

Brown University Program in Medicine
Brown U

SOUTH CAROLINA

Medical University of South Carolina College of Medicine
Med U SC, Charleston

University of South Carolina School of Medicine
U SC Sch Med, Columbia

SOUTH DAKOTA

University of South Dakota School of Medicine
U SD Sch Med

TENNESSEE

East Tennessee State University James H. Quillen College of Medicine
E Tenn State U

University of Tennessee Memphis College of Medicine
U Tenn Memphis Coll Med

Meharry Medical College School of Medicine
Meharry Med Coll

Vanderbilt University School of Medicine
Vanderbilt U

TEXAS

Texas A&M University Health Science Center College of Medicine
Texas A&M U

University of Texas
U Texas, Dallas

University of North Texas Health Science Center/College of Osteopathic Medicine
U of North TX Coll of Osteo Med

University of Texas Medical School at Galveston
U Texas Med Br, Galveston

Baylor College of Medicine
Baylor

University of Texas Medical School at Houston
U Texas, Houston

Texas Tech University Health Science Center School of Medicine
Tex Tech U Sch Med

University of Texas Medical School at San Antonio
U Tex San Antonio

UTAH

University of Utah School of Medicine
U Utah

VERMONT

University of Vermont College of Medicine
U Vt Coll Med

VIRGINIA

University of Virginia School of Medicine
U Va Sch Med

Eastern Virginia Medical School of the Medical College of Hampton Roads
Eastern VA Med Sch, Norfolk

Virginia Commonwealth University
Medical College of Virginia School of
Medicine
Med Coll Va

WASHINGTON

University of Washington
School of Medicine
U Wash, Seattle

WEST VIRGINIA

Marshall University School of Medicine
Marshall U

West Virginia School
of Osteopathic Medicine
WV Sch Osteo Med

Robert C. Byrd Health Sciences Center of
West Virginia University School of
Medicine
W Va U Sch Med

WISCONSIN

University of Wisconsin School of
Medicine
U Wisc Med Sch

Medical College of Wisconsin
Med Coll Wisc

CANADA

The University of Calgary Faculty of
Medicine
U Calgary

Faculty of Medicine University of Alberta
U Alberta

University of British Columbia Faculty of
Medicine
U British Columbia Fac Med

University of Manitoba Faculty of
Medicine
U Manitoba

Memorial University of Newfoundland
Faculty of Medicine
Meml U-St Johns, Newfoundland

Dalhousie University Faculty of Medicine
Dalhousie U

McMaster University Faculty of Health
Sciences
McMaster U

Queen's University Faculty of Medicine
Queens U

University of Western Ontario
Faculty of Medicine
U Western Ontario

University of Ottawa Faculty of Medicine
U Ottawa

University of Toronto
Faculty of Medicine
U Toronto

McGill University Faculty of Medicine
McGill U

Laval University Faculty of Medicine
Laval U, Quebec

APPENDIX G

SELECTED RESOURCES

American Ambulance Association (AAA)
1255 Twenty-Third Street, NW, Suite 200
Washington, DC 20037-1174
202-452-8888
fax 202-452-0005
www.the-aaa.org/
The American Ambulance Association represents emergency and non-emergency medical transportation providers, advocating high quality pre-hospital care and keeping these providers aware of legislation and news that may affect them.

American Association of Health Plans (AAHP)
1129 20th Street, NW, Suite 600
Washington, DC 20036-3421
202-778-3200
www.aahp.org/
The American Association of Health Plans is the national trade association that speaks on behalf of over 1,000 health plans regarding regulatory and legislative issues.

American Board of Medical Specialties (ABMS)
1007 Church Street, Suite 404
Evanston, Illinois 60201-5913
847-491-9091
fax 847-328-3596
www.abms.org
The ABMS is the authoritative body for the recognition of medical specialties, coordinating 24 medical specialty boards (including 25 medical specialties) and providing information on the board certification of doctors.

American Hospital Association (AHA)
1 North Franklin
Chicago, IL 60606
800-424-4301 or 312-422-2000
www.aha.org/
A national health advocacy organization, the AHA represents hospitals and healthcare networks in legislative and regulatory matters. In 1973 the AHA adopted the Patient Bill of Rights to help patients understand their rights and responsibilities.

American Medical Association (AMA)
515 North State Street
Chicago, IL 60610
312-464-5000
www.ama-assn.org/
The AMA is an association that maintains information on physicians practicing throughout the nation. Healthcare consumers can use their database to check the location, licensing, education and specialty of many doctors in the United States.

Center for Medical Consumers
130 Macdougal Street
New York, NY 10012
212-674-7105
fax 212-674-7100
www.medicalconsumers.org
Provides volume and outcome data on certain medical procedures performed in New York state.

Centers for Disease Control and Prevention (CDC)
1-800-311-3435
toll free number for international travelers 877 FYI-TRIP
fax information service for international travelers 888-232-3299
www.cdc.gov/netinfo.htm
Part of the Department of Health and Human Services, the CDC's mission is to prevent and manage diseases and illnesses. Its Web site contains information on a range of illnesses and the research being pursued to manage them. It also provides free faxed reports on disease risk and prevention in various parts of the world.

The CenterWatch Clinical Trials Listing Service
22 Thomson Place, 36T1
Boston, MA 02210-1212
617-856-5900
fax 617-856-5901
www.centerwatch.com
Profiles centers conducting clinical research by therapeutic area and geographic region, including more than 41,000 international industry and government-sponsored clinical trials and new FDA approved drug therapies, as well as 5,200 clinical trials that are actively recruiting patients.

Health Care Choices
P.O. Box 21039
Columbus Circle Station
New York, NY 10023
212-724-9395
www.healthcarechoices.org
Provides information on volume and outcomes of certain medical procedures performed in hospitals in various states throughout the country.

International Association for Medical Assistance To Travellers (IAMAT)
417 Center Street
Lewiston, New York 14092
716-754-4883
IAMAT is a non-profit organization that disseminates information on health and sanitary conditions worldwide. Membership is free but donations are appreciated. Members will receive a membership card making them eligible to access English speaking physicians all over the world. The organization also provides information on immunization requirements, malaria, and other tropical diseases, and sanitary and climactic conditions around the world. For information, send request in writing.

Medic Alert Foundation
2323 Colorado Avenue
Turlock, CA 95382
800-432-5378
The Medic Alert Foundation (a non-profit organization) provides an "ID tag" engraved with personal medical facts, as well as a 24-hour emergency response center which can release additional personal medical details. Membership is $15/year (waived for the first year) and members need to purchase the "ID tag" which sells for as low as $35.

Medline
One Medline Place
Mundelein, Illinois 60060
1-800-MEDLINE
fax 1-800-351-1512
www.medline.com
A medical database including millions of medical references and abstracts from thousands of scientific and medical journals.

The National Cancer Institute (NCI)
Clinical Studies Support Center (CSSC)
6116 Executive Boulevard
Bethesda, MD 20892-8329
800-4-CANCER (800-422-6237)
www.nci.nih.gov
Part of the NIH, the NCI sponsors cancer clinical trials at more than 100 sites in the United States. Trials are carried out in major medical research centers, such as teaching hospitals, as well as in community hospitals, specialized medical clinics and even in doctors' offices.

National Center for Complementary and Alternative Medicine
Clearinghouse (NCCAMC)
P.O. Box 7923
Gaithersburg, MD 20898-7923
888-644-6226
fax 866-464-3616
www.nccam.nih.gov website
nccamc@altmedinfo.org email
The NCCAMC facilitates the evaluation of alternative medical treatment modalities to help determine their effectiveness and bring alternative medicine into mainstream medicine. This agency does not provide referrals.

National Consumers League (NCL)
1701 K Street, NW, Suite 1200
Washington, DC 20006
202-835-3323
www.nclnet.org
NCL is a private, nonprofit consumer advocacy organization. NCL strives to investigate, educate, and advocate on a variety of issues including healthcare. Membership is $20 annually, but individuals can also write to the organization for a list of publications that non-members can purchase.

The National Institutes of Health (NIH)
Patient Recruitment Referral Center
10 Cloister Court
Bethesda, MD 20892-4754
800-411-1222
www.nih.gov
www.clinicaltrials.gov
*An organization operated by the U.S. government, the NIH operates its own hospital at
which the care provided is usually related to clinical studies its researchers are undertaking.
Information about the Warren G. Magnuson Clinical Center is also available.*

National Insurance Consumer Helpline
800-942-4242
www.iii.org
*The National Insurance Consumer Helpline advises consumers on how to choose an insur-
ance company or broker. It also offers an analysis of life insurance and assists in insurance
complaints.*

The Patient Advocate Foundation
753 Thimble Shoals Boulevard, Suite B
Newport News, VA 23606
800-532-5274
www.patientadvocate.org/
*A national non-profit organization that provides consultation, referrals and case management
to patients to ensure that they are not denied access to healthcare, insurance coverage,
employment and public assistance programs during an illness. In particular, the organization
maintains comprehensive information on cancer treatment options that are available to consumers through a separate Web site: www.oncology.com.*

People's Medical Society
462 Walnut Street
Allentown, PA 18102
610-770-1670
fax 610-770-0607
www.peoplesmed.org/index.html
*The People's Medical Society, a nonprofit organization, is focused on educating the healthcare
consumer about healthcare issues and medical rights. Their Web site provides information on
useful books and publications as well as the latest healthcare developments.*

Persons United Limiting Substandards and Errors in Healthcare (P.U.L.S.E.)
PO Box 353
Wantagh NY 11793-0353
516-579-4711
www.PULSEofNY.com
A support group for the survivors of medical malpractice and substandard healthcare, this nonprofit group also advocates patient education and patient-doctor communication.

Physicians Who Care
12125 Jones Maltsberger, Suite 607
San Antonio, Texas 78217
800-545-9305
fax 210-545-4475
www.pwc.org/
Physicians Who Care is a non-profit organization devoted to the doctor-patient relationship and maintaining high standards in healthcare.

Public Citizen's Health and Research Group
1600 20th Street NW
Washington, D.C. 20009
202-588-1000
www.citizen.org/hrg/
A non-profit organization, the Public Citizen's Group acts as a watchdog agency by advocating accountability and the open use of doctors' disciplinary backgrounds.

Veritas Medicine
238 Main Street Suite 501
Cambridge, Massachusetts 02142
617-234-1500
fax 617-234-1555
www.veritasmedicine.com
An organization that allows individuals to perform confidential, personalized searches of their clinical trials database and to access information on new treatment and drug options. The text is submitted by Harvard-affiliated doctors.

Appendix H

ADDITIONAL MEDICAL SPECIALTIES AND
SUBSPECIALTIES RECOGNIZED BY THE
ABMS

All specialties in this section are in capital letters and boldface type (e.g., **INTERNAL MEDICINE**). All subspecialties in this section are in initial capitals and boldface type (e.g., **Critical Care Medicine**).

Some specialties have a page number following the name of the specialty. This page number indicates where you will find a description of that specialty in this Guide.

Subspecialties require board certification in the specialty plus additional training and examination in the subspecialty.

ALLERGY-IMMUNOLOGY *(see page 93)*

Clinical & Laboratory Immunology: A subspecialist who utilizes various laboratory procedures to diagnose and treat disorders characterized by defective responses of the body's immune system. These results are used for patient management.

ANESTHESIOLOGY
An anesthesiologist is trained to provide pain relief and maintenance, or restoration, of a stable condition during and immediately following an operation, an obstetric or diagnostic procedure. The anesthesiologist assesses the risk of the patient undergoing surgery and optimizes the patient's condition prior to, during, and after surgery. In addition to these management responsibilities, the anesthesiologist provides medical management and consultation in pain management and critical care medicine. Anesthesiologists diagnose and treat acute, long-standing and cancer pain problems; diagnose and treat patients with critical illnesses or severe injuries; direct resuscitation in the care of patients with cardiac or respiratory emergencies, including the need for artificial ventilation; and supervise post anesthesia recovery.

Training required: Four years

Critical Care Medicine: An anesthesiologist who specializes in critical care medicine diagnoses, treats and supports patients with multiple organ dysfunction. This specialist may have administrative responsibilities for intensive care units and may also facilitate and coordinate patient care among the primary physician, the critical care staff, and other specialists.

DERMATOLOGY *(see page 189)*

Clinical and Laboratory Dermatological Immunology: A dermatologist who utilizes various specialized laboratory procedures to diagnose disorders characterized by defective responses of the body's immune system. *Immunodermatologists* also may provide consultation in the management of these disorders and administer specialized forms of therapy for these diseases.

EMERGENCY MEDICINE

An emergency physician focuses on the immediate decision making and action necessary to prevent death or any further disability both in the pre-hospital setting by directing emergency medical technicians and in the emergency department. The emergency physician provides immediate recognition, evaluation, care, stabilization and disposition of a generally diversified population of adult and pediatric patients in response to acute illness and injury.

Training required: Three years

Certification in one of the following subspecialties requires additional training and examination.

Medical Toxicology: An emergency physician who has special knowledge about the evaluation and management of patients with accidental or purposeful poisoning through exposure to prescription and nonprescription medications, drugs of abuse, household or industrial toxins and environmental toxins. Areas of medical toxicology include acute pediatric and adult drug ingestion; drug abuse, addiction and withdrawal; chemical poisoning exposure and toxicity; hazardous materials exposure and toxicity and occupational toxicology.

Pediatric Emergency Medicine: An emergency physician who has special qualifications to manage emergencies in infants and children.

Sports Medicine: An emergency physician with special knowledge in sports medicine is responsible for continuous care in the field of sports medicine, not only for the enhancement of health and fitness, but also for the prevention and management of injury and illness. A sports medicine physician has knowledge and experience in the promotion of wellness and the role of exercise in promoting a healthy lifestyle. Knowledge of exercise physiology, biomechanics, nutrition, psychology, physical rehabilitation and epidemiology is essential to the practice of sports medicine.

FAMILY PRACTICE

A family physician is concerned with the total healthcare of the individual and the family, and is trained to diagnose and treat a wide variety of ailments in patients of all ages. The family physician receives a broad range of training that includes internal medicine, pediatrics, obstetrics and gynecology, psychiatry and geriatrics. Special emphasis is placed on prevention and the primary care of entire families, utilizing consultations and community resources when appropriate.

Training required: Three years

Certification in one of the following subspecialties requires additional training and examination.

Geriatric Medicine: A family physician with special knowledge of the aging process and special skills in the diagnostic, therapeutic, preventive and rehabilitative aspects of illness in the elderly. This specialist cares for geriatric patients in the patient's home, the office, long-term care settings such as nursing homes and the hospital.

Sports Medicine: A family practice physician who is trained to be responsible for continuous care in the field of sports medicine, not only for the enhancement of health and fitness, but also for the prevention of injury and illness. A sports medicine physician must have knowledge and experience in the promotion of wellness and the prevention of injury. Knowledge about special areas of medicine such as exercise physiology, biomechanics, nutrition, psychology, physical rehabilitation, epidemiology, physical evaluation, injuries (treatment and prevention and referral practice) and the role of exercise in promoting a healthy life style are essential to the practice of sports medicine. The sports medicine physician requires special education to provide the knowledge to improve the healthcare of the individual engaged in physical exercise (sports) whether as an individual or in team participation.

INTERNAL MEDICINE (*see page 355*)

Clinical and Laboratory Immunology: An internist who uses laboratory tests and complex procedures to diagnose and treat disorders characterized by defective responses of the body's immune system.

Critical Care Medicine: An internist who diagnoses, treats and supports patients with multiple organ dysfunction. This specialist may have administrative responsibilities for intensive care units and may also facilitate and coordinate patient care among the primary physician, the critical care staff and other specialists.

APPENDIX H

MEDICAL GENETICS *(see Clinical Genetics page 165)*

The Board issues multiple general certificates in the following areas of genetics:

Clinical Biochemical Genetics: A clinical biochemical geneticist demonstrates competence in performing and interpreting biochemical analyses relevant to the diagnosis and management of human genetic diseases, and is a consultant regarding laboratory diagnosis of a broad range of inherited disorders.

Clinical Cytogenetics: A clinical cytogeneticist demonstrates competence in providing laboratory diagnostic and clinical interpretive services dealing with cellular components, particularly chromosomes, associated with heredity.

Ph.D. Medical Genetics: A medical geneticist works in association with a medical specialist, is affiliated with a clinical genetics program, and serves as a consultant to medical and dental specialists.

Molecular Genetic Pathology: A molecular genetic pathologist is expert in the principles, theory, and technologies of molecular biology and molecular genetics. This expertise is used to make or confirm diagnoses of Mendelian genetic disorders, of human development, infectious diseases and malignancies, and to assess the natural history of those disorders. A molecular genetic pathologist provides information about gene structure, function, and alteration and applies laboratory techniques for diagnosis, treatment, and prognosis for individuals with related disorders.

NEUROLOGY *(see page 423)*

Clinical Neurophysiology: A neurologist who specializes in the diagnosis and management of central, peripheral and autonomic nervous system disorders using a combination of clinical evaluation and electrophysiologic testing such as electroencephalography (EEG), electromyography (EMG) and nerve conduction studies (NCS), among others.

Neurodevelopmental Disabilities: A pediatrician or neurologist who specializes in the diagnosis and management of chronic conditions that affect the developing and mature nervous system such as cerebral palsy, mental retardation and chronic behavioral syndromes, or neurologic conditions.

OBSTETRICS AND GYNECOLOGY *(see page 467)*

Critical Care Medicine: An obstetrician-gynecologist who specializes in critical care medicine diagnoses, treats and supports female patients with multiple organ dysfunc-

1022

tion. This specialist may have administrative responsibilities for intensive care units and may also facilitate and coordinate patient care among the primary physician, the critical care staff, and other specialists.

OTOLARYNGOLOGY *(see page 537)*

Plastic Surgery within the Head and Neck: An otolaryngologist with additional training in plastic and reconstructive procedures within the head, face, neck and associated structures, including cutaneous head and neck oncology and reconstruction, management of maxillofacial trauma, soft tissue repair and neural surgery. The field is diverse and involves a wide age range of patients, from the newborn to the aged. While both cosmetic and reconstructive surgery are practiced, there are many additional procedures which interface with them.

Otology/Neurotology: An otolaryngologist who treats diseases of the ear and temporal bone, including disorders of hearing and balance. The additional training in otology and neurotology emphasizes the study of embryology, anatomy, physiology, epidemiology, pathophysiology, pathology, genetics, immunology, microbiology and the etiology of diseases of the ear and temporal bone.

PATHOLOGY *(see page 573)*

Blood Banking/Transfusion Medicine: A physician who specializes in blood banking/transfusion medicine is responsible for the maintenance of an adequate blood supply, blood donor and patient-recipient safety and appropriate blood utilization. Pretransfusion compatibility testing and antibody testing assure that blood transfusions, when indicated, are as safe as possible. This physician directs the preparation and safe use of specially prepared blood components, including red blood cells, white blood cells, platelets and plasma constituents.

Chemical Pathology: A chemical pathologist has expertise in the biochemistry of the human body as it applies to the understanding of the cause and progress of disease. This physician functions as a clinical consultant in the diagnosis and treatment of human disease. Chemical pathology entails the application of biochemical data to the detection, confirmation or monitoring of disease.

Cytopathology: A cytopathologist is an anatomic pathologist trained in the diagnosis of human disease by means of the study of cells obtained from body secretions and fluids, by scraping, washing or sponging the surface of a lesion, or by the aspiration of a tumor mass or body organ with a fine needle. A major aspect of a cytopathologist's practice is the interpretation of Papanicolaou-stained smears of cells from the female reproductive systems, the "Pap" test. However, the cytopathologist's expertise is applied to the diagnosis of cells from all systems and areas of the body. He/she is a consultant to all medical specialists.

Forensic Pathology: A forensic pathologist is expert in investigating and evaluating cases of sudden, unexpected, suspicious and violent death as well as other specific classes of death defined by law. The forensic pathologist serves the public as coroner or medical examiner, or by performing medicolegal autopsies for such officials.

Hematology: A physician who is expert in diseases that affect blood cells, blood clotting mechanisms, bone marrow and lymph nodes. He/she has the knowledge and technical skills essential for the laboratory diagnosis of anemias, leukemias, lymphomas, bleeding disorders and blood clotting disorders.

Medical Microbiology: A physician who is expert in the isolation and identification of microbial agents that cause infectious disease. Viruses, bacteria and fungi, as well as parasites are identified and, where possible, tested for susceptibility to appropriate antimicrobial agents.

Molecular Genetic Pathology: A molecular genetic pathologist is expert in the principles, theory and technologies of molecular biology and molecular genetics. This expertise is used to make or confirm diagnoses of Mendelian genetic disorders, disorders of human development, infectious diseases and malignancies, and to assess the natural history of those disorders. A molecular genetic pathologist provides information about gene structure, function and alteration and applies laboratory techniques for diagnosis, treatment and prognosis for individuals with related disorders.

Neuropathology: A neuropathologist is expert in the diagnosis of diseases of the nervous system and skeletal muscles and functions as a consultant primarily to neurologists and neurosurgeons. The neuropathologist is knowledgeable in the infirmities of humans as they affect the nervous and neuromuscular systems, be they degenerative, infectious, metabolic, immunologic, neoplastic, vascular or physical in nature.

Pediatric Pathology: A pediatric pathologist is expert in the laboratory diagnosis of diseases that occur during fetal growth, infancy and child development. The practice requires a strong foundation in general pathology and substantial understanding of normal growth and development, along with extensive knowledge of pediatric medicine.

PEDIATRICS *(see page 585)*

Clinical & Laboratory Immunology: A pediatrician who utilizes laboratory tests and complex procedures to diagnose and treat disorders characterized by defective responses of the body's immune system.

Medical Toxicology: A pediatrician who focuses on the evaluation and management of patients with accidental or intentional poisoning through exposure to prescription and non-prescription medications, drugs of abuse, household or industrial toxins and environmental toxins. Important areas of medical toxicology include acute pediatric and adult drug ingestion; drug abuse, addiction and withdrawal; chemical poisoning exposure and toxicity; hazardous materials exposure and toxicity and occupational toxicology.

Neurodevelopmental Disabilities: A pediatrician who treats children having developmental delays or learning disorders, including those associated with visual and hearing impairment, mental retardation, cerebral palsy, spina bifida, autism and other chronic neurologic conditions. This specialist provides medical consultation and education and assumes leadership in the interdisciplinary management of children with neurodevelopmental disorders. They may also focus on the early identification and diagnosis of neurodevelopmental disabilities in infants and young children as well as on changes that occur as the child with developmental disabilities grows.

Pediatric Critical Care Medicine: A pediatrician expert in advanced life support for children from the term or near-term neonate to the adolescent. This competence extends to the critical care management of life-threatening organ system failure from any cause in both medical and surgical patients, and to the support of vital physiological functions. This specialist may have administrative responsibilities for intensive care units and also facilitate patient care among other specialists.

Pediatric Emergency Medicine: A pediatrician who has special qualifications to manage emergencies in infants and children.

Sports Medicine: A pediatrician who is responsible for continuous care in the field of sports medicine, not only for the enhancement of health and fitness, but also for the prevention of injury and illness. A sports medicine physician must have knowledge and experience in the promotion of wellness and the prevention of injury. Knowledge about special areas of medicine such as exercise physiology, biomechanics, nutrition, psychology, physical rehabilitation, epidemiology, physical evaluation, injuries (treatment and prevention and referral practice) and the role of exercise in promoting a healthy life style are essential to the practice of sports medicine. The sports medicine physician requires special education to provide the knowledge to improve the healthcare of the individual engaged in physical exercise (sports) whether as an individual or in team participation.

PHYSICAL MEDICINE & REHABILITATION *(see page 673)*

Pain Management: A physician who provides a high level of care, either as a primary physician or consultant, for patients experiencing problems with acute, chronic or cancer pain in both hospital and ambulatory settings.

Pediatric Rehabilitation Medicine: A physiatrist who utilizes an interdisciplinary approach and addresses the prevention, diagnosis, treatment, and management of congenital and childhood onset physical impairments including related or secondary medical, physical, functional, psychosocial, and vocational limitations or conditions, with an understanding of the life course of disability.

PREVENTIVE MEDICINE

A preventive medicine specialist focuses on the health of individuals and defined populations in order to protect, promote and maintain health and well being, and to prevent disease, disability and premature death. The distinctive components of preventive medicine include:

1. Biostatistics and the application of biostatistical principles and methodology;
2. Epidemiology and its application to population-based medicine and research;
3. Health services management and administration including: developing, assessing and assuring health policies; planning, implementing, directing, budgeting and evaluating population health and disease management programs; and utilizing legislative and regulatory processes to enhance health;
4. Control of environmental factors that may adversely affect health;
5. Control and prevention of occupational factors that may adversely affect health safety;
6. Clinical preventive medicine activities, including measures to promote health and prevent the occurrence, progression and disabling effects of disease and injury; and
7. Assessment of social, cultural and behavioral influences on health.

A preventive medicine physician may be a specialist in general preventive medicine, public health, occupational medicine, or aerospace medicine. This specialist works with large population groups as well as with individual patients to promote health and understand the risks of disease, injury, disability and death, seeking to modify and eliminate these risks.

Training required: Three years

Certification in one of the following subspecialties requires additional training and examination.

Medical Toxicology: A specialist who is expert in the evaluation and management of patients with accidental or intentional poisoning through exposure to prescription and nonprescription medications, drugs of abuse, household or industrial toxins and environmental toxins. Important areas of medical toxicology include acute pediatric and adult drug ingestion; drug abuse, addiction and withdrawal; chemical poisoning exposure and toxicity; hazardous materials exposure and toxicity and occupational toxicology.

ADDITIONAL ABMS SPECIALTIES AND SUBSPECIALTIES

Undersea and Hyperbaric Medicine: A specialist who treats decompression illness and diving accident cases and uses hyperbaric oxygen therapy to treat such conditions as carbon monoxide poisoning, gas gangrene, non-healing wounds, tissue damage from radiation and burns and bone infections. This specialist also serves as consultant to other physicians in all aspects of hyperbaric chamber operations, and assesses risks and applies appropriate standards to prevent disease and disability in divers and other persons working in altered atmospheric conditions.

PSYCHIATRY *(see page 711)*

Clinical Neurophysiology: A psychiatrist with expertise in the diagnosis and management of central, peripheral, and autonomic nervous system disorders using a combination of clinical evaluation and electrophysiologic testing such as electroencephalography (EEG), electromyography (EMG), and nerve conduction studies (NCS).

Forensic Psychiatry: A psychiatrist who focuses on the interrelationships between psychiatry and civil, criminal and administrative law. This specialist evaluates individuals involved with the legal system and provides specialized treatment to those incarcerated in jails, prisons and forensic psychiatry hospitals.

Pain Management: A psychiatrist who provides a high level of care, either as a primary physician or consultant, for patients experiencing problems with acute, chronic or cancer pain in both hospital and ambulatory settings.

RADIOLOGY *(see page 781)*

Radiological Physics: A radiological physicist deals with the diagnostic and therapeutic applications of roentgen rays, gamma rays from sealed sources, ultrasonic radiation and radio-frequency radiation, as well as the equipment associated with their production and use, including radiation safety.

Nuclear Radiology: A radiologist who is involved in the analysis and imaging of radionuclides and radiolabeled substances in vitro and in vivo for diagnosis, and the administration of radionuclides and radiolabeled substances for the treatment of disease.

SURGERY *(see page 833)*

Surgical Critical Care: A surgeon with expertise in the management of the critically ill and postoperative patient, particularly the trauma victim, who specializes in critical care medicine diagnoses, treats and supports patients with multiple organ dysfunction. This specialist may have administrative responsibilities for intensive care units and may also facilitate and coordinate patient care among the primary physician, the critical care staff and other specialists.

INDICES

SUBJECT INDEX

SPECIAL EXPERTISE INDEX

Interchangeable Terms and Cross References
The following are terms that you may find helpful. These are medical synonyms or cross references that often are used interchangeably. While this list is not all-inclusive, it is offered to assist you both in understanding your medical records and in discussions you may have with your doctors.

If you are unable to find the term you are seeking in the **Special Expertise Index** that follows, we suggest looking under the synonym or cross reference for the term since it is likely that you will find what you need there.

Since this list contains only those terms that relate to the special expertise of doctors in this Guide, you may wish to consult a medical dictionary either in print format or online for other terms.

ACOUSTIC NEUROMA. . . . . ACOUSTIC NERVE TUMORS
AMYOTROPHIC LATERAL SCLEROSIS (ALS). . LOU GEHRIG'S DISEASE
ANXIETY DISORDERS. . . . . MOOD DISORDERS, DEPRESSION
AORTIC VALVE DISEASE. . . . . HEART VALVE DISEASE
BILIARY . . . . GALLBLADDER AND BILE DUCTS
CARDIAC . . . . HEART
CIRRHOSIS. . . . . LIVER DISEASE
CROHN'S DISEASE. . . . . INFLAMMATORY BOWEL DISEASE
DIPLOPIA . . . . DOUBLE VISION
EPILEPSY . . . . SEIZURE DISORDERS
ERECTILE DYSFUNCTION. . . . . IMPOTENCE
GYNECOMASTIA. . . . . MALE BREAST ENLARGEMENT
HEMATOLOGY . . . . BLOOD DISORDERS
HEPATIC DISEASE . . . . LIVER DISEASE
HEPATIC . . . . LIVER
KNEE/SHOULDER SURGERY. . . . . SHOULDER/KNEE SURGERY
LAPAROSCOPIC SURGERY . . . . MINIMALLY INVASIVE SURGERY
MITRAL VALVE DISEASE . . . . HEART VALVE DISEASE
MOHS' SURGERY . . . . MELANOMA/SKIN CANCER
NEPHROLOGY . . . . KIDNEY
OCULAR . . . . EYE
ONCOLOGY . . . . SOLID TUMORS
OPHTHALMIC . . . . EYE
PARKINSON'S DISEASE . . . . MOVEMENT DISORDERS
PEPTIC . . . . GASTRIC
PULMONARY . . . . LUNG

SPECIAL EXPERTISE INDEX

REFLEX SYMPATHETIC DYSTROPHY (RSD)... SHOULDER/HAND SYNDROME
RENAL.............................. KIDNEY
STRABISMUS........................ SQUINT, LAZY EYE
TRANSFUSION FREE SURGERY.......... BLOODLESS SURGERY
ULCERATIVE COLITIS................. INFLAMMATORY BOWEL DISEASE
VOIDING DYSFUNCTION .... INCONTINENCE (URINARY)

Some Common Medical Abbreviations and Acronyms

Following is a list of some commonly used medical abbreviations or acronyms that healthcare professionals frequently use as a "shorthand" way to record information. These sometimes make a medical record difficult for a non-professional to understand. Therefore, we are providing their complete meaning.

Abbreviation ..Medical Term
Acronym

ACL .... Anterior Cruciate Ligament
ADD .... Attention Deficit Disorder
ADHD .... Attention Deficit Hyperactivity Disorder
AIDS .... Acquired ImmunoDeficiency Syndrome
ALS .... Amyotrophic lateral sclerosis (Lou Gehrig's Disease)
ARDS .... Adult respiratory distress syndrome
BPH .... Benign prostatic hypertrophy
CABG .... Coronary artery bypass graft
CAD .... Coronary artery disease
CBC .... Complete blood count
CNS .... Central nervous system
COPD .... Chronic obstructive pulmonary disease
CSF .... Cerebrospinal fluid
CT .... Computerized tomography
ECG .... Electrocardiogram
EEG .... Electroencephalogram
EKG .... Electrocardiogram
ERCP .... Biliary/Pancreatic Endoscopy
EUS .... Endoscopic ultrasound
GERD .... Gastroesophageal reflux disease
HDL .... High density lipoprotein
HTN .... Hypertension
IBD .... Inflammatory Bowel Disease
IBS .... Irritable bowel syndrome
IVP .... Intravenous pyelogram
LDL .... Low density lipoprotein
LVAD .... Left ventricular assisted device (cardiac)

SPECIAL EXPERTISE INDEX

SPECIAL EXPERTISE INDEX

1043

SPECIAL EXPERTISE INDEX

SPECIAL EXPERTISE INDEX

SPECIAL EXPERTISE INDEX

SPECIAL EXPERTISE INDEX

SPECIAL EXPERTISE INDEX

SPECIAL EXPERTISE INDEX

SPECIAL EXPERTISE INDEX

SPECIAL EXPERTISE INDEX

SPECIAL EXPERTISE INDEX

SPECIAL EXPERTISE INDEX

SPECIAL EXPERTISE INDEX

SPECIAL EXPERTISE INDEX

Special Expertise	Spec	Name	Pg
Musculoskeletal Disorders	DR	Dalinka, M (PA)	785
Musculoskeletal Disorders	PMR	Ma, D (NY)	679
Musculoskeletal Disorders	PMR	Matthews, D (CO)	683
Musculoskeletal Disorders	Rhu	Bunning, R (DC)	816
Musculoskeletal Disorders	Rhu	Kagen, L (NY)	817
Musculoskeletal Infections	Inf	Wilson, W (MN)	351
Musculoskeletal Injuries	PMR	Press, J (IL)	682
Musculoskeletal Tumors	OrS	Benevenia, J (NJ)	517
Musculoskeletal Tumors	OrS	Gebhardt, M (MA)	515
Musculoskeletal Tumors	OrS	Luck Jr, J (CA)	536
Musculoskeletal Tumors	OrS	Neff, J (NE)	532
Myasthenia Gravis	N	Arnason, B (IL)	446
Myasthenia Gravis	N	Elias, S (MI)	447
Myasthenia Gravis	N	Garcia, C (LA)	452
Myasthenia Gravis	N	Lisak, R (MI)	448
Myasthenia Gravis	N	Reder, A (IL)	449
Myasthenia Gravis	N	Seybold, M (CA)	456
Myasthenia Gravis	N	Swerdlow, M (NY)	441
Myasthenia Gravis	N	Wright, R (IL)	451
Mycobacterial Infections	Pul	Iseman, M (CO)	759
Mycobacterial Infections	Pul	Reichman, L (NJ)	748
Myelodysplastic Syndromes	Hem	Adler, S (IL)	307
Myelodysplastic Syndromes	Hem	Nand, S (IL)	309
Myelodysplastic Syndromes	Onc	Gabrilove, J (NY)	317
Myelodysplastic Syndromes	Onc	Powell, B (NC)	324
Myeloma	Hem	Barlogie, B (AR)	310
Myeloma	Onc	Coleman, M (NY)	316
Myeloproliferative Disorders	Hem	Baron, J (IL)	308
Myeloproliferative Disorders	Hem	Nand, S (IL)	309
Myeloproliferative Disorders	Hem	Spivak, J (MD)	306
Myeloproliferative Disorders	Hem	Zuckerman, K (FL)	307
Myocardial Infarction	Cv	Borzak, S (FL)	139
Myocardial Infarction	Cv	Conti, C (FL)	140
Myocardial Infarction	Cv	Gibbons, R (MN)	144
Myocardial Infarction	IC	Holmes Jr, D (MN)	155
Myocardial Infarction	IC	Weaver, W (MI)	155
Myofacial Pain Syndrome	PM	Benzon, H (IL)	569
Myomectomy	RE	Wallach, E (MD)	803

N

Special Expertise	Spec	Name	Pg
Nail Diseases	D	Scher, R (NY)	197
Nail Surgery	D	Scher, R (NY)	197
Narcolepsy	Psyc	Kavey, N (NY)	731
Nasal & Eyelid Reconstruction	PlS	Miller, T (CA)	707
Nasal & Sinus Disorders	Oto	Benninger, M (MI)	554
Nasal & Sinus Disorders	Oto	Corey, J (IL)	555
Nasal & Sinus Disorders	Oto	Kuhn, F (GA)	551
Nasal & Sinus Disorders	Oto	Siegel, G (IL)	557
Nasal & Sinus Disorders	Oto	Sillers, M (AL)	553
Nasal & Sinus Disorders	Oto	Stankiewicz, J (IL)	558
Nasal & Sinus Disorders	Oto	Stringer, S (MS)	553
Nasal & Sinus Surgery	Oto	Blitzer, A (NY)	544
Nasal Allergy	Oto	Hurst, M (WV)	546
Nasal Reconstruction	Oto	Papel, I (MD)	547
Nasal Reconstruction	PlS	Burget, G (IL)	699
Nasal Reconstruction	PlS	Constantian, M (NH)	689
Nasal Reconstruction	PlS	Walton Jr, R (IL)	701
Nasal Surgery	PlS	Rohrich, R (TX)	704
Neck & Carotid Reconstruction	NS	Diaz, F (MI)	415
Neonatal Cardiology	NP	Bucciarelli, R (FL)	384
Neonatal Cardiology	PCd	Gewitz, M (NY)	621
Neonatal Genetics	Ped	McCabe, E (CA)	613
Neonatal Infections	PInf	Baker, C (TX)	650
Neonatal Neurology	ChiN	Lell, M (NY)	160

Special Expertise	Spec	Name	Pg
Neonatal Neurology	ChiN	Volpe, J (MA)	1
Neonatal Nutrition	NP	Neu, J (FL)	
Neonatal Respiratory Disease	NP	Martin, R (OH)	3
Neonatal Sepsis	NP	Polin, R (NY)	3
Neonatal Surgery	PS	Ginsburg, H (NY)	6
Neonatal Surgery	PS	Nakayama, D (NC)	6
Neonatal Surgery	PS	Oldham, K (WI)	6
Neonatal Surgery	PS	Sato, T (WI)	6
Neonatal Surgery	PS	Stolar, C (NY)	6
Neonatal Surgery	PS	Weinberger, M (FL)	6
Neonatal Surgery-Gastrointestinal	PS	Adkins, J (PA)	6
Neonatal-Perinatal Medicine	Ped	Regan, J (NY)	6
Neonatology	NP	Bancalari, E (FL)	3
Neonatology	NP	Boyle, R (VA)	3
Neonatology	NP	Cloherty, J (MA)	3
Neonatology	NP	Denson, S (TX)	3
Neonatology	NP	Ehrenkranz, R (CT)	3
Neonatology	NP	Escobedo, M (OK)	3
Neonatology	NP	Hurt, H (PA)	3
Neonatology	NP	Kitterman, J (CA)	3
Neonatology	NP	Lemons, J (IN)	3
Neonatology	NP	Martin, R (OH)	3
Neonatology	NP	Odom, M (TX)	3
Neonatology	NP	Stevenson, D (CA)	3
Neonatology	NP	Stiles, A (NC)	3
Neonatology	NP	Tyson, J (TX)	3
Neonatology	Ped	Miller, C (CA)	6
Neoromuscular Disorders	N	Glass, J (GA)	4
Nephrotic Syndrome	Nep	Black, H (IL)	3
Nephrotic Syndrome	Nep	Couser, W (WA)	3
Nephrotic Syndrome	Nep	Okusa, M (VA)	3
Nephrotic Syndrome	PNep	Alexander, S (CA)	6
Nephrotic Syndrome	PNep	Cohn, R (IL)	6
Nephrotic Syndrome	PNep	Nash, M (NY)	6
Nephrotic Syndrome	PNep	Zilleruelo, G (FL)	6
Nerve Compression	HS	McAuliffe, J (FL)	2
Nerve Reconstruction	HS	Wolfe, S (NY)	2
Nerve Regeneration	HS	Trumble, T (WA)	2
Nerve Surgery	HS	Greene, T (FL)	2
Nerve Transplantation	PlS	Mackinnon, S (MO)	7
Nerve/Muscle Disorders	N	Kurtzke, R (VA)	4
Neural Imaging	N	Burke, A (IL)	4
Neural Regulation of Mucosal Secretion	A&I	Baraniuk, J (DC)	
Neural Transplantation	NS	Freeman, T (FL)	4
Neuro-Behavioral Disorder	N	Jackson, J (LA)	4
Neuro-Endocrinology	ChiN	Ferriero, D (CA)	1
Neuro-Endocrinology	ObG	Naftolin, F (CT)	1
Neuro-Genetics	CG	Korf, B (MA)	1
Neuro-Genetics	CG	Northrup, H (TX)	1
Neuro-Immunology	N	Apatoff, B (NY)	4
Neuro-Immunology	N	Cohen, J (OH)	4
Neuro-Immunology	N	Coyle, P (NY)	4
Neuro-Immunology	N	Richert, J (DC)	4
Neuro-Oncology	N	Cloughesy, T (CA)	4
Neuro-Oncology	N	De Angelis, L (NY)	4
Neuro-Oncology	N	Greenberg, H (MI)	4
Neuro-Oncology	N	Hiesiger, E (NY)	4
Neuro-Oncology	N	Posner, J (NY)	4
Neuro-Oncology	N	Rogers, L (MI)	4
Neuro-Oncology	N	Sagar, S (OH)	4
Neuro-Oncology	N	Shapiro, W (AZ)	4
Neuro-Oncology	N	Spence, A (WA)	4
Neuro-Oncology	NS	Al-Mefty, O (AR)	4
Neuro-Oncology	NS	Piepmeier, J (CT)	4

SPECIAL EXPERTISE INDEX

SPECIAL EXPERTISE INDEX

SPECIAL EXPERTISE INDEX

SPECIAL EXPERTISE INDEX

Special Expertise	Spec	Name	Pg	Special Expertise	Spec	Name
Prostate Cancer	RadRO	Hilaris, B (NY)	771	Prostate Disease	U	Gribetz, M (NY)
Prostate Cancer	RadRO	Leibel, S (NY)	771	Prostate Disease	U	Lowe, F (NY)
Prostate Cancer	RadRO	Lichter, A (MI)	775	Prostate Disease	U	Macchia, R (NY)
Prostate Cancer	RadRO	Nori, D (NY)	772	Prostate Disease	U	Naslund, M (MD)
Prostate Cancer	RadRO	Petrovich, Z (CA)	778	Prostate Disease	U	Ross, L (IL)
Prostate Cancer	RadRO	Pollack, A (PA)	772	Prostate Disease	U	Seftel, A (OH)
Prostate Cancer	RadRO	Pollack, J (NY)	772	Prostate Disease	U	Vaughan, E (NY)
Prostate Cancer	RadRO	Rose, C (CA)	779	Prostate Disease	U	Waldbaum, R (NY)
Prostate Cancer	RadRO	Rosenman, J (NC)	774	Prostate Surgery	U	Albala, D (NC)
Prostate Cancer	RadRO	Schiff, P (NY)	772	Prostate Surgery	U	Thompson Jr, I (TX)
Prostate Cancer	RadRO	Shipley, W (MA)	769	Prosthetic Nose	PlS	Tabbal, N (NY)
Prostate Cancer	RadRO	Stock, R (NY)	772	Prosthetic Valves	Cv	Mehlman, D (IL)
Prostate Cancer	RadRO	Vicini, F (MI)	775	Pseudomyxoma Peritonei	S	Sugarbaker, P (DC)
Prostate Cancer	U	Bander, N (NY)	900	Pseudotumor Cerebri	N	Corbett, J (MS)
Prostate Cancer	U	Bardot, S (LA)	913	Pseudotumor Cerebri	Oph	Burde, R (NY)
Prostate Cancer	U	Basler, J (TX)	914	Psoriasis	D	Fenske, N (FL)
Prostate Cancer	U	Benson, M (NY)	901	Psoriasis	D	Freedberg, I (NY)
Prostate Cancer	U	Brendler, C (IL)	909	Psoriasis	D	Krueger, G (UT)
Prostate Cancer	U	Burnett II, A (MD)	901	Psoriasis	D	Lebwohl, M (NY)
Prostate Cancer	U	Catalona, W (MO)	910	Psoriasis	D	Lowe, N (CA)
Prostate Cancer	U	Chodak, G (IL)	910	Psoriasis	D	McDonald, C (RI)
Prostate Cancer	U	Danoff, D (CA)	916	Psoriasis	D	Menter, M (TX)
Prostate Cancer	U	Flanigan, R (IL)	910	Psoriasis	D	Shupack, J (NY)
Prostate Cancer	U	Huben, R (NY)	902	Psoriasis	D	Voorhees, J (MI)
Prostate Cancer	U	Jacobs, S (MD)	902	Psoriasis/Eczema	D	Orlow, S (NY)
Prostate Cancer	U	Jarow, J (MD)	902	Psoriasis/Lupus	D	Braverman, I (CT)
Prostate Cancer	U	Kirschenbaum, A (NY)	902	Psoriatic Arthritis	Rhu	Mitnick, H (NY)
Prostate Cancer	U	Klein, E (OH)	910	Psychiatric Aspects of GI Disorders	Ge	Drossman, D (NC)
Prostate Cancer	U	Kozlowski, J (IL)	911	Psychiatric Disorders of Young Children	ChAP	Luby, J (MO)
Prostate Cancer	U	Lepor, H (NY)	903	Psychiatric Neuro-Imaging	Psyc	Pearlson, G (MD)
Prostate Cancer	U	Libertino, J (MA)	899	Psychiatric Rehabilitation	Psyc	Liberman, R (CA)
Prostate Cancer	U	Lieskovsky, G (CA)	916	Psychiatry for Cancer	Psyc	Spiegel, D (CA)
Prostate Cancer	U	Macchia, R (NY)	903	Psychiatry in Chronic Medical Illness	GerPsy	Borson, S (WA)
Prostate Cancer	U	Marshall, F (GA)	907	Psychiatry of Cancer	Psyc	Holland, J (NY)
Prostate Cancer	U	Mc Vary, K (IL)	911	Psychiatry of Cancer	Psyc	Lederberg, M (NY)
Prostate Cancer	U	McConnell, J (TX)	914	Psychiatry of Illness	ChAP	Campo, J (PA)
Prostate Cancer	U	McDougal, W (MA)	899	Psychiatry-Adolescent/College Age	ChAP	Wiener, J (DC)
Prostate Cancer	U	McGovern, F (MA)	899	Psychiatry-Geriatric	GerPsy	Borson, S (WA)
Prostate Cancer	U	Menon, M (MI)	911	Psychiatry-Geriatric	GerPsy	Luchins, D (IL)
Prostate Cancer	U	Miles, B (TX)	914	Psychiatry-Geriatric	Psyc	Alexopoulos, G (NY)
Prostate Cancer	U	Montie, J (MI)	911	Psychiatry-Geriatric	Psyc	Blazer II, D (NC)
Prostate Cancer	U	Mostwin, J (MD)	903	Psychiatry-Geriatric	Psyc	Jenike, M (MA)
Prostate Cancer	U	Naslund, M (MD)	904	Psychiatry-Geriatric	Psyc	Nelson, J (CT)
Prostate Cancer	U	Nelson, J (PA)	904	Psychiatry-Geriatric	Psyc	Weiner, M (TX)
Prostate Cancer	U	Olsson, C (NY)	904	Psychoanalysis	ChAP	King, R (CT)
Prostate Cancer	U	Resnick, M (OH)	912	Psychoanalysis	Psyc	Altshuler, K (TX)
Prostate Cancer	U	Richie, J (MA)	900	Psychoanalysis	Psyc	Munich, R (KS)
Prostate Cancer	U	Sanders, W (GA)	908	Psychoanalysis	Psyc	Pomer, S (CA)
Prostate Cancer	U	Scardino, P (NY)	904	Psychoanalysis	Psyc	Samberg, E (NY)
Prostate Cancer	U	Schellhammer, P (VA)	908	Psychoanalysis	Psyc	Stone, M (NY)
Prostate Cancer	U	Schlegel, P (NY)	904	Psychoanalysis	Psyc	Zerbe, K (OR)
Prostate Cancer	U	Schmidt, J (CA)	917	Psychopharmacology	AdP	Schuckit, M (CA)
Prostate Cancer	U	Smith, J (TN)	908	Psychopharmacology	ChAP	Biederman, J (MA)
Prostate Cancer	U	Thompson Jr, I (TX)	915	Psychopharmacology	ChAP	Riddle, M (MD)
Prostate Cancer	U	von Eschenbach, A (TX)	915	Psychopharmacology	GerPsy	Friedman, B (CA)
Prostate Cancer	U	Waldbaum, R (NY)	905	Psychopharmacology	GerPsy	Schneider, L (CA)
Prostate Cancer	U	Walsh, P (MD)	905	Psychopharmacology	Psyc	Alexopoulos, G (NY)
Prostate Cancer	U	Wein, A (PA)	905	Psychopharmacology	Psyc	Bowers Jr, M (CT)
Prostate Cancer	U	Williams, R (IA)	913	Psychopharmacology	Psyc	Cohen, B (MA)
Prostate Cancer Pain	NuM	Silberstein, E (OH)	465	Psychopharmacology	Psyc	Greist, J (WI)
Prostate Disease	U	Alexander, R (MD)	900	Psychopharmacology	Psyc	Janicak, P (IL)
Prostate Disease	U	Bruskewitz, R (WI)	910	Psychopharmacology	Psyc	Klein, D (NY)
Prostate Disease	U	Chodak, G (IL)	910	Psychopharmacology	Psyc	Manevitz, A (NY)
Prostate Disease	U	Fuselier Jr, H (LA)	914	Psychopharmacology	Psyc	Marder, S (CA)

SPECIAL EXPERTISE INDEX

SPECIAL EXPERTISE INDEX

SPECIAL EXPERTISE INDEX

SPECIAL EXPERTISE INDEX

SPECIAL EXPERTISE INDEX

SPECIAL EXPERTISE INDEX

ALPHABETICAL LISTING OF DOCTORS

ALPHABETICAL LISTING OF DOCTORS

Name	Specialty	Page	Name	Specialty	Page
Bernstein, Daniel (CA)	PCd	626	Boniuk, Milton (TX)	Oph	500
Bernstein, Robert M (NJ)	D	194	Bonkovsky, Herbert (MA)	Ge	229
Bhan, Atul Kumar (MA)	Path	575	Bonner, James Ryan (AL)	A&I	97
Bieber, Eric J (PA)	ObG	472	Bonomi, Philip (IL)	Onc	327
Biederman, Joseph (MA)	ChAP	717	Bonow, Robert O (IL)	Cv	142
Bierbaum, Benjamin (MA)	OrS	515	Boone, Timothy Bolton (TX)	U	914
Biesecker, Leslie Glenn (MD)	CG	169	Booth, Robert (PA)	OrS	518
Biggs Jr, Thomas M (TX)	PlS	703	Borchert, Mark S (CA)	Oph	502
Biglan, Albert William (PA)	Oph	484	Borer, Jeffrey (NY)	Cv	133
Bigliani, Louis (NY)	OrS	517	Borgen, Patrick Ivan (NY)	S	846
Bilchik, Anton Joel (CA)	S	864	Borges, Lawrence F (MA)	NS	405
Bilezikian, John P (NY)	EDM	208	Borkowsky, William (NY)	PInf	647
Biller, Beverly M K (MA)	EDM	207	Boronow, John Joseph (MD)	Psyc	729
Billmire, David A (OH)	PlS	699	Borson, Soo (WA)	GerPsy	727
Binder, Perry Scott (CA)	Oph	502	Borzak, Steven (FL)	Cv	139
Bird, Hector (NY)	ChAP	718	Bosl, George (NY)	Onc	316
Bishop, Allen Thorp (MN)	HS	280	Bostwick, David (VA)	Path	578
Bissell Jr, Dwight Montgomery (CA)	IM	364	Boucek, Mark M (CO)	PCd	625
Bitran, Jacob (IL)	Onc	327	Boucek, Robert (FL)	PCd	622
Black, Henry R (IL)	Nep	394	Bourdette, Dennis (OR)	N	454
Black, Keith Lanier (CA)	NS	420	Bourge, Robert Charles (AL)	Cv	139
Black, Peter (MA)	NS	405	Bourgoignie, Jacques (FL)	Nep	392
Blackburn, George L (MA)	S	843	Boushey Jr, Homer A (CA)	Pul	762
Blackwell, Richard (AL)	RE	803	Bouwman, David L (MI)	S	856
Blaha, J David (WV)	OrS	518	Bove, Edward (MI)	PS	669
Blaivas, Jerry G (NY)	U	901	Bowden, Charles (TX)	Psyc	737
Bland, Kirby (AL)	S	853	Bowen, James (WA)	N	454
Blaser, Martin Jack (NY)	Inf	344	Bower, Charles (AR)	Oto	560
Blasko, John Charles (WA)	RadRO	778	Bowers Jr, Malcolm B (CT)	Psyc	728
Blass, John (NY)	Ger	251	Boxrud, Cynthia Ann (CA)	Oph	502
Blazer II, Dan G (NC)	Psyc	734	Boyajian, Michael (DC)	PlS	691
Bleday, Ronald (MA)	CRS	181	Boyce Jr, H Worth (FL)	Ge	234
Blei, Andres T (IL)	Ge	237	Boyce, John G (NY)	ObG	472
Bleiberg, Efrain (KS)	ChAP	722	Boyd, Robert (TX)	Ped	613
Bleifer, Selvyn Burton (CA)	Cv	149	Boyd, Stuart D (CA)	U	915
Bleyer, W Archie (TX)	PHO	645	Boyle, Robert John (VA)	NP	384
Blinder, Morey (MO)	Hem	308	Brackmann, Derald E (CA)	Oto	562
Blitzer, Andrew (NY)	Oto	544	Braddom, Randall L (IN)	PMR	680
Bloom, David A (MI)	U	909	Braden, Gregory Alan (NC)	IC	154
Bloom, Patricia (NY)	Ger	251	Bradford, David S (CA)	OrS	534
Bloomer, Joseph (AL)	Ge	234	Bradley, James P (PA)	OrS	518
Bluestone, Charles D (PA)	PO	656	Bradley, John S (CA)	PInf	651
Blum, Manfred (NY)	EDM	208	Brady III, Charles Elmer (TX)	Ge	243
Blum, Paul (MN)	PA&I	616	Brage, Michael (CA)	OrS	534
Blum, Robert W (MN)	AM	91	Braman, Sidney (RI)	Pul	745
Blume, Ralph (NY)	Rhu	816	Branch Jr, Charles L (NC)	NS	411
Blumenthal, David S (NY)	Cv	133	Brandt, Keith (MO)	PlS	699
Boachie, Oheneba (NY)	OrS	518	Brandt, Lawrence (NY)	Ge	230
Bobrove, Arthur M (CA)	Rhu	825	Branham, Gregory H (MO)	Oto	554
Bockenstedt, Paula (MI)	Hem	308	Brasington, Richard (MO)	Rhu	820
Bockman, Richard (NY)	EDM	209	Braun, Carl (NY)	N	435
Bodenheimer Jr, Henry (NY)	Ge	230	Braunstein, Seth N (PA)	IM	361
Boehm, Frank Henry (TN)	MF	373	Braunwald, Eugene (MA)	Cv	130
Bogrov, Michael (MD)	ChAP	718	Brause, Barry (NY)	Inf	344
Bohlman, Henry H (OH)	OrS	528	Braverman, Alan Charles (MO)	Cv	142
Boland Jr, Arthur L (MA)	OrS	515	Braverman, Irwin (CT)	D	193
Boles, Richard Gregory (CA)	CG	173	Braylan, Raul (FL)	Path	579
Bollen, Andrew W (CA)	Path	582	Brazer, Scott Robert (NC)	Ge	234
Bollinger, R Randal (NC)	S	853	Brazy, Peter C (WI)	Nep	394
Bolman III, Ralph Morton (MN)	TS	881	Bredenberg, Carl Eric (ME)	TS	871
Bolton, Warren Kline (VA)	Nep	392	Breidenbach, Warren C (KY)	HS	279

ALPHABETICAL LISTING OF DOCTORS

Name	Specialty	Page	Name	Specialty	Page
Caplan, Louis Robert (MA)	N	433	Chang-Miller, April (MN)	Rhu	821
Capo, Hilda (FL)	Oph	492	Chap, Linnea (CA)	Onc	335
Caprioli, Joseph (CA)	Oph	502	Chapman, Paul (NY)	Onc	316
Caputo, Anthony R (NJ)	Oph	484	Chapman, Paul H (MA)	NS	405
Caputo, Thomas A (NY)	GO	264	Char, Devron H (CA)	Oph	502
Caputy, Anthony J (DC)	NS	407	Charboneau, J William (MN)	Rad	795
Carbonell, Manuel (FL)	CRS	183	Charney, Jonathan (NY)	N	436
Cardenas, Diana (WA)	PMR	684	Charrow, Joel (IL)	CG	171
Carey, John (UT)	CG	172	Chatham, Walter W (AL)	Rhu	819
Carey, Larry C (FL)	S	853	Chatterjee, Kanu (CA)	Cv	150
Carey, Timothy Stephen (NC)	IM	363	Chen, David (IL)	PMR	681
Carlson, Grant W (GA)	S	853	Cheney, Mack Lowell (MA)	Oto	543
Carlson, John (PA)	GO	264	Chernoff, William Gregory (IN)	Oto	554
Carlson, Robert Wells (CA)	Onc	335	Cherry Jr, Kenneth J (MN)	GVS	933
Carmel, Peter (NJ)	NS	407	Cherry, James Donald (CA)	PInf	651
Carneiro, Ronaldo Dos Santos (FL)	HS	279	Chervenak, Francis Anthony (NY)	MF	371
Caronna, John J (NY)	N	436	Chescheir, Nancy Custer (NC)	MF	373
Carpenter Jr, William T (MD)	Psyc	730	Chiu, David (NY)	HS	277
Carpenter, Charles B (MA)	Nep	389	Chlebowski, Rowan Thomas (CA)	Onc	335
Carr, Bruce (TX)	ObG	477	Chodak, Gerald (IL)	U	910
Carr, Daniel B (MA)	PM	567	Choe, Soo-Sang (CA)	Cv	150
Carr, David Brian (MO)	Ger	254	Choi, Noah C (MA)	RadRO	769
Carr-Locke, David L (MA)	Ge	229	Chopra, Inder Jit (CA)	EDM	219
Carrasquillo, Jorge Amilcar (MD)	NuM	463	Choy, Andrew Eng (CA)	Oph	502
Carrau, Ricardo L (PA)	Oto	545	Christiani, David (MA)	Pul	745
Carraway, James Howard (VA)	PlS	695	Christiansen, Thomas (MN)	Oto	554
Carroll, Charles (IL)	HS	281	Christie, Dennis (WA)	PGe	639
Carroll, Peter Robert (CA)	U	916	Christie, John (FL)	CRS	183
Carroll, William L (UT)	PHO	644	Christman, Brian Wallace (TN)	Pul	750
Carson, Benjamin S (MD)	NS	407	Christman, Gregory (MI)	RE	805
Carson, Culley (NC)	U	906	Chrousos, George (MD)	PEn	630
Carter, Darryl (CT)	Path	575	Chui, Helena Chang (CA)	N	454
Carter, John E (TX)	N	452	Chung, Kevin (MI)	HS	281
Carter, William Jerry (AR)	Ger	256	Church, Joseph August (CA)	PA&I	618
Cartwright, Patrick (UT)	U	913	Chutorian, Abraham (NY)	ChiN	159
Casella, Samuel Joseph (NH)	PEn	630	Chuttani, Ram (MA)	Ge	229
Cassidy, Suzanne (CA)	CG	173	Cibis, Gerhard W (MO)	Oph	496
Cassisi, Nicholas J (FL)	Oto	550	Cicale, Michael Jon (FL)	Pul	751
Castell, Donald O (SC)	Ge	235	Cilo, Mark P (CO)	N	451
Castle, Valerie (MI)	PHO	643	Ciocon, Jerry (FL)	Ger	253
Catalona, William J (MO)	U	910	Cioffi, William (RI)	S	843
Catanzaro, Antonino (CA)	Pul	762	Cirigliano, Michael (PA)	IM	362
Cavallino, Robert (IL)	DR	787	Civin, Curt Ingraham (MD)	PHO	640
Cederbaum, Stephen D (CA)	CG	173	Clagett, George Patrick (TX)	GVS	935
Celli, Bartolome (MA)	Pul	745	Clairmont, Albert (OH)	PMR	681
Cello, John Patrick (CA)	Ge	244	Clark, Orlo H (CA)	S	864
Cerqueira, Manuel (DC)	Cv	134	Clark, Vivian (MI)	IC	155
Chaisson, Richard Ernest (MD)	Inf	344	Clarke-Pearson, Daniel L (NC)	GO	266
Chait, Alan (WA)	EDM	219	Clauw, Daniel J (DC)	Rhu	816
Chaitman, Bernard R (MO)	Cv	143	Clayman, Gary Lee (TX)	Oto	560
Chalas, Eva (NY)	GO	264	Clayman, Ralph V (CA)	U	916
Chambers, Richard Byron (CA)	OrS	534	Clements III, Dennis Alfred (NC)	PInf	648
Chan, Joseph (FL)	Inf	348	Clements Jr, Stephen (GA)	Cv	139
Chandar, Jayanthi (FL)	PNep	653	Clements, Philip Jordan (CA)	Rhu	825
Chandler, Michael (NY)	A&I	95	Cleveland, William (FL)	PEn	631
Chandler, William F (MI)	NS	414	Clifton, Guy (TX)	NS	418
Chandrasoma, Parakrama T (CA)	Path	582	Cloherty, John (MA)	NP	383
Chang, Alfred Edward (MI)	S	856	Cloninger, C Robert (MO)	Psyc	735
Chang, Helena (CA)	S	864	Close, Lanny Garth (NY)	Oto	545
Chang, Rowland Waton (IL)	Rhu	821	Cloughesy, Timothy Francis (CA)	N	454
Chang, Stanley (NY)	Oph	484			

ALPHABETICAL LISTING OF DOCTORS

Name	Specialty	Page	Name	Specialty	Page
Culbertson, William (FL)	Oph	492	Day, Arthur L (FL)	NS	411
Culkin, Daniel J (OK)	U	914	Day, Susan H (CA)	Oph	502
Cullen, Kevin (DC)	Onc	317	De Angelis, Lisa (NY)	N	436
Culp, Randall (PA)	HS	277	De Franco, Anthony (MI)	Cv	143
Cummings, Charles (MD)	Oto	545	De Fronzo, Ralph Anthony (TX)	IM	364
Cummings, Jeffrey Lee (CA)	N	455	De Fusco, Patricia A (CT)	Onc	313
Cundiff, Geoffrey Williams (MD)	ObG	472	De Geest, Koen (IL)	GO	268
Cunha, Burke A (NY)	Inf	344	De Giorgio, Christopher M (CA)	N	455
Cunniff, Christopher (AZ)	CG	172	De Groot, Leslie (IL)	EDM	215
Cunningham Jr, Joseph N (NY)	TS	874	De Juan Jr, Eugene (CA)	Oph	503
Cunningham, John (AZ)	Ge	243	de Kernion, Jean Bayhi (CA)	U	916
Cunningham-Rundles, Charlotte (NY)	A&I	95	De la Cruz, Antonio (CA)	Oto	562
Cupps, Thomas R (DC)	Rhu	816	De Lateur, Barbara J (MD)	PMR	678
Curl, Walton Wright (NC)	OrS	526	De Long, Mahlon R (GA)	N	442
Curley, Steven Alan (TX)	S	861	De Meester, Tom R (CA)	TS	888
Curran Jr, Walter J (PA)	RadRO	770	De Sanctis, Roman (MA)	Cv	130
Curran, James Joseph (IL)	Rhu	821	de Shazo, Richard Denson (MS)	A&I	97
Currie, John L (NH)	GO	263	De Simone, Philip A (KY)	Hem	307
Curry, Cynthia J (CA)	CG	173	De Vita Jr, Vincent T (CT)	Onc	313
Curtin, John P (NY)	GO	265	De Vivo, Darryl C (NY)	ChiN	160
Curtis, Anne B (FL)	CE	126	Dean, Richard H (NC)	GVS	932
Cushing, Gary W (MA)	EDM	207	DeCamp Jr, Malcolm M (OH)	TS	882
Cutilletta, Anthony F (IL)	PCd	623	DeCherney, Alan Hersh (CA)	ObG	478
Cutrer, F Michael (MN)	N	447	Deitch, Edwin (NJ)	S	847
Cutting, Court (NY)	PlS	691	DeKosky, Steven T (PA)	N	436
			Del Monte, Monte A (MI)	Oph	496
D			Del Negro, Albert Anthony (VA)	Cv	140
			Del Priore, Lucian (NY)	Oph	485
D'Alton, Mary Elizabeth (NY)	MF	372	Delahay, John Norris (DC)	OrS	519
D'Amico, Anthony V (MA)	RadRO	769	Deland, Jonathan T (NY)	OrS	519
Daar, Eric S (CA)	IM	365	DeLeo, Vincent A (NY)	D	195
Dabbagh, Shermine (DE)	PNep	652	Della Rocca, Robert (NY)	Oph	485
Dabezies, Eugene (TX)	OrS	533	Delmez, James Albert (MO)	Nep	394
Dacey Jr, Ralph Gerald (MO)	NS	414	Demer, Joseph L (CA)	Oph	503
Dahms, William (OH)	PEn	632	Dempsey, Robert J (WI)	NS	415
Dake, Michael David (CA)	Rad	796	Denenberg, Steven M (NE)	Oto	559
Dale, Lowell C (MN)	Ger	254	Dennis, Gary Creed (DC)	NS	407
Dalinka, Murray (PA)	DR	785	Denson, Susan Ellen (TX)	NP	385
Dalkin, Alan Craig (VA)	EDM	212	DePaulo, Jr, J Raymond (MD)	Psyc	730
Daniel, Rollin K (CA)	PlS	705	Deren, Julius J (PA)	Ge	230
Daniel, Thomas M (VA)	TS	878	Derman, Gordon Harris (IL)	HS	281
Daniels, Gilbert (MA)	EDM	207	Dershaw, D David (NY)	DR	785
Danielson, Gordon (MN)	TS	882	Deschamps, Claude (MN)	TS	882
Danoff, Dudley S (CA)	U	916	Desnick, Robert J (NY)	CG	170
Dardik, Herbert (NJ)	GVS	929	Desposito, Franklin (NJ)	CG	170
Darling, Ralph Clement (NY)	GVS	929	DeVane, Gary Williams (FL)	RE	803
Darras, Basil Theodore (MA)	ChiN	159	Devinsky, Orrin (NY)	N	436
Daspit, C Phillip (AZ)	Oto	560	Dewberry, Robert Gerard (MD)	N	437
Dattwyler, Raymond (NY)	A&I	96	Di Magno, Eugene (MN)	Ge	238
Davidson, Bruce J (DC)	Oto	545	Di Persio, John (MO)	Onc	327
Davidson, Jonathan (NC)	Psyc	734	Di Spaltro, Franklin (NJ)	PlS	691
Davidson, Joyce Eileen (KS)	Psyc	736	Diamond, Frank (FL)	PEn	632
Davidson, Nancy E (MD)	Onc	317	Diamond, Gary Richard (PA)	Oph	485
Davies, Terry (NY)	EDM	209	Diamond, Jeffrey (FL)	Ge	235
Davis Jr, James William (CA)	Ger	257	Diamond, Michael (MI)	RE	805
Davis, Gary L (FL)	Ge	235	Diao, Edward (CA)	HS	284
Davis, Ira D (OH)	PNep	654	Diaz, Angela (NY)	AM	91
Davis, Jessica S (NY)	CG	169	Diaz, Fernando G (MI)	NS	415
Davis, Kenneth (NY)	Psyc	730	Dichter, Marc A (PA)	N	437
Davis, R Kim (UT)	Oto	559	Dick, Macdonald (MI)	PCd	623
Davis, William Eugene (LA)	Rhu	824	Dienstag, Jules Leonard (MA)	Ge	229

ALPHABETICAL LISTING OF DOCTORS

Name	Specialty	Page
Eisendrath, Stuart James (CA)	Psyc	738
Eismont, Frank (FL)	OrS	526
El-Youssef, Mounif (MN)	PGe	638
Elefteriades, John (CT)	TS	871
Elias, Sherman (IL)	ObG	475
Elias, Stanton B (MI)	N	447
Elkayam, Uri (CA)	Cv	150
Ellenbogen, Kenneth A (VA)	CE	126
Ellenbogen, Richard (WA)	NS	420
Elliott, C Gregory (UT)	Pul	758
Elliott, David (IA)	Ge	238
Ellis III, George John (NC)	EDM	213
Ellis Jr, George S (LA)	Oph	500
Ellis, Jonathan C (CA)	Ge	244
Ellis, Stephen Geoffrey (OH)	IC	155
Ellison, David H (OR)	Nep	398
Ellison, Edwin Christopher (OH)	S	857
Ellman, Michael H (IL)	Rhu	821
Ellner, Jerrold Jay (NJ)	Inf	344
Elsas II, Louis Jacob (GA)	CG	171
Emami, Bahman (IL)	RadRO	774
Emans, Sarah Jean Herriot (MA)	AM	91
Emanuele, Mary Ann (IL)	EDM	215
Emanuele, Nicholas Victor (IL)	EDM	215
Emery, Helen Margaret (CA)	PRhu	665
Emmanuel, Patricia (FL)	PInf	648
Emond, Jean Crawford (NY)	S	847
Emslie, Graham J (TX)	ChAP	723
Enelow, Richard Ian (VA)	Pul	751
Engel, William King (CA)	N	455
Engstrom, John Walter (CA)	N	455
Enker, Warren (NY)	S	848
Ennis, Ronald (NY)	RadRO	770
Epstein, Andrew Ernest (AL)	CE	127
Epstein, Fred Jacob (NY)	NS	407
Epstein, Jonathan (MD)	Path	576
Epstein, Leon G (IL)	ChiN	161
Epstein, Michael (MI)	PCd	624
Epstein, Stuart Zane (CA)	PA&I	618
Eriksson, Elof (MA)	PlS	689
Errico, Thomas (NY)	OrS	519
Esch, Peter (OH)	IM	363
Eschenbach, David Arthur (WA)	ObG	478
Escobedo, Marilyn Barnard (OK)	NP	385
Esquenazi, Alberto (PA)	PMR	678
Esquivel, Carlos Orlando (CA)	S	864
Esserman, Laura J (CA)	S	865
Essner, Richard (CA)	S	865
Estabrook, Alison (NY)	S	848
Eth, Spencer (NY)	Psyc	730
Ettenger, Robert Bruce (CA)	PNep	655
Ettinger, David Seymour (MD)	Onc	317
Eustace, John C (FL)	IM	363
Eustis, Horatio Sprague (LA)	Oph	500
Evans III, Richard (IL)	PA&I	616
Evans, Douglas Brian (TX)	S	861
Evans, Mark Ira (PA)	ObG	472
Eviatar, Lydia (NY)	ChiN	160
Ezaki, Marybeth (TX)	HS	283

F

Name	Specialty	Page
Faber, L Penfield (IL)	TS	882
Fabian, Carol J (KS)	Onc	332
Fabian, Richard (MA)	Oto	543
Fagien, Steven (FL)	Oph	492
Fahey, Patrick J (IL)	Pul	755
Fahn, Stanley (NY)	N	437
Failla, Joseph M (MI)	HS	281
Faillace, Walter (FL)	NS	411
Falcone, Tommaso (OH)	RE	806
Falk, Rena Ellen (CA)	CG	173
Falk, Ronald J (NC)	Nep	392
Falletta, John (NC)	PHO	642
Fan, Leland Lane (TX)	PPul	662
Fang, Leslie (MA)	Nep	389
Fanous, Yvonne F (CA)	PA&I	618
Fanta, Christopher (MA)	Pul	745
Fantini, Gary A (NY)	GVS	929
Farber, Martin Stuart (NY)	Rhu	816
Farcy, Jean-Pierre (NY)	OrS	519
Farlow, Martin (IN)	N	447
Farmer, Joseph (NC)	Oto	550
Farmer, Richard G (DC)	Ge	231
Faro, Sebastian (TX)	ObG	477
Farrior, Edward (FL)	Oto	550
Farrior, Joseph Brown (FL)	Oto	551
Fauci, Anthony Stephen (MD)	Inf	344
Fawcett, Jan A (IL)	Psyc	735
Faxon, David P (IL)	Cv	143
Fazio, Victor (OH)	CRS	185
Feder, Robert S (IL)	Oph	496
Fee Jr, Willard E (CA)	Oto	563
Feig, Stephen A (CA)	PHO	645
Fein, William (CA)	Oph	503
Feinberg, Joseph Hunt (NY)	PMR	678
Feinglos, Mark (NC)	EDM	213
Feinstein, Donald I (CA)	Hem	311
Feinstein, Steven B (IL)	Cv	144
Feldman, David Steven (NY)	OrS	519
Feldman, Eva L (MI)	N	447
Feldman, Joel (MA)	PlS	689
Feldman, Mark (TX)	Ge	243
Feldman, Robert G (MA)	N	433
Feldman, Ted (IL)	IC	155
Feldmann, Edward (RI)	N	433
Feldon, Steven E (NY)	Oph	485
Felig, Philip (NY)	EDM	209
Fenichel, Gerald M (TN)	ChiN	161
Fennell III, Robert Samuel (FL)	PNep	653
Fenske, Neil (FL)	D	198
Ferguson II, James E (VA)	MF	373
Ferguson, Mark (IL)	TS	882
Ferguson, Ronald (OH)	S	857
Ferlic, Donald C (CO)	HS	283
Ferrante, F Michael (CA)	PM	571
Ferrara, James (MI)	PHO	643
Ferraz, Francisco M (VA)	NS	411
Ferree, Carolyn Ruth Black (NC)	RadRO	773
Ferrell, Linda (CA)	Path	582
Ferrendelli, James A (TX)	N	452

ALPHABETICAL LISTING OF DOCTORS

Name	Specialty	Page	Name	Specialty	Page
Funk, Gerry Franklin (IA)	Oto	555	Gershengorn, Kent N (CA)	Cv	150
Furlan, Anthony J (OH)	N	447	Gershenson, David Marc (TX)	GO	270
Furukawa, Satoshi (PA)	TS	874	Gershon, Anne (NY)	PInf	647
Fuselier Jr, Harold A (LA)	U	914	Gershwin, Merrill Eric (CA)	Rhu	825
Fuster, Carlos Daniel (CA)	AM	92	Gersony, Welton Mark (NY)	PCd	621
Fuster, Valentin (NY)	Cv	134	Gewertz, Bruce (IL)	GVS	934
			Gewitz, Michael (NY)	PCd	621
G			Gewurz, Anita (IL)	PA&I	616
Gabbard, Glen O (TX)	Psyc	737	Giangola, Gary (NY)	GVS	929
Gabbe, Steven G (TN)	MF	373	Giannotta, Steven L (CA)	NS	420
Gabram, Sheryl (IL)	S	857	Gianoli, Gerard (LA)	Oto	560
Gabrilove, Janice (NY)	Onc	317	Gianopoulos, John (IL)	MF	374
Gadacz, Thomas R (GA)	S	854	Gibbons, Gary William (MA)	GVS	927
Gage, James (MN)	OrS	529	Gibbons, Raymond John (MN)	Cv	144
Gagel, Robert F (TX)	EDM	218	Gibbs, John F (NY)	S	848
Gagner, Michel (NY)	S	848	Gibbs, Ronald Steven (CO)	MF	376
Galandiuk, Susan (KY)	CRS	184	Gilchrest, Barbara (MA)	D	193
Galante, Jorge O (IL)	OrS	529	Gill, Harcharan Singh (CA)	U	916
Galanter, Marc (NY)	AdP	715	Gillette, Paul Crawford (TX)	PCd	625
Galask, Rudolph P (IA)	ObG	475	Gills Jr, James P (FL)	Oph	493
Galati, Joseph Steven (TX)	Ge	243	Gilman, Sid (MI)	N	447
Galetta, Steven (PA)	N	437	Gingold, Bruce (NY)	CRS	182
Gallico, G Gregory (MA)	PlS	689	Ginsburg, Howard (NY)	PS	666
Galloway, Aubrey (NY)	TS	874	Ginzler, Ellen (NY)	Rhu	817
Gambert, Steven (MD)	Ger	252	Gitlin, Michael Jay (CA)	Psyc	738
Gamelli, Richard Louis (IL)	S	857	Gitlow, Stanley (NY)	IM	362
Gandara, David R (CA)	Onc	335	Gittler, Michelle (IL)	PMR	681
Gang, Eli Shimshon (CA)	CE	128	Giuliano, Armando E (CA)	S	865
Ganguli, Rohan (PA)	Psyc	730	Givner, Laurence Bruce (NC)	PInf	649
Gantz, Bruce (IA)	Oto	555	Gizzi, Martin (NJ)	N	437
Ganz, Patricia Anne (CA)	Onc	336	Glader, Bertil E (CA)	PHO	645
Garb, Leslie Julian (TX)	Ger	256	Glaser, Joel (FL)	Oph	493
Garber, Judy E (MA)	Onc	313	Glasgold, Alvin (NJ)	Oto	546
Garcia, Carlos (LA)	N	452	Glass, Jonathan (GA)	N	443
Garcia-Gonzalez, Efrain (TX)	Cv	148	Glassford Jr, David M (TN)	TS	878
Garcia-Prats, Joseph (TX)	NP	386	Glassroth, Jeffrey (WI)	Pul	755
Garden, Jerome (IL)	D	200	Glatstein, Eli (PA)	RadRO	770
Gardin, Julius Markus (MI)	Cv	144	Glick, John H (PA)	Onc	317
Gardner, Gregory (WA)	Rhu	825	Glickel, Steven (NY)	HS	278
Gardner, Timothy Joseph (PA)	TS	874	Gliklich, Jerry (NY)	Cv	135
Garfin, Steven R (CA)	OrS	535	Glisson, Bonnie S (TX)	Onc	333
Garin, Eduardo Humberto (FL)	PNep	653	Glogau, Richard Gordon (CA)	D	203
Garnick, Marc Bennett (MA)	Onc	313	Glombicki, Alan Paul (TX)	Ge	243
Garrett, William (NC)	OrS	526	Gloviczki, Peter (MN)	GVS	934
Garvey, Glenda Josephine (NY)	Inf	345	Gluck, Joan (FL)	A&I	98
Garvin, James (NY)	PHO	641	Gluck, Paul (FL)	ObG	474
Gass, John Donald (TN)	Oph	493	Gluck, Stephen (FL)	Nep	393
Gaynor, Ellen (IL)	Hem	308	Gluckman, Gordon (IL)	U	910
Gebhardt, Mark (MA)	OrS	515	Gluckman, Jack L (OH)	Oto	555
Geffner, Mitchell Eugene (CA)	PEn	634	Gockerman, Jon Paul (NC)	Onc	322
Gelberman, Richard (MO)	HS	281	Godine, John Elliott (MA)	EDM	207
Gelfand, Erwin (CO)	PA&I	617	Godwin, John (IL)	Hem	308
Geller, Kenneth Allen (CA)	Oto	563	Godzik, Cathleen (CA)	HS	284
Gendelman, Seymour (NY)	N	437	Goebel, Joel Alan (MO)	Oto	555
Gentile, Ronald (NY)	Oph	486	Goepfert, Helmuth (TX)	Oto	561
Georgeson, Keith E (AL)	PS	668	Goetz, Christopher (IL)	N	447
Georgiade, Gregory (NC)	PlS	696	Goffinet, Don R (CA)	RadRO	778
Geppert, Eugene (IL)	Pul	755	Goin, Marcia Kraft (CA)	Psyc	738
Germano, Isabelle M (NY)	NS	408	Goitz, Henry (OH)	OrS	529
Geronemus, Roy (NY)	D	195	Golbe, Lawrence (NJ)	N	438
			Gold, Alan (NY)	PlS	691

ALPHABETICAL LISTING OF DOCTORS

Name	Specialty	Page	Name	Specialty	Page
Grossman, Robert I (PA)	NRad	789	Hanel, Douglas (WA)	HS	284
Grossniklaus, Hans E (GA)	Oph	493	Haney, Arthur F (NC)	RE	804
Grotta, James (TX)	N	452	Hanke, C William (IN)	D	200
Grotting, James (AL)	PlS	696	Hankinson, Hal L (NM)	NS	418
Grubb Jr, Robert L (MO)	NS	415	Hanks, John B (VA)	S	854
Grubb, Blair Paul (OH)	Cv	144	Hanley, Frank Louis (CA)	TS	889
Grum, Cyril M (MI)	Pul	756	Hanna, Ehab (AR)	Oto	561
Grundfast, Kenneth (MA)	PO	656	Hannafin, Jo (NY)	OrS	520
Gruss, Joseph (WA)	PlS	705	Hansen Jr, Sigvard (WA)	OrS	535
Guerrant, Richard (VA)	Inf	348	Hansen, Kimberley J (NC)	GVS	932
Guidry, George Gary (LA)	Pul	760	Hansen, Lori Eldean (OK)	Oto	561
Guilleminault, Christian (CA)	Psyc	738	Hansen, Nora Marie (CA)	S	865
Gujral, Saroj K (MN)	U	910	Hansen, Ronald (AZ)	D	202
Gulotta, Stephen J (NY)	Cv	135	Hansen-Flaschen, John (PA)	Pul	747
Gunasekaran, T S (IL)	PGe	638	Hanson, Laura Catherine (NC)	Ger	253
Gunderson, Leonard (AZ)	RadRO	777	Haponik, Edward Francis (MD)	Pul	747
Gundry, Steven (CA)	TS	888	Har-El, Gady (NY)	Oto	546
Gunter, Jack (TX)	PlS	703	Harden, R Norman (IL)	PM	569
Gurevitch, Arnold William (CA)	D	203	Hardesty, Robert (CA)	PlS	705
Gutai, James (MI)	PEn	633	Hardt, Nancy S (FL)	Path	579
Gutierrez, Francisco A (IL)	NS	415	Hardy, Mark (NY)	S	849
Guyer, David (NY)	Oph	486	Hare, John W (MA)	EDM	207
Guyton, David Lee (MD)	Oph	486	Harkema, James M (MI)	S	858
Guyton, Robert A (GA)	TS	879	Harman, Eloise M (FL)	Pul	752
			Harmon, Gary (KS)	Pul	758
H			Harmon, William E (MA)	PNep	652
			Harper, Richard L (TX)	NS	418
Haas, Richard H (CA)	ChiN	163	Harrell Jr, James E (TX)	TS	886
Hadler, Nortin (NC)	Rhu	819	Harrington, Elizabeth (NY)	GVS	930
Hadley, Mark N (AL)	NS	412	Harrington, J Timothy (WI)	Rhu	822
Haffty, Bruce (CT)	RadRO	769	Harris Jr, Edward Day (CA)	Rhu	826
Hafler, David A (MA)	N	433	Harris, Burton H (NY)	PS	666
Hagan, Kevin Francis (TN)	PlS	696	Harris, Jay R (MA)	RadRO	769
Hager, William David (KY)	ObG	474	Harris, Nancy L (MA)	Path	575
Hahn, Bevra H (CA)	Rhu	825	Harris, Raymond C (TN)	Nep	393
Haig, Andrew (MI)	PMR	681	Harrison, John Kevin (NC)	Cv	140
Haik, Barrett (TN)	Oph	493	Harrison, Louis (NY)	RadRO	771
Haines, Kathleen (NY)	PRhu	663	Harrison, Lynn (LA)	TS	886
Hait, William (NJ)	Onc	318	Harrison, Michael R (CA)	PS	671
Halberg, Francine Erna (CA)	RadRO	778	Hart, Robert G (TX)	N	452
Haley Jr, Elliott Clarke (VA)	N	443	Hart, William (OH)	Path	580
Halff, Glenn Alexander (TX)	S	862	Hartman, Barry Jay (NY)	Inf	345
Hall, Bryan Davis (KY)	Ped	612	Hartmann, Lynn Carol (MN)	Onc	328
Hall, Jesse (IL)	Pul	756	Hartmann, Rene (FL)	CRS	184
Hall, Lisabeth (NY)	Oph	486	Harty, James (KY)	U	906
Halle, Jan (NC)	RadRO	773	Haskal, Ziv (NY)	Rad	793
Haller, Daniel (PA)	Onc	318	Hassenbusch, Samuel J (TX)	NS	418
Hallett Jr, John (ME)	GVS	927	Hastings II, Hill (IN)	HS	282
Halmi, Katherine (NY)	Psyc	731	Haughey, Bruce (MO)	Oto	556
Halperin, Jonathan (NY)	Cv	135	Hauser, Stephen Lawrence (CA)	N	456
Halter, Jeffrey Brian (MI)	Ger	255	Hausman, Michael R (NY)	OrS	521
Hamaker, Ronald (IN)	Oto	555	Hawes, Robert H (SC)	Ge	236
Hamilton, William (NY)	OrS	520	Hawkins Jr, Irvin (FL)	DR	786
Hammer, Glenn (NY)	Inf	345	Hayashi, Robert H (MI)	MF	374
Hammill, Stephen Charles (MN)	CE	127	Hayden, Richard Earle (PA)	Oto	546
Hammon Jr, John W (NC)	TS	879	Hayes, Daniel Fleming (MI)	Onc	328
Hammond, Charles B (NC)	RE	804	Haynes, Johnson (AL)	Pul	752
Hammond, Dennis (MI)	PlS	700	Healey, John (NY)	OrS	521
Hamra, Sameer T (TX)	PlS	703	Healy, Gerald (MA)	PO	656
Hanauer, Stephen (IL)	Ge	239	Hebert, James C (VT)	S	843
Hande, Kenneth (TN)	Onc	323	Heck, Louis William (AL)	Rhu	819

ALPHABETICAL LISTING OF DOCTORS

Name	Specialty	Page
Hunt, Sharon Ann (CA)	Cv	151
Hunter, Ellen B (ID)	Ge	242
Hunter, John G (OR)	S	865
Hurd, Eric (TX)	Rhu	824
Hurley, James R (NY)	EDM	210
Hurst, Michael K (WV)	Oto	546
Hurst, Robert W (PA)	NRad	789
Hurt, Hallam (PA)	NP	383
Hurtig, Howard (PA)	N	438
Hurwitz, Barrie (NC)	N	443
Hurwitz, Dennis (PA)	PlS	692
Hussein, Mohammed Ahmed (OH)	Onc	328
Hussey, Michael J (IL)	MF	375
Hutchins, Laura (AR)	Onc	333
Hutter Jr, Adolph M (MA)	Cv	131
Huvos, Andrew G (NY)	Path	576
Huynh, Phan Tuong (TX)	DR	787
Hyers, Thomas Morgan (MO)	Pul	756

I

Name	Specialty	Page
Iannaccone, Susan (TX)	ChiN	162
Iannettoni, Mark D (MI)	TS	883
Iannotti, Joseph (OH)	OrS	530
Idler, Richard S (IN)	HS	282
Iglehart, J Dirk (MA)	S	843
Illingworth, D Roger (OR)	IM	365
Ilowite, Norman T (NY)	PRhu	663
Infante, Ernesto (TX)	N	453
Ingle, James N (MN)	Onc	328
Inglis, Andrew (WA)	PO	658
Ingram, David (NC)	PInf	649
Interian Jr, Alberto (FL)	CE	127
Ipp, Eli (CA)	EDM	220
Irby III, Pierce B (NC)	U	907
Irvine, John Alexander (CA)	Oph	503
Irwin Jr, Charles Edwin (CA)	AM	92
Irwin, Richard Stephen (MA)	Pul	745
Irwin, Robert J (NJ)	U	902
Isaacson, Keith B (MA)	RE	801
Isaacson, Steven (NY)	RadRO	771
Iseman, Michael (CO)	Pul	759
Isenberg, Keith Eugene (MO)	GerPsy	726
Isenberg, Sherwin Jay (CA)	Oph	503
Ishak, Kamal G (DC)	Path	576
Ismail, Mahmoud (IL)	MF	375
Isom, O Wayne (NY)	TS	875
Ivanhoe, Cindy (TX)	PMR	683

J

Name	Specialty	Page
Jaafar, Mohamad S (DC)	Oph	487
Jackler, Robert K (CA)	Oto	563
Jackman, Warren (OK)	CE	128
Jackson, Amie Brown (AL)	PMR	680
Jackson, Gilchrist (TX)	S	862
Jackson, John Kevin (LA)	N	453
Jackson, Neil (RI)	ObG	471
Jacob, Molly (IL)	Ped	612
Jacobs, Alice K (MA)	IC	153
Jacobs, Charlotte DeCroes (CA)	Onc	336

Name	Specialty	Page
Jacobs, Elliot (NY)	PlS	692
Jacobs, Laurence (IL)	RE	806
Jacobs, Richard F (AR)	PInf	650
Jacobs, Stephen C (MD)	U	902
Jacobs, Thomas (NY)	EDM	210
Jacobson, Ira (NY)	Ge	231
Jacobson, Jeff (DC)	NS	408
Jaffe, Allan S (MN)	Cv	144
Jaffe, Elaine Sarkin (MD)	Path	577
Jaffe, Kenneth M (WA)	PMR	684
Jaffe, Robert B (CA)	RE	808
Jain, Subhash (NY)	PM	567
Jakobiec, Frederick A (MA)	Oph	483
Janicak, Philip G (IL)	Psyc	735
Jankovic, Joseph (TX)	N	453
Jarow, Jonathan (MD)	U	902
Jeevanandam, Valluvan (IL)	TS	883
Jelks, Glenn (NY)	PlS	692
Jenike, Michael Andrew (MA)	Psyc	728
Jenkins, Herman A (CO)	Oto	559
Jenkins, Roger L (MA)	S	843
Jenkinson, Stephen George (TX)	Pul	760
Jensen, Donald (IL)	Ge	239
Jensen, Michael D (MN)	EDM	216
Jenson, Hal B (TX)	PInf	650
Jewell, Mark L (OR)	PlS	706
Jho, Hae-Dong (PA)	NS	408
Jillella, Anand (GA)	Onc	323
Jobe, Alan Hall (OH)	NP	385
Jobe, Frank Wilson (CA)	SM	832
Jochimsen, Peter R (IA)	S	858
Johansen, Kaj (WA)	GVS	936
Johnson Jr, Calvin M (LA)	Oto	561
Johnson, Bruce Ellsworth (VA)	Pul	752
Johnson, Bruce Evan (MA)	Onc	314
Johnson, Carl A (MD)	OrS	521
Johnson, Darren Lee (KY)	OrS	526
Johnson, David H (TN)	Onc	323
Johnson, Jonas Talmadge (PA)	Oto	546
Johnson, Kenneth P (MD)	N	438
Johnson, Maryl R (IL)	Cv	144
Johnson, Timothy M (MI)	D	200
Johnson, Timothy RB (MI)	ObG	476
Johnson, Warren (NY)	Inf	345
Johnston, Carolyn Marie (MI)	GO	268
Johnston, James (PA)	Nep	390
Johr, Robert (FL)	D	199
Jokl, Peter (CT)	OrS	515
Jonas, Adam Jonathan (CA)	CG	174
Jonas, Richard A (MA)	TS	871
Jones III, Howard Wilbur (TN)	GO	266
Jones, Ellis (GA)	TS	879
Jones, Jacqueline (NY)	PO	656
Jones, James F (CO)	A&I	100
Jones, Kenneth L (CA)	Ped	613
Jones, Marilyn (CA)	CG	174
Jones, Neil (CA)	HS	284
Jones, Paul John (IL)	Oto	556
Jones, Stephen E (TX)	Onc	333
Jordan, Barry D (NY)	N	438
Jordan, Gerald (VA)	U	907

ALPHABETICAL LISTING OF DOCTORS

ALPHABETICAL LISTING OF DOCTORS

ALPHABETICAL LISTING OF DOCTORS

Name	Specialty	Page	Name	Specialty	Page
McGowan Jr, John E (GA)	Inf	349	Michler, Robert (OH)	TS	883
McGrath, Patrick C (KY)	S	854	Middleton, Richard (UT)	U	913
McGregor, Christopher (MN)	TS	883	Mih, Alexander (IN)	HS	283
McGuirt, W Fredrick (NC)	Oto	552	Mihm Jr, Martin C (MA)	D	194
McHugh, Paul (MD)	Psyc	732	Milad, Magdy P (IL)	RE	806
McKenna Jr, Robert J (CA)	TS	889	Milam, Douglas F (TN)	U	907
McKeown, Craig A (FL)	Oph	494	Mildvan, Donna (NY)	Inf	346
McKinney Jr, Ross E (NC)	PInf	649	Miles, Brian J (TX)	U	914
McKinney, Peter W (IL)	PlS	700	Milhorat, Thomas H (NY)	NS	410
McLaren, Rodney A (VA)	MF	374	Miller, Carol A (CA)	Ped	613
McLeod, Allan G W (FL)	ObG	474	Miller, Charles M (NY)	S	849
McMahon, Marion (MN)	EDM	216	Miller, David Craig (CA)	TS	889
McNeese, Marsha (TX)	RadRO	777	Miller, Douglas Kent (MO)	Ger	255
McNutt, N Scott (NY)	Path	577	Miller, Franklin (UT)	Rad	796
Meals, Roy Allen (CA)	HS	285	Miller, Joshua (FL)	S	855
Medbery, Clinton A (OK)	RadRO	777	Miller, Kenneth B (MA)	Hem	305
Medich, David (PA)	CRS	182	Miller, Marilyn T (IL)	Oph	498
Medina, Jesus (OK)	Oto	561	Miller, Neil (MD)	Oph	488
Medow, Norman (NY)	Oph	488	Miller, Norman S (IL)	AdP	716
Medsger Jr, Thomas A (PA)	Rhu	817	Miller, Robert P (IL)	PO	658
Meek, Rita (DE)	PHO	641	Miller, Sheldon I (IL)	AdP	716
Mehlman, David J (IL)	Cv	145	Miller, Stanley (MD)	D	196
Mehta, Atul Chandrakant (OH)	Pul	757	Miller, Timothy Alden (CA)	PlS	707
Meier, Diane (NY)	Ger	252	Millis, J Michael (IL)	S	858
Meiselman, Mick Scott (IL)	Ge	240	Millman, Richard P (RI)	Pul	746
Mellins, Robert (NY)	PPul	660	Mills, Monte D (PA)	Oph	488
Mellman, Thomas (FL)	Psyc	734	Mills, Stacey E (VA)	Path	579
Mellow, Alan M (MI)	GerPsy	726	Milmoe, Gregory J (DC)	PO	656
Melman, Arnold (NY)	U	903	Milsom, Jeffrey W (NY)	CRS	182
Melmed, Shlomo (CA)	EDM	220	Mims III, James Luther (TX)	Oph	501
Melone Jr, Charles P (NY)	HS	278	Minaker, Kenneth (MA)	Ger	251
Meltzer, Toby R (OR)	PlS	707	Minckler, Donald Saier (CA)	Oph	504
Melvin, W Scott (OH)	S	858	Mindich, Bruce (NJ)	TS	876
Mendell, Jerry R (OH)	N	448	Minervini, Donald (FL)	S	855
Mendelsohn, Janis (IL)	Ped	613	Minich, Lois LuAnn (UT)	PCd	625
Mendenhall, Nancy P (FL)	RadRO	773	Minkoff, Howard L (NY)	ObG	473
Mendenhall, William M (FL)	RadRO	773	Minkoff, Jeffrey (FL)	OrS	526
Menezes, Arnold (IA)	NS	416	Minor, Lloyd B (MD)	Oto	547
Menkes, John H (CA)	ChiN	163	Minsky, Bruce (NY)	RadRO	771
Menninger, W Walter (KS)	Psyc	736	Miro-Quesada, Miguel (TX)	Hem	311
Mennuti, Michael (PA)	MF	372	Miskovitz, Paul (NY)	Ge	233
Menon, Mani (MI)	U	911	Mitchell, Beverly (NC)	Onc	323
Menter, M Alan (TX)	D	202	Mitchell, Charles (FL)	PInf	649
Meredith, Travis (NC)	Oph	494	Mitchell, James E (ND)	Psyc	736
Merrick III, Hollis W (OH)	GVS	934	Mitchell, Paul Ralph (CT)	Oph	483
Merrill, Walter H (TN)	TS	879	Mitchell, Wendy Gayle (CA)	ChiN	163
Merritt, Diane (MO)	ObG	476	Mitnick, Hal J (NY)	Rhu	817
Mersey, James Harris (MD)	EDM	211	Mitnick, Julie (NY)	DR	786
Messer, Joseph V (IL)	Cv	145	Miyamoto, Richard (IN)	Oto	557
Mesulam, Marek Marsel (IL)	N	448	Mladick, Richard (VA)	PlS	697
Metcalfe, Dean D (MD)	A&I	96	Moawad, Atef H (IL)	ObG	476
Metersky, Mark Lewis (CT)	Pul	746	Mobley, William Charles (CA)	ChiN	163
Mets, Marilyn (IL)	Oph	498	Moder, Kevin Gerard (MN)	Rhu	823
Metson, Ralph (MA)	Oto	543	Modic, Michael (OH)	NRad	791
Metz, David C (PA)	Ge	232	Mohl, Paul C (TX)	Psyc	737
Metz, Henry (NY)	Oph	488	Mohr, Jay Preston (NY)	N	439
Meyer, Anthony A (NC)	S	855	Mohsenifar, Zab (CA)	Pul	763
Meyers, Bryan (MO)	TS	883	Molnar, Joseph (NC)	PlS	698
Meyers, Paul (NY)	PHO	641	Monaco, Anthony (MA)	S	844
Michalska, Margaret (IL)	Rhu	823	Moncure, Ashby (MA)	TS	871
Micheli, Lyle J (MA)	OrS	516	Mondino, Bartly John (CA)	Oph	504

1118

ALPHABETICAL LISTING OF DOCTORS

Name	Specialty	Page
Niederman, Michael (NY)	Pul	748
Nigra, Thomas P (DC)	D	196
Nigro, Michael A (MI)	ChiN	161
Niloff, Jonathan Mitchell (MA)	GO	263
Niparko, John (MD)	Oto	547
Nisonson, Barton (NY)	SM	831
Nissenblatt, Michael (NJ)	Onc	320
Nitti, Victor (NY)	U	904
Nivatvongs, Santhat (MN)	CRS	186
Nixon, Daniel (FL)	Onc	324
Nobunaga, Austin (OH)	PMR	682
Nocero, Michael (FL)	Cv	141
Noetzel, Michael (MO)	ChiN	161
Nogueras, Juan Jose (FL)	CRS	184
Nolan, Bruce A (FL)	N	444
Noon, George P (TX)	TS	887
Noone, R Barrett (PA)	PlS	693
Norenberg, Michael D (FL)	Path	579
Nori, Dattatreyudu (NY)	RadRO	772
Norman, Kim Peter (CA)	Psyc	739
Northrup, Hope (TX)	CG	173
Norton, Karen (NY)	Rad	794
Norton, Larry (NY)	Onc	320
Noseworthy, John (FL)	U	908
Novak, Donald A (FL)	PGe	637
Novick, Andrew (OH)	U	911
Novy, Miles (OR)	ObG	478
Noyes, Frank (OH)	SM	832
Nuber, Gordon (IL)	OrS	531
Numann, Patricia (NY)	S	850
Nunley, James (NC)	HS	280
Nussbaum, Julian (GA)	Oph	494
Nussbaum, Robert (MD)	CG	170
Nutt Jr, John G (OR)	N	456

O

Name	Specialty	Page
O'Brien, Mark S (GA)	NS	412
O'Brien, Richard (GA)	Pul	753
O'Brien, Susan M (TX)	Onc	334
O'Gara, Patrick Thomas (MA)	Cv	132
O'Laughlin, Martin P (NC)	PCd	622
O'Leary, Patrick (NY)	OrS	522
O'Neill, William (MI)	Cv	145
O'Reilly, Richard (NY)	PHO	642
O'Sullivan, Mary Jo (FL)	MF	374
Oakes, W Jerry (AL)	NS	413
Oates, Robert Davis (MA)	U	900
Oberfield, Sharon (NY)	PEn	631
Oddis, Chester (PA)	Rhu	818
Odem, Randall R (MO)	RE	806
Odom, Lorrie Furman (CO)	PHO	645
Odom, Michael W (TX)	NP	386
Offit, Kenneth (NY)	Onc	320
Ohl, Dana Alan (MI)	U	912
Ojemann, Robert G (MA)	NS	405
Oktay, Kutluk (NY)	RE	802
Okusa, Mark D (VA)	Nep	393
Olanow, C Warren (NY)	N	440
Oldham, Keith T (WI)	PS	670
Olitsky, Scott Eric (NY)	Oph	489

Name	Specialty	Page
Oliva-Hemker, Maria Magdalena (MD)	PGe	636
Olive, David (WI)	ObG	476
Olivero, Juan Jose (TX)	Nep	397
Olney, Richard Koch (CA)	N	456
Olopade, Olufunmilayo I F (IL)	Onc	329
Olson, Jack Conrad (IL)	Ger	255
Olsson, Carl (NY)	U	904
Omachi, Rodney S (CA)	Nep	398
Ondra, Stephen (IL)	NS	416
Ontjes, David A (NC)	EDM	213
Opelka, Frank (LA)	CRS	187
Orlow, Seth (NY)	D	196
Orobello Jr, Peter W (FL)	Oto	552
Orringer, Mark B (MI)	TS	884
Ory, Steven (FL)	RE	804
Osborn, Anne G (UT)	NRad	791
Osborne, Charles Kent (TX)	Onc	334
Osteen, Robert T (MA)	S	844
Oster, Martin (NY)	Onc	321
Osterman Jr, Arthur Lee (PA)	OrS	522
Ostroff, James Warren (CA)	Ge	245
Ostrom, Nancy Kay (CA)	PA&I	618
Ott, David A (TX)	TS	887
Otto, Pamela (TX)	DR	787
Otto, Randal A (TX)	Oto	561
Ouellette, Elizabeth Anne (FL)	HS	280
Ouriel, Kenneth (OH)	GVS	934
Ouslander, Joseph (GA)	Ger	253
Ovalle, Fernando (AL)	EDM	213
Owen, William F (IL)	Nep	395
Owsley, John Q (CA)	PlS	707
Owyang, Chung (MI)	Ge	240
Oz, Mehmet Cengiz (NY)	TS	876
Ozols, Robert Felix (PA)	Onc	321

P

Name	Specialty	Page
Pachter, H Leon (NY)	S	850
Pacifico, Albert D (AL)	TS	880
Pacin, Michael (FL)	A&I	98
Pack, Allan I (PA)	Pul	748
Packer, Milton (NY)	Cv	136
Packer, Roger (DC)	ChiN	160
Padma-Nathan, Harin (CA)	U	917
Pagani, Francis Domenic (MI)	TS	884
Paganini, Emil (OH)	Nep	395
Page, David L (TN)	Path	579
Paget, Stephen (NY)	Rhu	818
Pagon, Roberta Anderson (WA)	CG	174
Paidas, Charles Nicholas (MD)	PS	667
Pairolero, Peter (MN)	TS	884
Palacios, Igor F (MA)	Cv	132
Palascak, Joseph E (OH)	Hem	310
Paletta, George A (MO)	SM	832
Paller, Amy Susan (IL)	D	200
Palmaz, Julio C (TX)	Rad	796
Palmberg, Paul (FL)	Oph	494
Palmer, Andrew (NY)	OrS	522
Palmer, Earl A (OR)	Oph	505
Palmer, Robert (OH)	Ger	255
Panicek, David (NY)	DR	786

ALPHABETICAL LISTING OF DOCTORS

ALPHABETICAL LISTING OF DOCTORS

ALPHABETICAL LISTING OF DOCTORS

1126

ALPHABETICAL LISTING OF DOCTORS

ALPHABETICAL LISTING OF DOCTORS

...e	Specialty	Page	Name	Specialty	Page
...npson Jr, Ian M (TX)	U	915	Tychsen, Lawrence (MO)	Oph	499
...npson, Ann Ellen (PA)	PCCM	628	Tyson, Jon Edward (TX)	NP	386
...npson, John (FL)	PGe	637	Tzakis, Andreas (FL)	S	856
..., Ann D (OK)	Path	581			
...ne, Charles (NY)	PlS	694	**U**		
...nhill, Thomas S (MA)	OrS	516	Udelsman, Robert (CT)	S	845
...p Jr, John Mercer (NC)	MF	374	Uehling, David T (WI)	U	913
...son, Alan (NE)	CRS	187	Uhde, Thomas W (MI)	Psyc	736
...y, Nicholas (MA)	S	845	Ulshen, Martin H (NC)	PGe	637
...ti, Mary (CT)	Ger	251	Umans, Jason (DC)	Nep	391
..., Gregory (PA)	Pul	750	Umetsu, Dale T (CA)	PA&I	619
...ler, Henry (NY)	OrS	524	Underwood, Louis (NC)	Ped	612
...n, Gordon R (KY)	PlS	698	Underwood, Paul (SC)	ObG	475
...n, Martin (IL)	Pul	758	Ungerleider, Ross M (OR)	TS	890
...III, Robert F (MI)	Onc	331	Unni, K Krishnan (MN)	Path	580
..., George (NY)	GVS	931	Upton, Joseph (MA)	HS	277
..., Richard D (MO)	ChAP	722	Urba, Susan G (MI)	Onc	331
...as, Alkis George (MD)	A&I	97	Urba, Walter J (OR)	Onc	336
...Randall (IL)	ObG	477	Urbaniak, James R (NC)	HS	280
...off-Rubin, Nina (MA)	Nep	390	Uribe, John (FL)	OrS	528
...Vernon Thorpe (CA)	OrS	536	Urist, Marshall (AL)	S	856
...era, Kevin M (AK)	U	918	Urken, Mark (NY)	Oto	549
...ich, Paul (IL)	MF	375	Urschel Jr, Harold C (TX)	TS	888
...l, Eric Jeffrey (OH)	Cv	147			
...imi, Dean (IL)	Oto	558	**V**		
...es, Vincente Esbarranch (MN)	Nep	396	Vail, Thomas Parker (NC)	OrS	528
..., Frank M (NC)	Onc	325	Valenstein, Edward (FL)	N	445
...es, Phillip (FL)	Ge	237	Valentino, Joseph (KY)	Oto	553
...nchi, Emil (IL)	U	913	Valentino, Leonard A (IL)	PHO	644
...anian, Ahmad (FL)	PS	669	Valero, Vicente (TX)	Onc	335
...ne, Jonathan (WI)	GVS	935	Valji, Karim (CA)	Rad	796
...nsend, Raymond R (PA)	Nep	391	Van Der Horst, Charles (NC)	Inf	350
...oulsi, Elias Iskan (OH)	Oph	499	van der Kolk, Bessel (MA)	Psyc	729
...baugh, Robert (NY)	TS	877	Van Heerden, Jon (MN)	S	860
...tek, Victor (AZ)	TS	887	Van Heertum, Ronald Lanny (NY)	NuM	464
...iner, Doris Ann (CA)	ChiN	163	Van Nagell Jr, John R (KY)	GO	267
...nelis, Vincent C (IA)	NS	417	Van Thiel, David (IL)	Ge	242
...dwell, Marjorie Clarke (MI)	MF	376	Vance, Mary Lee (VA)	IM	363
...dwell, Patricia (IN)	D	201	Vander Ark, Condon R (WI)	Cv	147
...t, Joseph (PA)	Onc	321	Vander Kolk, Craig Alan (MD)	PlS	694
...m, William R (NC)	PGe	637	Vander Laan, Ronald Lee (MI)	Cv	147
...naine, William John (MN)	Ge	241	Vander Salm, Thomas (MA)	TS	872
...to, Alfredo (CA)	TS	890	Vapnek, Jonathan M (NY)	U	905
...e, Michael T (MI)	Oph	499	Vas, George A (NY)	N	441
...k, Lorence Wain (TX)	OrS	534	Vasconez, Luis O (AL)	PlS	698
...ier, Michael (FL)	Onc	326	Vaughan, Edwin D (NY)	U	905
...st, Bradley Todd (NC)	N	445	Vaughey, Ellen (VA)	Pul	754
...ock, Elbert (MO)	Pul	758	Veith, Frank James (NY)	GVS	931
...nble, Thomas (WA)	HS	285	Veith, Richard (WA)	GerPsy	727
..., Tsu-Min (KY)	HS	280	Velcek, Francisca (NY)	PS	668
...David (FL)	Oph	495	Veldhuis, Johannes D (VA)	EDM	214
...ci, Debara Lyn (NC)	Oto	553	Venkat, K K (MI)	Nep	396
...pan, Noel B (TN)	NS	413	Verrier, Edward (WA)	TS	890
...kel, David Eric (MD)	PO	657	Vetrovec, George (VA)	Cv	142
...k, William (FL)	ChiN	161	Vicini, Frank A (MI)	RadRO	775
...ner, James (NY)	GVS	931	Vicioso, Belinda Angelica (TX)	Ger	257
...ner, Roderick Randolph (CA)	Path	583	Vierling, John Moore (CA)	Ge	245
...ner, Stephen Gordon (CA)	Oph	506	Vignola, Paul (FL)	Cv	142
...ner, William F (TX)	TS	887	Vijayan, Nazhivath (CA)	N	457
...rentine, Mark W (IN)	TS	885			
...risi III, Andrew Thomas (SC)	RadRO	774			

ALPHABETICAL LISTING OF DOCTORS

Name	Specialty	Page	Name	Specialty	Page
Vining, Eugenia (CT)	Oto	543	Warady, Bradley (MO)	PNep	655
Vinuela, Fernando (CA)	NRad	792	Ward, Barbara (CT)	S	845
Vitek, Jerrold Lee (GA)	N	445	Ward, John Harris (UT)	Onc	332
Voelkel, Norbert F (CO)	Pul	760	Ward, Robert (NY)	Oto	549
Vogel, Stephen Burton (FL)	S	856	Waring III, George Oral (GA)	Oph	495
Vogelzang, Nicholas (IL)	Onc	331	Warnke, Roger Allen (CA)	Path	583
Vogt, Peter (MN)	PlS	701	Warren, Robert Hughes (AR)	PPul	662
Vokes, Everett Emmett (IL)	Onc	331	Warren, Robert Samuel (CA)	S	866
Volberding, Paul Arthur (CA)	Onc	337	Warren, Robert Wells (TX)	PRhu	664
Volkmar, Fred R (CT)	ChAP	718	Warren, Russell (NY)	OrS	525
Vollmer, Timothy Lee (CT)	N	434	Warshaw, Andrew L (MA)	S	845
Volpe, Joseph J (MA)	ChiN	159	Wartofsky, Leonard (DC)	EDM	212
Volpe, Peter Anthony (CA)	CRS	188	Wasserman, Stephen (CA)	A&I	102
Volshteyn, Oksana (MO)	PMR	682	Waters, Peter Michael (MA)	HS	277
von Eschenbach, Andrew C (TX)	U	915	Watkins, Robert Green (CA)	OrS	536
Von Sternberg, Thomas (MN)	Ger	256	Watkins, Sandra (WA)	PNep	655
Voorhees, John (MI)	D	201	Watts, Ray Lannon (GA)	N	445
			Waxman, Alan D (CA)	NuM	466
			Waye, Jerome (NY)	Ge	234
## W			Wazen, Jack (NY)	Oto	549
Waagner, David (TX)	PInf	650	Wazer, David E (MA)	RadRO	769
Wackym, Phillip (WI)	Oto	558	Weaver, David Dawson (IN)	CG	172
Waggoner, Steven (IL)	GO	270	Weaver, Wayne Douglas (MI)	IC	155
Wagner-Weiner, Linda (IL)	PRhu	664	Webb, Lawrence (NC)	OrS	528
Wahl, Richard L (MD)	NuM	464	Webb, Maurice James (MN)	GO	270
Wain, John (MA)	TS	872	Weber, Barbara L (PA)	Onc	321
Wait, Susan Braynard (MD)	Psyc	734	Weber, Randal Scott (PA)	Oto	549
Wajsman, Zew Lew (FL)	U	909	Webster Jr, Marshall W (PA)	GVS	931
Wald, Arnold (PA)	Ge	233	Webster, George David (NC)	U	909
Wald, Ellen (PA)	PInf	648	Wechsler, Lawrence Richard (PA)	N	441
Wald, Jeffrey A (KS)	A&I	101	Weder, Alan B (MI)	IM	364
Waldbaum, Robert (NY)	U	905	Weichselbaum, Ralph R (IL)	RadRO	776
Waldman, Steven D (KS)	PM	570	Weiland, Andrew J (NY)	HS	279
Waldo, Albert (OH)	CE	128	Wein, Alan J (PA)	U	905
Walker III, R Dixon (FL)	U	909	Weinberg, Andrew David (GA)	Ger	254
Walker, Alonzo P (WI)	S	860	Weinberg, Harold (NY)	N	442
Walker, David H (TX)	Path	581	Weinberger, Malvin (FL)	PS	669
Walker, Marion L (UT)	NS	418	Weinberger, Michael (NY)	PM	569
Walkup, John (MD)	ChAP	720	Weinblatt, Michael Eliot (MA)	Rhu	815
Wallace Jr, Richard James (TX)	Inf	352	Weiner, Bonnie H (MA)	IC	153
Wallace, Jeanne Marie (CA)	Pul	764	Weiner, Howard (MA)	N	434
Wallach, Edward Eliot (MD)	RE	803	Weiner, Irving David (FL)	Nep	393
Wallach, Robert C (NY)	GO	265	Weiner, Leslie P (CA)	N	457
Waller, John F (NY)	OrS	524	Weiner, Louis M (PA)	Onc	321
Walsh, B Timothy (NY)	Psyc	734	Weiner, Michael (NY)	PHO	642
Walsh, Christine A (NY)	PCd	621	Weiner, Myron (TX)	Psyc	737
Walsh, Edward Patrick (MA)	PCd	620	Weiner, Richard (FL)	OrS	528
Walsh, Joseph (NY)	Oph	491	Weiner, William J (MD)	N	442
Walsh, Nicolas E (TX)	PM	571	Weinstein, Arthur (DC)	Rhu	819
Walsh, Patrick (MD)	U	905	Weinstein, Gregory (PA)	Oto	549
Walters, Mark (OH)	ObG	477	Weinstein, Howard (MA)	PHO	640
Walters, Theodore (ID)	Onc	332	Weinstein, Stuart L (IA)	OrS	532
Walton Jr, Robert Lee (IL)	PlS	701	Weinstock, Robert (CA)	AdP	716
Walton, David S (MA)	Oph	483	Weisberg, Leon (LA)	N	453
Waner, Milton (AR)	Oto	562	Weisberg, Tracey (ME)	Onc	315
Wang, Frederick (NY)	Oph	491	Weisenburger, Dennis (NE)	Path	580
Wang, Winfred C (TN)	PHO	643	Weisman, Steven Jay (WI)	PM	570
Wanner, Adam (FL)	Pul	754	Weiss, Arnold Peter (RI)	HS	277
Wapner, Keith Leslie (PA)	OrS	525	Weiss, Arthur (CA)	Rhu	826
Wapner, Ronald (PA)	MF	373	Weiss, Avery (WA)	Oph	506
Wara, Diane W (CA)	PA&I	619	Weiss, Lawrence M (CA)	Path	583

ALPHABETICAL LISTING OF DOCTORS

Name	Specialty	Page
Wright, Harry (SC)	ChAP	721
Wright, Kenneth W (CA)	Oph	506
Wright, Robert B (IL)	N	451
Wunderink, Richard (TN)	Pul	754
Wylen, Michele (DC)	ObG	473
Wyllie, Elaine (OH)	ChiN	162
Wyllie, Robert (OH)	PGe	638

Y

Name	Specialty	Page
Yaffe, Bruce (NY)	IM	362
Yager, Joel (NM)	Psyc	737
Yancovitz, Stanley (NY)	Inf	347
Yannuzzi, Lawrence (NY)	Oph	491
Yao, James (IL)	GVS	935
Yates, Alayne (HI)	ChAP	724
Yee, Billy (CA)	RE	809
Yellin, Albert E (CA)	GVS	937
Yetman, Randall John (OH)	PlS	702
Yonkers, Kimberly A (CT)	Psyc	729
Yoon, Sydney (NY)	Rad	794
Yoshikawa, Thomas T (CA)	Inf	353
Yoshizumi, Marc Osamu (CA)	Oph	506
Young, Anne (MA)	N	435
Young, Bruce (NY)	ObG	473
Young, Iven (NY)	EDM	212
Young, James B (OH)	Cv	147
Young, Keith Randall (AL)	Pul	754
Young, Ming-Lon (FL)	PCd	623
Young, Robert Henry (MA)	Path	576
Young, Vernon Leroy (MO)	PlS	702
Younge, Brian R (MN)	Oph	499
Younger, J Benjamin (AL)	RE	805
Yousem, David Mark (MD)	NRad	790
Yousem, Samuel A (PA)	Path	578
Yu, Victor (PA)	Inf	347
Yurt, Roger (NY)	S	852

Z

Name	Specialty	Page
Zackai, Elaine (PA)	CG	170
Zacur, Howard A (MD)	RE	803
Zafonte, Ross (PA)	PMR	680
Zaidman, Gerald (NY)	Oph	491
Zalusky, Ralph (NY)	Hem	307
Zalzal, George (DC)	Oto	549
Zarem, Harvey Alan (CA)	PlS	709
Zaret, Barry L (CT)	Cv	132
Zarins, Bertram (MA)	OrS	517
Zarins, Christopher Kristaps (CA)	GVS	937
Zdeblick, Thomas (WI)	OrS	532
Zeanah Jr, Charles H (LA)	ChAP	723
Zeitels, Steven (MA)	Oto	544
Zeitlin, Pamela Leslie (MD)	PPul	660
Zelenetz, Andrew D (NY)	Onc	322
Zelickson, Brian D (MN)	D	201
Zeltzer, Lonnie Kaye (CA)	Ped	614
Zerbe, Kathryn J (OR)	Psyc	740
Ziegler, Moritz M (MA)	PS	666
Zilleruelo, Gaston E (FL)	PNep	653
Zimmerman, Donald (MN)	PEn	634

Name	Specialty	Page
Zimmerman, Earl Abram (NY)	N	44.
Zimmerman, Jerry John (WA)	PCCM	62.
Zimmerman, Robert A (PA)	NRad	79.
Zimmerman, Stephen W (WI)	Nep	39.
Zinaman, Michael (IL)	RE	80.
Zinner, Michael (MA)	S	84.
Zins, James (OH)	PlS	70.
Zipes, Douglas P (IN)	Cv	14.
Zisook, Sidney (CA)	Psyc	74.
Zitelli, John (PA)	D	19.
Zorn, George L (AL)	TS	88.
Zorumski, Charles F (MO)	Psyc	73.
Zuckerman, Joseph (NY)	OrS	52.
Zuckerman, Kenneth (FL)	Hem	30.

CASTLE CONNOLLY ORDER FORM

I want to order the following Castle Connolly Guides:

America's Top Doctors, 2nd edition   # ___ of books at $29.95 $_____

Top Doctors:
    New York Metro Area, 6th edition   # ___ of books at $24.95 $_____
    Chicago Metro Area, 2nd edition   # ___ of books at $24.95 $_____

How to Find the Best Doctors:
    Florida   # ___ of books at $24.95 $_____

The Buyer's Guide to Choosing
the Best Healthcare   # ___ of books at $12.95 $_____

The ABCs of HMOs: How To
Get The Best From Managed Care   # ___ of books at $11.95 $_____

    Subtotal $_____

*NY residents, please add 8.25% sales tax $_____
**NJ residents, please add 6% sales tax $_____

Add $3 per book for shipping and handling: # ___ of books x $3 $_____

    TOTAL $_____

Please fill in the following information (please print):

Name: _____

Address: _____

City: _____

State: _____ Zip: _____

Phone (day): _____ (eve): _____

E-mail: _____

___ Check or Money Order enclosed
    (payable to Castle Connolly Medical Ltd.)
___ Credit Card: please circle one   Amex   MC   Visa

Card #: _____

Exp. Date: _____ Today's Date: _____

Signature: _____

Mail to: Castle Connolly Medical Ltd. 42 West 24th Street, New York, NY 10010
or fax to: (212) 367-0964

Order online and save: www.castleconnolly.com   AOL keyword: Castle Connolly

RATE A PHYSICIAN

The purpose of this questionaire is to enable you to rate physicians who have cared for you. Please feel free to duplicate this form in order to rate multiple physicians.

Doctor's First Name:_____   Doctor's Last Name:_____

Specialty:_____   Hospital:_____

Phone:(_____)_____-_____   Doctor's Address:_____

City:_____   State:_____

Please rate your doctor in the following areas (leave blank if not applicable):

	Poor	Fair	Good	Very Good	Excellent
Overall quality of care	____	____	____	____	____
Doctor availability	____	____	____	____	____
Returns calls in a timely fashion	____	____	____	____	____
Personal attention during visit	____	____	____	____	____
Shows caring & compassion	____	____	____	____	____
Ability to communicate	____	____	____	____	____
Explanation/coordination of medications	____	____	____	____	____
Willingness to make referrals	____	____	____	____	____
Quality of referrals	____	____	____	____	____
Professionalism of staff	____	____	____	____	____
Accuracy of billing	____	____	____	____	____
Cleanliness of office	____	____	____	____	____
Waiting room time	____	____	____	____	____

Would you recommend this doctor to a friend or relative?   Yes____   No____

Mail or fax to:
Castle Connolly Medical Ltd. 42 West 24th Street, New York, NY 10010
Fax: (212) 367-0964   www.castleconnolly.com   AOL keyword: Castle Connolly

ACKNOWLEDGMENTS

The publishers would like to thank the entire staff for their many hours and days of intense and precise work on this guide in order to further its goal of assisting consumers in making the best healthcare choices.

Castle Connolly Management:

President & CEO:	John J. Connolly, Ed.D.
Vice President, Research	Jean Morgan, M.D.
Vice President, Business Development	William Liss-Levinson, Ph.D.
Director, Information Technology	Michael Pitkin
Director, Content Development	Arline Lane, J.D., M.P.S.
Research Coordinator	Maryann Hynd, M.S., M.A.

We also would like to extend our gratitude to the American Board of Medical Specialties (ABMS) for allowing us to use excerpts, especially the descriptions of medical specialties and subspecialties, from the text of their publication "Which Medical Specialist for You?"

OTHER PUBLICATIONS FROM CASTLE CONNOLLY MEDICAL LTD.:

Top Doctors: New York Metro Area
Top Doctors: Chicago Metro Area
How to Find the Best Doctors: Florida
The Buyer's Guide to Choosing the Best Healthcare
The ABCs of HMOs: How To Get The Best From Managed Care
The Best Senior Living & Eldercare Options

To order, see form on page 1133

DOCTOR-PATIENT ADVISOR

Doctor-Patient Advisor is a Castle Connolly Medical Resources, Inc. service providing one on one consultations with a Healthcare Advocate to individuals who have extremely serious or complex medical problems or to anyone who feels he/she needs assistance finding the right physician for any purpose. Each client will receive personalized assistance from these physician-supervised nurses in identifying the appropriate top specialists for his/her condition. The Healthcare Advocate will utilize the extensive Castle Connolly Medical Ltd. database of physicians and hospitals to locate, and facilitate access to, the best resources to meet the client's needs. Fee: $995.00. For further information call (212) 367-8400 x 16.

For further information on physicians and hospitals please visit the Castle Connolly Web site at
www.CastleConnolly.com   AOL keyword: Castle Connolly
or at
www.AmericasTopDoctors.com